A Case Oriented Approach Towards

BIOCHEMISTRY

A Case Oriented Approach Towards

BIOCHEMISTRY

Second Edition

Editors

Namrata Chhabra MBBS MD (Biochemistry)
MPhil Health Professions Education
CMCL FAIMER Fellow
PhD Medical Biochemistry (Scholar)

Principal-in-Charge,
Professor and Chair (Biochemistry)
Sir Seewoosagur Ramgoolam Medical College
Belle Rive, Mauritius

Sahil Chhabra MBBS MAS (Scholar)
Leadership of Health Care Organization
University of California
San Diego, The United States of America

Co-editors

Sahiba Kukreja MBBS MD (Biochemistry) CMCL-FAIMER Fellow
Professor and Head
Sri Guru Ram Das Institute of Medical Sciences and Research
Amritsar, Punjab, India

Sarah Chhabra MBBS Resident (Internal Medicine)
Mount Sinai Hospital and Research Centre
Miami Beach, The United States of America

Forewords

Sona Vasudevan
Binita Goswami
Navjot Bajwa
Ranjit Patil
Kuldeep Sodhi
AK Lavania
Nitin Wadhwa
Nitin Malhotra
Vijayasarathy S

JAYPEE

JAYPEE BROTHERS MEDICAL PUBLISHERS
The Health Sciences Publisher
New Delhi | London

JAYPEE **Jaypee Brothers Medical Publishers (P) Ltd**

Headquarters
Jaypee Brothers Medical Publishers (P) Ltd
EMCA House, 23/23-B
Ansari Road, Daryaganj
New Delhi 110 002, India
Landline: +91-11-23272143, +91-11-23272703
+91-11-23282021, +91-11-23245672
Email: jaypee@jaypeebrothers.com

Corporate Office
Jaypee Brothers Medical Publishers (P) Ltd
4838/24, Ansari Road, Daryaganj
New Delhi 110 002, India
Phone: +91-11-43574357
Fax: +91-11-43574314
Email: jaypee@jaypeebrothers.com

Overseas Office
J.P. Medical Ltd
83 Victoria Street, London
SW1H 0HW (UK)
Phone: +44 20 3170 8910
Fax: +44 (0)20 3008 6180
Email: info@jpmedpub.com

Website: www.jaypeebrothers.com
Website: www.jaypeedigital.com

Inquiries for bulk sales may be solicited at: jaypee@jaypeebrothers.com

A Case Oriented Approach Towards Biochemistry

First Edition : 2013
Second Edition : 2022
Reprint : **2023**

ISBN 978-93-90595-79-2

Printed at: Sterling Graphics Pvt. Ltd. India.

Dedicated to

My parents for their unconditional love, support and encouragement

Contributors and Reviewers

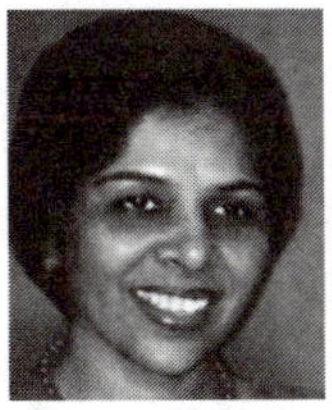

Namrata Chhabra
MPhil Health Professions Education
CMCL FAIMER Fellow
PhD Medical Biochemistry (Scholar)
Principal-in-charge,
Professor and Chair (Biochemistry)
Sir Seewoosagur Ramgoolam Medical College
Belle Rive, Mauritius
(Chapters 1, 2, 3, 4, 5, 6, 7, 8, 9, 10, 11, 12, 13, 14, 15, 16, 17, 18, 19, 20, 21, 22, 23, 24, 25, 26)

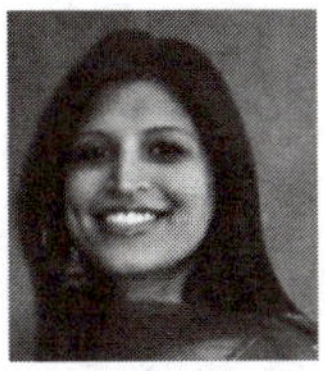

Jasdeep Gill
Dayanand Medical College
and Hospital
Ludhiana, Punjab, India
(Chapters 3, 11, 15, 16)

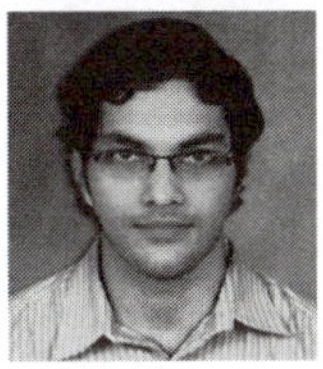

Bharath Raj Kidambi
Department of Cardiology
All India Institute of Medical Sciences
New Delhi, India
(Chapters 3, 4, 5, 6, 25, 26)

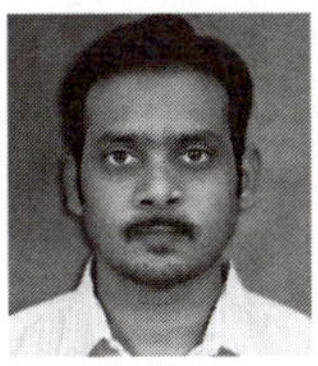

Vijayasarathy S
Surgical Resident
Regional Cancer Center
Thiruvananthapuram, Kerala, India
Government Medical College and Hospital
Chennai, Tamil Nadu, India
Ex-Student, Sir Seewoosagur Ramgoolam
Medical College
Belle Rive, Mauritius
(Chapters 13, 14, 18)

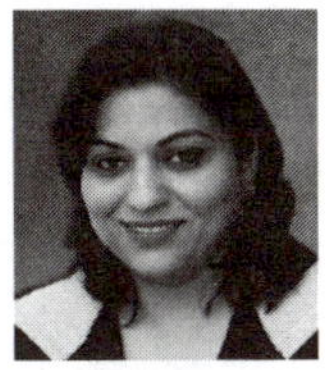

Sahiba Kukreja
Sri Guru Ram Das Institute of
Medical Sciences and Research
Amritsar, Punjab, India
(Chapters 4, 10, 21)

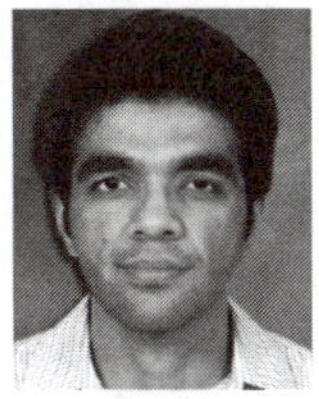

Sahil Chhabra
Leadership of Health Care Organization
University of California
San Diego, The United States of America
(Chapters 1, 2, 3, 4, 5, 6, 7, 8, 9, 10, 11, 12, 15, 16, 19, 21, 24, 25, 26)

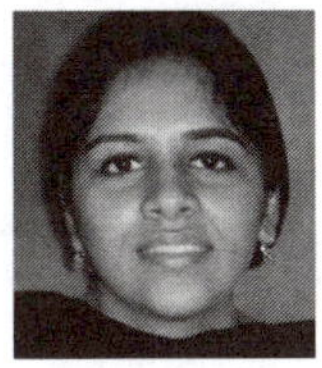

Sarah Chhabra
Resident (Internal Medicine)
Mount Sinai Hospital and Research Center
Miami Beach, The United States of America
(Chapters 2, 6, 11, 15, 17)

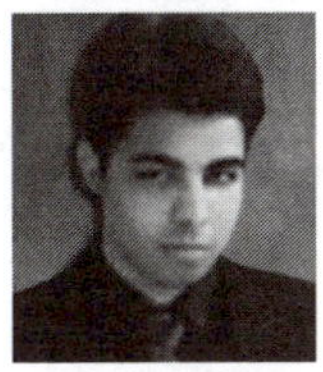

Kavish Ramessur
Sir Seewoosagur Ramgoolam
Medical College, Belle Rive
Mauritius
(Chapters 2, 4, 11, 17, 19)

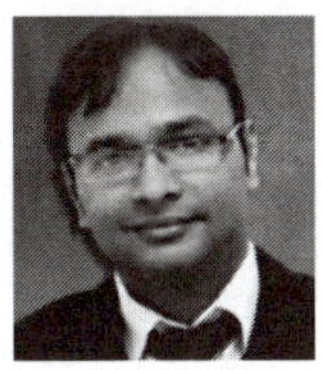

Robby Kumar
Sir Seewoosagur Ramgoolam
Medical College, Belle Rive
Mauritius
(Chapters 10, 11, 22, 25, 26)

Foreword

Biochemistry is fundamental to understanding the underlying causes of diseases and their treatments. A surface approach to biochemistry with memorization of material, rather than an in-depth approach to understanding the underlying concepts, leads to poor outcomes. The approach of case-based learning (CBL) has demonstrated that improvements in student learning and success in clinical practice can be achieved by CBL. In medical education, CBL aims at teaching content while engaging the students actively with real-life case-studies. The biggest challenge to realizing CBL in practice, is the lack of books that can help educators around the world to effectively adapt to bringing CBL into the classroom. This book addresses this challenge and demonstrates in a systematic manner the process of imparting knowledge about diseases to students. I am an educator myself, who directs a MS program in Systems Medicine at Georgetown University Medical Center. For more than a decade, I have searched for a book that can be used to teach my own graduate, and medical students via the CBL methodology. Fairly recently, I was fortunate to meet Dr Chhabra, an amazing modest, brilliant person. She has made the learning of biochemistry easy and fun by her unique approaches described in this book to impart much needed knowledge in this field. In fact, I have created a course called *The Case Oriented Approach to Biochemistry* for my graduate students. Dr Chhabra, in my opinion, is one of the best educators in the world with unique insights into many aspects of diseases covered in this book. I am looking forward to more books and resources from her in the years to come.

Sona Vasudevan PhD
Professor, Medical Education
Director, MD/MS Dual Degree Program in Systems Medicine
Director, MS Program in Systems Medicine
Biochemistry and Molecular & Cellular Biology
Georgetown University Medical Center
Washington, DC, USA

FOREWORD

It gives me immense pleasure to introduce the second edition of *A Case Oriented Approach Towards Biochemistry*.

I have known Dr Namrata Chhabra for many years. She is known for her impeccable writing skills, thorough knowledge of biochemistry, and exceptional teaching skills. She has authored many books dealing with the theoretical as well as practical aspects of biochemistry for undergraduate students. She also shares academic pearls through her website, which is very popular with students and teachers alike.

The first edition of her book has been a stupendous success among students with clinical scenarios and their detailed biochemical explanations. The second edition has many aha moments with:

- Thrust on biochemical techniques
- New CBME curriculum-based writeup with components of horizontal and vertical integration
- Self-directed learning through unsolved clinical cases
- Quick revision charts
- Multiple choice questions for self-assessment
- Moreover, many more.

I would like to congratulate Dr Namrata for the hard work put in for the compilation of such a masterpiece. I am looking forward to having the hard copy of this book on my table very soon.

Binita Goswami MD DNB MNAMS FIMSA FAIMER (CMCL)
Professor
Department of Biochemistry
Maulana Azad Medical College
New Delhi, India
Associate Editor, Indian Journal of Medical Biochemistry

Foreword

I am highly pleased to read the revised edition of, *A Case Oriented Approach Towards Biochemistry* by Dr Namrata Chhabra. All relevant points as per the revised curriculum have been incorporated very meticulously. Integrated learning and early clinical exposure have been dealt with excellent case studies. The book will undoubtedly help the aspiring students not only to prepare for pre-clinical years of MBBS course but would also work as a life-long companion in the entire medical continuum.

I wish Dr Namrata and the team, very good luck for their innovative venture to make the subject of extreme complexity meaningful, clinically contextual, and extremely conceptual. I am sure this book will create a benchmark in the field of biochemistry for its thoughtful discussions and logical clinical correlations.

Navjot Bajwa MBBS MD (Biochemistry)
Department of Biochemistry
Dayanand Medical College and Hospital
Ludhiana, Punjab, India

FOREWORD

Biochemistry is the primary language of biomedical science and essential for literacy in the field of medicine. All diseases have a biochemical basis, and this book helps you understand the importance of biochemistry in diagnosing and treating illness.

This edition has several significant changes and additions. Three new chapters have been included—biochemical techniques, multiple choice questions, and summary charts.

The book has 300 case studies and is based on the new CBME curriculum. Each case study has a theme, and new cases have been included. Many of the chapters are a real pleasure in themselves, and the book achieves the unenviable task of making biochemistry enjoyable to medical students.

When I think of precise knowledge, flawless teaching technique, and a knack of speaking the truth, I think of Dr Namrata Chhabra. There is a lot of information available in biochemistry, but the clarity and wisdom with which the material is presented in this book is a rarity. The style, content, and information contained in this book make it one of the most influential books in clinical biochemistry. The book provides a stunningly organized approach to the biochemical basis of medicine through case studies. Dr Namrata has a vast experience in the field of teaching and research, which is evident in the lucid manner in which the cases are presented and explained.

This work takes its place as one of the most comprehensive yet-readable books in biochemistry, and I am confident that it will continue to enjoy international success. I recommend *A Case Oriented Approach Towards Biochemistry* to be on the desk of every medical student. It has been my pleasure and privilege to write this foreword.

Ranjit Patil MBBS MD (Biochemistry)
Professor
Department of Biochemistry
Sir Seewoosagur Ramgoolam Medical College
Belle Rive, Mauritius

Foreword

A Case Oriented Approach Towards Biochemistry is truly a clinically-oriented, very thorough and extremely well-illustrated presentation of the essentials of biochemistry. The editors have provided an up-to-date and logical coverage of basic biochemistry with normal and abnormal aspects of physiological chemistry. The book emphasizes a problem-solving approach that illustrates the value of thinking in biochemical terms to understand clinical problems. The case studies are interesting and important part a of the text; they would allow the students to apply the learned principles of biochemistry. The book provides students with an in-depth look into the traditional domains of biochemistry in a very readable format with outstanding illustrations. The material is appropriate and relevant for medical and other health sciences students.

Kuldeep Sodhi MBBS MD (Biochemistry)
Professor, Department of Biochemistry
Maharishi Markandeshwar Institute of Medical Sciences
and Research
Ambala, Haryana, India

Foreword

The editors have focused towards a case-oriented approach to understand enigmatic biochemistry. This clinically-oriented book provides an excellent, updated and logical coverage of basic biochemistry. By means of case studies, the students would not only learn the principles themselves but would also understand why biochemistry is important in health sciences and how biochemical principles are involved in day-to-day professional practice.

The editors have rightfully justified the saying *The Biochemistry of Today is the Medicine of Tomorrow*. This book will encourage the students of medicine and life sciences to clad the thinking cap and facilitate the application of knowledge to demystify the clinical problems.

I recommend the book with utmost enthusiasm, it is a unique and an exceptionally intelligent work and highly appreciate the tremendous efforts, the authors have put in to provide students a convenient reading material and a complete understanding of the subject. I wish authors and contributors all the success and congratulate on this publication.

AK Lavania MBBS MD (Physiology)
Professor
Department of Physiology
Sir Seewoosagur Ramgoolam Medical College
Belle Rive, Mauritius

Foreword

Mastering the knowledge in a discipline such as biochemistry is a formidable task. It is even more difficult to retain this information and to recall it when the clinical setting is encountered. Clinicians, however, often wish they knew more about the basic sciences, because it is through this science that complexities of the human body can be better understood to have rational methods of diagnosis and treatment. The gulf between the basic sciences and the patient arena is wide. *A Case Oriented Approach Towards Biochemistry* has bridged this gulf with carefully constructed clinical cases. The explanations for these cases, emphasize the underlying mechanisms and perfectly relate the clinical setting to the basic science data. The book is extremely well organized to allow the student "in a rush" to go quickly through the scenarios, check the corresponding answers and also to provide more detailed information for those, who want thought-provoking explanations. This is a unique book and I am sure that the book will be successful in its mission to make *today's students tomorrow's good clinicians*.

Nitin Wadhwa MD (Neonatology)
9209 Springbrooke Circle
Louisville, Kentucky 40241
United States of America

FOREWORD

Rational understanding of disease and plans for treatment are best acquired by learning about the normal human processes on a basic science level. *A Case Oriented Approach Towards Biochemistry* has been written in an unconventional way to provide complete background knowledge of a disease process and at the same time, there is an excellent and updated correlation of the clinical database with the basic fundamental facts. Going through the history, clinical manifestations and laboratory findings, the students would learn to find out the underlying physiological and biochemical deviations and this would help them to frame a diagnosis and plan a suitable treatment.

Most commonly encountered cases in clinical practice have been emphasized in the book. I am confident, this pattern of learning will be most welcomed and enjoyed by the students to recall the learned facts later upon actual encounter with the patients.

I congratulate the authors on this novel and commendable publication.

Nitin Malhotra MD (Internal Medicine)
Ex-Professor
Department of Internal Medicine
Christian Medical College
Ludhiana, Punjab, India

FOREWORD

A determined mind, unwavering from the level of hard work and excellence is what would define Dr Namrata Chhabra, the teacher and a role model for many. Her self-persuasion to not compromise on the quality of content is reflected in this textbook.

She aims not only to teach but train the students to analyze and dissect a clinical problem, a very essential art required for the medical profession. We realize that when we do the ward rounds in the clinical subjects, the level of encroachment of biochemistry is in every area from pathophysiology to the investigations and treatment rationale. Thus, one's understanding of biochemistry concepts must be strong. Her untiring interest in advanced teaching and her enthusiasm is so infectious that one would develop instant energy to learn and accomplish tasks.

Her knowledge surpasses many textbooks and is now wielded into a form of a multifaceted textbook, a book which would soon go into the list of essentials of medical students. The well-crafted format of the book makes it different and advanced from the conventional textbooks, such that it can be utilized as a source for mainstream study, quick reference, symptomatology, high-yield facts, question bank and a lot more. I hope the building of a clinician could start with the book, with all the ingredients for problem-solving packed within. The book connects with students in every level of their academic study with its student-friendly approach, emphasis on essential facts with a diversity of case studies. The simple language and the simple construction of contents make it easy-to-access information quickly. The case studies are structured in such a way that it takes into an investigating atmosphere connecting from panel-to-panel and establishing links between the symptoms and the underlying disease. In this way, it becomes enjoyable to learn the art of diagnosis. The abundance of illustrations and clinical pearls adds on to the information wealth and makes the book an innovation.

I strongly believe that the knowledge and clinical wisdom which Professor Namrata has shared with us in the text is an indispensable asset to the medical community.

Vijayasarathy S MCH Surgical resident
Regional Cancer Centre
Thiruvananthapuram
Government Medical College and Hospital
Chennai, Tamil Nadu, India
Ex-Student, Sir Seewoosagur Ramgoolam Medical College
Belle Rive, Mauritius

PREFACE TO THE SECOND EDITION

I am honored to have been asked to revise the first edition of our book, *A Case Oriented Approach Towards Biochemistry*. The book is intended to promote critical thinking skills in students embarking on the journey of biochemistry. It had been gratifying to see that the book was recognized as a standard reference book by the reputed medical institutes across the world. The comments and recommendations of the readers have encouraged me to expand the horizons and improve the hallmark features of this book.

The revised edition contains illustrations of three hundred clinical cases. Each case has been carefully designed and described with a logical coverage of the fundamental aspects of biochemistry and the clinical implications of the underlying biochemical deviations. The efforts have been made to horizontally or vertically integrate the knowledge of biochemistry with the related subjects.

The original format of the description of clinical cases has been maintained in the revised edition. In each case, illustrations of the basic defect, the underlying pathophysiology, and the clinically relevant details have been provided. Each case study ends-up in a 'clinical note' and a summary in the form of essential points, titled as "clinical pearls."

The course contents have been spread out in twenty-nine chapters. Each chapter starts with a list of 'learning objectives.' The case descriptions relate to the learning objectives. Each case study has been assigned a 'theme' based on the contextual details, and three clinically relevant 'icons' for the depiction of theme, clinical note, and clinical pearls.

Three new chapters have been added including the details of biochemical and molecular techniques, case-based multiple choice questions, and quick revisions of significant biochemical deviations. Newborn screening due to its diagnostic and prognostic significance, and some topics of clinical concerns, such as heavy metal toxicity, tumor markers, mechanisms of enzyme action, and enzymes inhibition have also been included. Some redundant cases have been removed to reduce content load, and some have been updated to include the latest information and pictorial representations. Thirty-seven diagrams, tables, flowcharts, and nine new cases have been added to provide broad and conceptual coverage of the course contents.

Extreme care has been taken to constructively align the course contents with the latest *Competency-based Medical Curriculum*. Hopefully, the learners will be able to build up the core concepts and learn to apply knowledge in solving clinical problems. Students will be able to assess their problem-solving skills through partially explained cases and case-based multiple choice questions. Furthermore, the summary charts will help the learners to revise the learned contents quickly. I am hopeful that in this clinical environment of curiosity, the learners will be able to attain the desired learning goals.

I am grateful to the students and faculty of medical institutes for their valuable suggestions. No book is ever free from errors. I would be delighted to receive comments, positive or negative, and recommendations for future editions.

Thank you,

Namrata Chhabra
Email: *nam.chhabra@gmail.com*

Sahil Chhabra
Email: *doctorsahil@gmail.com*

Preface to the First Edition

Education is what we remember after we have forgotten all that we learnt

The vast medical ocean, consisting of diverse diseases and puzzling mechanisms, demands a very analytical type of approach towards learning. The immensity of the course often makes us skip the essentials, making the knowledge baseless. The application of the preacquired knowledge in the clinical arena requires cultivation of lateral thinking. The clinical case-oriented approach towards learning undoubtedly is the key to a better understanding of a subject.

In an attempt to facilitate the learning process of students, the book aims at bringing out the conceptual aspects of biochemistry in a magnified view with a complete picture of the context in a different style. The book provides a platform for an acquisition of knowledge of biochemistry through a case-oriented approach. It lays strong emphasis on the biochemical aspects of the medically important diseases. I hope that the new introduction would simulate a clinical environment and make the students' experience, the excitement that has yet to come in their careers.

Namrata Chhabra
Sahil Chhabra

Acknowledgments

The second edition of this book is the result of a team effort by many individuals, several of whom deserve special mention.

I am particularly indebted to Dr Sahiba Kukreja (Professor and Head, Sri Guru Ram Das Institute of Medical Sciences and Research, Amritsar, Punjab, India), who had been unfailing support throughout the preparation and revision of this manuscript.

It had been a great privilege to work under the guidance of a knowledgeable and conscientious professional, Dr Sona Vasudevan (Professor, Department of Biochemistry, Molecular Biology and Cellular Biology, Georgetown University, USA), who provided valuable suggestions for the improvement and presentation of the content. I extend my sincerest appreciation and heartfelt gratitude to her.

My gratitude goes to my loving kids, Dr Sahil Chhabra and Dr Sarah Chhabra for their tremendous support, love, care, and constructive criticism about the book. Their contemporary ideas brought life to this book. Their passion, enthusiasm, and diligence to introduce reality and innovation in each chapter motivated me to test my abilities to meet their expectations.

I shall fail from my duties, if I would not acknowledge the untiring efforts of Dr. Sarthak Virmani, my son-in-law, (Fellow, Yale New Haven Hospital, USA), for extending emotional support, suggestions and encouragement to exceed set boundaries.

Special recognition is extended to Shri Jitendar P Vij (Group Chairman), Mr Ankit Vij (Managing Director), and Mr MS Mani (Group President) of M/s Jaypee Brothers Medical Publishers (P) Ltd., New Delhi, India, for believing in the concept of teaching by clinical cases.

Above all, I am thankful to God, without the blessings of whom, this book would not have seen the light of the day.

Namrata Chhabra

CONTENTS

Introduction

This book summarizes the essentials of biochemistry with clinical correlations. The purpose of the book is to present a clear discussion of biochemistry in relation to physiological processes occurring at the cellular levels and to cite examples of deviant biochemical processes in different clinical conditions.

The book contains evaluations of clinical cases in sections, namely history, physical examination, laboratory workup and questions related to the diagnosis of the case. A reader shall go through the history to make a preliminary outline of the disorder, then follow the physical examination findings and investigation results to reach at a presumptive diagnosis. This will help sharpen the clinical skills by simulating a clinical "reaching at a diagnosis" experience.

In each case detail, fundamentals of the basic defect, entire format of pathophysiology and the clinically relevant details have been provided. Each case study ends-up in a clinical note and a short summary in the form of important points, titled as "clinical pearls". This will help the readers to quickly revise the contents.

Many alternative unsolved case studies have been provided at the end of the book which would help the students to evaluate their learning skills gained through the course of the book.

I hope that this work will be of immense value to those embarking on the exciting experience of learning biochemistry for the first time and to those who are returning to the subject in which the information is expanding in leaps and bounds. I would look forward to the comments, criticisms and suggestions from students, faculty and professionals who would use the book.

Chapter 1

Carbohydrate: Chemistry and Clinical Significance

LEARNING OBJECTIVES

To understand:
- ❖ Chemistry of glycosides
- ❖ Biological and clinical significance of glycosides
- ❖ Chemistry of glycosaminoglycans
- ❖ Functions and significance of glycosaminoglycans
- ❖ Clinical implications of nondegradation of glycosaminoglycans (mucopolysaccharidoses)

CASE STUDIES

CASE STUDY 1

Theme: Chemistry and Significance of Glycosides

A 62-year-old man suffered from congestive heart failure. He was hospitalized and was started with a loading dose of digitalis. Gross improvement was seen in his symptoms. He was discharged after a few days and was put on a maintenance dose of digitalis.

What is the chemical nature of digitalis?
How does it help in improving the symptoms of heart failure?

CASE DISCUSSION

Cardiac failure can be described as the inability of the heart to pump blood effectively at a rate that meets the needs of the metabolizing tissues. Cardiac failures primarily arise from the reduced contractility of heart muscles, especially the ventricles. Reduced contraction of heart leads to reduced cardiac output resulting in the increase in cardiac blood volume. The heart feels congested. Hence, the term congestive heart failure.

Congested heart leads to hypotension and poor renal perfusion. This results in the development of edema in the lower extremities, pulmonary edema, as well as renal failure.

Cardiac glycosides are used for the treatment of congestive heart failure and arrhythmias. Digitalis used in the given case is a cardiac glycoside.

BASIC CONCEPT

Glycosides are compounds containing a carbohydrate and a noncarbohydrate residue in the same molecule. In these compounds, the carbohydrate residue is attached by an acetal linkage of carbon-I to the noncarbohydrate residue. The noncarbohydrate residue present in the glycoside is called as **aglycone**. The aglycones present in the glycosides vary in complexity from simple substances as methyl alcohol, glycerol, phenol, or a base such as adenine to complex substances, such as sterols, hydroquinones, and anthraquinones. The glycosides are named according to the carbohydrate they contain. If it contains glucose then, it forms **"Glucoside"**. If it contains galactose then it forms **"Galactoside",** etc. The attached carbohydrate can be in the alpha or beta configuration **(Fig. 1.1)**

Glycosides are present in many drugs, spices, and in the constituents of animal tissues.

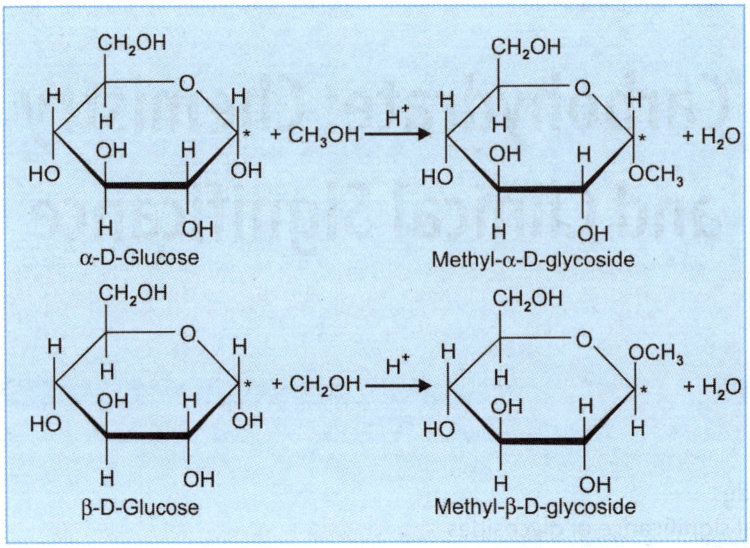

Fig. 1.1: Alpha and beta anomers of methyl glycoside.

Note: *indicates C-1 of glucose to which the aglycone (noncarbohydrate residue) is attached.

Cardiac Glycosides

Cardiac glycosides contain steroids as aglycone or genin component in combination with sugar molecules. These include derivatives of *digitalis* and *Strophanthus* such as ouabain.

Aglycone: The steroid nucleus has a unique set of fused ring system that makes the aglycone moiety structurally distinct from the other more common steroid ring systems. The steroid nucleus has hydroxyls at 3- and 14- positions of which the sugar attachment uses the 3-OH group. 14-OH is normally unsubstituted.

Sugar: One to four sugars are found to be present in most cardiac glycosides attached to the 3-OH group. The sugars most commonly used include L-rhamnose, D-glucose, D-digitoxose, D-digitalose, D-digginose, D-sarmentose, L-vallarose, and D-fructose. These sugars predominantly exist in the cardiac glycosides in the β-conformation **(Fig. 1.2)**.

The pharmacological activity is contained in the aglycone, which has, however, a less potent and shorter action than the parent glycoside. The sugar ensures increased water solubility, cell penetrability, and potency of the aglycone.

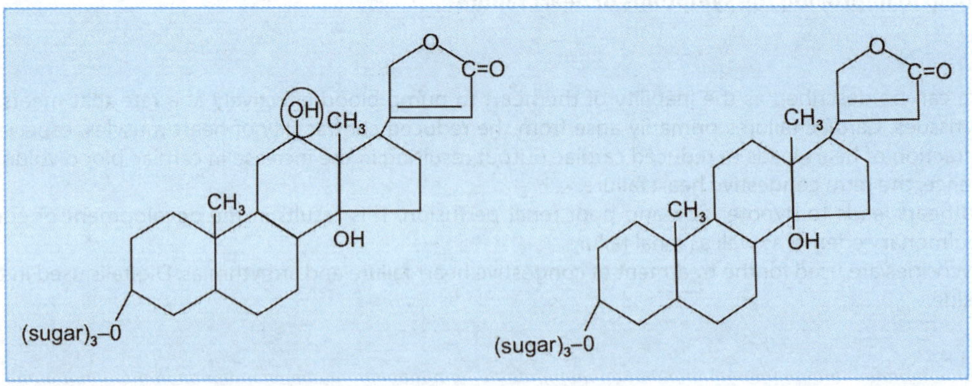

Fig. 1.2: Chemical structures of two digitalis glycosides. Each compound has 3 structural elements: an unsaturated lactone ring, a steroid nucleus, and several sugar moieties. Digoxin has an extrahydroxyl group compared to digitoxin. The sugar is attached at 3-OH group.

Digitalis

Digitalis was previously the drug of choice for treating congestive heart failure and arrhythmias. But its use in patients who are in sinus rhythm has declined since the therapeutic-to-toxic ratio is quite narrow.

This is a purified glycoside from European foxglove, *digitalis purpurea*.

A group of pharmacologically active compounds are extracted mostly from the leaves in pure form and are referred to by common chemical names such as *digitoxin* or *digoxin*.

Mechanism of Action of Digitalis

Direct action: The most probable mechanism of action for the positive inotropic effect of digitalis is inhibition of the membrane-bound Na^+/K^+-ATPase pump directly, which acts as the digitalis receptor; when this occurs, Na^+ increases in the cell, the exchange of Na^+ for Ca^{2+} is augmented, and calcium influx is increased. The increased intracellular calcium in turn leads to increased release of Ca^{2+} from the sarcoplasmic reticulum and increased contractility of the cardiac muscle. Changes in the ratio of intracellular and extracellular electrolytes can result in increased automaticity and cardiac arrhythmias. The inhibition of the Na^+/K^+-ATPase pump prevents the re-entry of potassium into the cell after the repolarization is complete, leading to depletion of the intracellular potassium. This potassium-depleting action of the digitalis is not confined to the cardiac muscle but also involves the skeletal muscle and the liver. By direct action, it increases the force of contraction of the heart muscle.

Digitalis also has a negative chronotropic effect due to decreased conduction velocity in the atrioventricular (AV) node. Therapeutically, it is very useful in heart failure associated with atrial fibrillation and rapid ventricular rate.

Ouabain

A glycoside obtained from *Strophanthus* species inhibits active transport of Na^+ in the cardiac muscle (sodium pump inhibitor). It also acts as a cardiac glycoside. It is now rarely used.

Other Glycosides of Clinical Importance

Many biologically active compounds are glycosides. **Glycosides comprise several important classes of compounds such as hormones, sweeteners, alkaloids, flavonoids, antibiotics, etc.** The glycosidic residue can be crucial for their activity or can only improve pharmacokinetic parameters.

Other glycosides such as streptomycin are used as antibiotics. Phloridzin is another glycoside, which is obtained from the root and bark of apple tree. It blocks the transport of sugar across the mucosal cells of small intestine and also renal tubular epithelium. It displaces Na^+ from the binding site of "carrier protein" and prevents the binding of sugar molecule and produces glycosuria.

Glycosides of vitamins, both hydrophilic and lipophilic, often occur in nature. Glycosylated vitamins have an advantage over the respective aglycone in their better solubility in water (especially the lipophilic ones), stability against Ultraviolet (UV) light, heat and oxidation, reduction of the bitter taste and odor (e.g., thiamine), and resistance to an enzymatic action. Some of the vitamin glycoconjugates have altered or improved pharmacokinetic properties.

CLINICAL NOTE

The inhibition of the Na^+/K^+-ATPase pump by digitalis prevents the re-entry of potassium into the cell after the repolarization is complete; this causes depletion of the intracellular potassium.

CLINICAL PEARLS

1. Glycosides are compounds containing a carbohydrate and a noncarbohydrate residue in the same molecule.
2. Cardiac glycosides contain steroids as aglycone component in combination with sugar molecules.
3. Glycosides comprise several important classes of compounds such as hormones, sweeteners, alkaloids, flavonoids, antibiotics, etc.
4. The most probable mechanism of action for the inotropic effect of digitalis is inhibition of the membrane-bound Na^+/K^+-ATPase pump.
5. Therapeutically, it is very useful in heart failure associated with atrial fibrillation and rapid ventricular rate.

CASE STUDY 2

Theme: Clinical Significance of Heparin and an Overview of Chemistry and Significance of Glycosaminoglycans

A 54-year-old woman who was bedbound in a nursing home began to develop swelling of her left leg. She was evaluated with venous Doppler ultrasound and was found to have a deep vein thrombosis. She was immediately started on heparin to prevent the clot from further enlarging.

What is the chemical nature of heparin?
How will it help in preventing the clot formation?

CASE DISCUSSION

Heparin is a highly sulfated GAG (glycosaminoglycan), see the details below.

Heparin

Heparin is also called α heparin. It is an anticoagulant widely used in clinical practice. It is present in liver, lungs spleen, and monocytes. Commercial preparations are from animal lung tissues. It contains repeating units of sulfated glucosamine and either of the two uronic acids—D-glucuronic acid and L-iduronic acid. In fully formed heparin molecules, 90% or more of uronic acid residues are L-iduronic acid **(Fig. 1.3)**. It is strongly acidic due to sulfuric acid groups and readily forms salts.

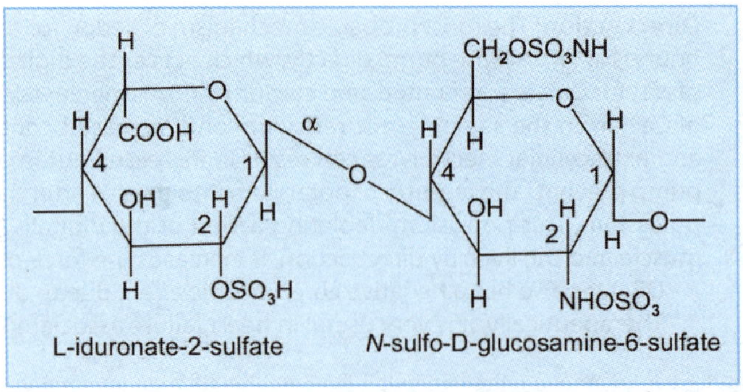

Fig. 1.3: Structure of heparin.

Clinical Role of Heparin

In vitro heparin is used as an anticoagulant while taking blood samples, in vitro heparin is used as an anticoagulant while taking blood samples. A concentration of 2 mg/10 mL of blood is used.. It is considered the most satisfactory anticoagulant as it does not produce a change in red cell volume or interfere with subsequent determinations.

In vivo heparin is used in suspected thromboembolic conditions to prevent intravascular coagulation.

Heparin is used for anticoagulation for the following conditions:

- Acute coronary syndrome
- Atrial fibrillation
- Deep-vein thrombosis and pulmonary embolism (heparin and its derivatives enoxaparin, dalteparin, and tinzaparin are effective at preventing deep-vein thromboses and pulmonary emboli in patients at risk)
- Cardiopulmonary bypass for heart surgery
- Extracorporeal membrane oxygenation (ECMO) circuit for extracorporeal life support.

Mechanism of Action

Role of heparin as an anticoagulant: The biological effect of heparin is to bind and activate antithrombin, which in turn inactivates thrombin and factor X. Binding of heparin to lysine residues in antithrombin III produces conformational changes, which promote the binding of the latter to serine protease "thrombin", which is inhibited; thus, fibrinogen is not converted to fibrin and the coagulation is inhibited.

Role of heparin as a coenzyme: Heparin acts in the body to potentiate the activity of the enzyme "lipoprotein lipase" **(Fig. 1.4)**. Heparin binds specifically to the enzyme present in capillary walls causing its release into the circulation. Hence, it is also called releasing factor.

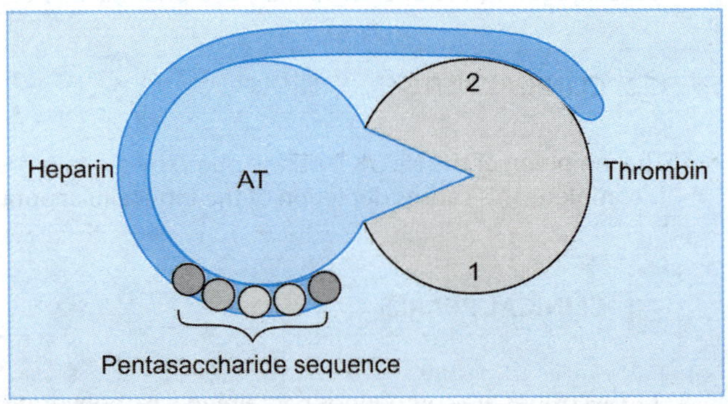

Fig. 1.4: Mechanism of action of heparin, AT (antithrombin). Heparin binds to AT through a high-affinity pentasaccharide.

Administration of Heparin

Heparin is given parenterally, as it is degraded when taken by mouth. It can be injected intravenously or subcutaneously. Intramuscular injections are avoided because of the potential for forming hematomas.

Because of its short biological half-life of approximately 1 hour, heparin must be given frequently or as a continuous infusion. However, the use of low-molecular-weight heparin (LMWH) has allowed once-daily dosing, thus not requiring a continuous infusion of the drug. If long-term anticoagulation is required, heparin is often used only to commence anticoagulation therapy until the oral anticoagulant warfarin shows its effects.

Adverse Effects

A serious side effect of **heparin is heparin-induced thrombocytopenia (HIT).** HIT is caused by an immunological reaction that makes platelets a target of immunological response, resulting in the degradation of platelets. This is what causes thrombocytopenia. This condition is usually reversed on discontinuation and can generally be avoided with the use of synthetic heparins. There is also a benign form of thrombocytopenia associated with early heparin use, which resolves without stopping heparin.

There are two nonhemorrhagic side effects of heparin treatment. The first is **elevation of serum aminotransferase levels**, which has been reported in as many as 80% of patients receiving heparin. This abnormality is not associated with liver dysfunction, and it disappears after the drug is discontinued. The other complication is **hyperkalemia**, which occurs in 5–10% of patients receiving heparin, and is the result of heparin-induced aldosterone suppression. The hyperkalemia can appear within a few days after the onset of heparin therapy.

CLINICAL NOTE

In vivo heparin is used in suspected thromboembolic conditions to prevent intravascular coagulation.

CLINICAL PEARLS

1. Heparin is component of intracellular granules of mast cells lining the arteries of the lungs, liver, and skin.
2. It contains repeating units of sulfated glucosamine and either of the two uronic acids—D-glucuronic acid and L-iduronic acid.
3. The biological effect of heparin is to bind and activate antithrombin, which in turn inactivates thrombin and factor X.
4. Heparin binds specifically to the lipoprotein lipase enzyme present in capillary walls causing its release into the circulation. Hence, it is also called releasing factor.
5. Heparin is given parenterally, as it is degraded when taken by mouth.

BASIC CONCEPT

Glycosaminoglycans

The most abundant heteropolysaccharides in the body are the glycosaminoglycans **(GAGs). GAGs are highly negatively charged molecules with extended conformation that imparts high viscosity to the solution.** GAGs are located primarily on the surface of cells or in the extracellular matrix (ECM). Along with the high viscosity of GAGs comes low compressibility, which makes these molecules ideal for a lubricating fluid in the joints. At the same time, their rigidity provides structural integrity to cells and provides passageways between cells, allowing for cell migration.

The specific GAGs of physiological significance are hyaluronic acid, dermatan sulfate, chondroitin sulfate, heparin, heparan sulfate, and keratan sulfate. Although each of these GAGs has a predominant disaccharide component, heterogeneity does exist in the sugars present in the make-up of any given class of GAG. These molecules are long unbranched polysaccharides containing a repeating disaccharide unit. The disaccharide units contain either of two modified sugars, N-acetylgalactosamine (GalNAc) or N-acetylglucosamine (GlcNAc), and a uronic acid such as glucuronate or iduronate.

Proteoglycans (mucoproteins) are formed of glycosaminoglycans (GAGs) covalently attached to the core proteins. They are found in all connective tissues, extracellular matrix (ECM), and on the surfaces of many cell types. Proteoglycans are remarkable for their *diversity* (different cores and different numbers of GAGs with various lengths and compositions).

The specific GAGs of physiological significance are:

Hyaluronic acid: (D-glucuronate + GlcNAc)n—

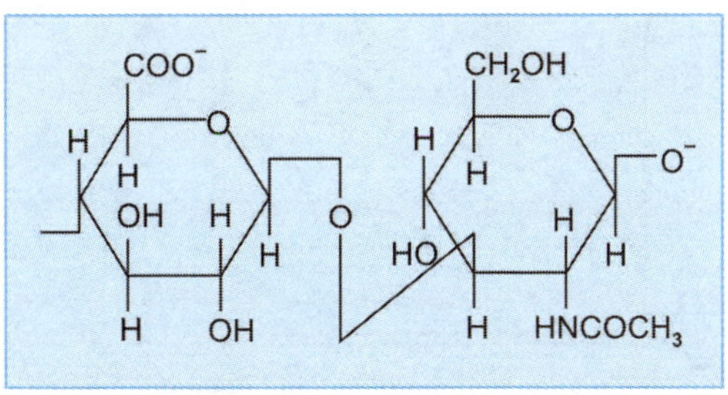

Occurrence: Synovial fluid and extracellular matrix (ECM) of loose connective tissue. It serves as a lubricant and shock absorber.

Hyaluronic acid is unique among the GAGs because it does not contain any sulfate and is not found covalently attached to proteins. It forms noncovalently linked complexes with proteoglycans in the ECM.

Hyaluronic acid polymers are very large (100–10,000 kDa) and can displace a large volume of water.

Dermatan sulfate: (L-iduronate + GalNAc sulfate)n—

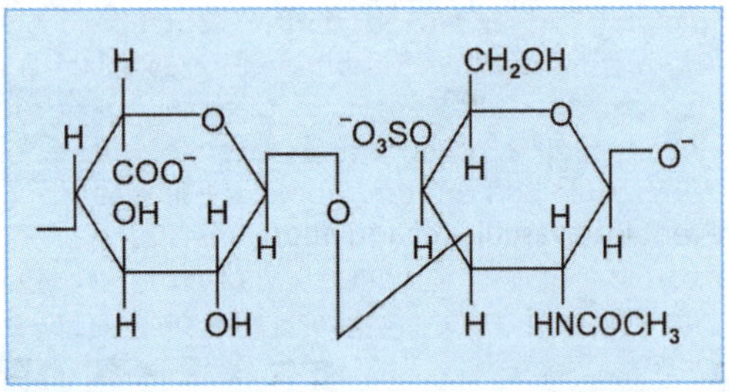

Occurrence: Skin, blood vessels, and heart valves

Chondroitin sulfate: (D-glucuronate + GalNAc sulfate) n—

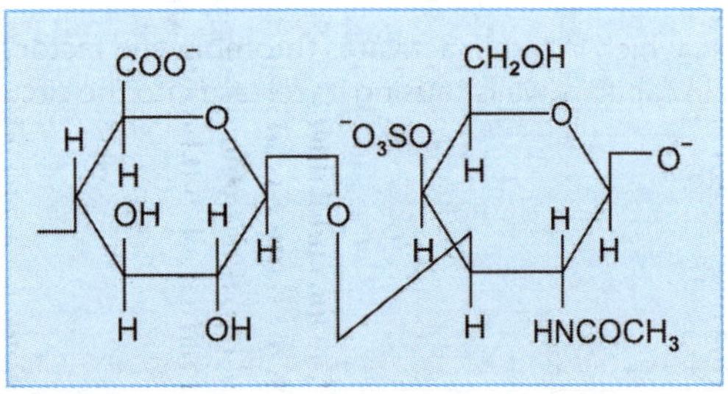

Occurrence: Cartilages, tendons, ligaments, heart valves, and aorta. It is the most abundant GAG.

Heparin and heparan sulfate: (D-glucuronate sulfate + N-sulfo-D-glucosamine)n—

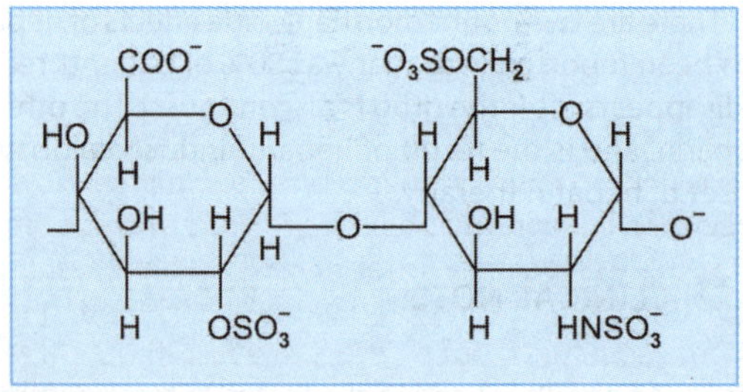

Heparans have less sulfate groups than heparins.

Occurrence:

- **Heparin:** Component of intracellular granules of mast cells lining the arteries of the lungs, liver, and skin (contrary to other GAGs that are extracellular compounds, it is intracellular).
- **Heparan sulfate:** Basement membranes and component of cell surfaces.

Keratan sulfate: (Gal + GlcNAc sulfate)n—

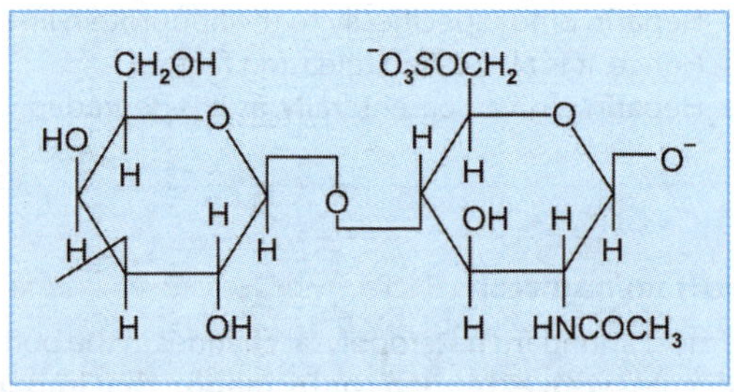

Occurrence: Cornea, bone, and cartilage.

Keratan sulfates are often aggregated with chondroitin sulfates.

Structure of Proteoglycans (Fig. 1.5)

The GAGs extend perpendicular from the core protein in a bottlebrush-like structure.

The linkage of GAGs such as (*heparan sulfates and chondroitin sulfates*) to the protein core involves a specific trisaccharide linker.

Some forms of *keratan sulfates* are linked to the protein core through an N-asparaginyl bond.

The protein cores of proteoglycans are rich in serine (Ser) and threonine (Thr) residues, which allow multiple GAG attachments.

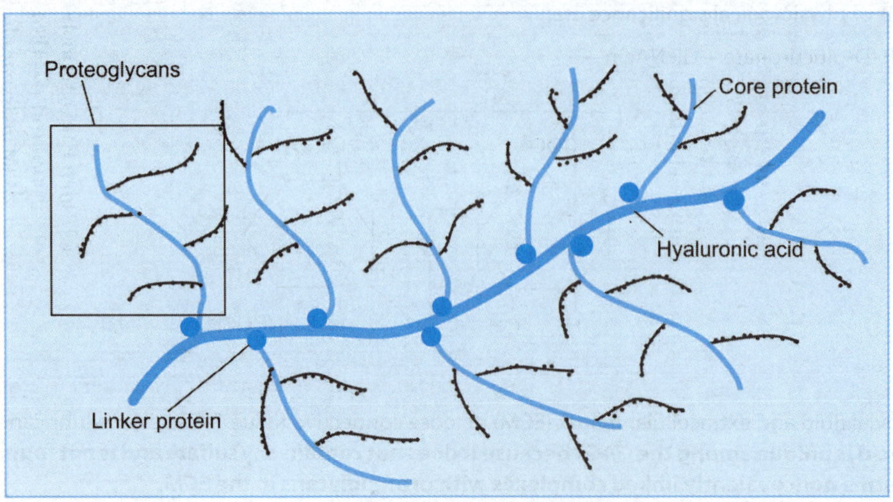

Fig. 1.5: Structure of proteoglycans.

Role of Proteoglycans and Glycosaminoglycans

They perform numerous vital functions within the body.

Glycosaminoglycan-dependent functions can be divided into two classes: the biophysical and the biochemical.

1. The biophysical functions depend on the unique properties of GAGs: the ability to fill the space, bind and organize water molecules, and repel negatively charged molecules. Because of high viscosity and low compressibility, they are ideal for a lubricating fluid in the joints. On the other hand, their rigidity provides structural integrity to the cells and allows the cell migration due to providing the passageways between cells.
2. The other, more biochemical functions of GAGs are mediated by specific binding of GAGs to other macromolecules, mostly proteins. Proteoglycans participate in cell and tissue development and physiology.

CASE STUDY 3

Theme: Mucopolysaccharidoses

A 10-year- old male child was brought to pediatric OPD. History revealed that the child was born normal, but he stopped developing after the age of 2 years. The skeletal deformities and coarse facial features appeared at the age of 3 years, and the child regressed to a vegetative state by age of 8 years. Examination revealed a nonresponsive child having constant dribbling of thick mucus from mouth. The history and clinical symptoms were suggestive of a metabolic disorder.

Complete urine analysis revealed the presence of heparan sulfate and dermatan sulfate.

What might be the probable diagnosis?

CASE DISCUSSION

The child is suffering from Hurler's syndrome ("gargoylism"). It is a type of mucopolysaccharidoses, which is caused due to nondegradation of glycosaminoglycans. Glycosaminoglycans are negatively charged, long, unbranched, and heteropolysaccharide chains and usually composed of a repeating disaccharide unit (acid sugar-amino sugar)n.

These chains are degraded by chain-specific lysosomal hydrolases. A deficiency of any of these hydrolases can result in mucopolysaccharidosis.

CASE DETAILS

Hurler's Syndrome

It is type-1 mucopolysaccharidoses (MPS 1).

Basic Defect

The disease is characterized by a deficiency of α-L-iduronidase enzyme, which removes iduronic acid residues from the heteropolysaccharide chains. A deficiency of this enzyme results in impaired degradation of dermatan and heparan sulfates. These undegraded GAGs (glycosaminoglycans) get accumulated in tissues (such as skin, blood vessels, heart valves, and basement membranes), producing a variety of symptoms characteristic of this disease. These GAGs are also excreted excessively in urine.

Inheritance

This disease is inherited in an autosomal recessive manner.

Frequency

Approximately 1 in 150,000 infants are affected.

Classification

The MPS I is divided into three subtypes based on severity of symptoms:

a. MPS IH or Hurler's syndrome—the most severe form
b. MPS IS or Scheie syndrome, and
c. MPS I-H/S or Hurler–Scheie syndrome.

All three types result from an absence of, or insufficient levels of, the enzyme α-L-iduronidase.

Clinical Manifestations

- The disease is characterized by progressive mental retardation, visual impairment, hearing loss, hepatosplenomegaly, dwarfism, and gargoyle-like faces. Death frequently occurs by the age of 10 years.
- The child may appear normal or larger than normal at the time of birth and may have inguinal or umbilical hernias. Developmental progression usually stops between 2 years and 4 years. Majority of children develop a short body trunk and a maximum stature of less than 4 feet.
- Speech difficulty is often observed due to an enlarged tongue.
- Coarse facial features (flat face, depressed nasal bridge, and bulging forehead) become more prominent in the second year **(Fig. 1.6)**
- Skeletal deformities appear at the age of 2 years. Carpal tunnel syndrome and restricted joint movement are commonly observed.
- Corneal clouding and conductive hearing loss are almost always present.
- **Miscellaneous symptoms:**
  - Noisy breathing, recurring upper respiratory tract, and ear infections.
  - Difficult feeding and frequent gastrointestinal infections.
  - Death occurs before the age of 10 years from obstructive lung disease, respiratory infections, or cardiac complications.

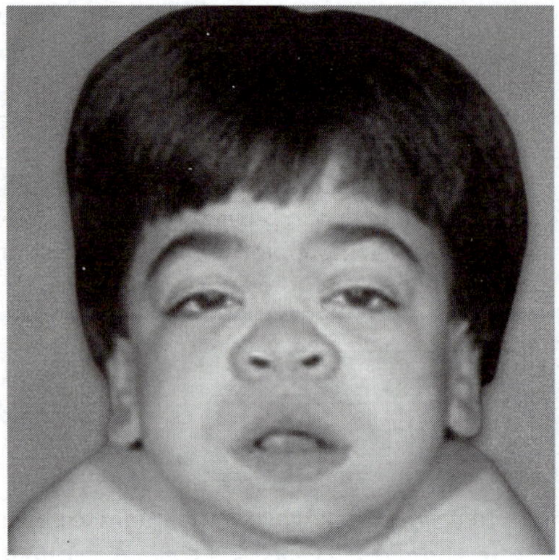

Fig. 1.6: Hurler's disease (distinct facial features).

Diagnosis

Diagnosis can be confirmed through clinical examination, laboratory investigations, and enzyme estimations.

Laboratory Investigations

1. **Urine examination** shows the excessive excretion of heparan and dermatan sulfate. Cetyltrimethylammonium bromide test is undertaken to confirm the presence of glycosaminoglycans in urine.
2. **Enzyme estimation:** The diagnosis can be confirmed by the absence of lysosomal alpha-L-iduronidase enzyme in cultured fibroblasts.
3. Prenatal testing: Culture of cells from amniotic fluid (obtained by amniocentesis) shows the absence of enzyme.
4. Molecular diagnosis using amniocentesis and chorionic villus sampling can confirm whether the fetus is a carrier of the mutated gene or has been affected by the disorder.

Radiology

X-rays of spine and chest show the characteristic skeletal deformities.

Treatment

- There is no cure for MPS I.
- With bone marrow transplantation (BMT) and umbilical cord blood transplantation (UCBT) preferably before the age of 18 months, abnormal physical characteristics, except for those affecting the skeleton and eyes, can be improved, and progression of neurologic degeneration can often be halted. BMT and UCBT are high-risk procedures with high rates of morbidity and mortality.

Advances in the management of Hurler's disease:

- Enzyme replacement therapy has been successfully employed in treating non-neurological symptoms.
- Gene therapy is under trial as a permanent cure.

Scheie Syndrome

This is a mild form of MPS I. The onset of symptoms occurs usually after the age of 5 years. The affected children manifest normal intelligence and stature. The disease is usually characterized by—joint stiffness, aortic valve disease, and corneal clouding. The diagnosis is made between 10 years and 20 years.

An overview of different mucopolysaccharidoses is shown in **Table 1.1** below.

AN OVERVIEW OF TYPES OF MUCOPOLYSACCHARIDOSES

Main Mucopolysaccharidoses

TABLE 1.1: An overview of types of mucopolysaccharidoses.

Type	*Main diseases*	*Deficient enzyme*	*Accumulated products*	*Symptoms*
MPS I	Hurler's syndrome	a-L-iduronidase	Heparan sulfate Dermatan sulfate	• Mental retardation • Micrognathia • Coarse facies • Macroglossia • Retinal degeneration • Corneal clouding • Cardiomyopathy
MPS II	Hunter syndrome	Iduronate sulfatase	• Heparan sulfate • Dermatan sulfate	• Mental retardation (similar, but milder, symptoms to Hurler's syndrome)
MPS III	Sanfilippo syndrome A Sanfilippo syndrome B Sanfilippo syndrome C Sanfilippo syndrome D	Heparan sulfamidase N-acetylglucosaminidase Acetyl-CoA: alpha-glucosaminide N-acetyltransferase N-acetylglucosamine-6-sulfatase	• Heparan sulfate	• Developmental delay • Severe hyperactivity • Spasticity • Motor dysfunction • Death by the second decade
MPS IV	Morquio syndrome A Morquio syndrome B	Galactose-6-sulfate sulfatase Beta-galactosidase	• Keratan sulfate • Chondroitin 6-sulfate • Keratan sulfate	• Severe skeletal dysplasia • Short stature • Motor dysfunction
MPS VI	Maroteaux–Lamy syndrome	N-acetylgalactosamine-4-sulfatase	• •Dermatan sulfate	• Severe skeletal dysplasia • Short stature • Motor dysfunction • Kyphosis • Heart defects
MPS VII	Sly syndrome	β-glucuronidase	• Heparan sulfate • Dermatan sulfate • Chondroitin 4,6-sulfate	• Hepatomegaly • Skeletal dysplasia • Short stature • Corneal clouding • Developmental delay
MPS IX	Natowicz syndrome	Hyaluronidase	• Hyaluronic acid	• Nodular soft-tissue masses around joints • Episodes of painful swelling of the masses • Short-term pain • Mild facial changes • Short stature • Normal joint movement • Normal intelligence

CLINICAL NOTE

Hurler's syndrome is marked by progressive deterioration, hepatosplenomegaly, dwarfism, and gargoyle-like faces.

CLINICAL PEARLS

1. The basic defect in Hurler's syndrome is deficiency of α-L-iduronidase enzyme.
2. Newborn infants with this defect appear normal at birth, developmental delay is evident by the end of the first year, and patients usually stop developing between ages 2 and 4.
3. Hurler's syndrome is marked by progressive deterioration, hepatosplenomegaly, dwarfism, and gargoyle-like faces.
4. Urine test, which shows the excessive excretion of heparan and dermatan sulfate.
5. This disease can be treated by bone marrow transplantation (BMT) and umbilical cord blood transplantation (UCBT).

Chapter 2

Carbohydrate: Metabolism and Related Disorders

LEARNING OBJECTIVES

To understand:

- ❖ Clinical implications of impaired digestion of carbohydrates
- ❖ Steps and significance of glycolysis
- ❖ Biological and clinical significance of reaction catalyzed by PDH complex
- ❖ Clinical significance of HMP pathway
- ❖ Causes and diagnosis of glycosuria
- ❖ Glucose homeostasis and causes; laboratory diagnosis and management of hypoglycemia
- ❖ Causes and consequences of hypoglycemia
- ❖ Galactose metabolism and clinical significance
- ❖ Chemistry and metabolism of glycogen
- ❖ Biochemical basis and clinical implications of glycogen storage diseases

CASE STUDIES

CASE STUDY 1

Theme: Clinical Implications of Impaired Digestion of Lactose

A newborn baby experienced abdominal distension, severe bowel cramps, and diarrhea after being fed milk.

A hydrogen analysis of his exhaled breath discovered an 80-fold increase in the production of hydrogen 90 minutes after milk feeding. The urine analysis revealed the presence of a reducing sugar.

What is the possible defect?
How can this be treated?

CASE DISCUSSION

This child is suffering from lactose intolerance. The abdominal distension and bowel cramps after being fed with milk are due to undigested lactose. **Some of the undigested lactose is absorbed by pinocytosis in the intestinal cell, which is ultimately excreted in urine; hence, it gives a positive test for reducing sugar.**

BASIC CONCEPT

Lactose Intolerance

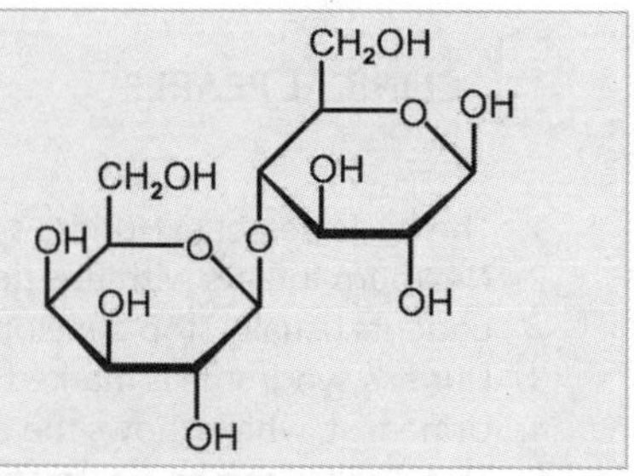

Fig. 2.1: Lactose (disaccharide of β-D-galactose and β-D-glucose) is normally split by lactase.

Lactose intolerance: Lactose intolerance is the inability or insufficient ability to digest lactose, a sugar found in milk and milk products **(Fig. 2.1)**. Lactase breaks down lactose into two simpler forms of sugar called glucose and galactose, which are then absorbed into the bloodstream. **Lactose intolerance is caused by a deficiency of the enzyme lactase, which is produced by the cells lining the small intestine.** Enzyme levels are highest shortly after birth and decline with aging, despite a continued intake of lactose.

Pathophysiology of Lactose intolerance

Disaccharides cannot be absorbed through the wall of the small intestine into the bloodstream, so in the absence of lactase, lactose present in ingested dairy products remains uncleaved and passes intact into the colon. The operons of enteric bacteria quickly switch over to lactose metabolism, and the resulting in vivo fermentation produces copious amounts of gas (a mixture of hydrogen, carbon dioxide, and methane).

This, in turn, may cause a range of abdominal symptoms, including abdominal cramps, bloating, and flatulence. In addition, as with other unabsorbed sugars (such as sorbitol, mannitol, and xylitol), the presence of lactose and its fermentation products raises the osmotic pressure of the colon contents.

The osmotic load of the unabsorbed lactose causes secretion of fluid and electrolytes until osmotic equilibrium is reached. Dilation of the intestine caused by the osmosis induces an acceleration of small intestinal transit, which increases the degree of maldigestion. The combined increase in fecal water, intestinal transit, and generated hydrogen gas accounts for the wide range of gastrointestinal symptoms.

Incidence

Some populations of the human species, including those of Asian, South American, and African descent, have a propensity for developing lactase deficiency. By contrast, races descended from northern Europe or from the northwestern Indian subcontinent are likely to retain the ability to absorb lactose till adulthood. **Of the world's population, 75% is estimated to be lactose deficient.**

Classification of Lactose Intolerance

There are three major types of lactose intolerance:

1. **Primary lactose intolerance:** Primary lactase deficiency develops overtime and begins after about age two when the body begins to produce less lactase. Most children who have lactase deficiency do not experience symptoms of lactose intolerance until late adolescence or adulthood.
2. **Secondary lactose intolerance:** Secondary, or acquired, lactase deficiency may develop in a person with a healthy small intestine during episodes of acute illness. This occurs because of mucosal damage or from medications resulting from certain gastrointestinal diseases, including exposure to intestinal parasites such as *Giardia lamblia*. In such cases, the production of lactase may be permanently disrupted. **A very common cause of temporary lactose intolerance is gastroenteritis, particularly when the gastroenteritis is caused by rotavirus. Another form of temporary lactose intolerance is lactose overload in infants.** Secondary lactase deficiency also results from injury to the small intestine that occurs with celiac disease, Crohn's disease, or chemotherapy. This type of lactase deficiency can occur at any age but is more common in infancy.
3. **Congenital lactase deficiency:** It is a genetic disorder, which prevents enzymatic production of lactase. It is present at birth and is diagnosed in early infancy.

Clinical Manifestations

People with lactose intolerance may feel uncomfortable 30 minutes to 2 hours after consuming milk and milk products. Symptoms range from mild to severe based on the amount of lactose consumed and the amount a person can tolerate. **Common symptoms include—abdominal pain, abdominal bloating, gas, diarrhea, and nausea.**

Diagnosis of Lactose Intolerance

Lactose intolerance can be hard to diagnose based on symptoms alone. Other conditions such as irritable bowel syndrome can cause similar symptoms. After taking a medical history and performing a physical examination, elimination of all milk and milk products is recommended from the person's diet for a short-time to see if the symptoms resolve. Tests may be necessary to provide more information.

Two tests are commonly used to measure the digestion of lactose.

Hydrogen breath test: The person drinks a lactose-loaded beverage and then the breath is analyzed at regular intervals to measure the amount of hydrogen. **Normally, very little hydrogen is detectable in the breath, but undigested lactose produces high levels of hydrogen.** The test takes about 2–3 hours.

Stool acidity test: The stool acidity test is used for infants and young children to measure the amount of acid in the stool. **Undigested lactose creates lactic acid and other fatty acids that can be detected in a stool sample.** Glucose may also be present in the stool as a result of undigested lactose.

Management of Lactose Intolerance

Although the body's ability to produce lactase cannot be changed, the symptoms of lactose intolerance can be managed with dietary changes. Most people with lactose intolerance can tolerate some amount of lactose in their diet. Gradually introducing small amounts of milk or milk products may help some people to adapt them with fewer symptoms. **Lactose-free or lactose-reduced milk, soy milk, and other products may be recommended.** Lactase enzyme drops or tablets can also be consumed. Getting enough calcium is important for people with lactose intolerance when the intake of milk and milk products is limited.

A balanced diet that provides an adequate amount of nutrients—including calcium and vitamin D—and minimizes discomfort is to be planned for the patients of lactose intolerance.

Complications

Osteopenia occurs in ignored and untreated cases.

Prognosis

The prognosis of patients with lactose intolerance is excellent with dietary restrictions.

CLINICAL NOTE

Resolution of symptoms with elimination of lactose-containing food products and resumption of symptoms with the reintroduction are findings suggestive of lactose intolerance.

CLINICAL PEARLS

1. Lactose intolerance is the inability or insufficient ability to digest lactose, a sugar found in milk and milk products.
2. The combined increase in fecal water, intestinal transit, and generated hydrogen gas accounts for the wide range of gastrointestinal symptoms.
3. Common symptoms include—abdominal pain, abdominal bloating, gas, diarrhea, and nausea.
4. Normally, very little hydrogen is detectable in the breath, but undigested lactose produces high levels of hydrogen. The test takes about 2–3 hours.
5. Lactose-free milk, lactose-reduced milk, or soy milk with calcium and vitamin D can be recommended.

CASE STUDY 2

Theme: Clinical Significance of Glycolysis

A 2-year-old African-American girl was referred to the hematologist after her pediatrician found her to be severely anemic with splenomegaly and jaundice. Her mother gave a possible history of a "blood problem" in her family but did not know for sure.

Her hemoglobin electrophoresis was normal, and the complete blood count (CBC) revealed a normocytic anemia. The platelet and white blood cell counts were normal. On the peripheral smear, there were many bizarre erythrocytes including spiculated cells. A diagnosis of pyruvate kinase deficiency was made.

What is the biochemical mechanism for this disorder?

How is this disorder inherited?

CASE DETAILS

The girl has hemolytic anemia and jaundice due to pyruvate kinase deficiency (PKD).

Pyruvate kinase deficiency, manifested as hemolytic anemia, is the most common enzymopathy in red blood cells (RBCs). Clinically, the symptoms are not as severe as indicated by the hematological indices, presumably due to enhanced oxygen delivery to the tissues resulting from the defect. The patients present with a wide spectrum of clinical severity. The disease may be as severe as to cause fetal death in utero, or the symptoms may be limited to early life or precipitated by physiological stress or infections. There may be mild asymptomatic compensated anemia or severe anemia requiring blood transfusion or splenectomy.

Inheritance

This disease is inherited in an autosomal recessive manner.

Pathophysiology

Pyruvate kinase deficiency (PKD) is an erythrocyte enzymopathy involving the Embden–Meyerhof pathway of anaerobic glycolysis. Erythrocytes have evolved without oxidative phosphorylation to form adenosine triphosphate (ATP), the compound is essential for providing the erythrocyte energy. **A discrepancy between erythrocyte energy requirements and ATP-generating capacity produces irreversible membrane injury, resulting in cellular distortion, rigidity, and dehydration.** This leads to premature erythrocyte destruction by the spleen and liver. Low ATP levels are responsible for erythrocyte intracellular electrolyte concentration disruption, due to failure of the adenosine triphosphatase cation pump.

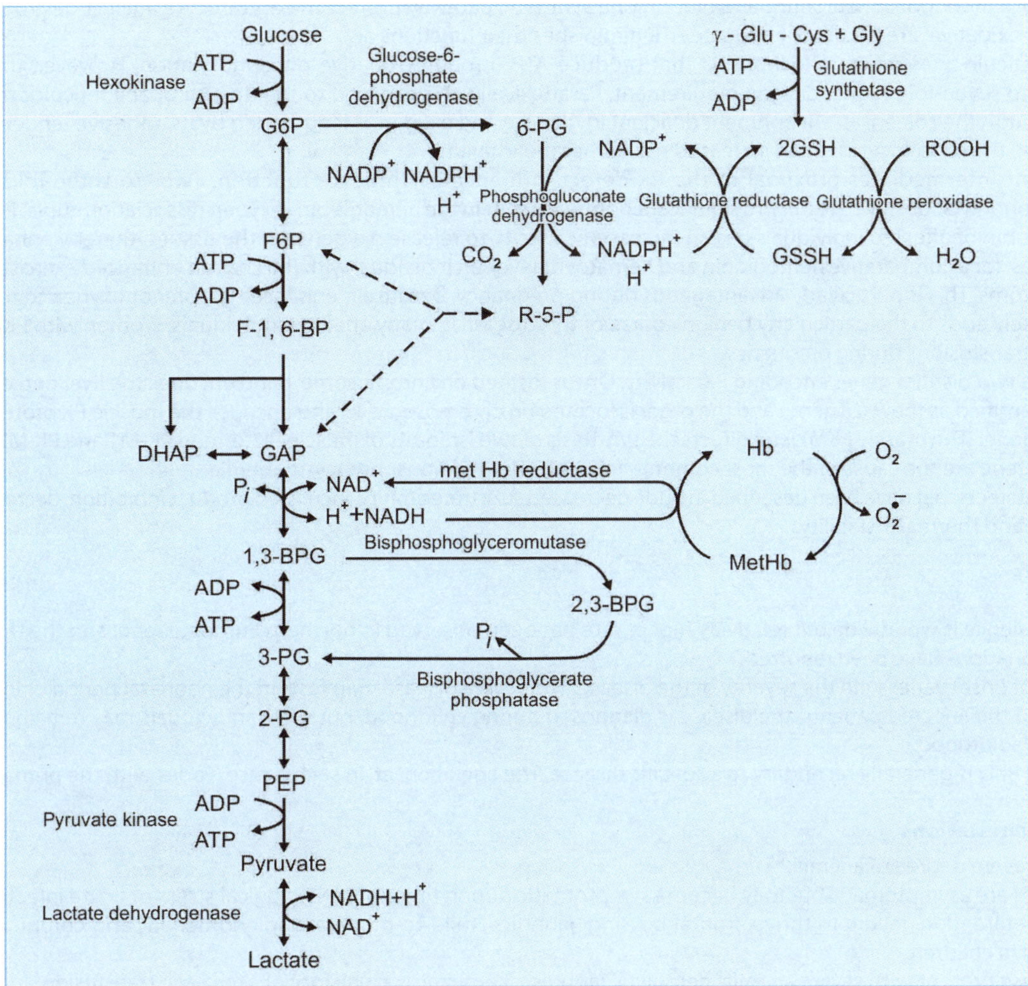

Fig. 2.2: Pathway of anaerobic glycolysis in red blood cells (RBCs).

Basic Concept

As shown in **Figure 2.2**, 1 mol of ATP is formed per mole of glucose metabolized by the glycolytic cycle. The primary final product of glucose metabolism by glycolysis in the RBC is not pyruvate, as in other tissues most of the time, but lactate. **Since RBCs have no mitochondria, NAD^+ cannot be regenerated by shuttling NADH produced in glycolysis into the mitochondrial electron transport system. Therefore, the only option to continue glycolysis is to regenerate NAD^+ from NADH by reducing pyruvate to lactate in the lactate dehydrogenase reaction.** But, lactate is not the sole product of RBC glycolysis. Methemoglobin reductase uses some of the NADH produced by glycolysis to reduce methemoglobin (Fe^{3+}) back to active hemoglobin (Fe^{2+}) capable of binding O_2 for transport to the tissues. Thus, the final products are a mixture of lactate and pyruvate with lactate being the primary product **(Fig. 2.2)**.

In tissues other than the RBC, pyruvate has alternative metabolic fates that, depending on the tissue, include gluconeogenesis, conversion to acetyl-CoA by pyruvate dehydrogenase for further metabolism to CO_2 in the tricarboxylic acid (TCA) cycle, transamination to alanine or carboxylation to oxaloacetate by pyruvate carboxylase. In the RBC, however, the restricted enzymatic endowment precludes all but the conversion to lactate. The pyruvate and lactate produced are end products of RBC glycolysis that are transported out of the RBC to the liver where they can undergo the alternative metabolic conversions described above.

How does compromise of pyruvate kinase (PK) activity lead to anemia? Pyruvate kinase lies at the end of the glycolytic pathway in RBCs followed only by lactate dehydrogenase. Pyruvate kinase activity is critical for the pathway and therefore critical for energy production. If ATP is not produced in amounts sufficient to meet the energy demand then those functions are compromised. **Energy is required to maintain the Na^+/K^+ balance within the RBC and to maintain the flexible discoid shape of the cell. In the absence of sufficient pyruvate kinase activity and therefore ATP, the ionic balance fails and the membrane becomes misshapen.** Cells reflecting pyruvate kinase insufficiency rather than a change in membrane composition are removed from the circulation by the macrophages of the spleen. This results in an increased number of circulating reticulocytes and possibly bone marrow hyperplasia, which is a biological response to lowered RBC count as a result of hemolysis of erythrocytes.

The hexose monophosphate shunt and glutathione synthetic pathway protect the erythrocyte against destruction from free radicals and oxidative stress. Loss of adequate ATP diminishes their functions also.

Young reticulocytes retain mitochondria that produce ATP through oxidative phosphorylation. However, this comes at a price, a six- to seven-fold higher oxygen requirement. Paradoxically, this can lead to the demise of any reticulocyte, because its journey through the spleen, an environment deficient in glucose and oxygen, is lengthened by its adhesive tendency. In such an environment, the reticulocyte is at an increased risk of metabolic failure.

Important intermediates proximal to the PK defect influence erythrocyte function. Two- to three-fold increases of 2,3-bisphosphoglycerate levels result in a significant rightward shift in the hemoglobin–oxygen dissociation curve. Physiologically, the hemoglobin of affected individuals has an increased capacity to release oxygen into the tissues, thereby enhancing oxygen delivery. Thus, for a comparative hemoglobin and hematocrit level, an individual with PKD has an enhanced exercise capacity and fewer symptoms. This is particularly advantageous during pregnancy, because it enhances transfer of oxygen to the fetal blood. This most likely adds to the particularly benign course of this disease in many affected individuals. Women with PKD typically do not require transfusions during pregnancy.

There are two distinct genes encoding PK activity. One is located on chromosome 1 and encodes the liver and erythrocyte PK proteins (identified as the *PKLR* gene) and the other is located on chromosome 15 and encodes the muscle PK proteins (identified as the *PKM* gene). The muscle PKM gene directs the synthesis of two isoforms of muscle PK termed PK-M1 and PK-M2. Deficiencies in the *PKLR* gene are the cause of the most common form of inherited nonspherocytic anemia.

Enzyme defects that have been described include decreased substrate affinity, increased product inhibition, decreased response to activator, and thermal instability.

Incidence

- The prevalence is worldwide but relatively higher rate has been observed in northern Europe, Japan, and the United States.
- No sex variations have been reported.
- The age of onset varies with the severity of the disease. The severe disease manifests in the neonatal period or in early infancy.
- In most of the affected patients, the disease is diagnosed during childhood, but some individuals may remain asymptomatic until late adulthood.
- Acquired PKD is generally secondary to a specific disease. The age of onset, in such a case, varies with the primary illness.

Clinical Manifestations

- Mild-to-severe degree of anemia.
- Mild cases are asymptomatic but may become symptomatic during times of physiological stress or acute infections.
- Growth retardation, failure to thrive, frontal bossing, jaundice, mild-to-moderate splenomegaly, and chronic leg ulcers are observed in children.
- Severe case present with severe anemia, hemolytic jaundice, kernicterus, or history of exchange transfusion.

Causes

- Acquired PKD can occur secondary to acute leukemia, refractory sideroblastic anemia, or as a complication of chemotherapy. The acquired PKD is more common and milder than the hereditary type.
- The hereditary type mostly occurs as a result of missense mutations; however, abnormal splicing, insertions, and deletions can also cause PKD. More than 100 genetic defects of the PK gene have been reported so far.
- The inheritance is autosomal recessive, and the affected individuals may be compound heterozygous for 2 different mutant alleles.

Treatment

In patients with mild-to-moderate disease, care is predominantly supportive in nature.

- **Red blood cell transfusion may be necessary, if the hemoglobin value falls significantly.** This tends to occur in early childhood and during periods when physiological stress is present, such as when an infection exists or during pregnancy.
- **Bone marrow transplantation** can be performed.

  Surgical care—splenectomy is indicated only for patients with severe anemia.

Prevention

- Monitor the hematocrit value carefully during times of physiological stress.
- If the defects in the parents are known, prenatal diagnosis using deoxyribonucleic acid (DNA) testing is possible.

Complications

- Cholecystolithiasis is common in the first decade of life for children with severe anemia.
- Splenectomy increases the risk of (1) sepsis by encapsulated bacteria for children and (2) thromboembolic disease for adults.
- Ischemic stroke has been reported in previously undiagnosed young adults with pyruvate kinase deficiency.

- Multiple-transfusion therapy can cause iron overload.
- Blood transfusions expose a person to the risk of contracting certain infections that are not well detected [e.g. human immunodeficiency virus (HIV) disease, hepatitis C].
- Repeated transfusions during pregnancy increase the risk of alloimmunization, which may lead to fetal complications.

Prognosis

- Mild-and-moderate forms of the disease are associated with an excellent prognosis.
- Severe forms of the disease are mostly symptomatic during early childhood. Following early childhood, the disorder is much better tolerated.
- Most morbidity develops from the above-mentioned complications.
- Hydrops fetalis has been reported in a severely affected fetus.

CLINICAL NOTE

Two- to three-fold increases of 2,3-bisphosphoglycerate levels result in a significant rightward shift in the hemoglobin–oxygen dissociation curve in pyruvate kinase deficiency.

CLINICAL PEARLS

1. Pyruvate kinase deficiency (PKD) is an erythrocyte enzymopathy involving the Embden–Meyerhof pathway of anaerobic glycolysis.
2. A discrepancy between erythrocyte energy requirements and ATP-generating capacity produces irreversible membrane injury, resulting in cellular distortion, rigidity, dehydration, and premature erythrocyte destruction by the spleen and liver.
3. Although inheritance is clinically autosomal recessive; most affected individuals are compound heterozygous for 2 different mutant alleles.
4. In patients with mild-to-moderate disease, care is predominantly supportive in nature.
5. Splenectomy is indicated only for patients with severe anemia.

CASE STUDY 3

Theme: Implications of Impaired Conversion of Pyruvate to Acetyl CoA

A full-term female infant failed to gain weight and showed metabolic acidosis in the neonatal period.

A physical examination at 6 months showed failure to thrive, hypotonia, small muscle mass, severe head lag, and a persistent acidosis (pH 7.0–7.2). Blood lactate, pyruvate, and alanine were greatly elevated. Treatment with thiamine did not alleviate the lactic acidosis.

What is the probable diagnosis of this patient?

CASE DETAILS

The child is most probably suffering from pyruvate dehydrogenase complex deficiency. **Metabolic acidosis, elevation of blood pyruvate, lactate, and alanine, all signify the nonconversion of pyruvate to acetyl-CoA .** The persistent metabolic acidosis is due to accumulation of lactates in blood.

BASIC CONCEPT

Pyruvate Dehydrogenase Complex Deficiency

Pyruvate dehydrogenase complex deficiency (PDCD) is one of the most common neurodegenerative disorders associated with abnormal mitochondrial metabolism. The citric acid cycle is a major biochemical process that derives energy from carbohydrates. Malfunction of this cycle deprives the body of energy. An abnormal lactate buildup results in nonspecific symptoms (e.g. severe lethargy, poor feeding, and tachypnea), especially during times of illness, stress, or high carbohydrate intake.

Progressive neurological symptoms usually start in infancy but may be evident at birth or in later childhood. These symptoms may include developmental delay, intermittent ataxia, poor muscle tone, abnormal eye movements, or seizures. Childhood-onset forms of this disorder are often associated with intermittent periods of decompensation but normal neurological development. The key feature of this condition is gray matter degeneration with foci of necrosis and capillary proliferation in the brainstem. The group of disorders that results in this pathology is termed Leigh syndrome.

Pathophysiology

Pyruvate dehydrogenase complex (PDC) converts pyruvate to acetyl-coenzyme A (CoA), which is one of the two essential substrates needed to produce citrate.

Oxidative metabolism requires the processing of pyruvate, a three-carbon product of glycolysis, to form the two-carbon compound acetyl-CoA, which is fed into the citric acid cycle. This conversion, an oxidative decarboxylation of pyruvate yielding a thioester product, is carried out by a complex and multienzyme complex known as the pyruvate dehydrogenase (PDH) complex **(Fig. 2.3).**

Multiple copies of three different enzymes—E1, E2, and E3—compose a supramolecular structure that coordinates a four-step process converting the α-keto acid pyruvate to the thioester (with coenzyme A) of acetate, as well as electron transfer (redox) reactions that yield NADH. Five cofactors participate in the reactions of the complex. E1 is pyruvate dehydrogenase (EC 1.2.4.1), which uses thiamine pyrophosphate (TPP) as a cofactor to decarboxylate pyruvate and transfer the remaining hydroxyethyl fragment to the lipoamide cofactor attached to E2. This results in the formation of acetyl-lipoamide, equivalent to reduction of lipoamide (and oxidation of the hydroxyethyl fragment), as becomes clear upon subsequent transfer of the acetyl residue to coenzyme A, catalyzed by E2, a acetyltransferase (EC 2.3.1.12) and E3, which regenerates lipoamide from dihydrolipoamide, is dihydrolipoyl dehydrogenase (EC 1.8.1.4).

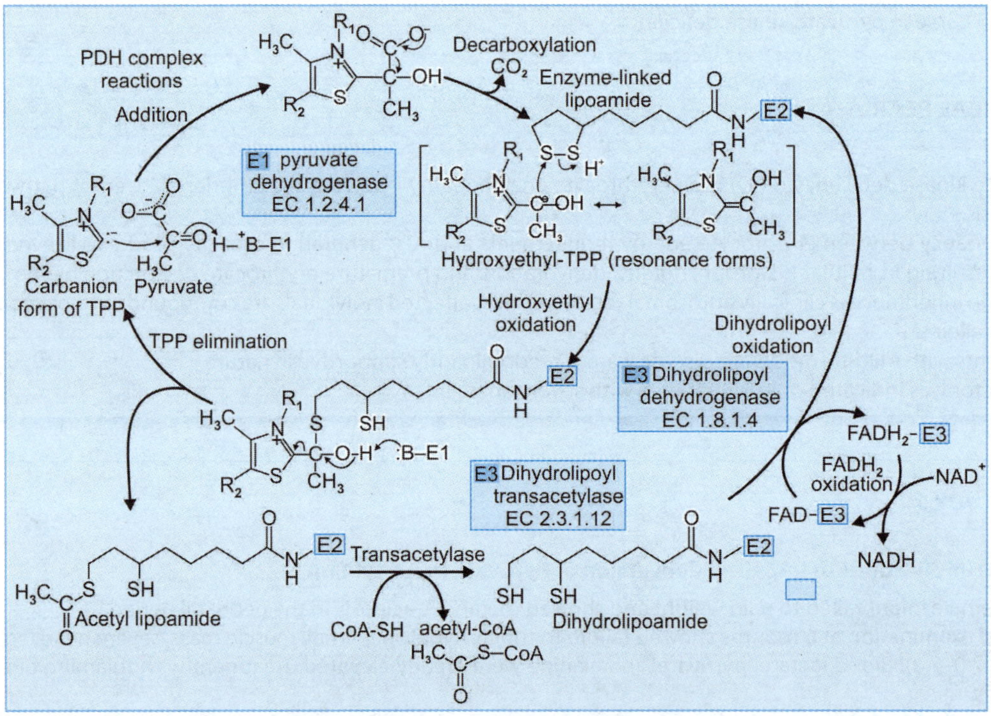

Fig. 2.3: Conversion of pyruvate to acetyl-coenzyme A (CoA).

The following features are characteristic of this disease:

1. **Energy deficit:** A deficiency in this enzymatic complex limits the production of citrate. Because citrate is the first substrate in the citric acid cycle, the cycle cannot proceed. Alternate metabolic pathways are stimulated in an attempt to produce acetyl-CoA; however, an energy deficit remains, especially in the CNS. The magnitude of the energy deficit depends on the residual activity of the enzyme.
2. **Neurological deficit:** Severe enzyme deficiencies may lead to congenital brain malformation because of a lack of energy during neural development. Underlying neuropathology is not usually observed in individuals whose onset of pyruvate dehydrogenase complex deficiency is in childhood.

Incidence

Pyruvate dehydrogenase complex deficiency is a rare disorder.

Inheritance

It most commonly follows an X-linked inheritance pattern, but is approximately equally prevalent in both males and females. This is because heterozygote females commonly manifest severe symptoms, an unusual situation in X-linked conditions.

Clinical Manifestations

Age of presentation varies from prenatal to early childhood and depends on the residual activity of the pyruvate dehydrogenase complex. Individuals with severe disease have prenatal onset with structural brain abnormalities. Moderate disease presents in infants as psychomotor delay. Individuals with less severe disease usually present in early childhood with intermittent lethargy or ataxia. The progression of pyruvate dehydrogenase complex deficiency (PDCD) widely varies.

- Nonspecific but common symptoms of metabolic illnesses include the following:
  - Poor feeding
  - Lethargy
  - Rapid breathing (i.e. tachypnea)
- Developmental nonspecific signs of metabolic disease include the following:
  - Mental delays
  - Psychomotor delays
  - Growth retardation
- Progressive neurological symptoms of pyruvate dehydrogenase complex deficiency usually start in infancy but may be evident at birth or in later childhood. The following are signs of poor neurological development or degenerative lesions:
  - Poor acquisition or loss of motor milestones
  - Poor muscle tone
  - New onset seizures
  - Periods of incoordination (i.e. ataxia)
  - Abnormal eye movements
  - Poor response to visual stimuli
  - *Episodic dystonia*: This is associated with a deficiency of the E2 subunit.
- Early childhood-onset pyruvate dehydrogenase complex deficiency typically presents with intermittent periods of incoordination, especially during mild illnesses.

Mortality/Morbidity

Individuals with neonatal-onset and infantile-onset types of pyruvate dehydrogenase complex deficiency usually die during the first year of life. Later childhood onset of the disease is usually, but not always, associated with survival into adulthood.

All children are born with some residual enzyme activity because a complete deficiency of pyruvate dehydrogenase complex is incompatible with life. Infants with 15% or less pyruvate dehydrogenase complex activity normally do not survive the newborn period. Pyruvate dehydrogenase complex activity greater than 25% is associated with less severe disease and is usually characterized by ataxia and mild psychomotor delay. Some therapies may extend the lives of individuals who are severely affected with pyruvate dehydrogenase complex deficiency; however, the progressive nature of the neurological deterioration results in significant morbidity.

Causes

Dysfunction in all 3 substrate—processing enzymes, regulatory protein, and thiamine dependence of the E1 alpha enzyme—has been described; however, dysfunction of the E1 alpha enzyme subunit is most common.

Laboratory Investigations

The following studies are indicated in pyruvate dehydrogenase complex deficiency (PDCD):

- **Lactate and pyruvate levels:**
  - High blood lactate and pyruvate levels with/without lactic acidemia
  - In mild cases of pyruvate dehydrogenase complex deficiency, these levels may be elevated only slightly under normal conditions; elevated levels may also be found during periods of crisis.
  - **Lactate-to-pyruvate ratio is diagnostically useful to differentiate pyruvate dehydrogenase complex deficiency from other forms of congenital lactic acidosis at higher lactate levels (>5 mmol/L).**
- **Serum and urine analysis:**
  - Serum and urine amino acid analyses reveal hyperalaninemia.
  - Deficiency of the E3 enzyme also causes an elevation in branched-chain amino acids in the serum and alpha-ketoglutarate in the serum and urine.
  - Hyperammonemia and nonspecific amino acid elevation are associated with E2 enzyme deficiency, which is more common during acute illnesses.
- **Other studies:**
  - Definitive diagnosis is made by showing abnormal enzyme function.
  - Functional assays can be performed on leukocytes, fibroblasts, or properly preserved tissue samples. Pyruvate dehydrogenase complex activity should be measured with and without thiamine in order to detect cases of thiamine-responsive pyruvate dehydrogenase complex deficiency.

Imaging Studies

- **MRI:**
  - Magnetic resonance imaging (MRI) shortly after birth may reveal ventricular dilation, cerebral atrophy.
  - MRI of infants with progressive neurological symptoms may reveal symmetric cystic lesions or generalized hypomyelination.

Treatment

Direct treatment that stimulates the pyruvate dehydrogenase complex (PDC) provides alternative fuels and prevents acute worsening of the syndrome. Correction of acidosis does not reverse all the symptoms. CNS damage is common and limits recovery of normal function.

- **Cofactor supplementation with thiamine, carnitine, and lipoic acid is the standard-of-care.** The cases of pyruvate dehydrogenase complex deficiency (PDCD) that are responsive to these cofactors respond to supplementation, especially thiamine. Some evidence suggests that high doses of thiamine may be most effective in some mutations causing thiamine-responsive pyruvate dehydrogenase complex deficiency. However, administration of all of these cofactors to all patients with pyruvate dehydrogenase complex deficiency is typical in order to optimize pyruvate dehydrogenase complex function.
- **Ketogenic diets** (with restricted carbohydrate intake) have been used to control lactic acidosis with minimal success.
- **Oral dichloroacetate** administered for 6 months was found to be well tolerated and blunted the postprandial increase in circulating lactate but did not improve neurological or other clinical measures.
- **Oral citrate** is often used to treat acidosis.

CLINICAL NOTE

Underlying neuropathology is not usually observed in individuals whose onset of pyruvate dehydrogenase complex deficiency is in childhood.

CLINICAL PEARLS

1. Pyruvate dehydrogenase complex (PDC) converts pyruvate to acetyl-coenzyme A (CoA), which is one of the two essential substrates needed to produce citrate.
2. All children are born with some residual enzyme activity because a complete deficiency of pyruvate dehydrogenase complex is incompatible with life.
3. Dysfunction in all 3 substrate—processing enzymes, regulatory protein, and thiamine dependence of the E1 alpha enzyme—has been described; however, dysfunction of the E1 alpha enzyme subunit is most common.
4. High blood lactate and pyruvate levels with/without lactic acidemia suggest an inborn error of metabolism at the mitochondrial level.
5. Ketogenic diets (with restricted carbohydrate intake) have been used to control lactic acidosis.

CASE STUDY 4

Theme: Clinical Significance of HMP Pathway

A 34-year-old African-American man was seen with fever and shortness of breath. Shortly afterwards, he developed pancreatitis and was treated with antibiotic—clindamycin and primaquine. After four days into this therapy, the onset of hematuria was noted.

The patient's hemoglobin (Hb) fell from 11.0 g/dL to 7.4 g/dL, his total bilirubin increased from 1.2 mg/dL to 4.3 mg/dL and his lactic dehydrogenase (LDH) increased from 248 IU/L to 612 IU/L.

What is the probable diagnosis?

What is the relationship of primaquine and hemolytic anemia?

CASE DETAILS

The patient is most probably suffering from glucose-6-phosphate dehydrogenase (G6PD) deficiency. The hemolysis is primaquine induced, which is an oxidant drug. The rise in bilirubin is due to hemolytic jaundice and the rise in lactic dehydrogenase (LDH) is commonly observed in hemolytic anemia.

Glucose-6-Phosphate Dehydrogenase Deficiency

Background

Glucose-6-phosphate dehydrogenase deficiency is the most common disease-producing enzymopathy in humans. Inherited as an X-linked disorder, G6PD deficiency affects 400 million people worldwide. The disease is highly polymorphic with more than 300 reported variants. It confers protection against malaria, which probably accounts for its high gene frequency.

Pathophysiology

Glucose 6-phosphate dehydrogenase is an enzyme critical in the redox metabolism of all aerobic cells. In red cells, its role is even more critical because it is the only source of reduced nicotinamide adenine dinucleotide phosphate (NADPH), which, directly and via reduced glutathione (GSH), defends these cells against oxidative stress **(Fig. 2.4)**.

Nicotinamide adenine dinucleotide phosphate is a required cofactor in many biosynthetic reactions, which also maintains glutathione in its reduced form. Reduced glutathione acts as a scavenger for dangerous oxidative metabolites in the cell. With the help of the enzyme glutathione peroxidase, reduced glutathione converts harmful hydrogen peroxide to water. **G6PD deficiency is a prime example of a hemolytic anemia due to interaction between an intracorpuscular and an extracorpuscular cause, because in the majority of cases, hemolysis is triggered by an exogenous agent.** People deficient in G6PD are not prescribed oxidative drugs, because their red blood cells undergo rapid hemolysis under this stress.

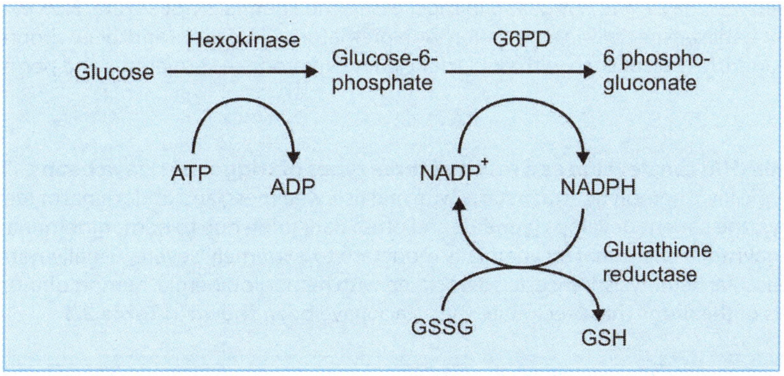

Fig. 2.4: Role of glucose-6-phosphate dehydrogenase (G6PD) in glucose metabolism.

Although in G6PD-deficient subjects, there is a decrease in G6PD activity in most tissues, this is less marked than in red cells, and it does not seem to produce symptoms.

Incidence

The highest prevalence rates with gene frequencies from 5% to 25% of (G6PD) deficiency are found in tropical Africa, the Middle East, tropical and subtropical Asia, and some areas of the Mediterranean.

In several of these areas, the frequency of a G6PD deficiency gene may be as high as 20% or more. It would be quite extraordinary for a trait that causes significant pathology to spread widely and reach high frequencies in many populations without conferring some biological advantage. **G6PD deficiency has been selected by *Plasmodium falciparum* malaria, by virtue of the fact that it confers a relative resistance against this highly lethal infection.** Whether this protective effect is exerted mainly in hemizygous males or in females heterozygous for G6PD deficiency is still not clear.

Inheritance

The ***G6PD* gene is X-linked**, and this has important implications. First, as males have only one G6PD gene (i.e. they are hemizygous for this gene), they must be either normal or G6PD deficient. By contrast, **females, having two G6PD genes, can be normal, deficient (homozygous), or intermediate (heterozygous).**

The enzymatically active form of G6PD is either a dimer or a tetramer of a single protein subunit of 514 amino acids. G6PD-deficient subjects have been found invariably to have mutations in the coding region of the G6PD gene. Almost all of the 140 different mutations known are single missense point mutations, entailing single amino acid replacements in the G6PD protein. In most cases, these mutations cause G6PD deficiency by decreasing the in vivo stability of the protein, and thus the physiological decrease in G6PD activity that takes place with red cell aging is greatly accelerated. In some cases, an amino acid replacement can also affect the catalytic function of the enzyme.

Classifications of G6PD Deficiency Disease

Glucose-6-phosphate dehydrogenase gene variants are currently divided into five classifications, depend on enzyme activity and clinical manifestations. In addition, the deficiencies are classified as to whether or not they are sporadic or polymorphic.
The five classifications are:

1. **Class 1:** Enzyme deficiency with chronic nonspherocytic hemolytic anemia
2. **Class 2:** Severe enzyme deficiency, less than 10% of normal activity
3. **Class 3:** Moderate-to-mild enzyme deficiency, 10–60% of normal activity
4. **Class 4:** Very mild or no enzyme deficiency, at least 60% percent of normal activity
5. **Class 5:** Increased enzyme activity.

Mutations in the G6PD gene that result in nonspherocytic hemolytic anemia have all been found to cluster near the carboxyl terminal end of the protein, whereas, the mutations that result in clinically mild symptoms are clustered near the amino terminal end of the protein.

Clinical Manifestations

1. The **vast majority of people with G6PD deficiency remain clinically asymptomatic throughout their lifetime.**
2. However, all of them have an increased risk of developing neonatal jaundice (NNJ) and a risk of developing acute HA when challenged by a number of oxidative agents. NNJ related to G6PD deficiency is very rarely present at birth: the peak incidence of clinical onset is between day 2 and day 3, and in most cases, the anemia is not severe. However, NNJ can be very severe in some G6PD-deficient babies, especially in association with prematurity, infection, and/or environmental factors. In these cases, if inadequately managed, NNJ associated with G6PD deficiency can produce kernicterus and permanent neurological damage.

Precipitating Factors

Acute hemolytic anemia (HA) can develop as a result of three types of triggers: (1) fava beans, (2) infections, and (3) drugs.
Sequence of events: Typically, a hemolytic attack starts with malaise, weakness, and abdominal or lumbar pain. After an interval of several hours to 2–3 days, the patient develops jaundice and often dark urine due to hemoglobinuria. The onset can be extremely abrupt, especially with favism in children. The anemia is moderate to extremely severe, usually normocytic and normochromic, and partly due to intravascular hemolysis; hence, it is associated with hemoglobinemia, hemoglobinuria, and low or absent plasma haptoglobin. The details of the drugs that precipitate the attack have been shown in **Table 2.1**.

TABLE 2.1: Drugs that precipitate the attack.

Definite risk		*Possible risk*	*Doubtful risk*
Antimalarials	Primaquine Dapsone/chlorproguanil	Chloroquine	Quinine
Sulfonamides/sulfones	Sulfamethoxazole Others Dapsone	Sulfasalazine Sulfadimidine	Sulfisoxazole Sulfadiazine
Antibacterial/antibiotics	Cotrimoxazole Nalidixic acid Nitrofurantoin Niridazole	Ciprofloxacin Norfloxacin	Chloramphenicol P-aminosalicylic acid
Antipyretic/analgesics	Acetanilide Phenazopyridine (Pyridium)	Acetylsalicylic acid high dose (>3 g/day)	Acetylsalicylic acid <3 g/day Acetaminophen Phenacetin
Other	Naphthalene Methylene blue	Vitamin K analogs Ascorbic acid >1 g	Doxorubicin Glucose-6-phosphate dehydrogenase

Laboratory Diagnosis

The laboratory workup for G6PD deficiency includes the following:

- Measure the actual enzyme activity of G6PD rather than the amount of G6PD protein.
- Obtain a complete blood cell (CBC) count with the reticulocyte count to determine the level of anemia and bone marrow function.

- Indirect bilirubinemia occurs with excessive hemoglobin degradation and can produce clinical jaundice.
- Serum haptoglobin levels serve as an index of hemolysis and will be decreased.
- LDH is high and so is the unconjugated bilirubin, indicating that there is also extravascular hemolysis.

Imaging Studies

Abdominal ultrasound may be useful in assessing for splenomegaly and gallstones in cases of G6PD deficiency.

Peripheral Blood Film

The blood film shows anisocytosis, polychromasia, and spherocytes. **The most typical feature is the presence of bizarre poikilocytes with red cells that appear to have unevenly distributed hemoglobin and red cells that appear to have had parts of them bitten away (bite cells or blister cells).** A classic test, now rarely carried out, is supravital staining with methyl violet, which, if done promptly, reveals the presence of Heinz bodies, consisting of precipitates of denatured hemoglobin and regarded as a signature of oxidative damage to red cells (except for the rare occurrence of an unstable hemoglobin) **(Fig. 2.5)**.

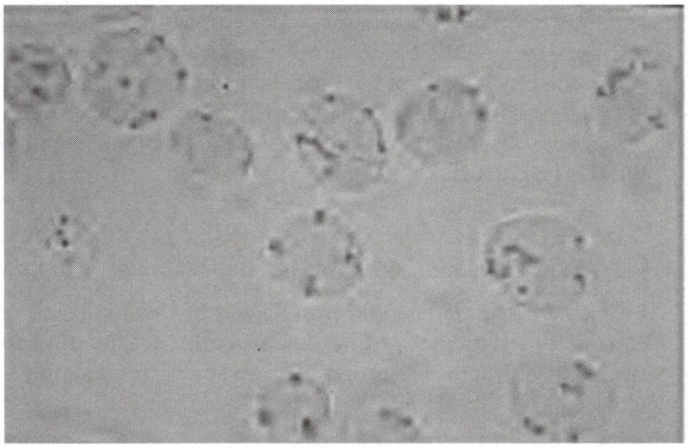

Fig. 2.5: Acute hemolysis from glucose-6-phosphate dehydrogenase deficiency is linked to the development of Heinz bodies, which are composed of denatured hemoglobin.

Treatment

Medical care: Identification and discontinuation of the precipitating agent are critical in cases of G6PD deficiency. Affected individuals are treated with oxygen and bed rest, which may afford symptomatic relief. Prevention of drug-induced hemolysis is possible in most cases by choosing alternative drugs. **When acute HA develops and once its cause is recognized, no specific treatment is needed in most cases. However, if the anemia is severe, it may be a medical emergency, especially in children, requiring immediate action, including blood transfusion.** If acute renal failure develops, hemodialysis may be necessary, but if there is no previous kidney disease, full recovery is the rule. The management of NNJ associated with G6PD deficiency is no different from that of NNJ due to other causes.

Diet: Patients must avoid broad beans (i.e. fava beans). Favism occurs only in the Mediterranean variety of G6PD deficiency.

Prognosis

Most individuals with G6PD deficiency do not need treatment.

CLINICAL NOTE

The disease is highly polymorphic, with more than 300 reported variants. It confers protection against malaria, which probably accounts for its high gene frequency.

CLINICAL PEARLS

1. Pyruvate dehydrogenase complex (PDC) converts pyruvate to acetyl-coenzyme A (CoA), which is one of the two essential substrates needed to produce citrate.
2. All children are born with some residual enzyme activity because a complete deficiency of pyruvate dehydrogenase complex is incompatible with life.
3. Dysfunction in all 3 substrate—processing enzymes, regulatory protein, and thiamine dependence of the E1 alpha enzyme—has been described; however, dysfunction of the E1 alpha enzyme subunit is most common.
4. High blood lactate and pyruvate levels with/without lactic acidemia suggest an inborn error of metabolism at the mitochondrial level.
5. Ketogenic diets (with restricted carbohydrate intake) have been used to control lactic idosis.

CASE STUDY 5

Theme: Glycosuria—Causes and Laboratory Diagnosis

A 32-year-old female visited the family physician for routine checkup. She was keeping well and was very much particular about her physical fitness. Her general physical examination was normal, but the urine test was positive for reducing sugar. There were no symptoms suggestive of diabetes mellitus. There was no family history of diabetes mellitus. There was no history of any drug intake.

Blood sample was drawn for random sugar estimation. It was normal. The patient was asked to report next day for oral glucose tolerance test. All the blood samples had glucose within normal limits, but the urine test was positive for nonglucose reducing sugar. The physician kept the probability of essential benign fructosuria and advised the patient to report again after 2 days and instructed her to totally abstain from fructose or fructose containing diet during those 2 days.

On her subsequent visit, urine test came out to be negative for reducing sugar. The diagnosis of fructosuria was confirmed.

What is fructosuria?

CASE DETAILS

Essential Fructosuria

Essential fructosuria, also known as hepatic fructokinase deficiency or ketohexokinase deficiency, is a hereditary metabolic disorder **caused by a deficiency of hepatic fructokinase, leading to fructose being excreted in the urine.** It is essentially a benign condition, as fructose cannot be broken down, so it is simply excreted in the urine.

Inheritance

This disease is inherited in an autosomal recessive manner.

Biochemical Defect

Normally, fructose is first metabolized in the body to fructose-1-phosphate by a specific enzyme called fructokinase **(Fig. 2.6)**. In fructosuria, this particular enzyme is defective, and the concentration of fructose increases in the blood and urine. **Essential fructosuria should not be confused with hereditary fructose intolerance, which is a very serious condition and is due to deficiency of aldolase B enzyme.** It causes a rise in uric acid, growth abnormalities, in severe cases hepatic or renal failure, and finally coma or death. (*See* the details in Hereditary Fructose Intolerance).

On the other hand, being symptomless, fructosuria is commonly left undetected or undiagnosed.

Symptoms

Fructosuria is generally asymptomatic; it may be a chance finding that urine test is positive for nonglucose-reducing sugar. Presence of fructose in urine can be confirmed by specific tests. The condition has to be differentiated from other causes of glycosuria, like Type 1 and Type 2 diabetes mellitus, and other conditions.

Differential Diagnosis

Fructosuria should be differentiated from the other causes of glycosuria.

Glycosuria

Although normal urine contains virtually no sugar but under certain circumstances, glucose or other sugars may be excreted in urine. This condition is called "melituria". The terms glycosuria, fructosuria, galactosuria, lactosuria, and pentosuria are applied specifically for urinary excretion of glucose, fructose, galactose, lactose, and pentose, respectively.

Types of Glycosuria

Glycosuria can be classified into two main groups:

a. Hyperglycemic glycosuria
b. Renal glycosuria.

a. Hyperglycemic glycosuria:

- Alimentary glycosuria (excessive ingestion of carbohydrates)
- Emotional glycosuria (excessive catecholamine release)
- Glycosuria due to endocrinal disorders, e.g.:
  - Diabetes mellitus
  - Hyperthyroidism
  - Epinephrine hypersecretion
  - Hyperactivity of anterior pituitary (acromegaly)
  - Hyperactivity of adrenal cortex (Cushing's syndrome/disease)
  - Increased secretion of glucagon

b. **Renal glycosuria:**
   i. **Renal causes of glucose in the urine:**
      - Signs suggestive of renal tubular disease:
        - Serum glucose <180 mg/dL
        - Glucose tolerance tests are normal ketosis absent
      - Specific causes:
        - Fanconi's syndrome
        - Toxic renal tubular disease:
          - Lead toxicity
          - Mercury toxicity
          - Degraded tetracycline
      - Inflammatory renal disease:
        - Acute glomerulonephritis
        - Nephrosis
      - Increased glomerular filtration rate (GFR) without tubular damage:
        - Hereditary renal glycosuria (carrier protein deficiency)
        - Lowering of renal threshold (pregnancy).
   ii. **Causes of false positive glucose on urinalysis:**
      - Ascorbic acid
      - Nalidixic acid
      - Cephalosporins
      - Probenecid
      - Ketones
      - Levodopa.
   iii. **Causes of false-negative glucose on urinalysis:**
      - Increased specific gravity
      - Uric acid
      - Vitamin C.
   iv. **Nonglucose-reducing sugars:**
      - Fructose
      - Galactose
      - Lactose
      - Pentose.

Laboratory Diagnosis of Fructosuria

Based on the history, positive urine test for reducing sugar and absence of clinical findings, **the confirmation of the diagnosis can be done by thin layer chromatography of the urine sample** to ensure the presence of fructose. Blood sugar can be estimated in doubtful cases to rule out the presence of diabetes mellitus.

Treatment

Since it is a benign condition, no treatment is required. Only fructose-containing foods have to be avoided.

CLINICAL NOTE

Essential fructosuria should not be confused with hereditary fructose intolerance, which is due to deficiency of aldolase B enzyme.

CLINICAL PEARLS

1. Essential fructosuria, also known as hepatic fructokinase deficiency or ketohexokinase deficiency, is a hereditary metabolic disorder caused by a deficiency in hepatic fructokinase.
2. It is essentially a benign condition, as fructose cannot be broken down, so it is simply excreted in the urine.
3. The condition has to be differentiated from other causes of glycosuria, like Type 1 and Type 2 diabetes mellitus, and other conditions.
4. Blood sugar can be estimated in doubtful cases to rule out the presence of diabetes mellitus.

Based on the history, positive urine test for reducing sugar and absence of clinical findings, the confirmation of the diagnosis can be done by thin layer chromatography of the urine sample to ensure the presence of fructose.

CASE STUDY 6

Theme: Clinical Implications of Impaired Fructose Metabolism

A 3-year-old boy was brought to the emergency department after several episodes of vomiting and lethargy. His pediatrician was concerned about his failure to thrive and possible hepatic failure along with recurrent episodes of the vomiting and lethargy. After a careful history, it was observed, that these episodes occur after ingestion of certain types of food, especially high in fructose. His blood sugar was checked in the emergency department and was extremely low (42 mg/dL). The test for reducing sugar in urine was positive.

What is the most likely diagnosis?
What is the biochemical basis for the clinical symptoms?
What is the treatment of the disorder?

CASE DETAILS

The child is most probably suffering from "hereditary fructose intolerance". **The onset of symptoms after ingestion of fructose or fructose-containing diet is a sign of "hereditary fructose intolerance".** All these symptoms of vomiting, lethargy, failure to thrive, hypoglycemia, and liver failure are characteristics of this disease.

BASIC CONCEPT

Hereditary Fructose Intolerance

In the liver, kidney, and intestine, fructose can be converted to glycolytic/gluconeogenic intermediates by the actions of three enzymes—fructokinase, aldolase B, and triokinase (also called triose kinase) **(Fig. 2.6)**. In these tissues, fructose is rapidly phosphorylated to fructose-1-phosphate (F1P) by fructokinase at the expense of a molecule of adenosine triphosphate (ATP). This has the effect of trapping fructose inside the cell. A deficiency in this enzyme leads to the rare but benign condition known as "essential fructosuria". In other tissues such as muscle, adipose, and red blood cells, hexokinase can phosphorylate fructose to the glycolytic intermediate fructose 6-phosphate (F6P). Fructose-1-phosphate is further metabolized to dihydroxyacetone phosphate (DHAP) and glyceraldehyde by the hepatic isoform of the enzyme aldolase, which catalyzes a reversible aldol condensation reaction. Aldolase is present in three different isoforms. Aldolase A is present in greatest concentrations in the skeletal muscle, whereas the B isoform predominates in the liver, kidney, and intestine. Aldolase C is the brain isoform. Aldolase B has similar activity for either fructose 1,6-bisphosphate (F16BP) or F1P; however, the A or C isoforms are only slightly active when F1P is the substrate. Glyceraldehyde may be converted to the glycolytic intermediate, glyceraldehyde 3-phosphate (GAP), by the action of the enzyme triokinase. This enzyme phosphorylates glyceraldehyde at the expense of another molecule of ATP. The GAP can then enter into the glycolytic pathway and be further converted to pyruvate, or recombine with DHAP to form F16BP by the action of aldolase.

Biochemical Defect

Hereditary fructose intolerance is caused by mutation in the gene encoding aldolase B enzyme.

Pathophysiology

A defect in the aldolase B gene results in a decrease in activity that is 15% or less than that of normal. This results in a build-up of F1P levels in the hepatocytes. **Because the maximal rate of fructose phosphorylation by fructokinase is so high (almost an order of magnitude greater than that of glucokinase), intracellular levels of both ATP and inorganic phosphate (Pi) are significantly decreased (Fig. 2.6)**. The drop in ATP concentration adversely affects a number of cellular events, including detoxification of ammonia, formation of cyclic AMP (cAMP), and ribonucleic acid (RNA) and protein synthesis. **The decrease in intracellular concentrations of Pi leads to a hyperuricemic condition as a result of an increase in uric acid formation.** AMP deaminase is inhibited by normal cellular concentrations of Pi. When these levels drop, the inhibition is released and AMP is converted to IMP and, ultimately, uric acid **(Fig. 2.7)**.

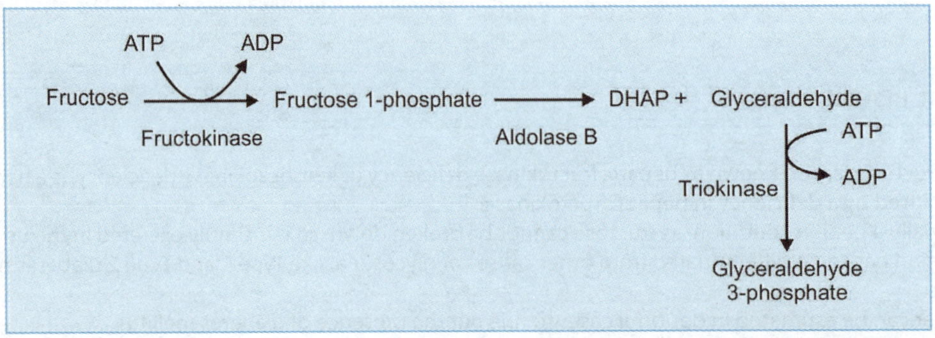

Fig. 2.6: Metabolic pathway for the entry of fructose into the glycolytic pathway. Fructokinase rapidly converts fructose to fructose 1-phosphate, which in the liver is cleaved by aldolase B to dihydroxyacetone phosphate (DHAP) and glyceraldehyde.

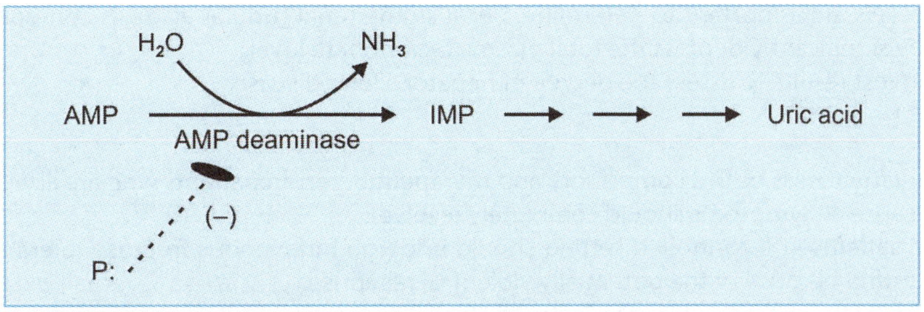

Fig. 2.7: Inhibition of adenosine monophosphate (AMP) deaminase by inorganic phosphate (Pi). A decrease in Pi increases the activity of AMP deaminase and leads to increased production of uric acid. Competition between urate and lactate for renal tubule excretion accounts for the lactic acidemia.

The toxic effects of F1P can also be exhibited in patients that do not have a deficiency in aldolase B, if they are parenterally fed with solutions containing fructose. Parenteral feeding with solutions containing fructose can result in blood fructose concentrations that are several times higher than can be achieved with an oral load. **Since the rate of entry into the hepatocyte is dependent on the fructose gradient across the cell, intravenous loading results in increased entry into the liver and increased formation of F1P. Since the rate of formation of F1P is much faster than its further metabolism, this can lead to hyperuricemia and hyperuricosuria by the mechanisms described above.**

The cause of severe hepatic dysfunction remains unknown but may be a manifestation of focal cytoplasmic degeneration and cellular fructose toxicity. The cause of renal tubular dysfunction also remains unclear; patients with renal tubular dysfunction primarily present with a proximal tubular acidosis complicated by aminoaciduria, glucosuria, and phosphaturia. Thus, in an infant who is homozygous for fructose 1-aldolase deficiency, fructose ingestion triggers a cascade of biochemical events that result in severe clinical disease.

Inheritance

Hereditary fructose intolerance is an autosomal recessive trait that is equally distributed between the sexes.

Age: In many infants, the age at symptom onset leads to the diagnosis. An accurate dietary history can indicate a link between the introduction of fruits into the diet and symptom onset.

Incidence

The incidence of hereditary fructose intolerance in the Caucasian population has been estimated at 1 in 20,000 births. Although the true prevalence has not been established, hereditary fructose intolerance may be more common than originally believed; many asymptomatic affected people may simply avoid the ingestion of most or all sweets.

Clinical Manifestations

These patients are healthy and asymptomatic until fructose or sucrose (table sugar) is ingested (usually from fruit, sweetened cereal, or sucrose-containing formula).

Clinical features include:

- Recurrent vomiting
- Abdominal pain
- Hypoglycemia that may be fatal
- Older patients who survive infancy develop a natural avoidance of sweets and fruits early in life and as a result frequently are without any dental caries.

Long-term exposure to fructose can result in:

- Liver failure
- Renal tubulopathy
- Growth retardation
- Progression of liver and kidney failure, eventually leading to death.

Laboratory Findings

- Based on the thorough dietary history of an ill child, the most straightforward approach to diagnosis of fructose 1-phosphate aldolase deficiency is to demonstrate the presence of a nonglucose-reducing sugar in the urine. This is readily accomplished with Clinitest. Then, if test results are positive, thin-layer chromatographic separation should be used for confirmation.
- Urine metabolic screening results may also provide evidence of glucosuria, proteinuria, and aminoaciduria, all of which are part of renal Fanconi syndrome.

- Plasma electrolyte levels are important to determine, because the renal tubular acidosis component of hereditary fructose intolerance (HFI) may significantly depress the total plasma bicarbonate level.
- Obtain liver function test results to assess the degree of hepatocellular disease.

Other Tests

- Elimination of dietary fructose is both a compulsory and therapeutic step. In patients who are ill, elimination may also serve as a diagnostic test because all symptoms should completely resolve.
- Only asymptomatic patients in a controlled setting should undergo intravenous fructose tolerance testing; do not use oral fructose tolerance testing because of the potentially violent GI response.
- The combination of a therapeutic response to fructose elimination and a positive response to the fructose tolerance test is sufficient to exclude obtaining a biopsy sample. However, a molecular analysis in leukocytes of the gene on chromosome 9 may provide definitive evidence of a mutation at the q22.3 band.

Treatment

Treatment consists of the complete elimination of all sources of sucrose, fructose, and sorbitol from the diet. With this treatment, liver and kidney dysfunction improve and catch-up growth is common. Intellectual development is usually unimpaired. As the patient matures, symptoms become milder, even after fructose ingestion, and the long-term prognosis is good. Hepatomegaly may require months to resolve. Prolonged delay in diagnosis may result in cirrhotic changes with subsequent degeneration of function.

Medication

Drug therapy is not a component of the standard-of-care for this condition.

Mortality/Morbidity

Morbidity is implicit in untreated patients. Hypoglycemia and acidosis may act together to cause organ shock or coma. Ongoing hepatocellular insult may result in cirrhosis and eventual hepatic failure. Failure to thrive progressing to cachexia is the rule. Mortality may result from any or all of the above conditions.

CLINICAL NOTE

Based on the thorough dietary history of an ill child, the most straightforward approach to diagnosis of fructose 1-phosphate aldolase deficiency is to demonstrate the presence of a nonglucose-reducing sugar in the urine.

CLINICAL PEARLS

1. Hereditary fructose intolerance is caused by mutation in the gene encoding aldolase B enzyme.
2. The maximal rate of fructose phosphorylation by fructokinase is so high (almost an order of magnitude greater than that of glucokinase), intracellular levels of both ATP and inorganic phosphate (Pi) are significantly decreased.
3. Vomiting, lethargy, failure to thrive, hypoglycemia, and liver failure are characteristic symptoms of this disease.
4. These patients are healthy and asymptomatic until fructose or sucrose (table sugar) is ingested (usually from fruit, sweetened cereal, or sucrose-containing formula).
5. Treatment consists of the complete elimination of all sources of sucrose, fructose, and sorbitol from the diet.

CASE STUDY 7

Theme: Glucose Homeostasis and Hypoglycemia

A 36-year-old woman was brought to the emergency room complaining of dizziness, she recalled getting up early that morning to do as much shopping as possible for her friend's wedding. In that hurry, she missed her breakfast. She had a cup of tea at lunchtime and again skipped the meals. She went to the party in the evening and soon after reaching there, she felt weakness and dizziness and was transported to the hospital.

Following examination, a random blood sugar was estimated and it was 43 mg%. The patient was given orange juice and she felt better.

What is the probable diagnosis?

CASE DETAILS

The patient had hypoglycemia. Prolonged fasting could be the cause for hypoglycemia.

Glucose Homeostasis

Glucose is an obligate metabolic fuel for the brain under physiologic conditions. **The brain cannot synthesize glucose or store more than a few minutes supply as glycogen and therefore requires a continuous supply of glucose from the arterial circulation.** As the arterial plasma glucose concentration falls below the physiologic range, blood-to-brain glucose transport becomes insufficient to support brain energy metabolism and function. However, redundant glucose counter-regulatory mechanisms normally prevent or rapidly correct hypoglycemia. Plasma glucose concentrations are normally maintained within a relatively narrow range, roughly 70–110 mg/dL (3.9–6.1 mmol/L) in the fasting state with transient higher excursions after a meal, despite wide variations in exogenous glucose delivery from meals and in endogenous glucose utilization by, for example, exercising muscle. Between meals and during fasting, plasma glucose levels are maintained by endogenous glucose production, hepatic (and renal) gluconeogenesis, and hepatic glycogenolysis. Although hepatic glycogen stores are usually sufficient to maintain plasma glucose levels for approximately 8 hours, this time period can be shorter, if glucose demand is increased by exercise or if glycogen stores are depleted by illness or starvation.

Gluconeogenesis requires a coordinated supply of precursors from muscle and adipose tissue to the liver (and kidneys). Muscle provides lactate, pyruvate, alanine, glutamine, and other amino acids. Triglycerides in adipose tissue are broken down into fatty acids and glycerol, which is a gluconeogenic precursor. Fatty acids provide an alternative oxidative fuel to tissues other than the brain (which requires glucose).

Systemic Glucose Balance

Maintenance of the normal plasma glucose concentration is accomplished by a network of hormones, neural signals, and substrate effects that regulate endogenous glucose production and glucose utilization by tissues other than the brain. Among the regulatory factors, insulin plays a dominant role. As plasma glucose levels decline within the physiological range in the fasting state, pancreatic β-cell insulin secretion decreases, thereby increasing hepatic glycogenolysis and hepatic (and renal) gluconeogenesis. Low-insulin levels also reduce glucose utilization in peripheral tissues, inducing lipolysis and proteolysis, thereby releasing gluconeogenic precursors. Thus, a decrease in insulin secretion is the first defense against hypoglycemia.

As plasma glucose levels decline just below the physiological range, glucose counter-regulatory (plasma glucose-raising) hormones are released. Among these, pancreatic α-cell glucagon, which stimulates hepatic glycogenolysis, plays a primary role. Glucagon is the second defense against hypoglycemia.

Adrenomedullary epinephrine, which stimulates hepatic glycogenolysis and gluconeogenesis (and renal gluconeogenesis), is not normally critical; however, it becomes critical when glucagon is deficient. Epinephrine is the third defense against hypoglycemia.

When hypoglycemia is prolonged, cortisol and growth hormone also support glucose production and limit glucose utilization.

As plasma glucose levels fall to lower levels, symptoms prompt the behavioral defense against hypoglycemia, including the ingestion of food.

The normal glycemic thresholds for these responses to decreasing plasma glucose concentrations do exist; however, these thresholds are dynamic. They shift to higher-than-normal glucose levels in people with poorly controlled diabetes who can experience symptoms of hypoglycemia when their glucose levels decline into the normal range. On the other hand, they shift to lower-than-normal glucose levels in people with recurrent hypoglycemia, e.g. those with aggressively treated diabetes or an insulinoma. Such patients have symptoms at glucose levels lower than those that cause symptoms in healthy individuals.

HYPOGLYCEMIA

Hypoglycemia is a laboratory "diagnosis", which is usually considered a blood glucose level below 60 mg/dL. Symptoms begin at plasma glucose levels in the range of 60 mg/dL and impairment of brain function at approximately 50 mg/dL.

Types of Hypoglycemia

Spontaneous hypoglycemia in adults is of two principal types: (1) fasting and (2) postprandial. Fasting hypoglycemia is often subacute or chronic and usually presents with neuroglycopenia as its principal manifestation. Postprandial hypoglycemia is relatively acute and is often heralded by symptoms of neurogenic autonomic discharge (sweating, palpitations, anxiety, and tremulousness).

Common Causes of Hypoglycemia in Adults

a. **Physiological:** Prolonged fasting or starvation.
b. **Pathological:**
   1. **Fasting hypoglycemia:**
      a. Drugs—especially insulin, sulfonylureas, ethanol, sometimes quinine, pentamidine, rarely salicylates, sulfonamides, others

b. Critical illnesses—hepatic, renal, or cardiac failure, sepsis, inanition
c. Hormone deficiencies—cortisol, growth hormone, or both, glucagon and epinephrine (in insulin-deficient diabetes)
d. Non-β-cell tumors
e. Endogenous hyperinsulinism
f. Insulinoma
g. Other β-cell disorders
h. Insulin secretagogue (sulfonylurea, other)
i. Autoimmune (autoantibodies to insulin or the insulin receptor)
j. Ectopic insulin secretion
k. Disorders of infancy or childhood—transient intolerance of fasting, congenital hyperinsulinism, and inherited enzyme deficiencies.

2. **Postprandial (reactive) hypoglycemia:**
   a. Alimentary (postgastrectomy)
   b. Noninsulinoma pancreatogenous hypoglycemia syndrome
   c. Other causes of endogenous hyperinsulinism
   d. Hereditary fructose intolerance and galactosemia
   e. Idiopathic.

Clinical Manifestations of Hypoglycemia

1. **Neuroglycopenic symptoms of hypoglycemia** are the direct result of central nervous system (CNS) glucose deprivation. They include behavioral changes, confusion, fatigue, seizure, loss of consciousness, and, if hypoglycemia is severe and prolonged, death.
2. **Neurogenic (or autonomic) symptoms of hypoglycemia** are the result of the perception of physiological changes caused by the CNS-mediated sympathoadrenal discharge triggered by hypoglycemia. They include:
   a. **Adrenergic symptoms** (mediated largely by norepinephrine released from sympathetic postganglionic neurons but perhaps also by epinephrine released from the adrenal medullae) such as palpitations, tremor, and anxiety.
   b. **Cholinergic symptoms** (mediated by acetylcholine released from sympathetic postganglionic neurons) such as sweating, hunger, and paresthesias. Clearly, these are nonspecific symptoms.

Common signs of hypoglycemia include diaphoresis and pallor. Heart rate and systolic blood pressure are typically raised, but these findings may not be prominent. Neuroglycopenic manifestations are often observable. Hypoglycemia is most convincingly documented by **Whipple's triad: (1) symptoms consistent with hypoglycemia, (2) a low plasma glucose concentration measured with a precise method (not a glucose monitor), and (3) relief of those symptoms after the plasma glucose level is raised.** The lower limit of the fasting plasma glucose concentration is normally approximately 70 mg/dL (3.9 mmol/L), but substantially lower venous glucose levels occur normally, late after a meal. Glucose levels <55 mg/dL (3.0 mmol/L) with symptoms that are relieved promptly after the glucose level is raised document hypoglycemia. Hypoglycemia can cause serious morbidity; if severe and prolonged, it can be fatal. It should be considered in any patient with episodes of confusion, an altered level of consciousness, or a seizure.

Diagnosis of the Hypoglycemic Mechanism

In a patient with documented hypoglycemia, a plausible hypoglycemic mechanism can often be deduced from the history, physical examination, and available laboratory data.

Laboratory Investigations

a. **Blood glucose estimation:** Blood should be drawn, whenever possible, before the administration of glucose to allow documentation of a low-plasma glucose concentration. Convincing documentation of hypoglycemia requires the fulfillment of Whipple's triad. Thus, the ideal time to measure the plasma glucose level is during a symptomatic episode. A normal glucose level excludes hypoglycemia as the cause of the symptoms. A low-glucose level confirms that hypoglycemia is the cause of the symptoms, provided the latter resolve after the glucose level is raised.
b. **Plasma insulin levels:** When the cause of hypoglycemia is obscure, plasma insulin is estimated to rule out the presence or absence of insulinoma. **A reliable serum insulin level (radioimmunoassay) of 6 µIU/mL or more in the presence of blood glucose values below 40 mg/dL is diagnostic of inappropriate hyperinsulinism.** Immunochemiluminometric assays (ICMA) have sensitivities of less than 1 µIU/mL, and with these assays, the cutoffs for insulinomas is insulin level 3 µIU/mL or higher. β-cell adenomas do not reduce secretion in the presence of hypoglycemia, and the critical diagnostic test is to demonstrate inappropriately elevated serum insulin levels at a time when hypoglycemia is present.
c. **Insulin/glucose ratio:** In order to make the diagnostic use of insulin estimation better, a ratio of insulin/glucose is estimated on the same sample.
d. **Plasma C-peptide:** Insulin measurement in insulin-treated diabetics cannot be done accurately, since insulin administered exogenously is also measured in the assay. Here, C-peptide estimation proves valuable since it differentiates between the

endogenously synthesized insulin and exogenously administered insulin. Insulin and C-peptide are secreted in the equimolar amounts **(Fig. 2.8)**. This helps in differentiating between hypoglycemia due to insulinoma and other causes. In insulinoma, the C-peptide level is high, while in other causes, the level of C-peptide is low.

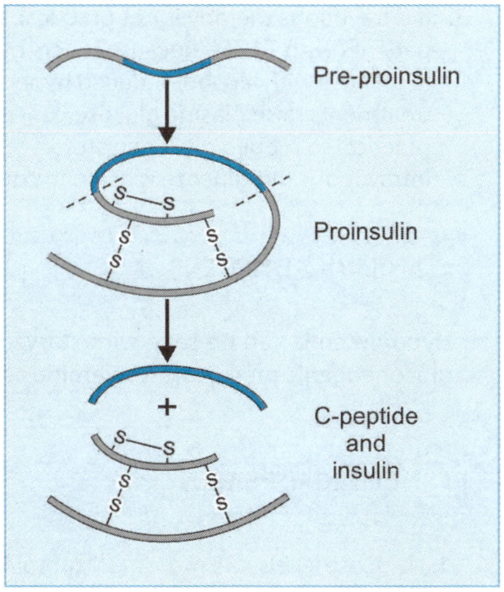

Fig. 2.8: Formation of mature insulin and C-peptide from preproinsulin. Insulin is synthesized in the form of preproinsulin, which is converted to proinsulin and then finally to mature insulin. C-peptide and mature insulin are synthesized in equimolar amounts.

Specific Hypoglycemic States

1. **Postprandial (reactive) hypoglycemia** may be classified as early (within 2–3 hours after a meal) or late (3–5 hours after eating). Early, or alimentary, hypoglycemia occurs when there is a rapid discharge of ingested carbohydrate into the small bowel followed by rapid glucose absorption and hyperinsulinism. It may be seen after gastrointestinal surgery and is particularly associated with the dumping syndrome after gastrectomy. In some cases, it is functional and may represent overactivity of the parasympathetic nervous system mediated via the vagus nerve. Rarely, it results from defective counter-regulatory responses such as deficiencies of growth hormone, glucagon, cortisol, or autonomic responses.
2. **Alcohol-related hypoglycemia** is due to hepatic glycogen depletion combined with alcohol-mediated inhibition of gluconeogenesis. It is most common in malnourished alcohol abusers but can occur in anyone who is unable to ingest food after an acute alcoholic episode followed by gastritis and vomiting.
3. **Immunopathologic hypoglycemia** is an extremely rare condition in which anti-insulin antibodies or antibodies to insulin receptors develop spontaneously. In the former case, the mechanism appears to relate to increasing dissociation of insulin from circulating pools of bound insulin. When antibodies to insulin receptors are found, most patients do not have hypoglycemia but rather severe insulin-resistant diabetes and acanthosis nigricans. However, during the course of the disease in these patients, certain anti-insulin receptor antibodies with agonist activity mimicking insulin action may develop, producing severe hypoglycemia.
4. **Factitious hypoglycemia** is self-induced hypoglycemia due to surreptitious administration of insulin or sulfonylureas.
5. **Insulinoma:** (See details)
6. **Hormone deficiencies:** Neither cortisol nor growth hormone is critical to the prevention of hypoglycemia, at least in adults. Nonetheless, hypoglycemia can occur with prolonged fasting in patients with primary adrenocortical failure (Addison's disease) or hypopituitarism. Anorexia and weight loss are typical features of chronic cortisol deficiency and likely result in glycogen depletion. Cortisol deficiency is associated with impaired gluconeogenesis and low levels of gluconeogenic precursors, suggesting that substrate-limited gluconeogenesis, in the setting of glycogen depletion, is the cause of hypoglycemia. Growth hormone deficiency can cause hypoglycemia in young children. In addition to extended fasting, high rates of glucose utilization (e.g. during exercise or in pregnancy) or low rates of glucose production (e.g. following alcohol ingestion) can precipitate hypoglycemia in adults with previously unrecognized hypopituitarism.
7. **Neonatal hypoglycemia:** The diagnosis and treatment of neonatal hypoglycemia is very important since if left untreated it can lead to brain damage. There are a number of important causes:
   a. **Babies of diabetic mothers:** The growing fetus of a diabetic mother is exposed to maternal hyperglycemia, which leads to hyperplasia of pancreatic islet cells. After delivery, the fetus fails to suppress the excessive insulin secretions and develops hypoglycemia.
   b. **Intrauterine growth retardation:** Small for date babies have inadequate glycogen stores, so at the time of need, there is diminished outpouring of glucose. The situation worsens further due to prematurity since the glycogen store is laid in the last months of pregnancy. Hence, a premature baby has diminished stores and frequently undergoes hypoglycemia.
   c. **Inborn errors of metabolism:** There are a number of causes for this category. The important out of these are glycogen storage diseases and galactosemia.

Treatment of Hypoglycemia

In addition to recognition and documentation of hypoglycemia, and often urgent treatment, diagnosis of the hypoglycemic mechanism is critical for choosing a treatment that prevents, or at least minimizes, recurrent hypoglycemia.

1. **Oral treatment** with glucose tablets or glucose-containing fluids, candy, or food is appropriate, if the patient is able and willing to take these. A reasonable initial dose is 20 g of glucose.
2. **Parenteral therapy:** If the patient is unable or unwilling, because of neuroglycopenia, to take carbohydrates orally, parenteral therapy is necessary. Intravenous glucose (25 g) should be given and followed by a glucose infusion guided by serial plasma glucose measurements.

3. If intravenous therapy is not practical, subcutaneous or intramuscular glucagon (1.0 mg in adults) can be used, particularly in patients with T1DM. Because it acts by stimulating glycogenolysis, glucagon is ineffective in glycogen-depleted individuals (e.g. those with alcohol-induced hypoglycemia). It also stimulates insulin secretion and is, therefore, less useful in T2DM. These treatments raise plasma glucose concentrations only transiently, and patients should therefore be urged to eat as soon as it is practical to rebuild glycogen stores.
4. Intravenous (IV) glucose is given in comatose patients.

CLINICAL NOTE

Hypoglycemia can be seen with starvation, perhaps because of loss of whole-body fat stores and subsequent depletion of gluconeogenic precursors (e.g. amino acids), necessitating increased glucose utilization.

CLINICAL PEARLS

1. Glucose levels <55 mg/dL (3.0 mmol/L) with symptoms that are relieved promptly after the glucose level is raised document hypoglycemia.
2. There are many causes of fasting (postabsorptive) hypoglycemia. However, drugs are the most common cause by far.
3. Reactive (postprandial) hypoglycemia occurs exclusively after meals. Its diagnosis requires documentation of Whipple's triad after a mixed meal.
4. When the cause of the hypoglycemic episode is obscure, additional measurements, while the glucose level is low and before treatment, should include plasma insulin, C-peptide, and ethanol concentrations, as well as levels of insulin secretagogues.
5. Hypoglycemia can cause serious morbidity; if severe and prolonged, it can be fatal. It should be considered in any patient with episodes of confusion, an altered level of consciousness, or a seizure.

CASE STUDY 8

Theme: Clinical Implications of Impaired Galactose Metabolism

The patient, a boy, was the first child of healthy parents. Delivery was normal and birth weight was 3.8 kg. From the 3rd day of life, the child developed an increasing degree of jaundice and at the same time became indolent and difficult to feed. No blood group incompatibility could be demonstrated. At 6 days of age, he had a serum bilirubin of 14 mg/dL, and his weight was 15% below the normal weight. He was readmitted to the hospital on the 7th day after birth. Muscular tonus was increased, and the patient later began to convulse. Between the 7th day and 9th day, exchanged blood transfusion was performed three times, but the serum bilirubin concentration still remained high. On the 9th day of life, the boy began vomiting, the liver enlargement was noted, and the cerebral symptoms became accentuated.

A positive test for reducing sugar had already been obtained on the 6th day after birth. A repeated test performed on the 7th day was positive, whereas at the same time, a test specific for glucose was negative. Hereditary galactosemia was then suspected; special tests performed on the 8th day confirmed the diagnosis.

- Hemoglobin (Hb)—10.4 g/dL
- AST—64 IU/L
- ALT—40 IU/L
- Bilirubin—14 mg/dL (at 7th day)
- Galactose-1–phosphate–uridy ltransferase

What are the biochemical effects of galactosemia?
What are the interpretations of laboratory results?

CASE DETAILS

Galactosemia

Hereditary galactosemia is among the most common carbohydrate metabolism disorders and can be a life-threatening illness during the newborn period. Galactose-1-phosphate uridyltransferase (GALT) deficiency is the most common enzyme deficiency that causes galactosemia. Removing lactose largely eliminates the toxicity associated with newborn disease, but long-term complications routinely occur.

BASIC CONCEPT

Galactose is metabolized from the milk sugar and lactose (a disaccharide of glucose and galactose). It gains entry into glycolysis by its conversion to glucose-1-phosphate (G1P). This occurs through a series of steps **(Fig. 2.9)**. First galactose is phosphorylated by galactokinase to yield galactose-1-phosphate. Epimerization of Galactose-1-P to Glucose-1-P requires the transfer of UDP from uridine diphosphoglucose (UDP-glucose) catalyzed by galactose-1-phosphate uridyltransferase. This generates UDP-galactose and G1P. The UDP-galactose is epimerized to UDP-glucose by UDP-galactose-4 epimerase. The UDP portion is exchanged for phosphate generating glucose-1-phosphate, which then is converted to G6P by phosphoglucose mutase (See the reactions).

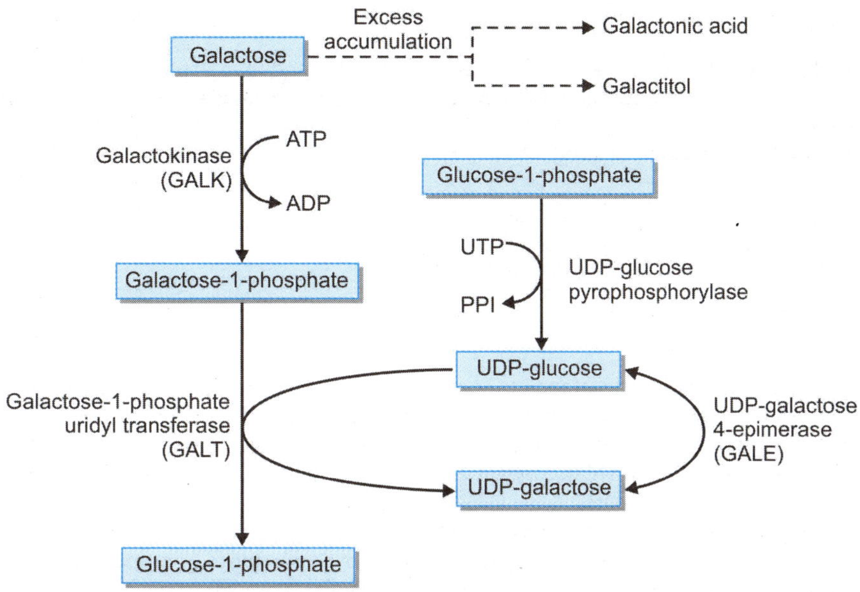

Fig. 2.9: Metabolism of galactose and the entry of galactose carbon atoms into the glycolytic pathway.

Pathophysiology

Galactosemia is associated with the following enzyme deficiencies:

- Galactokinase converts galactose to galactose-1-phosphate and it is not a common deficiency.
- Uridine diphosphate (UDP) galactose-4-epimerase epimerizes UDP galactose to UDP glucose and it is also an uncommon deficiency.
- Deficiency of galactokinase causes cataracts. Deficiency of uridine diphosphate galactose-4-epimerase can be benign when the enzyme deficiency is limited to blood cells but can be as severe as classic galactosemia when the enzyme deficiency is generalized.
- **GALT is responsible for hereditary or classical galactosemia and is the most common deficiency**. This enzyme catalyzes conversion of galactose-1-phosphate and UDP glucose to UDP galactose and glucose-1-phosphate. Individuals with GALT deficiency manifest abnormal galactose tolerance. Initially, galactose-1-phosphate accumulates in the tissues and blood, as more and more of galactose and galactose-1-phosphate accumulate, damage to the cells occurs. In this case, the major organ damaged by galactose accumulation is liver.
- *Biosynthesis of galactitol*: **Galactitol is an alcohol that is made from galactose.** The pathway is similar to that of formation of glucose. Because of the excessive quantity of galactose, some of it is converted to galactitol, which build-up in the body and is excessively excreted in urine. Since, it is an alcohol and not a reducing substance, therefore, the positive test for reducing substances in the urine is caused by galactose and not by galactitol. Galactitol appears to be toxic at high concentration and produces tissue injuries, especially cataract formation.

Incidence

In United State, incidence is approximately one case per 40,000 to 60,000 persons. The disorder is thought to be much less common in Asians.

Genetic Considerations

- Classic galactosemia is caused by a severe deficiency in GALT.

- The deficiency is an autosomal recessive genetic condition.
- The gene for GALT is located on chromosome 9p13.
- With the several mutations that have been identified at the GALT locus, the tendency for clinical complications to develop varies from apparent clinical normality in the relatively common Duarte type to perhaps mild symptoms in the S135L variant to the severe galactosemia syndrome in the "classic", Indiana, and Rennes variants. Neonates with Duarte variant may or may not have positive (i.e. abnormal) newborn screening test results, and most can tolerate normal diets. During infancy, but less so in childhood, these individuals may have elevated galactose metabolite levels.

CLINICAL MANIFESTATIONS

The cardinal features of classic galactosemia are hepatomegaly, cataracts, and mental retardation.

Untreated infants with severely deficient galactose-1-phosphate uridyltransferase (GALT) activity typically present with the following variable findings:

- Poor growth within the first few weeks of life
- Jaundice
- Bleeding from coagulopathy
- Liver dysfunction and/or hepatomegaly
- Cataracts (sometimes as early as the first few days of life)
- Lethargy
- Hypotonia
- Sepsis (*Escherichia coli*)
- Ascites may also be detected during early infancy. In some patients, ascites are detected as early as the first few days of life.
- Blindness is due to the conversion of circulating galactose to the sugar alcohol galactitol, by an NADPH-dependent galactose reductase that is present in neural tissue and in the lens of the eye. At normal circulating levels of galactose, this enzyme activity causes no pathological effects. However, a high concentration of galactitol in the lens causes osmotic swelling, with the resultant formation of cataracts and other symptoms.
- Learning problems, speech, and language deficits are common.
- The most common findings in adults include hypergonadotropic hypogonadism or primary ovarian insufficiency in women, although some women have become pregnant, most notably blacks who probably have variant disease.
- Short stature and neurological abnormalities (e.g. tremor, ataxia, and dystonia) also occur in a minority of patients.

Laboratory Investigations

- Urine test for reducing sugar is positive. **The confirmation for the presence of galactose can be done by thin layer chromatography.**
- **Galactose tolerance test:** A galactose tolerance test is abnormal in these patients. There is much higher than normal rise in blood galactose after the administration of galactose, and the elevation persists for a much longer time than normal. The galactose tolerance test in a normal person shows the level in the blood rising to a maximum at about half an hour after the galactose administration. It then returns to baseline value within 1 hour.
- **Serum transaminases:** Both the serum transaminases are elevated, suggesting the possibility of liver damage.
- **Serum bilirubin:** It is elevated. If the hemoglobin (Hb) level is normal, it is unlikely that the elevated Hb results from hemolysis. A more likely explanation is that the liver cannot handle normal amount of bilirubin because of the galactose and galactose-1-phosphate accumulation. A high proportion of the bilirubin is unconjugated; the bilirubin has difficulty in penetrating the hepatocytes. Also the function of the glucuronyl transferase is probably adversely affected by the liver cell damage.
- **Estimation of galactose-1-phosphate uridyltransferase:** Finally, the diagnosis can be made by demonstrating that the galactose-1-phosphate transferase is absent in the erythrocytes.

TREATMENT

The treatment of galactosemia to prevent long-term complications remains a challenge.

Long-term results of treatment have been disappointing; IQ is low in many despite early and seemingly adequate therapy. Widespread newborn screening for galactosemia identifies these infants early and allows them to be placed on dietary restriction.

Elimination of galactose from the diet reverses growth failure and renal and hepatic dysfunction, improving the prognosis. However, on long-term follow-up, these patients still have ovarian failure manifest as primary or secondary amenorrhea, as well as developmental delays and learning disabilities, which increase in severity with age.

Even on a galactose-restricted diet, transferase-deficient individuals exhibit urinary galactitol excretion and persistently elevated erythrocyte galactose-1-phosphate levels.

An alternative source of galactose exists even if the patient is fed on a galactose-free diet. Galactose can be formed from glucose. First, glucose is converted to glucose-1-phosphate and then to UDP-glucose. Next, an epimerase converts the UDP-glucose to UDP-galactose.

A galactosemic mother can produce milk-containing galactose. The galactose needed for lactose synthesis is formed from glucose by the pathway described above.

Prognosis

Patients with transferase deficiency, such as this infant, eventually have a less severe disease because an alternative enzyme for galactose utilization develops during childhood. This enzyme enables the galactose-1-phosphate to bypass the uridyltransferase step. Instead of reacting with UDP-glucose, the galactose-1-phosphate reacts with UTP to form UDP galactose. The alternative pathway can handle only a fraction of the galactose than the uridyltransferase reaction can. It handles enough, however, to enable the person to have some galactose in the diet. Therefore, a patient does not have to maintain as severely a restrictive diet as he/she grows older. If the galactokinase was deficient, alternate pathway could not function later in life because the patient could not produce galactose-1-phosphate in the diet. Therefore, the patient would have to remain on a much more restrictive diet throughout the life. Fortunately, very few cases of galactosemia are caused by galactokinase deficiency.

CLINICAL NOTE

The positive test for reducing substances in the urine is caused by galactose and not by galactitol.

CLINICAL PEARLS

1. Galactose-1-phosphate uridyltransferase (GALT) deficiency is the most common enzyme deficiency that causes galactosemia.
2. Initially galactose-1-phosphate accumulates in the tissues and blood, as more and more of galactose and galactose-1-phosphate accumulate, damage to the cells occurs.
3. Neonates with Duarte variant may/may not have positive newborn screening test results, and most can tolerate normal diets.
4. The cardinal features of classic galactosemia are hepatomegaly, cataracts, and mental retardation.
5. Elimination of galactose from the diet reverses growth failure and renal and hepatic dysfunction, improving the prognosis.

CASE STUDY 9

Theme: Biological and Clinical Significance of Glycogen Metabolism

The patient was a 12-year-old girl who had a grossly enlarged abdomen. She had a history of frequent episodes of weakness, sweating, and pallor that were eliminated by sweating, and pallor that were eliminated by eating. Her development had been slow, she sat at the age of 1 year, walked unassisted at the age of 2 years, and was doing poorly in the school. She sat at the age of 1 year, walked unassisted at the age of 2 years, and was doing poorly in the school.

Physical examination revealed normal blood pressure, temperature, and a normal pulse rate but a subnormal weight (23 kg). The liver was enlarged, firm, and was descended into pelvis. The spleen was not palpable, nor were the kidneys. The remainder of the physical examination was within the normal limits.

Laboratory investigation report revealed low blood glucose, low pH, high lactate, triglycerides, ketones, and high-free fatty acids. The liver biopsy revealed high glycogen content. Hepatic glycogen structure was normal. The enzyme assay performed on the biopsy tissue revealed very low glucose-6-phosphatase levels.

What is the probable diagnosis?
What is the possible treatment for this patient?

CASE DETAILS

The girl is suffering from von Gierke's disease. The clinical picture, biochemical findings, hypoglycemia, and increased hepatic glycogen stores are all characteristic of von Gierke's disease.

Von Gierke's Disease

Glycogen storage disease (GSD) Type I is also known as von Gierke's disease or hepatorenal glycogenesis. Von Gierke described the first patient with GSD Type I in 1929 under the name hepatonephromegalia glycogenica. GSD Type I is divided into GSD Type Ia caused by G6Pase deficiency and GSD Type Ib resulting from deficiency of a specific translocase T1. Apart from the substrate translocation defect, patients with GSD Type Ib have altered neutrophil functions predisposing them to gram-positive bacterial infections.

BASIC CONCEPT

Glycogen is a readily mobilized storage form of glucose. It is a very large and branched polymer of glucose residues that can be broken down to yield glucose molecules when energy is needed. Most of the glucose residues in glycogen are linked by α-1,4-glycosidic bonds. Branches at about every tenth residue are created by α-1,6-glycosidic bonds **(Fig. 2.10)**. The α-glycosidic linkages form open helical polymers, whereas β-linkages produce nearly straight strands that form structural fibrils, as in cellulose. Glycogen is not as reduced as fatty acids are and consequently not as energy rich. Why do animals store any energy as glycogen? Why not convert all excess fuel into fatty acids? Glycogen is an important fuel reserve for several reasons. The controlled breakdown of glycogen and release of glucose increase the amount of glucose that is available between meals. Hence, glycogen serves as a buffer to maintain blood–glucose levels. Glycogen's role in maintaining blood–glucose levels is especially important because glucose is virtually the only fuel used by the brain, except during prolonged starvation. Moreover, the glucose from glycogen is readily mobilized and is, therefore, a good source of energy for sudden and strenuous activity. Unlike fatty acids, the released glucose can provide energy in the absence of oxygen and can thus supply energy for anaerobic activity.

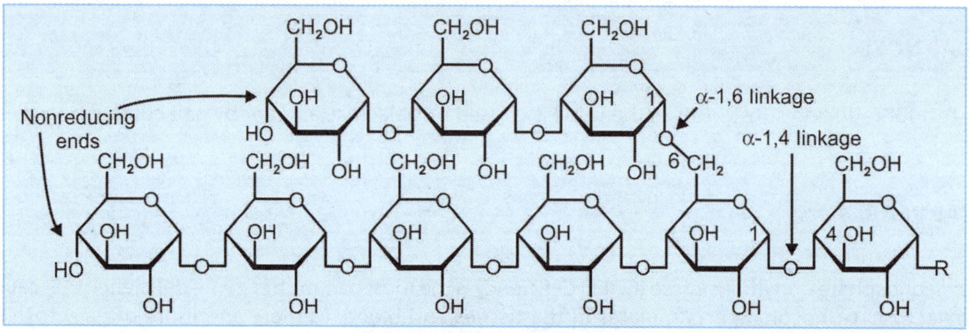

Fig. 2.10: Structure of glycogen.

The two major sites of glycogen storage are the liver and skeletal muscle. **The concentration of glycogen is higher in the liver than in muscle (10% versus 2% by weight), but more glycogen is stored in skeletal muscle overall because of its much greater mass.** Glycogen is present in the cytosol in the form of granules ranging in diameter from 10 nm to 40 nm **(Fig. 2.11)**. In the liver, glycogen synthesis and degradation are regulated to maintain blood–glucose levels as required to meet the needs of the organism as a whole. In contrast, in muscle, these processes are regulated to meet the energy needs of the muscle itself.

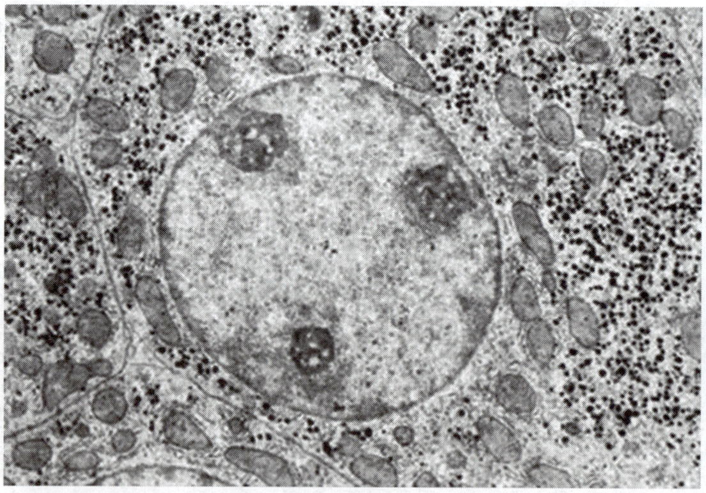

Fig. 2.11: Glycogen granules.

An Overview of Glycogen Metabolism

Glycogen degradation and synthesis are relatively simple biochemical processes. Glycogen degradation consists of three steps: (1) the release of glucose-1-phosphate from glycogen, (2) the remodeling of the glycogen substrate to permit further degradation, and (3) the conversion of glucose-1-phosphate into glucose-6-phosphate for further metabolism **(Fig. 2.12)**.

The glucose-6-phosphate derived from the breakdown of glycogen has three fates—(1) it is the initial substrate for glycolysis, (2) it can be processed by the pentose phosphate pathway to yield NADPH and ribose derivatives, and (3) it can be converted into free glucose for release into the bloodstream **(Fig. 2.12)**. This conversion takes place mainly in the liver and to a lesser extent in the intestines and kidneys.

Glycogen synthesis requires an activated form of glucose, uridine diphosphate glucose (UDP-glucose), which is formed by the reaction of UTP and glucose-1-phosphate. UDP-glucose is added to the nonreducing end of glycogen molecules. As is the case for glycogen degradation, the glycogen molecule must be remodeled for continued synthesis **(Fig. 2.13)**.

The regulation of these processes is quite complex. Several enzymes taking part in glycogen metabolism allosterically respond to metabolites that signal the energy needs of the cell. These allosteric responses allow the adjustment of enzyme activity to meet the needs of the cell in which the enzymes are expressed. Glycogen metabolism is also regulated by hormonally stimulated cascades that lead to the reversible phosphorylation of enzymes, which alters their kinetic properties. Regulation by hormones allows glycogen metabolism to adjust to the needs of the entire organism. By both these mechanisms, glycogen degradation is integrated with glycogen synthesis.

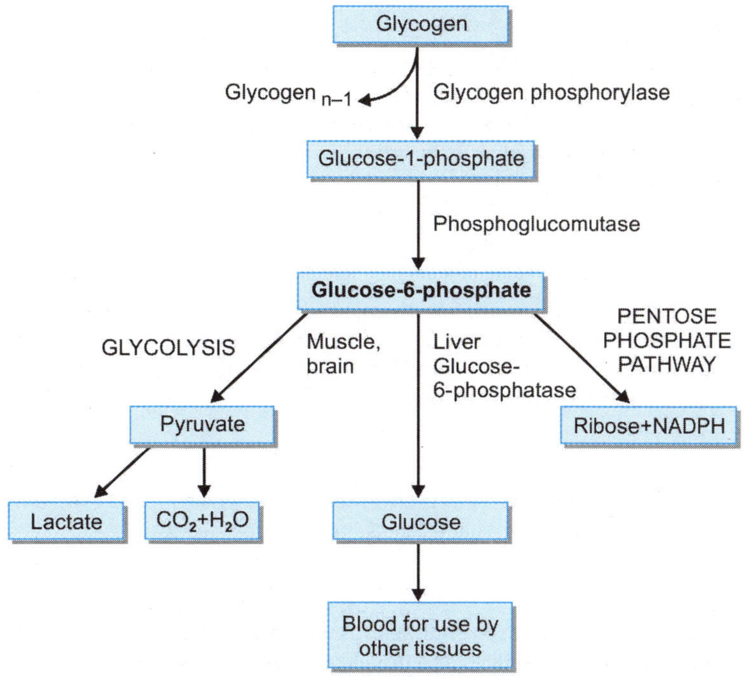

Fig. 2.12: Glycogen degradation and the fate of glucose-6-phosphate.

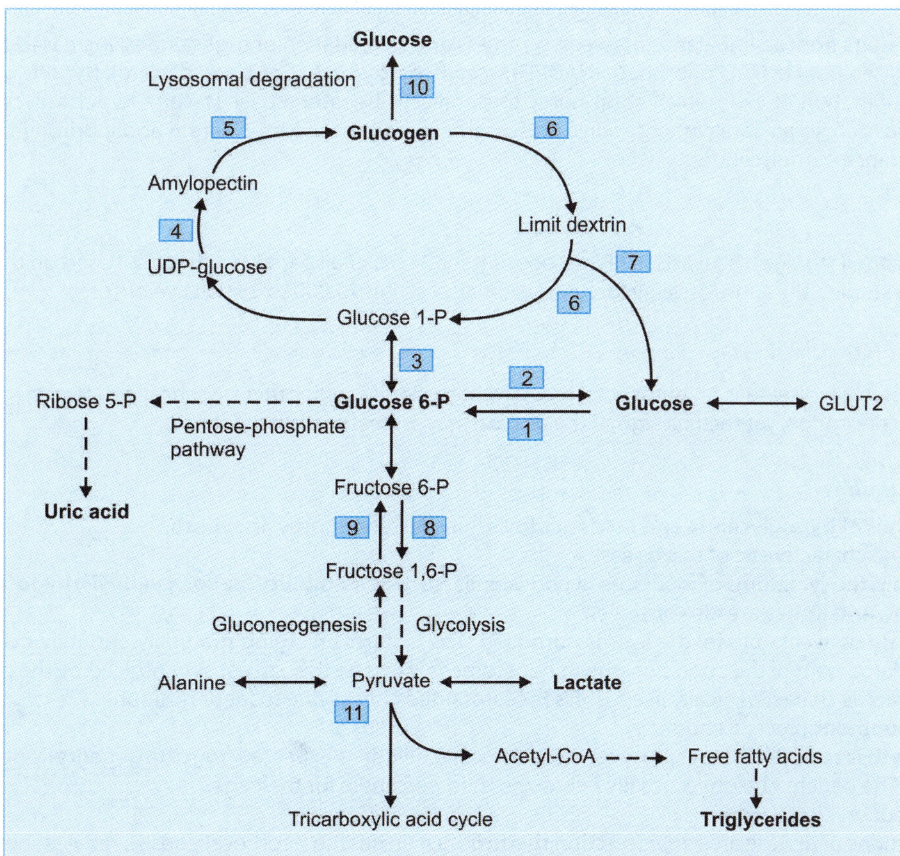

Fig. 2.13: An overview of glycogen metabolism—glucose is transported through GLUT2 transporters, converted to glucose-6-P and then to glucose-1-P, activated to UDP glucose, polymerized to form a straight polymer (amylopectin) initially and then branch points are created and polymerized to form glycogen. During degradation, initially glucose-1-P is formed by the action of phosphorylase enzyme and the resultant structure is limit dextrin; debranching takes place and free glucose is released by the action of debranching enzyme. Glucose-1-P is converted to glucose-6-phosphate and then to glucose. Glucose-6-phosphate can enter glycolytic pathway or pentose–phosphate pathway depending upon the need of the cell.

Pathophysiology of Von Gierke's Disease

In the absence of sufficient G6Pase activity, G6P fails to get converted into free glucose, therefore, it is either channeled into the pathway of glycolysis and metabolized to lactic acid or incorporated into glycogen. In this way, large amounts of glycogen are synthesized and stored in the cytoplasm of liver, kidney, and intestinal mucosa cells causing enlargement of liver and kidneys, which are the predominant features of this disease. The stored glycogen is though abundant, but it is normal in structure. The major biochemical alteration is hypoglycemia, while secondary alterations of varying degrees such as hyperlactacidemia, metabolic acidosis, hyperlipidemia, and hyperuricemia are also observed.

Hypoglycemia

The deficiency of G6Pase decreases the production of free glucose by blocking the process of glycogenolysis and gluconeogenesis in the liver. As a result, patients present with fasting hypoglycemia. The process of glucose production is not completely inhibited despite the block. The synthesis of free glucose can be half- or two-thirds of that of healthy individuals. Hypoglycemia inhibits secretion of insulin and stimulates glucagon and cortisol release.

Hyperlactatemia and Acidosis

The undegraded G6P is metabolized through glycolytic pathway to lactate, which is used as an alternative source of energy in the brain. The elevated blood lactate levels cause hyperlactatemia and metabolic acidosis.

Hyperuricemia

Serum uric acid levels are elevated both by increased endogenous synthesis and reduced urinary excretion caused by competition with the elevated concentrations of lactate. (lactates and urates compete with each other for the same transporter, lactates are excreted and urates are retained causing hyperuricemia).

Hyperlipidemia:

Hyperlipidemia results from an imbalance between synthesis and degradation of triglycerides. Increased triglycerides synthesis results from increased pool of NAD phosphate (NADPH), acetyl-coenzyme A (CoA), and glycerol. Hypertriglyceridemia increases the risk of fatty infiltration of liver, which contributes to significant hepatomegaly. Despite hypertriglyceridemia, the vascular lesions and atherosclerosis are rare complications, presumably due to the elevated serum apolipoprotein E concentrations that promote the clearance of triglycerides.

Incidence

Patients with glycogen storage disease (GSD) Type I account for 24.6% of all patients with GSD. Based on the results of combined US and European studies, the cumulative incidence is estimated at 1 in 20,000 to 25,000 live births.

Inheritance

Type I glycogen storage disease is an autosomal recessive disorder. As with other genetically determined diseases, GSD Type I develops during conception, yet the first sign of the disease may appear at birth or later.

Clinical Manifestations

- The earliest signs of **hypoglycemia and lactic acidosis** may develop shortly after birth.
- **Convulsions** are characteristic of this disease.
- Most commonly, the symptoms of moderate hypoglycemia, such as **irritability, pallor, cyanosis, hypotonia, tremors, loss of consciousness, and apnea** are also observed.
- During the first few weeks of life, the liver is normal in size. It starts enlarging gradually and may even reach up to public symphysis. Enlargement of the abdomen due to hepatomegaly can be the earliest sign noticed by the patient's mother.
- The patient's face is characteristically like a **doll's face** (rounded cheeks due to fat deposition).
- **Mental development** proceeds normally.
- **Physical growth is retarded**. The child never gains the same height as expected from the genetically determined potential of their families. The patient's height is usually below the third percentile for their age.
- The onset of puberty is delayed.
- Late complications of disease are **renal function disturbance** (including nephrocalcinosis), renal stones, tubular defects, and hypertension, mainly in patients older than 20 years. Renal function deterioration progresses to terminal insufficiency, requiring dialysis and transplantation.
- Skin and mucous membrane changes include the following:
    - **Eruptive xanthomas** develop on the extensor surfaces of the extremities.
    - **Tophi or gouty arthritis:** Uric tophi often have the same distribution as xanthomas.
    - **Spider angiomas** may be present.

- Many patients develop **bleeding tendencies, especially** from the nose. This tendency is a result of decreased adhesiveness of the platelets. Frequent and, occasionally, prolonged epistaxis may cause iron deficiency anemia. At times, the bleeding may be so severe that blood transfusions are required.

Laboratory Investigations

Glycogen storage disease (GSD) Type I: Serum glucose and blood pH levels are frequently decreased, while the serum lactate, uric acid, triglyceride, and cholesterol levels are elevated. Urea and creatinine levels might be elevated when renal function is impaired. The following laboratory values should be obtained:

- Serum glucose and electrolyte levels (higher anion gap may suggest lactic acidosis).
- Serum lactate level
- Blood pH
- Serum uric acid level
- Serum triglyceride and cholesterol levels
- Gamma-glutamyl transferase level
- CBC and differential (e.g. anemia, leukopenia, and neutropenia)
- Coagulation—bleeding and clotting time
- Urinalysis for aminoaciduria, proteinuria, and microalbuminuria in older patients
- Urinary excretion levels of uric acid and calcium
- Serum alkaline phosphatase, calcium, phosphorus, urea, and creatinine levels.

Imaging Studies

- In GSD Type I, liver and kidney ultrasonography should be performed for follow-up of organomegaly and detection of hepatic adenomas and nephrocalcinosis.
- Abdominal CT scanning or MRI is advised whenever the lesions are large, poorly defined, or are growing rapidly.

Other Tests

- Glucagon and epinephrine tests do not cause a rise in glucose levels, but plasma levels of lactic acid are raised.
- Orally administered galactose and fructose (1.75 g/kg) do not increase glucose levels, but plasma lactic acid levels do increase.
- Glucose tolerance test (1.75 g/kg PO) progressively lowers lactic acid levels over several hours after the administration of glucose.
- For diagnostic purposes, 13C nuclear magnetic resonance spectroscopy may be used for enzyme function assessment.
- Definitive diagnosis requires determination of G6Pase activity in fresh and frozen liver tissue specimens and/or DNA-based analysis. When assaying for translocases, an open surgical liver biopsy is needed for sampling an adequate tissue specimen.

TREATMENT

Most children with GSD Type I are admitted to the hospital to make a final diagnosis and to manage hepatomegaly or hypoglycemia.

- Because no specific treatment is available, symptomatic therapy is very important.
- **Diet: The primary goal of treatment is to correct hypoglycemia and maintain a normoglycemic state.** The normoglycemic state can be achieved with overnight nasogastric infusion of glucose, parenteral nutrition, or per oral administration of raw cornstarch. Glucose molecules are continuously released by hydrolysis of raw cornstarch in the digestive tract over 4 hours following its intake. The intake of fructose and galactose should be restricted because it has been shown that they cannot be converted to glucose but that they do increase lactate production. Limited intake of lipids is advisable for the existing hyperlipidemia.

Medication

- No specific drug treatment is recommended for GSD Type Ia. Appropriately treat concurrent infections with antibiotics.
- Allopurinol (Zyloprim), a xanthine oxidase inhibitor, therapy can reduce uric acid levels in the blood and prevent occurrence of gout and kidney stones in adult life.
- Hyperlipidemia can be reduced by lipid-lowering drugs [e.g. 3-hydroxy-3-methylglutaryl coenzyme A (HMG-CoA) reductase inhibitors and fibric acid derivatives].
- In patients with renal lesions, microalbuminuria can be reduced with angiotensin-converting enzyme (ACE) inhibitor therapy. In addition to their antihypertensive effects, ACE inhibitors are renoprotective and reduce albuminuria. Nephrocalcinosis and renal calculi can be prevented with citrate therapy.
- Severe infection and chronic inflammatory bowel disease in patients with GSD Type Ib should be treated with antibiotics and granulocyte-macrophage colony-stimulating factors (Neupogen).
- Additionally, for patients with GSD Type I, the future may bring adeno-associated virus vector-mediated gene therapy, which may result in curative therapy.

Complications

- **Bacterial infections and cerebral edema**
- **Long-term complications** include **growth retardation, hepatic adenomas with a high rate of malignant change, xanthomas, gout, and glomerulosclerosis.**
- Chronic metabolic lactic acidosis and changes in the proximal renal tubule cells can lead to **osteopenia and rickets with severe skeletal deformities or bone fractures.**
- **Acute hypoglycemia may be fatal**, and long-term complications include irreversible damage to the CNS.
- **Early death** usually caused by acute metabolic complications (e.g. hypoglycemia, acidosis), bleeding in the course of various surgical procedures (in all patients with GSD type I), and infections (in patients with GSD type Ib) is now uncommon with improving care and treatment.

MORTALITY/MORBIDITY

In GSD Type I, acute hypoglycemia may be fatal. Early death is now uncommon with improving care and treatment. Late complications, such as renal failure, hypertension, or malignant alteration of hepatic adenomas, may be responsible for mortality in adolescent and adult patients.

Prognosis

The prognosis is better than in the past provided that all the available dietary and medical measures are implemented.

CLINICAL NOTE

The chief biochemical alteration in von Gierke's disease is hypoglycemia, while secondary abnormalities are hyperlactatemia, metabolic acidosis, hyperlipidemia, and hyperuricemia.

CLINICAL PEARLS

1. Glycogen storage disease (GSD) Type I is divided into GSD Type Ia caused by G6Pase deficiency and GSD Type Ib resulting from deficiency of a specific translocase T1.
2. The earliest signs of the disease may develop shortly after birth and are caused by hypoglycemia and lactic acidosis.
3. Serum glucose and blood pH levels are frequently decreased, while the serum lactate, uric acid, triglyceride, and cholesterol levels are elevated. Urea and creatinine levels might be elevated when renal function is impaired.
4. The primary goal of treatment is to correct hypoglycemia and maintain a normoglycemic state.
5. Long-term complications encompass growth retardation, hepatic adenomas with a high rate of malignant change, xanthomas, gout, and glomerulosclerosis.

CASE STUDY 9

Theme: An Overview of Glycogen Storage Diseases

A baby girl was brought for consultation. She was born normal but developed muscular weakness at the age of 3 months. There were signs of liver dysfunction and her liver was also enlarged.

She showed hypoglycemia, hyperlipidemia, and ketoacidosis, blood pH was 7.25 and total CO_2 was 12 mmol/L. Serum transaminases were significantly elevated. A liver biopsy revealed an elevation of glycogen content, but the debranching enzyme was absent. Muscle biopsy also revealed the similar findings. Two brothers of the baby suffered from the same disease. Parents were normal but they were first cousins.

What is the probable diagnosis?

CASE DISCUSSION

The child is suffering from Cori's disease. GSD Type III is also known as Forbes–Cori disease or limit dextrinosis. In contrast to GSD Type I, liver and skeletal muscles are involved in GSD Type III. Glycogen deposited in these organs has an abnormal structure. Differentiating patients with GSD Type III from those with GSD Type I solely on the basis of physical findings is not easy.

BASIC CONCEPT

Glycogen Storage Diseases

"Glycogen storage disease" is a generic term to describe a group of inherited disorders characterized by deposition of an abnormal type or quantity of glycogen in tissues, or failure to mobilize glycogen.

An overview of the important glycogen storage diseases has been shown in **Table 2.2:**

TABLE-2.2: An overview of the important glycogen storage diseases.

Type	*Name*	*Enzyme deficiency*	*Clinical features*
0	—	Glycogen synthase	Hypoglycemia; hyperketonemia; early death
I	Von Gierke's disease	Glucose-6-phosphatase	Glycogen accumulation in liver and renal tubule cells; hypoglycemia; lactic acidemia; ketosis; hyperlipidemia
II	Pompe's disease	Lysosomal α1→4 and α1→6 Glucosidase (acid maltase)	Accumulation of glycogen in lysosomes: juvenile onset variant, muscle hypotonia; death from heart failure by age 2; adult onset variant, muscle dystrophy
III	Limit dextrinosis, Forbes or Cori's disease	Debranching enzyme	Fasting hypoglycemia; hepatomegaly in infancy; accumulation of characteristic branched polysaccharide
IV	Amylopectinosis, Andersen's disease	Branching enzyme	Hepatosplenomegaly; accumulation of polysaccharide with few branch points; death from heart or liver failure in first year of life
V	Myophosphorylase deficiency, McArdle's syndrome	Muscle phosphorylase	Poor exercise tolerance; muscle glycogen abnormally high (2.5–4%); blood lactate very low after exercise
VI	Hers' disease	Liver phosphorylase	Hepatomegaly; accumulation of glycogen in liver; mild hypoglycemia; generally good prognosis
VII	Tarui's disease	Muscle and erythrocyte phosphofructokinase 1	Poor exercise tolerance; muscle glycogen abnormally high (2.5–4%); blood lactate very low after exercise; also hemolytic anemia
VIII	—	Liver phosphorylase kinase	Hepatomegaly; accumulation of glycogen in liver; mild hypoglycemia; generally good prognosis
IX	—	Liver and muscle phosphorylase kinase	Hepatomegaly; accumulation of glycogen in liver and muscle; mild hypoglycemia; generally good prognosis
X	—	cAMP-dependent protein kinase A	Hepatomegaly; accumulation of glycogen in liver

Enzyme deficiency results in glycogen accumulation in tissues. In many cases, the defect has systemic consequences, but, in some cases, the defect is limited to specific tissues. Most patients experience muscle symptoms, such as weakness and cramps, although certain GSDs manifest as specific syndromes, such as hypoglycemic seizures or cardiomegaly.

These inherited enzyme defects usually present in childhood, although some, such as McArdle disease and Pompe's disease, have separate adult-onset forms. In general, GSDs are inherited as autosomal recessive conditions. Several different mutations recently have been reported for each disorder.

Diagnosis depends on patient history and physical examination, muscle biopsy, electromyelography, ischemic forearm test, and creatine kinase levels. Biochemical assay for enzyme activity is the method of definitive diagnosis. Unfortunately, no specific treatment or cure exists, although diet therapy may be highly effective at reducing clinical manifestations. In some cases, liver transplantation may abolish biochemical abnormalities. Active research continues.

Glycogen Storage Diseases

Although at least 14 unique glycogen storage diseases (GSDs) are discussed in the literature, the four that cause clinically significant muscle weakness are Pompe's disease (GSD Type II), Cori disease (GSD Type III), McArdle disease (GSD Type V), and Tarui disease (GSD Type VII). One form, von Gierke disease (GSD Type Ia, glucose-6-phosphatase deficiency), causes clinically significant end-organ disease with significant morbidity. The remaining GSDs are not benign but are less clinically significant; a GSD Type 0 also exists, which is due to defective glycogen synthase.

Cori's Disease

Pathophysiology of Type III Disease

In Type III disease, the enzyme amylo-1,6-glucosidase is deficient, leading to an accumulation of dextrin. The site of glycogen accumulation is primarily cytoplasmic. The enzyme is found in all tissues.

Debranching enzyme has two independent active sites, consisting of residues in different segments of a single polypeptide chain that catalyze (α1,6) glycosidase and transferase (transglycosylase) reactions.

The transferase of the debranching enzyme transfers three glucose residues from a 4-residue limit branch to the end of another branch, diminishing the limit branch to a single glucose residue.

The (α1,6) glycosidase moiety of the debranching enzyme then catalyzes hydrolysis of the (α1,6) linkage, yielding free glucose **(Fig. 2.14)**. This is a minor fraction of glucose released from glycogen.

Disease results from a pan-deficiency of the enzyme (GSD IIIa) or muscle-specific retention of glycogen debranching enzyme (GSD IIIb).

Clinical Manifestations

- History of infantile convulsions
- Growth retardation
- Hepatomegaly and splenomegaly
- Kidney enlargement is not observed
- In adults, hepatomegaly may progress to liver cirrhosis or hepatic adenomas
- Progressive weakness, however vigorous exercise, is not associated with cramping or tenderness
- Muscle wasting may occur.

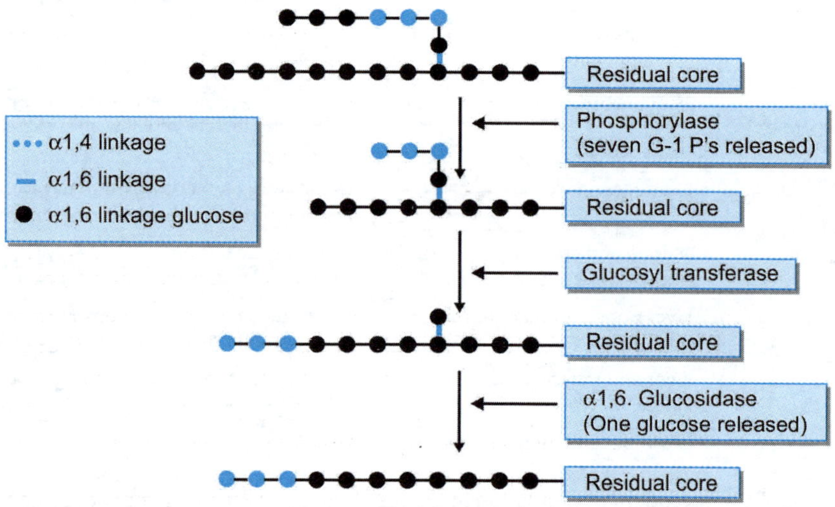

Fig. 2.14: Glycogenolysis and the role of debranching enzyme.

Mortality/Morbidity

- Hypoglycemic seizures occurring in the first decade of life may cause immediate mortality.
- Hepatic disease and progressive muscle weakness cause long-term morbidity.

Laboratory Investigations

- Fasting blood glucose estimation is indicated. Hypoglycemia is life-threatening and may lead to hypoglycemic seizures.
- Urinalysis is required because myoglobinuria may be present in some cases.
- Hepatic failure occurs in some cases of GSD. Liver function studies are indicated.
- Confirmation of diagnosis can be done by estimating debrancher enzyme activity, which may be reduced or absent.
- Hyperlipidemia is a common observation.
- Fasting ketonemia is observed due to enhanced rate of fatty acids oxidation.

Imaging Studies

- Imaging may reveal hepatomegaly.
- Cardiomegaly may be present, but heart failure is not typical of GSD II.

Other Tests

Ischemic forearm test: This is an important method for diagnosis of muscle disorders. The basic principle is to analyze normal chemical reactions and products of muscle activity. The patient is instructed to rest, and a loosened blood pressure cuff is placed on the arm. A venous line is placed in the antecubital vein to obtain blood samples. Blood samples are collecting for creatine kinase, ammonia, and lactate levels. The process is repeated in 5–10 minutes. Urine is analyzed for myoglobin. Blood pressure cuff is inflated above systolic blood pressure to induce ischemia, and the patient is instructed to repetitively grasp an object such as a dynamometer. After 2–3 minutes, the blood pressure cuff is released, and blood samples are collected for creatine kinase, ammonia, and lactate, immediately and at 5, 10, and 20 minutes. The urine sample is collected for myoglobin analysis.

Interpretation of ischemic forearm test results: Normally, exercise during ischemia results in lactate production. Lack of lactate production during exercise signifies a disturbance of metabolic pathway, and an enzyme deficiency is presumed. In such conditions, a muscle biopsy with biochemical estimations is recommended. Healthy individuals show a rise in lactate concentration of at least 5–10 mg/dL, ammonia of at least 100 µg/dL, and the levels revert to baseline. If neither level rises, it is assumed that the exercise was not strenuous enough and the test is considered invalid. Increased lactate production at rest (before exercise) signifies mitochondrial myopathy. Failure of rise of lactate with ammonia signifies a GSD causing block in the pathways of carbohydrate metabolism and the failure of rise of ammonia with lactate signifies myoadenylate deaminase deficiency. All GSDs do not show a positive result on ischemic test; however, test result is positive in Cori disease.

Electromyography: Electromyography patterns vary from patient to patient.

Treatment

Medical Care

- There is no permanent cure for GSDs.
- In some cases, diet therapy is helpful. Cornstarch therapy may be beneficial in reducing hypoglycemia. Strict adherence to a dietary regimen can reduce liver size, prevent hypoglycemia, provide symptomatic relief, and promote physical growth.

Surgical Care

Liver transplantation may be indicated for patients with hepatic malignancy.

Complications

- Hepatocellular carcinoma
- Hepatic failure.

Prognosis

Severe hepatic failure with malignant transformation can be fatal.

CLINICAL NOTE

The debranching enzyme deficiency leads to liver disease, with subsequent hypoglycemia and seizure.

CLINICAL PEARLS

1. GSD Type III is also known as Forbes–Cori disease or limit dextrinosis.
2. In Type III disease, the enzyme amylo-1-6-glucosidase is deficient, leading to an accumulation of dextrin.
3. The debranching enzyme deficiency leads to liver disease, with subsequent hypoglycemia and seizure. Progressive muscle weakness also occurs.
4. In Cori disease, the ischemic forearm test result is positive.
5. Meticulous adherence to a dietary regimen may reduce liver size, prevent hypoglycemia, allow for reduction in symptoms, and allow for growth and development.

Chapter 3

Lipid: Chemistry and Clinical Significance

LEARNING OBJECTIVES

To understand:
- Biochemical defect and clinical implications of lipid storage diseases
- Therapeutic significance of prostaglandins
- Role of aspirin in the prevention of ischemic heart disease

CASE STUDIES

CASE STUDY 1

Theme: Clinical significance of Cerebrosides (Glycolipids)

A 25-year-old woman presented with a history that includes:
a. Hepatosplenomegaly with eventual removal of spleen.
b. Bone and joint pains with several fractures of femur.
c. A liver biopsy that shows wrinkled looking cells with accumulation of glucosylceramide.
What would be the likely diagnosis for this patient?

CASE DISCUSSION

The patient is suffering from **Gaucher's disease**. It is an inherited disorder of cerebroside metabolism.

BASIC CONCEPT

Cerebrosides occur in large amount in the white matter of brain and in the myelin sheath of nerves. **Structurally, cerebrosides contain a carbohydrate, which is generally galactose or sometimes glucose, a high-molecular weight fatty acid, and an alcohol, which is sphingosine or dihydrosphingosine.** There is no glycerol, no phosphoric acid, and no nitrogenous base. Individual cerebrosides are differentiated by the type of fatty acid present in them.

CASE DETAILS

Gaucher's Disease

This disease is a multisystem lipidosis **characterized by hematological changes, organomegaly, and skeletal involvement**, the latter is usually manifested in the form of bone pains and multiple fractures. It is the most common genetic disorder among Ashkenazi Jews. It is the most common lysosomal storage disease.

Inheritance

It is autosomal recessive in nature.

Biochemical defect

Gaucher's disease results from **deficient activity of lysosomal hydrolase and β-glucocerebrosidase.** The enzyme defect results in accumulation of undegraded glycolipid in the form of glucosylceramide in the cells of reticuloendothelial system. This progressive accumulation results in infiltration of bone marrow, hepatosplenomegaly, and skeletal complications **(Fig. 3.1)**.

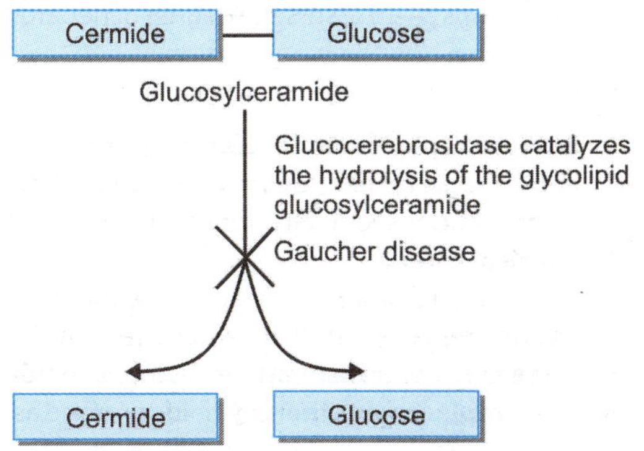

Fig. 3.1: Reaction catalyzed by β-glucocerebrosidase.

Clinical Features

There are three clinical subtypes depending upon the presence of, absence of, or progression of neurological complications:

1. **Type 1:** It accounts for 99% of cases. The age of onset is variable—from early childhood to late adulthood. The patients present with easy bruising due to thrombocytopenia, chronic fatigue due to anemia, and hepatomegaly with/without impaired liver functions. Progressive enlargement of spleen is there, which can become massive. Clinical bone involvement is apparent, which is manifested in the form of bone pains or pathological fractures. **The hallmark of Gaucher's disease is Gaucher cells in the reticuloendothelial system, particularly in the bone marrow.** These cells have a typical appearance, they are 20–100 µm in diameter, wrinkled looking due to the presence of intracytoplasmic inclusion bodies. The presence of these cells is highly diagnostic of Gaucher's disease **(Fig. 3.2)**.
2. **Type 2:** It is less common; it is **characterized by neurodegeneration, extreme visceral involvement, and death** within 2 years of life. The death is due to respiratory compromise.
3. **Type 3:** It is intermediate in presentation to Types 1 and 2. Neurological involvement is there but occurs later in life with **decreased severity** as compared to Type 2.

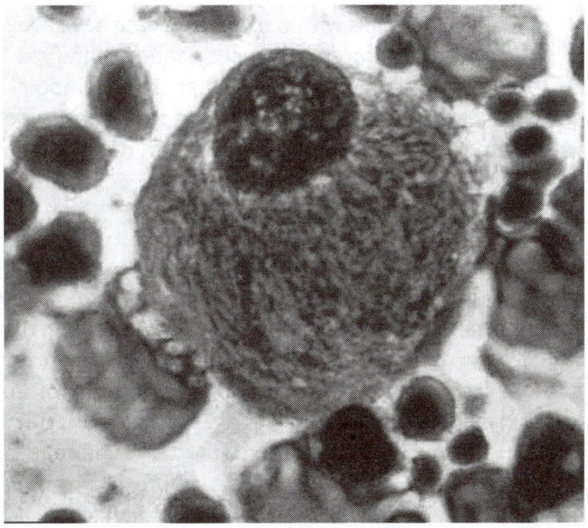

Fig. 3.2: Gaucher cells.

Laboratory Studies

The following studies are indicated in Gaucher's disease:

- **Enzyme activity testing:** Diagnosis can be confirmed through measurement of glucocerebrosidase activity in peripheral blood leukocytes. A finding of less than 15% of mean normal activity is diagnostic.
- **Genotype testing**: Molecular diagnosis can be helpful, especially in Ashkenazi patients, in whom 6 GBA mutations account for most disease alleles.
- **Complete blood count (CBC):** Obtain CBC count and differential to assess the degree of cytopenia.
- **Liver function enzyme testing:** Minor elevations of liver enzyme levels are common, even in patients who are mildly affected with Gaucher's disease; however, the presence of jaundice or impaired hepatocellular synthetic function merits a full hepatic evaluation. Coagulations studies should be monitored.
- **Associated marker testing:** Angiotensin-converting enzyme levels are typically elevated, as are total acid phosphatase and ferritin levels.

Imaging Studies

- Abdominal ultrasonography—to determine the extent of organomegaly.
- Magnetic resonance imaging (MRI) to determine:
  - Organ size
  - Early avascular necrosis (hip MRI)
  - Degree of marrow infiltration, and
  - Extent of spinal involvement.
- **Radiography:**
  - To diagnose skeletal deformities, and
  - To evaluate the degree of respiratory involvement.

- **Bone marrow examination:** The presence of typical Gaucher's cells (wrinkled looking cells) is diagnostic.
- **Liver biopsy**—to assess the degree of hepatomegaly.

Treatment

1. **Enzyme replacement therapy:** Recombinant β-glucocerebrosidase has been effectively used to reverse the visceral and hematologic manifestations of Gaucher's disease. The skeletal deformities, however, take longer to respond and respiratory complications seem refractory to treatment with enzyme replacement therapy.
2. **Surgical care:**
   Partial and total splenectomy can be undertaken depending upon the extent of splenomegaly, however, with the advent of enzyme replacement therapy, splenectomy is no longer a choice in majority of patients.
3. **Bone marrow transplant** can also help in treating the symptoms.
4. **Gene replacement therapy** holds promise as a permanent cure, but it is still under trial.

Prognosis

- Many individuals with Gaucher's disease have a few manifestations and a normal life expectancy without any intervention.
- The prognosis for symptomatic patients with Type 1 or Type 3 Gaucher's disease who receive treatment is very good, with a decrease in organomegaly and an eventual rise in hemoglobin levels and platelet counts.
- Skeletal disease is slow to respond to ERT and widely varies.
- Some patients describe symptomatic improvement within the first year of treatment, although a much longer period of ERT is required to achieve a radiologic response.

CLINICAL NOTE

The hallmark of Gaucher's disease is Gaucher cells in the reticuloendothelial system, particularly in the bone marrow.

CLINICAL PEARLS

1. Gaucher's disease is a multisystem lipidosis characterized by hematological changes, organomegaly, and skeletal involvement, the latter is usually manifested in the form of bone pains and multiple fractures.
2. It is the most common genetic disorder among Ashkenazi Jews.
3. It results from deficient activity of lysosomal hydrolase, β-glucocerebrosidase.
4. The enzyme defect results in accumulation of undegraded glycolipid in the form of glucosylceramide in the cells of reticuloendothelial system. This progressive accumulation results in infiltration of bone marrow, hepatosplenomegaly, and skeletal complications.
5. Enzyme replacement therapy by recombinant β-glucocerebrosidase is currently done. This preparation is highly effective in reversing the visceral and hematologic manifestations of Gaucher's disease.

OVERVIEW OF SPHINGOLIPIDOSES (LIPID STORAGE DISEASES)

The sphingolipidoses (lipid storage diseases) are a group of inherited diseases that are caused by a genetic defect in the catabolism of lipids containing sphingosine. They are part of a larger group of lysosomal disorders and exhibit several constant features: (1) complex lipids containing ceramide accumulates in cells, particularly neurons, causing neurodegeneration and shortening the lifespan. (2) The rate of synthesis of the stored lipid is normal. (3) The enzymatic defect is in the lysosomal degradation pathway of sphingolipids. (4) The extent to which the activity of the affected enzyme is decreased is similar in all tissues. There is no effective treatment for many of the diseases, although some success has been achieved with enzyme replacement therapy and bone marrow transplantation in the treatment of Gaucher's and Fabry's diseases. Other promising approaches are substrate deprivation therapy to inhibit the synthesis of sphingolipids and chemical chaperone therapy. Gene therapy for lysosomal disorders is also currently under investigation **(Table 3.1)**.

TABLE 3.1: Summary of lipid storage diseases.

Disease	*Enzyme deficiency*	*Lipid accumulating*	*Clinical symptoms*
Tay–Sachs disease	Hexosaminidase A	GM2 ganglioside	Mental retardation, blindness, muscular weakness
Fabry's disease	α-galactosidase	Globotriaosylceramide	Skin rash, kidney failure (full symptoms only in males; X-linked recessive)
Metachromatic leukodystrophy	Arylsulfatase A	Sulfogalactosylceramide	Mental retardation and psychological disturbances in adults; demyelination
Krabbe's disease	β-galactosidase	Galactosylceramide	Mental retardation; myelin almost absent
Gaucher's disease	β-glycosidase	Glucosylceramide	Enlarged liver and spleen, erosion of long bones, mental retardation in infants
Niemann–Pick disease	Sphingomyelinase	Sphingomyelin	Enlarged liver and spleen, mental retardation; fatal in early life
Farber's disease	Ceramidase	Ceramide	Hoarseness, dermatitis, skeletal deformation, mental retardation; fatal in early life

Multiple sulfatase deficiency results in accumulation of sulfogalactosylceramide, steroid sulfates, and proteoglycans owing to a combined deficiency of arylsulfatase A, B, and C and steroid sulfatase.

CASE STUDY 2

Theme: Clinical significance of "Gangliosides" (Glycolipids)

A boy was born normal but started flinching at loud noises (enhanced startle response) at the age of 6 months. The child initially could sit up, but then regressed, so that he could not roll over or recognize his parents.

Ophthalmological examination revealed a central red area of the retina surrounded by white tissue (cherry-red spot).

What is the possible defect?

What is the treatment for this disease?

CASE DISCUSSION

The child is suffering from Tay–Sachs disease (GM2 gangliosidosis). The disease is named after the British ophthalmologist Warren Tay who first described the red spot on the retina of the eye, and the American neurologist Bernard Sachs who described the cellular changes of Tay–Sachs and noted an increased prevalence in the Eastern European Jewish (Ashkenazi) population.

BASIC CONCEPT

Gangliosides have been isolated from the ganglion cells, neuronal bodies, dendrites, spleen, and RBC stroma. The highest concentration is found in the gray matter of brain. Structurally, they contain a long-chain fatty acid, alcohol sphingosine, a carbohydrate moiety, which is usually glucose and/or galactose, and at least one molecule of N-acetylneuraminic acid (NANA). Four important types of gangliosides are GM-1, GM-2, GM-3, and GD-3. GM-1 is more complex ganglioside and is known to be the receptor for cholera toxin in human intestine. Gangliosides are mainly components of membranes. They also serve as receptors for circulating hormones and thereby influence various biochemical processes in the cells.

CASE DETAILS

The GM2 gangliosidosis includes Tay–Sachs disease and Sandhoff disease; each results from the deficiency of β-hexosaminidase activity and the lysosomal accumulation of GM2 gangliosides, particularly in the central nervous system, causing severe effects (neurodegeneration) **(Fig. 3.3A)**. The child in the given case was born normal, but developed progressive deterioration of the neurological functions. This is characteristic of this disease.

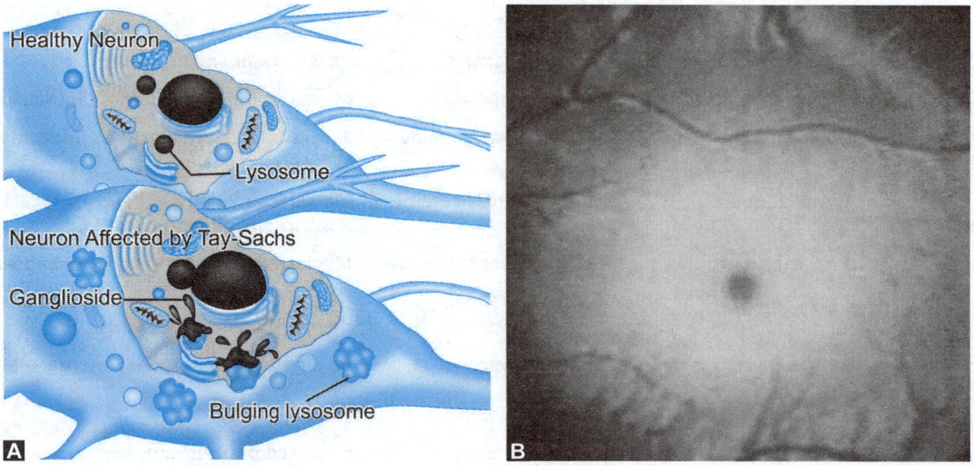

Figs. 3.3A and B: (A) Neuronal degeneration in Tay–Sachs disease. (B) Retina of the patient affected with Tay–Sachs disease.

Tay–Sachs Disease

Biochemical defect: There is deficiency of β-hexosaminidase A enzyme. This lysosomal enzyme removes amino hexose groups from gangliosides; subsequently, the other components are hydrolyzed by other specific enzymes. In its deficiency, the ganglioside is not degraded, so it accumulates in various tissues especially nervous tissue **(Fig. 3.4)**.

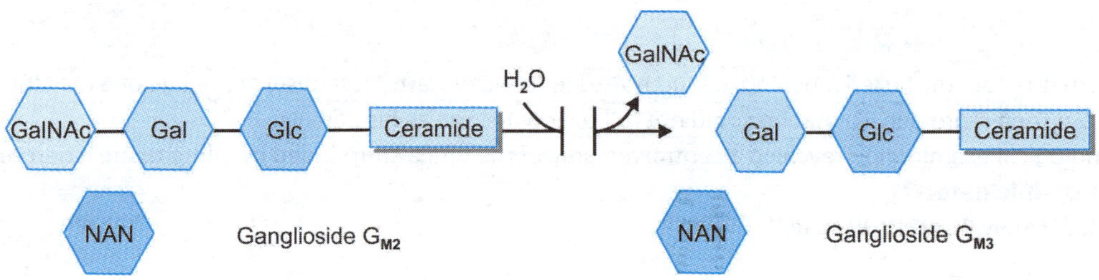

Fig. 3.4: Reaction catalyzed by hexosaminidase. (GalNAc: N-acetylgalactosamine; Gal: galactose; Glc: glucose; NAN: N-acetylneuraminic acid)

β-hexosaminidase occurs as two isozymes: β-hexosaminidase A, which is composed of one alpha and one beta subunit, and β-hexosaminidase B, which has two beta-subunits. β-hexosaminidase deficiency results from mutations in the alpha subunit and causes Tay–Sachs disease, whereas mutations in the beta subunit gene result in the deficiency of both β-hexosaminidase A and B and cause Sandhoff disease.

Inheritance

Both are autosomal recessive traits, with Tay–Sachs disease, having a predilection in the Ashkenazi Jewish population, where the carrier frequency is about 1/25.

More than 50 mutations have been identified; most are associated with the infantile forms of disease. Three mutations account for more than 98% of mutant alleles among Ashkenazi Jewish carriers of Tay–Sachs disease, including one allele associated with the adult-onset form. Mutations that cause the subacute or chronic forms result in enzyme proteins with residual enzymatic activities, the levels of which correlate with the severity of the disease.

Clinical Symptoms and Classification

Tay–Sachs disease is classified in variant forms, based on the time of onset of neurological symptoms. The variant forms reflect diversity in the mutation base.

- **Infantile Tay–Sachs disease (TSD):** Patients with this disease are **born normal, but they develop loss of motor skills, increased startle reaction, macular pallor, and retinal cherry-red spot**. Affected children develop normally till the age of 5–6 months, then decreased eye contact and hyperacusis (exaggerated startle response) to noise are noted. **Progressive development of idiocy and blindness are diagnostic of this disease** and they are due to wide spread injury to ganglion cells, in brain and retina **(Fig. 3.3B)**. The cherry-red spot about the macula is due to destruction of retinal ganglion cells exposing the underlying vasculature. Macrocephaly not associated with hydrocephalus may be there. Convulsions are seen in severe cases.

The clinical manifestations of Sandhoff disease are similar to those for Tay–Sachs disease. However, infants with Sandhoff disease have hepatosplenomegaly, cardiac involvement, and mild bony abnormalities.

- **Juvenile TSD:** Extremely rare, juvenile Tay-Sachs disease usually presents itself in children between 2 years and 10 years of age. They develop **cognitive, motor, speech difficulties (dysarthria), swallowing difficulties (dysphagia), unsteadiness of gait (ataxia), and spasticity.** Patients with juvenile TSD usually die between 5 years and 15 years.
- **Adult/late-onset TSD:** A rare form of the disorder, known as adult-onset Tay–Sachs disease or late–onset Tay-Sachs disease (LOTS), occurs in patients in their 20s and early 30s. LOTS is frequently misdiagnosed, and is usually nonfatal. It is characterized by unsteadiness of gait and progressive neurological deterioration. **Symptoms of LOTS, which present in adolescence or early adulthood, include speech and swallowing difficulties, unsteadiness of gait, spasticity, cognitive decline, and psychiatric illness, particularly schizophrenic-like psychosis.**

Diagnosis

The diagnosis of infantile Tay–Sachs disease and Sandhoff disease is usually suspected in an infant with neurological features and a cherry-red spot.

- **Enzymatic assays**: Definitive diagnosis is by determination of the level of β-hexosaminidase A and B in isolated blood leukocytes. The two disorders are distinguished by the enzymatic assay, because in Tay–Sachs disease, only the β-hexosaminidase A isozyme is deficient, whereas in Sandhoff disease, both the β-hexosaminidase A and B isozymes are deficient.
- **Fine-needle aspiration cytology (FNAC) of brain tissue**—can show the degree of neuronal degeneration. FNAC has a great potential for diagnosis and follow-up of Tay–Sachs disease.
- **Prenatal screening:** Future at-risk pregnancies for both disorders can be monitored by prenatal diagnosis by amniocentesis or chorionic villus sampling.
- **Carrier screening:** Identification of carriers within families is also possible by β-hexosaminidase A and B determination. Indeed, for Tay–Sachs disease, carrier screening of all couples in whom at least one member of Ashkenazi Jewish descent is recommended before the initiation of pregnancy to identify couples at risk. These studies can be conducted by the determination of the level of β-hexosaminidase A activity in peripheral leukocytes or plasma.
- **Molecular studies** to identify the exact molecular defect in enzymatically identified carriers should also be performed to permit more specific identification of carriers in the family, and for at-risk couples to allow prenatal diagnosis by both enzymatic and genotype determinations. The incidence of Tay–Sachs disease has been markedly reduced since the introduction of carrier screening programs in the Ashkenazi Jewish population.

Treatment

No cure for this disease. Symptomatic treatment is given. Enzyme replacement therapy and gene therapy are under trial. Although experimental work is underway, no current medical treatment exists for infantile TSD. Patients receive palliative care to ease the symptoms. Infants are given feeding tubes when they can no longer swallow. Improvements in palliative care have somewhat lengthened the survival of children with TSD, but no current therapy is able to reverse or delay the progress of the disease.

Prognosis

Prognosis is bad and death occurs in early years of life.

CLINICAL NOTE

The clinical manifestations of Sandhoff disease are similar to those for Tay–Sachs disease. However, infants with Sandhoff disease have hepatosplenomegaly, cardiac involvement, and mild bony abnormalities.

CLINICAL PEARLS

1. The GM2 gangliosidosis includes Tay–Sachs disease and Sandhoff disease; each results from the deficiency of β-hexosaminidase activity and the lysosomal accumulation of GM2 gangliosides, particularly in the central nervous system, causing severe effects (neurodegeneration).
2. More than 50 mutations have been identified; most are associated with the infantile forms of disease. Three mutations account for more than 98% of mutant alleles among Ashkenazi Jewish carriers of Tay–Sachs disease.
3. Tay–Sachs disease is classified into three variant forms, based on the time of onset of neurological symptoms—infantile, juvenile, and adult-onset TSD.
4. The diagnosis of infantile Tay–Sachs disease and Sandhoff disease is usually suspected in an infant with neurological features and a cherry-red spot.
5. No cure for this disease. Symptomatic treatment is given. Enzyme replacement therapy and gene therapy are under trial.

CASE STUDY 3

Theme: Chemistry and significance of Prostaglandins and NSAIDs versus Celecoxib

A 63-year-old female presented to the clinic with recurrent midepigastric pain over the last 3 months. She also reported feeling tired and had to increase the amount of ibuprofen needed for relief of her arthritis. She reported some relief of epigastric pain shortly after eating, but then the discomfort returned. She had tried various over-the-counter medications without relief. She denied nausea, vomiting, and diarrhea.

On examination, she was pale with no jaundice; pulse and blood pressure were normal. She was found to have mild midepigastric tenderness. A complete blood count (CBC) revealed normal white blood cell count and a microcytic anemia consistent with iron deficiency. The patient was referred to a gastroenterologist who performed an upper GI endoscopy that identified gastric ulcers. He stated that he suspected that the ibuprofen, a nonsteroidal anti-inflammatory drug (NSAID) was the causative agent and suggested switching from ibuprofen to a coxibs, such as celecoxib.

What is the likely biochemical etiology of the disorder?
Why NSAID was changed to celecoxib?

CASE DETAILS

The NSAIDs include a wide variety of medications including aspirin, ibuprofen, naproxen, and indomethacin. These medications are used for pain, inflammation, dysmenorrhea, headache, arthritis, or fever. These compounds act as anti-inflammatory and antipyretic agents by inhibiting cyclooxygenase (COX) catalysis by prostaglandin H synthase (PGHS). Side effects and complications due to NSAIDs are considered the most common drug-related toxicities in the United States. The spectrum of NSAID-induced morbidity ranges from nausea and dyspepsia (prevalence reported as high as 50–60%) to a serious gastrointestinal complication such as endoscopy-documented peptic ulceration (15–30% of individuals taking NSAIDs regularly) complicated by bleeding or perforation in as many as 1.5% of users per year. About 20,000 patients die each year from serious gastrointestinal complications from NSAIDs.

Pathophysiology

Prostaglandins play a critical role in maintaining gastroduodenal mucosal integrity and repair. It, therefore, follows that interruption of prostaglandin synthesis can impair mucosal defense and repair, thus facilitating mucosal injury via a systemic mechanism. Injury to the mucosa also occurs as a result of the topical encounter with NSAIDs. Aspirin and many NSAIDs are weak acids that remain in a nonionized lipophilic form when found within the acid environment of the stomach. Under these conditions, NSAIDs migrate across lipid membranes of epithelial cells, leading to cell injury once trapped intracellularly in an ionized form. Topical NSAIDs can also alter the surface mucous layer, permitting back diffusion of H^+ and pepsin, leading to further epithelial cell damage. Moreover, enteric-coated or buffered preparations are also associated with risk of peptic ulceration.

BASIC CONCEPT

Steps of Prostanoids Synthesis

- The binding of a ligand to a cell surface receptor triggers the process of prostanoids biosynthesis by activating phospholipase A2.
- Phospholipase A2 catalyzes the release of arachidonic acid from membrane phospholipids, such as phosphatidylethanolamine and phosphatidylinositol .
- One of the isoforms of PGH synthase (PGHS-1 or -2), located in the endoplasmic reticulum membrane and the nuclear envelope, further converts arachidonate to PGH_2.
- PGH2 is subsequently metabolized to either of PGD_2, PGE_2, $PGF_2\alpha$, PGH_2, PGI_2, or TXA_2 by one of the secondary enzymes.
- The synthesis of a specific prostanoids is determined by downstream enzyme present in a specific cell.

  For example, **in platelets thromboxane synthase predominates, therefore, thromboxane is synthesized;** whereas in **vascular endothelial cells, due to predominance of prostacyclin (PGI) synthase enzyme, prostacyclins are synthesized.**
- Conversion of arachidonate to PGH_2 by PGH synthase **is a rate-limiting step in the pathway of prostanoids biosynthesis.**

Isoforms of PGH Synthase

Each PGHS isoform catalyzes two separate reactions:

a. **Cyclooxygenase (COX) activity:**

   The conversion of **arachidonate** to PGG_2 involves insertion of two molecules of oxygen and cyclization of the fatty acid backbone. This reaction is catalyzed by the **cyclooxygenase** activity of PGHS-1 or -2. These cyclooxygenase activities (also called COX-1 and COX-2) are **inhibited by nonsteroidal anti-inflammatory drugs** (NSAIDs) **(Fig. 3.5).**

b. **Peroxidase activity:**
The conversion of PGG_2 to PGH_2 involves the **reduction of the hydroperoxide** on C15 to an alcohol. This reaction is **catalyzed by the peroxidase activity of PGHS-1 or -2 (Fig. 3.5)**

Significance of PGH Synthase

Both PGHS isoforms (-1 and -2) have cyclooxygenase and peroxidase activities, nevertheless, they perform distinct cellular functions.

- **Functions of PGH-1 synthase (noninducible-basal form):** The platelets and gastric mucosal cells have moderate levels of PGHS-1. The prostaglandins thus produced and help in maintaining—(i) hemostasis, (ii) vascular tone, (iii) renal function, (iv) platelet function, and (v) integrity of gastric mucosal cells **(Fig. 3.5)**.
- **Functions of PGH-2 synthase (inducible form):** In certain cells, such as macrophages, vascular endothelial cells, and fibroblasts, the PGHS-2 (inducible isoform) levels are upregulated upon exposure to microbial infections, cytokines, or mitogens. PGHS-2 levels have, therefore, been implicated in cellular proliferation, inflammation, and carcinogenesis.

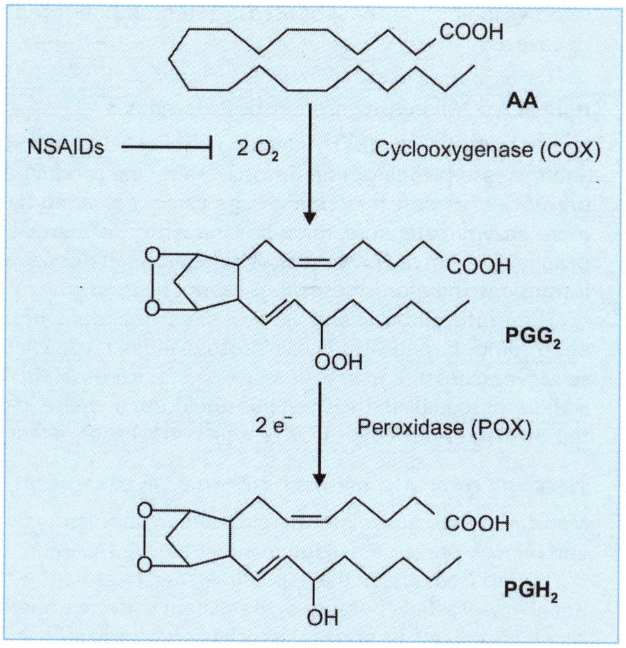

Fig. 3.5: Cyclooxygenase and peroxidase activities of prostaglandin H (PGH) synthase. (NSAID: nonsteroidal anti-inflammatory drugs; PGG_2: prostaglandin G_2; PGH_2: prostaglandin H_2)

Prostaglandin Inhibitors

- **Aspirin: Aspirin irreversibly inhibits the enzyme cyclooxygenase** by covalent modification and is widely used as an analgesic and anti-inflammatory drug. Aspirin is also used as an **antithrombotic agent** due to its inhibitory effect on **platelet cyclooxygenase activity.** Low dose of aspirin is used prophylactically to prevent ischemic heart disease in high-risk individuals **(Fig. 3.6)**
- **Flurbiprofen and indomethacin** inhibit both PGHS-1 and -2. The inhibition is reversible, enzyme is not covalently altered, and only transient complexes are formed.

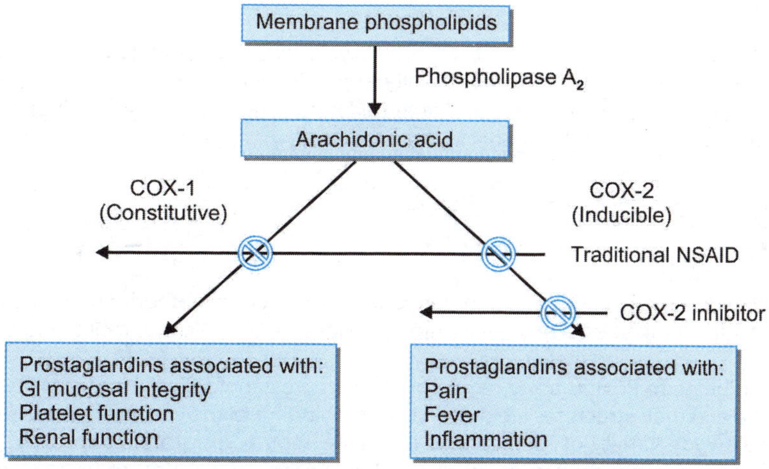

Fig. 3.6: The mechanism of action of traditional versus selective cyclooxygenase (COX) inhibitors. (NSAID: nonsteroidal anti-inflammatory drug; GI: gastrointestinal)

Selective COX inhibitors

Celecoxib and Rofecoxib

These drug selectively inhibit inducible form of PGH synthase (PGH synthase-2) by covalent modification, therefore, these drugs are effectively used as anti-inflammatory agents with minimal gastrointestinal side effects **(Fig. 3.6)**. In contract to aspirin, these selective inhibitors cannot be used in antithrombotic prophylaxis, consequently, their prolonged use can enhance cardiovascular disease risk.

Role of Aspirin in Antithrombotic Prophylaxis

Aspirin and other NSAIDs by inhibiting platelet COX-1 in concert with thromboxane synthase in platelets cause platelet dysfunction and increase bleeding time. Thromboxane, the product of thromboxane synthase activity, is prothrombotic in nature. In the presence of aspirin, the enzyme is irreversibly affected by covalent modification, the non-nucleated platelets fail to synthesize more enzyme, therefore, thromboxane synthesis is impaired. Due to this reason, low dose of aspirin is used in antithrombotic prophylaxis as in the prevention of ischemic heart disease, stroke, etc. NSAIDs cause reversible inhibition of the enzyme, the affect is transient, therefore, these drugs cannot be used effectively as antithrombotic drugs.

The prothrombotic and vasoconstrictive actions of COX-1-derived thromboxane in the vasculature are opposed by an antithrombotic and vasodilative prostaglandin, prostacyclin, that originates from COX-2 in vascular endothelial cells. The COX-2 selective coxibs thus tend to decrease prostacyclin levels in the vasculature without reducing the thromboxane levels. This tendency is thought to explain the small but significant increase in cardiovascular risk that recently led to withdrawal of two coxibs from the US market. Moreover, COX protein is irreversibly affected by aspirin but only temporarily affected by other NSAIDs.

THERAPY OF NSAID-RELATED GASTRIC OR DUODENAL INJURY

Medical intervention for nonsteroidal anti-inflammatory drug (NSAID)-related mucosal injury includes treatment of an active ulcer and primary prevention of future injury. Ideally, the injurious agent should be stopped as the first step in the therapy of an active NSAID-induced ulcer. If that is possible, then treatment with one of the acid inhibitory agents is indicated. Cessation of NSAIDs is not always possible because of the patient's severe underlying disease. Primary prevention of NSAID-induced ulceration can be accomplished by misoprostol, which is a prostaglandin analog.

Prostaglandin Analogs

In view of their central role in maintaining mucosal integrity and repair, stable prostaglandin analogs were developed for the treatment of peptic ulcers. The mechanism by which this rapidly absorbed drug provides its therapeutic effect is through enhancement of mucosal defense and repair. Prostaglandin analogs enhance mucous bicarbonate secretion, stimulate mucosal blood flow, and decrease mucosal cell turnover. The most common toxicity noted with this drug is diarrhea (10–30% incidence). Other major toxicities include uterine bleeding and contractions; misoprostol is contraindicated in women who may be pregnant, and women of childbearing age must be made clearly aware of this potential drug toxicity.

CLINICAL NOTE

The recently developed coxibs (such as celecoxib and rofecoxib) derive their exquisitely selective inhibition of PGHS-2 cyclooxygenase from their ability to bring about noncovalent modification of PGHS-2 and not of PGHS-1. This selectivity has made the coxibs very useful for anti-inflammatory and antiproliferative therapy with reduced gastrointestinal side effects, but it also makes them ineffective as antiplatelet agents and consequently can increase cardiovascular risks.

CLINICAL PEARLS

1. Prostaglandins play a critical role in maintaining gastroduodenal mucosal integrity and repair. It, therefore, follows that interruption of prostaglandin synthesis can impair mucosal defense and repair, thus facilitating mucosal injury via a systemic mechanism.
2. Conversion of arachidonate to PGH_2 is a key regulatory step in prostanoid biosynthesis. Many cyclooxygenase inhibitors have been developed and their structures are quite varied for binding to the cyclooxygenase site on the enzyme.
3. The NSAIDs include a wide variety of medications including aspirin, ibuprofen, naproxen, and indomethacin. These medications are used for pain, inflammation, dysmenorrhea, headache, arthritis, or fever. These compounds act as anti-inflammatory and antipyretic agents by inhibiting COX catalysis by prostaglandin H synthase (PGHS).
4. Aspirin has emerged as a very useful antithrombotic agent because of its action against platelet cyclooxygenase activity. Aspirin brings about inhibition of the enzyme by covalent modification making the transition irreversible.
5. Thromboxane produced by platelet COX-1 in concert with a downstream enzyme is prothrombotic, so aspirin and other NSAIDs cause platelet dysfunction and increase bleeding time.

CASE STUDY 4

Theme: Significance of Low-dose Aspirin in Preventing Ischemic Heart Disease

A 45-year-old man was brought to casualty complaining of chest pain radiating toward left arm. Electrocardiogram (ECG) did not reveal ischemic changes. He was admitted and his blood sample was sent for investigations. History revealed that his both parents died of heart attack and his elder brother also had an attack of myocardial infarction a month ago.

Patient was kept under observation although pain had already subsided. Blood biochemistry revealed normal enzyme profile but dyslipidemia was there. The patient was discharged after two days as there were no more symptoms suggestive of ischemic heart disease. He was advised to go for regular exercises and to start statins and low dose aspirin.

What is the significance of using low-dose aspirin for this patient?

CASE DISCUSSION

Aspirin (acetylsalicylic acid) has been found to be most effective drug in preventing platelet aggregation. It is antithrombogenic in nature. Platelets attempting to stick to blood vessel walls release "endoperoxides", which are converted to prostacyclins (PGI_2) by endothelial cells of blood vessel wall. **Prostacyclins by vasodilatation and by the property of inhibition of platelet aggregation prevent clot formation**. On the other hand, **thromboxane (TxA_2) has opposing effect. It is produced by activated platelets. It enhances platelet aggregation and produces vasoconstriction**. The above two actions promote thrombus formation. A balance between the two biochemical processes is critical for thrombus formation. Both prostacyclins and thromboxanes are produced from cyclic endoperoxide PGH_2. Cyclic endoperoxide first formed in PG synthesis is PGG_2, which is converted to PGH_2 **(Fig. 3.7)**, an immediate precursor of PGI_2 and thromboxane (TxA_2). Both these metabolites are biologically very active and have a very short half life.

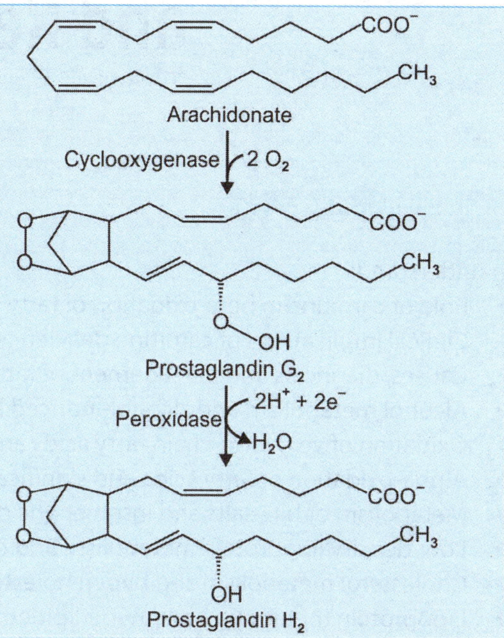

Fig. 3.7: Synthesis of prostaglandin H_2 (PGH_2) from arachidonic acid.

Role of Aspirin

Aspirin irreversibly acetylates cyclooxygenase-1 of platelets and inhibits the enzyme **(Fig. 3.8)**, so that thromboxane (TxA_2) is not formed. So, there is no vasoconstriction and no platelet aggregation and hence the thrombus formation is prevented.

At the same time, aspirin also inhibits production of prostacyclin (PGI_2) by endothelial cells, which prevents platelet aggregation and produces vasodilatation. But **unlike platelets, the endothelial cells regenerate cyclooxygenase within a few hours. Thus, the overall balance shifts toward prevention of thrombus formation by promoting the prostacyclin formation. Aspirin is clinically used for the prevention and management of angina, myocardial infarction, stroke, and transient ischemic attacks (TIA).**

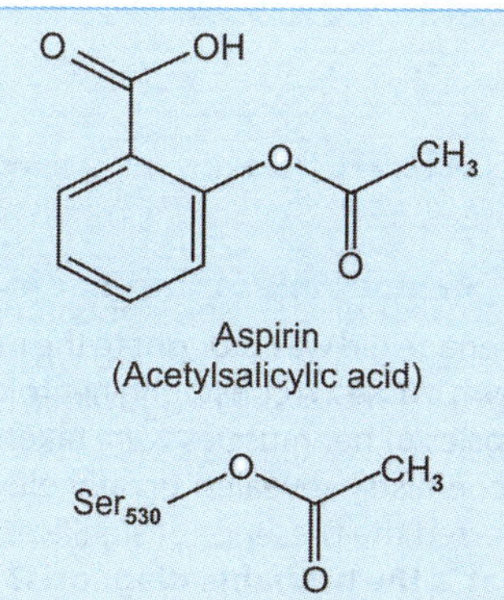

Fig. 3.8: Aspirin's effects on cyclooxygenase-1. Aspirin acts by transferring an acetyl group to a serine residue in cyclooxygenase-1. After acetylation, the enzyme is inhibited.

CASE DETAILS

In the present case, although the biochemical findings and ECG are not suggestive of IHD, but the patient has dyslipidemia and a strongly positive family history of IHD. Hence, the attempt is toward improving lipid levels and prevention of platelet aggregation, so that there is no clot formation. Thus, the ischemia due to atherosclerosis can be prevented. Platelets are extremely sensitive to aspirin and a very small amount can act as antiplatelet aggregator for 24 hours. A dose of 75–300 mg of aspirin is prescribed to the high-risk patients for the life time, unless it produces dyspepsia or other side effects.

Chapter 4

Lipid: Metabolism and Related Disorders

LEARNING OBJECTIVES

To understand:
- ❖ Role of carnitine in beta-oxidation of fatty acids
- ❖ Clinical implications of carnitine deficiency
- ❖ Causes, diagnosis and management of fatty liver
- ❖ Alcohol metabolism and alcohol-induced liver cell injury
- ❖ Oxidation of very long-chain fatty acids and clinical significance
- ❖ Alpha-oxidation of fatty acids and significance
- ❖ Metabolism of bile salts and intrahepatic cholestasis
- ❖ Low-density lipoprotein metabolism and clinical implications
- ❖ Cholesterol metabolism and hypercholesterolemia
- ❖ Lipoprotein metabolism and hyperlipidemia

CASE STUDIES

CASE STUDY 1

Theme: Role of Carnitine in Beta-oxidation of Fatty Acids and Clinical Implications of Carnitine Deficiency

A teenage girl was brought to the medical center because of her complaints that she used to get too tired when asked to participate in gym classes. A consulting neurologist found muscle weakness in girl's arms and legs. When no obvious diagnosis could be made, biopsies of her muscles were taken for test.

Biochemistry revealed greatly elevated amounts of triacylglycerides esterified with primary long-chain fatty acids. Pathology reported the presence of significant numbers of lipid vacuoles in the muscle biopsy.

What is the probable diagnosis?

What is the cause for these symptoms?

CASE DETAILS

The most likely cause of these symptoms is carnitine deficiency.

CARNITINE DEFICIENCY

The amino acid carnitine **(Fig. 4.1)** is required for the transport of long-chain fatty acyl-coenzyme A (CoA) esters into myocyte mitochondria, where they are oxidized for energy. Carnitine is obtained from foods, particularly animal-based foods, and via endogenous synthesis.

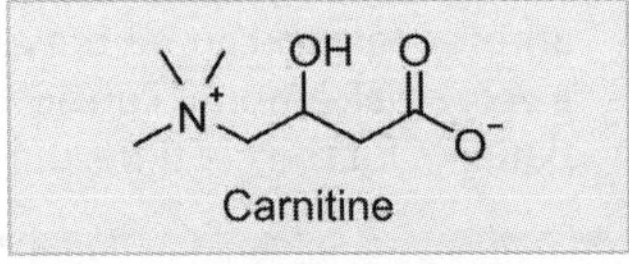

Fig. 4.1: Structure of carnitine.

Carnitine deficiency results from inadequate intake of or inability to metabolize the amino acid carnitine. It can cause a heterogeneous group of disorders. Muscle metabolism is impaired, causing myopathy, hypoglycemia, or cardiomyopathy. Infants typically present with hypoglycemic, hypoketotic encephalopathy. Most often, treatment consists of dietary L-carnitine.

BASIC CONCEPT

Fatty acids are activated on the outer mitochondrial membrane, whereas they are oxidized in the mitochondrial matrix. A special transport mechanism is needed to carry long-chain acyl-CoA molecules across the inner mitochondrial membrane. Activated long-chain fatty acids are transported across the membrane by conjugating them to carnitine, a zwitterionic alcohol. The acyl group is transferred from the sulfur atom of CoA to the hydroxyl group of carnitine to form acylcarnitine. This reaction is catalyzed by carnitine acyltransferase I (also called carnitine palmitoyltransferase I), which is bound to the outer mitochondrial membrane.

Acylcarnitine is then shuttled across the inner mitochondrial membrane by a translocase.

The acyl group is transferred back to CoA on the matrix side of the membrane. This reaction, which is catalyzed by carnitine acyltransferase II (carnitine palmitoyltransferase II), is simply the reverse of the reaction that takes place in the cytosol.

Finally, the translocase returns carnitine to the cytosolic side in exchange for an incoming acylcarnitine **(Fig. 4.2)**.

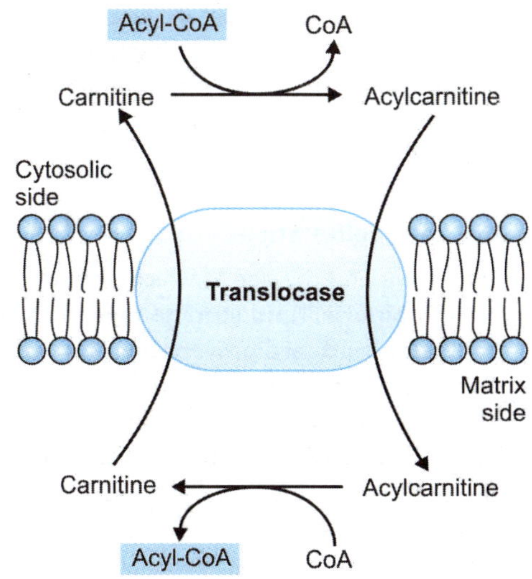

Fig. 4.2: Role of carnitine in transporting the activated fatty acids into the mitochondria.

Pathogenesis

A number of diseases have been traced to a deficiency of carnitine, the transferase or the translocase. **The symptoms of carnitine deficiency range from mild muscle cramping to severe weakness and even death.** The muscle, kidney, and heart are the tissues primarily affected. Muscle weakness during prolonged exercise is an important characteristic of a deficiency of carnitine acyltransferase because muscle relies on fatty acids as a long-term source of energy. **Medium-chain (C8–C10) fatty acids, which do not require carnitine to enter the mitochondria, are oxidized normally in these patients (Fig. 4.3).** These diseases illustrate that the impaired flow of a metabolite from one compartment of a cell to another can lead to a pathological condition.

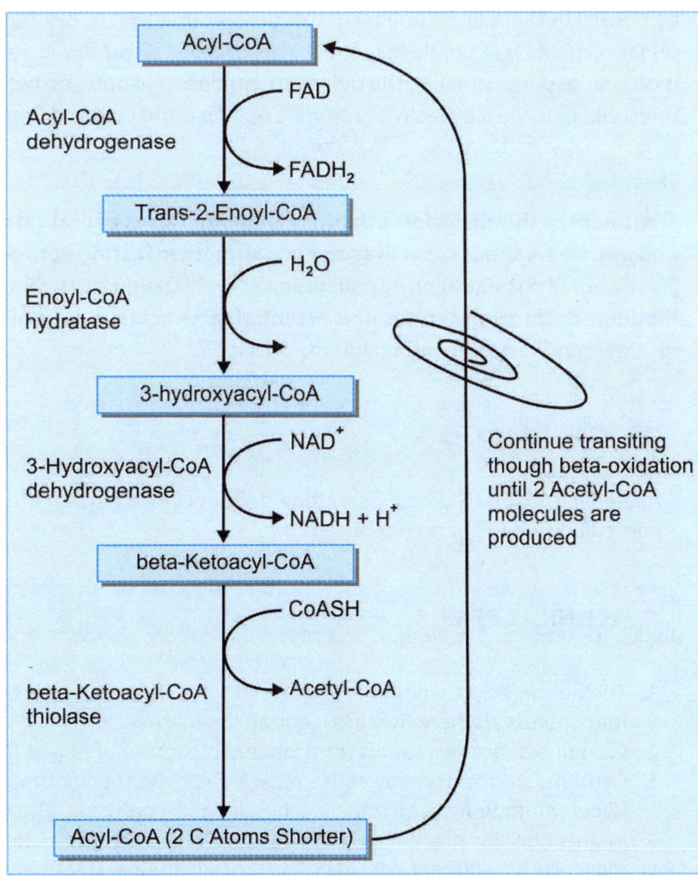

Fig. 4.3: Acyl-CoA transported in mitochondrial matrix undergoes cycles of beta-oxidation until two Acetyl-CoA molecules are produced. In this way, a long-chain fatty acid with an even number of carbons can be degraded completely to acetyl-CoA (C2 units). Acyl-CoA dehydrogenase catalyzes the first step of beta-oxidation. There are three chain specific dehydrogenases: short-, medium- and long-chain Acyl-CoA dehydrogenases.

Causes of Carnitine Deficiency

Causes of carnitine deficiency include the following:

- **Inadequate intake** (e.g. due to fad diets, lack of access, or long-term TPN)
- **Inability to metabolize carnitine** due to enzyme deficiencies (e.g. carnitine palmitoyltransferase deficiency, methylmalonic aciduria, propionic acidemia, isovaleric acidemia)
- **Decreased endogenous synthesis** of carnitine due to a severe liver disorder
- **Excess loss of carnitine** due to diarrhea, diuresis, or hemodialysis
- A hereditary disorder in which **carnitine leaks from renal tubules** (primary carnitine deficiency)
- **Increased requirements for carnitine** when ketosis is present or demand for fat oxidation is high (e.g. during a critical illness such as sepsis or major burns; after major surgery of the GI tract)
- Decreased muscle carnitine levels due to **mitochondrial impairment** (e.g. due to use of zidovudine)
- Use of valproate.

Primary Carnitine Deficiency

The underlying defect involves the plasma membrane sodium gradient-dependent carnitine transporter that is present in heart, muscle, and kidney. This transporter is responsible both for maintaining intracellular carnitine concentrations 20- to 50-fold higher than plasma concentrations and for renal conservation of carnitine. Primary carnitine deficiency has an autosomal recessive pattern of inheritance. Mutations in the SLC22A5 gene lead to the production of defective carnitine transporters. As a result of reduced transport function, carnitine is lost from the body and cells are not supplied with an adequate amount of carnitine.

Clinical Manifestations

Symptoms and the age at which symptoms appear depend on the cause. **Carnitine deficiency may cause muscle necrosis, myoglobinuria, lipid storage myopathy, hypoglycemia, fatty liver, and hyperammonemia with muscle aches, fatigue, confusion, and cardiomyopathy.** The most common presentation is progressive cardiomyopathy with/without skeletal muscle weakness beginning at 2–4 years of age. A smaller number of patients may present with fasting hypoketotic hypoglycemia during the 1st year of life before the cardiomyopathy becomes symptomatic. **Blockage of the transport of long-chain fatty acids into mitochondria not only deprives the patient of energy production, but also disrupts the structure of the muscle cells with the accumulation of lipid droplets.** Serious complications such as heart failure, liver problems, coma, and sudden unexpected death are also a risk. Acute illness due to primary carnitine deficiency can be triggered by periods of fasting or illnesses such as viral infections, particularly when eating is reduced. Deficiencies in the carnitine acyltransferase enzymes I and II can cause similar symptoms.

Diagnosis

Diagnosis of the carnitine transporter defect is aided by the fact that patients have extremely reduced carnitine levels in plasma and muscle (1–2% of normal). Heterozygote parents have plasma carnitine levels approximately 50% of normal. Fasting ketogenesis may be normal because liver carnitine transport is normal, but it may be impaired if dietary carnitine intake is interrupted. The fasting urinary organic acid profile may show a hypoketotic dicarboxylic aciduria pattern if hepatic fatty acid oxidation is impaired, but it is otherwise unremarkable. The defect in carnitine transport can be demonstrated clinically by severe reduction in renal carnitine threshold or in vitro by assay of carnitine uptake using cultured fibroblasts or lymphoblasts.

Treatment

Treatment of this disorder with pharmacologic doses of oral carnitine is highly effective in correcting the cardiomyopathy and muscle weakness as well as any impairment in fasting ketogenesis. Muscle total carnitine concentrations remain less than 5% of normal on treatment. All patients must avoid fasting and strenuous exercise. **Some patients require supplementation with medium-chain triglycerides and essential fatty acids (e.g. linoleic acid, linolenic acid).** Patients with a fatty acid oxidation disorder require a high-carbohydrate, low-fat diet.

CLINICAL NOTE

Acute illness due to primary carnitine deficiency can be triggered by periods of fasting or illnesses such as viral infections, particularly when eating is reduced.

CLINICAL PEARLS

1. The amino acid carnitine is required for the transport of long-chain fatty acyl-coenzyme A (CoA) esters into myocyte mitochondria, where they are oxidized for energy.
2. Carnitine deficiency results from inadequate intake of or inability to metabolize the amino acid carnitine.
3. Carnitine deficiency may cause muscle necrosis, myoglobinuria, lipid storage myopathy, hypoglycemia, fatty liver, and hyperammonemia with muscle aches, fatigue, confusion, and cardiomyopathy.
4. Infants typically present with hypoglycemic, hypoketotic encephalopathy.
5. Most often, treatment consists of dietary L-carnitine. Treatment of this disorder with pharmacologic doses of oral carnitine is highly effective in correcting the cardiomyopathy and muscle weakness as well as any impairment in fasting ketogenesis.

CASE STUDY 2

Theme: Fatty Liver—Causes and Clinical Implications

A 20-year-old primigravid female at 36 weeks of gestation presented to the hospital with nausea, vomiting, and malaise over the last several days. Patient had also noticed that her eyes were turning yellow in color. Her prenatal course had otherwise been unremarkable.

On examination, she was found to have elevated blood pressure (190/110 mm Hg). The laboratory investigation report revealed proteinuria, impaired liver function tests, prolonged clotting time, hyperbilirubinemia, hypofibrinogenemia, and hypoglycemia. A pelvic ultrasound identified a viable intrauterine pregnancy measuring approximately 36-week gestation. After reviewing all, the laboratory results and her clinical picture, the patient was diagnosed with acute fatty liver of pregnancy. The patient was immediately admitted and an emergency cesarean delivery was planned. After surgery, the patient developed a worsening hypoglycemia, coagulopathy, renal failure and went into hepatic coma.

What is the cause of acute fatty liver of pregnancy?
What is the etiology of the hypoglycemia?

CASE DETAILS

The patient developed symptoms of hepatic dysfunction at 36 weeks of gestation. **Short history of illness, hypoglycemia, liver failure, renal failure, and coagulopathy** all are suggestive of onset of acute fatty liver of pregnancy. The condition usually manifests in the second half of pregnancy, usually close to term, but may also develop in the postpartum period. Typically, diagnosis is made based on an incidental finding of abnormal liver enzyme levels. Affected patients may become jaundiced or develop encephalopathy from liver failure, usually reflected by an elevated ammonia level. Profound hypoglycemia is common.

ACUTE FATTY LIVER OF PREGNANCY

Prevalence: Acute fatty liver of pregnancy (AFLP) is a rare (occurring in 1 in 7,000–16,000 deliveries), but potentially fatal disease that typically develops during the third trimester.

Pathogenesis

Fatty liver (steatosis): Fatty liver (steatosis) is an abnormal accumulation of certain fats (triglycerides) inside liver cells. For a variety of reasons, lipid—mainly as triacylglycerol—can accumulate in the liver. Extensive accumulation is regarded as a pathologic condition. When accumulation of lipid in the liver becomes chronic, fibrotic changes occur in the cells that progress to cirrhosis and impaired liver function.

Biochemically, Fatty livers fall into two main categories. The first type is associated with raised levels of plasma free fatty acids resulting from mobilization of fat from adipose tissue or from the hydrolysis of lipoprotein triacylglycerol by lipoprotein lipase in extrahepatic tissues. The production of VLDL does not keep pace with the increasing influx and esterification of free fatty acids, allowing triacylglycerol to accumulate, causing a fatty liver. This occurs during starvation and the feeding of high-fat diets. The ability to secrete VLDL may also be impaired (e.g. in starvation). In uncontrolled diabetes mellitus, fatty infiltration is sufficiently severe to cause visible pallor (fatty appearance) and enlargement of the liver with possible liver dysfunction **(Fig. 4.4)**.

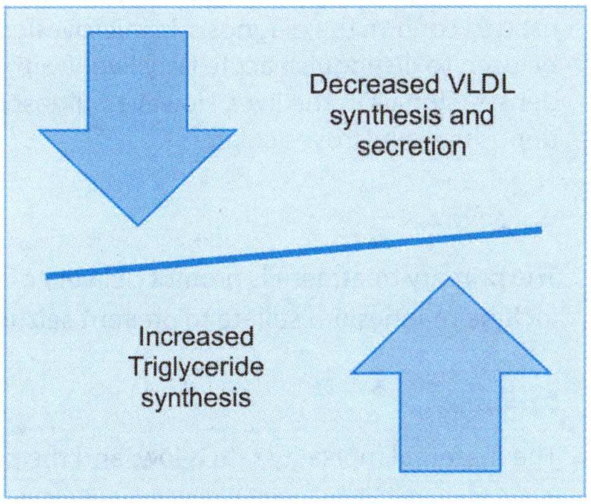

Fig. 4.4: Imbalance in the rate of triacylglycerol formation and export (impaired VLDL formation or secretion) causes fatty liver.

The second type of fatty liver is usually due to a metabolic block in the production of plasma lipoproteins, thus allowing triacylglycerol to accumulate. Theoretically, the lesion may be due to (1) a block in apolipoprotein synthesis, (2) a block in the synthesis of the lipoprotein from lipid and apolipoprotein, (3) a failure in provision of phospholipids that are found in lipoproteins, or (4) a failure in the secretory mechanism itself.

Fatty liver (with/without fibrosis) due to any condition except alcoholism is called nonalcoholic steatohepatitis (macrovesicular steatosis).

Clinical causes of nonalcoholic steatosis or NAFLD are:

- Obesity
- Diabetes mellitus
- Hypertriglyceridemia

- Drugs—corticosteroids, amiodarone, diltiazem, tamoxifen, highly active antiretroviral therapy
- Poisons (carbon tetrachloride and yellow phosphorus)
- Endocrinopathies such as Cushing's syndrome and hypopituitarism, hypobetalipoproteinemia and other metabolic disorders
- Obstructive sleep apnea
- Starvation
- Refeeding syndrome, and total parenteral nutrition.

Steatosis is nearly universal in obese alcoholic patients and is a hallmark of insulin resistance (metabolic syndrome), which is characterized by obesity, diabetes, hypertriglyceridemia, and hypertension. The risk of fatty liver in persons with metabolic syndrome is 4 to 11 times higher than that of persons without insulin resistance. In addition to macrovesicular steatosis, histologic features are indistinguishable from that of alcoholic hepatitis and referred to as nonalcoholic steatohepatitis (NASH). In patients with NAFLD, older age, obesity, and diabetes are risk factors for advanced hepatic fibrosis and cirrhosis.

Microvesicular steatosis is seen with Reye's syndrome, valproic acid toxicity, high-dose tetracycline, or acute fatty liver of pregnancy and may result in fulminant hepatic failure. Women in whom fatty liver of pregnancy develops often have a defect in fatty acid oxidation due to reduced long-chain 3-hydroxyacyl-CoA dehydrogenase activity.

Although the etiology of the AFLP syndrome is unclear, it does appear to be a defect affecting mitochondrial processes. Liver biopsy usually will show mitochondrial disruption and microvesicular fat deposits, indicating decreased β-oxidation of fatty acids. The fatty acids, since they cannot be efficiently oxidized in the mitochondria, are converted to triglycerides, which build up in the hepatocyte. The fat infiltration decreases the amount of glycogen that can be stored and mobilized to maintain blood glucose levels. Gluconeogenesis is also depressed because ATP is not available from the oxidation of fatty acids. Thus, blood glucose levels decline.

Symptoms

Patients most commonly present with clinical and laboratory evidence of acute hepatic failure with decreased hepatic metabolic activity.

Symptoms include nausea, vomiting, lethargy, abdominal pain, jaundice, bleeding, and mental status changes.

Transient polyuria and polydipsia may also occur. Acute renal failure occurs in 60% of patients.

Hypoglycemia, elevated blood pressure, disseminated intravascular coagulation, infection, and encephalopathy are also the common clinical findings.

Diagnosis

Serum aminotransferase levels are usually only moderately elevated (typically <500 U/L). Mild neutrophilia, as well as hypoglycemia and elevated ammonia levels, may be noted.

The diagnosis is made based on clinical grounds. Liver biopsy, although rarely needed, reveals microvesicular steatosis and is used to confirm the diagnosis. In microvesicular steatosis, fat droplets surround a centrally placed nucleus. Biopsy samples cannot be used to distinguish acute fatty liver from valproic acid toxicity. Imaging findings such as CT scanning demonstrate diffuse low-density signals in the liver. However, ultrasonography of the liver usually yields findings that are read as normal because the fat deposits are microvesicular.

Treatment

The primary treatment is prompt delivery of the fetus with supportive measures to stabilize the mother. The supportive measures include magnesium sulfate to prevent seizures, replacement of blood or clotting factors, and management of the hypertension.

Prognosis

The maternal mortality rate is low, and the prognosis is good.

Risk Factors

Acute fatty liver can recur in subsequent pregnancies. The incidence of acute fatty liver of pregnancy is increased in mothers who carry a fetus deficient in the liver isoform of carnitine palmitoyltransferase (L-CPT I). Affected mothers and their newborn infants should be assessed. Studies have revealed a higher incidence of AFLP in women who (1) have a genetic mutation that affects their mitochondrial fatty acid oxidation pathway and (2) carry a fetus with a long-chain 3-hydroxyacyl coenzyme A dehydrogenase (LCHAD) deficiency. This deficiency is associated with a higher mortality rate in affected children; therefore, affected mothers and their newborn infants should be assessed for this deficiency.

CLINICAL NOTE

Acute fatty liver of pregnancy usually manifests in the second half of pregnancy, usually close to term, but may also develop in the postpartum period.

CLINICAL PEARLS

1. Fatty liver (steatosis) is an abnormal accumulation of certain fats (triglycerides) inside liver cells.
2. Affected patients may become jaundiced or develop encephalopathy from liver failure, usually reflected by an elevated ammonia level. Profound hypoglycemia is common.
3. Management is delivery, with supportive measures such as magnesium sulfate to prevent seizures, replacement of blood or clotting factors, and management of the blood pressure.
4. The pathophysiology may be related to fetal deficiencies of long-chain 3-hydroxyacyl coenzyme A dehydrogenase (LCHAD).
5. The maternal mortality rate is low, and the prognosis is good.

CASE STUDY 3

Theme: Alcoholic Liver Disease

A 42-year-old executive complained of fatigue and some recent alterations in mental status, such as forgetting appointments. He traveled outside the United States 2 months ago on a business meeting.

He had vague right upper quadrant pain on deep palpation and borderline enlargement of the liver. Important laboratory findings are listed below:

Serum AST = 120 U/L, Serum ALT = 80 U/L

Serum ALP = 68 U/L, Serum GGT = 170 U/L

Serum total bilirubin = Normal serum glucose = 60 mg/dL

Serum uric acid = 9.8 mg/dL

CBC and urinalysis results are normal.

What is the clinical significance of the abnormal liver function tests?

Why does the patient have hypoglycemia?

Does the patient have gout?

CASE DETAILS

The patient is suffering from alcohol-related liver disease. Hypoglycemia and hyperuricemia are also due to alcoholism.

ALCOHOLIC LIVER DISEASE

Excessive alcohol intake can lead to fatty liver, hepatitis, and cirrhosis. Alcoholic hepatitis is characterized by acute or chronic inflammation and parenchymal necrosis of the liver induced by alcohol. Alcoholic hepatitis is often a reversible disease, is the most common precursor of cirrhosis in the United States, and is associated with four to five times the number of hospitalizations and deaths.

Pathogenesis

Alcoholism leads to fat accumulation in the liver, hyperlipidemia, and ultimately cirrhosis. **The fatty liver is caused by a combination of impaired fatty acid oxidation and increased lipogenesis,** which is thought to be due to changes in the [NADH]/[NAD+] redox potential in the liver, and also to interference with the action of transcription factors regulating the expression of the enzymes involved in the pathways. Oxidation of ethanol by alcohol dehydrogenase leads to excess production of NADH **(Fig. 4.5)**.

$$\underset{\text{Ethanol}}{CH_3-CH_2-OH} + NADPH + H^+ + O_2 \xrightarrow{\text{MEOS}} \underset{\text{Acetaldehyde}}{CH_3-CHO} + NADP^+ + 2H_2O$$

Fig. 4.5: Conversion of ethanol to acetaldehyde by alcohol dehydrogenase.

The NADH generated competes with reducing equivalents from other substrates, including fatty acids, for the respiratory chain, inhibiting their oxidation and causing increased esterification of fatty acids to form triacylglycerol, resulting in the fatty liver. Oxidation of ethanol, leads to the formation of acetaldehyde, which is oxidized by aldehyde dehydrogenase, producing acetate.

The increased [NADH]/[NAD$^+$] ratio also causes increased [lactate]/[pyruvate], resulting in hyperlactacidemia, which decreases excretion of uric acid, aggravating gout. Some metabolism of ethanol takes place via a cytochrome P450-dependent microsomal ethanol-oxidizing system (MEOS) involving NADPH and O_2. This system increases in activity in chronic alcoholism and may account for the increased metabolic clearance in this condition. Ethanol also inhibits the metabolism of some drugs, e.g. barbiturates, by competing for cytochrome P450-dependent enzymes **(Fig. 4.6)**.

In some Asian populations and Native Americans, alcohol consumption results in increased adverse reactions to acetaldehyde owing to a genetic defect of mitochondrial aldehyde dehydrogenase.

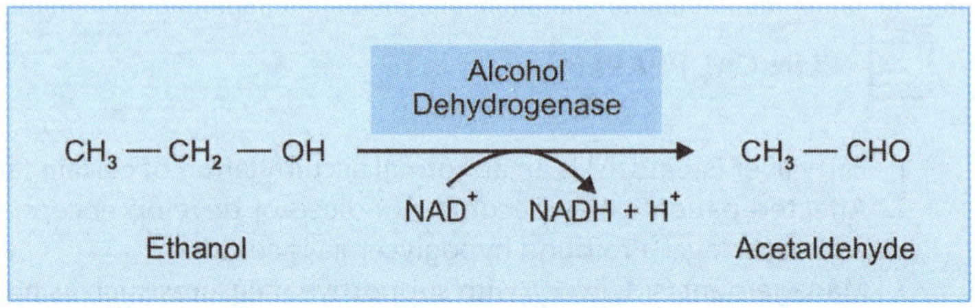

Fig. 4.6: Metabolism of ethanol by microsomal ethanol-oxidizing system.

Frequency

The frequency of alcoholic cirrhosis is estimated to be 10–15% among persons who consume over 50 g of alcohol (4 oz of 100-proof whiskey, 15 oz of wine, or four 12-oz cans of beer) daily for over 10 years (although the risk of cirrhosis may be lower for wine than for a comparable intake of beer or spirits). The risk of cirrhosis is lower (5%) in the absence of other cofactors such as chronic viral hepatitis and obesity. Genetic factors may also account for differences in susceptibility. Women appear to be more susceptible than men, in part because of lower gastric mucosal alcohol dehydrogenase levels. Over 80% of patients with alcoholic hepatitis have been drinking 5 years or more before symptoms that can be attributed to liver disease develop; **the longer the duration of drinking (10–15 or more years) and the larger the alcoholic consumption, the greater the probability of developing alcoholic hepatitis and cirrhosis.** In individuals who drink alcohol excessively, the rate of ethanol metabolism can be sufficiently high to permit the consumption of large quantities without raising the blood alcohol level over 80 mg/dL.

Deficiencies in vitamins and calories probably contribute to the development of alcoholic hepatitis or its progression to cirrhosis. Many adverse effects of alcohol on the liver are thought to be mediated by tumor necrosis factor-α and by the oxidative metabolite acetaldehyde, which contributes to lipid peroxidation and induction of an immune response following covalent binding to proteins in the liver.

Clinical Manifestations

The clinical presentation of alcoholic liver disease can vary from an asymptomatic hepatomegaly to a rapidly fatal acute illness or end-stage cirrhosis. A recent period of heavy drinking, complaints of anorexia and nausea, and the demonstration of hepatomegaly and jaundice strongly suggest the diagnosis. Abdominal pain and tenderness, splenomegaly, ascites, fever, and encephalopathy may be present.

Laboratory Findings

In patients with steatosis, mild liver enzyme elevations may be the only laboratory abnormality. Anemia (usually macrocytic) may be present. Leukocytosis with shift to the left is common in patients with severe alcoholic hepatitis. Leukopenia is occasionally seen and resolves after cessation of drinking. **About 10% of patients have thrombocytopenia related to a direct toxic effect of alcohol on megakaryocytic production or to hypersplenism.**

- **Enzyme profile:** The transaminases are markers of cell necrosis, and in normal health, the serum alanine aminotransferase (ALT) is higher than the aspartate aminotransferase (AST). However, this patient's serum AST is higher than the serum ALT, and his serum gamma-glutamyltransferase (GGT) is disproportionately elevated over the serum alkaline phosphatase (AP). AST is usually elevated but rarely above 300 units/L. **AST is greater than ALT, usually by a factor of 2 or more. This enzyme relationship is characteristic of alcohol-related liver disease.** Alcohol is a mitochondrial poison, and AST is primarily located in the mitochondria, hence, it is preferentially elevated over the ALT. Serum alkaline phosphatase is generally elevated, but seldom more than three times the normal value. **Alcohol also stimulates the cytochrome P450 system, increasing the synthesis of γ-glutamyltransferase (GGT).** Thus, the patient has alcohol-related liver disease rather than a viral hepatitis secondary to HAV (most common cause of traveler's hepatitis).
- **Serum bilirubin:** Serum bilirubin is increased in 60–90% of patients with alcoholic hepatitis. Serum bilirubin levels greater than 10 mg/dL and marked prolongation of the prothrombin time (>6 seconds above control) indicate severe alcoholic hepatitis with a mortality rate as high as 50%.
- **Serum proteins:** The serum albumin is depressed, and the γ-globulin level is elevated in 50–75% of individuals, even in the absence of cirrhosis.
- **Iron indices:** Increased transferrin saturation, hepatic iron stores, and sideroblastic anemia are found in many alcoholic patients. Folic acid deficiency may coexist.

- **Hypoglycemia:** Alcohol intake also explains the patient's hypoglycemia and memory problems. In the metabolism of alcohol, NADH is increased, which results in the reversal of all the normal NAD:NADH reactions, one of which is pyruvate to lactate. Since pyruvate is an intermediate in gluconeogenesis, its conversion to lactate reduces its concentration, so fasting hypoglycemia may occur. Brain requires glucose for fuel; therefore, fasting hypoglycemia results in mental status abnormalities (neuroglycopenia) in these patients.
- **Hyperuricemia:** Hyperuricemia in this patient is likely due to the increase in lactic acid and β--OH butyrate competing with uric acid for excretion in the proximal tubule. Hyperuricemia is not a criterion for the diagnosis of gout. The presence of monosodium urate crystals in the synovial fluid must be documented to diagnose gout. Furthermore, hyperuricemia is not always present even in acute attacks of gout.
- **Ketosis:** The synthesis of β-OH butyrate is increased in alcoholism owing to the increase in acetyl-CoA as the end product of alcohol metabolism and its conversion into ketone bodies by the liver. The increase in NADH drives the reaction from acetoacetic acid to β-OH butyrate.
- **Metabolic acidosis:** People with alcoholism commonly have two causes for increased anion gap metabolic acidosis: lactic acidosis and ketoacidosis. Approximately 20% of patients with hyperuricemia will develop gout.
- **Liver biopsy:** Liver biopsy, if done, demonstrates macrovesicular fat and the findings are identical to those of nonalcoholic steatohepatitis.
- **Other studies:** Imaging studies are used to exclude other diagnoses. Ultrasound helps exclude biliary obstruction and identifies subclinical ascites. Computed tomography (CT) scanning with intravenous contrast or MRI may be indicated in selected cases to evaluate patients for collateral vessels, space-occupying lesions of the liver or concomitant disease of the pancreas.

Differential Diagnosis

Alcoholic hepatitis may be closely mimicked by cholecystitis and cholelithiasis and by drug toxicity. Other causes of hepatitis or chronic liver disease may be excluded by serologic or biochemical testing, by imaging studies, or by liver biopsy. A formula based on the AST/ALT ratio, body mass index, mean corpuscular volume, and gender has been reported to reliably distinguish alcoholic liver disease from nonalcoholic fatty liver disease (NAFLD).

Treatment

General Measures

Abstinence from alcohol is essential. **Fatty liver is quickly reversible with abstinence.** Every effort should be made to provide sufficient amounts of carbohydrates and calories in anorectic patients to reduce endogenous protein catabolism, promote gluconeogenesis, and prevent hypoglycemia. Nutritional support (40 kcal/kg with 1.5–2 g/kg as protein) improves survival in patients with malnutrition. The administration of vitamins, particularly folic acid and thiamine, is indicated, especially when deficiencies are noted; **glucose administration increases the vitamin B1 requirement and can precipitate Wernicke-Korsakoff syndrome if thiamine is not coadministered.**

Pharmacologic Measures

Methylprednisolone may reduce short-term mortality in patients with alcoholic hepatitis.
Pentoxifylline: An inhibitor of tumor necrosis factor-α decreases mortality rates in patients with severe alcoholic hepatitis, primarily by decreasing the risk of hepatorenal syndrome. Other experimental therapies include propylthiouracil, oxandrolone, S-adenosyl-L-methionine, infliximab, antioxidants, and extracorporeal liver support. Colchicine does not reduce mortality in patients with alcoholic cirrhosis.

Prognosis

Short-term: Individuals in whom the prothrombin time prohibits liver biopsy have a 42% mortality rate at 1 year. Other unfavorable prognostic factors are a serum bilirubin greater than 10 mg/dL, hepatic encephalopathy, azotemia, leukocytosis, lack of response to corticosteroid therapy.

Long-term: The 3-year mortality rate of persons who recover from acute alcoholic hepatitis is ten times greater than that of control individuals of comparable age. Complications of portal hypertension (ascites, variceal bleeding, hepatorenal syndrome), coagulopathy, and severe jaundice following recovery from acute alcoholic hepatitis also suggest a poor long-term prognosis.

The most important prognostic consideration is continued excessive drinking.

Other Effects of Ethanol

- Between one-half and two-thirds of alcoholics have skeletal muscle weakness caused by acute alcoholic myopathy.
- Hormonal changes include:
  - An increase in cortisol levels
  - Inhibition of vasopressin secretion at rising blood alcohol concentrations and enhanced secretion at falling blood alcohol concentrations (with the final result that most alcoholics are likely to be slightly overhydrated)
  - A modest and reversible decrease in serum thyroxine (T_4); and a more marked decrease in serum triiodothyronine (T_3).

- **Alcohol intake can result in inflammation of the esophagus and stomach causing epigastric distress and gastrointestinal bleeding. Alcohol is one of the most common causes of hemorrhagic gastritis.** Violent vomiting can produce severe bleeding through a **Mallory-Weiss lesion, a longitudinal tear** in the mucosa at the gastroesophageal junction.
- **Acute pancreatitis** is almost three-fold higher in alcoholics than in the general population.
- Chronic high doses cause **peripheral neuropathy** in 5–15% of alcoholics.
- Few alcoholics develop **Wernicke-Korsakoff syndromes.** These occur as a result of thiamine deficiency, especially in predisposed individuals, e.g., those with transketolase deficiency.
- While alcohol supplies calories (a drink contains ~300 kJ, or 70–100 kcal), these are devoid of nutrients such as minerals, proteins, and vitamins. Alcohol can also interfere with absorption of vitamins in the small intestine and decreases their storage in the liver with modest effects on folate (Folacin or folic acid), pyridoxine (B_6), thiamine (B_1), nicotinic acid (niacin, B_3), and vitamin A.
- Chronic intake of modest doses of alcohol can have some beneficial effects. **A maximum of one to two drinks per day may decrease the risk for cardiovascular death, perhaps through an increase in high-density lipoprotein (HDL) cholesterol or changes in clotting mechanisms.**

CLINICAL NOTE

The administration of vitamins, particularly folic acid and thiamine, is indicated, in alcoholics, especially when deficiencies are noted; glucose administration increases the vitamin B_1 requirement and can precipitate Wernicke-Korsakoff syndrome if thiamine is not coadministered.

CLINICAL PEARLS

1. Excessive alcohol intake can lead to fatty liver, hepatitis, and cirrhosis.
2. The clinical presentation of alcoholic liver disease can vary from an asymptomatic hepatomegaly to a rapidly fatal acute illness or end-stage cirrhosis.
3. Anemia, hyperlipidemia, hypoglycemia, hyperuricemia, abnormal liver functions and high anion gap acidosis are characteristic of alcoholic liver disease.
4. Abstinence from alcohol is essential. Fatty liver is quickly reversible with abstinence. Every effort should be made to provide sufficient amounts of carbohydrates and calories in anorectic patients to reduce endogenous protein catabolism, promote gluconeogenesis, and prevent hypoglycemia.
5. Methylprednisolone and pentoxifylline (an inhibitor of tumor necrosis factor-α) may reduce short-term mortality in patients with alcoholic hepatitis.

CASE STUDY 4

Theme: Alcohol-induced Liver Cirrhosis

A 60-year-old man who has a history of chronic alcoholism comes to the hospital with complaints of protuberant abdomen (ascites) and edema feet. He also has history of hemorrhages.

The investigation report of this patient reveals:

Total serum protein 4.8 g/dL
Serum albumin 2.4 g/dL
Prothrombin time 30 seconds
Urine protein Nil

What is the probable diagnosis of this patient?

How will you explain the biochemical changes reported here?

The patient is suffering from cirrhosis of liver. History of alcoholism, hemorrhages, low protein levels, edema, prolonged prothrombin time all signify alcoholic cirrhosis. Absence of urinary proteins signifies that the cause of hypoproteinemia is impaired endogenous protein synthesis and not the renal loss.

BASIC CONCEPT

CIRRHOSIS OF LIVER

Cirrhosis is a consequence of chronic liver disease characterized by replacement of liver tissue by fibrous scar tissue as well as regenerative nodules, leading to progressive loss of liver function. **Excessive chronic alcohol use can cause several different**

types of chronic liver disease, including alcoholic fatty liver, alcoholic hepatitis, and alcoholic cirrhosis. Chronic alcohol use can produce fibrosis in the absence of accompanying inflammation and/or necrosis. When fibrosis reaches a certain degree, there is disruption of the normal liver architecture and replacement of liver cells by regenerative nodules. **In alcoholic cirrhosis, the nodules are usually <3 mm in diameter; this form of cirrhosis is referred to as micronodular. With cessation of alcohol use, larger nodules may form, resulting in a mixed micronodular and macronodular cirrhosis.**

Pathogenesis

Intake of ethanol increases intracellular accumulation of triglycerides by increasing fatty acid uptake, by reducing fatty acid oxidation and lipoprotein secretion. Protein synthesis, glycosylation, and secretion are impaired. Oxidative damage to hepatocyte membranes occurs due to the formation of reactive oxygen species; acetaldehyde (the majority of ethanol oxidation occurs via alcohol dehydrogenase to form acetaldehyde) is a highly reactive molecule that combines with proteins to form protein-acetaldehyde adducts. These adducts may interfere with specific enzyme activities. Hepatocyte loss occurs, and with increased collagen production and deposition, together with continuing hepatocyte destruction, the liver contracts and shrinks in size. This process generally takes from years to decades to occur.

Clinical Manifestations

Patients with alcoholic liver disease can present with nonspecific symptoms such as vague right upper quadrant pain, fever, nausea and vomiting, diarrhea, anorexia, and malaise. Alternatively, they may present with more specific complications of chronic liver disease, including ascites, edema, or upper gastrointestinal (GI) hemorrhage. Other clinical manifestations include the development of jaundice or encephalopathy.

On physical examination, the liver and spleen may be enlarged, with the liver edge being firm and nodular. Other frequent findings include **scleral icterus, palmar erythema, spider angiomas, parotid gland enlargement, digital clubbing, muscle wasting, or the development of edema and ascites. Men may have decreased body hair and gynecomastia as well as testicular atrophy,** which may be a consequence of hormonal abnormalities or a direct toxic effect of alcohol on the testes. In women with advanced alcoholic cirrhosis, menstrual irregularities usually occur, and some women may be amenorrheic. These changes are often reversible following cessation of alcohol.

Laboratory Diagnosis

Laboratory tests may be completely normal in patients with early compensated alcoholic cirrhosis. Alternatively, in advanced liver disease, many abnormalities are usually present. The following findings are typical in cirrhosis:

- *Aminotransferases*—AST and ALT are moderately elevated, with AST > ALT. However, normal aminotransferases do not preclude cirrhosis.
- *Alkaline phosphatase*—usually slightly elevated.
- GGT—correlates with AP levels. Typically much higher in chronic liver disease from alcohol.
- *Bilirubin*—may elevate as cirrhosis progresses.
- *Albumin*—levels fall as the synthetic function of the liver declines with worsening cirrhosis since albumin is exclusively synthesized in the liver.
- *Prothrombin time*—increases since the liver synthesizes clotting factors.
- *Globulins*—increased due to shunting of bacterial antigens away from the liver to lymphoid tissue.
- *Serum sodium*—hyponatremia due to inability to excrete free water resulting from high levels of ADH and aldosterone.
- *Thrombocytopenia*—due to both congestive splenomegaly as well as decreased thrombopoietin from the liver. However, this rarely results in platelet count <50,000/mL.
- *Leukopenia and neutropenia*—due to splenomegaly with splenic margination.
- *Coagulation defects*—the liver produces most of the coagulation factors and thus coagulopathy correlates with worsening liver disease.
- Liver biopsy can be helpful to confirm a diagnosis.

Imaging: Ultrasound is helpful for assessing liver size and detecting ascites or hepatic nodules, including small hepatocellular carcinomas. Together with a Doppler study, it may establish patency of the splenic, portal, and hepatic veins. Hepatic nodules are characterized further by contrast-enhanced computed tomography (CT) scan or magnetic resonance imaging (MRI). Nodules suspicious for malignancy may be biopsied under ultrasound or CT guidance.

Differential Diagnosis

The most common causes of cirrhosis are chronic hepatitis C and B and alcohol. Many cases of cirrhosis are "cryptogenic," in which unrecognized NAFLD (nonalcoholic fatty liver disease) may play a role. Hemochromatosis is the most commonly identified genetic disorder that causes cirrhosis. Other metabolic diseases that may lead to cirrhosis include Wilson's disease and α1-antiprotease (α1-antitrypsin) deficiency. Primary biliary cirrhosis occurs more frequently in women than men. Secondary biliary cirrhosis may result from chronic biliary obstruction due to a stone, stricture, or neoplasm. Congestive heart failure and constrictive pericarditis may lead to hepatic fibrosis ("cardiac cirrhosis") complicated by ascites and may be mistaken for other causes of cirrhosis.

Complications

Upper gastrointestinal tract bleeding may occur from varices, portal hypertensive gastropathy, or gastroduodenal ulcer. Varices may also result from portal vein thrombosis. Liver failure may be precipitated by alcoholism, surgery, and infection. The risk of carcinoma of the liver is increased greatly in patients with cirrhosis.

Treatment

Abstinence is the cornerstone of therapy for patients. Patients require good nutrition and long-term medical supervision in order to manage underlying complications that may develop. Complications such as the development of ascites and edema, variceal hemorrhage, or portosystemic encephalopathy all require specific management and treatment. **Glucocorticoids are occasionally used in patients with severe alcoholic hepatitis in the absence of infection.**

CLINICAL NOTE

The clinical features of cirrhosis result from hepatic cell dysfunction, portosystemic shunting, and portal hypertension.

CLINICAL PEARLS

1. Cirrhosis is a consequence of chronic liver disease characterized by replacement of liver tissue by fibrous scar tissue as well as regenerative nodules, leading to progressive loss of liver function.
2. Excessive chronic alcohol use can cause several different types of chronic liver disease, including alcoholic fatty liver, alcoholic hepatitis, and alcoholic cirrhosis.
3. Intake of ethanol increases intracellular accumulation of triglycerides by increasing fatty acid uptake, by reducing fatty acid oxidation and lipoprotein secretion. Protein synthesis, glycosylation, and secretion are impaired.
4. Patients with alcoholic liver disease can present with nonspecific symptoms such as vague right upper quadrant pain, fever, nausea and vomiting, diarrhea, anorexia, and malaise. Alternatively, they may present with more specific complications of chronic liver disease, including ascites, edema, or upper gastrointestinal (GI) hemorrhage.
5. Abstinence is the cornerstone of therapy for patients. Patients require good nutrition and long-term medical supervision in order to manage underlying complications that may develop.

CASE STUDY 5

Theme: Clinical Implications of Impaired Peroxisomal Fatty Acid Oxidation

A newborn infant had abnormal facial features, severe muscle weakness, hypotonia and refusal to feeds.

There was inability to suck and/or swallow. A diagnosis of Zellweger syndrome was made.

What is the probable defect in this disorder?

CASE DETAILS

Zellweger syndrome, also called cerebrohepatorenal syndrome, is a rare, congenital disorder (present at birth), characterized by the reduction or absence of peroxisomes in the cells of the liver, kidneys, and brain.

Biochemical Defect

Zellweger syndrome is one of a group of four related diseases called **peroxisome biogenesis disorders (PBDs),** which are part of a larger group of diseases known as the leukodystrophies. These are inherited conditions that damage the white matter of the brain and also affect how the body metabolizes particular substances in the blood and organ tissues. It is characterized by an individual's **inability to beta-oxidize very-long chain fatty acids in the peroxisomes of the cell (Fig. 4.7)**, due to a genetic disorder in one of the several genes involved with peroxisome biogenesis. Zellweger syndrome is the most severe of the PBDs. Infantile Refsum disease (IRD) is the mildest and neonatal adrenoleukodystrophy and rhizomelic chondrodysplasia have similar but less severe symptoms.

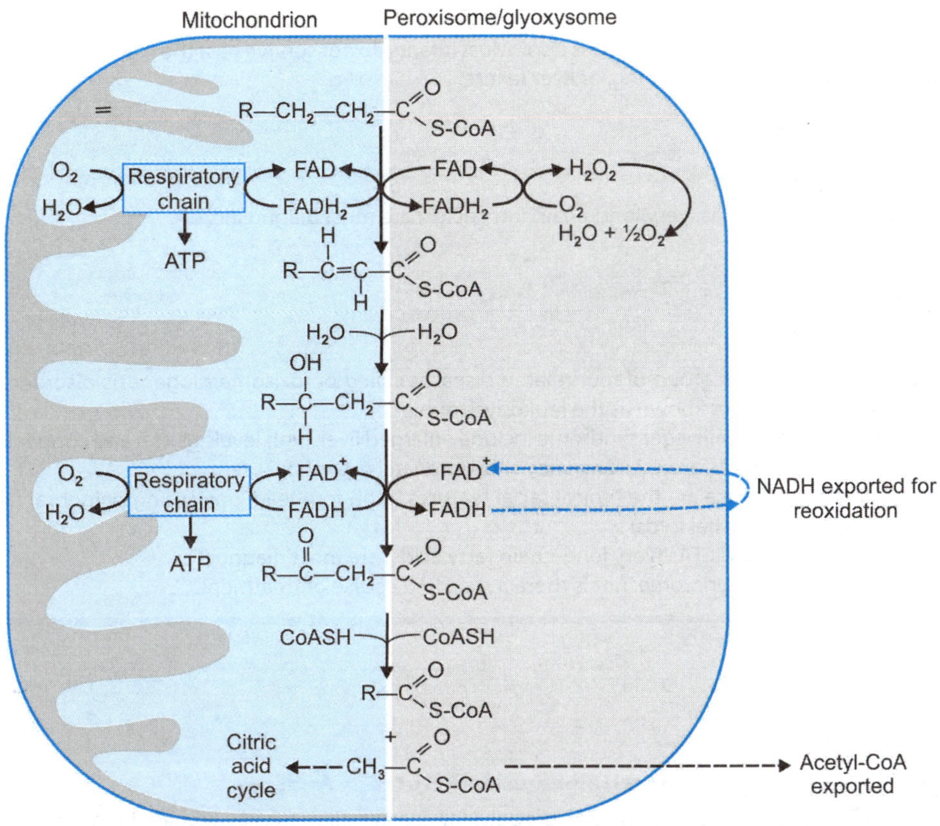

Fig. 4.7: A modified form of β-oxidation is found in peroxisomes and leads to the formation of acetyl-CoA and H_2O_2 (from the flavoprotein-linked dehydrogenase step), which is broken down by catalase. Thus, the dehydrogenation in peroxisomes is not linked directly to phosphorylation and the generation of ATP. The system facilitates the oxidation of very long-chain fatty acids (e.g. C20, C22). The enzymes in peroxisomes do not attack shorter chain fatty acids; the β-oxidation sequence ends at octanoyl-CoA. Octanoyl and acetyl groups are both further oxidized in mitochondria.

Clinical Manifestations

The most common features of Zellweger syndrome include **enlarged liver, high levels of iron and copper in the bloodstream, and vision disturbances.** Some affected infants may show prenatal growth failure. Symptoms at birth may include a lack of muscle tone, an inability to move and glaucoma. Other symptoms may include **unusual facial characteristics, mental retardation, seizures, and an inability to suck and/or swallow. Jaundice and gastrointestinal bleeding** may also occur. Of central diagnostic importance are the typical facial features (high forehead, unslanting palpebral fissures, hypoplastic supraorbital ridges, and epicanthal folds). More than 90% show postnatal growth failure **(Fig. 4.8)**.

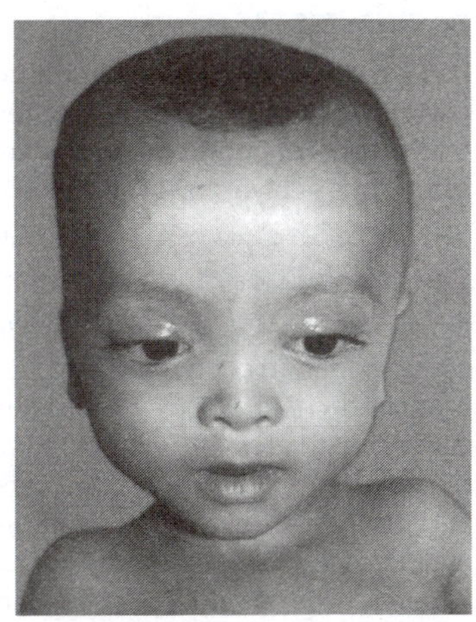

Fig. 4.8: Typical facial appearance of a child suffering from Zellweger syndrome (high forehead, unslanting palpebral fissures, hypoplastic supraorbital ridges, and epicanthal folds).

Laboratory Diagnosis

There are several noninvasive laboratory tests that permit precise and early diagnosis of peroxisomal disorders. The abnormally high levels of VLCFAs (very long-chain fatty acids) are most diagnostic.

Treatment

There is no cure for Zellweger syndrome, nor is there a standard course of treatment. Since the metabolic and neurological abnormalities that cause the symptoms of Zellweger syndrome are caused during fetal development, treatments to correct these abnormalities after birth are limited. Most treatments are symptomatic and supportive.

Prognosis

The prognosis for infants with Zellweger syndrome is poor. Most infants do not survive past the first 6 months, and usually succumb to respiratory distress, gastrointestinal bleeding, or liver failure.

CLINICAL NOTE

The abnormally high levels of VLCFAs (very long-chain fatty acids) are most diagnostic.

CLINICAL PEARLS

1. Zellweger syndrome is one of a group of four related diseases called peroxisome biogenesis disorders (PBDs), which are part of a larger group of diseases known as the leukodystrophies.
2. The most common features of Zellweger syndrome include enlarged liver, high levels of iron and copper in the bloodstream, and vision disturbances. Some affected infants may show prenatal growth failure.
3. Of central diagnostic importance are the typical facial features (high forehead, unslanting palpebral fissures, hypoplastic supraorbital ridges, and epicanthal folds) .
4. The abnormally high levels of VLCFAs (very long-chain fatty acids) are most diagnostic.
5. There is no cure for Zellweger syndrome, nor is there a standard course of treatment.

CASE STUDY 6

Theme: Clinical Implications of Impaired Alpha-oxidation of Fatty Acids

A 6-year-old child with progressive hearing loss was brought for consultation. History revealed that the child was born normal but progressively developed loss of hearing and loss of smell. From the past few months, the child was finding it difficult to locate the things at nighttime.

The child had dysmorphic features, a flat bridge of nose, and low-set ears.

On examination, pulse was irregular and the liver was enlarged. Laboratory investigations revealed low levels of plasma cholesterol, HDL and LDL. A diagnosis and Refsum disease was made.

What is the defect in this disease?

BASIC CONCEPT

REFSUM DISEASE

Refsum disease (RD) is a **neurocutaneous syndrome** that is characterized biochemically by the accumulation of phytanic acid in plasma and tissues. Refsum first described this disease.

Peripheral polyneuropathy, cerebellar ataxia, retinitis pigmentosa, and ichthyosis are the major clinical components. The symptoms evolve slowly and insidiously from childhood through adolescence and early adulthood.

Biochemical Defect

Refsum disease is a recessive disorder characterized by defective peroxisomal alpha-oxidation of phytanic acid. Consequently, this unusual, exogenous C20-branched-chain (3,7,11,15-tetramethyl-hexadecanoic acid) **(Fig. 4.9)** fatty acid accumulates in brain, blood and other tissues. It is almost exclusively of exogenous origin and is delivered mainly from dietary plant chlorophyll and, to a lesser extent, from animal sources. Blood levels of phytanic acid are increased in patients with Refsum disease. These levels are 10–50 mg/dL, whereas normal values are less than or equal to 0.2 mg/dL, and account for 5–30% of serum lipids. **Phytanic acid replaces other fatty acids, including such essential ones as Linoleic and Arachidonic acids, in lipid moieties of various tissues. This situation leads to an essential fatty acid deficiency, which is associated with the development of ichthyosis.**

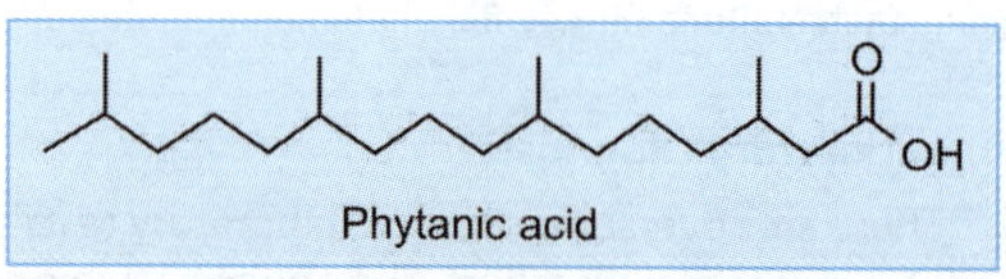

Fig. 4.9: Structure of phytanic acid.

An infantile form of Refsum disease also exists and is an autosomal recessive disorder of peroxisomal biogenesis, leading to many biochemical abnormalities, including elevated plasma concentration of phytanic acid, pristanic acid, very long-chain fatty acids, and C27 bile acids. The disease presents in the first year of life and manifests with developmental delay, visual and hearing disturbances, and dysmorphic features. Ichthyosis is an unusual symptom.

Reaction

Phytol (from chlorophyll in plant foods) phytanic acid → Pristanic acid → Propionyl-CoA

Frequency

Refsum disease is rare, with just 60 cases observed so far.

Clinical Manifestations

Classic Refsum disease manifests in children aged 2–7 years; however, diagnosis usually is delayed until early adulthood. Infantile Refsum disease makes its appearance in early infancy. Symptoms develop progressively and slowly with neurologic and ophthalmic manifestations. The disease is characterized by:

- Night blindness due to degeneration of the retina (retinitis pigmentosum)
- Loss of the sense of smell (anosmia)
- Deafness
- Concentric constriction of the visual fields
- Cataract
- Signs resulting from cerebellar ataxia:
  - Progressive weakness
  - Foot drop
  - Loss of balance
- Cardiac arrhythmias
- Some individuals will have shortened bones in their fingers or toes.
- The children usually have moderately dysmorphic features that may include epicanthal folds, a flat bridge of the nose, and low-set ears **(Figs. 4.10A and B)**.

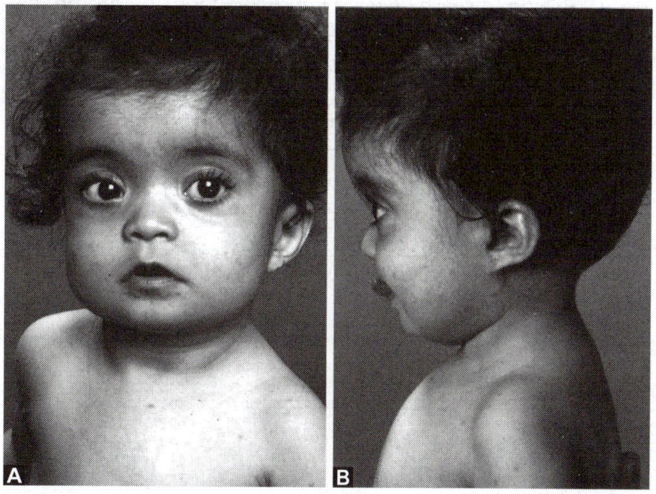

Figs. 4.10A and B: Refsum disease. The child has dysmorphic features, a flat bridge of nose, and low-set ears.

Laboratory Diagnosis

- Levels of plasma cholesterol and high- and low-density lipoprotein are often moderately reduced.
- Blood phytanic acid levels are elevated.
- Cerebrospinal fluid (CSF) shows a protein level of 100–600 mg/dL.
- Routine laboratory investigations of blood and urine do not reveal any consistent diagnostic abnormalities.
- Phytanic oxidase activity estimation in skin fibroblast cultures is important.

Imaging: Skeletal radiography is required to estimate bone changes.

Treatment

- Eliminate all sources of chlorophyll from the diet.
  - The major dietary exclusions are green vegetables (source of phytanic acid) and animal fat (phytol).
  - The aim of such dietary treatment is to reduce daily intake of phytanic acid from the usual level of 50 mg/day to less than 5 mg/day.
- Plasmapheresis

  Patients may also require plasma exchange (plasmapheresis) in which blood is drawn, filtered, and reinfused back into the body, to control the buildup of phytanic acid.
  - The main indication for plasmapheresis in patients with Refsum disease is a severe or rapidly worsening clinical condition.
  - A minor indication is failure of dietary management to reduce a high plasma phytanic acid level.

Prognosis

Prognosis in untreated patients generally is poor. Dysfunction of myelinated nerve fibers and the cardiac conduction system leads to central and peripheral neuropathic symptoms, impaired vision, and cardiac arrhythmias. The latter frequently is the cause of death.

In early diagnosed and treated cases, phytanic acid decreases slowly, followed by improvement of the skin scaling and, to a variable degree, reversal of recent neurological signs. Retention of vision and hearing are reported.

Pharmacological upregulation of the omega-oxidation of phytanic acid may form the basis of the new treatment strategy for adult Refsum disease in the near future.

CLINICAL NOTE

Blood phytanic acid levels in Refsum disease are 10–50 mg/dL, whereas normal values are less than or equal to 0.2 mg/dL, and account for 5–30% of serum lipids.

CLINICAL PEARLS

1. Refsum disease (RD) is a neurocutaneous syndrome that is characterized biochemically by the accumulation of phytanic acid in plasma and tissues.
2. Refsum disease is a recessive disorder characterized by defective peroxisomal alpha-oxidation of phytanic acid. Consequently, this unusual, exogenous C20-branched-chain (3,7,11,15-tetramethyl-hexadecanoic acid) fatty acid accumulates in brain, blood and other tissues to produce toxic effects.
3. The disease is characterized by night blindness due to degeneration of the retina (retinitis pigmentosum), loss of the sense of smell (anosmia), deafness, cataract and cerebellar ataxia.
4. Levels of plasma cholesterol and high- and low-density lipoprotein are often moderately reduced. Blood phytanic acid levels are elevated.
5. Treatment involves elimination of all sources of chlorophyll from the diet. Prognosis in untreated patients generally is poor.

CASE STUDY 7

Theme: Clinical Implications of Impaired Metabolism of Bile Salts

A 25-year-old female at 34 weeks of gestation presented to the clinic with complaints of generalized itching. Patient reported no rash or skin changes. She denied any changes in detergent, soaps, or perfumes. She denied nausea and vomiting. There was no history of any drug intake or previous allergies. There was no fever or any other medical illness.

What is the patient's likely diagnosis?

What is the cause of the patient's generalized itching?

CASE DETAILS

The patient is most probably having intrahepatic cholestasis of pregnancy.

Generalized pruritus in pregnancy and a characteristic enzyme profile; it is a typical picture of intrahepatic cholestasis of pregnancy. High alkaline phosphatase is a maker of cholestasis. (It is also high late in normal pregnancy due to the influx of placental alkaline phosphatase, But in cholestasis the level may be four times the normal reference range). Slightly high transaminases differentiate it from viral hepatitis in which very high levels are found and are due to bile salts induced toxic damage to the liver cells. Bilirubin is high due to intrahepatic obstruction as result of cholestasis. This is conjugated type. Increased serum bile salts and accumulation of bile salts in the dermis of the skin are responsible for generalized itching.

BASIC CONCEPT

INTRAHEPATIC CHOLESTASIS OF PREGNANCY

Intrahepatic cholestasis of pregnancy (ICP) is a benign disorder that occurs in the second or third trimester and resolves spontaneously after delivery. **Cholestasis of pregnancy is a condition in which the normal flow of bile from the gallbladder is impeded, leading to accumulation of bile salts in the body.**

Bile salt molecules secreted by the gallbladder are essential for the emulsification and absorption of fats. They are the salt forms of bile acids, which are the major product of cholesterol catabolism in the liver. Bile salts form micelles as their hydrophobic face contacts the fat (triacylglycerol), and their polar face maintains contact with the aqueous environment. This micelle formation allows water-soluble digestive enzymes to digest the entrapped triacylglycerol molecules, releasing fatty acids that are readily absorbed by the digestive system.

There are two primary bile acids formed in the liver from cholesterol: (1) cholic acid and (2) chenodeoxycholic acid. **The formation of bile acids prevents cholesterol accumulation in organs;** the body cannot break down the steroid ring of cholesterol. At physiologic pH, bile acids will always be in the form of bile salts. Bile salts are conjugated with glycine or taurine in the liver prior to excretion, forming glyco- or tauroconjugates. Bacterial enzymes present in the intestine produce the secondary bile salts, deoxycholate and lithocholate, by reducing the primary bile salts **(Fig. 4.11)**. Bile salts perform an important function and are recycled by the body. The body produces 400 mg of bile salts per day from cholesterol; this represents the fate of half of the cholesterol used daily in metabolism (800 mg). However, 20–30 g of bile acids is maintained in the enterohepatic circulation. Less than 0.5 g/day is lost to excretion. **Bile salts are produced in the liver, stored in the gallbladder, and secreted through the bile duct into the duodenum where they act on triacylglycerol molecules in the intestines. In the gut, the glycine or taurine moiety is removed from the bile salt.** It is reabsorbed in the small intestine and returned to the liver for reuse via the portal vein. Bile salts are absorbed by passive diffusion along the entire small intestine, and a specialized Na^+-bile salt cotransporter is present in the lower ileum.

Intrahepatic cholestasis of pregnancy is a syndrome of unknown etiology characterized by a 100-fold increase in maternal and fetal blood bile salt levels. Bile salts are produced in both the fetal and maternal liver. The fetus transfers the bile salts across the placenta for disposal. When the function of the maternal gallbladder is slowed, bile salts can accumulate in the liver and bloodstream, ultimately resulting in the classical pruritus symptom. It is believed that pregnancy-related hormones may slow bile salt excretion from the gallbladder.

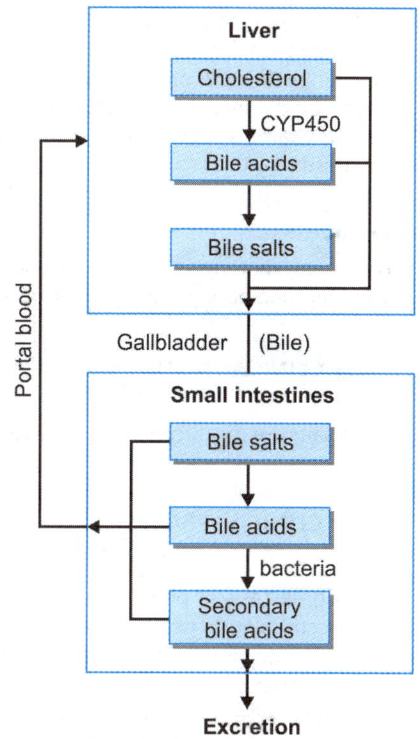

Fig. 4.11: Synthesis and enterohepatic recirculation of bile salts.

Incidence

Prevalence varies among countries. The prevalence in North America is 1–2/10,000 pregnancies. The condition occurs in all ages and in both primiparous and multiparous women. It can recur in subsequent pregnancies and is more common in the presence of multiple gestations.

Etiology

The etiology is unknown but may be multifactorial. Possible causes include genetic abnormalities, increased hormonal exposure, abnormal sulfotransferase activity, and endogenous opioids. Intrahepatic cholestasis of pregnancy has been found more frequently in certain ethnic groups, suggesting that the genetic factors are involved.

It is speculated that the **hormones such as estrogen and progesterone, which are elevated in pregnancy, cause a slowing of the gallbladder function, leading to this disorder. The incidence of intrahepatic cholestasis of pregnancy is highest during the third trimester, when estrogen levels peak.** Formation of large amounts of sulfated progesterone metabolites due to the abnormal sulfotransferase activity also results in saturation of the hepatic transport system used for biliary excretion.

Symptoms

Generalized pruritus is the main symptom of intrahepatic cholestasis of pregnancy. The itching may be more intense over the palms and soles but can extend to the trunk, extremities, eyelids, and, in rare cases, the oral cavity. The pruritus is worse at night. Jaundice is uncommon (10–25%); when it occurs, jaundice follows the onset of pruritus.

Diagnosis

The serum bilirubin level is usually lower than six times the upper limit of reference range and is usually conjugated. Fever is rare. Steatorrhea may be present, which may lead to deficiency of fat-soluble vitamins, especially vitamin K. **Aminotransferase levels are less than 1,000 U/L, which distinguishes intrahepatic cholestasis (IHC) from viral hepatitis. Alkaline phosphatase is four times higher than the reference range (44–147 U/L).** Interestingly, gamma-glutamyl transpeptidase levels are within the reference range or only mildly elevated. Liver biopsy is rarely needed for diagnosis but reveals cholestasis with minimal hepatocellular necrosis.

Treatment

Medical treatment is directed at relieving maternal symptoms and improving fetal outcome. Pruritus can be controlled with antihistamines and ursodeoxycholic acid.

More severe cases may require bile salt binders such as cholestyramine or corticosteroids. Fetal outcome is improved with early diagnosis and prompt treatment.

The most successful therapy for cholestasis of pregnancy has been ursodeoxycholic acid. Ursodeoxycholic acid is a naturally occurring bile acid, which, when administered, relieves both pruritus and liver function abnormalities. When administered orally, it helps to dissolve cholesterol gallstones. Experimental evidence suggests that it protects hepatocytes and cholangiocytes from bile acid-induced cytotoxicity and improves hepatobiliary excretion. Additionally, it decreases bile salt transfer to the fetus and improves the secretory function of placental trophoblastic cells. Ursodeoxycholic acid is recycled through the enterohepatic circulation. Cholestyramine is another treatment option for cholestasis of pregnancy. It is an oral medication that binds bile salts in the intestine and promotes their excretion in the feces. As this drug is not absorbed, it most likely has little effect on the fetus. Effects on the fetus are still under evaluation. However, cholestyramine can interfere with the absorption of fat-soluble vitamins, such as vitamins A, D, E, and K. In rare cases, drug-induced vitamin K deficiency is believed to contribute to hemorrhaging during childbirth.

Prognosis

Long-term maternal outcome is good. Intense pruritus can cause severe fatigue and distress for the mother. Anorexia, nausea, vomiting, and poor weight gain can occur. The risk of postpartum cholelithiasis is increased, as is the risk of postpartum hemorrhage.

CLINICAL NOTE

Bile salts are produced in both the fetal and maternal liver. The fetus transfers the bile salts across the placenta for disposal.

CLINICAL PEARLS

1. Cholestasis of pregnancy is a condition in which the normal flow of bile from the gallbladder is impeded, leading to accumulation of bile salts in the body.
2. Possible causes include genetic abnormalities, increased hormonal exposure, decreased sulfotransferase activity, and endogenous opioids.
3. Generalized pruritus is the main symptom of intrahepatic cholestasis of pregnancy. The itching may be more intense over the palms and sole but can extend to the trunk, extremities, eyelids, and, in rare cases, the oral cavity.
4. The serum bilirubin level is usually lower than six times the upper limit of reference range and is usually conjugated; aminotransferase levels are less than 1,000 U/L, which distinguishes intrahepatic cholestasis (IHC) from viral hepatitis. Alkaline phosphatase is four times higher than the reference range (44–147 U/L) and gamma-glutamyl transpeptidase levels are within the reference range or only mildly elevated.
5. Medical treatment is directed at relieving maternal symptoms and improving fetal outcome. Pruritus can be controlled with antihistamines and ursodeoxycholic acid. More severe cases may require bile salt binders such as cholestyramine or corticosteroids.

CASE STUDY 8

Theme: Gallstones—Causes and Clinical Implications

A 44-year-old female presented to the clinic with concerns over occasional midepigastric discomfort and nausea/vomiting after eating "greasy meals". She reported that the symptoms gradually disappear with no lasting discomfort. She denied and hematemesis, but complained that the pain was worst after eating heavy food. She further mentioned that she had elevated cholesterol levels in the past and was on an exercise program, but not anymore.

On examination, she was afebrile with normal vital signs. Her physical examination was completely normal with no evidence of abdominal pain. An abdominal ultrasound was performed which revealed a few gallstones in the gallbladder but no thickening of the gallbladder wall.

What are gallstones made of?
What is the biochemical basis for the formation of gallstones?
What is the cause of pain in such patients?

CASE DISCUSSION

This patient fits the "classic" criteria of gallbladder disease: female, middle-aged, overweight. Gallstones are collections of solid material (predominantly crystals of cholesterol) in the gallbladder. The liver can secrete too much cholesterol, which precipitates from bile in the gallbladder. Gallstones sometimes cause upper abdominal pain that can last for hours. Ultrasonography is quite accurate in detecting gallstones. If gallstones cause recurrent pain or other problems, the gallbladder is removed.

CHOLELITHIASIS (GALLSTONES)

Incidence

Gallstones are more common in women than in men and increase in incidence in both sexes and all races with aging. In the United States, over 10% of men and 20% of women have gallstones by age 65 years; the total exceeds 20 million people. Although cholesterol gallstones are less common in black people, cholelithiasis attributable to hemolysis occurs in over a third of individuals with sickle cell anemia.

Risk Factors

Genetic mutations that predispose persons to gallstones have been identified. **Obesity** is a risk factor for gallstones, especially in women. **Rapid weight loss** also increases the risk of symptomatic gallstone formation. There is evidence that **glucose intolerance and elevated serum insulin levels (insulin resistance syndrome)** are risk factors for gallstones, and a **high intake of carbohydrate** and high-dietary glycemic load increase the risk of cholecystectomy in women. A low-carbohydrate diet and physical activity may help prevent gallstones. Consumption of caffeinated coffee appears to protect against gallstones in women, and a high intake of polyunsaturated and monounsaturated fats reduces the risk of gallstones in men on an energy-balanced diet. A high-fiber diet reduces the risk of cholecystectomy in women. **Hypertriglyceridemia** may promote gallstone formation by impairing gallbladder motility. The incidence of gallstones is high in individuals with Crohn's disease; approximately one-third of those with inflammatory involvement of the terminal ileum have gallstones due to disruption of bile salt resorption that results in decreased solubility of the bile. The incidence of cholelithiasis is also increased in patients with diabetes mellitus and the prevalence of gallbladder disease is increased in men (but not women) with **cirrhosis and hepatitis C virus infection.**

Pathophysiology

The gallstones are mainly of two types: (1) cholesterol and (2) pigmented stones.

1. **Cholesterol stones:** Eighty percent of gallstones are cholesterol stones, resulting from precipitation of cholesterol in gallbladder (cholelithiasis). Cholelithiasis is caused due to an imbalance between the ratios of cholesterol and cholesterol solubilizers in bile. Bile contains variable concentrations of cholesterol, bile acids/salts, bile pigments and phospholipids. Bile salts (ionized) and bile acids (neutral) maintain the solubility of cholesterol in the aquatic medium of bile and facilitate its excretion, therefore, the conditions causing elevation of cholesterol or lowering of bile acids/bile salts may result in cholelithiasis.

   Elevated cholesterol concentration can occur due to:
   - Increased activity of HMG-CoA reductase, the key regulatory enzyme of cholesterol biosynthetic pathway. This condition is typically observed in obesity.
   - Decreased activity of acyl-CoA:cholesterol acyltransferase (ACAT), the enzyme that catalyzes intercellular esterification of cholesterol.
   - Decreased activity of 7α-hydroxylase, the first and the rate-limiting enzyme of bile acid biosynthetic pathway. Cholesterol is oxidized to 7α-hydroxycholesterol by 7α-hydroxylase (CYP7A1), the mixed-function oxidase of the cytochrome P450 superfamily.
   - High level of deoxycholate, a secondary bile acid synthesized by intestinal bacteria action, can inhibit 7α-hydroxylase enzyme. Therefore, elevated levels of deoxycholate resulting from chronic exposure of bile acids to intestinal bacteria might cause elevated cholesterol levels in bile.

   In conditions, when the bile becomes supersaturated with cholesterol, the excess crystallizes forming solid particles, which eventually clump together and grow into gallstones.
2. **Pigmented stones:** These stones appear darker and are made up of bilirubin. The pigment stones are usually observed in chronic hemolytic anemias. Mixed stones (mixture of cholesterol and bilirubin) are also observed in certain clinical conditions. The gallstones may remain in gallbladder, pass into bile ducts, or may obstruct the flow of bile, either by obstructing the cystic duct, common bile duct, or ampulla of Vater. Bile duct strictures can also promote the blockage of ducts by stones. Stasis of bile due to obstruction can result in bacterial infections. Prolonged stasis of bile in gallbladder, as in pregnancy, can result in forming "biliary sludge", which is composed of cholesterol, calcium compounds, bilirubin and other similar substances. The biliary sludge resolves itself with the disappearance of primary cause; however, it can develop into gallstones, or obstruct the flow of bile by passing into the ducts.

Clinical Manifestations

The gallstones may remain silent for years together without causing any signs or symptoms. Approximately 80% of people with gallstones do not manifest any symptoms; however, gallstones may cause pain, which develops when the stones descend and obstruct the bile ducts. The dilatation of the gallbladder resulting from obstruction is the real cause of **"biliary colic".** The pain is typically experienced in the epigastrium or right hypochondrium. A heavy fatty meal can trigger the biliary colic which is accompanied by nausea or vomiting. Most of the episodes of biliary colic resolve spontaneously, and the patients remain asymptomatic between the episodes. The pain is felt each year in 20–40% of people.

Complications

1. **Persistent bile duct obstruction** can cause infection and inflammation of gallbladder.
2. **Acute cholangitis** manifested by fever, chills and jaundice, results from bacterial infection in the obstructed bile ducts. Acute cholangitis can even cause septicemia, or liver abscess.
3. **Pancreatitis:** The stones that obstruct the ampulla of Vater, can obstruct the pancreatic duct, causing **pancreatitis.**
4. **Perforation of the gallbladder:** The gallstones can erode the walls of the inflamed gallbladder resulting in perforation, which may progress to peritonitis due to leakage of gallbladder contents throughout the peritoneal cavity.
5. **Gallstone Ileus:** The intestinal obstruction resulting from a large stone is called gallstone ileus. This complication is mostly observed in elderly individuals.

Diagnosis

A provisional diagnosis can be made by the characteristic signs and symptoms. In asymptomatic individuals, gallstones may be detected as a chance finding when ultrasonography is conducted for some other clinical reasons. Ultrasonography is less accurate in detecting stones in bile ducts; however, it has 95% accuracy in diagnosing stones in the gallbladder. The dilatation of the ducts caused by obstruction can be diagnosed by ultrasonography. Other imaging techniques, such as magnetic resonance imaging (MRI) of the bile and pancreatic ducts, computed tomography (CT), and endoscopic retrograde cholangiopancreatography can help in the confirmation of the diagnosis.

Blood chemistry remains unaltered until the obstruction of the bile ducts. High serum bilirubin levels and alteration of liver enzymes are usually observed in "cholestasis" resulting from obstruction of the bile ducts.

Treatment

No treatment is required for silent gallstones. Conservative treatment is offered to treat pain and infections. The surgical removal of the gallbladder (cholecystectomy) is recommended in symptomatic gallbladder diseases. Laparoscopic cholecystectomy remains the treatment of choice. Bile salts, such as cheno-and ursodeoxycholic acids, when given orally for 2 years help in dissolving some cholesterol stones and may be considered in patients unfit for surgery.

Gallstones in the bile ducts: Stones in the bile ducts are removed during endoscopic retrograde cholangiopancreatography (ERCP).

Prognosis

Prognosis is good in the treated cases.

CLINICAL NOTE

Eating a heavy meal can trigger biliary colic, but simply eating fatty foods does not.

CLINICAL PEARLS

1. Gallstones are collections of solid material (predominantly crystals of cholesterol) in the gallbladder.
2. Gallstones sometimes cause upper abdominal pain that can last for hours.
3. Ultrasonography is quite accurate in detecting gallstones.
4. If gallstones cause recurrent pain or other problems, the gallbladder is removed.
5. Cheno- and ursodeoxycholic acids are bile salts that when given orally for up to 2 years dissolve some cholesterol stones and may be considered in occasional, selected patients who refuse cholecystectomy.

CASE STUDY 9

Theme: Clinical Implications of Impaired Cholesterol Uptake

A 48-year-old male presented to the clinic because of concerns about heart disease.

He reported that his father died from a heart attack at age of 46, and his older brother also had a heart attack at the same age but survived and was on medications for elevated cholesterol. The patient reported chest pain occasionally with ambulation and was not able to climb stairs without significant chest pain and shortness of breath.

The physical examination was normal, and the physician ordered an electrocardiogram (ECG), exercise stress test, and blood biochemistry tests. The patient's cholesterol was 350 mg/dL (normal 200).

The physician prescribed medication, which he stated was directed at the rate-limiting step of cholesterol biosynthesis.

What is the problem with the patient?
What is the rate-limiting step of cholesterol metabolism?
What is the class of medication prescribed?

CASE DETAILS

The patient is suffering from familial hypercholesterolemia.

FAMILIAL HYPERCHOLESTEROLEMIA

Familial hypercholesterolemia (FH) is an **autosomal dominant** disorder that causes severe elevations in total cholesterol and low-density lipoprotein cholesterol (LDL-C). Although moderate hypercholesterolemia is a common finding in industrialized countries, heterozygous FH occurs in approximately 1 per 500 persons worldwide.

Because FH is associated with a high risk for premature coronary artery disease (CAD), early detection and aggressive management to lower the LDL-C level helps prevent or slows the progression of coronary atherosclerosis. Moreover, if the first-degree relatives of a patient with FH are screened, other gene carriers can be identified and treated. Exercise, dietary adjustments, and weight loss are the initial therapy of hyperlipidemia. If these are not sufficient, then pharmacologic therapy is required.

BASIC CONCEPT

Cholesterol is present in tissues and in plasma either as free cholesterol or as a storage form, combined with a long-chain fatty acid as cholesteryl ester. In plasma, both forms are transported in lipoproteins. Cholesterol is an amphipathic lipid and as such is an essential structural component of membranes and of the outer layer of plasma lipoproteins. It is synthesized in many tissues from acetyl-CoA and is the precursor of all other steroids in the body, including corticosteroids, sex hormones, bile acids, and vitamin D. As a typical product of animal metabolism, cholesterol occurs in foods of animal origin such as egg yolk, meat, liver, and brain. **Plasma low-density lipoprotein (LDL) is the vehicle of uptake of cholesterol and cholesteryl ester into many tissues. Free cholesterol is removed from tissues by plasma high-density lipoprotein (HDL), in the process known as reverse cholesterol transport,** and transported to the liver, where it is eliminated from the body either unchanged or after conversion to bile acids. Cholesterol is a major constituent of gallstones. However, its chief role in pathologic processes is as a factor in the genesis of atherosclerosis of vital arteries, causing cerebrovascular, coronary, and peripheral vascular disease.

The normal range for total plasma cholesterol in humans is considered to be <5.2 mmol/L, with the greater part found in the esterified form. Cholesterol is transported in plasma in lipoproteins, and in humans the highest proportion is found in low-density lipoprotein (LDL). Dietary cholesterol equilibrates with plasma cholesterol in days and with tissue cholesterol in weeks. Cholesteryl ester in the diet is hydrolyzed to cholesterol, which is then absorbed by the intestine together with dietary unesterified cholesterol and other lipids. With cholesterol synthesized in the intestines, it is then incorporated into chylomicrons. **Of the cholesterol absorbed, 80–90% is esterified with long-chain fatty acids in the intestinal mucosa.** Ninety-five percent of the chylomicron cholesterol is delivered to the liver in chylomicron remnants, and most of the cholesterol secreted by the liver in VLDL is retained during the formation of IDL and ultimately LDL, which is taken up by the LDL receptor in liver and extrahepatic tissues.

Uptake of LDL cholesterol: The LDLs (containing cholesteryl esters) are taken up by cells by a process known as receptor-mediated endocytosis. The LDL receptor mediates this endocytosis and is important to cholesterol metabolism. The LDL receptor gene is located on the short arm of chromosome 19, and the protein is composed of 860 amino acids. It is the primary determinant of hepatic LDL uptake, which normally processes approximately 70% of circulating LDL. **Two ligands on LDL bind to the receptor, apolipoprotein B-100 (apoB-100) and apoE and is, therefore, more accurately termed the B, E receptor.** ApoE is found on most lipoproteins other than LDL, including very low-density lipoprotein (VLDL) and chylomicrons and their remnants, intermediate-density lipoprotein (IDL), and a subclass of high-density lipoprotein (HDL). The LDL receptor binds apoE with higher affinity than apoB-100, and some mutations in the receptor may spare uptake of LDL by allowing binding to apoE.

After LDL binding to the LDL receptor, the ligand-receptor complexes cluster on the plasma membrane in coated pits, which then invaginate forming coated vesicles. These coated vesicles are internalized and clathrin, the protein composing the lattice in membrane coated pits, is removed. These vesicles are now called endosomes and these endosomes fuse with the lysosome. The LDL receptor-containing membrane buds off and is recycled to the plasma membrane. Fusion of the lysosome and endosome releases lysosomal proteases that degrade the apoproteins into amino acids. Lysosomal enzymes also hydrolyze the cholesteryl esters to free cholesterol and fatty acids. The free cholesterol is released into the cell's cytoplasm, and this free cholesterol is then available to be used by the cell. **Excess cholesterol is re-esterified by acyl-CoA:cholesterol acyltransferase (ACAT),** which uses fatty acyl-CoA as the source of activated fatty acid. Free cholesterol affects cholesterol metabolism by inhibiting cholesterol biosynthesis. Cholesterol inhibits the enzyme hydroxymethylglutaryl-CoA reductase (HMG-CoA reductase), which catalyzes an early rate-limiting step in cholesterol biosynthesis. **HMG-CoA reductase is the target of the statin drugs in wide use for treating patients with elevated cholesterol levels.** In addition, free cholesterol inhibits the synthesis of the LDL receptor, thus limiting the amount of LDLs that are taken up by the cell **(Fig. 4.12)**.

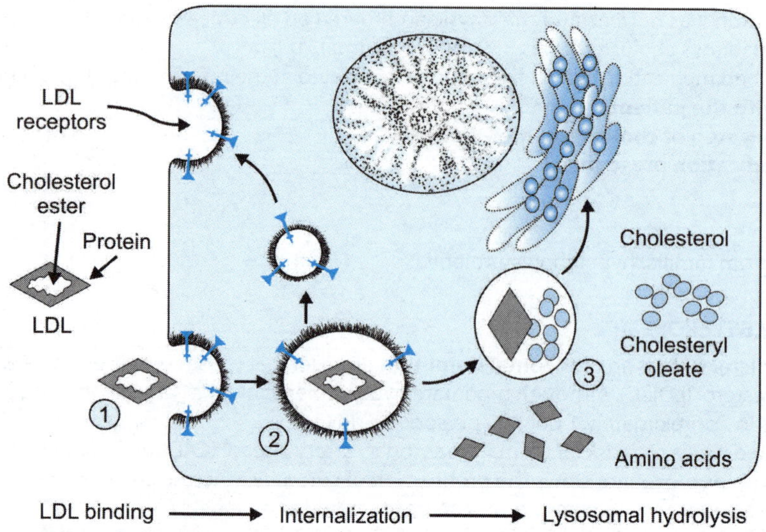

Fig. 4.12: Receptor-mediated endocytosis of LDL cholesterol.

Pathophysiology of Familial Hypercholesterolemia

Familial hypercholesterolemia (FH) is a disorder of absent or grossly malfunctioning low-density lipoprotein (LDL) receptors. LDL receptor function ranges from completely absent to approximately 25% of normal receptor activity.

Although more than 700 mutations have been described but three types of mutations are of prime importance.

- In the first type, the LDL receptor is not produced.
- The second type is a result of a mutation in the terminal region of the receptor that results in an LDL receptor unable to bind LDL.
- The third type is caused by a mutation in the C-terminal region that prevents the LDL-receptor complex from undergoing endocytosis.

In the absence of a functioning LDL receptor, LDL cholesterol levels are greatly elevated in individuals with this disease.

Also, when LDL is not internalized by hepatocytes, hepatic synthesis of cholesterol is not suppressed. This leads to further cholesterol production despite high levels of circulating cholesterol. Therefore, circulating cholesterol levels are increased dramatically. **The total and LDL-C levels of infants and children with homozygous FH are higher than 600 mg/dL.** In patients with heterozygous FH, half the LDL receptors are normal and half are rendered ineffective by the mutation. These patients' total cholesterol and LDL-C levels are twice as high as the population average. LDL-C levels of 200–400 mg/dL are common.

High levels of LDL-C increase cholesterol uptake in nonhepatic cells that is independent of LDL receptors. These scavenger pathways allow cholesterol uptake by monocytes and macrophages, leading to foam cell formation, plaque deposition in the endothelium of coronary arteries, and premature CAD. Cholesterol also accumulates in other areas, particularly the skin, causing xanthelasmas and a variety of xanthomas. Early corneal arcus is frequent, and, in patients with the homozygous condition, valvular abnormalities, most frequently aortic stenosis, are common secondary to the deposition of cholesterol.

Genetic defects in apoprotein B-100, the protein in the LDL recognized by the LDL receptor, also exist and lead to elevated LDL because the LDL complex is not recognized by the LDL receptor (familial ligand-defective apoB-100).

Frequency

- The global prevalence of familial hypercholesterolemia is about 10 million people.
- Heterozygous familial hypercholesterolemia occurs in about 1:500 people
- Homozygous familial hypercholesterolemia occurs in about 1:1,000,000 people.

Clinical Manifestations

Homozygous FH

- The children with severe hypercholesterolemia present with symptoms of ischemic heart disease, peripheral vascular disease, cerebrovascular disease, or aortic stenosis. The additional symptoms such as tendonitis, arthralgias and cutaneous xanthomas may also be present.
- The xanthomas appear in the first decade of life. The planar xanthomas are earlier to appear and are diagnostic of homozygous state. The other xanthomas such as tuberous or tendon appear late in life.
- The children may present with a circumferential corneal arcus which is otherwise an unusual finding, this observation, therefore, should raise an alarm for a complete laboratory workup.

Heterozygous FH

- The children with heterozygous FH do not develop symptoms of CHD. However, the symptoms are commonly observed in adults, even the first-degree relatives may also present with severe hypercholesterolemia and premature IHD.
- The implications of severe hypercholesterolemia are delayed in women until menopause due to protective effects of female sex hormones.
- Xanthomas and corneal arcus are rare findings in children.
- The tendon xanthomas may appear by the third decade of life in more than 60% of untreated patients.

Laboratory Investigations

- **Lipid profile**
  - In children and adults with homozygous FH, severe hypercholesterolemia (total cholesterol >600 mg/dL) with normal triglyceride levels are diagnostic.
  - In adults, LDL-C levels higher than 290–300 mg/dL are diagnostic of heterozygous FH.
  - In children, LDL-C levels higher than 200 mg/dL are diagnostic of heterozygous FH.
  - Lipoprotein(a) levels help to determine prognosis. The levels of lipoprotein(a) >30 mg/dL are suggestive of worst prognosis in patients with heterozygous FH.
- Additional tests to rule out secondary hypercholesterolemia can also be carried out.

Treatment

Treatment for Homozygous FH

General recommendations

Lifestyle changes

- Balanced diet, regular physical exercise and maintenance of body weight are strongly encouraged.
- In patients with moderate degree of hypercholesterolemia, dietary modifications, high doses of HMG-CoA reductase inhibitors, bile acid sequestrants, ezetimibe, and niacin can be effective.
- In postmenopausal women, hormone replacement therapy (HRT) can be recommended; however, it may be contraindicated in older women because of its adverse side effects.

LDL apheresis

LDL apheresis involves selective extraction of apoB containing lipoproteins. This technique effectively lowers lipoprotein(a), VLDL, triglycerides and more than 50% of LDL levels. HDL levels remain unaffected. This is an extremely expensive procedure, applied only in patients with absent or nonfunctional LDL receptors.

Other treatments for homozygous FH

- Probucol is recommended to cause regression of cutaneous and tendon xanthomas.
- Gene therapy is still under trial.
- Liver transplantation and ileal bypass surgery are undertaken in patients with severe familial hypercholesterolemia.

Treatment for Heterozygous FH

In patients with heterozygous FH, lifestyle modifications are although recommended but they are less likely to cause desirable LDL-C levels; therefore, cholesterol-lowering drugs (usually more than one) are prescribed.

Recommendations

- The diet should be low in saturated fats, trans fats, and cholesterol.
- Weight reduction is highly encouraged in obese patients to improve all lipid parameters.
- Physical exercise improves blood lipid levels if performed for longer than 30 minutes, 4 or more days per week.
- Heterozygous FH patients with 50% functional LDL receptors can be treated with usual cholesterol-lowering drugs, but treatment still remains difficult.
- In order to achieve the desired LDL-C levels, a high dose of one of the three HMG-CoA reductase inhibitors (statins), simvastatin, atorvastatin, or rosuvastatin, and one or more other LDL-lowering drugs, bile acid sequestrants, ezetimibe, or niacin, is recommended. Fibrates are ineffective unless triglyceride levels are elevated.
- Hormone replacement therapy helps in lowering LDL-C levels in postmenopausal women but this therapy is avoided in older women because of its adverse effects, although the benefits may sometimes outweigh risks.
- In patients with CHD whose LDL-C levels cannot be reduced below 200 mg/dL by conventional therapy, LDL apheresis can be undertaken.

Prevention

- In carriers of FH, early diagnosis and treatment can prevent the risk of CAD.
- In addition to treating hypercholesterolemia, cardiovascular risk factors should be identified and treated aggressively.

Prognosis

- Prognosis depends on the extent to which LDL-C levels are lowered.
- Majority of the patients with homozygous FH survive only up to the age of 30 years, unless treated with unconventional methods.
- Treatment of other modifiable risk factors such as smoking, hypertension, and diabetes further decreases the risk of CAD.

CLINICAL NOTE

An LDL-C level higher than 200 mg/dL in a patient younger than 20 years is highly suggestive of heterozygous FH.

CLINICAL PEARLS

1. Familial hypercholesterolemia (FH) is an autosomal dominant disorder that causes severe elevations in total cholesterol and low-density lipoprotein cholesterol (LDL-C).
2. Familial hypercholesterolemia is a disorder of absent or grossly malfunctioning low-density lipoprotein (LDL) receptors. LDL receptor function ranges from completely absent to approximately 25% of normal receptor activity.
3. Homozygous children may have symptoms consistent with ischemic heart disease, peripheral vascular disease, cerebrovascular disease, or aortic stenosis.
4. Healthy diet, regular exercise, and maintenance of desirable weight along with pharmacological intervention are required for treating hypercholesterolemia.
5. Prognosis depends on the extent to which LDL-C levels can be reduced. Patients with homozygous FH have extremely limited life expectancy without major medical intervention.

CASE STUDY 10

Theme: Regulation of Cholesterol Biosynthesis and Management of Hyperlipidemia

A 45-year-old man presented to the emergency center with chest pain. The chest pain lasted for approximately 15 minutes then subsided on its own. He also noticed that he was nauseated and was sweating during the pain episode. He had no medical problems and had not been to a physician for several years.

On examination, he was in no acute distress with normal vital signs. His lungs were clear to auscultation bilaterally, and his heart had a regular rate and rhythm with no murmurs. An electrocardiogram (ECG) revealed slight ischemic changes. The blood biochemistry revealed raised serum total cholesterol and LDL cholesterol levels. He was placed on a low-fat diet and lovastatin therapy.

He was without complaints and was feeling well on his subsequent follow-up visit. On repeat serum cholesterol screening, a decrease in the cholesterol level was noted.

What is the mechanism of action of this drug?
What are the potential side effects?
What are the alternative options to treat this patient?

CASE DETAILS

The patients had an episode of IHD (ischemic heart disease), and had hyperlipidemia.

HYPERLIPIDEMIA

Hyperlipidemia is one of the most treatable risk factors of coronary heart disease. Initially, when the fasting low-density lipoprotein (LDL) cholesterol is measured and is found to be elevated, lifestyle modification is recommended such as dietary adjustments, exercise, and weight loss. If the LDL cholesterol level is again found to be above threshold, then pharmacologic therapy is entertained. Since this patient had a mild attack of IHD, so without trial he had been put on low-fat diet and statins.

BASIC CONCEPT

A little more than half the cholesterol of the body arises by synthesis (about 700 mg/day), and the remainder is provided by the average diet. The liver and intestine account for approximately 10% each of total synthesis in humans. Virtually all tissues containing nucleated cells are capable of cholesterol synthesis, which occurs in the endoplasmic reticulum and the cytosol.

Biosynthesis of Cholesterol

The biosynthesis of cholesterol may be divided into five steps: (1) Synthesis of mevalonate from acetyl-CoA. (2) Formation of isoprenoid units from mevalonate by loss of CO_2. (3) Condensation of six isoprenoid units forms squalene. (4) Cyclization of squalene gives rise to the parent steroid, lanosterol. (5) Formation of cholesterol from lanosterol.

Regulation of Cholesterol synthesis

Regulation of cholesterol synthesis is exerted near the beginning of the pathway, at the HMG-CoA reductase step. HMG-CoA reductase in liver is inhibited by mevalonate, the immediate product of the pathway, and by cholesterol, the main product. Cholesterol and metabolites repress transcription of the HMG-CoA reductase via activation of a sterol regulatory element-binding protein (SREBP) transcription factor. SREBPs are a family of proteins that regulate the transcription of a range of genes involved in the cellular uptake and metabolism of cholesterol and other lipids. A diurnal variation occurs in both cholesterol synthesis and reductase activity. In addition to these mechanisms regulating the rate of protein synthesis, the enzyme activity is also modulated more rapidly by post-translational modification. Insulin or thyroid hormone increases HMG-CoA reductase activity, whereas glucagon or glucocorticoids decrease it. Activity is reversibly modified by phosphorylation-dephosphorylation mechanisms, some of which may be cAMP-dependent and therefore immediately responsive to glucagon. Attempts to lower plasma cholesterol in humans by reducing the amount of cholesterol in the diet produce variable results. Generally, a decrease of 100 mg in dietary cholesterol causes a decrease of approximately 0.13 mmol/L of serum.

Hypercholesterolemia and the Consequences

Atherosclerosis is characterized by the deposition of cholesterol and cholesteryl ester from the plasma lipoproteins into the artery wall. Diseases in which prolonged elevated levels of VLDL, IDL, chylomicron remnants, or LDL occur in the blood (e.g. diabetes mellitus, lipid nephrosis, hypothyroidism, and other conditions of hyperlipidemia) are often accompanied by premature or more severe atherosclerosis. There is also an inverse relationship between HDL (HDL2) concentrations and coronary heart disease, making the LDL:HDL cholesterol ratio a good predictive parameter. This is consistent with the function of HDL in reverse cholesterol transport.

Diet can Play an Important Role in Reducing Serum Cholesterol

Hereditary factors play the greatest role in determining individual serum cholesterol concentrations; however, dietary and environmental factors also play a part, and the most beneficial of these is the substitution in the diet of polyunsaturated and monounsaturated fatty acids for saturated fatty acids. Plant oils such as corn oil and sunflower seed oil contain a high proportion of polyunsaturated fatty acids, while olive oil contains a high concentration of monounsaturated fatty acids. On the other hand, butter fat, beef fat, and palm oil contain a high proportion of saturated fatty acids. Sucrose and fructose have a greater effect in raising blood lipids, particularly triacylglycerols, than do other carbohydrates.

The reason for the cholesterol-lowering effect of polyunsaturated fatty acids is still not fully understood. It is clear, however, that one of the mechanisms involved is the upregulation of LDL receptors by poly- and monounsaturated as compared with saturated fatty acids, causing an increase in the catabolic rate of LDL, the main atherogenic lipoprotein. In addition, saturated fatty acids cause the formation of smaller VLDL particles that contain relatively more cholesterol, and they are utilized by extrahepatic tissues at a slower rate than are larger particles—tendencies that may be regarded as atherogenic.

Lifestyle and the Serum Cholesterol Level

Additional factors considered to play a part in coronary heart disease include high blood pressure, smoking, male gender, obesity (particularly abdominal obesity), lack of exercise, and drinking soft as opposed to hard water. Premenopausal women appear to be protected against many of these deleterious factors, and this is thought to be related to the beneficial effects of estrogen. There is an association between moderate alcohol consumption and a lower incidence of coronary heart disease. This may be due to elevation of HDL concentrations resulting from increased synthesis of apoA-I and changes in activity of cholesteryl ester transfer protein. It has been claimed that red wine is particularly beneficial, perhaps because of its content of antioxidants. Regular exercise lowers plasma LDL but raises HDL. Triacylglycerol concentrations are also reduced, due most likely to increased insulin sensitivity, which enhances the expression of lipoprotein lipase.

HYPOLIPIDEMIC DRUGS

When diet changes fail, hypolipidemic drugs are prescribed to reduce serum cholesterol and triacylglycerol levels. Few of the commonly used drugs to lower cholesterol level are as follows:

Statins (Lovastatin)

A family of drugs, known as statins, has proved highly efficacious in lowering plasma cholesterol and preventing heart disease .

- **Mechanism of action of drug:** Lovastatin is a member of a class of drugs (atorvastatin, fluvastatin, pravastatin and simvastatin are others in this class) called statins that are used to treat hypercholesterolemia. The statins act as competitive inhibitors of the enzyme HMG-CoA reductase.
  3-hydroxy-3-methylglutaryl CoA + 2NADPH + 2H+ Mevalonate + 2NADP+ + CoA-SH
  These molecules mimic the structure of the normal substrate of the enzyme (HMG-CoA) and act as transition state analogs. While the statins are bound to the enzyme, HMG-CoA cannot be converted to mevalonic acid, thus inhibiting the whole cholesterol biosynthetic process. Effective treatment with lovastatin, along with low-fat diet, decreases levels of blood cholesterol. The lowering of cholesterol also lowers the amounts of the lipoproteins that transport cholesterol to peripheral tissues, i.e. low-density lipoproteins (LDLs).

  Side effects of therapy: The potential side effects include elevated liver function tests, increased muscle creatine phosphokinase (CPK) secondary to myopathy and rarely rhabdomyolysis.

  Alternative treatment options: Other agents that may be considered include bile acid sequestrants, niacin, fibric acid, and fish oils.
- **Niacin** is a vitamin that is used in high doses to treat hypercholesterolemia. Niacin acts to decrease VLDL and LDL plasma levels. Its mechanism of action is not clearly understood but probably involves inhibition of VLDL secretion, which in turn decreases the production of LDL. Niacin inhibits the release of free fatty acids from adipose tissue which leads to a decrease of free fatty acids entering the liver and decreased VLDL synthesis in the liver. This decreases the availability of VLDL for conversion to LDL (containing cholesterol esters). Niacin also increases high-density lipoprotein (HDL) (the "good cholesterol") by an unknown mechanism.
- **Fibrates** such as clofibrate and gemfibrozil act mainly to lower plasma triacylglycerols by decreasing the secretion of triacylglycerol and cholesterol-containing VLDL by the liver.
- **Ezetimibe**—a new drug, ezetimibe, which reduces blood cholesterol levels by inhibiting the absorption of cholesterol by the intestine, has recently been introduced. Ezetimibe belongs to the azetidinone class of cholesterol absorption inhibitors.
- **Bile acid sequestrants (resins)**—bile acid sequestrants bind bile acids in the intestine and promote their excretion in the stool. To maintain the bile acid pool size, the liver diverts cholesterol to bile acid synthesis. The decreased hepatic intracellular cholesterol content results in upregulation of the LDL receptor and enhanced LDL clearance from the plasma. Bile acid sequestrants, including cholestyramine, colestipol, and colesevelam.
- **Omega-3 fatty acids (fish oils)**—N-3 polyunsaturated fatty acids (n-3 PUFAs) are present in high concentration in fish and in flax seeds. The most widely used n-3 PUFAs for the treatment of hyperlipidemias are the two active molecules in fish oil: (1) eicosapentaenoic acid (EPA) and (2) decosahexaenoic acid (DHA). Fish oils can result in an increase in plasma LDL-C levels in some patients. Fish oil supplements can be used in combination with fibrates, niacin, or statins to treat hypertriglyceridemia. In general, fish oils are well tolerated and appear to be safe, at least at doses up to 3–4 g. A lower dose of omega-3 (about 1 g) has been associated with reduction in cardiovascular events in CHD patients and is used by some clinicians for this purpose.

Management of low HDL-C

Causes of low HDL levels:

- Severely reduced plasma levels of HDL-C (<20 mg/dL) accompanied by triglycerides <400 mg/dL usually indicate the presence of a genetic disorder, such as a mutation in apoA-I, LCAT deficiency, or Tangier disease.
- HDL-C levels <20 mg/dL are common in the setting of severe hypertriglyceridemia, in which case the primary focus should be on the management of the triglycerides.
- HDL-C levels <20 mg/dL also occur in individuals using anabolic steroids.
- Secondary causes of more moderate reductions in plasma HDL (20–40 mg/dL) should be considered like smoking, diabetes mellitus type 2, Gaucher's disease, and malnutrition.

Management

Smoking should be discontinued, obese persons should be encouraged to lose weight, sedentary persons should be encouraged to exercise, and diabetes should be optimally controlled. When possible, medications associated with reduced plasma levels of HDL-C should be discontinued. The presence of an isolated low plasma level of HDL-C in a patient with a borderline plasma level of LDL-C should prompt consideration of LDL-lowering drug therapy in high-risk individuals. Statins increase plasma levels of HDL-C only modestly (~5–10%). Fibrates also have only a modest effect on plasma HDL-C levels (increasing levels ~5–15%), except in patients with coexisting hypertriglyceridemia, where they can be more effective. Niacin is the most effective available HDL-C-raising therapeutic agent and can be associated with increases in plasma HDL-C by up to approximately 30%, although some patients do not respond to niacin therapy.

CLINICAL NOTE

Generally, a decrease of 100 mg in dietary cholesterol causes a decrease of approximately 0.13 mmol/L of serum.

CLINICAL PEARLS

1. Regulation of cholesterol synthesis is exerted near the beginning of the pathway, at the HMG-CoA reductase step.
2. The statins act as competitive inhibitors of the enzyme HMG-CoA reductase.
3. Niacin inhibits the release of free fatty acids from adipose tissue which leads to a decrease of free fatty acids entering the liver and decreased VLDL synthesis in the liver.
4. Fibrates such as clofibrate and gemfibrozil act mainly to lower plasma triacylglycerols by decreasing the secretion of triacylglycerol and cholesterol-containing VLDL by the liver.
5. Bile acid sequestrants bind bile acids in the intestine and promote their excretion in the stool. To maintain the bile acid pool size, the liver diverts cholesterol to bile acid synthesis.

CASE STUDY 11

Theme: Metabolism of Lipoproteins and Hyperlipoproteinemia

Two sisters, aged 19 and 17 years, were referred to the dermatologist because they had large number of yellowish spots on the exposed parts of the body.

What is the cause of yellow spots?
How are the medical advices going to help these patients?

CASE DETAILS

Both the sisters are having xanthomas, xanthomas are lesions characterized by accumulations of lipid-laden macrophages. Xanthomas can develop in the setting of altered systemic lipid metabolism or as a result of local cell dysfunction. Most of the disorders of hyperlipidemias are associated with xanthomas.

XANTHOMAS

Pathophysiology

Altered Lipoprotein Metabolism (Hyperlipoproteinemia)

Lipoproteins: Lipids are insoluble in water; therefore, they are transported as complexes of lipoproteins with specific apoproteins. These proteins also serve as ligands to specific receptors, they facilitate transmembrane transport, and they regulate enzymatic activities. Lipoproteins may be classified according to their density, as follows: chylomicrons, very low-density lipoproteins (VLDLs), intermediate-density lipoproteins (IDLs), low-density lipoproteins (LDLs), and high-density lipoproteins (HDLs). Lipoproteins may also be separated by electrophoresis into beta (LDL), prebeta (VLDL), and alpha (HDL) lipoproteins. Beta-VLDL (IDL) can be determined by ultracentrifugation and electrophoresis.

Metabolism of Lipoproteins

The triglycerides of VLDL (the lipoproteins secreted by the liver) and the chylomicrons (secreted by the intestinal cells) are hydrolyzed by the action of lipoprotein lipase (LPL). The lipoprotein lipase is present anchored to the endothelial lining of the blood vessels by the negatively charged heparan sulfate. It is found in the adipose tissue, skeletal muscle, lung, spleen, renal medulla, aorta, and lactating mammary glands. Lipoprotein lipase requires phospholipids and apoC-II as cofactors for its activations, whereas its activity is inhibited by apoA-II and apoC-III. Its activity is increased by insulin in adipose tissue.

The hydrolysis of triglycerides by LPL proceeds through stages forming diacylglycerol, monoacylglycerol and finally free fatty acids and glycerol. The released free fatty acids are mainly transported into the tissues; however, some of them bind with albumin and return to the circulation. The glycerol component of the triglycerides is mobilized to liver and utilized, either as a source of energy or substrate for gluconeogenesis. The action of lipoprotein lipase, extracting approximately 90% of the triacylglycerol of chylomicrons and VLDL, results in the formation of chylomicron and VLDL remnants or IDL (intermediate-density lipoprotein). The chylomicron and VLDL remnants can be taken up by the liver through specialized receptors. IDL that contains apoproteins B-100 and E can be taken up either by the liver through LDL receptor, or be converted to the cholesterol-rich LDL that contains apoprotein B-100. LDL can be removed from the circulation either through hepatic or extrahepatic LDL receptors. HDL particles interact with other lipoproteins for the exchange of cholesterol and triglycerides. The HDL particles extract cholesterol from peripheral cells and transport it back to liver for degradation (reverse cholesterol transport). The extraction of cholesterol is mediated by the action of LCAT (lecithin-cholesterol acyltransferase).

Lipoprotein(a) [Lp(a)], another lipoprotein, that contains an apoprotein B, and a side chain of highly glycosylated protein, is both atherogenic and thrombogenic because of its structural homology with LDL and plasminogen.

Hyperlipoproteinemia

Depending upon the cause, hyperlipoproteinemia may be primary or secondary. Primary hyperlipoproteinemias are inherited disorders, caused due to defective apoprotein synthesis resulting from mutated genes; whereas secondary hyperlipoproteinemias result from metabolic alterations of other systemic diseases such as diabetes mellitus, hypothyroidism, or nephrotic syndrome.

Fredrickson's classification of Primary Hyperlipoproteinemia

Conventionally, five types of hyperlipidemias, based on the electrophoretic patterns of elevated lipoproteins, have been described by Fredrickson:

1. **Type I hyperlipidemia (familial lipoprotein lipase deficiency):** Type I hyperlipidemia is characterized by excessive accumulation of chylomicrons in the plasma (chylomicronemia). It results from primary deficiency of lipoprotein lipase. The onset of the disease occurs in early childhood, often with symptoms of acute pancreatitis. "Eruptive xanthomas" are characteristically present in this disorder. This defect is associated with severe hypertriglyceridemia, but the serum total cholesterol levels are usually normal.
2. **Type II hyperlipidemia (familial hypercholesterolemia):** There are two variants of this disorder.
   Type IIa pattern of hyperlipidemia results from primary LDL receptor deficiency or defective apoB-100 protein. In this disorder, plasma cholesterol levels are severely elevated, but plasma triglyceride levels are typically normal. The delivery of cholesterol to cells is mediated by LDL that binds to specific LDL receptors through its apoB-100 protein. Defective apoB-100 or LDL receptor deficiency results in the accumulation of LDL in the plasm, characterized by severe hypercholesterolemia. Patients with type IIa present with severe atherosclerosis and tendinous or tuberous xanthomas as well as xanthelasmas.
   Type IIb pattern of hyperlipidemia is manifested in adults by *tendinous or tuberous xanthomas as well as xanthelasmas*. **The underlying defect is not known, but the disorder is characterized by** familial combined hyperlipidemia. The levels of both LDL and VLDL are elevated, and some variations in the levels of serum total cholesterol and triglyceride levels are also observed.
3. **Type III hyperlipidemia:** Type III hyperlipidemia is characterized by the accumulation of IDL (beta-VLDL), which is manifested by increases in both triglyceride levels and cholesterol levels in the plasma. A genetic basis for the primary disorder, familial dysbetalipoproteinemia, has been well established. Various mutations of apoprotein E impair its ability to bind to the IDL receptor. Patients with type III present as adults with premature atherosclerosis and xanthomas, particularly plane (palmar) xanthomas.
4. **Type IV hyperlipidemia:** Familial hypertriglyceridemia is an example of a primary defect resulting in type IV hyperlipidemia. Accumulation of VLDL causes severe elevations of plasma triglyceride levels. Plasma cholesterol levels are typically normal. A definitive molecular defect has not been established. Patients with type IV may present with *eruptive xanthomas*. This type of pattern is commonly associated with coronary heart disease, type II diabetes mellitus, obesity, alcoholism, and administration of progestational hormones.
5. **Type V hyperlipidemia:** Genetic defects of the apolipoprotein C-II gene result in the accumulation of chylomicrons and VLDL, which is the type V pattern of hyperlipidemia. Patients with this type have severe elevations of triglyceride levels in the plasma. These patients, like those with lipoprotein lipase deficiency, may present in early childhood with acute pancreatitis and eruptive xanthomas.
6. Decreased synthesis of HDL due to decreased formation of apoprotein A-I and apoprotein C-III leads to decreased reversed cholesterol transport, resulting in increased LDL levels, premature coronary artery disease, and plane xanthomas.
7. **Hepatic lipase deficiency:** Deficiency of the enzyme leads to accumulation of large triacylglycerol-rich HDL and VLDL remnants. Patients have xanthomas and coronary heart disease.

Secondary Hyperlipidemia

Hyperlipidemia is also related to a variety of secondary causes. Secondary hypercholesterolemia can be found in pregnancy, hypothyroidism, cholestasis, and acute intermittent porphyria. Secondary hypertriglyceridemia can be associated with oral contraceptive use, diabetes mellitus, alcoholism, pancreatitis, gout, sepsis due to Gram-negative bacterial organisms, and type I glycogen storage disease. Combined hypercholesterolemia and hypertriglyceridemia can be found in nephrotic syndrome, chronic renal failure, and steroid immunosuppressive therapy.

Incidence of Xanthomas

Equal prevalence is reported in males and females. Xanthomas can occur in persons of any age. Xanthelasmas usually occur in people older than 50 years. Xanthomas are a common manifestation of lipid metabolism disorders.

Clinical Manifestations

Hyperlipidemia are usually associated with "Cutaneous xanthomas" which can be clinically subclassified as follows:

- **Xanthelasma palpebrarum** is the most common, usually asymptomatic, bilateral and symmetric. The lesions are found around the eyelids as soft, flat, polygonal, yellow velvety patches. They may be associated with any type of primary or secondary hyperlipidemia.

- **Tuberous xanthomas** are found in or around the pressure areas, such as the extensor surfaces of the knees, elbows, and the buttocks **(Figs. 4.13A and B)**. They appear as painless, firm, red- or yellow-colored nodules which may coalesce to form multilobed tumors. Tuberous xanthomas are associated with hypercholesterolemia and elevated LDL levels. They are commonly observed in patients with familial dysbetalipoproteinemia and familial hypercholesterolemia. They may also be present in some of the secondary hyperlipidemias (e.g. nephrotic syndrome or hypothyroidism).
- **Tendinous xanthomas** are found as slow growing subcutaneous nodules on the ligaments and extensor tendons of hands and feet. The lesions usually develop after a trauma and are associated with severe hypercholesterolemia and elevated LDL levels. They are typically found in type IIa hyperlipidemia but can also be associated with secondary hyperlipidemia.

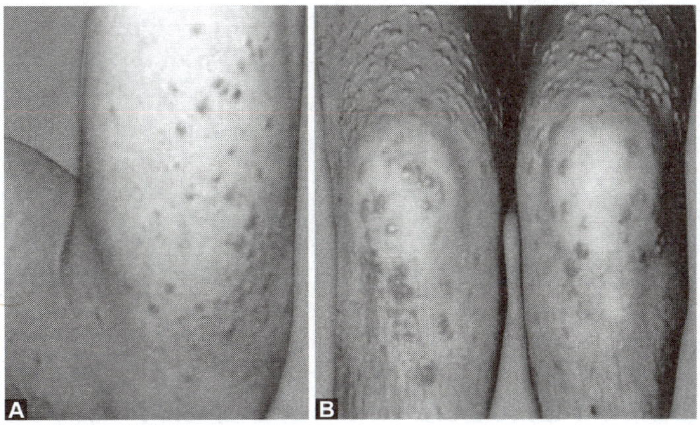

Figs. 4.13A and B: Tuberous xanthomas.

- **Eruptive xanthomas** appear as tiny, red-yellow papules on an erythematous base. They are commonly observed over the buttocks, shoulders, and the extensor surfaces of the extremities. Although they are self-resolving, yet they are commonly associated with primary hyperlipidemia (type I, IV, and V) or some of the secondary hyperlipidemia especially in diabetes mellitus.
- **Plane xanthomas** can be observed anywhere, generalized plane xanthomas are found covering the large areas of face, neck, and the thorax. They are usually associated with secondary hyperlipidemia (especially cholestasis), type III dysbetalipoproteinemia, monoclonal gammopathy, and hypertriglyceridemia.

Laboratory Investigations

Blood chemistry, complete urinalysis, and radiological investigations are undertaken to differentiate between primary and secondary hyperlipidemia; diagnosis of metabolic disorders, and to assess the cardiovascular risk.

Treatment

Xanthomas are not always associated with underlying hyperlipidemia, but when they are, diagnosing and treating underlying lipid disorders is necessary to decrease the size of the xanthomas and to prevent the risks of atherosclerosis. Treatment of the hyperlipidemia initially consists of diet and lipid-lowering agents such as statins, fibrates, bile acid-binding resins, probucol, or nicotinic acid. The lipid-lowering effects of these agents have been well documented, but few studies mention the efficacy of these drugs for resolving xanthomas. Eruptive xanthomas usually resolve within weeks of initiating systemic treatment and tuberous xanthomas usually resolve after months, but tendinous xanthomas take years to resolve or may persist indefinitely.

Prognosis

Prognosis is good if the underlying cause is treated.

CLINICAL NOTE

Xanthomas are not always associated with underlying hyperlipidemia, but when they are, diagnosing and treating underlying lipid disorders is necessary to decrease the size of the xanthomas and to prevent the risks of atherosclerosis.

CLINICAL PEARLS

1. Xanthomas are lesions characterized by accumulations of lipid-laden macrophages. Xanthomas are a common manifestation of lipid metabolism disorders.
2. Xanthomas can occur in persons of any age. Xanthelasmas usually occur in people older than 50 years.
3. Appropriate blood, urine, and radiographic workups are required to rule out a secondary cause of hyperlipidemia.
4. Xanthomas are not always associated with underlying hyperlipidemia, but when they are, diagnosing and treating underlying lipid disorders is necessary to decrease the size of the xanthomas and to prevent the risks of atherosclerosis.
5. Treatment of the hyperlipidemia initially consists of diet and lipid-lowering agents such as statins, fibrates, bile acid-binding resins, probucol, or nicotinic acid.

Chapter 5

Protein: Chemistry and Significance

LEARNING OBJECTIVES

To understand:

- Protein structure and function relationship
- Implications of protein misfolding
- Clinical significance of abnormal gamma-globulins
- Collagen structure
- Clinical implications of abnormal collagen structure
- Structure and significance of dystrophin protein
- Clinical significance of alpha-1-antitrypsin

CASE STUDIES

CASE STUDY 1

Theme: Clinical Implications of Protein Misfolding

An 80-year-old man presented with impairment of brain functions, alterations of mood and behavior.

His family reported that he was having progressive disorientation and memory loss over the past 6 months. He had trouble handling money and paying bills. He repeated questions, took longer to complete normal daily tasks, had poor judgment, and had developed mood and personality changes.

There was no family history of dementia.

The routine blood, urine and cerebrospinal fluid (CSF) analysis did not reveal much.

After a computerized tomography (CT) scan and the histopathological examination of the brain tissue, the patient was diagnosed to be having Alzheimer's disease.

What is the defect in this disease?

How is the diagnosis done and what is its prognosis?

CASE DISCUSSION

Alzheimer's disease.

BASIC CONCEPT

Alzheimer's disease (AD) is defined as **premature aging of the brain**, usually beginning in mid-adult life and progressing rapidly to extreme loss of mental powers—similar to those, seen in very, very old age.

Clinical Features

Alzheimer's disease is a progressive and fatal neurodegenerative disorder that results in impairment of a person's ability to perform routine activities and the patient finally enters into a vegetative state with no comprehension to the outside world. **The disease runs in four stages: (1) predementia, (2) mild dementia, (1) moderate dementia, and (1) advanced dementia.**

Although the course of Alzheimer's disease is unique for every individual, there are many common symptoms.

- The earliest observable symptoms are often mistakenly thought to be "age-related" concerns, or manifestations of stress. In the early stages, the most commonly recognized symptom is memory loss, such as difficulty in remembering recently learned facts.
- As the disease advances, symptoms include confusion, irritability and aggression, mood swings, language breakdown, long-term memory loss, and the general withdrawal of the sufferer as their senses decline.
- Gradually, bodily functions are lost, ultimately leading to death.

Incidence

Alzheimer's disease is the most common form of dementia in the elderly and about 5 million people in the United States are estimated to be afflicted by this disorder. The percentage of persons with Alzheimer's disease approximately doubles with every 5 years of age, with about 1% of 60-year-old and about 30% of 85-year-old having the disease.

Biochemical Defect

Alzheimer's disease has been identified as a protein misfolding disease, caused by accumulation of abnormally folded A-beta and tau proteins in the brain. Plaques are made-up of small peptides, 39 to 43 amino acids in length, called beta-amyloid (also written as A-beta or Aβ). Beta-amyloid is a fragment from a larger protein called amyloid precursor protein (APP), a transmembrane protein that penetrates through the neuron's membrane.

Amyloid precursor protein is critical to neuron growth, survival and postinjury repair.

In Alzheimer's disease, an unknown process causes APP to be divided into smaller fragments by enzymes through proteolysis. One of these fragments gives rise to fibrils of beta-amyloid, which form clumps that deposit outside neurons in dense formations known as senile plaques.

Alzheimer's disease is also considered a tauopathy due to abnormal aggregation of the tau protein. Every neuron has a cytoskeleton, an internal support structure partly made-up of structures called microtubules. These microtubules act like tracks, guiding nutrients and molecules from the body of the cell to the ends of the axon and back. A protein called tau stabilizes the microtubules when phosphorylated, and is therefore called a microtubule-associated protein. **In AD, tau undergoes chemical changes, becoming hyperphosphorylated; it then begins to pair with other threads, creating neurofibrillary tangles and disintegrating the neuron's transport system (Fig. 5.1).**

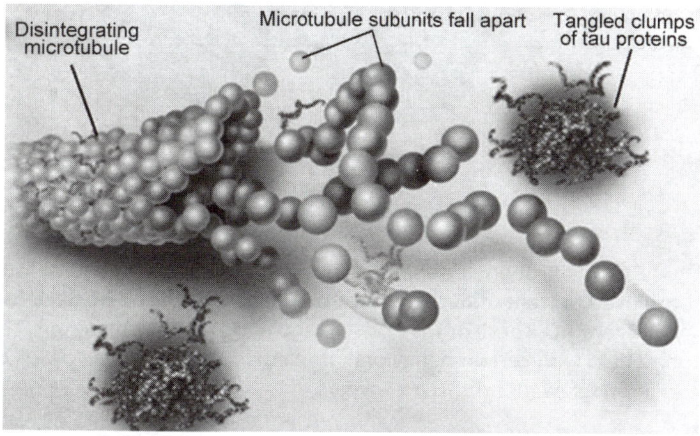

Fig. 5.1: Changes in tau protein lead to the disintegration of microtubules in brain cells of a patient suffering from Alzheimer's disease.

Alzheimer's disease is also associated with a decrease in the cerebral cortical levels of several proteins and neurotransmitters, especially acetylcholine; there is reduction in norepinephrine levels also in brainstem nuclei.

Apolipoprotein E4 (ApoE4) allele has a strong association with AD in the general population, ApoE is present in the neuritic amyloid plaques of AD, and it may also be involved in neurofibrillary tangle formation, because it binds to tau protein. Accumulation of aggregated amyloid fibrils, which are believed to be the toxic form of the protein responsible for disrupting the cell's calcium ion homeostasis, induces programmed cell death (apoptosis). Aβ selectively builds up in the mitochondria in the cells of Alzheimer's-affected brains, and it also inhibits certain enzyme functions and the utilization of glucose by neurons.

Inheritance

The vast majority of cases of Alzheimer's disease are **sporadic**, meaning that they are not genetically inherited although some genes may act as risk factors. On the other hand, around 0.1% of the cases are familial forms of autosomal-dominant inheritance, which usually have an onset before age 65.

The best known genetic risk factor is the inheritance of the ε4 allele of the apolipoprotein E (ApoE). Between 40% and 80% of patients with AD possess at least one ApoE4 allele. The ApoE4 allele increases the risk of the disease by 3 times in heterozygotes and by 15 times in homozygotes.

Diagnosis

Alzheimer's disease is usually diagnosed clinically from the patient's history, collateral history from relatives, and clinical observations, based on the presence of characteristic neurological and neuropsychological features and the absence of alternative conditions.

Assessment of intellectual functioning including memory testing can further characterize the state of the disease. Advanced medical imaging with computed tomography (CT) or magnetic resonance imaging (MRI), and with single-photon emission computed tomography (SPECT) or positron emission tomography (PET) can be used to help exclude other cerebral pathology or subtypes of dementia.

Alzheimer's disease is characterized by loss of neurons and synapses in the cerebral cortex and certain subcortical regions. This loss results in gross atrophy of the affected regions, including degeneration in the temporal lobe and parietal lobe, and parts of the frontal cortex and cingulate gyrus (Figs. 5.2A and B). Studies using MRI and PET have documented reductions in the size of specific brain regions in patients as they progressed from mild cognitive impairment to Alzheimer's disease, and in comparison with similar images from healthy older adults.

A histopathological confirmation including a microscopic examination of brain tissue is required for a definitive diagnosis. Both amyloid plaques and neurofibrillary tangles are clearly visible by microscopy in brains of those afflicted by AD.

Treatment

There is no cure for Alzheimer's disease; available treatments offer relatively small symptomatic benefit but remain palliative in nature. **Current treatments can be pharmaceutical, psychosocial and care giving.**

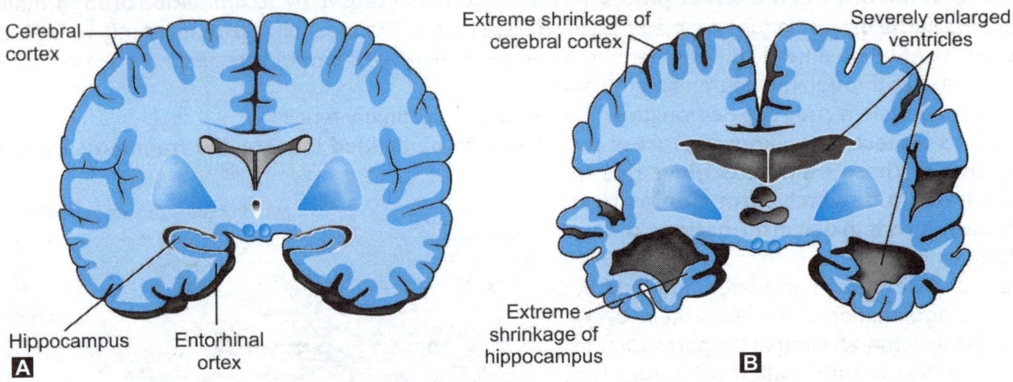

Figs. 5.2A and B: Comparison of a normal aged brain (A) and an Alzheimer's patient's brain (B).

Four medications are approved by the US Food and Drug Administration to treat AD. **Donepezil, rivastigmine, and galantamine are used to treat mild to moderate AD (Donepezil can be used for severe AD as well). Memantine is used to treat moderate to severe AD.** These drugs work by regulating neurotransmitters. They may help maintain thinking, memory, and speaking skills, and help with certain behavioral problems. However, these drugs do not change the underlying disease process and may help only for a few months to a few years.

Prognosis

Individual prognosis is difficult to assess, as the duration of the disease varies. AD develops for an indeterminate period of time before becoming fully apparent, and it can progress undiagnosed for years. The mean life expectancy following diagnosis is approximately 7 years. The earlier the age at onset the higher the total survival years, life expectancy is part, men have a less favorable survival prognosis than women.

CLINICAL NOTE

In the early stages of Alzheimer's disease, the most commonly recognized symptom is memory loss, such as difficulty in remembering recently learned facts.

CLINICAL PEARLS

1. Alzheimer's disease is a progressive and fatal neurodegenerative disorder that results in impairment of a person's ability to perform routine activities and the patient finally enters into a vegetative state with no comprehension to the outside world.
2. The disease runs in four stages: (1) predementia, (2) mild dementia, (3) moderate dementia, and (4) advanced dementia.
3. The disease has been identified as a protein misfolding disease, caused by accumulation of abnormally folded A-beta and tau proteins in the brain.
4. It is usually diagnosed clinically from the patient's history, collateral history from relatives, and clinical observations, based on the presence of characteristic neurological and neuropsychological features and the absence of alternative conditions.
5. Four medications are approved by the US Food and Drug Administration to treat AD. Donepezil, rivastigmine, and galantamine are used to treat mild to moderate AD (Donepezil can be used for severe AD as well).

CASE STUDY 2

Theme: Clinical Implications of Abnormal Gamma-globulins

A 45-year-old man presented with severe back pain and weakness. He had lost 8 kg weight in 3 months. There was apparent loss of appetite. History revealed that he suffered from facial palsy 2 months back for which he was taking treatment, but there was no visible improvement. There was no history of any fever or any illness. He reported that he was having constant body aches and was too tired to do the routine work.

The X-ray skull revealed punched out lesions. His bone marrow biopsy showed an excess of plasma cells. Serum electrophoresis showed an abnormal band between β-globulin and γ-globulins. Urine test for Bence Jones proteins was positive.

What is the probable diagnosis?

What are Bence Jones proteins?

CASE DISCUSSION

The patient is suffering from multiple myeloma.

Multiple myeloma represents a malignant proliferation of plasma cells derived from a single clone. The plasma cells in a normal individual are end-stage cells that secrete specific antibody for a few days and then die. In contrast, the plasma cells in an individual with multiple myeloma have escaped normal control over their life span and proliferation and are not end-stage cells; rather they divide over and over in an unregulated way without requiring any activation by any antigen to induce proliferation. Although such a plasma cell, called myeloma cell, has been transformed, its protein synthesizing machinery and secretory functions are not altered thus the cells continue to secrete specific antibodies. **The tumor, its products, and the host response to it result in a number of organ dysfunctions and symptoms of bone pain or fracture, renal failure, susceptibility to infection, anemia, hypercalcemia, and occasionally clotting abnormalities, neurological symptoms, and manifestations of hyperviscosity.**

Pathophysiology

Multiple myeloma can cause a wide variety of problems. The proliferation of plasma cells may interfere with the normal production of blood cells, resulting in leukopenia, anemia, and thrombocytopenia. The cells may cause soft tissue masses (plasmacytomas) or lytic lesions in the skeleton. Feared complications of multiple myeloma are bone pain, hypercalcemia, renal failure, and spinal cord compression. The aberrant antibodies that are produced lead to impaired humoral immunity, and patients have a high prevalence of infection, especially with encapsulated organisms such as *Pneumococcus*. The overproduction of these antibodies may lead to hyperviscosity, amyloidosis, and renal failure.

Incidence

About 19,900 cases of myeloma were diagnosed in 2007, and 10,790 people died from the disease in the United States. Myeloma increases in incidence with age. The median age at diagnosis is 68 years; it is uncommon under age 40.

Clinical Features

- **Bone pain** is the most common symptom in myeloma affecting nearly 70% of patients. The lumbar spine is one of the most common sites of pain.
- **Pathologic fractures** are very common in multiple myeloma; 93% of patients have more than one site of bony involvement. A severe bony event is a common presenting issue.
- **Spinal cord compression**—this complication occurs in approximately 10–20% of patients with multiple myeloma at sometime during the course of disease.

  The symptoms that should alert physicians to consider spinal cord compression are back pain, weakness, numbness, or dysesthesias in the extremities. It is common for spinal cord compressions in multiple myeloma to occur at multiple levels, so comprehensive evaluation of the spine is warranted.
- There is **increased susceptibility to bacterial infections.**
- **Renal failure** occurs in nearly 25% of patients, many factors contribute to this. **Hypercalcemia** is the most common cause of renal failure. Confusion, somnolence, bone pain, constipation, nausea, and thirst are the presenting symptoms of hypercalcemia.
- **Anemia** occurs in about 80% of patients. It is usually normocytic and normochromic and related both to the replacement of normal marrow by expanding tumor cells and to the inhibition of hematopoiesis by factors made by the tumor. In addition, mild hemolysis may contribute to the anemia. A larger than expected fraction of patients may have megaloblastic anemia due to either folate or vitamin B_{12} deficiency.
- **Clotting abnormalities** may be seen due to the failure of antibody-coated platelets to function properly. Occasionally, a patient may come to medical attention for bleeding resulting from thrombocytopenia.
- Besides these, **neurological symptoms** are also seen in some of the patients. Carpal tunnel syndrome is a common complication of myeloma. Meningitis (especially that resulting from pneumococcal or meningococcal infection) is more common in patients with multiple myeloma. Some peripheral neuropathies have been attributed to multiple myeloma.

- **Total Ig content may be very high but useful antibodies are low**, so the general immunity is low and the susceptibility to infections is increased. About 53% of cases have IgG and 25% have IgA paraproteins. However, IgD variety, comprising about 2% of myeloma have poor prognosis with survival only for about 1 year. Twenty percent of the patients have only light chain immunoglobulins in serum and urine. Abnormal humoral immunity and leukopenia may lead to infection.

Hyperviscosity

Due to high volume of monoclonal antibodies, serum viscosity rises in patients with multiple myeloma. The clinical symptoms appear when the serum viscosity rises 4 times of that of normal serum. The common symptoms include: headaches, somnolence, easy bruising, hazy vision, epistaxis, stroke, myocardial ischemia or infarction.

Physical Examination

- Pallor (due to anemia).
- Ecchymoses or purpura (due to thrombocytopenia).
- Bony tenderness (resulting from bone lesions or pathologic fracture).
- Pain without tenderness is a characteristic finding.
- Neurologic findings include: sensory deficit (loss of sensation below a dermatome corresponding to a spinal cord compression), weakness, or carpal tunnel syndrome.
- Extramedullary plasmacytomas consisting of soft tissue masses of plasma cells are found almost everywhere in the body.
- Amyloidosis may develop in some patients with multiple myeloma. Amyloidosis may also be associated with carpal tunnel syndrome and subcutaneous nodules. Macroglossia is a common finding in patients with amyloidosis **(Fig. 5.3)**.

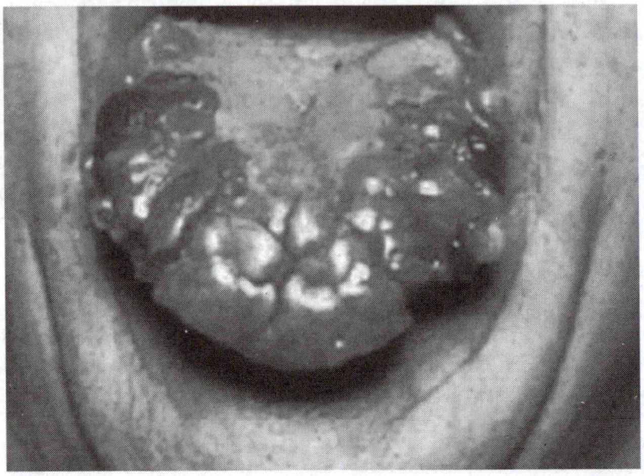

Fig. 5.3: Amyloidosis infiltrating the tongue in multiple myeloma (macroglossia).

Diagnosis

The classic triad of multiple myeloma is marrow plasmacytosis (>10%), lytic bone lesions, and a serum and/or urine M component. The confirmation of the diagnosis is done as follows:

1. Electrophoresis—the Igs of the same type (monoclonal antibodies) are produced in large amount. This is seen in electrophoresis as the myeloma band or M band with a sharp spike **(Fig. 5.4)**.
2. Bone marrow examination—reveals a large number of malignant plasma cells.
3. X-ray shows punched out lesions **(Fig. 5.5)**.
4. Hypercalcemia and hypercalciuria are present.
5. Proteinuria is essentially present. In 20–50% of patients of multiple myeloma, Bence Jones proteins are excreted in urine.
6. Beta-2-microglobulin—the level of beta-2-microglobulin is increased in patients with renal insufficiency without multiple myeloma, which is one reason that it is a useful prognosticator in multiple myeloma. The prognosis of patients with multiple myeloma and impaired renal function is reduced.
7. Histologic findings—in patients with multiple myeloma, plasma cells proliferate within the bone marrow.

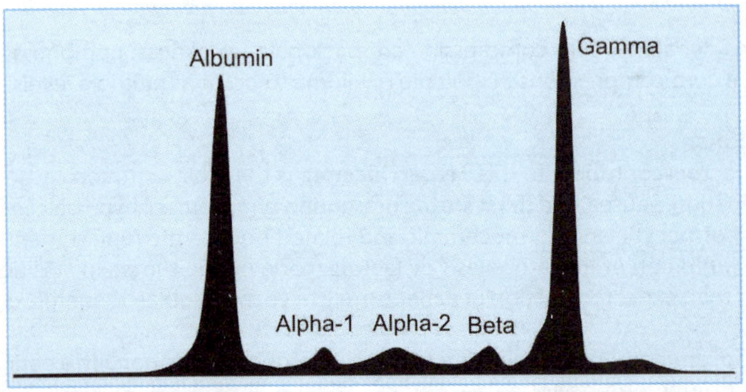

Fig. 5.4: Protein electrophoresis showing monoclonal gammopathy (paraprotein, M-peak) in a patient with multiple myeloma.

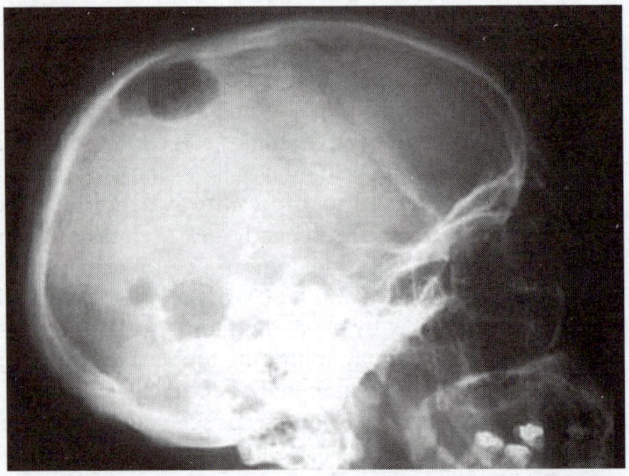

Fig. 5.5 Radiograph of skull showing punched out lesions.

Treatment

Chemotherapy and local irradiation is undertaken.

Prognosis

Prognosis is generally good, and average survival is more than 5 years. The major causes of death are progressive myeloma, renal failure, sepsis, or therapy-related acute leukemia. Nearly a quarter of patients die of myocardial infarction, chronic lung disease, diabetes, or stroke, all intercurrent illnesses related more to the age of the patient group than to the tumor.

IDENTIFICATION OF BENCE JONES PROTEINS

BENCE JONES PROTEINS

In most patients of multiple myeloma, the myeloma cells also secrete excessive amount of light chains of immunoglobulins. These excess light chains were first discovered in the urine of myeloma patients and were named **Bence Jones proteins on the name of their discoverer. These are either kappa (κ) or lambda (λ) light chains.** Sometimes, the chains are excreted in the form of a dimer of light chains. Normally, only very small amounts of "κ" or "λ" chains are excreted in urine. They pass through glomerular filter but are reabsorbed by kidney tubules and are degraded in the lining cells thus they do not appear in urine in normal health.

Heat Coagulation Test

The proteins are identified in the urine by a simple heat test. **On heating the urine to 50–60°C, the Bence Jones proteins are precipitated, but when heated further they are dissolved again. Reverse occurs on cooling.**

Electrophoresis

These are best detected by zone electrophoresis or immunoelectrophoresis.

CLINICAL NOTE

The classic triad of multiple myeloma is marrow plasmacytosis (>10%), lytic bone lesions, and a serum and/or urine M component.

CLINICAL PEARLS

1. Multiple myeloma represents a malignant proliferation of plasma cells derived from a single clone.
2. The tumor, its products, and the host response to it result in a number of organ dysfunctions and symptoms of bone pain or fracture, renal failure, susceptibility to infection, anemia, hypercalcemia, and occasionally clotting abnormalities, neurological symptoms, and manifestations of hyperviscosity.
3. The classic triad of multiple myeloma is marrow plasmacytosis (>10%), lytic bone lesions, and a serum and/or urine M component.
4. The confirmation is done by electrophoresis. This is seen in electrophoresis as the myeloma band or M band with a sharp spike.
5. Chemotherapy and local irradiation are undertaken as a part of treatment.

CASE STUDY 3

Theme: Clinical Significance of Disruption of Normal Collagen Structure

A 65-year-old man with a history of type 2 diabetes mellitus reported to the emergency complaining of severe pain and blackening of the right foot. He had an infected nonhealing ulcer on the same foot from the last 3 months, for which he was regularly taking treatment in the form of local dressings and antibiotic supplementations. History revealed that the patient met with a roadside accident a week back and ever since the condition of the foot worsened.

Culture of wound exudates, revealed the presence of *Clostridium perfringens*. A diagnosis of diabetic foot with gas gangrene was made and the patient was admitted for further treatment.

The highly pathogenic anaerobic bacterium *C. perfringens* is responsible for gas gangrene, a condition in which animal tissue structure is destroyed. This bacterium secretes an enzyme that efficiently catalyzes the hydrolysis of the peptide bond indicated.

$$—X\text{-Gly-Pro-Y}\xrightarrow{H_2O} \text{à } X\text{-}COO^- + H_2N\text{-Gly-Pro-Y-}$$

Where X and Y are any of the 20 standard amino acids.

How does the secretion of this enzyme contribute to the invasiveness of this bacterium in the human tissues?

Why does this enzyme not affect the bacterium itself?

CASE DISCUSSION

The structure shown below is that of collagen tissue, here X and Y are glycine and proline, which are the most abundant amino acids in collagen **(Fig. 5.6)**.

The bacterial enzyme (a collagenase) can destroy the connective tissue barrier of the host, allowing the bacterium to invade the host tissues. Bacteria themselves do not contain collagen, so they are not affected by the enzyme.

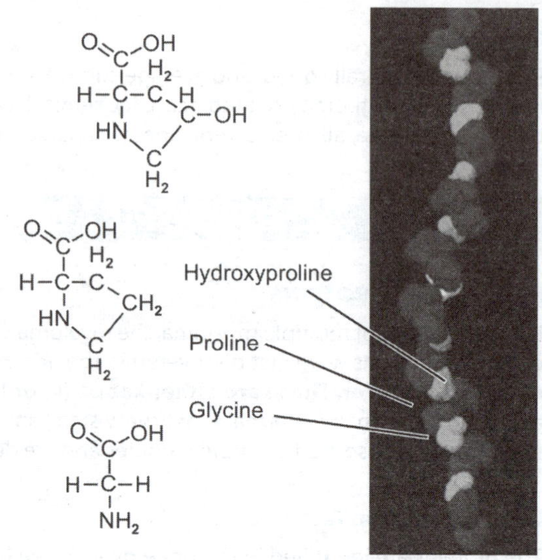

Fig. 5.6: Structure of collagen (triple-helical structure).

CASE DETAILS

Gangrene of Foot

Gangrene of the foot is a common complication of untreated diabetes mellitus.

Gangrene is a condition of decay and death of living tissues caused by **poor circulation** or invasion by pathogenic bacteria (through an open wound or sore).

The commonly affected areas are feet, toes, hands, and fingers **(Fig. 5.7)**; however, internal organs such as intestines can also get affected.

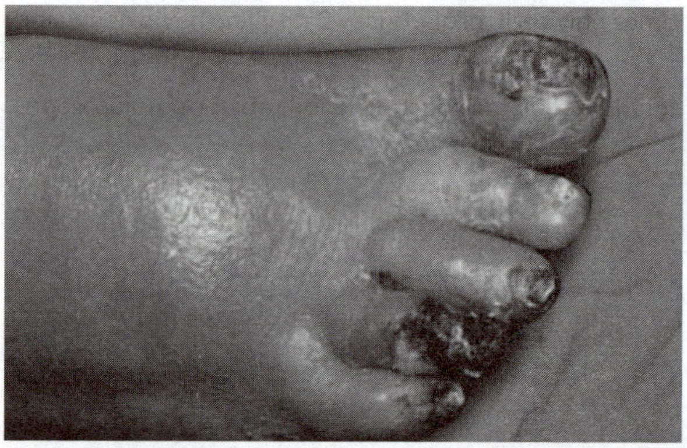

Fig. 5.7: Gangrene of foot.

Types of Gangrene

There are three major types of gangrene: (1) dry, (2) wet, and (3) gas gangrene.

Dry Gangrene

Causes

It usually occurs as a **complication of diabetes mellitus, arteriosclerosis, or frostbite.**

Clinical Features

- Dry gangrene develops slowly and may even go unnoticed for weeks or months.
- Causes blackening/darkening of the affected areas.
- It is not a life-threatening condition but has to be treated expeditiously.

Surgical removal of the dead tissue is the mainstay of treatment.

Wet Gangrene

Causes

The causes include:

- **Bacterial infections** *(Streptococcus* or *Staphylococcus)* **from severe wounds or burns**
- **Crush injuries** that impede the blood flow of certain areas.

Clinical Features

- Pain, swelling, and blistering of the skin
- Foul odor from the open wound.

Prognosis is bad without treatment.

Gas Gangrene

It is a form of wet gangrene.

Causes

Infection of body tissue by anaerobic bacteria (such as *C. perfringens*). These bacteria release toxins and gases.

Clinical Features

This rarest form of gangrene is characterized by:

- High fever
- Brown-colored pus
- Gas bubbles underneath the skin
- Discoloration of skin and a foul odor.

Gas gangrene can be fatal if left untreated.

Diagnosis

The diagnosis of gangrene is based on history, **physical examination** and the results of laboratory tests. **Culture from the gangrenous area** can be helpful to identify the type and extent of bacterial infection.

Treatment

Debridement: Dead gangrenous tissue is removed surgically. Healthy new tissue grows, and the wound heals after debridement.

Antibiotics: Gangrene caused by bacterial infections can be treated with **antibiotics.**

Amputation: In more severe cases, **amputation of a finger, toe, or part of a limb** may be necessary.

Hyperbaric chamber: Sometimes patients with gangrene are exposed to oxygen at a high pressure in hyperbaric chambers to help the affected tissue heal.

Prognosis

The prognosis is usually favorable if the condition is diagnosed and treated early. Complete recovery and tissue regeneration can take several weeks to months.

In the untreated cases, **sepsis from wet and gas gangrene can result in shock or death.**

CLINICAL NOTE

Organisms that are commonly involved in wet gangrene include *Streptococcus* and *Staphylococcus* bacteria. Without treatment, wet gangrene can be fatal.

CLINICAL PEARLS

1. Gangrene of the foot is a common complication of untreated diabetes mellitus. Gangrene is not a contagious disease. It is a condition in which living tissue (e.g. skin, muscle, or bone) begins to decay and die because blood flow (and oxygen) to an area is blocked or because harmful bacteria invade the body's tissues after entering through a wound or sore.
2. There are three major forms of gangrene: (1) dry, (2) wet, and (3) gas gangrene.
3. Gas gangrene, which is a form of wet gangrene, involves infection of body tissue by certain types of bacteria (such as *C. perfringens* (that are capable of thriving in anaerobic) conditions.
4. Gas gangrene is marked by a high fever, brownish pus, gas bubbles under the skin, skin discoloration, and a foul odor.
5. Treatment with antibiotics before and after abdominal surgery has been shown to reduce the rate of infection and the possibility of developing wet or gas gangrene.

CASE STUDY 4

Theme: Clinical Implications of Genetically Altered Type I Collagen Structure

A 7-month-old child fell over while crawling and presented with a swollen leg. History revealed that at the age of 1 month the baby had multiple fractures in various stages of healing (right clavicle, right humerus, right radius).

An X-ray taken from the affected leg revealed a fracture of a bowed femur. The bones were thin, had few trabeculae and thin cortices. History of child abuse was ruled out by careful questioning from the parents.

What is the possible diagnosis for this child?

Is there any treatment of this defect?

CASE DISCUSSION

The child most likely has **osteogenesis imperfecta (OI)**. This disease is also known as **"brittle bone syndrome"**. It is a heterogeneous group of inherited disorders distinguished by bones that easily bend and fracture. Bones in affected patients are thin, osteoporotic, with thin cortices and deficient trabeculae.

Delayed wound healing, a rotated and a twisted spine leading to a "humped back appearance" are common features of this disease. The disorder is frequently associated with blue sclerae, dental abnormalities progressive hearing loss, and a positive family history.

OSTEOGENESIS IMPERFECTA

Biochemical Defect

Most cases arise from a mutation in the gene encoding type I collagen. **The most common mutations cause the substitutions of single amino acid with bulky side chain for the glycine residues that appear as every third amino acid in the triple helix.** The structural abnormality affects the proper folding of the protein into a triple helical conformation.

Classification

Based on severity of symptoms, osteogenesis imperfecta can be classified into four types. Types I and II account for the majority of the cases. Types III and IV are intermediate in severity between types I and II. The child in the given case has type I OI.

Incidence

Although the frequency of type I OI is about 1 in 30,000 but the combined incidence of the three severe forms recognizable at birth (types II, III, and IV) may be much higher.

Clinical Manifestations

The clinical presentation is variable.

Skeletal Effects

- In type I OI, the bones are fragile. The bone fragility may be so mild to cause no disability or severe enough to hamper physical activity. X-ray skull in patients with mild disease may show a **mottled appearance** due to small deposits of irregular ossification.
- In type II OI, bones and other connective tissues are highly fragile and may cause massive injuries in utero or during delivery. **Continuously beaded, fractured ribs and crumpled long bones (accordion femora)** are characteristic of this disease. Many bones are incompletely ossified.
- In types III and IV, multiple fractures from minor physical trauma can produce severe deformities. Kyphoscoliosis, which is a usual finding, can cause cor pulmonale and predispose to pulmonary infections. The **"popcorn-like"** appearance in X-rays of the ends of long bones due to deposits of mineral is a diagnostic sign. Progressive neurologic symptoms may result from associated hydrocephalus.
- In all forms of OI, bone mass and mineral density is decreased.

Ocular Features

The sclerae can be normal, slightly bluish, or bright blue. The discoloration is caused by exposure of underlying choroids layers due to thinning of the collagen layers of the sclerae. Blue sclerae, however, are an inherited trait in some families who do not have increased bone fragility.

Dentinogenesis

The teeth may be normal, moderately discolored, or grossly abnormal. In some patients, the teeth readily fracture and need to be extracted. The enamel usually appears normal, but the teeth may have characteristic amber, yellowish brown, or translucent bluish gray color because of improper deposition or deficiency of dentin. The defect in dentin is directly attributable to abnormal type I collagen in these patients.

Hearing Loss

Hearing loss usually begins during the second decade of life and occurs in more than 50% of patients over the age of 30 years. The middle ear shows abnormal development, persistence of cartilages and deficient ossification.

Miscellaneous Features

Thin skin that scars extensively, joint laxity with permanent dislocations, cardiovascular manifestations such as aortic regurgitation, floppy mitral valves, mitral incompetence, and fragility of large blood vessels are also observed in patients with OI.

Diagnosis

Easy fractures, blue sclerae, dentinogenesis or family history of the disease are characteristic of OI.

Differential diagnosis: Other causes of pathologic fractures such as battered child syndrome, nutritional deficiencies, malignancies, and other inherited disorders should be excluded. The absence of superficial bruises helps in differentiating OI from battered child syndrome.

Radiology: A decrease in bone density revealed by X-ray can be verified by photon or X-ray absorptiometry.

Molecular techniques:

a. *Polyacrylamide gel electrophoresis (PAGE)*: A molecular defect in type I procollagen can be confirmed in over two-thirds of patients by polyacrylamide gel electrophoresis.
b. *Polymerase chain reaction (PCR)*: Analysis of collagen genes is usually performed by PCR.
c. *DNA sequencing*: DNA sequencing can be carried out in chorionic villus biopsies at 8–12 weeks of pregnancy.

Treatment

- Patients with mild disorder may require less treatment as the fractures generally decrease after puberty.
- Women, however, require special care during pregnancy and after menopause, as the fractures tend to increase again.
- In severely affected children, physical therapy, surgical management of fractures and skeletal deformities, and vocational training are required.
- In moderate to severe forms of OI, treatment with bisphosphonates is helpful to decrease bone loss.
- Bone marrow transplant and stem cell therapy are under trial.
- Many patients with OI do well despite severe deformities.

CLINICAL NOTE

In all forms of OI, bone mineral density is decreased. However, the fractures appear to heal normally.

CLINICAL PEARLS

1. Osteogenesis imperfecta (OI) is predominantly characterized by a generalized decrease in bone mass (osteopenia) and by brittle bones.
2. Most cases arise from a mutation in the gene encoding type I collagen.
3. There are four types, but types I and II account for the majority of the cases. Types III and IV are intermediate in severity between types I and II.
4. The presence of fractures together with blue sclerae, dentinogenesis or family history of the disease is usually sufficient to make the diagnosis.
5. Patients with mild disorder may need little treatment; women require special attention during pregnancy and after menopause. More severely affected children require physical therapy, surgical management of fractures and skeletal deformities.

CASE STUDY 5

Theme: Clinical Implications of Genetically Altered Type II Collagen Structure

A child with tall stature, loose joints, and detached retinas is found to have mutation in type II collagen. Collagen consists of a repeating tripeptide motif where the first amino acid of each tripeptide is same.

Which amino acid is the recurring amino acid most likely to be altered in mutations that distort collagen molecule?
What is this defect?
What are the other associated symptoms? How can this be treated?

CASE DISCUSSION

Basic Concept

The primary structure of collagen peptides consists of repeating tripeptides with Gly-X-Y motif, where Gly is glycine and X and Y are any amino acid. The small CH2 group connecting the amino and carboxyl groups of glycine contrasts with the larger connecting groups and side chains of other amino acids. The small volume of glycine molecules is crucial for alpha-helix secondary structure of collagen peptides. This in turn is necessary for their tertiary helical structure and their assembly into quaternary tripeptides, triple-helix structures (see Fig. 5.6). The most severe clinical phenotype caused by amino acid substitutions in collagen peptides is those affecting glycine that prevents alpha-helix formation. The child in the present case has a disorder called Stickler skeletal dysplasia syndrome.

CASE DETAILS

STICKLER SYNDROME

Inheritance

Autosomal dominant.

Incidence

The prevalence of Stickler syndrome is estimated to be 1 in 7,500, but it is thought to be frequently undiagnosed or misdiagnosed. When a mother or father has Stickler syndrome, there is a 50% chance that the Stickler-causing gene will be passed on to a child, with each pregnancy. **Unlike some genetic syndromes, a person will not have a "carrier" gene for this disorder that can be passed on to the next generation without the parent having Stickler syndrome themselves.** Occasionally, though, a person will have a spontaneous genetic mutation that will cause Stickler syndrome without either parent having the disorder.

Clinical Features

Stickler syndrome is an underdiagnosed disorder because a patient can be affected in only certain areas. It is possible for other family members to be affected differently and even more or less severely. **Families are frequently not aware that they have Stickler syndrome until a child is born with a palate abnormality, has early degenerative joint changes or a retinal detachment.**

The following is a brief summary of the symptoms as they affect patients in five different areas. The premature degenerative change in weight-bearing joints is one of the most consistent features of Stickler syndrome. The number and severity of symptoms will vary greatly from person to person, within families and with the aging process.

Auditory

- Sensor neural hearing loss and a conductive hearing loss are frequently present in patients with a cleft palate due to fluid in the ear.
- Children with a cleft palate are also prone to frequent ear infections and swallowing difficulties.

Cardiovascular

Mitral valve prolapse is a common finding.

Ocular

- Retinal degeneration, including retinal detachments
- Holes and slits
- Cataracts
- Myopia
- Severe or mild glaucoma and
- Vitreous degeneration.

Musculoskeletal

- Bony enlargement of joints
- Hypermobility of joints
- Ankle joint instability
- Kyphosis and scoliosis
- Joint pain and stiffness
- Arachnodactyly (long and slender fingers)
- Pectus excavatum (sunken chest) and
- Slender tubular bones.

Orofacial

- Flat mid-face; flat nasal bridge
- Long philtrum (area between nose and upper lip)
- Micrognathia (small jaw)

- Large and prominent eyes; cleft of hard/soft palate
- High-arched palate
- Submucous cleft palate; bifid uvula.

The characteristic feature of Stickler syndrome is a somewhat flattened facial appearance. This is caused by underdeveloped bones in the middle of the face, including the cheekbones and the bridge of the nose. A particular group of physical features, called the Pierre Robin syndrome, is common in children with Stickler syndrome. Robin sequence includes a U-shaped or sometimes V-shaped cleft palate (an opening in the roof of the mouth) **(Figs. 5.8A and B)** with a tongue that is too large for the space formed by the small lower jaw.

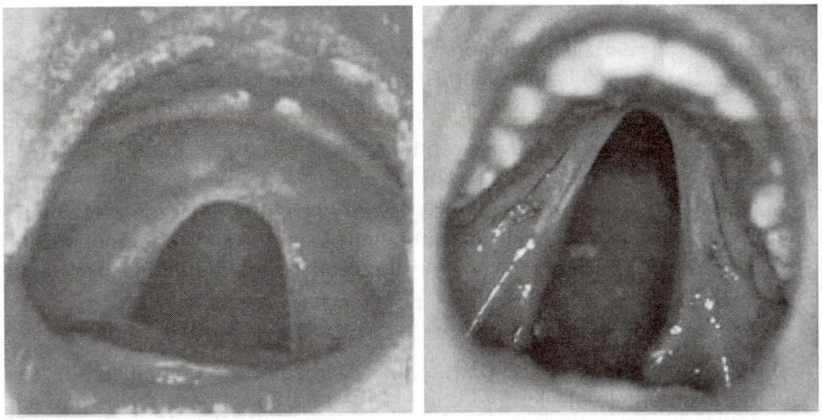

A U-shaped cleft palate B V-shaped cleft palate

Figs. 5.8A and B: U-shaped or V-shaped cleft palate—a characteristic finding in Stickler syndrome.

Diagnosis

Diagnosis of Stickler syndrome can be made two ways. The first method is clinical diagnosis using the diagnostic criteria**. The diagnostic criterion is a 12-point system which measures abnormalities in the following systems: eyes, ears, bones/joints, and face/palate, as well as family history or gene data. A score of 5 or more indicates Stickler syndrome.**

Stickler syndrome can also be diagnosed by using genetic testing.

Treatment

Mainly symptomatic, special attention is required for the eye complications during childhood. Careful evaluation of breathing and feeding is very important.

Some infants must have a surgical tracheotomy (a breathing tube placed in the trachea).

Infants with Pierre Robin sequence often have a hard time taking all of their nutrition by bottle because of breathing problems. Sometimes a feeding tube from the nose to the stomach is needed. Often infants with Pierre Robin sequence do not have their cleft palate repaired until they are 15–18 months old so their jaw has more time to grow and their breathing symptoms improve. Some children with Pierre Robin sequence may have the option of surgery to move the lower jaw forward.

Prognosis

A person with Stickler syndrome can live a long, happy and healthy life—it is a disorder, not a disease, unless some complications are there.

CLINICAL NOTE

A particular group of physical features, called the Pierre Robin syndrome, is common in children with Stickler syndrome. Robin sequence includes a U-shaped or sometimes V-shaped cleft palate (an opening in the roof of the mouth) with a tongue that is too large for the space formed by the small lower jaw.

CLINICAL PEARLS

1. Stickler skeletal dysplasia syndrome is due to a mutation that distorts collagen molecule.
2. The premature degenerative change in weight-bearing joints is one of the most consistent features of Stickler syndrome. The number and severity of symptoms will vary greatly from person to person, within families and with the aging process.
3. The characteristic feature of Stickler syndrome is a somewhat flattened facial appearance. This is caused by underdeveloped bones in the middle of the face, including the cheekbones and the bridge of the nose.
4. The diagnostic criterion is a 12-point system which measures abnormalities in the following systems: eyes, ears, bones/joints, and face/palate, as well as family history or gene data. A score of 5 or more indicates Stickler syndrome.
5. Mainly symptomatic, special attention is required for the eye complications during childhood. Careful evaluation of breathing and feeding is very important.

CASE STUDY 6

Theme: Clinical Implications of Genetically Altered Dystrophin

A 4-year-old boy was brought to a children's hospital clinic. His mother was concerned because she had noticed that her son was walking awkwardly, fell over frequently and had difficulty in climbing stairs. There were no other affected children but the mother had a brother who died at the age of 19 suffering from muscular dystrophy. The examining physician noticed

1. Muscle weakness in both the pelvic and shoulder girdle.
2. Modest enlargement of the calf muscles.

   Because of the muscle weakness and its distribution, a tentative diagnosis of Duchenne muscular dystrophy (DMD) was made.

What is the defect in this disease?

How can this be treated?

DUCHENNE MUSCULAR DYSTROPHY

Muscular dystrophy itself implies genetically inherited progressive muscle disease.

Duchenne muscular dystrophy (DMD) is caused by mutations in the DMD gene. This gene encodes a protein called dystrophin.

BASIC CONCEPT

Dystrophin

1. Acts as mechanical link between actin in the cytoskeleton and the extracellular matrix. It helps anchor the muscle fiber to the extracellular matrix thus helping in subsequent contractions and relaxations **(Fig. 5. 9)**.
2. **Dystrophin and its isoforms are found in skeletal muscles, smooth muscles and the brain.**

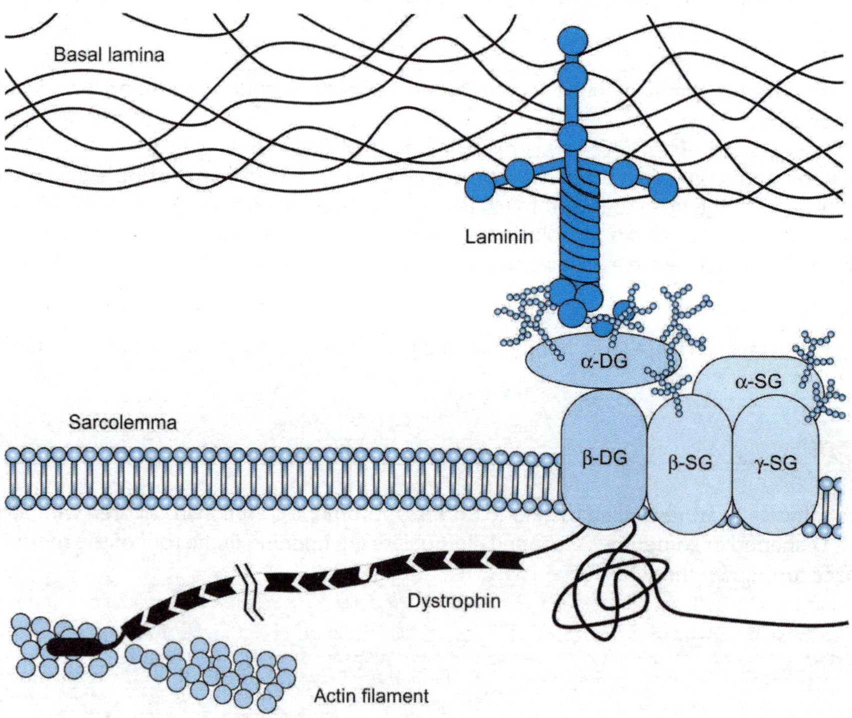

Fig. 5.9: Dystrophin-sarcoglycan complex protein.

Inheritance

Location: Xp21.

Transmission: X-linked recessive (affects only males that is the reason for the brother's death and her son getting affected. The mother was the carrier).

Clinical Features

Age group: Usually presents during 3–5 years. The most frequent presenting symptoms are:

- Motor delay or an abnormal gait.

- Affected child may present with difficulty in running or getting-up from the ground, frequent falls, or toe walking.
- Less frequent presentations include language or generalized developmental delay.
- Incidentally raised serum creatine kinase or transaminase levels when these investigations are performed for other reasons.

Muscle Weakness

- Proximal muscles affected first (quadriceps and shoulder girdle) due to the deficient dystrophin protein which they usually have in abundance.
- Progresses to upper extremities—wheelchair dependence by the age of 12 years.
- **Gowers' sign—"child climbs up on himself" while trying to standing-up.**
- Pseudohypertrophy—the calf enlargement is called pseudohypertrophy because it is not the true enlargement of the muscle fiber rather its fibrofatty replacement of the degenerating muscle tissue.

Cardiac Involvement

- Cardiomyopathy.
- Rhythm disturbances.

Respiratory Involvement Usually by the Age of 16 to 18

- Scoliosis impairs pulmonary functions.
- Respiratory failure due to progressive weakness of respiratory muscles (intercostal muscles).
- They are prone to get hypercapnia, followed by severe pulmonary infections in the last stages.

Intellectual Ability Affects One-third of Cases

- Affects the verbal ability more than performance ability.
- Mental retardation may be seen.

Orthopedic Complications

- Scoliosis.
- Lordotic posture.
- Tip toe walking.
- Easy fractures.

Investigations
1. Serum enzymes: CK (increases 10–100 times normal)
   AST, ALT, LDH (but nonspecific)
2. Electromyography
3. Muscle biopsy: Immunostaining for dystrophin protein. Dystrophin will be deficient in DMD
4. Molecular genetic testing (PCR)

Treatment

General Measures

1. Symptomatic treatment of systemic manifestations.
   Example: Wheelchair support
2. Ventilatory support.

Pharmaceutical Approaches

Corticosteroids therapy: Corticosteroids such as prednisolone, prednisone, and deflazacort have been successfully used to improve muscle strength in DM. The corticosteroids act by decreasing rate of skeletal muscle degradation, increasing myogenic repair and lowering cytosolic concentrations of calcium and Tc-cells in muscle fibers. Corticosteroids also appear to have a positive effect on the complications associated with Duchenne muscular dystrophy (DMD).

Molecular Approaches

1. ***Viral vectors:*** Adeno-associated viral (AAV) vectors that carry critical regions of the DMD gene have been tried to create microdystrophin and minidystrophin genes in mouse models.
2. ***Antisense oligonucleotide exon skipping:*** In order to restore the reading frame and produce a partially functioning dystrophin, antisense oligonucleotides have been used to redirect splicing and induce exon skipping.
3. ***Readthrough stop codon strategies:*** The drugs such as PTC124 and gentamicin that promote ribosomal readthrough of stop codons, allowing continuation of translation and production of a functioning protein have been tried.
4. ***Stem cell therapy:*** The results have not been very promising in patients with DMD.

5. ***Utrophin:*** Utrophin, a protein homologue of dystrophin in the sarcolemma, if upregulated may compensate for dystrophin deficiency.
6. ***Prevention and genetic counseling:*** A family having a male with DMD should be referred for genetic counseling.
7. **Prenatal diagnosis** should be carried out in all carrier mothers.

CLINICAL NOTE

The DMD patients are prone to get hypercapnia and severe pulmonary infections in the last stages due to weakness of the respiratory muscles.

CLINICAL PEARLS

1. Duchenne muscular dystrophy is caused by mutations in the DMD gene. This gene encodes a protein called dystrophin.
2. Dystrophin acts as mechanical link between actin in the cytoskeleton and the extracellular matrix. It helps anchor the muscle fiber to the extracellular matrix thus helping in subsequent contractions and relaxations.
3. Proximal muscles are affected first by weakness due to deficient but abundant dystrophin protein, wheelchair dependence by the age of 12 years.
4. Diagnosis is made by serum enzymes estimations, electromyography, muscle biopsy and by genetic testing.
5. Treatment is symptomatic. Corticosteroids such as prednisolone, prednisone and deflazacort have been the only drugs shown to be effective to date in DMD.

CASE STUDY 7

Theme: Biological Role of Alpha-1-antitrypsin and Clinical Implications of its Deficiency

A severe form of obstructive lung disease starting with dyspnea and leading progressively toward emphysema was found in several members of the family. One brother had died earlier of lung disease.

Blood plasma from his surviving brother and sister showed abnormally low concentration of α1-antitrypsin (5.5 μm, normal is 20–48 μm), the α1-plasma fraction also moved abnormally on isoelectric focusing gel electrophoresis.

What is the relationship of emphysema with α1-antitrypsin?
What is the cause of abnormal movement during electrophoresis?
What are the prospects for treatment of this emphysema?

CASE DISCUSSION

Emphysema is a lung disease characterized by destruction of the alveolar walls. Its causes are complex but airway infection, cigarette smoking, air pollution and familial factors are involved. A deficiency in plasma α1-antitrypsin leads to the development of emphysema and less frequently hepatic disease.

ALPHA-1-ANTITRYPSIN

It was so named because it is a good inhibitor in vitro of pancreatic protease trypsin. It is synthesized primarily in the liver and is secreted into the bloodstream. The inhibitor makes up most of the proteins in the α1-globulin band following the electrophoresis of plasma.

Pathogenesis of α1-Antitrypsin Deficiency

In healthy individuals, the lungs contain a natural enzyme called neutrophil elastase that, under normal circumstances, helps the lungs by digesting damaged, aging cells and bacteria. This process promotes healing of the lung tissue. Unfortunately this enzyme is nonspecific in nature and eventually attacks the lung tissue instead of helping it heal. That is where alpha-antitrypsin (AAT) comes into action, by destroying the enzyme before it can cause actual damage to healthy lung tissue. It promotes the lungs to function normally. When there is not enough AAT, however, the lung tissue will continue to be destroyed, which may lead to the chronic lung disease, emphysema.

Inheritance

The two patients described in this case are male and female, suggesting that the deficiency is inherited as an autosomal trait. The genetics has been studied in large number of patients and family members. Analysis suggests that two independent alleles exist on chromosome 14. The deficiency is inherited as a codominant trait; that is, both alleles contribute to the disease and neither is dominant over the other. The two genes that each person carries for α1-antitrypsin may be diverse, more than 100 variants are known.

The two common deficiency variants of α1-antitrypsin, S and Z, result from point mutations in the α1-antitrypsin gene and are named on the basis of their slower electrophoretic mobility on isoelectric focusing analysis compared with the normal M allele. S α1-antitrypsin (^{264}Glu→Val) is found in up to 28% of Southern Europeans and, although it results in plasma α1-antitrypsin levels that are 60% of the M allele, it is not associated with any pulmonary sequelae. This is usually sufficient to protect the lungs from the effects of elastase in people who do not smoke. The Z variant (^{342}Glu→Lys) results in a more severe deficiency that is characterized, in the homozygote, by plasma α1-antitrypsin less than 15% of normal, and patients are likely to develop panacinar emphysema at a young age; 50% of these patients will develop liver cirrhosis, because the A1AT is not secreted properly and instead accumulates in the liver.

Clinical Manifestations

The first signs and symptoms of lung disease caused by alpha-1-antitrypsin deficiency usually appear between ages 20 and 50. The earliest symptoms are:

- Shortness of breath following mild activity
- Reduced ability to exercise, and
- Wheezing.

Other signs and symptoms can include:

- Unintentional weight loss
- Recurring respiratory infections
- Fatigue, and
- Rapid heartbeat upon standing.

Advanced lung disease leads to emphysema, in which small air sacs in the lungs (alveoli) are damaged. **Characteristic features of emphysema include:**

- Difficulty breathing
- A hacking cough, and
- A barrel-shaped chest.

Smoking or exposure to tobacco smoke accelerates the appearance of symptoms and damage to the lungs. About 10% of infants and 15% of adults with alpha-1-antitrypsin deficiency have liver damage. Signs of liver disease can include:

- Ascites
- Edema feet or legs, and
- Jaundice.

Diagnosis

The following tests may also help with diagnosis:

- Alpha-1-antitrypsin estimation
- Arterial blood gases
- Chest X-ray **(Fig. 5.10)**
- CT scan of the chest
- Genetic testing
- Pulmonary function tests.

Measurement of alpha-1-antitrypsin: Isoelectric focusing on polyacrylamide gel is useful in distinguishing specific variants to establish the specific phenotype.

Effect of smoking on antitrypsin levels: Smoking greatly exacerbates antitrypsin deficiency. A methionyl-seryl group (position 358 and 359) is present at the point where the inhibitor binds to the active site of elastase. The smoke promotes the oxidation of methionine residues to the corresponding sulfoxide. This results in inactivation of the protein which fails to bind elastase. The active elastase then destroys the lung tissue.

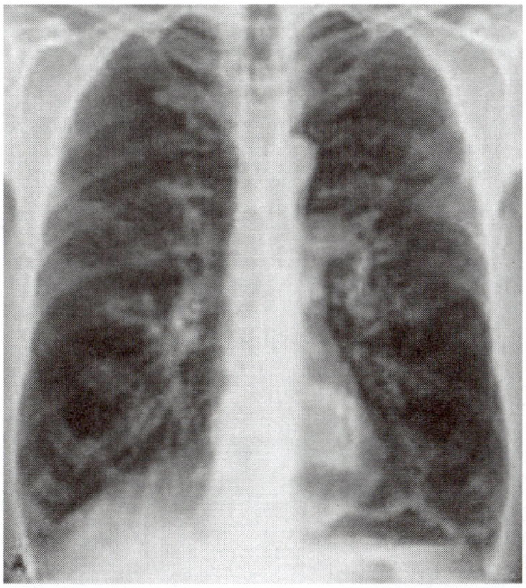

Fig. 5.10: Hyperinflation due to panacinar emphysema. Posteroanterior chest radiograph shows that the dome of the right hemidiaphragm is below the level of the anterior right 7th rib consistent with increased lung volumes. Also noted is decrease in the peripheral vascular markings. The patient had severe panacinar emphysema due to alpha-1-antitrypsin deficiency.

Treatment

Treatment involves replacing the missing AAT protein. The protein derived from donated human plasma is given intravenously each week. This augmentation therapy is thought to arrest the course of the disease and halt any further damage to the lungs. Long-term studies of the effectiveness of A1AT replacement therapy are not available. It is currently recommended that patients begin augmentation therapy only after the onset of emphysema symptoms.

Quitting smoking is crucial.
Other treatments specifically for emphysema and cirrhosis are also used.
Treatments currently being studied include recombinant and inhaled forms of A1AT.
Antioxidants are also supplemented.

CLINICAL NOTE

Measurement of alpha-1-antitrypsin by isoelectric focusing on polyacrylamide gel is useful in distinguishing specific variants to establish the specific phenotype.

CLINICAL PEARLS

1. A deficiency in plasma α1-antitrypsin leads to the development of emphysema and less frequently hepatic disease.
2. The earliest symptoms are shortness of breath following mild activity, reduced ability to exercise, and wheezing.
3. About 10% of infants and 15% of adults with alpha-1-antitrypsin deficiency have liver damage. Signs of liver disease can include: ascites, edema feet or legs, and jaundice.
4. Alpha-1-antitrypsin estimation, arterial blood gas measurements, chest X-ray, CT scan of the chest, genetic testing, and pulmonary function tests can be carried out for the confirmation of the diagnosis.
5. Treatment involves replacing the missing AAT protein. The protein derived from donated human plasma is given intravenously each week. This augmentation therapy is thought to arrest the course of the disease and halt any further damage to the lungs.

Chapter 6

Amino Acid Metabolism and Related Disorders

LEARNING OBJECTIVES

To understand biochemical deviations and clinical implications in:
- ❖ Urea cycle disorders
- ❖ Disorders of phenylalanine metabolism
- ❖ Disorders of tryptophan metabolism
- ❖ Disorders of cysteine, cystine, and homocysteine metabolism
- ❖ Disorders of metabolism of branched-chain amino acids
- ❖ Impaired nitric oxide synthesis

CASE STUDIES

CASE STUDY 1

Theme: Urea Cycle Disorders

A 6-month-old infant began to vomit occasionally and ceased to gain weight. At 9 months of age, he was readmitted to the hospital.

Routine examination and laboratory tests were normal but after 1 week, he became drowsy, his temperature rose to 39.4°C, his pulse was elevated, and his liver was enlarged. The electroencephalogram (EEG) was grossly abnormal. Since the infant could not retain milk by gavage feeding, intravenous glucose was administered. Urine analysis showed abnormally high amount of glutamine and uracil. This suggested high amount of ammonia concentration, which was confirmed by laboratory test.

What is the cause of hyperammonemia in this patient?

Why were the urine glutamine and uracil levels elevated?

How can such a patient be treated?

CASE DISCUSSION

The child is most probably suffering from hyperammonemia due to impaired urea formation. **Hyperammonemia in a newborn or very young infant is the characteristic sign of inherited defect in a gene for urea cycle enzymes,** but the most frequent abnormality is in ornithine transcarbamoylase, a mitochondrial enzyme encoded by a nuclear gene on the X-chromosome. The enzyme affected in this patient is ornithine transcarbamoylase because of the excretion of uracil. Excessive excretion of uracil or its precursor orotic acid, results from an accumulation of carbamoyl phosphate in the mitochondria. In the absence of ornithine transcarbamoylase, carbamoyl phosphate accumulates and leaks in to the cytoplasm, where it can be used to make carbamoyl aspartate, the first intermediate in the pathway of pyrimidine nucleotide biosynthesis. This case is unusual, in that, the symptoms took longer to appear. Urine glutamine excretion has increased because it has exceeded the capacity of the kidney to hydrolyze glutamine to glutamate and ammonia. It is excreted in compensation for the inoperative urea cycle.

ORNITHINE TRANSCARBAMOYLASE DEFICIENCY

Inheritance

- The disease is characterized as **X-linked dominant** because most females are also somewhat affected. Females usually respond well to treatment. A significant number of carrier females have hyperammonemia and neurologic compromise presumed to be secondary to skewed X-chromosome inactivation. The risk for hyperammonemia is particularly high in pregnancy and the postpartum period. Drugs such as valproic acid and corticosteroids may also trigger a hyperammonemia crisis in a carrier.
- The disease is much more severe in males than in females.
- The enzyme activity can range from 0% to 30% of the normal.

BASIC CONCEPT

Urea Cycle Disorders

The urea cycle is composed of five catalytic enzymes, a cofactor producer, and at least two transport proteins. The urea cycle is the sole source of endogenous production of arginine, and it is the principal mechanism for the clearance of waste nitrogen resulting from protein turnover, the metabolism of other compounds like adenosine monophosphate, and dietary intake. This extra nitrogen is converted into ammonia (NH3) and transported to the liver, where it is processed. The urea cycle disorders (UCDs) result from inherited molecular defects which compromise this clearance.

Reactions of Urea Cycle

Synthesis of 1 mol of urea requires 3 mol of ATP plus 1 mol each of ammonium ion and of the α-amino nitrogen of aspartate. Five enzymes catalyze the reactions of urea cycle **(Fig. 6.1)**. Of the six participating amino acids, **N-acetyl glutamate functions solely as an enzyme activator (*see* Fig. 6.3)**. The others serve as carriers of the atoms that ultimately become urea. The major metabolic role of ornithine, citrulline, and argininosuccinate in mammals is urea synthesis. Urea synthesis is a cyclic process. Since the ornithine is consumed in 2nd reaction and is regenerated in last reaction, so there is no net loss or gain of ornithine, citrulline, argininosuccinate, or arginine. Ammonium ion, CO_2, ATP, and aspartate are, however, consumed. Some reactions of urea synthesis occur in the matrix of the mitochondrion, other reactions in the cytosol **(Fig. 6.1)**.

Carbamoyl Phosphate Synthase I initiates Urea Biosynthesis

Condensation of CO_2, ammonia, and ATP to form carbamoyl phosphate (2) is catalyzed by mitochondrial carbamoyl phosphate synthase I (CPS-I). A cytosolic form of this enzyme, carbamoyl phosphate synthase II, uses glutamine rather than ammonia as the nitrogen donor and functions in pyrimidine biosynthesis.

Carbamoyl phosphate synthase I, the rate-limiting enzyme of the urea cycle, is active only in the presence of its allosteric activator N-acetyl glutamate, which enhances the affinity of the synthase for ATP. Formation of carbamoyl phosphate requires 2 mol of ATP, one of which serves as a phosphoryl donor. Conversion of the second ATP to AMP and pyrophosphate, coupled to the hydrolysis of pyrophosphate to orthophosphate, provides the driving force for synthesis of the amide bond and the mixed acid anhydride bond of carbamoyl phosphate.

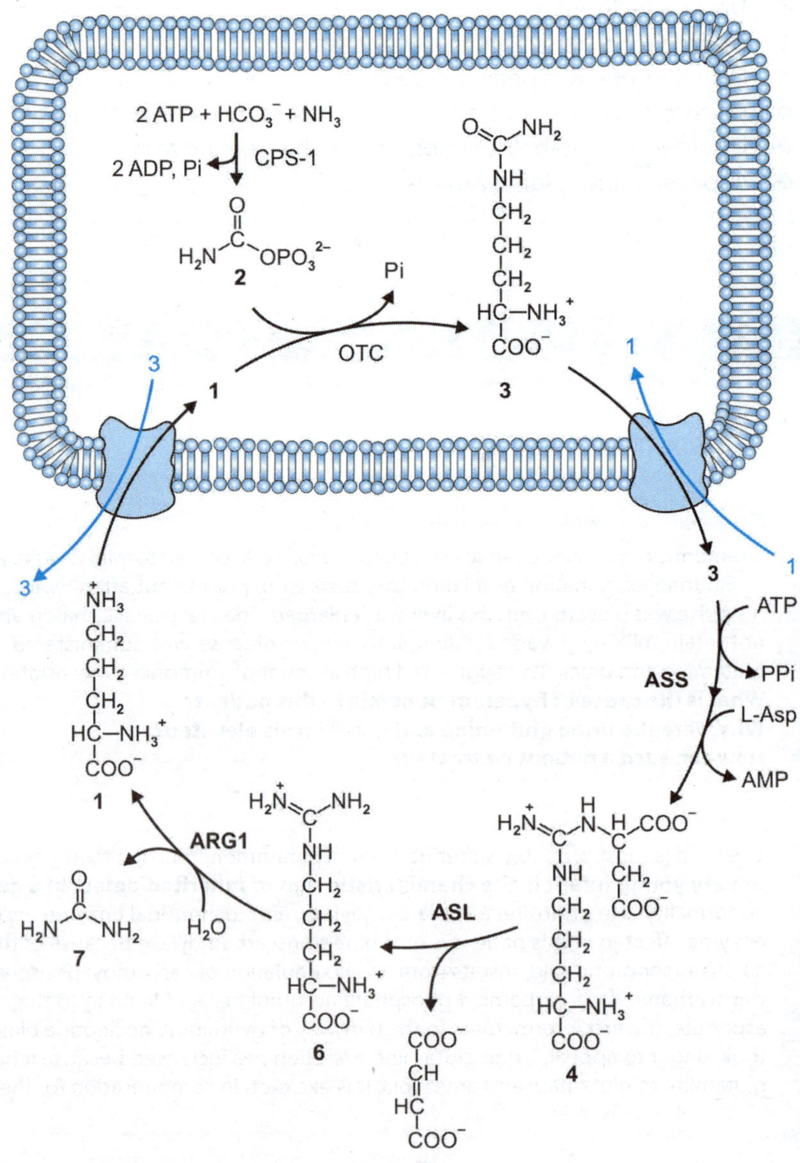

Fig. 6.1: Reactions of urea cycle; 1 L-ornithine; 2 Carbamoyl phosphate; 3 L-Citrulline; 4 Argininosuccinate; 5 Fumarate; 6 L-Arginine; 7 Urea L-Asp L-aspartate.

Carbamoyl Phosphate Plus Ornithine forms Citrulline

L-ornithine transcarbamoylase (OTC) catalyzes transfer of the carbamoyl group of carbamoyl phosphate to ornithine (1), forming citrulline (3) and orthophosphate (see the numbered products in the **Figure 6.1**). While the reaction occurs in the mitochondrial matrix, both the formation of ornithine and the subsequent metabolism of citrulline take place in the cytosol. Entry of ornithine into mitochondria and exodus of citrulline from mitochondria, therefore involve mitochondrial inner membrane transport systems **(Fig. 6.1)**.

Citrulline Plus Aspartate forms Argininosuccinate

Argininosuccinate synthase (ASS) links L-aspartate and citrulline via the amino group of aspartate and provides the second nitrogen of urea. The reaction requires ATP and involves intermediate formation of citrullyl-AMP. Subsequent displacement of AMP by aspartate then forms argininosuccinate (4).

Cleavage of Argininosuccinate forms Arginine and Fumarate

Cleavage of argininosuccinate (4), catalyzed by argininosuccinate lyase (ASL), proceeds with retention of nitrogen in arginine, (6) and release of the aspartate skeleton as fumarate (5). Addition of water to fumarate forms L-malate, and subsequent NAD^+-dependent oxidation of malate forms oxaloacetate. These two reactions are analogous to reactions of the citric acid cycle, but are catalyzed by cytosolic fumarase and malate dehydrogenase. Transamination of oxaloacetate by glutamate aminotransferase then reforms aspartate. The carbon skeleton of aspartate-fumarate thus acts as a carrier of the nitrogen of glutamate into a precursor of urea.

Cleavage of Arginine releases Urea and reforms Ornithine

Hydrolytic cleavage of the guanidino group of arginine, catalyzed by liver arginase (ARG1), releases urea (7) and the other product, ornithine (1), reenters liver mitochondria for additional rounds of urea synthesis. Ornithine and lysine are potent inhibitors of arginase, competitive with arginine. Arginine also serves as the precursor of the potent muscle relaxant nitric oxide (NO) in a Ca^{2+}-dependent reaction catalyzed by NO synthase.

Carbamoyl Phosphate Synthase I is the Pacemaker Enzyme of the Urea Cycle

The activity of carbamoyl phosphate synthase I is determined by N-acetyl glutamate, whose steady-state level is dictated by its rate of synthesis from acetyl-CoA and glutamate, and its rate of hydrolysis to acetate and glutamate. These reactions are catalyzed by N-acetyl glutamate synthase and N-acetyl glutamate hydrolase, respectively. Major changes in diet can increase the concentrations of individual urea cycle enzymes 10–20-folds. Starvation, for example, elevates enzyme levels, presumably to cope with the increased production of ammonia that accompanies enhanced protein degradation.

Causes of Urea Cycle Disorders

Carbamoyl Phosphate Synthetase I Deficiency

Along with OTC deficiency, deficiency of CPS-I is the most severe of the urea cycle disorders. Individuals with complete carbamoyl phosphate synthetase I (CPS-I) deficiency rapidly develop hyperammonemia in the newborn period. Children who are successfully rescued from crisis are chronically at risk for repeated bouts of hyperammonemia.

Ornithine Transcarbamoylase Deficiency

Absence of OTC activity in males is as severe as CPS-I deficiency. Approximately 15% of carrier females develop hyperammonemia during their lifetime and many require chronic medical management.
The components of the pathway are:

- Carbamoyl phosphate synthase I (CPS-I)
- Ornithine transcarbamoylase (OTC)
- Argininosuccinic acid synthetase (ASS)
- Argininosuccinic acid lyase (ASL)
- Arginase (ARG).

Citrullinemia Type I (ASS Deficiency)

The hyperammonemia in this disorder is quite severe. Affected individuals are able to incorporate some waste nitrogen into urea cycle intermediates, which makes treatment slightly easier.

Argininosuccinic Aciduria (ASL Deficiency)

This disorder also presents with rapid-onset hyperammonemia in the newborn period. This enzyme defect is past the point in the metabolic pathway at which all the waste nitrogen has been incorporated into the cycle. Treatment of affected individuals often requires only supplementation of arginine. ASL deficiency is marked by chronic hepatic enlargement and elevation of transaminases. Biopsy of the liver shows enlarged hepatocytes, which may over time progress to fibrosis, the etiology of which is unclear. Affected individuals can also develop trichorrhexis nodosa, a node-like appearance of fragile hair, which usually responds to arginine supplementation. Affected individuals who have never had prolonged coma but nevertheless have significant developmental disabilities have been reported.

Arginase Deficiency (Hyperargininemia; ARG Deficiency)

This disorder is not typically characterized by rapid-onset hyperammonemia. Affected individuals develop progressive spasticity and can also develop tremor, ataxia, and choreoathetosis. Growth is affected.

NAG Synthase Deficiency

Deficiency of this enzyme has been described in a number of affected individuals. Symptoms mimic those of CPS-I deficiency; since CPS-I is rendered inactive in the absence of NAG **(*see* Fig. 6.3)**.

Prevalence

The incidence of UCDs is estimated to be at least 1:25,000 births; partial defects may make the number much higher.

Clinical Manifestations

Infants with a urea cycle disorder often appear normal initially, but rapidly develop cerebral edema and the related signs of lethargy, anorexia, hyperventilation or hypoventilation, hypothermia, seizures, neurologic posturing, and coma. In milder (or partial) urea cycle enzyme deficiencies, ammonia accumulation may be triggered by illness or stress at almost any time of life, resulting in multiple mild elevations of plasma ammonia concentration; the hyperammonemia is less severe and the symptoms are more subtle. In individuals with partial enzyme deficiencies, the first recognized clinical episode may be delayed for months or years.

Diagnosis/Testing

The diagnosis of a urea cycle disorder is based on evaluation of clinical, biochemical, and molecular genetic data.

- A plasma ammonia concentration of 150 mmol/L or higher, associated with a normal anion gap and a normal serum glucose concentration, is a strong indication for the presence of a UCD.
- Plasma quantitative amino acid analysis can be used to diagnose a specific urea cycle disorder. Plasma concentration of arginine may be reduced in all urea cycle disorders, except ARG deficiency, in which it is elevated five- to seven-fold.
- Plasma concentration of citrulline helps discriminate between the proximal and distal urea cycle defects, as citrulline is the product of the proximal enzymes (OTC and CPS-I) and a substrate for the distal enzymes (ASS, ASL, and ARG).
- Urinary orotic acid is measured to distinguish CPS-I deficiency and NAGS deficiency from OTC deficiency.
- A definitive diagnosis of CPS-I deficiency, OTC deficiency, or NAGS deficiency depends on determination of enzyme activity from a liver biopsy specimen.
- However, the combination of family history, clinical presentation, amino acid and orotic acid testing, and, in some cases, molecular genetic testing is often sufficient for diagnostic confirmation, eliminating the risks of liver biopsy.
- Molecular genetic testing for OTC deficiency is clinically available in the US. Molecular genetic testing for CPS-I deficiency, NAGS deficiency, citrullinemia type I, arginase deficiency, and argininosuccinic aciduria is clinically available in laboratories outside the US.

Management

The mainstays of treatment for urea cycle disorders include:

- **Dialysis to reduce plasma ammonia concentration**
- **Intravenous administration of arginine chloride** and nitrogen scavenger drugs to allow alternative pathway excretion of excess nitrogen. Excess nitrogen is removed by intravenous phenyl acetate and benzoate (0.25 g/kg for the priming dose and subsequently as an infusion over 24 hours) that conjugate with glutamine and glycine, respectively, to form phenylacetylglutamine and hippuric acid, which are water-soluble molecules efficiently excreted in urine. Arginine (200 mg/kg/day) becomes an essential amino acid (except in arginase deficiency) and should be provided intravenously to resume protein synthesis. If these measures fail to reduce ammonia, hemodialysis should be initiated promptly. Restriction of protein for 24–48 hours to reduce the amount of nitrogen in the diet, providing calories as carbohydrates (intravenously as glucose) and fat (intralipid or as protein-free formula) to reduce catabolism.
- Physiologic stabilization with intravenous fluids and cardiac pressors (while avoiding over hydration and resulting cerebral edema) to reduce the risk of neurologic damage.
- Chronic therapy consists of a protein-restricted diet, phenylbutyrate (a more palatable precursor of phenyl acetate), arginine, or citrulline supplements, depending on the specific diagnosis. Liver transplantation should be considered in patients with severe urea cycle defects that are difficult to control medically.

Genetic Counseling

Deficiencies of CPS-I, ASS, ASL, NAGS, and ARG are inherited in an autosomal recessive manner. OTC deficiency is inherited in an X-linked manner. Prenatal testing using molecular genetic testing is available for five of the six urea cycle disorders if the disease-causing mutations have been identified in an affected family member. For families in which the disease-causing mutations have not been identified, prenatal testing may be available by linkage analysis for families with OTC deficiency or CPS-I deficiency, and biochemical testing for families with ASS, ASL, or ARG deficiency.

Newborn Screening

- Current extended newborn screening panels, using tandem mass spectrometry, detect abnormal concentrations of analytes associated with ASS deficiency and ASL deficiency, although the sensitivity and specificity of such screening for these disorders are unknown.
- CPS-I deficiency, OTC deficiency, and NAGS deficiency cannot be detected using tandem mass spectrometry.
- Although argininemia has been detected by these methods, newborn screening cannot be expected to reliably detect all cases.

Differential Diagnosis

A number of other disorders that perturb the liver can result in hyperammonemia and mimic the effects of a urea cycle disorder. The most common/significant ones are viral infection of the liver and vascular bypass of the liver.

Defects in the transporter proteins for ornithine (HHH syndrome) and aspartate (citrin deficiency) are clinically different from the classic urea cycle disorders.

Citrin Deficiency

The two phenotypes of citrin deficiency are citrullinemia type II (CTLN2) and neonatal intrahepatic cholestasis caused by citrin deficiency (NICCD).

Citrullinemia type II (CTLN2) is characterized by adult-onset, recurring episodes of hyperammonemia, and associated neuropsychiatric symptoms including nocturnal delirium, aggression, irritability, hyperactivity, delusions, disorientation, restlessness, drowsiness, loss of memory, flapping tremor, convulsive seizures, and coma; death can result from brain edema. Onset is sudden and usually between the ages of 20 years and 50 years. Pathologic findings include fatty infiltration and mild fibrosis of the liver despite little or no liver dysfunction.

Children younger than 1 year of age with NICCD have transient intrahepatic cholestasis, diffuse fatty liver and parenchymal cellular infiltration associated with hepatic fibrosis, low birth weight, growth retardation, hypoproteinemia, decreased coagulation factors, hemolytic anemia, hepatomegaly, variable liver dysfunction, and/or hypoglycemia; NICCD is generally not severe. Symptoms disappear by age 1 year with fat-soluble vitamin supplementation and lactose-free formulas or formulas containing medium chain triglycerides. One or more decades later, some individuals develop severe CTLN2 with neuropsychiatric symptoms; the transition from NICCD to the onset of CTLN2 is gradual.

Affected individuals have the dietary peculiarity of avoiding carbohydrate rather than protein.

Citrin is an aspartate glutamate transporter across the mitochondrial membrane. Citrin deficiency limits the activity of the enzyme argininosuccinic acid synthase, which combines aspartate and citrulline to make argininosuccinic acid **(Fig. 6.2)**. The diagnosis of CTLN2 and NICCD is based on biochemical findings, including increase of blood or plasma concentration of ammonia, increased plasma or serum concentrations of citrulline and arginine; citrin deficiency is inherited in an autosomal recessive manner.

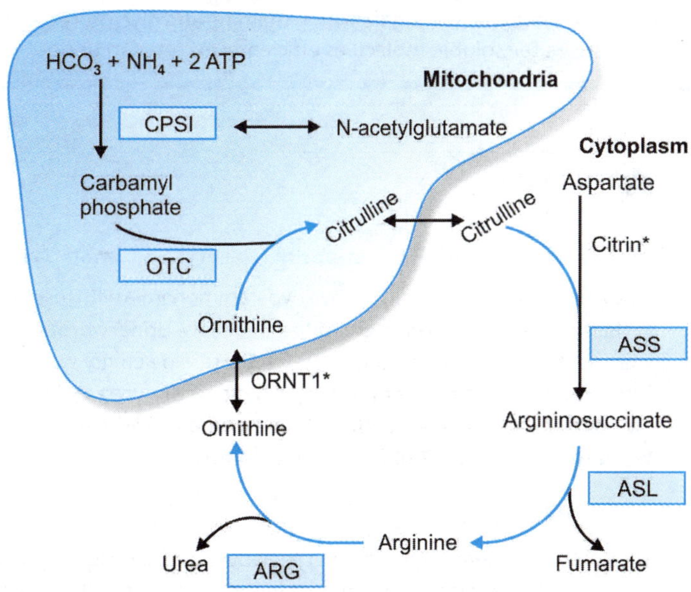

Fig. 6.2: Reactions of urea cycle. The sites for citrin and ornithine deficiency are marked (*).

Ornithine Translocase Deficiency (HHH Syndrome)

The HHH (hyperornithinemia, hyperammonemia, homocitrullinuria) syndrome is an autosomal recessive disorder described in more than 50 individuals.

Symptoms result from hyperammonemia and resemble those of the urea cycle disorders. Most affected individuals have intermittent hyperammonemia accompanied by vomiting, lethargy, and coma (in extreme cases). Growth is abnormal and intellectual development is affected. Spasticity and seizures are common. Adults with partial activity of the enzyme typically self-select low-protein diets.

Ornithine translocase deficiency results in diminished ornithine transport into the mitochondria; reduced intramitochondrial ornithine causes orotic aciduria and impaired ureagenesis. Plasma ornithine concentrations are extremely high, but diagnosis can be complicated because plasma ornithine concentrations can normalize on a protein-restricted diet. The presence of hyperammonemia and homocitrullinuria is helpful in diagnosis. Homocitrulline is thought to originate from the transcarbamylation of lysine.

Prevention of Primary Manifestations of Hyperammonemia

The prevention of catabolism is a key goal of treatment to prevent hyperammonemic episodes. Long-term management is focused on restriction of dietary protein through use of specialized formulas and administration of oral nitrogen-scavenging drugs.

Prognosis

Prognosis is bad in the undiagnosed and untreated cases.

CLINICAL NOTE

Plasma concentration of citrulline helps discriminate between the proximal and distal urea cycle defects, as citrulline is the product of the proximal enzymes (OTC and CPS-I) and a substrate for the distal enzymes (ASS, ASL, and ARG).

CLINICAL PEARLS

1. Complete absence of any of the enzymes of urea cycle usually causes severe hyperammonemia in newborns, while milder variants can be seen in adults.
2. The accumulation of ammonia and glutamine leads to brain edema and direct neuronal toxicity.
3. Deficiencies in urea cycle enzymes are individually rare, but as a group they affect about 1:25,000 individuals.
4. They are all transmitted as autosomal recessive traits, with the exception of ornithine transcarbamoylase deficiency, which is X-linked.
5. Therapy is aimed at stopping catabolism and ammonia production by providing adequate calories (as intravenous glucose and lipids in the comatose patient) and, if needed, insulin. Excess nitrogen is removed by intravenous phenylacetate and benzoate that conjugate with glutamine and glycine, respectively, to form phenylacetylglutamine and hippuric acid, which are water-soluble molecules efficiently excreted in urine.

CASE STUDY 2

Theme: Clinical Implications of N-Acetyl Glutamate Synthase Deficiency

A newborn infant was found to have hyperammonemia with respiratory alkalosis. An inherited defect in the urea cycle was suspected.

Plasma citrulline levels were found to be low. Urinary orotate concentration was found to be normal. Extracts of a liver biopsy were assayed for N-acetyl glutamate synthase. No activity was found.

What relationship does this enzyme have to the urea cycle?

The patient was treated with sodium benzoate and sodium phenyl acetate.

What is the rationale behind this treatment?

CASE DISCUSSION

The cause of hyperammonemia in the baby is due to N-acetyl glutamate synthase deficiency **(Fig. 6.3)**. Since the plasma citrulline levels are low, this indicates a defect in the urea cycle rather than transient hyperammonemia. It also rules out the involvement of certain other urea cycle enzymes. Urinary orotic acid concentration is normal, so this also rules out the deficiency of carbamoyl phosphate synthase I and other subsequent enzymes of urea cycle, because in defects of urea cycle enzymes, orotic acid concentration rises in urine. So most probably, the cause of hyperammonemia is N-acetyl glutamate synthase deficiency.

N-Acetyl Glutamate Synthase Deficiency

It is an autosomal recessive urea cycle disorder. The cause for this disorder is a single base deletion that leads to frame shift mutation, and thus the error in gene's coding for this specific enzyme.

Pathogenesis

Carbamoyl phosphate synthase I is an enzyme found in mitochondrial matrix and it catalyzes the very first reaction of the urea cycle, in which carbamoyl phosphate is produced.

Carbamoyl phosphate synthase I, abbreviated as CPS-I, is activated by its natural activator N-acetyl glutamate, which in turn is synthesized from acetyl-CoA and glutamic acid in the reaction catalyzed by N-acetyl glutamate synthase, commonly called NAGS. N-acetyl glutamate is required for the urea cycle to take place. **(Fig. 6.3)**

Deficiency in N-acetyl glutamate synthase or a genetic mutation in the gene coding for the enzyme, will lead to urea cycle failure in which ammonia is not converted to urea, but rather accumulated in blood leading to the condition called type I hyperammonemia. This is a severe neonatal disorder with fatal consequences, if not detected immediately upon birth.

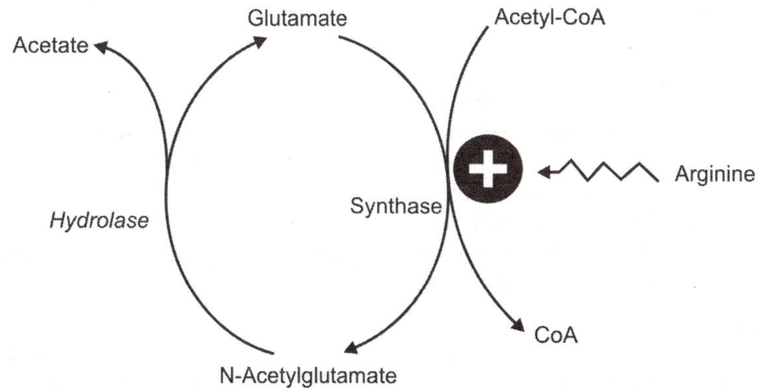

Fig. 6.3: Reaction catalyzed by N-Acetyl glutamate synthase (NAG synthase) and NAG hydrolase-6.

Clinical Manifestations

The symptoms are visible within the 1st week of life and early symptoms include lethargy, vomiting, and deep coma. The other symptoms are hypotonia, convulsions, and later coma. If not detected and diagnosed correctly immediately, the consequences are fatal.

Novel Treatment

Although there is currently no cure, treatment includes injections of structurally similar compound, N-carbamoyl-L-glutamate, an analog of N-acetylglutamate. This analog likewise activates CPS-I. This treatment mitigates the intensity of the disorder.

If symptoms are detected early enough and the patient is injected with this compound, levels of severe mental retardation can be slightly lessened, but brain damage is irreversible.

Sodium benzoate and phenyl acetate are given to treat hyperammonemia. These substances act to trap ammonium ions as glycine and glutamine and convert them to forms that are readily excreted by the kidney.

Reactions

Benzoate + Glycine → Hippuric acid

Phenylacetic acid+ Glutamine → Phenylacetylglutamine

Both glycine and glutamine are nonessential amino acids that can be synthesized by the human body from nonprotein metabolites. Glycine eliminates one nitrogen molecule per mole. These two substances have proven to be useful in the treatment of hyperammonemia.

PROGNOSIS

Prognosis is bad, if the diagnosis is delayed.

CLINICAL NOTE

Carbamoyl phosphate synthase I is an enzyme found in mitochondrial matrix and it catalyzes the very first reaction of the urea cycle, in which carbamoyl phosphate is produced.

CLINICAL PEARLS

1. The cause for this disorder is a single base deletion that leads to frame shift mutation, and thus the error in gene's coding for this specific enzyme.
2. Deficiency in N-acetyl glutamate synthase or a genetic mutation in the gene coding for the enzyme, will lead to urea cycle failure in which ammonia is not converted to urea, but rather accumulated in blood leading to the condition called type I hyperammonemia.
3. Sodium benzoate and phenyl acetate are given to treat hyperammonemia. These substances act to trap ammonium ions as glycine and glutamine and convert them to forms that are readily excreted by the kidney.
4. Both glycine and glutamine are nonessential amino acids that can be synthesized by the human body from nonprotein metabolites. Glycine eliminates one nitrogen molecule per mole. These two substances have proven to be useful in the treatment of hyperammonemia.
5. Prognosis is bad, if the diagnosis is delayed.

CASE STUDY 3

Theme: Clinical Significance of Impaired Tyrosine Metabolism

A 2-week-old child was brought to the emergency. The parents were fearful that the child had been given some poison as they noted black discoloration on the diaper. They had delayed disposing one of the child's diapers and noted black discoloration where the urine had collected. Later, they realized that all of the child's diapers would turn black if kept unwashed for a longer time.

The attending pediatrician examined the child and explained them that it was due to an amino acid disorder.

Which amino acid pathway is implicated in this phenomenon? What is the cause of blackening of the diapers? How can this defect be treated?

CASE DISCUSSION

The baby is suffering from alkaptonuria/black urine disease. This disease was first identified by Archibald Garrod (Garrod first coined the term "inborn error in metabolism" to describe this and other congenital, inherited disorders that affect metabolic pathways).

Alkaptonuria: Alkaptonuria is a rare genetic disease that is characterized by passing urine that becomes black when left standing. The earliest sign of the condition is usually dark staining found in nappies or diapers of infants.

The most obvious sign in adults is a thickening and blue-black discoloration of the ear cartilage. **This blue-black discoloration of connective tissue (including bone, cartilage, and skin) is caused by deposits of yellow or ochre-colored pigment, and is called ochronosis (Fig. 6.4).**

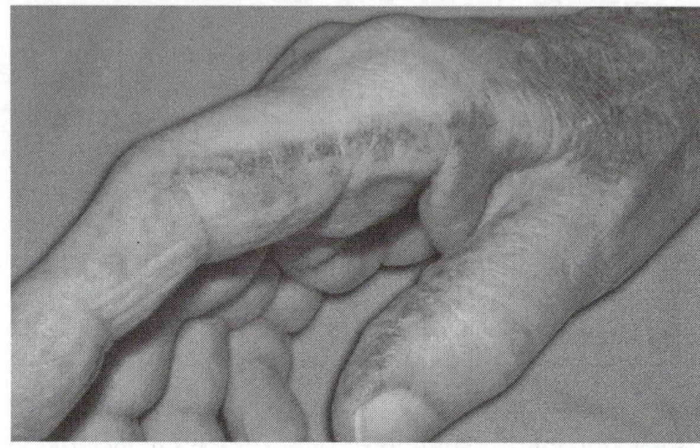

Fig. 6.4: Ochronosis—The blue-black discoloration of connective tissue (including bone, cartilage, and skin) is caused by deposits of yellow or ochre-colored pigment.

Biochemical Defect

Alkaptonuria is an autosomal recessive inherited disorder that is **caused by a defect in the enzyme homogentisic acid oxidase.** The enzyme normally breaks down a toxic tyrosine by-product, homogentisic acid (also called alkapton), which is harmful to bones and cartilages. The defect causes the body not to produce enough of the enzyme as a result, homogentisic acid remains in the body, and slowly and progressively get deposited in bones and cartilage where it turns into a pigmented polymeric material.

These polymerized homogentisic acid products are excreted in large amounts in urine and impart the black color to baby's diapers.

Clinical Manifestations

Most patients do not have any symptoms throughout childhood or early adult life, and it is not until they reach their 40's that other signs of the disease start appearing.

- One of the earliest signs is thickening of the ear cartilage (the pinna feels noticeably thickened and flexible).
  In addition, the skin turns to blue-black color **(Fig. 6.5)**.
- Earwax is often reddish-brown or jet-black. Gradually patients will suffer sore joints, leading to arthropathy (joint disease characterized by swelling and enlarged bones). Many body parts become affected due to the buildup of pigment deposits in bones and cartilage.
- Bones and cartilage of the lower back, knees, shoulders, and hips are most affected. Firstly, patients suffer low back pain with stiffness, followed by knee, shoulder, and hip pain over the next 10 years. Cartilage becomes brittle and can break apart easily. In some cases, this leads to spinal injuries such as prolapsed intervertebral disks.
- Deposits around the trachea, larynx, and bronchi may cause shortness of breath and difficulty in breathing.
- Deposits around the heart and blood vessels can calcify and lead to atherosclerotic plaques.

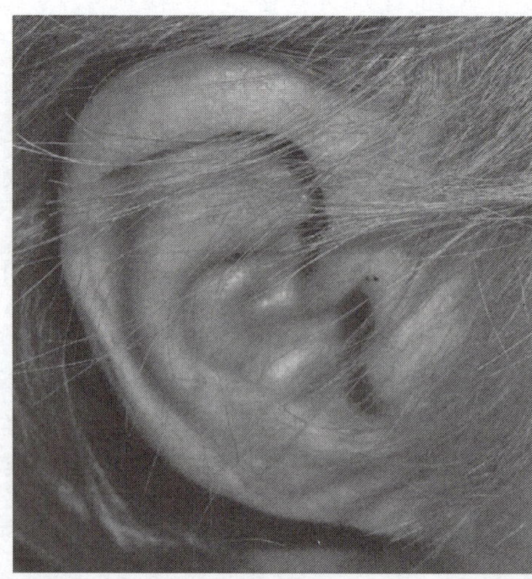

Fig. 6.5: Showing blackening of the ear cartilage.

- Pigmentation of the sclera of the eye usually occurs early on **(Fig. 6.7)**. This does not affect vision but appears as brown or gray deposits on the surface of the eye.
- Skin color changes are most apparent on areas exposed to the sun and where sweat glands are found.
- Urine exposed to air can become dark **(Figs. 6.6A and B)**; this is useful for diagnosing young children using diapers.

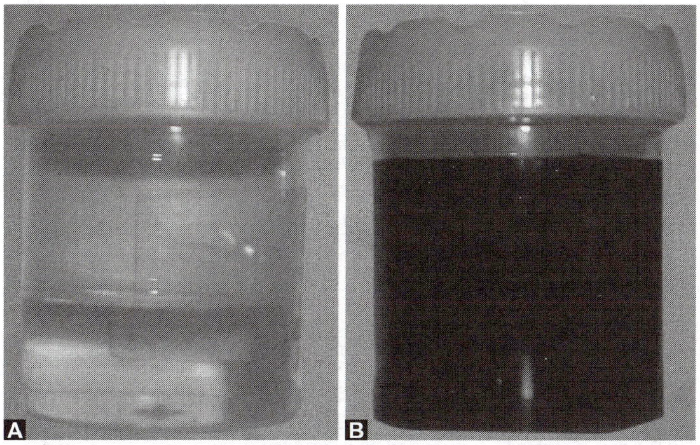

Figs. 6.6A and B: Darkening of urine on standing.

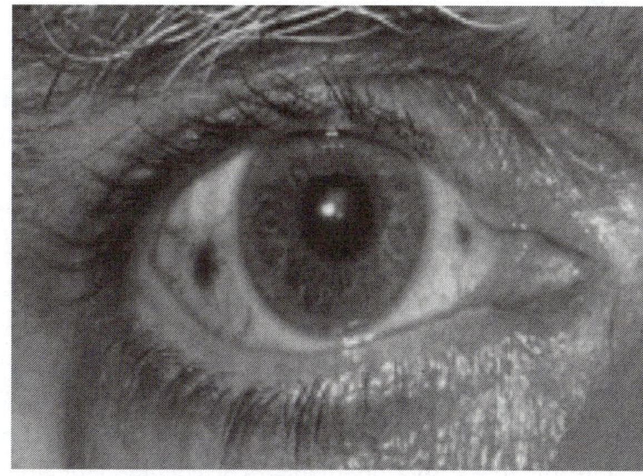

Fig. 6.7: Pigmentation of the sclera.

- In adulthood, but usually not before age of 40, persons suffering from alkaptonuria develop progressive arthritis (especially of the spine), due to the long-term buildup of homogentisate in bones and cartilage. The urine is malodorous.

Diagnosis

Presumptive diagnosis can be made by adding sodium or potassium hydroxide to urine and observing the formation of a dark brown to black pigment on the surface layer of urine within 30 minutes to 1 hour.

Diagnosis can be confirmed by demonstrating the presence of homogentisic acid in the urine. This may be done by paper chromatography and thin-layer chromatography.

Treatment

Alkaptonuria is a lifelong disease. There is no cure for the condition. Prevention is not possible and the treatment is aimed at ameliorating symptoms. **Reducing intake of the amino acids like phenylalanine and tyrosine to the minimum required to sustain health (phenylalanine is an essential amino acid) can help slow the progression of the disease. Vitamin C has been found to slow down the conversion of homogentisic acid to the polymeric deposits in cartilage and bone. A dose of up to 1 g/day is recommended for older children and adults.**

Prognosis

Life expectancy is normal, although patients may be at increased risk of heart conditions and may require surgical treatments for spine, hip, knee, and shoulder joint problems. Exogenous cutaneous ochronosis has been successfully treated by laser.

CLINICAL NOTE

The most obvious signs in adults are thickening and blue-black discoloration of the ear cartilage. This blue-black discoloration of connective tissue (including bone, cartilage, and skin) is caused by deposits of yellow or ochre-colored pigment and is called ochronosis.

CLINICAL PEARLS

1. Alkaptonuria is a rare genetic disease that is characterized by passing urine that becomes black when left standing.
2. It is an autosomal recessive disorder that is caused by a defect in the enzyme homogentisic acid oxidase.
3. One of the earliest signs is thickening of the ear cartilage (the pinna feels noticeably thickened and flexible). In addition, the skin turns to blue-black color.
4. Diagnosis can be confirmed by demonstrating the presence of homogentisic acid in the urine. This may be done by paper chromatography and thin-layer chromatography.
5. Reducing intake of the amino acids phenylalanine and tyrosine to the minimum required to sustain health can help slow the progression of the disease. Vitamin C has been found to slow down the conversion of homogentisic acid to the polymeric deposits in cartilage and bone.

CASE STUDY 4

Theme: Clinical Implications of Impaired Melanin Synthesis

A 2-month-old baby girl was brought by her parents for consultation. She had pale skin, blonde hair, and pink iris. The baby girl was otherwise healthy, feeding well but was unable to fix the gaze. Parents revealed that their first two children, a boy and a girl, had complete albinism, but the parents themselves were normal.

The eye examination of the child showed absence of pigment in the retina. A diagnosis of albinism was made for the child.

What is the defect in albinism?
What is the pattern of inheritance?
How can this disease be treated?

CASE DISCUSSION

Normal parents having two affected children, male and female, is suggestive of autosomal recessive inheritance of oculocutaneous albinism. The baby has defect in the synthesis of melanin. Pale skin, blonde hair, and pink color of iris, are due to the absence of melanin. The visual impairment is also typical of albinism.

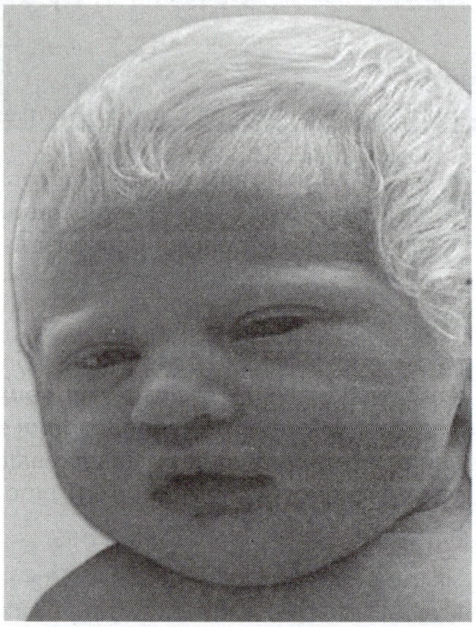

Fig. 6.8: A child with oculocutaneous albinism.

Albinism

Albinism is a defect of melanin production that results in little or no color (pigment) in the skin, hair, and eyes.

Biochemical Defect

Albinism was formerly categorized as tyrosinase-positive or -negative. In cases of tyrosinase-positive albinism, the enzyme tyrosinase is present. The melanocytes (pigment cells) are unable to produce melanin for any one of a variety of reasons that do not directly involve the tyrosinase enzyme. In tyrosinase-negative cases, either the tyrosinase enzyme is not produced or a nonfunctional version is produced. This classification has been rendered obsolete by recent research.

Classification

There are two main categories of albinism in humans:

- **In oculocutaneous albinism,** pigment is lacking in the eyes, skin, and hair **(Fig. 6.8)**. (The equivalent mutation in nonhumans also results in lack of melanin in the fur, scales or feathers.) People with oculocutaneous albinism can have anywhere from no pigment at all to almost normal levels.
- **In ocular albinism**, only the eyes lack pigment. People who have ocular albinism have generally normal skin and hair color, although it is typically lighter than either parent. Many even have a normal eye appearance.

Hermansky–Pudlak syndrome (HPS) is a form of albinism caused by a single gene. It can occur with a bleeding disorder, as well as with lung and bowel diseases.

Other complex diseases may lead to loss of coloring in only a certain area (localized albinism). These conditions include:

- **Chediak–Higashi syndrome (lack of coloring all over the skin, but not complete)**
- **Tuberous sclerosis** (small areas without skin coloring)
- **Waardenburg syndrome** (often a lock of hair that grows on the forehead, or no coloring in one or both irises).

Inheritance

Most forms of albinism are the result of the biological inheritance of genetically recessive alleles (genes) passed from both parents of an individual, though some rare forms are inherited from only one parent.

There are other genetic mutations which are proven to be associated with albinism. All alterations, however, lead to changes in melanin production in the body.

Albinism usually occurs with equal frequency in both genders. An exception to this is ocular albinism, because it is passed on to offspring through X-linked inheritance. Thus, males more frequently have ocular albinism as they do not have a second X chromosome.

Frequency

Overall, an estimated 1 in 20,000 people worldwide are born with oculocutaneous albinism. The condition affects people in many ethnic groups and geographical regions.

Clinical Manifestations

A person with albinism will have one of the following symptoms:
- Absence of coloring from the hair, skin, or iris of the eye.
- Lighter than normal skin and hair.
- Patchy areas of depigmentation.
- Long-term sun exposure greatly increases the risk of skin damage and skin cancers, including an aggressive form of skin cancer called melanoma, in people with this condition.

Many forms of albinism are associated with the following symptoms:
- Crossed eyes (strabismus)
- Light sensitivity (photophobia)
- Rapid eye movements (nystagmus)
- Refractive errors such as myopia or hyperopia, and especially astigmatism are more likely
- Functional blindness can also occur.

Diagnosis

The diagnosis of the condition is based on the appearance of skin, hair, and eyes.

Genetic testing offers the most accurate way to diagnose albinism and its type. Such testing is helpful, if there is a family history of albinism, and is also useful for certain populations known to get the disease.

Treatment

The goal of treatment is to relieve symptoms. Treatment involves protecting the skin and eyes from the sun:
- To reduce sunburn risk by avoiding the sun, using sunscreen, and covering up completely with clothing when exposed to the sun.
- Sunscreen should have a high sun protection factor (SPF).
- Sunglasses (UV protected) may relieve light sensitivity.
- Optical correction of refractive errors, tinted or pinhole contact lenses, absorptive lenses optical aids, and lowered illumination if needed.

Prevention

Genetic counseling is recommended.

Prognosis

It is nonprogressive. Albinism does not usually affect lifespan. Hermansky–Pudlak syndrome can, however, shorten lifespan due to lung disease or bleeding problems.

People with albinism may be limited in their activities because they cannot tolerate the sun.

CLINICAL NOTE

In tyrosinase-negative cases, either the tyrosinase enzyme is not produced or a nonfunctional version is produced

CLINICAL PEARLS

1. Albinism is a defect of melanin production that results in little or no pigment in the skin, hair, and eyes.
2. Albinism usually occurs with equal frequency in both genders. An exception to this is ocular albinism, because it is passed on to offspring through X-linked inheritance. Thus, males more frequently have ocular albinism as they do not have a second X chromosome.
3. In oculocutaneous albinism, pigment is lacking in the eyes, skin, and hair while in ocular albinism, only the eyes lack pigment. People who have ocular albinism have generally normal skin and hair color, although it is typically lighter than either parent.
4. The diagnosis of the condition is based on the appearance of skin, hair, and eyes. Genetic testing offers the most accurate way to diagnose albinism and its type.
5. Treatment involves protecting the skin and eyes from the sun.

CASE STUDY 5

Theme: Clinical Implications of Impaired Tyrosine Synthesis

A 2-week-old infant with refusal to feeds, lethargy, excessive cry, and irritability, responded positively to a test for phenylketonuria. A diagnosis of classical phenylketonuria (PKU) was made and the child was maintained on a low phenylalanine diet.

Serum phenylalanine was 30 mg/dL and tyrosine was 2 mg/dL. Ferric chloride test was positive for urine. A diagnosis of classical phenylketonuria (PKU) was made and the child was maintained on a low phenylalanine diet.

What enzymatic reactions are defective in the patient with PKU?
What are the physiological consequences of PKU and why it should be detected as early as possible?
What is the treatment for this disease?

CASE DISCUSSION

Phenylketonuria

Phenylketonuria (PKU) is an inherited error of metabolism caused by deficiency of the enzyme phenylalanine hydroxylase. Loss of this enzyme results in mental retardation, organ damage, and unusual posture and in cases of maternal PKU, it can result in severely compromised pregnancy.

Incidence

Classic PKU and the other causes of hyperphenylalaninemia affect about one of every 10,000–20,000 Caucasian or Oriental births. The incidence in African-Americans is far less. These disorders are equally frequent in males and females.

Biochemical Defect

Deficiency of the enzyme phenylalanine hydroxylase or of its cofactor tetrahydrobiopterin causes accumulation of phenylalanine in body fluids and the central nervous system (CNS) (Fig. 6.9).

The severity of hyperphenylalaninemia depends on the degree of enzyme deficiency and may vary from very high plasma concentrations (>20 mg/dL, or >1200 μM, "classic PKU") to mildly elevated levels (2–6 mg/ dL or 120–360 μM). In affected infants with plasma concentrations over 20 mg/dL, excess phenylalanine is metabolized to phenylketones (phenylpyruvate) and phenyl acetate; that are excreted in the urine, giving rise to the term phenylketonuria (PKU). These metabolites have no role in pathogenesis of CNS damage in patients with PKU, and their presence in body fluids simply signifies the severity of the condition.

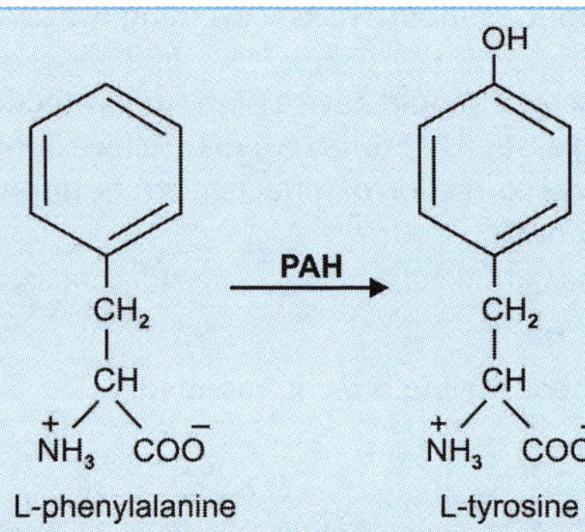

The enzyme phenylalanine hydroxylase converts the amino acid phenylalanine to tyrosine

Fig. 6.9: Conversion of phenylalanine to tyrosine.

The brain is the main organ affected by hyperphenylalaninemia. **The CNS damage in affected patients is caused by the elevated concentration of phenylalanine in brain tissue, which interferes with the transport of other large neutral amino acids (tyrosine, tryptophan) into the brain.**

Clinical Manifestations

Classical Phenylketonuria

The affected infant is normal at birth. **Mental retardation** may develop gradually and may not be evident for the first few months. It is usually severe, and most patients require institutional care if the condition remains untreated. **Vomiting**, sometimes severe enough to be misdiagnosed as pyloric stenosis, may be an early symptom. Older untreated children become hyperactive with purposeless movements, rhythmic rocking, and athetosis.

On physical examination, these infants are fairer in their complexion than unaffected siblings. Some may have a **seborrheic or eczematous rash,** which is usually mild and disappears as the child grows older. These children have an **unpleasant odor** of phenylacetic acid, which has been described as musty or mousy. There are no consistent findings on neurologic examination. However, most infants are hypertonic with hyperactive deep tendon reflexes. About 25% of children have seizures, and more than 50% have electroencephalographic abnormalities. **Microcephaly, prominent maxilla with widely spaced teeth, enamel hypoplasia, and growth retardation** are other common findings in untreated children.

Milder forms of PKU

1. **Non-PKU hyperphenylalaninemia:** In any screening program for PKU, a group of infants are identified in whom initial plasma concentrations of phenylalanine are above normal (2 mg/dL, 120 μM) but less than 20 mg/dL (1,200 μM). These infants do not

excrete phenylketones. Clinically, these infants may remain asymptomatic but progressive brain damage may occur gradually with age. **These patients have milder deficiencies of phenylalanine hydroxylase or its cofactor tetrahydrobiopterin (BH4) than those with classic PKU.** As with classic PKU, deficiency of BH4 should be investigated in all infants with milder forms of hyperphenylalaninemia.

2. **Hyperphenylalaninemia from deficiency of the cofactor tetrahydrobiopterin (BH4):** In 1–2% of infants with hyperphenylalaninemia, the defect resides in one of the enzymes necessary for production or recycling of the cofactor BH4. These infants are diagnosed as having PKU, but they deteriorate neurologically despite adequate control of plasma phenylalanine. BH4 is the cofactor for phenylalanine, tyrosine, and tryptophan hydroxylase. The latter two hydroxylase are essential for biosynthesis of the neurotransmitters, dopamine and serotonin.
   Plasma phenylalanine levels may be as high as those in classic PKU or in the range of milder forms of hyperphenylalaninemia. Neurologic manifestations, such as loss of head control, truncal hypotonia (floppy baby), drooling, swallowing difficulties, and myoclonic seizures, develop after 3 months of age despite adequate dietary therapy.
3. **Maternal phenylketonuria:** A number of women with phenylketonuria who have been treated since infancy will reach adulthood and become pregnant. If maternal phenylalanine levels are not strictly controlled before and during pregnancy, their offspring are at increased risk for congenital defects and microcephaly. After birth, these children have severe mental and growth retardation. Pregnancy risks can be minimized by continuing lifelong phenylalanine-restricted diets and assuring strict phenylalanine restriction 2 months prior to conception and throughout gestation.

Diagnosis

Because of gradual development of clinical manifestations of hyperphenylalaninemia, early diagnosis can only be achieved by mass screening of all newborn infants.

Neonatal Screening for Hyperphenylalaninemia

The bacterial inhibition assay of Guthrie, which was the first and still the most widely used method for the purpose, is being replaced by more precise and quantitative methods (fluorometric and tandem mass spectrometry). **Blood phenylalanine in affected infants with PKU may rise to diagnostic levels as early as 4 hours after birth, even in the absence of protein feeding.** It is recommended, however, that the blood for screening be obtained in the first 24–48 hours of life after feeding protein to reduce the possibility of false-negative results, especially in the milder forms of the condition.

Plasma phenylalanine levels: In infants with positive results from the screen for hyperphenylalaninemia, diagnosis should be confirmed by quantitative measurement of plasma phenylalanine. A normal blood phenylalanine level is about 1 mg/dL. In classic PKU, levels may range from 6 mg/dL to 80 mg/dL, but are usually greater than 30 mg/dL. Levels are somewhat less in the other disorders of hyperphenylalaninemia.

Identification and measurement of phenylketones in the urine has no place in any screening program. However, in countries and places where such programs are not in effect, identification of phenylketones in the urine by ferric chloride may offer a simple test for diagnosis of infants with developmental and neurologic abnormalities.

Once the diagnosis of hyperphenylalaninemia is established, deficiency of cofactor (BH4) should be ruled out in all affected infants.

BH4 loading test: An oral dose of BH4 (20 mg/kg) normalizes plasma phenylalanine in patients with BH4 deficiency within 4 to 8 hours.

Enzyme assay: The activity of dihydropteridine reductase can be measured in the dry blood spots on the filter paper, used for screening purposes. The other enzymes required for the synthesis of BH4 can also be similarly estimated.

Treatment

The goal of PKU treatment is to maintain the blood level of phenylalanine between 2 mg/dL and 10 mg/dL. Some phenylalanine is needed for normal growth. This requires a diet that has some phenylalanine but in much lower amounts than normal.

High-protein foods, such as meat, fish, poultry, eggs, cheese, milk, dried beans, and peas are avoided. Instead, measured amounts of cereals, starches, fruits, and vegetables, along with a milk substitute are usually recommended.

In some clinics, a phenylalanine "challenge" may be suggested to evaluate whether or not the child continues to require a low phenylalanine diet. This test identifies those few persons with a transient or "variant" form of the disorder.

No dietary restriction is currently recommended for infants whose phenylalanine levels are between 2 mg/dL and 6 mg/dL. Plasma concentrations of phenylalanine in treated patients should be maintained as close to normal as possible.

Because phenylalanine is not synthesized by the body, "over treatment" may lead to phenylalanine deficiency manifested by lethargy, failure to thrive, anorexia, anemia, rashes, diarrhea, and even death; moreover, tyrosine becomes an essential amino acid in this disorder and its adequate intake must be ensured.

The current recommendation is that all patients be kept on a phenylalanine-restricted diet for life, in order to promote maximal development and cognitive abilities.

Oral administration of the cofactor (BH4) to patients with milder forms of hyperphenylalaninemia from phenylalanine hydroxylase deficiency may produce significant reductions.

CLINICAL NOTE

In infants with positive results from the screening for hyperphenylalaninemia, diagnosis should be confirmed by quantitative measurement of plasma phenylalanine.

CLINICAL PEARLS

1. Phenylketonuria (PKU) is an inherited error of metabolism caused by deficiency of the enzyme phenylalanine hydroxylase.
2. Loss of this enzyme results in mental retardation, organ damage, and unusual posture and in cases of maternal PKU, it can result in severely compromised pregnancy.
3. However, most infants are hypertonic with hyperactive deep tendon reflexes. About 25% of children have seizures, and more than 50% have electroencephalographic abnormalities. Microcephaly, prominent maxilla with widely spaced teeth, enamel hypoplasia, and growth retardation are other common findings in untreated children.
4. Blood phenylalanine in affected infants with PKU may rise to diagnostic levels as early as 4 hours after birth even in the absence of protein feeding.
5. The goal of PKU treatment is to maintain the blood level of phenylalanine between 2 and 10 mg/dL. Some phenylalanine is needed for normal growth. This requires a diet that has some phenylalanine but in much lower amounts than normal.

CASE STUDY 6

Theme: Clinical Implications of Tryptophan Absorption Defect

A 12-year-old boy was admitted to the hospital with a red scaly rash and mild cerebellar ataxia. His mother thought that the boy is suffering from pellagra because the same symptoms in her older daughter had been diagnosed earlier. The boy did not have the usual dietary deficiency form of pellagra, but large amounts of free amino acids were found in his urine. When the older daughter had a recurrent attack of ataxia, it was found that her urine also contained excessive amount of amino acids. Two other siblings had the same aminoaciduria; however, four others were normal. The parents were asymptomatic, but a family history revealed that they were first cousins.

Assuming that this defect is inherited, what abnormality could account for the unusual amount of amino acids in urine and what is its relationship with pellagra-like rashes?

How can this defect be treated?

CASE DISCUSSION

The boy is suffering from Hartnup disease.

Hartnup disease is an autosomal recessive disorder caused by impaired neutral (i.e. monoamino monocarboxylic) amino acid transport in the apical brush border membrane of the small intestine and the proximal tubule of the kidney. Patients present with pellagra-like skin eruptions, cerebellar ataxia, and gross aminoaciduria.

The disorder was first observed in the Hartnup family of London; 4 of the 8 family members presented with aminoaciduria, a rash resembling pellagra, and cerebellar ataxia.

Hartnup Disease

Inheritance

Hartnup disease is inherited as an autosomal recessive trait. Heterozygotes are normal. Consanguinity is common. The causative gene, *SLC6A19* is defective. **Mutations in the *SLC6A19* gene, which encodes the B0 AT1, sodium-dependent, chloride-independent, neutral amino acid transporter, cause a failure of the transport of neutral amino acids in the small intestine and the renal tubules.**

Pathogenesis

A person with Hartnup disease cannot absorb amino acids properly from the intestine and tubules in the kidneys. Excessive amounts of amino acids, such as tryptophan, are excreted in the urine. The body is thus left with inadequate amounts of amino acids, which are the building blocks of proteins.

With too little tryptophan in the blood, the body is unable to make a sufficient amount of the B complex vitamin niacinamide, particularly under stress when more vitamins are needed. As a result, tryptophan and niacin deficiencies generate similar symptoms.

Amino acids are retained within the intestinal lumen, where they are converted by bacteria to indolic compounds that can be toxic to the CNS. Tryptophan is converted to indole in the intestine. Following absorption, indole is converted to 3-hydroxyindole (i.e. indoxyl, indican) in the liver, where it is conjugated with potassium sulfate or glucuronic acid. Subsequently, it is transported to the kidneys for excretion (i.e. Indicanuria).

Other tryptophan degradation products, including kynurenine and serotonin, are also excreted in the urine. Tubular renal transport is also defective, contributing to gross aminoaciduria. Neutral amino acids are also found in the feces.

Frequency

With an overall prevalence of 1 case per 24,000 population (range, 1 case per 18,000–42,000 population), Hartnup disease ranks among the most common amino acid disorders in humans.

Clinical Manifestations

Hartnup disease manifests during infancy with variable clinical presentation: failure to thrive, photosensitivity, intermittent ataxia, nystagmus, and tremor. **Symptoms may be triggered by sunlight, fever, drugs, or emotional or physical stress. A period of poor nutrition nearly always precedes an attack. Most symptoms occur sporadically and are caused by a deficiency of niacinamide.**

A rash develops on parts of the body exposed to the sun. Mental retardation, short stature, headaches, unsteady gait, and collapsing or fainting are common. Psychiatric problems (such as anxiety, rapid mood changes, delusions, and hallucinations) may also result. Cutaneous signs usually precede the neurological manifestations.

Diagnosis

Urine analysis: Neutral amino acids, tryptophan, indole derivatives, and tryptophan degradation products are present in urine.

Treatment

A high-protein diet can overcome the deficient transport of neutral amino acids in most patients. Poor nutrition leads to more frequent and more severe attacks of the disease, which is otherwise asymptomatic. Avoiding excessive exposure to sunlight, wearing protective clothing, and using physical and chemical sunscreens are mandatory. Advise patients to avoid other aggravating factors, such as photosensitizing drugs, as much as possible. In patients with niacin deficiency and symptomatic disease, daily supplementation with nicotinic acid or nicotinamide reduces both number and severity of attacks. Neurological and psychiatric treatment is needed in patients with severe CNS involvement.

Prognosis

Hartnup disease is manifested by a wide clinical spectrum. Most patients remain asymptomatic, but, in a minority of patients, skin photosensitivity, and neurological and psychiatric symptoms may have a considerable influence on quality of life. Rarely, severe CNS involvement may lead to death.

CLINICAL NOTE

Symptoms of Hartnup disease may be triggered by sunlight, fever, drugs, emotional or physical stress. A period of poor nutrition nearly always precedes an attack. Most symptoms occur sporadically and are caused by a deficiency of niacinamide.

CLINICAL PEARLS

1. Hartnup disease is an autosomal recessive disorder caused by impaired neutral (i.e. monoamino monocarboxylic) amino acid transport in the apical brush border membrane of the small intestine and the proximal tubule of the kidney.
2. Patients present with pellagra-like skin eruptions, cerebellar ataxia, and gross aminoaciduria.
3. A rash develops on parts of the body exposed to the sun. Mental retardation, short stature, headaches, unsteady gait, and collapsing or fainting are common. Psychiatric problems (such as anxiety, rapid mood changes, delusions, and hallucinations) may also result. Cutaneous signs usually precede the neurological manifestations.
4. Neutral amino acids, tryptophan, indole derivatives, and tryptophan degradation products are present in urine.
5. A high-protein diet can overcome the deficient transport of neutral amino acids in most patients.

CASE STUDY 7

Theme: Clinical Implications of Hyperactive Serotonin Pathway

A 54-year-old postmenopausal woman, presented to internist for care of hot flashes that have returned 2 years after menopause. The symptoms occurred mostly after meals, when she drank wine, or when she went for running. There was history of hypertension and frequent diarrheas also. The patient was referred to gynecologist. The general physical examination was entirely normal. Hormone-replacement therapy (HRT) was prescribed to the patient and she was referred to gastroenterologist (GI) for irritable bowel syndrome (IBS) treatment. She experienced 2 hot flashes with no sweating during the examination.

Patient returned 3 months later with no improvement in hot flashes. A different formulation of HRT was prescribed. Patient returned to GI doctor 1 year later with worsening of her IBS. Patient reported cramping, abdominal pain, and increased episodes of diarrhea. She had to wake up at night with diarrhea. Patient discontinued her HRT although they were ineffective. After 1 year, patient was in need of emergency care. She presented with acute bowel obstruction and was taken to the operating room.

There was marked fibrosis of the terminal ileum with multiple hairpin turns of the bowel and a small tumor in the terminal ileum. Pathological report concluded that the patient had carcinoid syndrome.

What is the probable defect in carcinoid syndrome?
How can this be diagnosed at the earliest possible? What is the biochemical basis for all the clinical manifestations?
What is the prognosis of this disease?

CASE DISCUSSION

Carcinoid Syndrome

Carcinoid syndrome refers to the array of symptoms that occur secondary to carcinoid tumors.

Carcinoid tumors are discrete, yellow, well-circumscribed tumors that can occur anywhere along the gastrointestinal tract and in the lung. They most commonly affect the appendix, ileum, and rectum. Carcinoids are tumors of neuroendocrine nature that originate in the cells of the neuroendocrine system and are characterized by production of serotonin (5-hydroxytryptamine; 5-HT).

Incidence

Although quite rare with 15 cases/1,000,000 population, carcinoid tumors account for 75% of gastrointestinal endocrine tumors.

Clinical Presentation

Although it is the most common systemic clinical manifestation of **carcinoid tumors, carcinoid syndrome occurs in fewer than 10% of patients with carcinoid tumors, and becomes manifested when vasoactive substances from the tumors enter the systemic circulation escaping hepatic degradation.** This is the case when carcinoid tumors metastasize to the liver or they arise, for example in the bronchus.

The most important clinical finding is **flushing of the skin**, usually of the head and the upper part of thorax. **Secretory diarrhea and abdominal cramps** are also characteristic features of the syndrome. When the diarrhea is intensive, it may lead to electrolyte disturbance and dehydration. Other associated symptoms are nausea and vomiting. **Bronchoconstriction** affects a smaller number of patients and often accompanies flushing.

About 50% of patients have cardiac abnormalities, caused by **serotonin-induced fibrosis of the tricuspid and pulmonary valves**. Elevated levels of circulating serotonin have been associated with cardiac failure, due to fibrous deposits on the endocardium. These deposits are thought to be responsible for the fibrous degeneration of the valve apparatus. "TIPS" is an acronym for tricuspid insufficiency and pulmonary stenosis (fibrosis of tricuspid and pulmonary valves).

The likelihood of occurrence and the associated severity of carcinoid syndrome depend on several factors: tumor size, whether its location is in an area draining into the systemic circulation, and the degree of metastasis.

Carcinoid syndrome exhibits slow growth with early ill-defined symptoms, and is frequently misdiagnosed as "irritable bowel syndrome" or "spastic colon".

Carcinoid syndrome has an insidious progression, with recognition of the disease frequently occurring in late disease stages.

Pathophysiology

Malignant carcinoid syndrome, the predominant clinical feature of carcinoid tumors, results from excessive secretion of hormone products into the systemic circulation. These hormones (peptides and amines) cause the extreme symptoms of the disease, and a reduction in their circulating blood concentrations through targeted treatment is the therapeutic goal.

Gastrointestinal Peptides and Amines Secreted by Carcinoid Tumors

- Adrenocorticotropic hormone (ACTH)
- Gastrin

- Pancreatic polypeptide
- Insulin
- Bradykinin
- Vasoactive intestinal polypeptide (VIP)
- Serotonin
- 5-hydroxyindoleacetic acid (5-HIAA).

Many of the symptoms of carcinoid syndrome are produced by serotonin or its metabolites.

Biochemical Basis for Symptoms

- The flushing results from secretion of kallikrein, the enzyme that catalyzes the conversion of kininogen to lysyl-bradykinin. The latter is further converted to bradykinin, one of the most powerful vasodilators known.
- Other components of the carcinoid syndrome are diarrhea (probably caused by serotonin).
- A pellagra-like syndrome (probably caused by diversion of large amounts of tryptophan from synthesis of the vitamin B3, niacin, to the synthesis of 5-hydroxyindoles including serotonin).
- Fibrotic lesions of the endocardium, particularly on the right side of the heart, result in insufficiency of the tricuspid valve and, less frequently, the pulmonary valve and, uncommonly, bronchoconstriction. The pathogenesis of the cardiac lesions and the bronchoconstriction is unknown, but the former probably involves activation of serotonin 5-HT2B receptors by serotonin. When the primary tumor is in the gastrointestinal tract, as it is in the great majority of cases, the serotonin and kallikrein are inactivated in the liver; manifestations of carcinoid syndrome do not occur until there are metastases to the liver or when the cancer is accompanied by liver failure (cirrhosis). Carcinoid tumors arising in the bronchi may be associated with manifestations of carcinoid syndrome without liver metastases because their biologically active products reach the systemic circulation before passing through the liver and being metabolized.

In most patients, there is an **increased urinary excretion of 5-HIAA (5-hydroxyindoleacetic acid),** a degradation product of serotonin **(Fig. 6.10)**.

Steps of synthesis and degradation of serotonin have been shown in **Figure 6.10.**

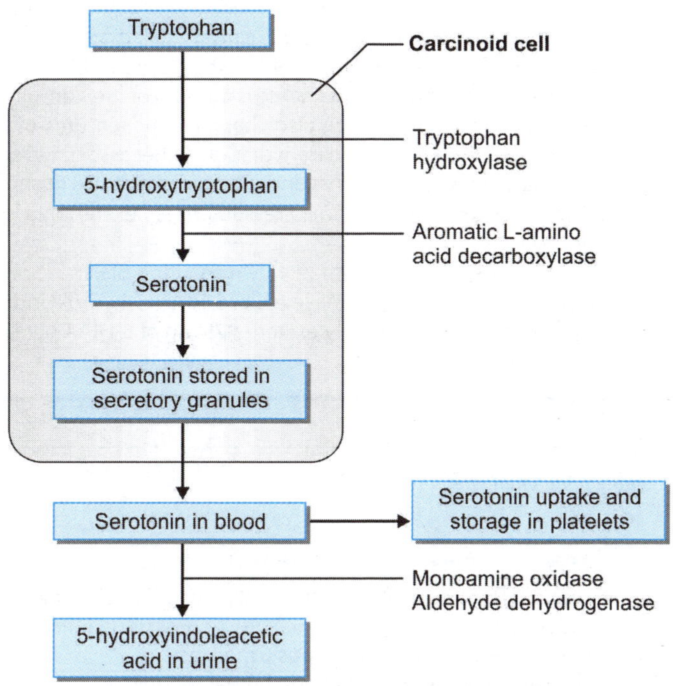

Fig. 6.10: Serotonin pathway of tryptophan metabolism.

Diagnosis

With a certain degree of clinical suspicion, diagnosis is made primarily by measuring plasma levels of the secreted glycoprotein chromogranin A, supported by measuring the 24-hour urine levels of 5-HIAA (5-hydroxyindoleacetic acid), a breakdown product of serotonin. Patients with carcinoid syndrome usually excrete >25 mg of 5-HIAA per day.

For localization of both primary lesions and metastasis, the initial imaging method is octreoscan. Median detection rates with octreoscan are about 89%, in contrast to other imaging techniques such as CT scan and MRI with detection rates of about 80%. Usually on CT scan, one will note a spider-like/crab-like change in the mesentery due to the fibrosis from the release of serotonin. PET scans, which evaluate for increased metabolism of glucose, may also aid in localizing the carcinoid lesion or evaluating for metastases.

Treatment

For symptomatic relief of carcinoid syndrome:

- **Octreotide** (a somatostatin analog that neutralizes serotonin and decreases urinary 5-HIAA)
- **Methysergide** maleate (antiserotonin agent, but not used because of serious side effect of retroperitoneal fibrosis)
- **Cyproheptadin**e (an antihistamine drug).

Alternative treatment for qualifying candidates:

- **Surgical resection of tumor and chemotherapy (5-FU and doxorubicin).**

Prognosis

Overall, the prognosis for patients with carcinoid tumors is relatively good compared with other malignancies. The average survival time from the start of octreotide treatment has increased to about 12 years.

CLINICAL NOTE

Carcinoid syndrome exhibits slow growth with early ill-defined symptoms and is frequently misdiagnosed as "irritable bowel syndrome" or "spastic colon".

CLINICAL PEARLS

1. Carcinoids are tumors of neuroendocrine nature that originate in the cells of the neuroendocrine system and are characterized by production of serotonin (5-hydroxytryptamine; 5-HT).
2. The most important clinical finding is flushing of the skin, usually of the head and the upper part of thorax. Secretory diarrhea and abdominal cramps are also characteristic features of the syndrome. When the diarrhea is intensive, it may lead to electrolyte disturbance and dehydration. Other associated symptoms are nausea and vomiting. Bronchoconstriction affects a smaller number of patients and often accompanies flushing.
3. In most patients, there is an increased urinary excretion of 5-HIAA (5-hydroxyindoleacetic acid), a degradation product of serotonin.
4. The diagnosis is made primarily by measuring plasma levels of the secreted glycoprotein chromogranin A, supported by measuring the 24-hour urine levels of 5-HIAA (5-hydroxyindoleacetic acid), a breakdown product of serotonin. Patients with carcinoid syndrome usually excrete >25 mg of 5-HIAA per day.
5. Treatment is symptomatic.

CASE STUDY 8

Theme: Cystine Absorption Defect

A 38-year-old female reported with a dull pain in the left flank. The pain was radiating towards left leg. She was in real agony. She reported that there was fever and inability to pass urine from the last few days. History revealed that she was admitted twice with the similar symptoms in the previous 6 months.

On general physical examination, she was found to be anemic, pulse was 80/min, BP was 130/90 mm Hg, and the abdomen was tender to touch. The patient was admitted for observation and treatment. There was costovertebral angle tenderness on Murphy's punch.

Routine urine analysis revealed the presence of RBCs, pus cells, WBC casts, characteristic hexagonal crystals, and amino acids. A diagnosis of aminoaciduria was made.

What is the probable defect? Which amino acid is expected to be there in urine?
What is the possible treatment?

CASE DISCUSSION

The diagnosis in this case is cystinuria.

BASIC CONCEPT

Cystinuria

Cystine is a sulfur containing amino acid. It is formed by the combination of 2 cysteine molecules. It is usually absorbed from intestine and reabsorbed from the proximal convoluted tubule in nephrons by a dibasic amino acid transporter.

Pathophysiology

Cystinuria is characterized by the buildup of cystine crystals or stones in the kidneys and bladder. As the kidneys filter blood to create urine, cystine is normally absorbed back into the bloodstream. Patients with cystinuria cannot properly reabsorb cystine into their bloodstream and the amino acid accumulates in their urine.

As urine becomes more concentrated in the kidneys, the excess cystine forms crystals in acidic pH. As these crystals become larger, they form stones that may lodge in the kidneys or in the bladder. Sometimes cystine crystals combine with calcium molecules in the kidneys to form larger stones. These crystals and stones can create blockages in the urinary tract and reduce the ability of the kidneys to eliminate waste through urine. The stones also provide sites where bacteria may cause infections.

CLASSIFICATION

Urine cystine excretion allows separation of homozygous cystinuria subjects into three groups.

In type 1, the most common form, there is no active transport of cystine or dibasic amino acids across the mucosal gradient, and heterozygous subjects show normal urine cystine values.

Type 2 is characterized by markedly reduced or absent intestinal transport of cystine. Heterozygotes for type 2 show significantly elevated urine cystine but less than that as seen in homozygotes.

In type 3, there is diminished, although demonstrable, intestinal absorption of cystine and dibasic amino acids. Urine cystine in heterozygotes is intermediate between types 1 and 2.

Clinical Features

Recurrent nephrolithiasis: Age of onset depends on the excretion rates. Type 1 cystinuria have symptoms in 1st decade. The frequency of recurrent stones in an individual can range from only a few stones in a lifetime to many stones each year. Similarly, the size of stones ranges from "gravel" passed frequently and with little discomfort, to "**stag horn**" calculi. These relatively massive stones fill the collecting system of the kidney, with branches extending into the calyces to resemble a deer's antler. Possible complications of all stones include obstruction of the urinary tract, which usually presents with severe, sudden onset of flank pain. Blood in the urine may be noted, and on occasion, obstruction can predispose to infection of the urine as well. In such cases, fever may be apparent, and white blood cells are noted in the urine. Unrelieved obstruction leads to renal dysfunction, but since this rarely affects both kidneys simultaneously, renal failure and the need for dialysis are quite rare.

Constant colicky type of pain and costovertebral angle tenderness are characteristics signs of renal stones.

Biochemical Defect

In the intestine: The high-affinity cystine transporter composed is present in the apical brush border membranes of the jejunum where it mediates absorption of cystine, dibasic amino acids, and some neutral amino acids as well. Although cystine absorption by the intestine is impaired in most patients with cystinuria, cystine deficiency is not clinically significant. This is because the intestine's absorption of oligopeptides, short amino acid chains, is intact. **Adequate cystine, as well as the other affected dibasic amino acids (ornithine, lysine, and arginine), can be absorbed in this form, combined with other amino acids.** Plasma levels of these amino acids may be normal, or slightly reduced. Dietary methionine, the absorption of which is not affected by cystinuria, serves as a precursor for the body's cystine requirement.

In the kidney: The amino acid transporters, *SLC7A9* and *SLC3A1*, are defective, both in the intestine and in proximal convoluted tubule (PCT) of nephron. This leads to retention of cystine in urine, which gets precipitated in acidic pH **(Fig. 6.11)**.

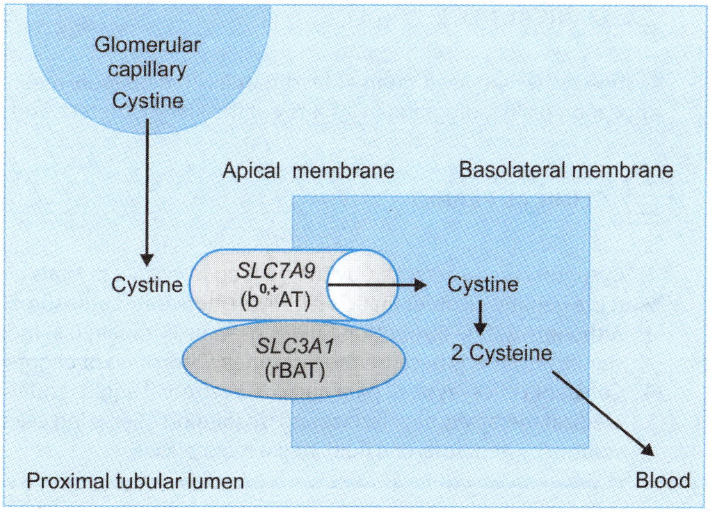

Fig. 6.11: Defective transporter in cystinuria.

Inheritance

Cystinuria is a genetic disorder that classically demonstrates autosomal recessive inheritance.

Two of the genes responsible for the disorder, *SLC3A1* and *SLC7A9*, have been identified. The identification of *SLC3A1* made cystinuria the first disorder of amino acid transport with an identified gene.

There are some more unusual cases, with mutations in *SLC7A9*, that manifest autosomal dominant inheritance with one defective gene sufficient for cystine stone formation.

Diagnosis

1. **Sodium cyanide nitroprusside test:** All patients who experience an episode of nephrolithiasis, but particularly children and those with a first episode before the age of 30, should be screened for cystinuria. This is conveniently accomplished by the addition to urine of sodium cyanide and sodium nitroprusside, which in the presence of cystine forms a purple-red color.
2. **X-ray:** Cystine stones are most often at least partially radiopaque, meaning that they do not allow full penetration of X-rays and do appear on plain radiographs. Flat X-ray of the kidney, ureters, and bladder (KUB), is undertaken.

3. Some cystine stones are better demonstrated by ultrasound of the kidneys or by helical computed tomography (CT).
4. The traditional intravenous pyelogram (IVP), which requires injection of a potentially nephrotoxic radiocontrast agent, is still used for demonstrating the anatomy of the urinary tract, particularly if a surgical procedure is likely to be needed.

General Urine Examination

Microscopic examination: Reveals flat hexagonal crystals of cysteine **(Fig. 6.12)**.

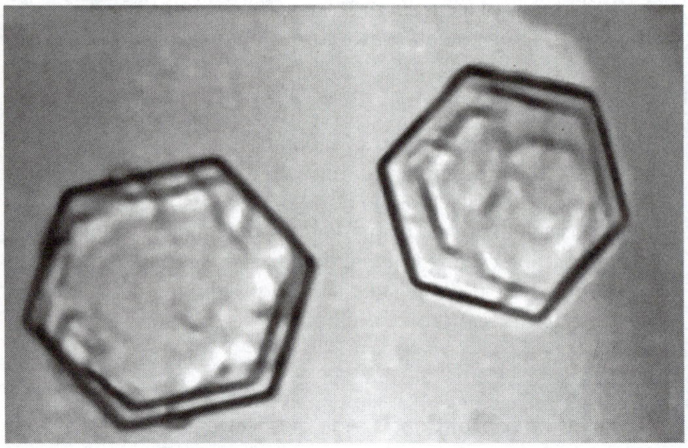

Fig. 6.12: Cystine crystals in urine.

Treatment

1. Medical therapy will be directed toward dissolution of existing calculi and prevention of new stone formation. Increasing urine volume by generous oral fluid intake is beneficial.
2. Dietary sodium and protein restriction has a favorable effect on urinary cystine excretion.
3. Cystine solubility can be improved by urinary alkalinization and where necessary by the administration of thiol chelators, particularly D-penicillamine or mercaptopropionyl glycine. Because these chelators have significant adverse effects, they should be reserved for patients who do not respond to a more conservative program.
4. Patients with infected, symptomatic, or obstructing stones require surgical intervention.

CLINICAL NOTE

Cystine stones are most often at least partially radiopaque, meaning that they do not allow full penetration of X-rays and do appear on plain radiographs. Flat X-ray of the kidney, ureters, and bladder (KUB), is undertaken.

CLINICAL PEARLS

1. Cystinuria is characterized by the buildup of cystine crystals or stones in the kidneys and bladder.
2. It is a genetic disorder that classically demonstrates autosomal recessive inheritance.
3. Although cystine absorption by the intestine is impaired in most patients with cystinuria, cystine deficiency is not clinically significant. This is because the intestine's absorption of oligopeptides, short amino acid chains, is intact.
4. Constant colicky type of pain and costovertebral angle tenderness are characteristics signs of renal stones.
5. Medical therapy is directed toward dissolution of existing calculi and prevention of new stone formation. Increasing urine volume by generous oral fluid intake is beneficial.

CASE STUDY 9

Theme: Clinical Implications of Abnormal Lysosomal Storage of Cystine

A 2-year-old child was brought to the pediatrics department for consultation. Mother of the child reported that the child was born normally; there was no complication during delivery of the child, and her other two children were also normal. The child was not feeding properly and was also not growing well. There was history of increased frequency of urination from the last few months for which the mother was very much apprehensive. The child avoided going to the sun and there was apparent visual impairment. On general physical examination, the child was found to be pale, thin, and small for his age. There was slight hepatomegaly. The child looked slightly dehydrated.

A urine sample was sent for complete analysis. The urine examination revealed the presence of excessive amount of phosphates and amino acid in urine.

A thorough examination of the eye was also done to know the cause of visual impairment. On slit lamp microscopic examination, characteristic crystals were found to be deposited in the cornea.

What could be the possible defect?
What is the biochemical basis for phosphate and amino acids in urine?
How can this defect be prevented?

CASE DISCUSSION

The child is suffering from cystinosis.

Cystinosis

Cystinosis is a lysosomal storage disease characterized by the abnormal accumulation of the amino acid cystine. Excess cystine forms crystals that can build up and damage cells. These crystals negatively affect many systems in the body, especially the kidneys and eyes.

Inheritance

Cystinosis is an autosomal recessive genetic disease. This means that both parents are carriers of the abnormal gene that leads to this condition. The parents do not exhibit any of the symptoms of cystinosis.

Frequency

Cystinosis is an "orphan" disease with about 500 people, mostly children, stricken with the disease in the United States and approximately 2,000 worldwide. Cystinosis affects approximately 1 in 100,000–200,000 newborns. The incidence is higher in the province of Brittany, France, where the disorder affects 1 in 26,000 individuals.

Biochemical Defect

The accumulation is caused by abnormal transport of cystine from lysosomes, resulting in a massive intralysosomal cystine accumulation in tissues. Via an as yet unknown mechanism, lysosomal cystine appears to amplify and alter apoptosis in such a way that cells die inappropriately, leading to loss of renal epithelial cells. This results in renal Fanconi syndrome and similar loss in other tissues can account for the short stature, retinopathy, and other features of the disease.

SIGNS AND SYMPTOMS

Cystinosis occurs due to a mutation in the gene CTNS, located on chromosome 17, which codes for cystinosin, the lysosomal cystine transporter. Symptoms are first seen at about 3–18 months of age with profound polyuria (excessive urination), followed by poor growth, photophobia, and ultimately kidney failure by age of 6 years in the nephropathic form.
There are three distinct types of cystinosis. In order of decreasing severity, they are:

1. Nephropathic cystinosis (Infantile)
2. Intermediate cystinosis (Juvenile)
3. Non-nephropathic or ocular cystinosis (Adult).

1. **Nephropathic cystinosis:** Infants affected by nephropathic cystinosis initially exhibit poor growth and a particular type of kidney damage (renal Fanconi syndrome) that causes the kidneys to eliminate certain molecules that should be reabsorbed into the bloodstream. The kidney problems lead to the loss of important minerals, salts, fluids, and other nutrients. The loss of nutrients impairs growth and may result in soft, bowed bones (hypophosphatemic rickets), especially in the legs. The nutrient imbalances in the body lead to increased urination, thirst, dehydration, and abnormally acidic blood (acidosis). By about the age of 2, cystine crystals may be present in the cornea **(Fig. 6.13)**. The buildup of these crystals in the eye causes an increased sensitivity to light (photophobia). Untreated children will experience complete kidney failure by about the age of 10. Other signs and symptoms that may occur in untreated people, especially after adolescence, include muscle deterioration, blindness, inability to swallow, diabetes, and thyroid and nervous system problems.

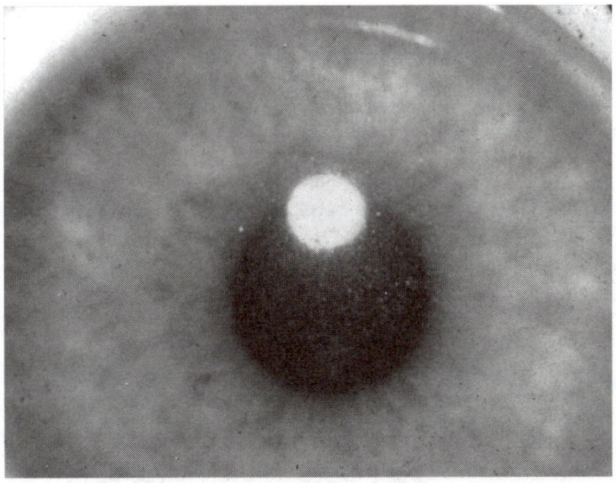

Fig. 6.13: Cystine deposition in cornea.

2. **Intermediate cystinosis:** The signs and symptoms of intermediate cystinosis are the same as nephropathic cystinosis, but they occur at a later age. Intermediate cystinosis typically becomes apparent in affected individuals in adolescence. Malfunctioning kidneys and corneal crystals are the main initial features of this disorder. If intermediate cystinosis is left untreated, complete kidney failure will occur, but usually not until the late teens to mid-twenties.
3. **Non-nephropathic or ocular cystinosis:** People with non-nephropathic or ocular cystinosis usually do not experience growth impairment or kidney malfunction. In most cases, the only symptom is photophobia due to cystine crystals in the cornea.

Diagnosis

Definitive diagnosis and treatment monitoring are most often performed through measurement of white blood cell cystine level using tandem mass spectrometry.

Treatment

Cystinosis is a common cause of the Fanconi syndrome, a renal tubular disease. By about 1 year of age, patients eliminate large volumes of urine and lose large amounts of salt and other minerals in their urine.

Without specific treatment, these children progress to end-stage renal failure by an average age of 9 years. These patients can receive renal dialysis or transplantation, but even with successful transplantations, they develop abnormalities in other organs.

The drug cysteamine slows the progression of cystinosis by removing the cystine from cells, but for the drug treatment to be effective, it must be taken every 6 hours. When administered regularly, cysteamine decreases the amount of cystine stored in lysosomes and correlates with conservation of renal function and improved growth. **Cysteamine eye drops remove the cystine crystals in the cornea** that can cause photophobia, if left unchecked. Patients with cystinosis are also often given sodium citrate to treat the blood acidosis, as well as potassium and phosphorus supplements. High doses of vitamin D and phosphate are required to replace the lost nutrients and minerals. Although this has led to a much better future for these children, but there is no cure for the disease.

CLINICAL NOTE

Cystinosis is a common cause of the Fanconi syndrome, a renal tubular disease. By about 1 year of age, patients eliminate large volumes of urine and lose large amounts of salt and other minerals in their urine.

CLINICAL PEARLS

1. Cystinosis is a lysosomal storage disease characterized by the abnormal accumulation of the amino acid cystine.
2. Excess cystine forms crystals that can build up and damage cells. These crystals negatively affect many systems in the body, especially the kidneys and eyes.
3. The accumulation is caused by abnormal transport of cystine from lysosomes, resulting in a massive intralysosomal cystine accumulation in tissues.
4. Definitive diagnosis and treatment monitoring are most often performed through measurement of white blood cell cystine level using tandem mass spectrometry.
5. The drug cysteamine slows the progression of cystinosis by removing the cystine from cells, but for the drug treatment to be effective, it must be taken every 6 hours.

CASE STUDY 10

Theme: Disorders of Homocysteine Metabolism

An adolescent girl develops hemiballismus (repetitive throwing motions of the arm) after anesthesia for a routine operation. She is tall and lanky, and it is noted that she and her sister both had previous operations for dislocated lenses of the eyes.

The symptoms are suspicious for the disease homocystinuria.

What is the nature of disease, how can this be treated?

CASE DETAILS

Homocystinuria (Homocysteinemia)

BASIC CONCEPT

Most homocysteine, an intermediate compound of methionine degradation, is normally remethylated to methionine. This methionine-sparing reaction is catalyzed by the enzyme methionine synthase, which requires a metabolite of folic acid (5-methyltetrahydrofolate) as a methyl donor and a metabolite of vitamin B_{12} (methylcobalamin) as a cofactor. Only 20–30% of total homocysteine (and its dimer homocystine) is in free form in the plasma of normal individuals. The rest is bound to protein.

Classification

Following major forms of homocysteinemia and homocystinuria have been identified:
Homocystinuria due to cystathionine beta synthetase deficiency
(Classical Homocystinuria)
In the synthesis of cysteine, the following sequence of steps occur,
Methionine $\rightarrow$ SAM $\rightarrow$ homocysteine + adenosine
Homocysteine + serine $\rightarrow$ cystathionine $\rightarrow$ cys + α-ketoglutarate + NH_4^+ (CS, B6)
(Where SAM is S-adenosyl methionine, CS is cystathionine synthetase, cys is cysteine).

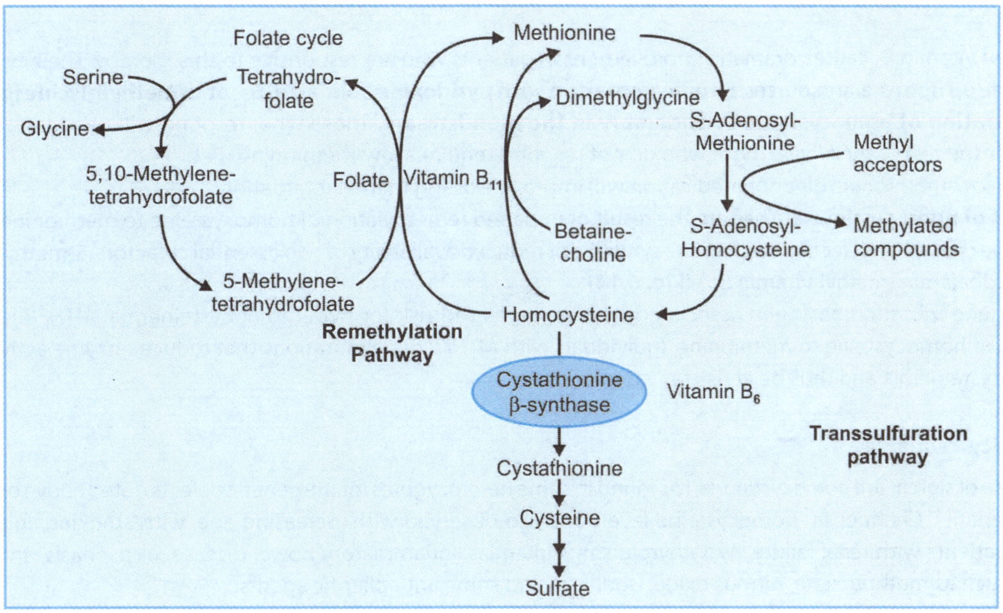

Fig. 6.14: Metabolism of methionine.

Cystathionine synthetase, a pyridoxal phosphate (Vitamin B_6) enzyme, catalyzes the condensation of serine and homocysteine to form cystathionine.
(*See* the reactions in **Figure 6.14**)

A deficiency of this enzyme leads to a buildup of homocysteine, which oxidizes to form homocystine. This is the most common inborn error of methionine metabolism.

Inheritance

Homocystinuria is inherited in families as an autosomal recessive trait. This means that the child must inherit the defective gene from both parents to be seriously affected.

Clinical Manifestations

- Infants with this disorder are normal at birth.
- Clinical manifestations during infancy are nonspecific and may include failure to thrive and developmental delay.
- The diagnosis is usually made after 3 years of age, when subluxation of the ocular lens (ectopia lentis) occurs. This causes severe myopia and iridodonesis (quivering of the iris), astigmatism, glaucoma, cataracts, retinal detachment, and optic atrophy may develop later in life.
- Progressive mental retardation is common. Normal intelligence, however, has been reported.
- Affected individuals with homocystinuria manifest skeletal abnormalities resembling those of Marfan syndrome; they are usually tall and thin with elongated limbs and arachnodactyly. Scoliosis, pectus excavatum, genu valgum, pes cavus, high arched palate, and crowding of the teeth are common.
- Patients usually have fair complexions, blue eyes, and a peculiar malar flush. Generalized osteoporosis, especially of the spine, is the main radiographic finding.
- Thromboembolic episodes involving both large and small vessels, especially those of the brain, are common and may occur at any age.

Laboratory Findings

- **Amino acid screening of blood and urine—elevations of both methionine and homocystine in body fluids are the diagnostic laboratory findings.** Total plasma homocysteine is extremely elevated (usually >100 M). Cystine is low or absent in plasma.
- Liver biopsy and enzyme assay
- Skeletal X-ray
- Skin biopsy with a fibroblast culture (The diagnosis may be established by assay of the enzyme in liver biopsy specimens, cultured fibroblasts)
- Standard ophthalmic exam
- Genetic testing.

Treatment

High doses of vitamin B_6 causes dramatic improvement in patients who are responsive to this therapy. Their cysteine deficiency must be made up from dietary sources. **Supplementation with pyridoxine, folic acid, B_{12} or trimethylglycine (betaine) reduces the concentration of homocysteine considerably in the bloodstream.** Those who respond will need to take supplemental vitamin B_6 for the rest of their lives. Those who do not respond require a low-methionine diet.

Neither a low-methionine diet nor medication will improve existing mental retardation.

Other forms of homocystinuria: They are the result of impaired remethylation of homocysteine to methionine.

This can be caused by defective methionine synthase or reduced availability of two essential cofactors, 5-methyltetrahydrofolate and methylcobalamin (methyl-vitamin B_{12}) **(Fig. 6.14)**.

MTHFR gene mutation has been associated with an increased risk for hyperhomocysteinemia. *MTHFR* is involved in the methylation of homocysteine to methionine. Individuals with *MTHFR* gene mutations that reduce enzyme activity may develop hyperhomocysteinemia and thus be at risk for vascular disease.

Hyperhomocysteinemia

In the absence of significant homocystinuria, it is found in some heterozygotes for the genetic defects noted above or in homozygotes for milder variants. Changes in homocysteine levels are also observed with increasing age, with smoking, in postmenopausal women, in patients with renal failure, hypothyroidism, leukemias, inflammatory bowel disease, or psoriasis, and during therapy with drugs such as methotrexate, nitrous oxide, isoniazid, and some antiepileptic agents.

Consequences of hyperhomocysteinemia: Homocysteine acts as an atherogenic and thrombophilic agent. An increase in total plasma homocysteine represents an independent risk factor for coronary, cerebrovascular, and peripheral arterial disease as well as for deep vein thrombosis. Homocysteine is synergistic with hypertension and smoking, and it is additive with other risk factors that predispose to peripheral arterial disease. In addition, hyperhomocysteinemia and folate and vitamin B_{12} deficiency have been associated with an increased risk of neural tube defects in pregnant women. Vitamin supplements are effective in reducing plasma homocysteine levels in these cases.

Prognosis

Although no cure exists for homocystinuria, vitamin B_6 therapy can help about half of people affected by the condition.

If the diagnosis is made while a patient is young, starting a low-methionine diet quickly can prevent some mental retardation and other complications of the disease. For this reason, some states screen for homocystinuria in all newborns.

Patients with persistent rise in blood homocysteine levels are at increased risk for thromboembolic episodes which can cause significant medical problems and shorten lifespan.

CLINICAL NOTE

Elevations of both methionine and homocystene in body fluids are the diagnostic laboratory findings. Total plasma homocysteine is extremely elevated (usually >100 M). Cystine is low or absent in plasma.

CLINICAL PEARLS

1. Homocystinuria is inherited in families as an autosomal recessive trait.
2. The diagnosis is usually made after 3 years of age, when subluxation of the ocular lens (ectopia lentis) occurs. This causes severe myopia and iridodonesis (quivering of the iris), astigmatism, glaucoma, cataracts, retinal detachment, and optic atrophy may develop later in life.
3. Infants with this disorder are normal at birth. Clinical manifestations during infancy are nonspecific and may include failure to thrive and developmental delay.
4. Elevations of both methionine and homocystine in body fluids are the diagnostic laboratory findings. Total plasma homocysteine is extremely elevated (usually >100 M). Cystine is low or absent in plasma.
5. Supplementation with pyridoxine, folic acid, B_{12} or trimethylglycine (betaine) reduces the concentration of homocysteine considerably in the bloodstream. Those who respond will need to take supplemental vitamin B_6 for the rest of their lives. Those who do not respond require a low-methionine diet.

CASE STUDY 11

Theme: Metabolic Disorder of Branched-Chain Amino Acids.

A child presented with severe vomiting, dehydration, and fever. History revealed that the child was born normal but was not growing well from the last few months. There was progressive mental retardation. Urine analysis revealed the presence of branched amino acids and their keto acids in high amount. Preliminary results from the blood amino acid screening showed two elevated amino acids with nonpolar side chains.

Blood studies showed acidosis with a low bicarbonate concentration. The urine of the patient had a smell of burnt sugar. Urine analysis revealed the presence of branched amino acids and their keto acids in high amount. Preliminary results from the blood amino acid screening showed two elevated amino acids with nonpolar side chains.

What is the probable defect?

What is the basis for these symptoms?

CASE DISCUSSION

The child is suffering from **maple syrup urine disease.** The signs and symptoms and the typical smell of urine, suggest the presence of maple syrup urine disease. Fever in this patient suggests that the metabolic imbalance was worsened by an infection. Blood and urine in this disease have elevated levels of branched amino acids and their keto derivatives. The keto derivatives cause acidosis as is evident in this patient; low bicarbonate levels are due to depletion of alkali reserve.

BASIC CONCEPT

MAPLE SYRUP URINE DISEASE

Maple syrup urine disease (MSUD), also called branched-chain ketoaciduria, is an autosomal recessive metabolic disorder affecting branched-chain amino acids. It is one type of organic acidemia. The condition gets its name from the distinctive sweet odor of affected infants' urine.

Biochemical Defect

Maple syrup urine disease (MSUD) is caused by a deficiency of the branched-chain alpha-keto acid dehydrogenase complex (BCKDH), leading to a buildup of the branched-chain amino acids (leucine, isoleucine, and valine) and their toxic by-products in the blood and urine.

Classification

Maple syrup urine disease can be classified by its pattern of signs and symptoms, or by its genetic cause. The most common and severe form of the disease is the classic type, which appears soon after birth. Variant forms of the disorder may appear later in infancy or childhood and are typically less severe, but still involve mental and physical problems if left untreated.

There are several variations of the disease:

- Classic severe MSUD
- Intermediate MSUD
- Intermittent MSUD
- Thiamine-responsive MSUD.

Clinical Manifestations

From early infancy, symptoms of the condition include **poor feeding, vomiting, dehydration, lethargy, hypotonia, seizures, ketoacidosis, opisthotonus, pancreatitis, coma, and neurological decline.** The disease is characterized in an infant by the presence of sweet-smelling urine, with an odor similar to that of maple syrup. Infants with this disease seem healthy at birth, but if left untreated, suffer severe brain damage, and eventually die.

Management

A diet with minimal levels of the amino acids such as leucine, isoleucine, and valine must be maintained in order to prevent neurological damage. As these three amino acids are required for proper metabolic functions, specialized protein preparations containing substitutes and adjusted levels of the amino acids have been synthesized and tested, allowing MSUD patients to meet normal nutritional requirements without causing harm. A careful monitoring of blood chemistry and frequent testing is required.

CLINICAL NOTE

Variant forms of the maple syrup urine disease may appear later in infancy or childhood and are typically less severe, but still involve mental and physical problems if left untreated.

CLINICAL PEARLS

1. Maple syrup urine disease (MSUD), also called branched-chain ketoaciduria, is an autosomal recessive metabolic disorder affecting branched-chain amino acids.
2. It is caused by a deficiency of the branched-chain alpha-keto acid dehydrogenase complex (BCKDH), leading to a buildup of the branched-chain amino acids (leucine, isoleucine, and valine) and their toxic by-products in the blood and urine.
3. The disease can be classified by its pattern of signs and symptoms, or by its genetic cause. The most common and severe form of the disease is the classic type, which appears soon after birth.
4. It is characterized in an infant by the presence of sweet-smelling urine, with an odor similar to that of maple syrup. Infants with this disease seem healthy at birth, but if left untreated, suffer severe brain damage, and eventually die.
5. A diet with minimal levels of the amino acids leucine, isoleucine, and valine must be maintained in order to prevent neurological damage.

CASE STUDY 12

Theme: Synthesis and Significance of Nitric Oxide.

An obese, middle-aged man was brought to the emergency room after an automobile accident. The patient stated that he had been short of breath and dizzy just before the accident. There was chest discomfort also.

The patient was admitted for observation and blood samples for enzyme assays were collected periodically. A chest X-ray was taken and a 12-lead ECG was recorded.

On general examination, his blood pressure was 150/90 mm Hg, pulse was 60/minute and he was sweating profusely. There was no evidence of cardiac failure. His initial ECG showed changes in certain leads, indicative of myocardial ischemia. Enzyme profile was normal. The patient was diagnosed to be having angina. He was immediately shifted to the cardiac care unit. Treatment with nitroglycerine was started to dilate his coronaries.

What is the rationale behind this treatment with nitroglycerine?

CASE DISCUSSION

Nitroglycerin, amyl nitrite (isobutyl nitrite or similar), and other nitrite derivatives are used in the treatment of heart disease. The compounds are converted to nitric oxide, which in turn dilates the coronary artery, thereby increasing its blood supply. These drugs, however, are predominantly vasodilators, dilating peripheral veins and hence reducing venous return and preload to the heart. This reduces the oxygen requirement of the myocardium and subsequently lessens the anginal pain felt with myocardial ischemia.

Nitric oxide: Nitric oxide is a highly reactive gas. It participates in many chemical reactions. Endothelium-derived relaxing factor was originally the name given to several proposed factors causing vasodilatation. The major endothelial-derived relaxing factor was later discovered to be nitric oxide (NO).

NITRIC OXIDE SYNTHESIS

Nitric oxide is synthesized by nitric oxide synthase (NOS). There are three isoforms of the NOS enzyme:

1. Endothelial (eNOS)
2. Neuronal (nNOS)
3. Inducible (iNOS)—each with separate functions.

The neuronal enzyme (NOS-1) and the endothelial isoform (NOS-3) are calcium-dependent and produce low levels of gas as a cell signaling molecule. The inducible isoform (NOS-2) is calcium-independent and produces large amounts of gas which can be cytotoxic.

Nitric oxide synthase (NOS) oxidizes the guanidine group of L-arginine in a process that consumes five electrons and results in the formation of NO with stoichiometric formation of L-citrulline. The process involves the oxidation of NADPH and the reduction of molecular oxygen. The transformation occurs at a catalytic site adjacent to a specific binding site of L-arginine **(Fig. 6.15)**.

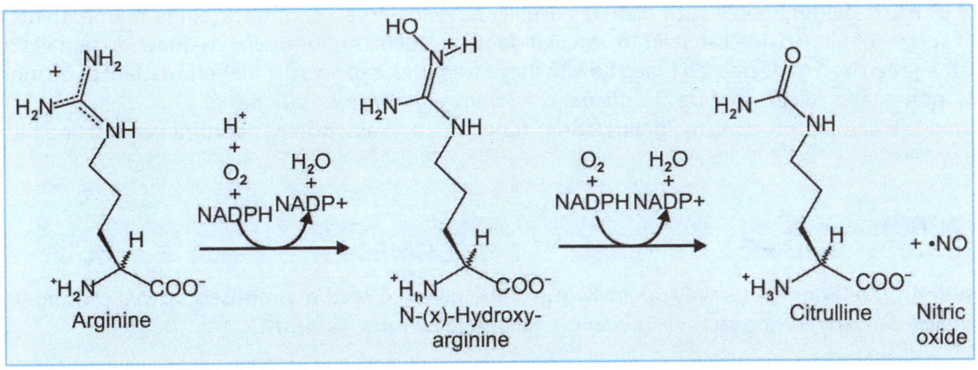

Fig 6.15: Formation of nitric oxide from arginine, the enzyme is nitric oxide synthase.

FUNCTIONS OF NITRIC OXIDE

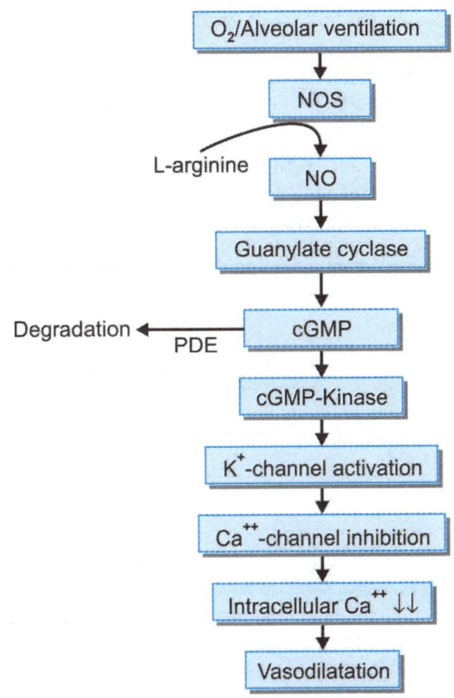

Fig. 6.16: Mechanism of vasodilatation by nitric oxide (NO).

Nitric oxide (NO) is an important regulator and mediator of numerous processes in the nervous, immune, and cardiovascular systems, including smooth muscle relaxation. The various functions are as follows:

1. **Vasodilatation:** Nitric oxide (NO) is of critical importance as a mediator of vasodilatation in blood vessels. It is induced by several factors, and once synthesized by eNOS, it results in activation of guanylate cyclase to form cGMP, which in turn causes phosphorylation of several proteins through activation of cGMP-dependent protein kinases that cause smooth muscle relaxation by decreasing the intracellular Ca^{++} concentration **(Fig. 6.16)**. The vasodilator action of nitric oxide plays a key role in renal control of extracellular fluid homeostasis and is essential for the regulation of blood flow and blood pressure. Nitric oxide (NO) also inhibits the aggregation of platelets and thus keeps inappropriate clotting from interfering with blood flow.
   Nitric oxide also acts on cardiac muscle to decrease contractility and heart rate. NO contributes to the regulation of cardiac contractility. Emerging evidence suggests that coronary artery disease (CAD) is related to defects in generation or action of NO. Adequate availability of NO prevents the coronary artery disease.
2. **Erection:** The vasodilatatory effect of NO, in turn, also plays a role in development and maintenance of erection. Vasodilatation of blood vessels supplying the corpus cavernosum results in more blood flowing in and hence, erection. This is the biological basis of sildenafil (Viagra), which works to inhibit the enzyme phosphodiesterase PDE5 that lowers the cGMP concentration by converting it back to GMP.
3. Other actions on smooth muscles:
   - The peristaltic movements are aided by the relaxing effect of NO on the smooth muscle in its walls.
   - NO also inhibits the contractility of the smooth muscle wall of the uterus. Near term, the production of NO decreases.
   - Release of NO around the glomeruli of the kidneys increases blood flow through them, thus increasing the rate of filtration and urine formation.
4. **Immune system:** Macrophages, certain cells of the immune system, produce nitric oxide in order to kill invading bacteria. In this case, the nitric oxide synthase is inducible NOS.
   Under certain conditions, there is excess production of nitric oxide by macrophages (e.g. during fulminant infections), leading to vasodilatation, probably one of the main causes of hypotension in sepsis. The inducible isoform of nitric oxide synthase is expressed and produces cytotoxic levels of nitric oxide.
5. **Neurotransmitter:** Nitric oxide also serves as a neurotransmitter between nerve cells. Unlike, most other neurotransmitters that only transmit information from a presynaptic to a postsynaptic neuron, the small nitric oxide molecule can diffuse all over and can thereby, act on several nearby neurons, even on those not connected by a synapse. It is conjectured that this process may be involved in memory through the maintenance of long-term potentiation. Nitric oxide is an important nonadrenergic, noncholinergic (NANC) neurotransmitter in various parts of the gastrointestinal tract. It causes relaxation of the gastrointestinal smooth muscle. In the stomach, it increases the capacity of the fundus to store food/fluids.

6. **Deficiency of nitric oxide:** People with diabetes usually have lower levels of nitric oxide than patients without diabetes. Diminished supply of nitric oxide can lead to vascular damage, such as endothelial dysfunction and vascular inflammation. Vascular damage can lead to decreased blood flow to the extremities, causing the diabetic patient to be more likely to develop neuropathy, non-healing ulcers, and be at a greater risk for lower limb amputation.

Thus, nitric oxide is cardioprotective, maintains kidney functions, acts as a potent neurotransmitter and has an important role in immune system.

CLINICAL NOTE

Endothelium-derived relaxing factor was originally the name given to several proposed factors causing vasodilatation. The major endothelial-derived relaxing factor was later discovered to be nitric oxide (NO).

CLINICAL PEARLS

1. Nitric oxide is a highly reactive gas. It participates in many chemical reactions.
2. Nitric oxide is synthesized by nitric oxide synthase (NOS). There are three isoforms of the NOS enzyme, endothelial, neuronal, and inducible.
3. NO is an important regulator and mediator of numerous processes in the nervous, immune, and cardiovascular systems, including smooth muscle relaxation.
4. Nitric oxide is an important nonadrenergic, noncholinergic (NANC) neurotransmitter in various parts of the gastrointestinal tract. It causes relaxation of the gastrointestinal smooth muscle. In the stomach, it increases the capacity of the fundus to store food/fluids.
5. Diminished supply of nitric oxide can lead to vascular damage, such as endothelial dysfunction and vascular inflammation.

Chapter 7

Nucleotide: Chemistry and Significance

LEARNING OBJECTIVES

To understand
- Biological significance of G-proteins
- Clinical significance of cAMP

CASE STUDIES

CASE STUDY 1

Theme: Significance of cAMP in the Causation of Cholera

A 21-year-old female working in a rural school suddenly began to pass profuse watery stools almost continuously. She soon started to vomit, her general condition declined abruptly, and she was rushed to the general hospital.

On admission, she was cyanotic, skin turgor was poor, blood pressure was 70/50 mm Hg, and her pulse was rapid and weak. The doctor on duty diagnosed cholera. The stool sample was taken for culture and the treatment was started immediately.

What is the biochemical basis for watery diarrhea and other symptoms in this patient?

CASE DETAILS

The patient is suffering from cholera. **Cholera is an acute diarrheal disease that can, in a matter of hours, result in profound, rapidly progressive dehydration, and death**. Cholera is caused by the bacteria *Vibrio cholerae*. People are infected when they consume contaminated food, often seafood, or water. Cholera is rare except in areas where sanitation is inadequate. **Patients present with watery diarrhea and vomiting, usually with no fever**. Identifying the bacteria in a stool sample confirms the diagnosis. Replacing lost fluids and giving antibiotics effectively treat the infection.

CHOLERA

Members of the genus *Vibrio* cause a number of important infectious syndromes. Classic among them is cholera, a devastating diarrheal disease caused by *V. cholerae* that has been responsible for seven global pandemics and much suffering over the past two centuries. Epidemic cholera remains a significant public health concern in the developing world today. **Cholera is caused by *V. cholerae* O1 or, more recently, by *V. cholerae* O139**. Cholera can spread as an endemic, epidemic, or pandemic disease. Despite all the major advances in research, the condition still remains a challenge to the modern medical world.

The appellation for cholera probably derives from the Greek word for the gutter of a roof, comparing the deluge of water following a rainstorm to that of the anus of an infected person. The hallmark for the disease is profuse secretory diarrhea.

BASIC CONCEPT

The recognition of a chemical signal by some membrane receptors, such as the β- and α2-adrenergic receptors, triggers either an increase or decrease in the activity of adenylate cyclase. The adenylate cyclase is a membrane protein that converts (Adenosine triphosphate) to cAMP. The chemical signals are most often hormones or neurotransmitters, each of which binds to a unique type of receptor. Certain toxins, such as produced by *Vibrio cholerae*, can also activate the adenylyl cyclase cascade, with potential disastrous consequences. These receptors are characterized by an extracellular ligand-binding region. Seven transmembrane helices and an intracellular domain interact with G-proteins.

G-proteins (GTP-dependent regulatory protein)

The effect of the occupied receptor on the second messenger formation is not direct but, rather, is mediated by specialized trimeric protein in the cell membrane.

A guanyl nucleotide-binding protein is an intermediary in signal transduction from the transmembrane receptors. This signal-coupling protein is termed a G-protein (G for guanyl nucleotide). It forms a link in the chain of communication between the receptor and adenylyl cyclase **(Fig. 7.1)**.

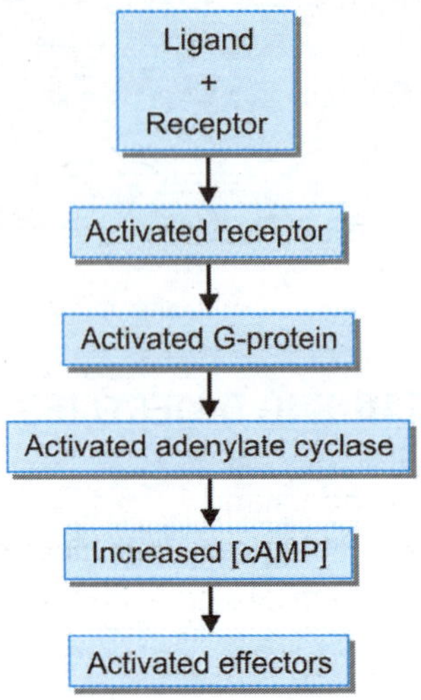

Fig. 7.1: Flow of information through G-proteins.

Activation of G-Proteins

In the inactivated state, the guanyl nucleotide bound to the G-protein is GDP. In this form, the G-protein exists as a heterotrimer consisting of α, β, and γ subunits; the α subunit (referred to as Gα) binds the nucleotide. The role of the hormone-bound receptor is to catalyze the exchange of GTP for bound GDP. The ligand/hormone–receptor complex interacts with the heterotrimeric G-protein and opens the nucleotide-binding site, so that GDP can depart and GTP from solution can bind. The α subunit simultaneously dissociates from the dimer (Gα and γ). The structure of the Gα subunit conforms tightly to the GTP molecule. These structural changes are responsible for the reduced affinity of Gα for Gβ and the dissociation of the G-protein heterotrimer into Gα, β, and γ units transmits the signal that the receptor has bound its ligand. Moreover, the surfaces of Gα and Gβ and γ that had formed the trimer interface are now exposed to interact with other proteins. A single hormone–receptor complex can stimulate nucleotide exchange in many G-protein heterotrimer. Thus, hundreds of Gγ molecules are converted from their GDP into their GTP forms for each bound molecule of hormone, giving an amplified response. The ability of a hormone or a neurotransmitter to stimulate or inhibit adenylate cyclase enzyme depends upon the type of G-protein that is linked to the receptor. One family of G-protein designated as Gs is specific for stimulation of adenylate cyclase; another family designated as Gi causes inhibition of the enzyme.

G-Proteins spontaneously reset themselves through GTP Hydrolysis

The ability to shut down signal transduction pathways is as critical as the ability to turn them on. Gα subunits have intrinsic GTPase activity, hydrolyzing bound GTP to GDP and Pi. This hydrolysis reaction is slow, however, requiring from seconds to minutes and thus allowing the GTP form of Gα to activate downstream components of the signal transduction pathway before GTP hydrolysis deactivates the subunit. In essence, the bound GTP acts as a built-in clock that spontaneously resets the Gα subunit after a short-time period. After GTP hydrolysis and the release of Pi, the GDP-bound form of Gα then reassociates with Gβ and γ to reform the heterotrimeric inactive G-protein **(Fig. 7.2)**.

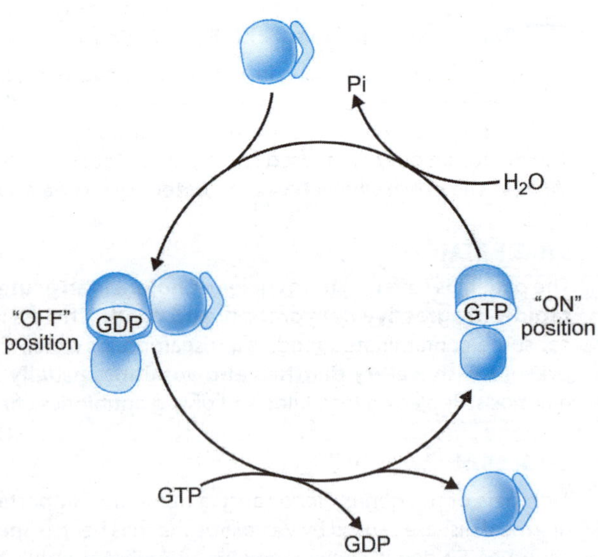

Fig. 7.2: Activation and inactivation of G-proteins.

Activated G-Proteins transmit Signals by Binding to Other Proteins

The G-protein binds to adenylate cyclase through the surface that had bound the βγ dimer when the G-protein was in its GDP form. The activation of the G-protein exposes this surface and subtly changes it, so that it now binds the surface of adenylate cyclase in preference to Gβγ. The interaction of Gαs with adenylate cyclase favors a more catalytically active conformation of the enzyme, thus stimulating cAMP production. The net result is that the binding of ligand to the receptor on the cell surface increases the rate of cAMP production inside the cell. **The increased concentration of cAMP can affect a wide range of cellular processes. For example, it enhances the degradation of storage fuels, increases the secretion of acid by the gastric mucosa, leads to the dispersion of melanin pigment granules, diminishes the aggregation of blood platelets, and induces the opening of chloride channels.**

Protein kinases

Most effects of cyclic AMP in eukaryotic cells are mediated by activation of a single protein kinase. This key enzyme is called protein kinase A (PKA). PKA consists of two regulatory (R) chains and two catalytic (C) chains. In the absence of cAMP, the

R2C2 complex is catalytically inactive. The binding of cAMP to the regulatory chains releases the catalytic chains, which are enzymatically active on their own. Activated PKA then phosphorylates specific serine and threonine residues in many targets to alter their activity. The phosphorylated proteins may act directly on the cell's ion channels, or become activated or inhibited enzymes. PKA can also phosphorylate specific proteins that bind to certain regions on the DNA causing increased expression of certain specific genes.

Dephosphorylation of Proteins

The phosphate groups added to proteins by protein kinases are removed by protein phosphatases enzymes that hydrolytically cleave phosphate esters. This ensures that the change in enzyme activity induced by protein phosphorylation is not permanent.

Hydrolysis of Cyclic Adenosine Monophosphate (cAMP)

cAMP is rapidly hydrolyzed to 5-AMP by cAMP phosphodiesterase. 5-AMP is not intracellular signaling molecule. Thus, the effects of neurotransmitter or hormone-mediated increase in cAMP are rapidly terminated, if the extracellular signal is removed.

PATHOGENESIS OF CHOLERA

Cholera is due to altered G-protein activity: Cholera is a toxin-mediated disease. Its characteristic watery diarrhea is due to the action of cholera toxin, a potent protein enterotoxin elaborated by the organism after it colonizes the small intestine. The cholera toxin, choleragen, is a protein composed of two functional units a β subunit and α subunit. The β pentamer binds to **GM1 ganglioside, a glycolipid on the surface of epithelial cells that serves as the toxin receptor** and makes possible the delivery of the α subunit to its cytosolic target. The α subunit catalyzes the covalent modification of Gs protein: the α subunit is modified by the attachment of an ADP-ribose to an arginine residue. This modification stabilizes the GTP-bound form of Gs in the active conformation. The ADP-ribosylated G-protein upregulates the activity of adenylate cyclase; the result is the intracellular accumulation of high levels of cyclic AMP **(Fig. 7.3)**. Since GTP hydrolysis is the event that inactivates the adenylate cyclase, the enzyme remains continually activated. The active Gs protein, in turn, continuously activates protein kinase A. PKA opens a chloride channel (a CFTR channel) and inhibits the Na^+–H^+ exchanger by phosphorylation **(Fig. 7.4)**.

The net result of the phosphorylation of these channels is inhibition of the absorptive sodium transport system in villus cells and activation of the secretory chloride transport system in crypt cells, and these events lead to the accumulation of sodium chloride in the intestinal lumen. Since water moves passively to maintain osmolality, isotonic fluid accumulates in the lumen. Watery diarrhea results, when the volume of the fluid exceeds the capacity of the rest of the gut to resorb it. Unless the wasted fluid and electrolytes are adequately replaced, shock (due to profound dehydration) and acidosis (due to loss of bicarbonate) follow. **Although perturbation of the adenylate cyclase pathway is the primary mechanism by which cholera toxin causes excess fluid secretion, increasing evidence indicates that cholera toxin also enhances intestinal secretion via prostaglandins and/or neural histamine receptors.**

Patients suffering from cholera for 4–6 days may pass as much as twice their body weight in fluid.

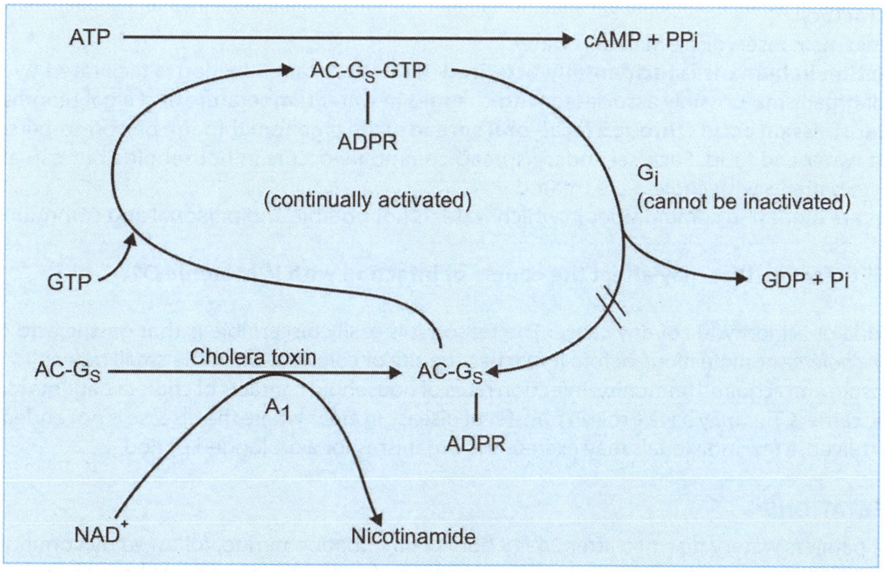

Fig. 7.3: Inactivation of guanosine triphosphatase (GTPase) enzyme by ADP-ribosylation, as a result, there is constant activation of adenylate cyclase to produce cyclic adenosine monophosphate (cAMP).

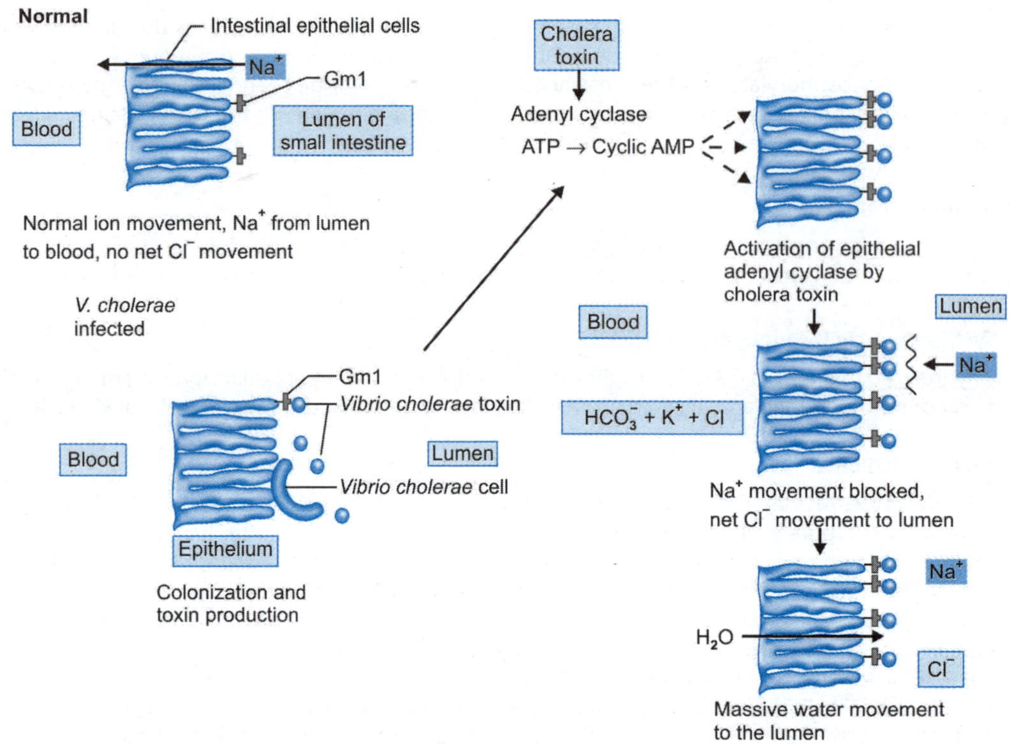

Fig. 7.4: Cholera toxin, mechanism of action.

INCIDENCE

It is common (endemic) in parts of Asia, the Middle East, Africa, and South and Central America. In endemic areas, outbreaks usually occur when war or civil unrest disrupts public sanitation services. Infection is most common during warm months and among children. In newly affected areas, outbreaks may occur during any season and affect all ages equally.

CAUSES

Certain environmental and host factors appear to play a role in the spread of *V. cholerae*.

- **Environmental factors:**
  - Cholera has two main reservoirs—man and water.
  - **Primary infection in humans is incidentally acquired**. Risk of primary infection is facilitated by seasonal increases in the number of organisms, possibly associated with changes in water temperature and algal blooms.
  - **Secondary transmission occurs through fecal–oral spread** of the organism through person-to-person contact or through contaminated water and food. Such secondary spread commonly occurs in households but can also occur in clinics or hospitals where patients with cholera are treated.
  - Infection rates are highest in communities in which water is not potable and personal and community hygiene standards are low.
- **Host susceptibility factors that may affect the course of infection with *V. cholerae* O1:**
  - Malnutrition
  - Hypochlorhydria or achlorhydria of any cause: The reason it is easily discernible is that gastric acid can quickly render an inoculum of *V. cholerae* noninfectious before it reaches the site of colonization in the small bowel.
  - Previous exposure and acquired immunity: Infection rates of household contacts of cholera patients range from 20% to 50%.
  - Asymptomatic carriers: This may have a role in transfer of disease in areas where the disease is not endemic. Although carriage usually is short-lived, a few individuals may excrete the organisms for a prolonged period.

CLINICAL MANIFESTATIONS

- Sudden onset of painless watery diarrhea after 24–48 hours of incubation period, followed by vomiting.
- Stool volume increases quickly and in severe cases, it can exceed 250 mL/kg in the first 24 hours causing **hypovolemic shock** and death in untreated cases.

- The stool has a typical "rice–water" appearance.
- Fever is generally absent but muscle cramps due to electrolyte imbalance are very common.
- The clinical features vary with the degree of dehydration:
  - Excessive thirst—at losses ranging between 3% and 5% of normal body weight.
  - Decreased skin elasticity, postural hypotension, tachycardia, and weakness—at 6–8% of losses.
  - Oliguria, weak or absent pulses, sunken eyes (and, in infants, sunken fontanelles), wrinkled skin, somnolence, and coma—above 9–10% of losses.

COMPLICATIONS

- Dehydration
- Electrolyte imbalance
- Acute tubular necrosis.

Cholera resolves itself in a few days, with adequate fluid and electrolyte replacement complications can be averted.

LABORATORY INVESTIGATIONS

The diseases is characterized by:

- High hematocrit (due to hemoconcentration) in nonanemic patients
- Mild leukocytosis
- High blood urea nitrogen (BUN) and creatinine due to prerenal azotemia
- Normal sodium, potassium, and chloride levels
- Reduced bicarbonate level (<15 mmol/L), and
- High-anion gap metabolic acidosis: Arterial pH is usually low (~7.2), high-anion gap (due to increases in serum lactate, protein, and phosphates).

DIAGNOSIS

The clinical suspicion of cholera can be confirmed by the identification of *V. cholerae* in stool. In endemic areas, there is little need for biochemical confirmation and characterization, although these tasks may be worthwhile in places where *V. cholerae* is an uncommon isolate.

The yield of stool cultures for the diagnosis of *V. cholerae* infection declines late in the course of the illness or when effective antibacterial therapy is initiated. **Monoclonal antibody-based diagnostic kits and methods based on the polymerase chain reaction and on DNA probes have been developed for detection of *V. cholerae* O1 and O139.**

TREATMENT

Rapid replacement of lost body water and salts is lifesaving. Fluid replacement may be given orally, but oral rehydration is not always feasible in the presence of significant vomiting. Oral rehydration takes advantage of the hexose-Na^+ cotransport mechanism to move Na^+ across the gut mucosa together with an actively transported molecule such as glucose. For the sake of simplicity, the WHO advises routine use of a single solution of oral rehydration salts (ORS) for diarrheal disease rather than encouraging attempts to choose among multiple formulations according to etiology. A simple oral replacement fluid can be made from 1 teaspoon of table salt and 4 heaping teaspoons of sugar added to 1 liter of water. Intravenous fluids are indicated for persons with signs of severe hypovolemia and those who cannot take adequate fluids orally. Lactated Ringer's infusion is satisfactory. Solid foods can be eaten after vomiting stops and appetite returns.

People are usually given an antibiotic to reduce the severity of diarrhea and make it stop sooner. Also, people who take an antibiotic are slightly less likely to spread the infection during an outbreak. Tetracycline or doxycycline is effective in adults, unless the bacteria in the area are resistant to tetracycline. Then, ciprofloxacin can be used. Because tetracycline and doxycycline discolor the teeth in children under 8 years old, azithromycin, erythromycin, or trimethoprim-sulfamethoxazole more than 50% of untreated people with severe cholera die. Less than 1% of people who receive prompt and adequate fluid replacement die.

PREVENTION

Purification of water supplies and appropriate disposal of human waste are essential. Other precautions include using boiled or chlorinated water and avoiding uncooked vegetables and undercooked fish or shellfish. Shellfish tend to carry other forms of *Vibrio* as well.

Several vaccines for cholera are available outside the United States. These vaccines provide only partial protection for a limited time and, therefore, are not generally recommended. New vaccines are currently being tested.

CLINICAL NOTE

Unless the wasted fluid and electrolytes are adequately replaced, shock (due to profound dehydration) and acidosis (due to loss of bicarbonate) can follow in cholera.

CLINICAL PEARLS

1. Cholera is caused by *Vibrio cholerae* O1 or, more recently, by *V. cholerae* O139.
2. Cholera is a toxin-mediated disease. Its characteristic watery diarrhea is due to the action of cholera toxin, a potent protein enterotoxin elaborated by the organism after it colonizes the small intestine.
3. Patients present with watery diarrhea and vomiting, usually with no fever.
4. Identifying the bacteria in a stool sample confirms the diagnosis.
5. Replacing lost fluids and giving antibiotics effectively treat the infection.

SUMMARY OF PATHOGENESIS OF CHOLERA

1. Normally Na^+ is absorbed from the intestinal lumen through Na^+/H^+ exchange system.
2. In the infected cells, β subunit of cholera toxin binds to GM1 ganglioside and α subunit brings about covalent modification of Gs protein. As a result, there is accumulation of cAMP.
3. There is constant activation of protein kinase A enzyme.
4. Protein kinase A (PKA) opens the chloride channel but inhibits Na^+/H^+ exchange. In these events, there is accumulation of Na^+ and Cl^- in the lumen. Water moves out as an osmotic effect.

Chapter 8

Nucleotide—Metabolism and Related Disorders

LEARNING OBJECTIVES

To understand the disorders of:

- Pathway of purine nucleotide degradation,
- Salvage pathway of purine nucleotide biosynthesis, and
- Pathway of *de novo* synthesis of pyrimidine nucleotides

CASE STUDIES

CASE STUDY 1

Theme: Biochemical Basis of Severe Combined Immunodeficiency in Adenosine Deaminase Enzyme Defect

A 17-month-old girl was found to have a severe combined immunodeficiency disease. This resulted in recurring respiratory infections. Injection of Diphtheria-Pertussis-Tetanus (DPT) and Typhoid vaccine produced only a minimal response.

The lysates of girl's erythrocytes were found to lack detectable adenosine deaminase activity. Her mother and father both showed approximately 50% of the normal red cell adenosine deaminase activity.

How is this deficiency related with immunodeficiency?
What is the reaction catalyzed by adenosine deaminase?
What is the possible treatment for this deficiency disease?

CASE DETAILS

Adenosine deaminase deficiency, also called ADA deficiency or ADA-SCID, is an autosomal recessive disorder that causes immunodeficiency. It accounts for about 15% of all cases of severe combined immunodeficiency (SCID). The SCID syndrome is characterized by gross functional impairment of both humoral and cell-mediated immunity and by susceptibility to devastating fungal, bacterial, and viral infections.

ADENOSINE DEAMINASE DEFICIENCY

Inheritance

The SCID syndrome is inherited either as an X-linked or autosomal recessive defect, and affected infants rarely survive beyond 1 year without treatment. The syndrome has been associated with mutations in one of several genes whose products are necessary for the normal differentiation of T, B, and sometimes, NK cells.

About half of patients with autosomal recessive SCID are deficient in an enzyme involved in Purine metabolism, adenosine deaminase (ADA), due to mutations in the ADA gene. The abortive lymphoid differentiation associated with ADA deficiency is due to intracellular accumulation of adenosine and deoxyadenosine nucleotides that trigger apoptosis of immature T and B lineage cells.

Severe combined immunodeficiency (SCID) may also occur with an X-linked inheritance pattern. Aborted thymocyte differentiation and an absence of peripheral T cells and NK cells are seen in X-linked SCID.

Incidence

The overall incidence of SCID is 1 in 100,000 to 1 in 1,000,000.

Adenosine deaminase: Catalyzes the conversion of adenosine to inosine and deoxyadenosine to deoxyinosine. Purine nucleoside phosphorylase catalyzes the phosphorolytic cleavage of inosine and deoxyinosine to yield hypoxanthine and either ribose-1-phosphate or deoxyribose-1-phosphate **(Fig. 8.1)**.

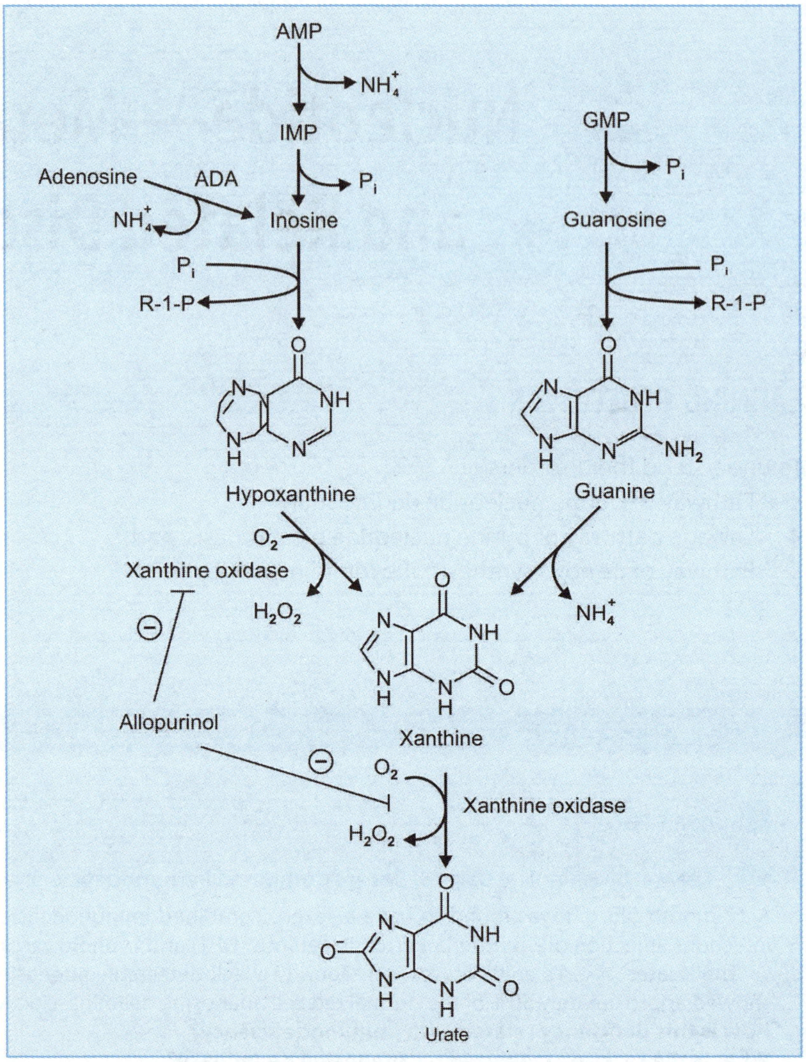

Fig. 8.1: Reaction catalyzed by adenosine deaminase.

Pathogenesis

Defects in this enzyme result in the accumulation of adenosine and deoxyadenosine, as well as inosine, if the purine nucleoside phosphorylase is also deficient. Excessive adenosine can be deaminated through a different route through conversion to AMP and then catabolized by adenylate deaminase. Excessive deoxyadenosine, however, accumulates and is either excreted or is converted to dATP. High concentrations of dATP are found in the lymphocytes of patients with adenosine deaminase deficiency. The enzyme ribonucleotide reductase is inhibited by the abnormally high concentration of dATP. As a result, the concentration of other deoxyribonucleotides is also reduced, and this inhibits DNA synthesis. The actively proliferating cells like T and B lymphocytes are most affected by impaired DNA synthesis. Accumulation of deoxyadenosine causes an increase in S-adenosyl homocysteine; by the back reaction of *S-adenosyl homocysteine hydrolase*, both substances are toxic to immature lymphocytes, which thus fail to mature. Intracellular accumulation of adenosine and deoxyadenosine nucleotides triggers the apoptosis of immature T and B lineage cells. Thus, the proliferation, differentiation, and the maturation of T and B lymphocytes are most affected; as a result, the immune response is grossly decreased and the affected person becomes highly susceptible to infections.

Clinical Manifestations

Adenosine deaminase (ADA) deficiency may present in infancy, childhood, adolescence, or adulthood. The disease is characterized by unusual susceptibility to infection. Patients have recurrent or chronic sinopulmonary infections, meningitis, and bacteremia, most commonly caused by pyogenic bacteria such as *Haemophilus influenzae*, *Streptococcus pneumoniae*, and *Staphylococcus aureus*. Individuals with severe combined immunodeficiency (SCID) are susceptible to the whole range of infectious agents including organisms not ordinarily considered pathogenic. Multiple infections with viruses, bacteria, and fungi occur, often simultaneously. Because donor lymphocytes cannot be rejected by these recipients, blood transfusions can produce fatal graft-versus-host disease.

Laboratory Diagnosis

The following investigations are carried out:
- Complete blood count with differential smear
- Serum immunoglobulin levels: IgM, IgG, IgA, IgD, IgE
- Delayed hypersensitivity skin tests
- Proliferative response to mitogens
- Response to immunization with protein (tetanus toxoid) and carbohydrate (pneumococcal vaccine, *H. influenzae* B vaccine) antigens
- Quantitative IgG subclass determinations.

Treatment

Symptomatic only, permanent cure is possible by any of the following methods:

- **Bone marrow transplant**
- **Enzyme replacement therapy:** Transfusions of red blood cells (containing high levels of ADA) from a healthy donor
- **Gene therapy:** The best current therapy introduces the normal adenosine deaminase enzyme gene into the white cells of the immune system that have been removed from the patient. The corrective gene is encapsulated in to empty viral shells so that the gene can bind to the appropriate target cells, condense with the target cell membrane, and deliver the gene into the cell. All the viral nucleic acid has been removed from the viral shells, so this therapy does not infect the cells with the virus. The viral protein coat that makes up the viral shells protects the corrective gene from breakdown and has surface proteins that bind specifically to receptor proteins on the target cells. After delivering the genes to the cells in the laboratory, the cells are returned to the patient. Since these cells have a short life span, so the therapy has to be repeated. If the stem cells from the bone marrow could be used as receptor cells for the corrective gene, repeated therapy might not be needed; however, the use of the stem cells is under trial.

Prognosis

Prognosis is bad in the untreated cases.

CLINICAL NOTE

Because donor lymphocytes cannot be rejected by these recipients, blood transfusions can produce fatal graft-versus-host disease.

CLINICAL PEARLS

1. Adenosine deaminase deficiency, also called ADA deficiency or ADA-SCID, is an autosomal recessive disorder that causes immunodeficiency.
2. The syndrome has been associated with mutations in one of several genes whose products are necessary for the normal differentiation of T, B, and, sometimes, NK cells.
3. The disease is characterized by unusual susceptibility to infection. Patients have recurrent or chronic sinopulmonary infections, meningitis, and bacteremia, most commonly caused by pyogenic bacteria.
4. Multiple infections with viruses, bacteria, and fungi occur, often simultaneously.
5. Treatment is symptomatic only. Gene therapy can be undertaken for permanent cure.

CASE STUDY 2

Theme: Clinical Significance of Pathway of Purine Nucleotide Degradation

A 46-year-old male presented to the emergency department with severe right toe pain. The patient was in usual state of health until early in the morning when he woke up with severe pain in his right big toe. The patient denied any trauma to the toe and no previous history of such pain in other joints. He did say that he had a "few too many" beers with the guys last night. Patient's past medical history was significant for hypertension, diabetes mellitus, chronic alcoholism, and renal stones for which he underwent left nephrectomy about 25 years ago. Family history was noncontributory.

On examination, he was found to have a temperature of 38.2°C (100.8°F) and in moderate distress secondary to the pain in his right toe. The right big toe was swollen, warm, red, and exquisitely tender. The remainder of the examination was normal. Synovial fluid was obtained and revealed rod- or needle-shaped crystals that were negatively birefringent under polarizing microscopy, consistent with gout. The laboratory investigation report revealed.

Hemoglobin (8.9 g/dL, ESR 124 mm) at the end of first hour, leukocyte count 7,400/mm^3 with normal differential count. Random blood sugar was 139 mg/dL, serum creatinine (1.6 mg/dL; serum uric acid level was 10.9 mg/dL). His 24-hour urinary uric acid excretion was 446 mg/dL. Serum calcium, phosphorus, LFT, electrolytes, and lipid profile were normal.

What is the likely diagnosis?
How would you make a definite diagnosis?
What is the pathophysiology of this disorder?

CASE DETAILS

The patient is suffering from gouty arthritis. The patient reported with pain in the big toe. Pain in the big toe precipitated by alcohol is very typical of history of gout. The patient had past history of alcoholism and renal stones. High serum urate levels and synovial fluid analysis are diagnostic of gout.

Gout is a metabolic disease most often affecting middle-aged to elderly men and postmenopausal women. It is the result of an increased body pool of urate with hyperuricemia. It is typically characterized by episodic acute and chronic arthritis, due to deposition of monosodium urate crystals in joints and connective tissues with the risk for deposition in kidney interstitium or uric acid nephrolithiasis.

Acute arthritis is initially monarticular and often involves the first metatarsophalangeal joint. Symptoms include acute pain, tenderness, warmth, redness, and swelling.

Diagnosis requires identification of crystals in synovial fluid. Treatment of acute attacks is with anti-inflammatory drugs. The frequency of attacks can be reduced by regular use of nonsteroidal anti-inflammatory drugs (NSAIDs), colchicine, or both and by treating hyperuricemia with allopurinol or uricosuric drugs.

Gout

Overview of uric acid metabolism: Uric acid is the final breakdown product of purine degradation in humans.

Purine bases are used in many important biological processes including the formation of nucleic acids [ribonucleic acid (RNA) and deoxyribonucleic acid (DNA)], energy currency [adenosine triphosphate (ATP)], cofactors [nicotinamide adenine dinucleotide (NAD), flavin adenine dinucleotide (FAD)], and cellular signaling [guanosine triphosphate (GTP), ATP, adenosine]. Purines are both synthesized *de novo* and taken in through the diet. Their degradation is a ubiquitous process; however, increased levels of the enzymes that carry out the metabolism of purine bases suggest that purine catabolism is higher in the liver and the gastrointestinal tract. Abnormalities in purine biosynthesis and degradation are associated with numerous disorders suggesting that the regulation of purine levels is essential.

Degradation of purine nucleotides, nucleosides, and bases follows a common pathway **(Fig. 8.1)**. During purine catabolism, the purine nucleotides adenosine monophosphate (AMP) and GMP are generated from the dephosphorylation of ATP and GTP, respectively. AMP is then deaminated to IMP by AMP deaminase. Subsequently, GMP and IMP are dephosphorylated by specific nucleotidases to produce the nucleosides guanosine and inosine, respectively.

Alternatively, AMP can be dephosphorylated to form adenosine, which is then deaminated by adenosine deaminase (ADA) to form inosine **(Fig. 8.1)**. Inosine and guanosine are further broken down by the cleavage of the purine base from the ribose sugar to yield ribose 1-phosphate and hypoxanthine and guanine, respectively. Similar reactions are carried out for the degradation of purine deoxyribonucleotides and deoxyribonucleoside. Guanine is deaminated to form xanthine, whereas hypoxanthine is oxidized to form xanthine by the enzyme xanthine oxidase. Xanthine is further oxidized, again by xanthine oxidase, to form uric acid, which is excreted in the urine.

Uric acid has a pKa of 5.4 and is in the ionized urate form at physiologic pH. Urate is not very soluble in an aqueous environment and the concentration of urate in human blood is very close to saturation. Therefore, conditions that lead to excessive degradation of purine bases can lead to the formation of urate crystals.

Hyperuricemia

Hyperuricemia can result from increased production or decreased excretion of uric acid or from a combination of the two processes. Sustained hyperuricemia predisposes some individuals to develop clinical manifestations including gouty arthritis, urolithiasis, and renal dysfunction.

Hyperuricemia is defined as a plasma (or serum) urate concentration >408 mol/L (6.8 mg/dL). The risk of developing gouty arthritis or urolithiasis increases with higher urate levels and escalates in proportion to the degree of elevation.

Incidence

Hyperuricemia is present in between 2.0% and 13.2% of ambulatory adults and is even more frequent in hospitalized individuals.

Causes of Hyperuricemia

Hyperuricemia may be classified as primary or secondary depending on whether the cause is innate or is the result of an acquired disorder. However, it is more useful to classify hyperuricemia in relation to the underlying pathophysiology, i.e. whether it results from increased production, decreased excretion, or a combination of the two.

1. **Increased urate production**
    - Diet contributes to the serum urate in proportion to its purine content. Strict restriction of purine intake reduces the mean serum urate level by about 60 µmol/L (1.0 mg/dL) and urinary uric acid excretion by ~1.2 mmol/day (200 mg/day). Foods high in nucleic acid content include liver, "sweetbreads" (i.e. thymus and pancreas), kidney, and anchovy. Excessive consumption leads to hyperuricemia.
    - Endogenous sources of purine production also influence the serum urate level. *De novo* purine biosynthesis is an 11-step process that forms inosine monophosphate (IMP). The rates of purine biosynthesis and urate production are determined,

for the most part, by amidophosphoribosyltransferase (amidoPRT), which combines phosphoribosylpyrophosphate (PRPP) and glutamine. Metabolic abnormalities that lead to the overproduction of purine nucleotides through the *de novo* pathway lead to increased purine degradation and subsequent hyperuricemia. An example of this is an increase in the activity of 5-phosphoribosyl-1-pyrophosphate (PRPP) synthetase. This enzyme is responsible for the production of PRPP, which is an important precursor of both purine and pyrimidine *de novo* biosynthesis. Elevations in PRPP lead to increased purine nucleotide production that can in turn increase the rate of degradation and hence increased uric acid production. Similarly, increased activity of amidophosphoribosyltransferase also leads to similar effects of increased uric acid production.

- Hyperuricemia can also result from defects in the purine salvage pathway. The enzyme hypoxanthine-guanine phosphoribosyltransferase (HGPRT) is responsible for reforming IMP and GMP from hypoxanthine and guanine, respectively. In this manner, purine bases are salvaged back into the purine nucleotide pool **(Fig. 8.2)**. Lesch-Nyhan syndrome results from an inherited deficiency in HGPRT. This syndrome is associated with mental retardation and self-destructive behavior, which may be associated with inadequate production of purine nucleotides through the salvage pathway in certain neuronal cells. In addition, Lesch-Nyhan patients have gout resulting from the inability to salvage purine bases, which leads to increased levels of uric acid.

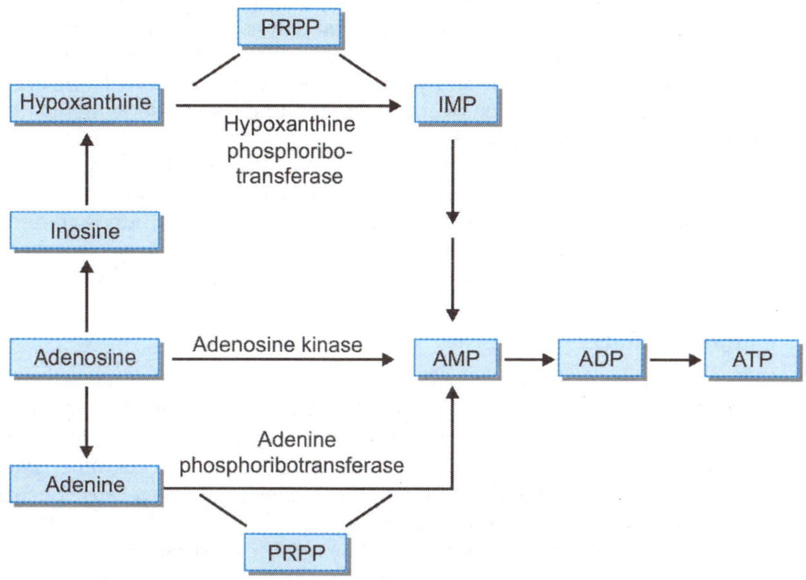

Fig. 8.2: Salvage pathway of purine nucleotide biosynthesis.

- Serum urate levels are closely coupled to the rates of *de novo* purine biosynthesis, which is driven in part by the level of PRPP, as evidenced by two X-linked inborn errors of purine metabolism. Both increased PRPP synthetase activity and HPRT deficiency are associated with overproduction of purines, hyperuricemia, and hyperuricaciduria.
- Overproduction of urate may also be due to glucose-6-phosphatase deficiency (von Gierke disease). In von Gierke disease, its both overproduction and decreased excretion are responsible for hyperuricemia. Overproduction is due to over active HMP pathway to utilize the excess load of glucose-6-phosphate and decreased excretion is due to lactate accumulation as a result of anaerobic glycolysis in muscles. Lactate is excreted while uric acid is reabsorbed through anion exchange transporters.
- Accelerated purine nucleotide degradation can also cause hyperuricemia, i.e. with conditions of rapid cell turnover, proliferation, or cell death, as in leukemic blast crises, cytotoxic therapy for malignancy, hemolysis, or rhabdomyolysis. Hyperuricemia can result from excessive degradation of skeletal muscle ATP after strenuous physical exercise or status epilepticus and in glycogen storage diseases Types III, V, and VII. The hyperuricemia of myocardial infarction, smoke inhalation, and acute respiratory failure may also be related to accelerated breakdown of ATP. Fructose-1-phosphate aldolase deficiency also causes excessive degradation of ATP resulting in hyperuricemia.
- Overproduction of uric acid may also occur, hemolytic anemias, pernicious anemia, ineffective erythropoiesis (as in B-12 deficiency), and obesity.

2. **Decreased uric acid excretion**
   - Over 90% of individuals with sustained hyperuricemia have a defect in the renal handling of uric acid. Gouty individuals excrete ~40% less uric acid than nongouty individuals for any given plasma urate concentration. Common causes of secondary gout due to underexcretion of uric acid include renal insufficiency, lead nephropathy (saturnine gout), starvation or dehydration, hypothyroidism, hyperparathyroidism, drugs (including diuretics and cyclosporine A), and chronic ethanol (especially beer and hard liquor) abuse. These disorders should be identified and corrected, if possible.

Altered uric acid excretion could theoretically result from:

- Decreased glomerular filtration,
- Decreased tubular secretion, or
- Enhanced tubular reabsorption.

Decreased urate filtration does not appear to cause primary hyperuricemia but does contribute to the hyperuricemia of renal insufficiency. Although hyperuricemia is invariably present in chronic renal disease, the correlation between serum creatinine, urea nitrogen, and urate concentration is poor. Uric acid excretion per unit of glomerular filtration rate increases progressively with chronic renal insufficiency, but tubular secretory capacity tends to be preserved, tubular reabsorptive capacity is reduced, and extrarenal clearance of uric acid increases as renal damage becomes more severe.

Many agents that cause hyperuricemia exert their effects by stimulating reabsorption rather than inhibiting secretion.

The kidneys clear urate from the plasma and maintain physiologic balance by utilizing specific organic anion transporters (OATs) including urate transporter 1 (URAT1) and human uric acid transporter (hUAT). URAT1 and other OATs carry urate into the tubular cells from the apical side of the lumen. Once inside the cell, urate must pass to the basolateral side of the lumen in a process controlled by the voltage-dependent carrier hUAT.

Urate transporter (URAT1) is a novel transporter expressed at the apical brush border of the proximal nephron. Uricosuric compounds directly inhibit URAT1 on the apical side of the tubular cell (so-called *cis*-inhibition). In contrast, antiuricosuric compounds, those that promote hyperuricemia, such as nicotinate, pyrazinoate, lactate, and other aromatic organic acids, serve as the exchange anion inside the cell, thereby stimulating anion exchange and urate reabsorption (trans-stimulation). They act through OATs; these anions are exchanged for urates, causing hyperuricemia.

These monovalent anions are also substrates for URAT1. Thus, increased blood levels of these substances result in their increased glomerular filtration and greater reabsorption by proximal tubular cells. The increased intraepithelial cell concentrations lead to increased reabsorption of urate by promoting URAT1-dependent anion exchange. Low doses of salicylates also promote hyperuricemia by this mechanism.

Alcohol promotes hyperuricemia because of increased urate production and decreased uric acid excretion. Excessive alcohol consumption accelerates hepatic breakdown of ATP to increase urate production. Alcohol consumption can also induce hyperlactacidemia, which blocks uric acid secretion. The higher purine content in some alcoholic beverages such as beer may also be a factor.

Decreased renal excretion is by far the most common cause of hyperuricemia. (*See* the causes of hyperuricemia later.)

Pathophysiology

Urate precipitates as needle-shaped monosodium urate (MSU) crystals, which are deposited extracellularly in avascular tissues (e.g. cartilage) or in relatively avascular tissues (e.g. tendons, tendon sheaths, ligaments, walls of bursae) and skin around cooler distal joints and tissues, e.g. ears. In severe, long-standing hyperuricemia, MSU crystals may be deposited in larger central joints and in the parenchyma of organs such as the kidney. At the acid pH of urine, urate precipitates readily as small plate like or irregular crystals that may aggregate to form gravel or stones, which may cause obstruction. Tophi are MSU crystal aggregates that most often develop in joint and cutaneous tissue.

Acute gouty arthritis may be triggered by trauma, medical stress (e.g. pneumonia or other infection), and especially vascular occlusions (e.g. stroke or MI), or by surgery, use of thiazide diuretics or drugs with uricosuric activity (e.g. allopurinol) or indulgence in purine-rich food or alcohol. Attacks are often precipitated by a sudden increase or, more commonly, a sudden decrease in serum urate levels. Why acute attacks follow some of these precipitating conditions is unknown. Tophi in and around joints can limit motion and cause deformities, called chronic tophaceous gouty arthritis.

Symptoms and Signs

Acute gouty arthritis is characterized by sudden onset of pain (usually nocturnal), which typically becomes progressively severe over a few hours, and is usually very intense. The first metatarsophalangeal joint is the first joint to be involved (podagra). The other joints such as ankle, knee, wrist, and **elbow joints are also commonly involved. However, the hip, shoulder, sacroiliac, sternoclavicular, or cervical spine joints are rarely involved. Heat, redness, swelling, and extreme tenderness may indicate** infection **(Fig. 8.3)**. The pain is accompanied by fever, tachycardia, chills, and general malaise. Obesity, hypertension, dyslipidemia, and chronic alcoholism often coexist with gouty arthritis.

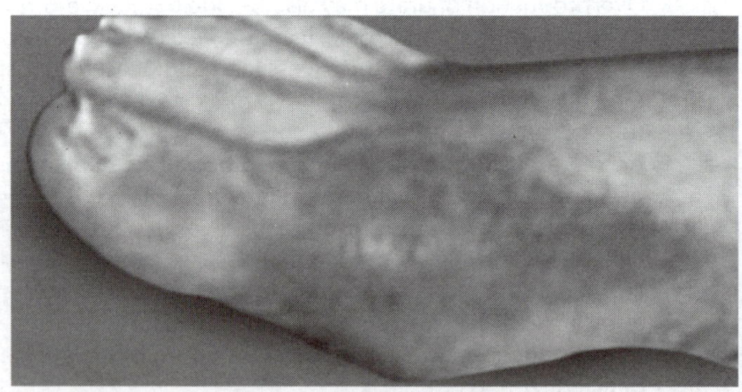

Fig. 8.3: Gout in the foot.

The initial few attacks are monoarticular, lasting only for a small number of days. The subsequent attacks, however, involve multiple joints. The joints may be simultaneously involved or over a period of time. The untreated attacks may last up to 3 weeks. The patients may remain symptoms free in between the attacks but the attacks occur more frequently. Ultimately, many attacks occur each year.

Tophi

Tophi are firm, yellow or white, papules or nodules. They may be single or multiple, and are found mostly on the fingers, hands, feet, ears, olecranon, or Achilles tendons, or even in the kidneys **(Fig. 8.4)**. They can cause deformities; generally, they erupt through the skin discharging urate crystals of chalky consistency.

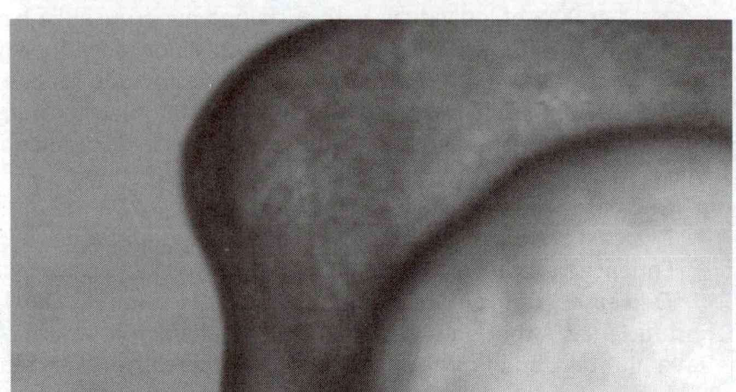

Fig. 8.4: Tophi in chronic arthritis.

Chronic gout: Chronic gout is characterized by a triad of: pain, deformity, and joint stiffness. Degree of joint Inflammation is variable; in some joints, it may be active or intense, while in others, it may be subsiding. Urolithiasis is very common in patients with chronic gout. Chemically, the stones may be uric acid or Ca oxalate stones. Obstruction and infection of the urinary tract with secondary tubulointerstitial disease are a common finding in patients with urolithiasis. The untreated kidney dysfunction, associated with hypertension, or some other cause of nephropathy can further impair the excretion of uric acid, causing deposition of urate crystals in tissues. Gout can also be associated with cardiovascular disease or the metabolic syndrome.

Diagnosis is made from clinical symptomatology and synovial fluid analysis. Clinically, the possibility of gout should be considered in patients with acute monoarticular arthritis, especially in older individuals or those with additional risk factors. Podagra and recurrent instep inflammation are specifically suggestive.

Synovial fluid analysis: Arthrocentesis and synovial fluid analysis are recommended in patients suspected of acute gouty arthritis. The diagnosis can be confirmed upon synovial fluid examination by identifying needle-shaped, strongly negative birefringent urate crystals that are free in the fluid or engulfed by phagocytes.

Serum urate level: Hyperuricemia supports the diagnosis of gout; however, it is neither specific nor sensitive. Serum uric acid level may be normal in around 30% of patients at the time of acute attack. Nonetheless, the size of the extracellular soluble urate pool is gauged by serum urate levels. In order to establish a baseline, the serum urate levels should be estimated on two or three occasions in newly diagnosed patients, and to support the diagnosis, 24-hour urinary urate excretion can also be measured, if serum urate levels are found >7 mg/dL. On a regular diet, 24-hour urinary urate excretion ranges between 600 and 900 mg in normal healthy individuals. The estimation of urinary uric acid concentration can signify whether hyperuricemia results from impaired elimination or increased production. This can help in formulating the therapeutic strategies to lower serum urate levels. The risk of urolithiasis increases in patients with high urinary urate excretion.

X-rays: X-rays of the affected joint may not be required if the diagnosis has already been confirmed by synovial fluid analysis. It may be undertaken to locate the bony tophi.

Diagnosis of chronic gouty arthritis

Chronic gouty arthritis can be suspected in patients with bony tophi and long-standing joint diseases. Since the bony lesions precede the development of subcutaneous tophi, plain X-rays of the first metatarsophalangeal joint or other affected joint can help in the framing the diagnosis.

Prognosis

Early diagnosis can help to improve the quality of life. In advanced cases, abrupt lowering of serum urate levels can improve the joint functions and resolve tophi. Gout is generally more severe in patients whose early symptoms appear before the age of 30 years. The coexisting metabolic syndrome and cardiovascular disease increase the mortality in patients with gout. Small majority of patients do not improve adequately with treatment, presumably due to noncompliance, alcoholism, and under treatment by physicians.

Treatment

- Termination of an acute attack with NSAIDs or corticosteroids
- Prevention of recurrent acute attacks with daily colchicine or an NSAID
- Prevention of further deposition of monosodium urate crystals and resolution of existing tophi by lowering the serum urate level
- Treatment of coexisting hypertension, hyperlipidemia, and obesity.

1. **Treatment of acute attacks:**
   The acute attack can be effectively treated by NSAIDs; however, to prevent relapse, the treatment has to be continued for several days after the pain and signs of inflammation have subsided.
   Oral colchicine produces a quick response if begun shortly after the onset of symptoms. **IV colchicine** is much less likely to cause GI symptoms, therefore, it is highly recommended in postoperative patients or those with GI disorders. IV colchicine is contraindicated in patients with renal or liver diseases or those receiving prophylactic oral colchicine. It may cause severe bone marrow suppression, shock, or even death.
   The use of corticosteroids is controversial; they are known to mask symptoms while inflammation may continue; however, they can be used to treat acute attacks.
   Additionally, for pain relief, analgesics, rest, application of ice, and splinting of the inflamed joints can be recommended. In order to prevent the relapse or prolongation of the attack, the uric acid lowering drugs are not recommended until the complete control of acute symptoms.
2. **Prevention of recurrent attacks:**
   The frequency of acute attacks can be reduced either by taking daily low dose of NSAIDs or colchicine (depending on tolerance and severity).

3. **Lowering the serum urate level:**
The progressive joint damage caused by tophi can be prevented or reversed by urate-lowering drugs. The drugs such as colchicine, NSAIDs, or corticosteroids are ineffective in decreasing the progression of joint damage. Lowering serum urate levels decrease the frequency of acute arthritic attacks as well as resolve tophaceous deposits.
The serum urate levels can be decreased by:
a. **Inhibiting** urate production through allopurinol
b. **Promoting urate excretion with uricosuric drugs**
c. Using a combination of drugs in severe tophaceous gout.
Uricase is not routinely used. Uricase converts urate to allantoin, which is more soluble and can be easily excreted out. IV uricase although transiently lowers serum urate by a large amount.
Hypouricemic therapy is indicated for patients with
- Tophaceous deposits
- Frequent or disabling attacks of gouty arthritis (e.g. more than 2 attacks/year or very severe attacks) despite prophylactic colchicine, an NSAID, or both
- Gout with persistent serum urate ≥9 mg/dL
- Urolithiasis
- Multiple comorbidities (e.g. peptic ulcer disease, chronic kidney disease) that are relative contraindications to the drugs used to treat acute attacks (NSAIDs or corticosteroids).

Allopurinol, that inhibits urate synthesis, is the most commonly prescribed hypouricemic drug. It is especially helpful in treating patients with urolithiasis or severe renal dysfunction. Uric acid stones or gravel can dissolve during allopurinol treatment.
Uricosuric therapy is preferred to allopurinol as early therapy for patients ≤60 years with normal renal function, no history of urolithiasis, and decreased renal urate excretion. Probenecid and sulfinpyrazone can also be tried. Salicylates at low doses antagonize both drugs and can increase urate levels.

Other treatments:

- **Fluid intake** ≥3 L/day is recommended to all patients, especially those who chronically pass urate gravel or stones.
- **Alkalinization of urine** (with K citrate, or acetazolamide) is also occasionally effective for those with persistent uric acid urolithiasis despite hypouricemic therapy and adequate hydration. However, excessive urine alkalinization may cause deposition of Ca oxalate crystals.
- **Extracorporeal shock wave lithotripsy** may be needed to disintegrate renal stones.
- Large tophi in areas with healthy skin may be removed surgically.
- Dietary restriction of purines is less effective, but high intake of **high-purine food and alcohol (beer in particular) should be avoided.**
- **Carbohydrate restriction and weight loss** can lower serum urate in patients with insulin resistance because high insulin levels suppress urate excretion.

4. **Asymptomatic Hyperuricemia**
Hyperuricemia is not usually treated in the absence of gout. Asymptomatic hyperuricemia is elevation of serum urate >7 mg/dL (>0.42 mmol/L) in the absence of clinical gout. Generally, treatment is not required. However, patients with over excretion of urate who are at risk of urolithiasis may receive allopurinol.

CLINICAL NOTE

An elevated serum urate level supports the diagnosis of gout but is neither specific nor sensitive; at least 30% of patients have normal serum urate at the time of an acute attack.

CLINICAL PEARLS

1. Gout is a metabolic disease as a result of an increased body pool of urate with hyperuricemia.
2. Hyperuricemia is defined as a plasma (or serum) urate concentration >408 mol/L (6.8 mg/dL). The risk of developing gouty arthritis or urolithiasis increases with higher urate levels and escalates in proportion to the degree of elevation.
3. Hyperuricemia in relation to the underlying pathophysiology results from increased production, decreased excretion, or a combination of the two.
4. Gout should be suspected in patients with acute monoarticular or oligoarthritis, particularly older adults or those with other risk factors. Podagra and recurrent instep inflammation are particularly suggestive.
5. Treatment consists of treatment of an acute attack with NSAIDs or corticosteroids, prevention of recurrent acute attacks with daily colchicine or an NSAID, prevention of further deposition of MSU crystals, and resolution of existing tophi by lowering the serum urate level and by treatment of coexisting hypertension, hyperlipidemia, and obesity.

Causes of Hyperuricemia

1. Urate overproduction
   - Primary idiopathic
   - HPRT deficiency
   - PRPP synthetase over activity
   - Hemolytic processes
   - Lymphoproliferative diseases
   - Myeloproliferative diseases
   - Polycythemia vera
   - Psoriasis
   - Paget's disease
   - Glycogen storage disease III, V, and VII
   - Rhabdomyolysis
   - Exercise
   - Alcohol
   - Obesity
   - Purine-rich diet.
2. **Decreased uric acid excretion**
   - Primary idiopathic
   - Renal insufficiency
   - Polycystic kidney disease
   - Diabetes insipidus
   - Hypertension
   - Acidosis
   - Lactic acidosis
   - Diabetic ketoacidosis
   - Starvation ketosis
   - Sarcoidosis
   - Lead intoxication
   - Hyperthyroidism
   - Hypothyroidism
   - Toxemia of pregnancy
   - Down syndrome
   - Low dose salicylates
   - Diuretics
   - Alcohol
   - Levodopa
   - Ethambutol
   - Pyrazinamide
   - Nicotinic acid
   - Cyclosporine
3. **Combined mechanism**
   - Alcohol
   - Glucose-6-phosphatase deficiency
   - Shock.

CASE STUDY 3

Theme: Clinical Significance of Salvage Pathway of Purine Nucleotide Biosynthesis

At the age of 11 months, a boy showed signs of delayed motor development and was brought for consultation. His mother had noticed sand-like crystals on the diaper of the baby but reported only when asked particularly about it. History revealed that the child had a compulsive urge to bite his lips and fingers. Upon questioning the mother revealed that she had a brother with similar symptoms.

The Lesch-Nyhan syndrome was suspected; urinary and serum uric acid levels were estimated. Both were abnormally high for the boy's age. The diagnosis was confirmed by estimating enzyme levels in skin fibroblasts; the enzyme activity was 50% of the normal.

Which enzyme is deficient in Lesch-Nyhan syndrome?
What is the basis for hyperuricemia, hyperuricosuria, and self-mutilation in this disorder?

CASE DISCUSSION

Lesch–Nyhan Syndrome

Lesch–Nyhan syndrome (LNS), also known as Nyhan's syndrome, Kelley-Seegmiller syndrome, and Juvenile gout, is a rare, inherited disorder.

Biochemical Defect

Lesch–Nyhan syndrome (LNS) is an X-linked recessive disorder, caused by a deficiency of the enzyme hypoxanthine-guanine phosphoribosyltransferase (HGPRT), and produced by mutations in the HGPRT gene. This enzyme is normally present in each cell in the body, but its highest concentration is in the brain, especially in the basal ganglia. The HGPRT gene has been localized to the long arm of the X chromosome (q26-q27). The disorder appears in males; occurrence in females is extremely rare and ascribed to nonrandom inactivation of the X chromosome. One-third of all cases arise *de novo* (from new mutations) and do not have a family history. The mutations are heterogeneous, including single base substitutions, deletions, insertion, or substitutions.

Pathogenesis

Formation of DNA (during cell division) requires nucleotides, molecules that are the building blocks for DNA. The purine bases (adenine and guanine) and pyrimidine bases (thymidine and cytosine) are bound to deoxyribose and phosphate and incorporated as necessary. Normally, the nucleotides are synthesized *de novo* from amino acids and other precursors **(Fig. 8.5)**. A small part, however, is "recycled" from degraded DNA of broken-down cells. This is termed the "salvage pathway" **(Fig. 8.2)**.

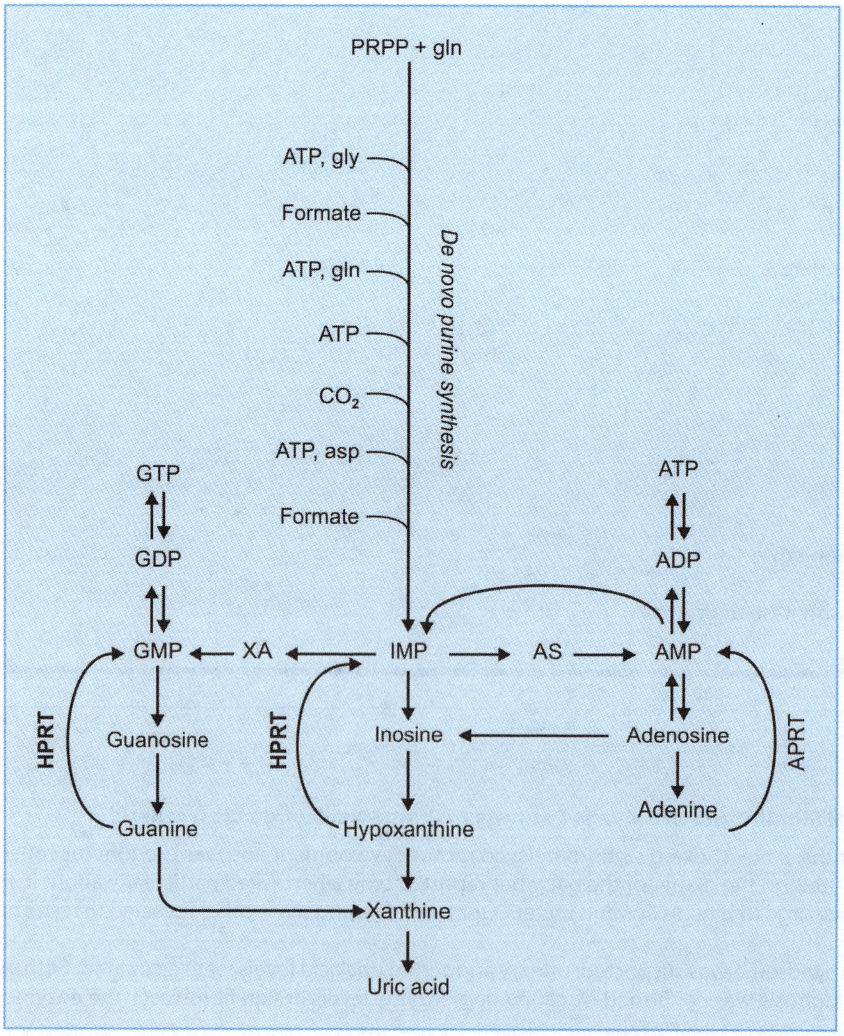

Fig. 8.5: Pathways of purine synthesis (*de novo* and salvage) and degradation to form uric acid.

Hypoxanthine-guanine phosphoribosyltransferase (HGPRT) is the "salvage enzyme" for the purines: it channels hypoxanthine and guanine back into DNA synthesis. Failure of this enzyme has two results:

1. Cell breakdown products cannot be reused, and are therefore degraded. This gives rise to increased uric acid, a purine breakdown product.
2. The *de novo* pathway is stimulated due to an excess of PRPP (5-phospho-D-ribosyl-1-pyrophosphate or simply phosphoribosyl-pyrophosphate).

In the absence of HGPRT, these purine bases cannot be salvaged, and instead are degraded and excreted as uric acid. In addition to the failure of purine recycling, the synthetic rate for purines is accelerated, presumably to compensate for purines lost by the failure of the salvage process. The failure of recycling together with the increased synthesis of purines is the basis for the overproduction of uric acid.

The increased production of uric acid leads to hyperuricemia. Since uric acid is near its physiological limit of solubility in the body, the persistent hyperuricemia increases the risk of uric acid crystal precipitation in the tissues to form tophi. Uric acid crystal deposition in the joints produces an inflammatory reaction and gouty arthritis. The kidneys respond to the hyperuricemia by increasing its excretion into the urogenital system, increasing the risk of forming urate stones in the urinary collecting system. These stones may be passed as a sandy sludge or as larger particles that may obstruct urine flow and increase the risk for hematuria and urinary tract infections.

The pathogenesis of the neurological and behavioral features is incompletely understood. Neurochemical and neuroimaging studies have demonstrated significant abnormalities of dopamine neuron function in the basal ganglia that might account for the abnormal extrapyramidal neurological signs and many of the behavioral anomalies. However, the mechanism by which HGPRT deficiency influences the basal ganglia, and particularly the dopamine systems, remains unknown. However, both hypoxanthine and guanine metabolism is affected and guanosine triphosphate and adenosine have substantial effects on neural tissues.

Frequency

The reported worldwide prevalence is 1 case per 380,000 population.

CLINICAL MANIFESTATIONS

Lesch–Nyhan syndrome (LNS) is characterized by three major hallmarks: neurological dysfunction, cognitive and behavioral disturbances including self-mutilation, and uric acid overproduction (hyperuricemia). Some may also be afflicted with macrocytic anemia. Virtually all patients are males; males suffer delayed growth and puberty, and most develop shrunken testicles or testicular atrophy. Female carriers are at an increased risk for gouty arthritis, but are usually otherwise unaffected.

There are several clinical presentations of HGPRT deficiency:

- The majority of individuals with classic LNS have low or undetectable levels of the HGPRT enzyme.
- Partial deficiency in HPRT (Kelley-Seegmiller syndrome) with more than 1.5 to 2.0% enzyme is associated with hyperuricemia and variable neurological dysfunction (neurological HPRT deficiency).
- HPRT deficiency with levels over 8% leads to a severe form of gout, with apparently normal cerebral functioning (HPRT-related hyperuricemia), although cognitive deficits may occur.

1. **Overproduction of uric acid**

   One of the first symptoms of the disease is the presence of sand-like crystals of uric acid in the diapers of the affected infant.

   The overproduction of uric acid is present at birth, but may not be recognized by routine clinical laboratory testing methods. The serum uric acid concentration is often normal initially **(Fig. 8.6)**, as the excess purines are promptly eliminated in the urine. But as the disease progresses, the hyperuricemia may be observed.

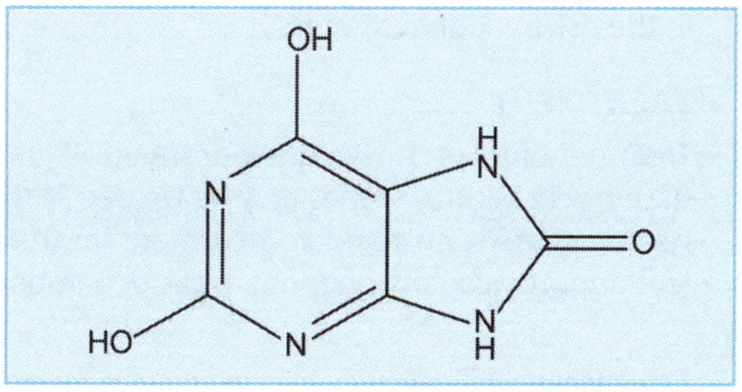

Fig. 8.6: Uric acid.

   The crystals usually appear as an orange grainy material, or they may coalesce to form either multiple tiny stones or distinct large stones that are difficult to pass. The stones, or calculi, usually cause hematuria (blood in the urine) and increase the risk of urinary tract infection. Some victims suffer kidney damage due to such kidney stones. Stones may be the presenting feature of the disease, but can go undetected for months or even years.

2. **Nervous system impairment**

   The most common presenting features are abnormally decreased muscle tone (hypotonia) and developmental delay, which are evident by three to six months of age. Affected individuals are late in sitting up, while most never crawl or walk. Lack of speech is also a very common trait associated with Lesch-Nyhan syndrome (LNS).

Irritability is most often noticed along with the first signs of nervous system impairment. Within the first few years of life, extrapyramidal involvement causes abnormal involuntary muscle contractions such as loss of motor control (dystonia), writhing motions (choreoathetosis), and arching of the spine (opisthotonus). Signs of pyramidal system involvement, including spasticity, overactive reflexes (hyper-reflexia), and extensor plantar reflexes, also occur. The resemblance to athetoid cerebral palsy is apparent in the neurologic aspects of LNS. As a result, most individuals are initially diagnosed as having cerebral palsy. The motor disability is so extensive that most individuals never walk, and are confined to a wheelchair for life.

3. **Self-injuring behavior**
   The age at onset of self-injury may be as early as 1 year and occasionally as late as the teens. The self-injury begins with biting of the lips and tongue; as the disease progresses, affected individuals frequently develop finger biting and head banging. The self-injury can increase during times of stress. Self-mutilation is a distinguishing characteristic of the disease and is apparent in 85% of affected males.

Diagnosis

The gross overproduction of uric acid is often evident in routine blood and urine studies.

- Uric acid levels in the blood typically are elevated, a helpful clue that can be obtained by routine clinical testing; however, hyperuricemia has many different causes, and some patients with Lesch-Nyhan syndrome have serum uric acid levels in the normal range. As a result, serum uric acid levels do not provide reliable diagnostic information.
- Urinary uric acid excretion is also increased typically. A 24-hour urine sample typically demonstrates a marked increase over normative values, particularly if corrected for patient weight. Calculation of the urinary uric acid to creatinine value in a spot urine specimen provides an alternative method, though less information is available concerning normative values. Hyperuricosuria is neither sensitive nor specific enough to provide reliable diagnostic information.
  - Definitive diagnosis is obtained most often by measurement of HGPRT enzyme activity in blood or tissue. Blood samples often are used, though intact fibroblasts or lymphocytes provide more precise information with prognostic implications.
  - Diagnosis is confirmed by identifying a molecular genetic mutation in the HGPRT gene. Molecular genetic diagnosis provides an ideal tool for carrier detection and prenatal screening of at-risk pregnancies.
  - Macrocytic anemia, sometimes profound, is relatively common. Vitamin B_{12}, folate, and iron results are typically normal.

Imaging Studies

- Neuroimaging studies of the brain, both CT scan and MRI, generally do not reveal obvious structural malformations or signal changes. They may reveal mild loss of brain volume, but this loss is often so small that it escapes notice in routine imaging studies.
- Neuroimaging studies of the spinal cord, particularly the cervical portions, may reveal early degenerative joint disease that can damage the spinal cord or emerging nerve roots.

Other Tests

Noninvasive imaging studies of the kidneys and other parts of the urogenital system are warranted because of the marked increase in the risk for kidney stones.

TREATMENT

Treatment for Lesch-Nyhan syndrome (LNS) is symptomatic. Gout can be treated with allopurinol to control excessive amounts of uric acid. Kidney stones may be treated with lithotripsy, a technique for breaking up kidney stones using shock waves or laser beams. There is no standard treatment for the neurological symptoms of LNS. Some may be relieved with the drugs carbidopa/levodopa, diazepam, phenobarbital, or haloperidol.

Prognosis

The prognosis for individuals with severe LNS is poor. Death is usually due to renal failure or complications from hypotonia, in the first or second decade of life. Less severe forms have better prognoses.

CLINICAL NOTE

Uric acid levels in the blood typically are elevated in Lesch-Nyhan syndrome; however, hyperuricemia has many different causes, and some patients with Lesch-Nyhan syndrome have serum uric acid levels in the normal range.

CLINICAL PEARLS

1. LNS is an X-linked recessive disorder, caused by a deficiency of the enzyme hypoxanthine-guanine phosphoribosyltransferase (HGPRT), and produced by mutations in the HGPRT gene.
2. LNS is characterized by three major hallmarks: neurological dysfunction, cognitive and behavioral disturbances including self-mutilation, and hyperuricemia. Some may also be afflicted with macrocytic anemia.
3. Uric acid levels in the blood and urine are typically are elevated; definitive diagnosis is obtained most often by measurement of HGPRT enzyme activity in blood or tissue.
4. Treatment for LNS is symptomatic. Gout can be treated with allopurinol to control excessive amounts of uric acid. Kidney stones may be treated with lithotripsy. There is no standard treatment for the neurological symptoms of LNS.
5. The prognosis for individuals with severe LNS is poor.

CASE STUDY 4

Theme: Clinical Significance of Pathway of *De Novo* Synthesis of Pyrimidine Nucleotides

A 4-year-old girl presented to the clinic with megaloblastic anemia and failure to thrive. History revealed that the child was born normally. The red blood cell count was 2.55 million/mm^3 and hemoglobin was 6 g/dL. He was given antibiotics and transfusions. Despite this, the anemia worsened. There was no response following treatment with B_{12}, folic acid, or pyridoxine.

A prominent feature of the child's urine was a crystalline sediment, which was found to be orotic acid.

Orotic acid in amounts as high as 1,500 mg (9.6 mmol) was excreted daily (normal 1.4 mg/day, 9 µmol). Enzyme measurements of white blood cells revealed a deficiency of the pyrimidine biosynthesis enzyme orotate phosphoribosyltransferase and abnormally high activity of enzyme aspartate transcarbamoylase.

What is the disease?
How can this be treated?

CASE DISCUSSION

The child is suffering from orotic aciduria.

BASIC CONCEPT

Orotic Aciduria

Orotic aciduria refers to an excessive excretion of orotic acid in urine **(Fig. 8.7)**.

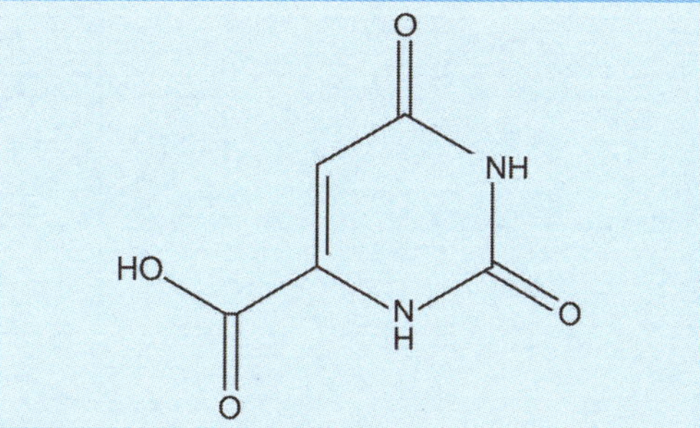

Fig. 8.7: Orotic acid.

Biochemical Defect

Orotic aciduria is a rare autosomal recessive disorder. The usual form of hereditary orotic aciduria is the build-up of orotic acid due to the deficiency in one or both of enzymes that convert it to UMP. Either orotate phosphoribosyltransferase and orotidylate decarboxylase both are defective, or the decarboxylase alone is defective. It can also arise secondary to blockage of the urea cycle, particularly ornithine transcarbamoylase deficiency.

Pathway of Pyrimidine Biosynthesis

The first step in *de novo* pyrimidine biosynthesis is the synthesis of carbamoyl phosphate from bicarbonate and ammonia in a multistep process, requiring the cleavage of two molecules of ATP. This reaction is catalyzed by carbamoyl phosphate synthetase (CPS). Carbamoyl phosphate synthetase primarily uses glutamine as a source of ammonia.

Carbamoyl phosphate reacts with aspartate to form carbamoyl aspartate in a reaction catalyzed by *aspartate transcarbamoylase*. Carbamoyl aspartate then cyclizes to form dihydro-orotate, which is then oxidized by NAD$^+$ to form orotate. At this stage, orotate couples to ribose, in the form of 5-phosphoribosyl-1-pyrophosphate (PRPP), a form of ribose activated to accept nucleotide bases. Orotate reacts with PRPP to form orotidylate, a pyrimidine nucleotide. This reaction is driven by the hydrolysis of pyrophosphate. The enzyme that catalyzes this addition, pyrimidine phosphoribosyl transferase, is homologous to a number of other phosphoribosyl transferases that add different groups to PRPP to form the other nucleotides. Orotidylate is then decarboxylated to form *uridylate (UMP)*, a major pyrimidine nucleotide that is a precursor to RNA. This reaction is catalyzed by orotidylate decarboxylase. This enzyme is one of the most proficient enzymes known. In its absence, decarboxylation is extremely slow and is estimated to take place once every 78 million years; with the enzyme present, it takes place approximately once per second, a rate enhancement of 1017-fold! **(Fig. 8.8)**

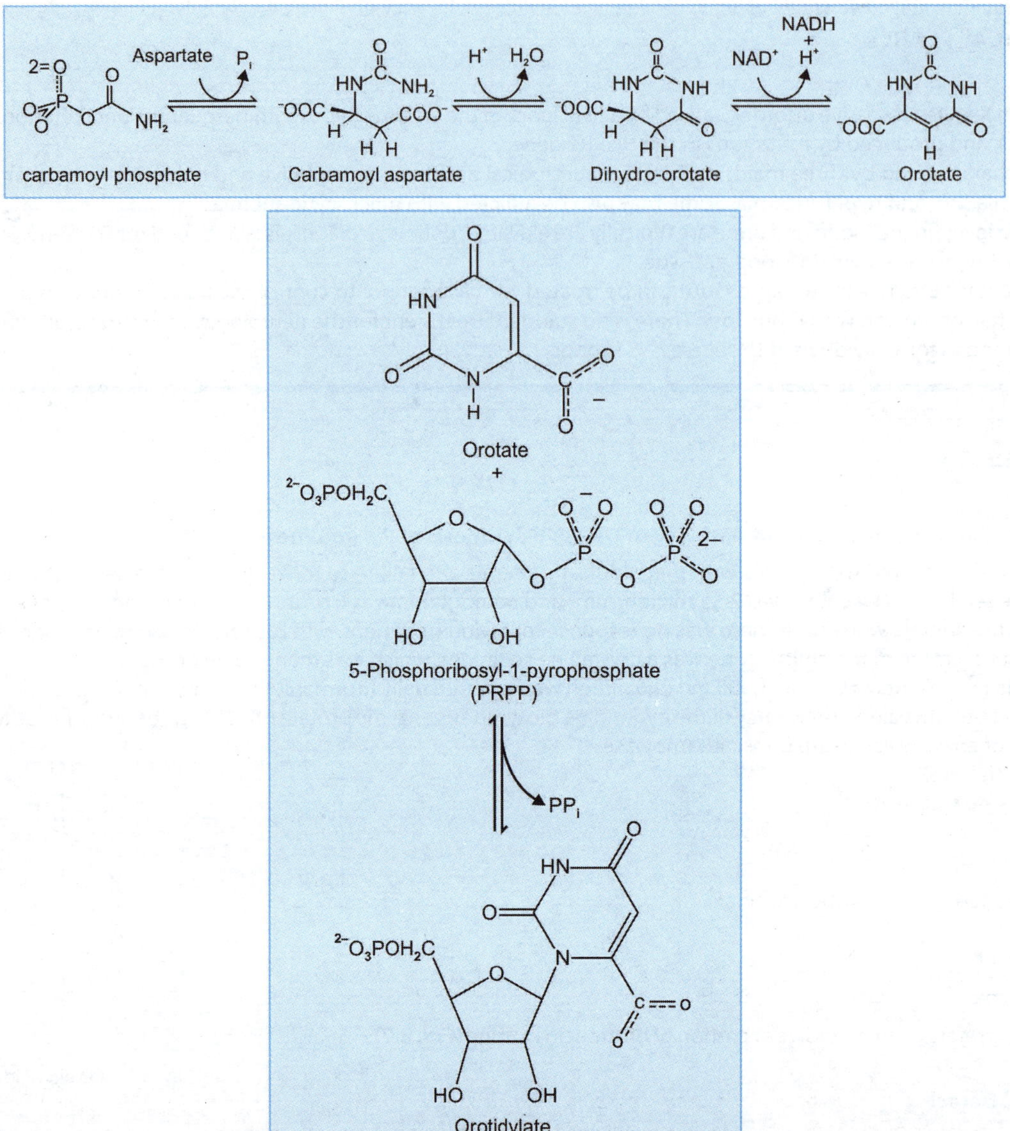

Fig. 8.8: *De novo* synthesis of pyrimidine nucleotide.

Uridylate (UMP) is the parent nucleotide; the other pyrimidine nucleotides are formed from UMP only but UMP is converted into UTP before the synthesis can take place as shown in **Figure 8.9**.

CLINICAL MANIFESTATIONS

This disorder usually appears in the first year of life and is characterized by growth failure, developmental retardation, megaloblastic anemia, and increased urinary excretion of orotic acid.

Uridylate (UMP), the end product of this pathway, is the precursor of UTP, CTP, and TMP. All of these end products normally act in some way to feedback inhibit the initial reactions of pyrimidine synthesis. Specially, the lack of CTP inhibition allows aspartate transcarbamoylase to remain highly active. This results in more and more production of orotic acid which gets accumulated and is excreted in urine excessively.

Lack of CTP, TMP, and UTP leads to a decreased nucleic acid synthesis and decreased erythrocyte formation resulting in megaloblastic anemia. Physical and mental retardation is frequently present. The anemia is refractory to vitamin B_{12} or folic acid.

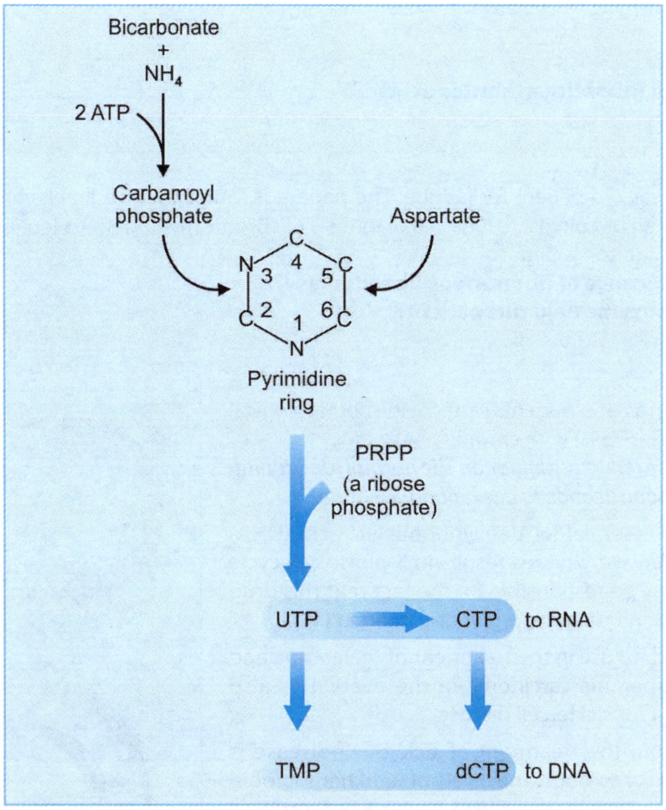

Fig. 8.9: *De novo* pyrimidine biosynthesis.

Laboratory Diagnosis

The diagnosis of this disorder is suggested by the presence of severe megaloblastic anemia with normal serum B_{12} and folate levels and no evidence of TC-II deficiency (Transcobalamin-II). A presumptive diagnosis is made by finding increased urinary orotic acid. Confirmation of the diagnosis, however, requires assay of the transferase and decarboxylase enzymes in the patient's erythrocytes.

TREATMENT

Uridine treatment is effective because uridine can easily be converted into UMP by omnipresent tissue kinases, thus allowing UTP, CTP, and TMP to be synthesized and feedback inhibit further orotic acid production.

CLINICAL NOTE

The megaloblastic anemia in orotic aciduria is refractory to vitamin B_{12} or folic acid.

CLINICAL PEARLS

1. Orotic aciduria refers to an excessive excretion of orotic acid in urine.
2. Orotic acid due to the deficiency in one or both of enzymes that convert it to UMP. Either orotate phosphoribosyltransferase and orotidylate decarboxylase both are defective, or the decarboxylase alone is defective. It can also arise secondary to blockage of the urea cycle, particularly ornithine transcarbamoylase deficiency.
3. This disorder usually appears in the first year of life and is characterized by growth failure, developmental retardation, megaloblastic anemia, and increased urinary excretion of orotic acid.
4. A presumptive diagnosis is made by finding increased urinary orotic acid. Confirmation of the diagnosis, however, requires assay of the transferase and decarboxylase enzymes in the patient's erythrocytes.
5. Uridine treatment is effective because uridine can easily be converted into UMP by omnipresent tissue kinases, thus allowing UTP, CTP, and TMP to be synthesized and feedback inhibit further orotic acid production.

CASE STUDY 5

Theme: Clinical Role of Ribonucleotide Reductase

CASE DETAILS

A physician evaluates a 32-year-old patient for fatigue. The patient is found to have an elevated white blood cell count and an enlarged spleen. A referral to an oncologist results in a diagnosis of chronic myelogenous leukemia. Treatment with hydroxyurea, a ribonucleotide reductase inhibitor, is begun.

What is the biological significance of ribonucleotide reductase?
How will inhibition of this enzyme help this patient?

CASE DISCUSSION

Either hydroxyurea or Busulfan as single agents can provide hematological control in majority of patients (>75%) with chronic phase CML. *Hydroxyurea is a ribonucleotide reductase inhibitor. The normal functioning of this enzyme is to convert ribonucleotide to deoxyribonucleotide.*

Ribonucleotide reductase is essential for deoxyribonucleic acid (DNA) synthesis, and its inhibition by hydroxyurea results in S-phase cell cycle arrest. Other mechanisms may be responsible for the fact that this drug acts as a radiation sensitizer, inhibiting the repair of damaged DNA.

Hydroxyurea is also approved for use in the treatment of melanoma and recurrent, metastatic, or inoperable carcinoma of the ovary. It is also recommended as a treatment for sickle-cell disease.

The efficacy of hydroxyurea in the treatment of sickle-cell disease is generally attributed to its ability to boost the levels of fetal hemoglobin (Hb F, $\alpha 2\gamma 2$). This lowers the concentration of Hb S within a cell resulting in less polymerization of the abnormal hemoglobin.

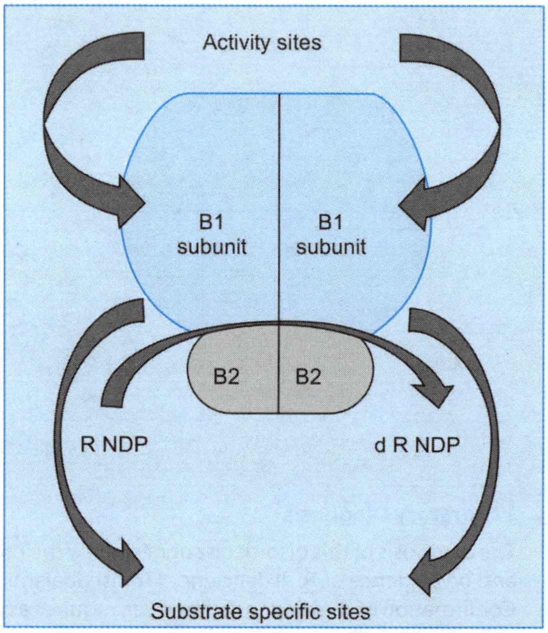

Fig. 8.10: Ribonucleotide reductase enzyme; the activity and substrate sites are for the regulation of enzyme activity.

BASIC CONCEPT

Ribonucleotide Reductase

The reduction of the 2′-hydroxyl of purine and pyrimidine ribonucleotides to deoxyribonucleoside diphosphates (dNDPs) is catalyzed by **ribonucleotide reductase enzyme complex. This is the rate-limiting step of DNA biosynthesis.**

Ribonucleotide reductase is a multi-subunit enzyme having each of two identical B1 and B2 subunits **(Fig. 8.10)**. ADP, GDP, CDP, and UDP are converted to dADP, dGDP, dCDP, and dUDP (their deoxy forms) respectively as a result of its action.

Reaction catalyzed can be represented as in **Figure 8.11**:

The immediate donors of the hydrogen atoms needed for the reduction of the 2′-hydroxyl are two sulfhydryl groups on the enzyme itself, which, during the reaction, form a disulfide bond.

In order for the enzyme to continue its action, the disulfide bond created during the process of catalysis must be reduced back. The process of reduction is carried out by thioredoxin, a peptide coenzyme of ribonucleotide reductase. Thioredoxin contains two cysteine residues separated by two amino acids in the peptide chain. These two sulfhydryl groups of thioredoxin donate their hydrogen atoms to ribonucleotide reductase, in the process forming a disulfide bond. The reduction of Thioredoxin itself is carried out by Thioredoxin reductase. The necessary reducing equivalents are provided by $NADPH^{+}$ H^{+} **(Fig. 8.11)**.

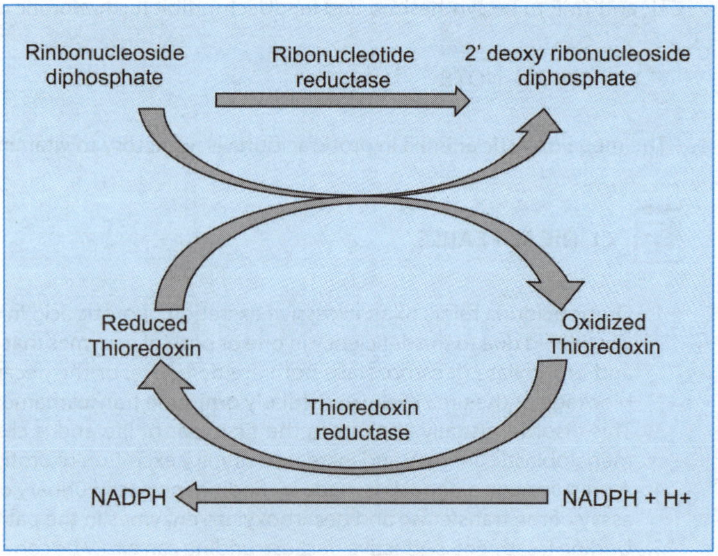

Fig. 8.11: The reaction catalyzed by ribonucleotide reductase; the enzyme complex requires reduced Thioredoxin for its action.

REGULATION OF RIBONUCLEOTIDE REDUCTASE

Reduction of ribonucleoside diphosphates (NDPs) to deoxyribonucleoside diphosphates (dNDPs) is subjected to complex regulatory controls that achieve balanced production of deoxyribonucleotides for the synthesis of DNA. The enzyme has an active site and additionally possesses two allosteric sites. The regulation at these sites can be explained as follows:

1. **Activity site:** The binding of ATP increases the net rate, whereas dATP binding to this allosteric site inhibits the overall catalytic activity of the enzyme, thus the reduction of all the ribonucleotides is inhibited. This effectively prevents DNA synthesis.
   Clinical significance: In "Adenosine deaminase" deficiency, DNA synthesis is inhibited due to inhibitio n of ribonucleotide reductase by excess dATP. The impact is mainly observed in the rapidly dividing cells, especially the proliferation of B and T lymphocytes, which is one of the reasons for reduced immunity in the affected patients.
2. **Substrate specific site:** The binding of specific nucleoside triphosphates to substrate specific site regulates substrates specificity causing an increase in the conversion of specific ribonucleotides to deoxyribonucleotides as required for DNA synthesis.

CLINICAL NOTE

Ribonucleotide reductase is essential for deoxyribonucleic acid (DNA) synthesis, and its inhibition by hydroxyurea results in S-phase cell cycle arrest.

CLINICAL PEARLS

1. The normal function of ribonucleotide reductase is to convert ribonucleotide to deoxyribonucleotide.
2. The immediate donors of the hydrogen atoms needed for the reduction of the 2′-hydroxyl are two sulfhydryl groups on the enzyme itself, which, during the reaction, form a disulfide bond.
3. The enzyme has an active site and additionally possesses two allosteric sites.
4. The binding of ATP increases the net rate, whereas dATP binding to this allosteric site inhibits the overall catalytic activity of the enzyme.
5. In "Adenosine deaminase" deficiency, DNA synthesis is inhibited due to the inhibition of ribonucleotide reductase by excess dATP.

Chapter 9

Clinical Enzymology

LEARNING OBJECTIVES

To understand the disorders of:
- ❖ Diagnostic significance of isoenzymes
- ❖ Clinical significance of serum enzymes
- ❖ Mechanism of enzyme inhibition
- ❖ Mechanism of enzyme action

CASE STUDIES

CASE STUDY 1

Theme: Diagnostic Significance of Isoenzymes

A 46-year-old businessman was admitted to the hospital complaining of severe retrosternal pain of 2-hour duration. He was admitted to the hospital previously also for the treatment of a small myocardial infarction. He was a chronic smoker.

On general examination, his blood pressure was 150/90 mm Hg, pulse 60/min and he was sweating profusely. There was no evidence of cardiac failure. His initial ECG showed ST segment elevation and other changes in certain leads, indicative of an acute anterior transmural infarction. Blood was taken at 4 hours and subsequently at regular intervals for measurement of CPK-MB isoenzymes. He was given injection morphine to relieve his pain and apprehension and was immediately shifted to the cardiac care unit.

What would be the status of CPK enzymes?
What are the other enzymes of importance to detect the presence of acute MI?

CASE DISCUSSION

Enzyme assays routinely carried out for the diagnosis of acute myocardial infarction (MI)—are creatine phosphokinase (CPK), aspartate transaminase and lactate dehydrogenase.

Creatine Kinase (CK, CPK)

It is an enzyme found primarily in the heart and skeletal muscles, and to a lesser extent in the brain but not found at all in liver and kidney. Small amounts are also found in lungs, thyroid and adrenal glands. Significant injury to any of these structures will lead to a measurable increase in CK levels. It is not found in red blood cells and its level is not affected by hemolysis.

Normal value serum activity varies from 10 IU/L to 50 IU/L at 30°C.

Elevations are found in:
- Myocardial infarction
- Crushing muscular trauma
- Any cardiac or muscle disease, but not myasthenia gravis or multiple sclerosis
- Brain injury

- Hypothyroidism
- Hypokalemia.

After myocardial infarction, serum value is found to increase within 3–6 hours, reaches a peak level in 24–30 hours and returns to normal level in 2–4 days (usually in 72 hours). Creatine kinase (CK) is a sensitive indicator in the early stages of myocardial ischemia. No increase in activity is found in heart failure and coronary insufficiency. In acute MI, CPK usually rises faster than serum glutamate-oxaloacetate transaminase (SGOT) and returns to normal faster than the SGOT.

CK/CPK Isoenzymes: There are three isoenzymes. Measuring them is of value in the presence of elevated levels of CK or CPK to determine the source of the elevation. Each isoenzyme is a dimer composed of two protomers "M" (for muscles) and "B" (for brain). These isoenzymes can be separated by electrophoresis or by ion exchange chromatography (**Table 9.1**).

The three possible isoenzymes are: (1) MM (CK3), (2) MB (CK2) and (3) BB (CK1).

TABLE 9.1: Isoenzymes of creatine phosphokinase (CPK).

Isoenzyme	*Electrophoretic mobility*	*Tissue of origin*	*Mean percentage in blood*
MM (CK3)	Least	Skeletal muscle	97–100%
MB (CK2)	Intermediate	Heart muscle	0–3%
BB (CK1)	Maximum	Brain	0%

- Normal levels of CK/CPK are almost entirely MM, from skeletal muscle.
- **Elevated levels of CK/CPK resulting from acute myocardial infarction are about half MM and half MB.** Myocardial muscle is the only tissue that contains more than 5% of the total CK activity as the CK2 (MB) isoenzyme.
- Following an attack of acute myocardial infarction, this isoenzyme appears within 4 hours following onset of chest pain, reaches a peak of activity at approximately 24 hours and falls rapidly. MB accounts for 4.5–20% of the total CK activity in the plasma of the patients with recent myocardial infarction and the total isoenzyme is elevated up to 20-folds above the normal **(Fig. 9.1)**.

Atypical isoenzymes: In addition, to the above three isoenzymes two atypical isoenzymes of CPK have been reported. They are: (1) Macro CK (CK-Macro) and (2) mitochondrial CK (CK-Mi).

- **Macro CK (CK-Macro):** It is formed by the aggregation of CK-BB with immunoglobulins usually with IgG but sometimes IgA. It may also be formed by complexing CK-MM with lipoproteins. No specific disease has been found to be associated with this isoenzyme.
- **Mitochondrial CK (CK-Mi):** It is present bound to the exterior surface of the inner mitochondrial membrane of muscle, liver and brain. It can exist in dimeric form or as oligomeric aggregates having molecular weight of approximately 35,000. It is only present in serum when there is extensive tissue damage causing breakdown of mitochondrial membrane and cell membrane. Thus, its presence in serum indicates severe illness and cellular damage. It is not related with any specific disease states but it has been detected in certain cases of malignant tumors.

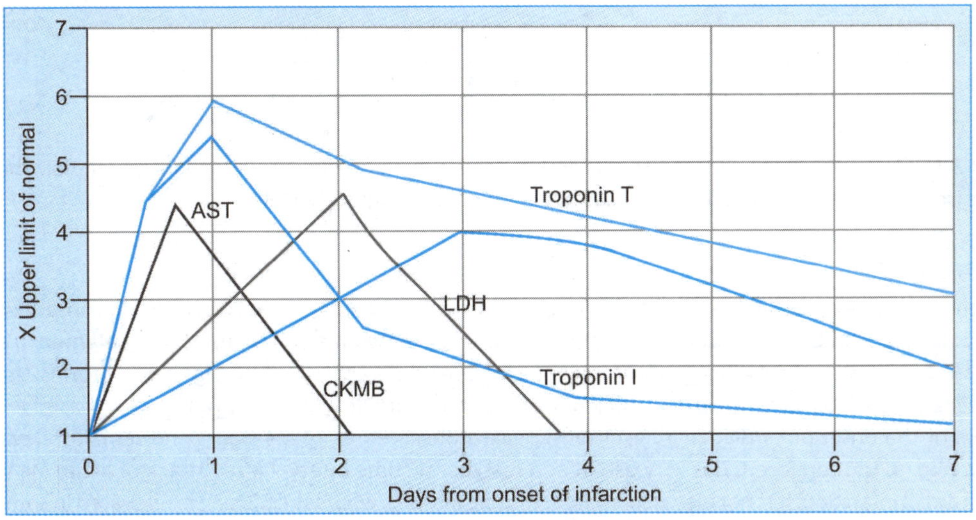

Fig. 9.1: Cardiac markers.

Aspartate Aminotransferase

It is also called as serum glutamate-oxaloacetate transaminase (SGOT). The level is significantly elevated in acute MI.

Normal value: 0–41 IU/L at 37°C.

Acute MI: In acute MI, the serum activity rises sharply within the first 12 hours, with a peak level at 24 hours or over and returns to normal within 3–5 days. The rise depends on the extent of infarction. Reinfarction results in secondary rise of SGOT **(Fig. 9.1)**.

Prognostic significance: Levels >350 IU/L are due to massive infarction (fatal), >150 IU/L are associated with high mortality and levels <50 IU/L are associated with low mortality.

Other diseases: The rise in activity is also observed in muscle and hepatic diseases. These can be well differentiated from simultaneous estimations of other enzyme activities like serum glutamate-pyruvate transaminase (SGPT), etc. which do not show and rise in activity in acute MI.

Dehydrogenase

Lactate dehydrogenase catalyzes the reversible conversion of pyruvate and lactate.

Normal level: 55–140 IU/L at 30°C. The levels in the upper range are generally seen in children. Lactate dehydrogenase (LDH) level is 100 times more inside the RBCs than in plasma, and therefore minor amount of hemolysis results in false-positive result.

Acute MI: In acute MI, the serum activity rises within 12–24 hours, attains a peak at 48 hours (2–4 days) reaching about 1,000 IU/L and then returns gradually to normal from 8th to 14th day. The magnitude of rise is proportional to the extent of myocardial infarction. Serum LDH elevation may persist for more than a week after CPK and SGOT levels have returned to normal levels **(Fig. 9.1)**.

Other diseases: The increase in serum activity of LDH is also seen in hemolytic anemias, hepatocellular damage, muscular dystrophies, carcinoma, leukemias, and any condition which causes necrosis of the body cells. Since the total LDH is increased in many diseases, so the study of isoenzymes of LDH is of more significance.

Isoenzymes of Lactate Dehydrogenase

Lactate dehydrogenase (LDH) enzyme is tetramer with four subunits. The subunit may be either H (heart) or M (muscle) polypeptide chains. These two chains are the product of two different genes. Although both of them have the same molecular weight, there are minor amino acid variations. There can be five possible combinations: (1) H4, (2) H3M1, (3) H2M2, (4) H1M3, and (5) M4, these are five different types of isoenzymes seen in all individuals (**Table 9.2**).

TABLE 9.2: Isoenzymes of lactate dehydrogenase.

No. of isoenzyme	*Subunit make of enzymes*	*Electrophoretic mobility at pH 8.6*	*Activity at 60° for 30 minutes*	*Tissue origin*	*Percentage in human serum (mean)*
LDH-1	H4	Fastest	Not destroyed	Heart muscle	30%
LDH-2	H3M1	Faster	Not destroyed	RBC	35%
LDH-3	H2M2	Fast	Partly destroyed	Brain	20%
LDH-4	H1M3	Slow	Destroyed	Liver	10%
LDH-5	M4	Slowest	Destroyed	Skeletal muscles	5%

Normally LDH-2 (H3M1) level in blood is greater than LDH-1, but this pattern is reversed in myocardial infarction, this is called "flipped pattern". These isoenzymes are separated by cellulose acetate electrophoresis at pH 8.6.

Cardiac Troponins

They are not enzymes; however, they are accepted as markers of myocardial infarction. **The troponin complex consists of three components: (1) troponin C (calcium binding), (2) troponin I (actomyosin ATPase inhibitory element), and (3) troponin T (tropomyosin-binding element).** Troponin I is encoded by three different genes, giving three isoforms; the "slow" and "fast" moving fractions are skeletal variety. Cardiac isoform is specific for cardiac muscle. Troponin I is released into the circulation within 4 hours of the onset of cardiac manifestations, peak is observed at 14–24 hours and remains elevated for 3–5 days postinfarction **(Fig. 9.1)**. Therefore, CTI is very useful as a marker any time interval after attack of acute MI. It is 75% sensitive index for myocardial infarction. It is not elevated in other muscle injuries, whereas CK2 may be elevated in some muscle injuries. CTI level greater than 1.5 mg/dL is indicative of myocardial damage. It is usually assayed by ELISA or RIA techniques.

Two isoforms of troponin T (TnT1 and TnT2) are present in adult cardiac tissue. Serum level of TnT increases within 6 hours of myocardial infarction, peaks at 72 hours and then remains elevated up to 7–10 days. The TnT2 estimation is 100% sensitive index for myocardial infarction.

CLINICAL NOTE

Normally LDH-2 (H3M1) level in blood is greater than LDH-1, but this pattern is reversed in myocardial infarction, this is called "flipped pattern".

CLINICAL PEARLS

1. Enzyme assays routinely carried out for the diagnosis of acute myocardial infarction are creatine phosphokinase, aspartate transaminase and lactate dehydrogenase.
2. Following an attack of acute myocardial infarction, CK-MB isoenzyme appears within 4 hours following onset of chest pain, reaches a peak of activity at approximately 24 hours and falls rapidly.
3. Serum activity of AST rises sharply within the first 12 hours, with a peak level at 24 hours or over and returns to normal within 3–5 days.
4. The serum activity of LDH rises within 12–24 hours, attains a peak at 48 hours (2–4 days) reaching about 1,000 IU/L and then returns gradually to normal from 8th to 14th day.
5. Troponins are not enzymes; however, they are accepted as markers of myocardial infarction. Troponin I is released into the circulation within 4 hours of the onset of cardiac manifestations, peak is observed at 14–24 hours and remains elevated for 3–5 days postinfarction. Serum level of TnT increases within 6 hours of myocardial infarction, peaks at 72 hours and then remains elevated up to 7–10 days. The TnT2 estimation is 100% sensitive index for myocardial infarction.

CASE STUDY 2

Theme: Clinical Significance of Enzymes in Acute Pancreatitis

A 42-year-old obese female presented to the emergency center with complaints of worsening nausea, vomiting, and abdominal pain. Her pain was located in the midepigastric area and right upper quadrant. She reported a low-grade fever and denied diarrhea. Her pain was constantly present and sharp in nature. History revealed that previously also intermittent and cramping pain was there but only after eating "greasy" foods.

On examination, she had a temperature of 37.8°C (100°F) with otherwise normal vital signs. She appeared ill and in moderate distress. She had significant midepigastric and right upper quadrant tenderness. Some guarding was present but no rebound. Her abdomen was otherwise soft with no distention and active bowel sounds. Laboratory values were normal except for increased liver function tests, white blood cell count, and serum amylase. Ultrasound of the gallbladder revealed numerous gallstones and a thickening of the gallbladder wall. A surgical consultation was immediately sought.

What is the most likely diagnosis?

CASE DISCUSSION

The patient probably has acute pancreatitis due to the presence of gallstones. Fat, fertile, female of 40 years and a typical history of pain abdomen after taking fatty foods is suggestive of gallstones. (Ultrasound of the gallbladder also reveals the presence of gallstones). The clinical signs during the acute episode and the laboratory findings (elevated liver function tests, WBC with high-serum amylase) are suggestive of acute pancreatitis.

ACUTE PANCREATITIS

Acute pancreatitis is inflammation of the pancreas (and, sometimes, adjacent tissues) caused by the release of activated pancreatic enzymes.

Etiology

Biliary tract disease and alcoholism account for ≥80% of acute pancreatitis cases. The remaining 20% result from different causes:

Causes of acute pancreatitis:

a. Drugs—ACE inhibitors, asparaginase, azathioprine, 2',3'-dideoxyinosine, furosemide, 6-mercaptopurine, pentamidine sulfa drugs, valproate.
b. Infectious diseases—coxsackie B virus, cytomegalovirus, mumps.
c. Inherited disorders—multiple known gene mutations, including a small percentage of cystic fibrosis patients.
d. Mechanical/structural—gallstones, Endoscopic retrograde cholangiopancreatography (ERCP), trauma, pancreatic or periampullary cancer, choledochal cyst and sphincter of Oddi stenosis.
e. Metabolic—hypertriglyceridemia, hypercalcemia (including hyperparathyroidism), estrogen use associated with high-lipid levels.
f. Toxins—alcohol, methanol.
g. Others—pregnancy, ischemia from hypotension.

Pathophysiology

Acute pancreatitis is a result of anatomical changes that arise from two events. The first is the autodigestion of the acinar cells by inappropriate activation of the pancreatic enzymes (especially trypsinogen) within the cell. The second is the cellular injury response that is mediated by proinflammatory cytokines. The mechanisms by which the digestive enzymes become activated within the acinar cell are unclear. However, such inappropriate activation of pancreatic enzymes leads to destruction of the acinar cell and surrounding fat deposits, and it weakens the elastic fibers of the blood vessels, resulting in leakage.

Obstruction of the main pancreatic duct as a result of a gallstone lodged in or near to the hepatopancreatic ampulla can result in acute pancreatitis. One theory is that obstruction increases the pressure in the main pancreatic duct. The increase in pressure causes interstitial edema, which impairs the blood flow to the acinus. The lack of blood flow leads to ischemic injury of the acinar cell, resulting in release of the digestive enzymes into the interstitial space. How this leads to premature activation of the proenzyme stored in the acinar cell is unclear.

Prolonged alcohol intake (>100 g/day for >3–5 years) may cause the protein of pancreatic enzymes to precipitate within small pancreatic ductules. Ductal obstruction by these protein plugs may cause premature activation of pancreatic enzymes. An alcohol binge in such patients can trigger pancreatitis, but the exact mechanism is not known.

A number of genetic mutations predisposing to pancreatitis have been identified. One, an autosomal dominant mutation of the cationic trypsinogen gene, causes pancreatitis in 80% of carriers; an obvious familial pattern is present. The genetic abnormality responsible for cystic fibrosis increases the risk of recurrent acute as well as chronic pancreatitis.

Irrespective of the cause, pancreatic enzymes (including trypsin, phospholipase A_2, and elastase) get prematurely activated within the gland itself. The activated enzymes trigger the cascades of complement and inflammation, and produce cytokines causing inflammation, edema, necrosis and tissue damage. The systemic inflammatory responses triggered by activated enzymes and cytokines, result in peritoneal irritation, acute respiratory distress syndrome, and renal failure. The enzyme-rich pancreatic fluid and cellular debris can collect in or around the pancreas in about 30–40% of the patients. The collections may resolve spontaneously, or become infected, or may even develop as pseudocysts. The encapsulated pseudocysts have the tendency to hemorrhage, rupture, or become infected.

Clinical Manifestations

- In about 50% of the patients, an acute attack starts with excruciating upper abdominal pain radiating to the back. In rare circumstances, pain can be first felt in the lower abdomen. The onset of pain varies with etiology; in alcoholic pancreatitis, pain develops over a few days, whereas, in gallstone pancreatitis, the pain develops suddenly. Pain persists for several days and is usually accompanied by nausea and vomiting.
- General physical examination reveals a critically-ill patient in an unconscious or semiconscious state. The pulse rate ranges between 100–140 beats/min with a shallow and rapid breathing. Variations in blood pressure are very common, transient hyper- or hypotension may be observed. Postural hypotension is invariably present. Body temperature may be subnormal or normal in the beginning but may rise up to 37.7–38.3°C (100–101°F) within first few hours.
- Mild jaundice is occasionally present.
- Abdomen appears markedly tender and rigid; the tenderness is usually confined to upper abdomen, rarely, mild tenderness and rigidity may be felt in the lower abdomen, rectal tenderness, however, is not observed. Rarely though, severe peritoneal irritation may result in a board-like rigidity over the abdomen.
- Extravasation of hemorrhagic exudate can be indicated by positive "Grey Turner's" sign (ecchymoses of the flanks) and "Cullen's" sign (ecchymoses of the umbilical region).
- Generally critical or toxic appearance of the patient, high body temperature and elevated WBC counts; or worsening of the clinical state following an initial state of stability can arouse suspicion of infection in the pancreas.

Morbidity and Mortality

Cardiovascular instability (with shock and renal failure) or respiratory failure (with hypoxia and adult respiratory distress syndrome) might lead to death in the first few days of illness. However, multiorgan system failure might be the cause of death after the first week of attack.

Diagnosis

Pancreatitis can be suspected in patients with significant alcohol use or previous history of gallstones, whenever they present with severe abdominal pain. Diagnosis can be confirmed by eliminating other causes for symptoms and measuring serum markers (including amylase and lipase).

Laboratory Tests

- A wide range of tests can be included such as complete blood count, serum electrolytes, calcium, magnesium, glucose, blood urea nitrogen (BUN), creatinine, amylase, and lipase.
- ECG and an abdominal series (chest, flat, and upright abdomen) to rule out associated complications. Ultrasound and CT are not generally recommended specifically to diagnose pancreatitis; however, they can be used for the differential diagnosis of acute abdominal pain.
- A urine dipstick for trypsinogen-2 has sensitivity and specificity of >90% for acute pancreatitis.
  1. Serum amylase and lipase levels rise on the first day of acute pancreatitis and return to normal in 3–7 days. Lipase is more specific for pancreatitis, but both enzymes may be increased in renal failure and various abdominal conditions such as perforated ulcer, mesenteric vascular occlusion, or intestinal obstruction. Amylase may rise in salivary gland dysfunction, macroamylasemia, and in amylase-secreting tumors.
  2. Amylase: Creatinine clearance ratio is generally used to diagnose macroamylasemia in the absence of pancreatitis. It lacks sufficient sensitivity or specificity to diagnose pancreatitis. In macroamylasemia, amylase bound to serum immunoglobulin falsely elevates the serum amylase level.
  3. Fractionation of total serum amylase into pancreatic type (p-type) and salivary-type (s-type) isoamylases increases the diagnostic accuracy of serum amylase. However, the level of p-type may also increases in renal failure and in other severe abdominal conditions in which amylase clearance is altered.
  4. WBC count usually increases to 12,000–20,000/μL. Third space fluid losses may increase the Hct to as high as 50–55%, indicating severe inflammation.
  5. Hyperglycemia may occur.
  6. Serum Ca concentration falls as early as the first day due to the formation of Ca "soaps" secondary to excess generation of free fatty acids, especially by pancreatic lipase.
  7. Serum bilirubin increases in 15–25% of patients because of the compression of the common bile duct by pancreatic edema.
  8. In patients with clear evidence of acute pancreatitis, a serum ALT level of more than 150 units/L is suggestive of biliary pancreatitis.

Imaging

- **Plain X-rays of the abdomen** for the diagnose calcifications within pancreatic ducts (evidence of prior inflammation and hence chronic pancreatitis) and calcified gallstones
- **Chest X-ray** may reveal atelectasis or a pleural effusion (usually left-sided or bilateral but rarely confined to the right pleural space).
- **Ultrasound** for the diagnosis of gallstone pancreatitis or when other etiology is not obvious.
- **CT with IV contrast** is generally done to identify necrosis, fluid collections, or pseudocysts once pancreatitis has been diagnosed.
- **Magnetic resonance cholangiopancreatography (MRCP)** can also be used to confirm the diagnosis.

Treatment

- Fluid resuscitation.
- Drugs, including analgesics and antacids.
- Antibiotics.
- Drainage of infected pseudocysts or areas of necrosis.
- Severe acute pancreatitis is treated in an ICU.

Prognosis

In pancreatitis with infection, mortality is about 100%; however, it is 10–50% in pancreatitis with necrosis and hemorrhage, and <5% in edematous pancreatitis.

CLINICAL NOTE

Pancreatitis is suspected whenever severe abdominal pain occurs, especially in a patient with significant alcohol use or known as gallstones.

CLINICAL PEARLS

1. Acute pancreatitis is inflammation of the pancreas (and, sometimes, adjacent tissues) caused by the release of activated pancreatic enzymes.
2. The most common triggers are biliary tract disease and chronic heavy alcohol intake.
3. The condition ranges from mild (abdominal pain and vomiting) to severe (pancreatic necrosis and a systemic inflammatory process with shock and multiorgan failure).
4. Diagnosis is based on clinical presentation and serum amylase and lipase levels.
5. Treatment is supportive with IV fluids, analgesics, and fasting.

CASE STUDY 3

Theme: Mechanism of Enzyme Inhibition

CASE DETAILS

A 56-year-old female presents with difficulty opening her eyelids, as well as inability to raise herself from sitting position. She is diagnosed with "myasthenia gravis", a disease of extreme fatigue, due to decreased concentration of acetylcholine in her muscles. She has been prescribed physostigmine, a drug that increases the amount of available acetylcholine, by competitively inhibiting acetylcholinesterase.

What is the exact mechanism of action of acetylcholinesterase?

How does it help in managing myasthenia gravis?

CASE DISCUSSION

Myasthenia gravis (MG) is a neuromuscular disorder characterized by weakness and fatigability of skeletal muscles.

Biochemical Defect

The major defect in **myasthenia gravis** is a marked reduction in number of acetylcholine receptors on the motor endplate where cranial nerves form a neuromuscular junction with muscle. Normally acetylcholine released by the nerve terminal binds to the receptor on the muscle endplate, resulting in the stimulation of the muscle contraction by depolarizing the muscle membrane, but in these patients, autoantibodies are found against the acetylcholine receptors, which effectively reduce the receptor numbers. Some forms of the antibodies impair the ability of acetylcholine to bind to receptors. Others lead to the destruction of receptors, either by complement fixation or by inducing the muscle cell to eliminate the receptors through endocytosis.

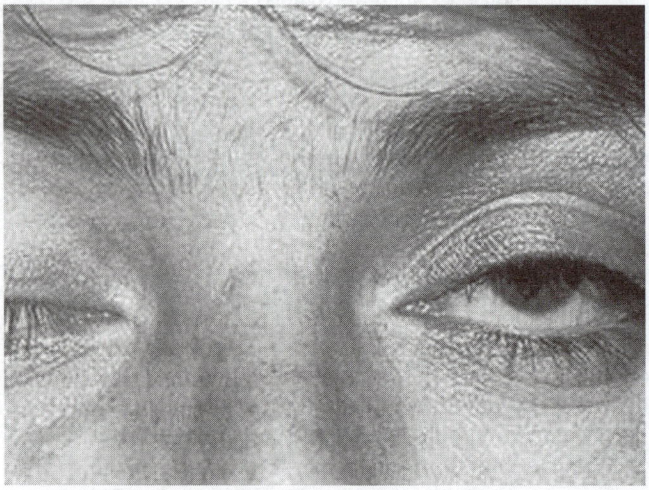

Fig. 9.2: Weakness of bulbar muscle in myasthenia gravis.

Clinical Features

Myasthenia gravis is not rare, having a prevalence of 1–7 in 10,000. It affects individuals in all age groups, but peaks of incidence occur in women in their twenties and thirties and in men in their fifties and sixties. Overall, women are affected more frequently than men.

The cardinal features are weakness and fatigability of muscles. The weakness increases during repeated use (fatigue) and may improve following rest or sleep. The cranial muscles, particularly the lids and extraocular muscles, are often involved early in the course of MG, and diplopia and ptosis are common initial complaints **(Fig. 9.2)**.

Difficulty in swallowing may occur as a result of weakness of the palate, tongue, or pharynx, giving rise to nasal regurgitation or aspiration of liquids or food. In about 85% of patients, the weakness becomes generalized, affecting the limb muscles as well. If weakness remains restricted to the extraocular muscles for 3 years, it is likely that it will not become generalized, and these patients are said to have ocular MG.

Diagnosis

If the diagnosis is suspected,

i. Serology can be performed in a blood test to identify certain antibodies.
ii. Muscle fibers of patients with MG are easily fatigued, and thus do not respond as well as muscles in healthy individuals to repeated stimulation. By repeatedly stimulating a muscle with electrical impulses, the fatigability of the muscle can be measured. This is called the **repetitive nerve stimulation test.**
iii. **Electromyography** is considered to be the most sensitive test.
iv. The **"edrophonium test"** is infrequently performed to identify MG; its application is limited to the situation when other investigations do not yield a conclusive diagnosis. This test requires the intravenous administration of edrophonium chloride.
v. Chest X-ray, CT scan, MRI and muscle biopsy can also be considered in doubtful cases.

Treatment

The prognosis has improved strikingly as a result of advances in treatment; virtually all myasthenic patients can be returned to full productive lives with proper therapy. The most useful treatments for MG include **anticholinesterase medications**, immunosuppressive agents, thymectomy, and plasmapheresis or intravenous immunoglobulin (IVIG). For emergency treatment, plasmapheresis or IVIG is used as a temporary measure to remove antibodies from the blood circulation.

Anticholinesterase agents include physostigmine, pyridostigmine, neostigmine, and edrophonium while immunosuppressive agents include corticosteroids, azathioprine, cyclosporine A, etc.

Anticholinesterase agents act by competitive inhibition of acetylcholinesterase, thereby spare acetylcholine from degradation.

Competitive Inhibition

In *competitive inhibition*, an enzyme can bind substrate (S) or inhibitor (I) but not both. The competitive inhibitor resembles the substrate and binds to the active site of the enzyme **(Fig. 9.3)**. The substrate is thereby prevented from binding to the same active site.

A competitive inhibitor diminishes the rate of catalysis by reducing the proportion of enzyme molecules bound to a substrate. *The hallmark of competitive inhibition is that it can be overcome by a sufficiently high concentration of substrate.* Under these conditions, the substrate "outcompetes" the inhibitor for the active site. However, the apparent value of Km is altered; the effect of a competitive inhibitor is to increase the apparent value of Km. As the value of inhibitor (I) increases, the value of *Km* increases **(Fig. 9.4)**. In the presence of a competitive inhibitor, an enzyme will have the same V_{max} as in the absence of an inhibitor. The inhibitor does not bind covalently to the enzyme to bring about irreversible changes.

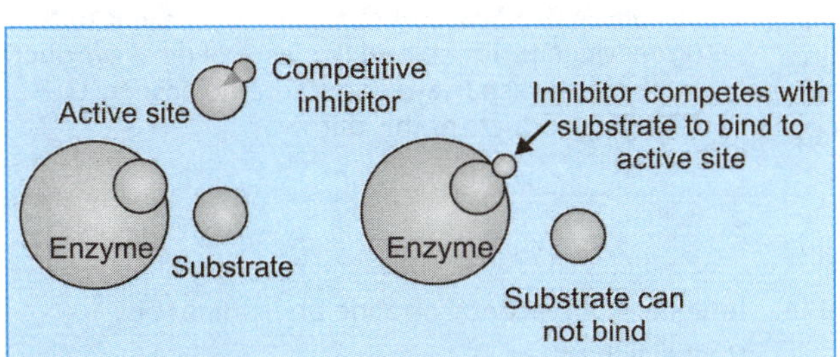

Fig. 9.3: Competitive inhibition. The competitive inhibitor resembles the substrate and binds to the active site of the enzyme. The substrate is thereby prevented from binding to the same active site.

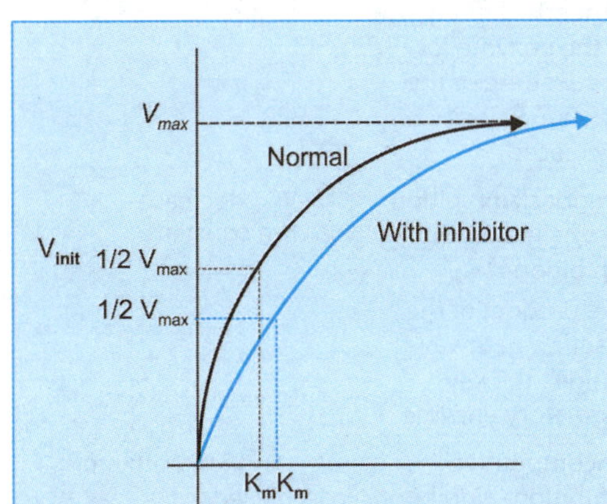

Fig. 9.4: As the concentration of a competitive inhibitor increases, higher concentrations of substrate are required to attain a particular reaction velocity. A sufficiently high concentration of substrate can completely relieve competitive inhibition.

Summary of Enzyme Inhibition (Table 9.3)

TABLE 9.3: Summary of enzyme inhibition.

Type of inhibition	*Effect on maximum reaction velocity (V_{max}) and Km*	*Reversible/ Irreversible*	*Examples*
Competitive inhibition (inhibitor—a structural analog) A competition between substrate and the inhibitor for the active site	1. V_{max} remains unchanged 2. Km increases	Reversible	1. HMG-CoA reductase inhibited by **Statins—**used as cholesterol lowering drugs 2. Epoxide reductase inhibited by **Dicoumarol—**used as an anticoagulant 3. Dihydrofolate reductase inhibited by **Methotrexate—**used as anticancer drug 4. Pteroyl synthase inhibited by **PABA** (para-aminobenzoic acid) used as antibiotic 5. Angiotensin-converting enzyme Inhibitor—inhibited by **Captopril—**used as an antihypertensive drug 6. Succinate dehydrogenase inhibited by **Malonate—**a poison 7. Lactate dehydrogenase inhibited by **Oxamate—**a poison
Noncompetitive (inhibitor binds at a site other than the active site)	1. V_{max} decreases 2. Km remains unchanged	Can be reversible or irreversible	1. Enolase is inhibited by **Fluoride,** used for sample collection for glucose estimation 2. PDH complex, alpha-ketoglutarate dehydrogenase complex, glyceraldehyde-3-P dehydrogenase (-SH group containing enzymes) are inhibited by **Arsenate**, a slow poison 3. Cytochrome oxidase inhibited by **cyanide**, a poison
Suicidal inhibition, also called mechanism-based inhibition Inhibitor gets activated by host enzyme to inhibit the subsequent enzyme	1. V_{max} decreases 2. Km increases	Irreversible	1. Inhibition of xanthine oxidase by **Allopurinol,** used for the treatment of gout 2. Inhibition of aconitase by **fluoroacetate**—a rat poison 3. Inhibition of thymidylate synthase by **5-FU (5-Fluorouracil)** used as an anticancer drug 4. Inhibition of ornithine decarboxylase by difluoromethylornithine (DFMO) used in sleeping sickness 5. Monoamine oxidase is inhibited by **Deprenyl** used to treat Parkinson disease and depression
Allosteric inhibition (binding of the inhibitor alters either the affinity of the enzyme for its substrate or the reaction velocity is decreased)	1. V_{max} is decreased in V-type enzymes 2. Km is increased in K-type enzymes	Reversible	Most of them are physiological inhibitors. 1. ATP and citrate are allosteric inhibitors of PFK-1 2. Fr 2,6 bisphosphate is an allosteric inhibitor of Fr 1,6 bisphosphatase enzyme
Feedback inhibition, also called product inhibition The product of the reaction pathway inhibits the key regulatory enzyme	1. V_{max} decreases 2. Km constant	Reversible depending upon the need of the product	1. Inhibition of HMG-CoA reductase by **Mevalonate** (immediate product) and cholesterol (final product) 2. Inhibition of aspartate transcarbamoylase by UTP and CTP, the products of this pathway
Uncompetitive inhibition—inhibitor binds to the enzyme-substrate complex	V_{max} and Km both are decreased	Irreversible	Inhibition of placental alkaline phosphatase by phenylalanine

CLINICAL NOTE

Myasthenia gravis is one of the most treatable neurologic disorders. Pharmacologic therapy includes anticholinesterase medication and immunosuppressive agents.

CLINICAL PEARLS

1. There is a competition between substrate and inhibitor for the active site in competitive inhibition. Km increases but V_{max} remains unchanged.
2. In noncompetitive inhibition, the inhibitor binds at a site other than the active site, Km remains unchanged but V_{max} decreases.
3. In suicidal inhibition, also called mechanism-based inhibition, inhibitor gets activated by host enzyme to inhibit the subsequent enzyme.
4. Allosteric inhibition involves binding of the inhibitor at a site other than the active site that alters either the affinity of the enzyme for its substrate (K-type enzyme) or the decreases the reaction velocity (V-type enzyme).
5. In feedback inhibition, also called product inhibition, the product of the reaction pathway inhibits the key regulatory enzyme.
6. In uncompetitive inhibition, the inhibitor binds to the enzyme substrate complex.

CASE STUDY 4

Theme: Mechanism of Enzyme Action

CASE DETAILS

A 55-year-old male presents with difficult breathing and swollen ankles. He is found to have a failing heart, resulting in blood backing up into his lungs (pulmonary congestion) and making it difficult for him to breathe. He is administered a drug that inhibits angiotensin-converting enzyme (ACE). By inhibiting this enzyme, which of the following will change about the reaction it catalyzes?

a. Energy of activation
b. Net free energy change
c. Equilibrium concentration of substrate
d. Equilibrium concentration of product
e. Thermodynamics

Answer: The right answer is—a. Energy of activation. The enzymes decrease the energy of activation for a reaction and speed up the reaction by many folds. The thermodynamics of a reaction, such as the free energy change and the equilibrium concentrations of the substrate and product remain unchanged.

General Mechanism of Action of Enzymes

Enzymes are catalysts and increase the speed of a chemical reaction without themselves undergoing any permanent chemical change. They are neither used up in the reaction nor do they appear as reaction products.
The basic enzymatic reaction can be represented as follows:

$$S + E \longrightarrow P + E$$

Where E represents the enzyme catalyzing the reaction, S the substrate, the substance being changed, and P the product of the reaction.

Enzymes employ multiple mechanisms to facilitate catalysis. The mechanism of action of enzymes can be explained by two perspectives:

1. Thermodynamic changes
2. Processes at the active site.

1. **Thermodynamic changes:** All enzymes accelerate reaction rates by providing **transition states** with a lowered G for formation of the transition states. However, they may differ in the way this is achieved.

   A chemical reaction of substrate S to form product P goes through a *transition state* S‡ that has a higher free energy than does either S or P. (The double dagger denotes a thermodynamic property of the transition state).

   The difference in free energy between the transition state and the substrate is called the *Gibbs free energy of activation* or simply the *activation energy*, symbolized by $\Delta G‡$.

   The activation energy barrier suggests how enzymes enhance reaction rate without altering ΔG of the reaction: enzymes function to lower the activation energy, or, in other words, *enzymes facilitate the formation of the transition state*. The combination of substrate and enzyme creates a new reaction pathway whose transition-state energy is lower than that of the reaction in the absence of enzyme **(Fig. 9.5)**. The lower activation energy means that more molecules have the required energy to reach the transition state. Decreasing the activation barrier is analogous to lowering the height of a high-jump bar; more athletes will be able to clear the bar. *The essence of catalysis is specific binding of the transition state.*

2. **Processes at the active site:** Enzymes use various combinations of four general mechanisms to achieve dramatic catalytic enhancement of the rates of chemical reactions. These are as follows:
   a. **Catalysis by bond strain:** In this form of catalysis, the induced structural rearrangements that take place with the binding of substrate and enzyme ultimately produce strained substrate bonds, which more easily attain the transition state. Enzymes that catalyze lytic reactions that involve breaking a covalent bond typically bind their substrates in a conformation slightly unfavorable for the bond that will undergo cleavage. The resulting strain stretches or distorts the targeted bond, weakening it and making it more vulnerable to cleavage.
   b. **Catalysis by proximity and orientation:** For molecules to react, they must come within bond-forming distance of one another. The higher their concentration, the more frequently they will encounter one another and the greater will be the rate of their reaction. When an enzyme binds substrate molecule at its active site, it creates a region of high local substrate concentration. Enzyme-substrate interactions orient reactive groups and bring them into proximity with one another.
   c. **Catalysis involving proton donors (acids) and acceptors (bases):** Other mechanisms also contribute significantly to the completion of catalytic events initiated by a strain mechanism, for example, the use of glutamate as a general acid catalyst (proton donor). The ionizable functional groups of aminoacyl side chains and (where present) of prosthetic groups contribute to catalysis by acting as acids or bases. Acid-base catalysis can be either specific or general. By "specific" we mean only protons (H_3O^+) or OH^- ions. In **specific acid** or **specific base catalysis,** the rate of reaction is sensitive to changes in the concentration of protons but independent of the concentrations of other acids (proton donors) or bases (proton acceptors) present in solution or at the active site. Reactions whose rates are responsive to *all* the acids or bases present are said to be subject to **general acid** or **general base catalysis.**
   d. **Covalent catalysis:** In catalysis that takes place by covalent mechanisms, the substrate is oriented to active sites on the enzymes in such a way that covalent intermediate forms between the enzyme or coenzyme and the substrate. One of the best-known examples of this mechanism is that involving proteolysis by serine proteases, which include both digestive enzymes (trypsin, chymotrypsin, and elastase) and several enzymes of the blood clotting cascade. These proteases contain an active site serine whose R group hydroxyl forms a covalent bond with a carbonyl carbon of a peptide bond, thereby causing hydrolysis of the peptide bond. Covalent catalysis introduces a new reaction pathway whose activation energy is lower—and therefore is faster—than the reaction pathway in homogeneous solution. The chemical modification of the enzyme is, however, transient. On completion of the reaction, the enzyme returns to its original unmodified state. Its role thus remains catalytic. Covalent catalysis is particularly common among enzymes that catalyze group transfer reactions.

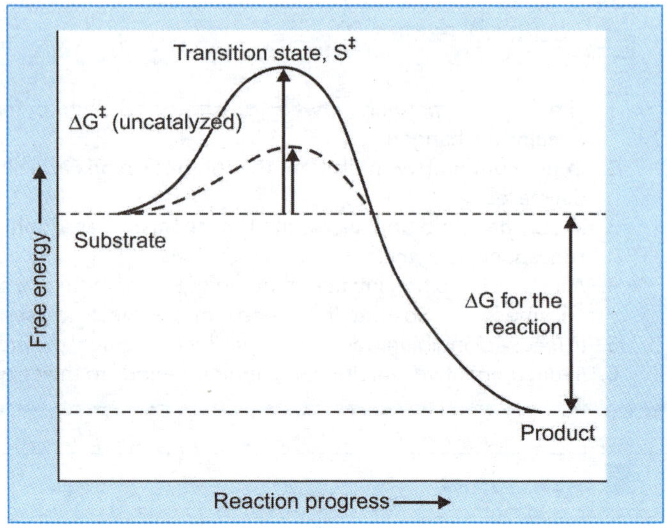

Fig. 9.5: Enzymes decrease the activation energy. Enzymes accelerate reactionsby decreasing ΔG, the free energy of activation.

CASE DISCUSSION

It is a case of cardiac failure. **The renin-angiotensin-aldosterone system (RAAS)** plays an important role in regulating blood volume and systemic vascular resistance, which together influence cardiac output and arterial pressure.

Basic Concept of Renin-Angiotensin-Aldosterone System

As the name implies, there are three important components to this system: (1) renin, (2) angiotensin, and (3) aldosterone. Renin, which is primarily released by the kidneys, stimulates the formation of angiotensin in blood and tissues, which in turn stimulates the release of aldosterone from the adrenal cortex. It is called a system because each part influences the other parts, and all are necessary for the whole to function correctly.

Renin is a proteolytic enzyme that is released into the circulation primarily by the kidneys. Its release is stimulated by:

1. Sympathetic nerve activation (acting via β1-adrenoceptors)
2. Renal artery hypotension (caused by systemic hypotension or renal artery stenosis)
3. Decreased sodium delivery to the distal tubules of the kidney.

When renin is released into the blood, it acts upon a circulating substrate, **angiotensinogen**, that undergoes proteolytic cleavage to form the decapeptide **angiotensin I**. Vascular endothelium, particularly in the lungs, has an enzyme,

angiotensin-converting enzyme (ACE), that cleaves off two amino acids to form the octapeptide, **angiotensin II** (AII), although many other tissues in the body (heart, brain, vascular) also can form AII **(Fig. 9.6)**.

Angiotensin I is able to alter the blood pressure to some degree, but it is not strong enough to cause large changes. Instead, most angiotensin I is converted to angiotensin II, a much more powerful hormone that does cause large changes in blood pressure. (This conversion is shut down by drugs called ACE inhibitors, an important type of high blood pressure medication.)

Angiotensin II is a strong hormone and can act directly on blood vessels to cause blood pressure increases. It also has another even more important function—stimulating the release of aldosterone. Aldosterone is a very powerful vasoconstrictor that causes large increases in blood pressure but is more important because it can actually change the baseline filtering activity of the kidneys. Aldosterone causes the kidneys to retain both salt and water, which—over time—increases the amount of water in the body. This increase, in turn, raises blood pressure.

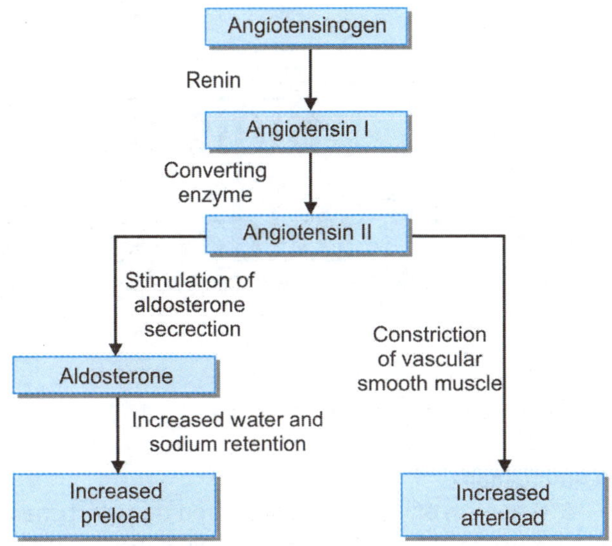

Fig. 9.6: Renin-angiotensin system.

Activation of the renin-angiotensin-aldosterone (RAA) system rapidly kicks in with heart failure, due to decreased renal perfusion caused by both a reduction in cardiac output and redistribution of blood away from nonessential organs (kidney). The kidney retains sodium and water in response to the perception of ineffective blood volume. The perception of decreased blood volume and the increase in sympathetic nervous activity stimulates renin release from the juxtaglomerular cells in the kidneys.

The compensatory mechanisms in heart failure eventually initiate a vicious cycle which leads to continued worsening and downward spiraling of the heart failure state. The peripheral vasoconstriction mediated by increased sympathetic activity, angiotensin II, and other possible mechanisms causes an increase in systemic vascular resistance or afterload. Afterload resists myocardial fiber shortening and further decreases cardiac output, which leads to further increases in sodium and water retention and sympathetic nervous activity **(Fig. 9.7)**.

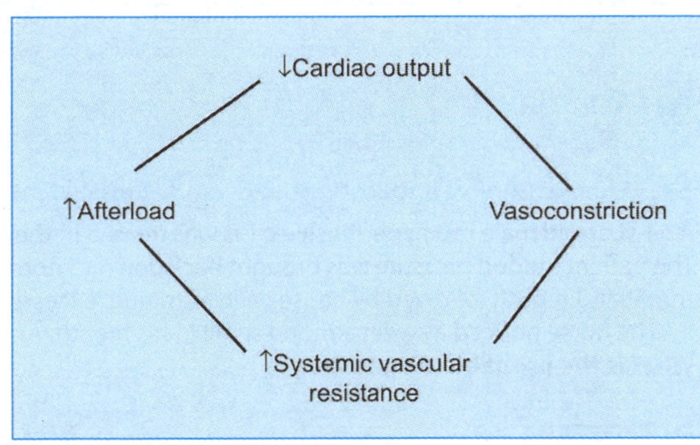

Fig. 9.7: Vicious cycle of cardiac failure.

Therapeutic manipulation of this pathway is very important in treating hypertension and heart failure. **ACE inhibitors, Angiotensin II receptor blockers and aldosterone receptor blockers**, for example, are used to decrease arterial pressure, ventricular afterload, blood volume and hence ventricular preload, as well as inhibit and reverse cardiac and vascular hypertrophy.

Mechanism of action of ACE inhibitors: Frequently prescribed ACE inhibitors include perindopril, captopril, enalapril, lisinopril, and ramipril. ACE inhibitors block the conversion of angiotensin I to angiotensin II. They act by competitive inhibition.

CLINICAL NOTE

ACE inhibitors, angiotensin II receptor blockers and aldosterone receptor blockers, are used to decrease arterial pressure, ventricular afterload, blood volume and hence ventricular preload, as well as inhibit and reverse cardiac and vascular hypertrophy.

CLINICAL PEARLS

1. Enzymes are catalysts and increase the speed of a chemical reaction without themselves undergoing any permanent chemical change.
2. The mechanism of action of enzymes can be explained by two perspectives: (1) thermodynamic changes and (2) processes occurring at the active site.
3. All enzymes accelerate reaction rates by providing transition states with a lowered G for formation of the transition states.
4. Enzymes use various combinations of four general mechanisms, viz.: catalysis by bond strain, proximity and orientation, acid-base catalysis and covalent catalysis to achieve dramatic catalytic enhancement of the rates of chemical reactions.

Chapter 10

Biological Oxidation and Oxidative Phosphorylation

LEARNING OBJECTIVES

To understand:

- Mechanism of inhibition of electron transport chain and the resultant clinical implications
- Process of ATP synthesis by oxidative phosphorylation
- Mechanism of action of uncouplers of oxidative phosphorylation
- Significance of uncoupling of oxidative phosphorylation.

CASE STUDIES

CASE STUDY 1

Theme: Clinical Implications of Cyanide Induced Inhibition of Electron Transport Chain

A 64-year-old male in a hypertensive crisis was treated in the intensive care unit (ICU) with intravenous nitroprusside for 48 hours. The patient's blood pressure was brought back down to normal levels; however, he was complaining of a burning sensation in his throat and mouth followed by nausea and vomiting, excessive sweating, agitation, and dyspnea.

The nurse noticed a sweet almond smell in his breath. An arterial blood gas revealed a significant metabolic acidosis.

What is the probable diagnosis?

CASE DETAILS

The patient is most probably suffering from cyanide poisoning. Cyanide inhibits mitochondrial cytochrome oxidase, blocks electron transport, and prevents oxygen utilization. Lactic acidosis results secondary to anaerobic metabolism. The oxygen metabolism at the cell level is grossly hampered. Fatality is induced in seconds to minutes.

BASIC CONCEPT

Hypertensive emergencies are defined as episodes of severely elevated blood pressure, such as a systolic blood pressure of 220 mm Hg and/or diastolic blood pressures exceeding 120 mm Hg with symptoms of end-organ dysfunction. Hypertensive emergencies require immediate lowering of the blood pressure. In contrast, hypertensive urgencies are circumstances of markedly elevated blood pressures in the absence of symptoms; lowering the blood pressure over 24–48 hours is reasonable in these cases.

In hypertensive individuals, the upper and lower limits of autoregulation of cerebral blood flow are shifted to higher levels of arterial pressure, and rapid lowering of blood pressure to below the lower limit of autoregulation may precipitate cerebral ischemia or infarction as a consequence of decreased cerebral blood flow. Renal and coronary blood flows may also decrease with overly aggressive acute therapy. The initial goal of therapy is to reduce mean arterial blood pressure by no more than 25% within minutes to 2 hours or to a blood pressure in the range of 160/100–110 mm Hg. This may be accomplished with IV nitroprusside, a short-acting vasodilator with a rapid onset of action that allows for minute-to-minute control of blood pressure. One side effect of sodium nitroprusside is that with prolonged use, cyanide poisoning may result, which inhibits the electron transport chain. Thus, in clinical practice, short-term nitroprusside is used.

CYANIDE POISONING

Cyanide ion (CN-): Cyanide is generally considered to be a rare source of poisoning; however, cyanide exposure occurs relatively frequently in patients with smoke inhalation from residential or industrial fires. Cyanide poisoning may also occur in industry, particularly in the metal trades, mining, electroplating, jewelry manufacturing, and X-ray film recovery. It is also encountered in fumigation of ships, warehouses, and other structures. Cyanides are also used as suicidal agents, particularly among healthcare and laboratory workers, and they can potentially be used in a terrorist attack.

Pathophysiology

Cyanide is a potent inhibitor of metalloenzymes; therefore, it affects almost all the body tissues. The major toxicity occurs as a result of inhibition of cytochrome aa3 oxidase enzyme complex (complex-IV) of electron transport chain **(Fig. 10.1)**. This results in uncoupling of oxidative phosphorylation, and inhibition of cellular respiration despite the availability of sufficient oxygen. Hence, the mode of cellular metabolism switches from aerobic to anaerobic, with the resultant production of lactic acid. Therefore, the tissues with the highest oxygen demands, such as brain and heart are the most significantly affected by acute cyanide poisoning.

Chronic consumption of cyanide-containing foods can cause ataxia and optic neuropathy.

Impaired cyanide metabolism due to rhodanese deficiency is known to cause Leber's optic atrophy which may progress to subacute blindness (reaction). The adverse effects of cyanide can also be observed in chronic smokers (tobacco amblyopia).

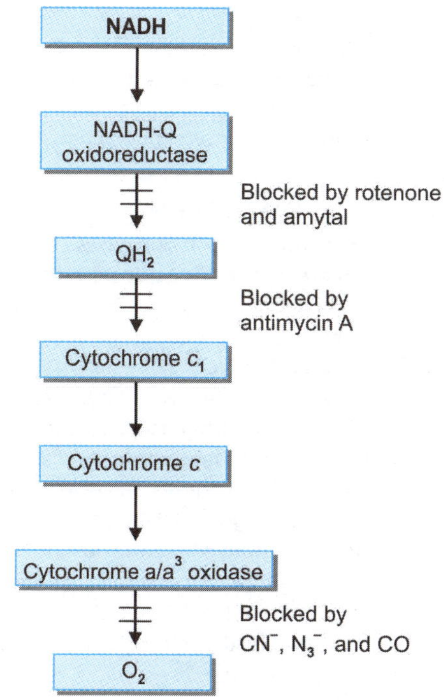

Fig. 10.1: Site of action of various inhibitors of electron transport chain. Cyanide inhibits cytochrome oxidase, the fourth complex of mitochondrial electron transport chain, and thereby inhibits cellular respiration. Similarly, CO also inhibits electron transport chain at the level of cytochrome oxidase to produce toxic effects.

Frequency

Smoke inhalation is an important source of cyanide poisoning.

Clinical Manifestations

A history of recent depression or altered mental status, acidosis, and tachyphylaxis, should evoke suspicion of the diagnosis in a patient on nitroprusside in the intensive care unit (ICU).

- Generalized weakness, malaise, and collapse
- Neurologic symptoms (reflect progressive hypoxia):
  - Headache, vertigo, dizziness
  - Giddiness, confusion
  - Generalized seizures
  - Coma
- **Gastrointestinal symptoms:** Abdominal pain, nausea, vomiting
- Cardiopulmonary symptoms:
  - Shortness of breath, possibly associated with chest pain
  - Apnea

  Physical findings of cyanide exposure are generally nonspecific, yet the onset of illness may be dramatic.
- Vital signs are variable.
  - Initial bradycardia and hypertension may rapidly give way to hypotension with reflex tachycardia, with resulting final bradycardia and hypotension.
  - Tachypnea may generally precede apnea.
- **General:** Cherry-red skin color, soot in the mouth and nose, and bitter almonds like smell of breath can suggest the possibility of cyanide poisoning.
- **Cardiopulmonary:**
  - Pulmonary edema is a frequent finding.
  - Aspiration can occur in comatose patients.
- Neurologic:
  - Mental confusion,
  - Ataxia,
  - Bizarre or drunken behavior,
  - Generalized convulsions, or
  - Coma in severe cases.

Mortality/morbidity

- Cyanide poisoning is highly fatal. The effects are observed in seconds to minutes following inhalation or intravenous injection; in minutes following ingestion of soluble salts, or minutes to several hours after skin absorption.
- Residual neurological effects, such as "Anoxic encephalopathy" or "Parkinson like syndrome," are observed in survivors.
- Early aggressive intervention comprising of supportive care and antidote therapy can be lifesaving.

Laboratory Investigations

- Arterial and venous blood gases
    - **Severe metabolic acidosis associated with reduced** arterial-venous oxygen saturation difference (<10%) is suggestive of cyanide poisoning.
    - Combined metabolic and respiratory acidosis resulting in apnea is also common.
- **Blood lactate level**
    - A plasma lactate level higher than 6 mmol/L suggests significant cyanide exposure.
- **Red blood cell and plasma cyanide concentration**
    - Blood cyanide levels are not reliable, falsely elevated levels may be observed after sodium nitrite administration during the analytical procedures. The levels are generally not available to help in the management of acute poisoning.
- **Carboxyhemoglobin (HbCO)** or blood carbon monoxide concentration can rule out simultaneous exposure.
- **Methemoglobin concentrations** identify the need for continuation of therapy with methemoglobin-inducing antidotes, such as sodium nitrite. Since methemoglobin strongly binds cyanide to form cyanmethemoglobin, the presence of methemoglobin is suggestive of small amount or absence of free cyanide for binding. However, elevated levels of methemoglobin (>10%) suggest that further nitrite therapy is not required, rather, may be dangerous.

Other Tests

- **ECG** may be suggestive of nonspecific changes, such as atrioventricular (AV) blocks, supraventricular or ventricular arrhythmias, and ischemic changes with subsequent asystole.

Treatment

Administer cyanide antidote kit (CAK) or hydroxocobalamin (Cyanokit) if the diagnosis is strongly suspected, without waiting for laboratory confirmation.

- Cyanide Antidote Kit contains amyl nitrite pearls, sodium nitrite, and sodium thiosulfate (see the reactions shown below). Cyanide ion competes effectively with oxygen for binding to cytochrome oxidase at the oxygen-binding site. Cyanide binding and therefore cyanide poisoning is reversible if treated properly and early. The treatment strategy depends on dissociation of cyanide from cytochrome a/a3 (Fe^{+3}).
- Increasing the percentage of oxygen breathed will increase the competition of oxygen over cyanide for the cytochrome a/a3 (Fe^{+3}).
- Amyl-and sodium nitrites induce methemoglobin formation in red blood cells which combines with cyanide, thus releasing cytochrome oxidase enzyme. Sodium thiosulfate enhances the conversion of cyanide to thiocyanate, which is excreted through kidneys.

$$\mathrm{Hb(Fe^{+2})O_2 + NO^{2-} \longrightarrow MetHb(Fe^{+3})OH + NO_3^-}$$
$$\mathrm{MetHb(Fe^{+3})OH + cyt\ a/a3(Fe^{+3}) - CN^- \longrightarrow cyt\ a/a3(Fe^{+3}) + MetHb(Fe^{+3}) - CN^-}$$
$$\mathrm{MetHb(Fe^{+3}) - CN^- + S_2O_3^{-2} \xrightarrow[\textit{rhodanese}]{} SCN^- + SO_3^{-2} + MetHb(Fe^{+3})OH}$$

Thiocyanate is incapable of inhibiting cytochrome oxidase and is excreted. The methemoglobin can be reconverted to oxyhemoglobin by NADH and methemoglobin reductase.

- Hydroxocobalamin (Cyanokit), which has been routinely used in Europe, has been approved by the US Food and Drug Administration (FDA) for treating known or suspected cyanide poisoning.
    - Hydroxocobalamin combines with cyanide to form cyanocobalamin (vitamin B_{12}), which is renally cleared.
    - Coadministration of sodium thiosulfate (through a separate line or sequentially) has been suggested to have a synergic effect on detoxification.
- Sodium bicarbonate is administered in severe poisoning because of marked lactic acidosis.

Prognosis

- Prognosis is reasonably good if rapid supportive intervention and effective antidotal therapy are provided.
- Suicidal poisonings tend to have severe outcomes because large doses are often involved.

CLINICAL NOTE

Individuals with smoke inhalation from enclosed space fires who have soot in the mouth or nose, altered mental status, or hypotension may have significant cyanide poisoning (blood cyanide concentrations >40 mmol/L or approximately 1 mg/L).

CLINICAL PEARLS

1. Cyanide (CN) toxicity principally results from the inactivation of cytochrome oxidase (at cytochrome a3), thus uncoupling mitochondrial oxidative phosphorylation and inhibiting cellular respiration, even in the presence of adequate oxygen stores.
2. Cherry-red skin color, soot in the mouth and nose after smoke inhalation, altered mental status, hypotension, and the smell of bitter almonds on the breath suggest the possibility of cyanide poisoning.
3. Metabolic acidosis, often severe, combined with reduced arterial-venous oxygen saturation difference (<10%) suggests diagnosis. Apnea may result in combined metabolic and respiratory acidosis. A plasma lactate concentration greater than10 mmol/L in smoke inhalation strongly suggests cyanide poisoning.
4. Treatment is in the form of supportive therapy, gastrointestinal (GI) decontamination, oxygen, and antidotal therapy with amyl nitrite, sodium nitrite, and sodium thiosulfate.
5. Prognosis is reasonably good if rapid supportive intervention and effective antidotal therapy are provided.

CASE STUDY 2

Theme: Implications of Carbon Monoxide Induced Inhibition of Electron Transport Chain

An elderly couple was brought by ambulance to the emergency department after their son noticed that they were both acting "strangely." The couple had been in good health prior to the weekend. Their son had gone out to spend the weekend with his friends.

The couple had been snowed in at their house until the snowplows cleared the roads.

They had plenty of food and were kept warm by a furnace and blankets. On reaching home after 2 days, their son noticed that they both were complaining of bad headaches, confusion, fatigue, and some nausea.

On arrival to the emergency department, both patients were afebrile with normal vital signs and O_2 saturation of 99% on 2 L of O_2 by nasal cannula. Their lips appeared to be very red. Both patients were slightly confused but otherwise oriented. The physical examinations were within normal limits. Carboxyhemoglobin levels were drawn and were elevated.

What is the most likely cause of these patients' symptoms?

CASE DETAILS

The elderly couple is most probable surfing from Carbon monoxide poisoning (CO). The cause might be the accidental exposure to CO by the burning of the furnace in the closed room. The symptoms, headache, confusion, fatigue, nausea, and red lips are suggestive of CO poisoning. Since the level of carboxyhemoglobin is also high, so the diagnosis is confirmed that the couple is suffering from CO poisoning.

BASIC CONCEPT

Carbon Monoxide poisoning

Carbon monoxide (CO) poisoning, one of the most common fatal poisonings, occurs by inhalation.

Carbon monoxide is a colorless, odorless gas produced by the combustion of carbon-containing materials; poisoning may occur as a result of suicidal or accidental exposure to automobile exhaust, smoke inhalation in a fire, or accidental exposure to an improperly vented gas heater or other appliance. Inhaling tobacco smoke results in CO in the blood but not enough to cause poisoning. Carbon monoxide avidly binds to hemoglobin, with an affinity approximately 250 times that of oxygen; this results in reduced oxygen-carrying capacity and altered delivery of oxygen to cells.

Pathophysiology

Mechanisms of CO toxicity are not completely understood. They appear to involve:

- Displacement of O_2 from Hb (because CO has a greater affinity for Hb than does O_2)
- Shifting of the O_2-Hb dissociation curve to the left (decreasing release of O_2 from Hb to tissues)
- Inhibition of mitochondrial respiration
- Possibly direct toxic effects on brain tissue **(Fig. 10.1)**.

CO toxicity causes impaired oxygen delivery and utilization at the cellular level. CO disrupts the O_2-dependent steps of the electron transport chain, leading to the unavailability of ATP. In the electron transport chain, only complex IV (cytochrome oxidase) interacts directly with O_2. As with hemoglobin, CO has a higher affinity for cytochrome oxidase than O_2.Thus, CO binds tightly to cytochrome oxidase and inhibits the transfer to O_2 **(Fig. 10.1)**. In tightly coupled mitochondria, the binding of CO to cytochrome oxidase also results in the inhibition of the phosphorylation of adenosine diphosphate (ADP), reducing the production of adenosine triphosphate (ATP) **(Fig. 10.2)**. This becomes more profound as additional molecules of cytochrome oxidase are bound by CO. Similarly, myoglobin also binds CO more avidly than O_2, and the transfer of O_2 to enzymes requiring O_2 is inhibited. The binding of CO to hemoglobin is fully dissociable, and dissociation requires ventilation. After removal from exposure to CO, administration of O_2 reverses CO binding to hemoglobin. Utilization of 100% O_2, accelerates the washout of CO. Use of hyperbaric chambers with pressures up to 2 atmospheres speeds up the CO washout process even more. Addition of 5–7% CO_2 to the O_2 is sometimes used as a prompt to ventilatory exchange. One disadvantage of the addition of CO_2 is the serious acidosis that results when the respiratory acidosis produced by CO_2 inhalation is added to the metabolic acidosis produced by O_2 deprivation in the tissues because of CO poisoning.

Toxicity primarily results from cellular hypoxia caused by impedance of oxygen delivery.

Several different sites within the body get affected but its most profound impact is on the organs (e.g., brain, heart) with the highest oxygen requirement.

Reversible binding of CO to hemoglobin results in relative functional anemia. Because it binds hemoglobin 230–270 times more avidly than oxygen, even small concentrations can result in significant levels of carboxyhemoglobin (HbCO).

An ambient CO level of 100 ppm produces an HbCO of 16% at equilibration, which is enough to produce clinical symptoms. Binding of CO to hemoglobin causes an increased binding of oxygen molecules at the three other oxygen-binding sites, resulting in a leftward shift in the oxyhemoglobin dissociation curve and decreasing the availability of oxygen to the already hypoxic tissues.

CO binds to cardiac myoglobin with an even greater affinity than to hemoglobin; the resulting myocardial depression and hypotension exacerbate the tissue hypoxia. Decrease in oxygen delivery is insufficient, however, to explain the extent of the CO toxicity. Clinical status often does not correlate well with HbCO level, leading some to postulate an additional impairment of cellular respiration.

Following severe intoxication, patients display central nervous system (CNS) pathology, including white matter demyelination.

CLINICAL MANIFESTATIONS

Symptoms tend to correlate well with the patient's peak blood carboxyhemoglobin levels. Many symptoms are nonspecific.

- Headache and nausea can begin when levels are 10–20%.
- Levels >20% commonly cause vague dizziness, generalized weakness, difficulty concentrating, and impaired judgment.
- Levels >30% commonly cause dyspnea during exertion, chest pain (in patients with coronary artery disease), and confusion.
- Higher levels can cause syncope, seizures, and obtundation.

Hypotension, coma, respiratory failure, and death may occur, usually when levels are >60%.

Patients may also have many other symptoms including visual deficits, abdominal pain, and focal neurologic deficits. If poisoning is severe, neuropsychiatric symptoms and signs (e.g., dementia, psychosis, parkinsonism, chorea, amnestic syndromes) can develop days to weeks after exposure and become permanent. Because CO poisoning often results from house fires, patients may have concomitant airway injuries which may increase risk of respiratory failure.

Causes

- Malfunctioning exhaust systems, inadequately ventilated passenger compartments, operation in an enclosed space, and utilization of auxiliary fuel-burning heaters inside a car or camper.
- Unvented cook stoves, furnaces, burning wood, charcoal, animal dung, or agricultural wastes.

Laboratory investigations

Diagnosis depends on specific measurement of the arterial or venous carboxyhemoglobin saturation, although the level may have declined if high-flow oxygen therapy has already been administered, and levels do not always correlate with clinical symptoms. Routine arterial blood gas testing and pulse oximetry are not useful because they give falsely normal PaO_2 and oxyhemoglobin saturation determinations, respectively.

TREATMENT

Emergency and Supportive Measures

- If necessary, a patent airway and assist ventilation should be maintained. Patients should be removed from the source of CO and stabilized as necessary. They are given 100% O_2 (by nonrebreather mask) and treated supportively. Hyperbaric O_2 therapy typically should be considered for patients who have any of the following:
- Life-threatening cardiopulmonary complications
- Ongoing chest pain

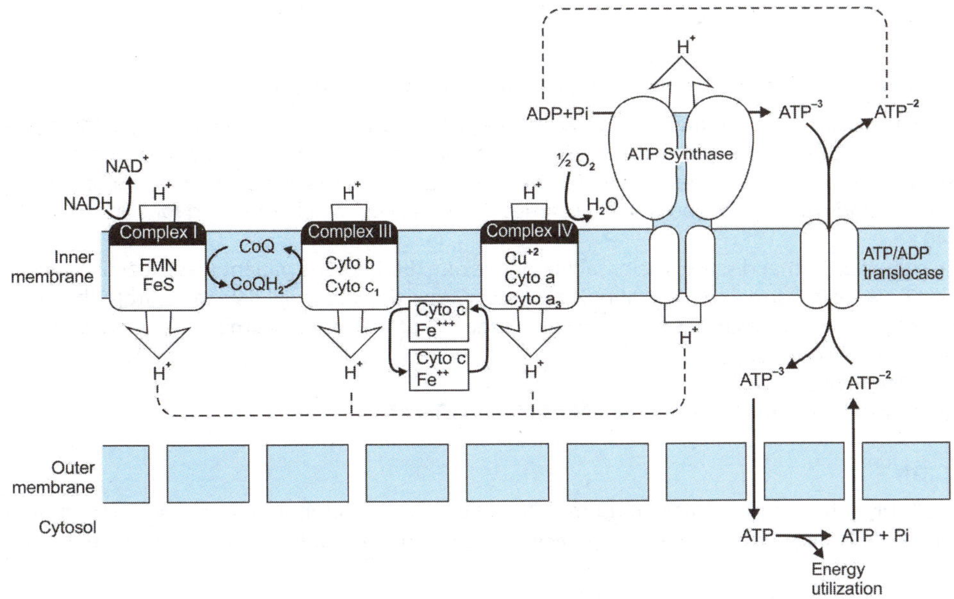

Fig. 10.2: Coupling of oxidation with phosphorylation. The chemiosmotic theory of oxidative phosphorylation—complexes I, III, and IV act as proton pumps creating a proton gradient across the membrane, which is negative on the matrix side. The proton motive force created drives the synthesis of ATP as the protons flow back into the matrix through the ATP synthase enzyme. Uncouplers increase the permeability of the membrane to ions, collapsing the proton gradient by allowing the H+ to pass across without going through the ATP synthase and thus uncouple electron flow through the respiratory complexes from ATP synthesis.

- Altered consciousness
- Loss of consciousness (no matter how brief)
- A carboxyhemoglobin level > 25%.

  Hyperbaric O_2 therapy should also be considered for pregnant patients.

  Hyperbaric O_2 therapy may decrease the incidence of delayed neuropsychiatric symptoms.

Prevention

Prevention involves checking sources of indoor combustion to make sure they are correctly installed and vented to the outdoors. Exhaust pipes should be inspected periodically for leaks. CO detectors should be installed because they provide early warning that CO is free in a dwelling's atmosphere. If CO is suspected in a dwelling, windows should be opened, and the dwelling should be evacuated and evaluated for the source of CO.

Prognosis

Prognosis is good if detected earlier and treated immediately with oxygen.

CLINICAL NOTE

Hyperbaric O_2 therapy may decrease the incidence of delayed neuropsychiatric symptoms; however, this therapy may cause barotrauma.

CLINICAL PEARLS

1. CO poisoning, one of the most common fatal poisonings, occurs by inhalation. Common sources of CO in poisonings include house fires and improperly vented automobiles, gas heaters, furnaces, hot water heaters, wood- or charcoal-burning stoves, and kerosene heaters.
2. Carbon monoxide poisoning causes acute symptoms, such as headache, nausea, weakness, angina, dyspnea, loss of consciousness, and coma. Neuropsychiatric symptoms may develop weeks later.
3. Diagnosis is by measuring arterial and venous carboxyhemoglobin levels. ABGs, which are pulse oximetry, are not useful.
4. Treatment is with supplemental O_2.
5. Prevention is often possible with household carbon monoxide detectors.

CASE STUDY 3

Theme: Mechanism of Action of "Uncouplers of Oxidative Phosphorylation"

A 30-year-old patient reported to the medical outpatient department (OPD) complaining of generalized weakness, excessive perspiration, and high caloric intake without increase in body weight. From the age of seven, she had suffered from profuse sweating that forced her to change clothes about 10 times a day. To compensate the loss of liquid, she had to drink water many liters every day. Her calorie intake was about 3,500 calories a day, approximately the need for a manual laborer, despite a body weight of only 40 kg.

There was no sign of any other disease. The basal metabolic rate (BMR) of the patient was excessively elevated but the thyroid hormones (T_3 and T_4) were in normal concentration. Laboratory tests showed small deviations from the normal picture, with the exception of her blood volume, which was about twice as large as normal, as well as the total amount of hemoglobin. There was also an increase in creatine excretion.

What is the probable diagnosis?
What is the biochemical basis for the elevated BMR in this patient?

CASE DISCUSSION

The patient is probably suffering from Luft's syndrome also called a hypermetabolic mitochondrial syndrome.

It is a case of severe hypermetabolism of nonthyroid origin with a defect in the maintenance of mitochondrial respiratory control.

LUFT'S SYNDROME

Pathophysiology

Mitochondria play a major role in human energy dynamics (ATP synthesis and related reactions), and a functional deficit may be expected to result in diminished supply of high-energy phosphate bonds. In mitochondria, electron transfer is coupled to oxidative phosphorylation via a proton gradient, and the energy released from oxidation is transferred to the ATP synthase trapping system. A class of compounds called uncouplers can block electron-transfer-linked phosphorylation at any of the three stages (energy production, transfer, or trapping). Redox reactions may release free energy (delta G negative). Such energy may be dissipated as heat, or be trapped as a proton gradient. Whether energy is dissipated or trapped depends on the characteristics of biologic membranes rather than on the reaction itself. Any substance that allows protons to leak across membranes will play an uncoupling role, since it will block the transfer of energy between electron flow and ATP synthesis.

Uncouplers dissociate oxidation in the respiratory chain from phosphorylation **(Fig. 10.2)**. These compounds are toxic in vivo, causing respiration to become uncontrolled, since the rate is no longer limited by the concentration of ADP or Pi. The uncoupler that has been used most frequently is 2,4-dinitrophenol, but other compounds act in a similar manner. Thermogenin (or the uncoupling protein) is a physiological uncoupler found in brown adipose tissue that functions to generate body heat, particularly for the newborn and during hibernation in animals. The antibiotic oligomycin completely blocks oxidation and phosphorylation by blocking the flow of protons through ATP synthase.

More than 90% of the oxygen used in the human body is utilized by mitochondrial cytochrome oxidase, which transfers four electrons into an oxygen molecule to produce two molecules of water. Under ordinary circumstances, reduction of oxygen by cytochrome oxidases in the above reaction does not release reactive oxygen radicals. This is assured by transitional metal ions, such as iron, copper, vanadium, and titanium, which are carried in the active sites of cytochrome oxidases.

Deficits in mitochondrial function arise by two mechanisms: (1) a block in electron flow or ATP synthesis which results in lactic acidosis and (2) uncoupling electron flow from ATP synthesis (Luft's syndrome) in which oxidation occurs at a rapid rate but without a concomitant increase in ATP synthesis (energy released is dissipated as heat). In both conditions, mitochondria increase in numbers and are often deformed, and the muscle cells show ragged red fibers. Surprisingly, ATP measured in muscle tissue in such cases is often near normal; however, there is a marked reduction in creatine phosphate Pi ratio—from a normal value of 9:1 to 1:1 in some affected individuals.

ETIOLOGY OF LUFT'S SYNDROME

Exact etiology is unknown. It is caused by abnormality in the mitochondrial membrane. Electron transport is only loosely coupled to ATP production, thus the extra energy evolves in the form of heat. There is a genetic mutation in the mitochondrial DNA of the mother and this can be passed to the children. It is a very rare genetic disorder.

CLINICAL MANIFESTATIONS

It is a syndrome characterized by:
- Severe hypermetabolism,
- Heat intolerance,

- Profuse perspiration,
- Polyphagia,
- Polydipsia without polyuria,
- Muscular wasting and weakness,
- Absent deep reflexes, and
- Resting tachycardia.
- At the cellular level, the mitochondria respire wildly and waste the excess energy as heat, elevation of body temperature up to 38.4°C.
- There is progressive weight loss despite increased food intake.
- Thyroid function is normal.
- Onset is in childhood.
- The rise in BMR is also due to the partial uncoupling of oxidative phosphorylation. Since there is less ATP production and the extra energy is lost in the form of heat, that is why the patient does not put on weight despite a good diet.

Laboratory Investigations

Routine investigations can be undertaken for differential diagnosis. BMR, thyroid function tests, blood glucose, etc., can be measured to rule out the presence of other conditions with similar symptoms.

TREATMENT

There is no permanent cure for this disease. Symptomatic treatment can only be given. Vitamin therapy in the form of vitamins C, K, and E, along with coenzyme Q10 and a high-caloric diet is recommended. Protection from heat is advised.

Prevention

Genetic counseling can be done, but it is not widely available because of the rarity of this condition.

CLINICAL NOTE

More than 90% of the oxygen used in the human body is utilized by mitochondrial cytochrome oxidase, which transfers four electrons into an oxygen molecule to produce two molecules of water.

CLINICAL PEARLS

1. Luft's syndrome is due to severe hypermetabolism of nonthyroid origin with a defect in the maintenance of mitochondrial respiratory control.
2. The defect is uncoupling of electron flow from ATP synthesis, oxidation occurs at a rapid rate but without a concomitant increase in ATP synthesis (energy released is dissipated as heat).
3. The syndrome is characterized by severe hypermetabolism, heat intolerance, profuse perspiration, polyphagia, polydipsia without polyuria, muscular wasting, and weakness, absent deep reflexes, and resting tachycardia.
4. There is no permanent cure for this disease. Symptomatic treatment can only be given.
5. Genetic counseling can be done, but it is not widely available.

CASE STUDY 4

Theme: Role of Calcium as an Uncoupler of Oxidative Phosphorylation

A 25-year-old male presented to the emergency department with acute abdominal pain accompanied by vomiting. Signs and symptoms were suggestive of acute appendicitis. He was promptly sent to the operating room for an emergency appendectomy. The patient was prepared and draped for the surgery, and halothane was given as an inhalation anesthetic. 2 minutes after the anesthetic was given, the patient was noted to have an extremely elevated temperature, muscle rigidity, and tachypnea.

An arterial blood gases test revealed a metabolic acidosis, and the serum electrolytes demonstrated hyperkalemia.

History revealed that previously also one of patient's uncles had a similar reaction during surgery and died. The surgeon made a diagnosis of malignant hyperthermia (MH).

What is the biochemical basis of this disease?
What is the best treatment for this condition?

MALIGNANT HYPERTHERMIA

Malignant hyperthermia is an unusual adverse response to some inhalation anesthetics, such as halothane in which there is an acute dramatic elevation in body temperature as well as tachypnea, muscle rigidity, and hyperkalemia.

Incidence

There is increased predominance in young males, children, and patients with musculoskeletal disorders. Overall the incidence is 1:50,000 and 1 in 100,000 adults.

Biochemical Defect and Inheritance

The exact cause is unknown but the primary defect may be related to a calcium release channel receptor known as ryanodine. In 50% of families, there is a genetic mutation on the short arm of chromosome 19, but multiple other chromosomal abnormalities have been detected. The disease is of heterogeneous etiology. Inheritance is autosomal dominant.

Pathophysiology

Most of the evidence points to the ryanodine receptor (chromosome 19q13.1) as the defective gene product. This receptor is the Ca^{2+} release channel of muscle sarcoplasmic reticulum. Stimulation of this channel leads to excessive Ca^{2+} release from the cisternae of the sarcoplasmic reticulum. Increased Ca^{2+} release triggers the binding of ATP charged myosin to actin to initiate muscle contraction. This muscle contraction may be repeated to the point of muscle rigidity with resultant muscle damage and release of myoglobin. The sustained muscle contraction uses increased amounts of ATP increasing demands on glycolysis, tricarboxylic acid (TCA) cycle, and oxidative phosphorylation. Ca^{2+} release serves to activate, at least partially, phosphorylase kinase, which speeds the mobilization of glycogen stores for ATP generation. Sympathetic outflow (catecholamines) triggered by these changes leads to increased activation of glycogen breakdown and lipolysis. Fatty acids serve as a signal to increase the levels of uncoupling proteins in various tissues. The uncoupling proteins form channels in the mitochondrial membrane allowing proton re-entry into the mitochondrial matrix. Because the phosphorylation of adenosine diphosphate (ADP) to ATP depends on the proton gradient through the ATP synthase, these channels collapse the proton gradient allowing electron transport to occur without the phosphorylation of ADP. Since ATP is being consumed at an elevated rate and mitochondrial production of ATP is compromised, glycolysis increases to compensate for the shortfall in ATP production. Pyruvate and lactate, the end products of glycolysis, increases in concentration, giving rise to the metabolic acidosis observed.

The uncoupling proteins (UCP 1 to 5) are a physiologic mechanism for maintaining body temperature through selective uncoupling of electron transport from ATP synthesis. The free energy release normally captured in the formation of the high-energy phosphate bond when phosphorylating ADP to ATP is lost as heat and changes body temperature. Physiologically, sympathetic outflow and catecholamine hormone release prompt new synthesis of the uncoupling proteins in response to the hypothalamus sensing lowered body temperature. In the case of malignant hyperthermia, this mechanism is triggered by anesthetic challenge to the calcium release channel and the subsequent metabolic and signaling changes.

Clinical Manifestations

There are three main underlying phenomena: Heat production, glycogenolysis progressing to lactic acidosis, and muscular rigidity. These are manifested as:

- Tachycardia
- Increase in body temperature
- Muscle rigidity
- Tachypnea, hypertension, and cardiac arrhythmias

Laboratory Investigations

- Blood gas analysis—metabolic acidosis, hyperlacticacidemia, decreased bicarbonate
- Electrolytes—hyperkalemia
- Urine analysis—myoglobinuria
- Renal function test—renal failure.

Diagnosis

- There may be a family history of malignant hyperthermia or unexplained death during anesthesia.
- Genetic testing to look for defects in the *RYR1* gene
- Muscle biopsy
- Myoglobin in the urine.

Treatment

Treatment involves, on the one hand, reversal of the primary disorder with dantrolene, and on the other, general resuscitative measures:

1. The volatile agent is stopped.
2. 100% oxygen is given.
3. The patient is manually hyperventilated.
4. A clean breathing system is used.
5. Surgery should be aborted.
6. Unconsciousness is maintained with an appropriate sedative-hypnotic.
7. Dantrolene 1 mg/kg is given intravenously, and then 1–2.5 mg/kg every 10 minutes until MH is under control (to a maximum dose of 10 mg/kg).
8. Measure core temperature.
9. Intravenous fluids are given to maintain a steady urinary output; insulin and dextrose may be given to reverse hyperkalemia.
10. Cardiac arrhythmias are treated as appropriate.
11. The patient is cooled by tepid sponging, cooled fluids, cooling blanket, cool nasogastric lavage, etc., as necessary.

Dantrolene acts by impairing calcium-dependent muscle activity. Dantrolene brings about the reduction in contraction of skeletal muscles by decreasing the amount of Ca^{2+} released from the sarcoplasmic reticulum. A serious side effect of dantrolene use is its potential hepatotoxicity. The hepatotoxicity is fatal to 0.1–0.2% of patients treated for 60 days or longer. Thus, use of dantrolene for longer than 45 days requires monitoring of hepatic markers.

Prevention

By taking a good preoperative history, one should be able to establish a family history of malignant hyperthermia (MH)—look for evidence of problems or even death among family (extended) during anesthesia. The best way of determining true susceptibility is to perform a muscle biopsy (quadriceps under local/regional blockade). The muscle is exposed to halothane and caffeine.

Prognosis

Repeated episodes or untreated episodes can cause kidney failure. Untreated episodes can be fatal.

Possible Complications

- Rhabdomyolysis
- Renal failure
- Myopathy or muscular dystrophy
- Death

CLINICAL NOTE

Prevention is the key in malignant hyperthermia in that every patient should be queried about personal or family history of complications during surgery. Once a patient is found to have MH, the clinician should alert other family members to the same possibility.

CLINICAL PEARLS

1. Malignant hyperthermia is an untoward response of susceptible individuals to preoperative anesthesia utilizing halothane and succinylcholine.
2. The frequency of occurrence is 1 in 15,000 children and 1 in 100,000 adults.
3. The clinical findings are muscle rigidity, hyperthermia, seizure, cardiac arrhythmias, and sometimes death.
4. Treatment of MH depends on cessation of anesthesia, mechanical means to reduce the temperature, and the correction of blood electrolyte and gas parameters to normal.
5. Even with prompt recognition and therapy, mortality is as high as 5%.

CASE STUDY 5

Theme: Salicylate-induced Hyperthermia and Respiratory Alkalosis

A 62-year-old male was brought to the emergency room with extreme weakness, mental confusion, and respiratory distress. For 2 days, he had experienced mild respiratory difficulty and shortness of breath. Intermittent vertigo and tinnitus had been present for 3 days, and his children had complained to him that "he was getting deaf." The past medical history included sciatica and depression. For his sciatica, the patient had been taking up to 10 aspirin tablets (325 mg each) per day, along with ibuprofen, 400 mg three times daily, and indomethacin (Indocin), 25 mg three times daily.

On examination, the patient was awake and alert but was in moderate respiratory distress and appeared restless and diaphoretic. The body temperature was 98.6°F. Pulse 80 beats/minute and blood pressure was 100/60 mm Hg. Diffuse rales were heard bilaterally. Heart rhythm was regular; there were no murmurs or gallops. Abdominal and neurologic findings were normal.
The electrocardiogram revealed sinus tachycardia.

Laboratory results included a hemoglobin level of 14 g per dL (140 g per L); serum sodium, 145 mEq per L (145 mmol per L); potassium, 3.6 mEq per L (3.6 mmol per L); chloride, 109 mEq per L (109 mmol per L) and carbon dioxide content, 17 mEq per L (17 mmol per L). An arterial blood gas determination, obtained while the patient was breathing 2 L of oxygen per minute, showed a pH of 7.47, PO_2 of 123 mmHg, PCO_2 of 19, and serum bicarbonate level of 14 mEq per L (14 mmol per L). Salicylate level at the time of admission was 38.2 mg per dL (2.75 mmol per L).

What is the probable diagnosis?

CASE DETAILS

The patient is suffering from salicylate toxicity. Salicylate toxicity can cause vomiting, tinnitus, confusion, hyperthermia, respiratory alkalosis, metabolic acidosis, and multi-organ failure. Diagnosis is clinical, supplemented by measurement of the anion gap, ABGs, and serum salicylate levels. Treatment is with activated charcoal and alkaline diuresis or hemodialysis.

BASIC CONCEPT

Salicylate Toxicity

Salicylate toxicity can result from chronic or acute ingestion. Acute ingestion of >150 mg/kg can cause severe toxicity. Acute intoxication is more likely to be the result of deliberate self-poisoning. Chronic intoxication is seen less frequently and generally has a poorer outcome, because of a low index of suspicion and delay in proper treatment. Chronic toxicity can occur after several days of high therapeutic doses. Most commonly, this is seen in elderly patients with arthritis or other musculoskeletal problems.

In general, the toxic effects of salicylates are seen at serum levels above 30 mg per dL (2.15 mmol per L). Therapeutic levels needed for the anti-inflammatory effects of salicylates range from 15 to 30 mg per dL (1.10–2.15 mmol per L). The Food and Drug Administration recommends that the maximum dose of salicylate in a 70-kg person does not exceed 3,900 mg in 24 hours for more than 10 days.

Pathophysiology

Salicylates impair cellular respiration by uncoupling oxidative phosphorylation. They stimulate respiratory centers in the medulla, causing primary respiratory alkalosis, which is often unrecognized in young children. Salicylates simultaneously and independently cause primary metabolic acidosis. Eventually, as salicylates disappear from the blood, enter the cells, and poison mitochondria, metabolic acidosis becomes the primary acid–base abnormality.

Salicylate poisoning also causes ketosis, fever, and, even when systemic hypoglycemia is absent, low brain glucose levels. Renal Na, K, and water loss and increased but imperceptible respiratory water loss due to hyperventilation lead to dehydration.

Salicylates are weak acids that cross cell membranes relatively easily; thus, they are more toxic when blood pH is low. Dehydration, hyperthermia, and chronic ingestion increase salicylate toxicity because they result in greater distribution of salicylate to tissues. Excretion of salicylates increases when urine pH increases.

Clinical Manifestations

Salicylate toxicity should be suspected in any patient with fever, hyperventilation, seizures, or coma of uncertain etiology. It is not uncommon for salicylate poisoning to be misdiagnosed initially as diabetic ketoacidosis.

Initial symptoms of salicylate toxicity include tinnitus (followed by hearing loss), vertigo, nausea, vomiting, hyperventilation, and agitation. As the serum level rises, metabolic acidosis ensues, resulting in more severe hyperpnea. This is followed by central nervous system deterioration (lethargy, confusion, delirium, convulsions, and, eventually, coma). Fever, due to uncoupling of oxidative phosphorylation, is also a common symptom.

Other manifestations of salicylate toxicity include noncardiogenic pulmonary edema, renal tubular damage, bleeding disorders, and hemolysis. The pathophysiology of salicylate damage to the lungs and kidneys is still unclear, but a central factor seems to be a disruption of capillary permeability to protein, producing high concentrations of protein in both pulmonary edema fluid and urine. A similar phenomenon occurs in cerebral membranes and may produce cerebral edema.

Laboratory Diagnosis

Salicylate poisoning is generally suspected in patients with any of the following:
- History of a single overdose,
- Long-term ingestion of therapeutic dosages (particularly in patients with fever and dehydration),
- Unexplained metabolic acidosis,
- Unexplained mental confusion and high fever (in elderly patients).

In suspected cases, serum salicylate levels (few hours after ingestion), urine pH, ABGs, serum electrolytes, serum creatinine, plasma glucose, and BUN are measured. If rhabdomyolysis is suspected, serum CK and urine myoglobin can be estimated.
- **Serum salicylate levels:** The levels above the therapeutic range (10-20 mg/dL), especially, 6 hours after ingestion are suggestive of salicylate toxicity.
- **Arterial blood gas analysis:** During the initial hours of ingestion, respiratory alkalosis is observed, later, however, compensated metabolic acidosis or mixed metabolic acidosis/respiratory alkalosis sets in. Subsequently, as the salicylate levels fall, partially compensated or uncompensated metabolic acidosis can be observed. In conditions of salicylates-induced respiratory failure, combined metabolic and respiratory acidosis may be observed.
- Variations in plasma glucose levels are also common. The levels can be normal, low, or high.
- High serum CK and urine myoglobin levels are suggestive of rhabdomyolysis.

Treatment

Activated charcoal is given as early as possible and in the presence of bowel sounds, may be repeated every 4 hours until charcoal appears in the stool.

Alkaline diuresis: After maintaining fluid and electrolyte balance, alkaline diuresis can be induced to raise the urinary pH to ≥ 8. The alkaline diuresis promotes salicylate excretion, therefore, can be safety recommended. Even in patients with rhabdomyolysis, alkaline diuresis can help prevent renal failure. As a caution, serum potassium is regularly monitored, as hypokalemia can interfere with alkaline diuresis; these patients are usually given a mixture of $NaHCO_3$ and KCl.

Metabolic acidosis can worsen with drugs that promote urinary bicarbonate excretion; hence, these drugs should be avoided. Similarly, drugs that suppress respiration should also be avoided as these can impair compensatory hyperventilation or respiratory alkalosis.

Fever: The use of antipyretics is avoided. Fever can be treated with physical measures, such as cold sponging.

Seizures are treated with benzodiazepines.

Hemodialysis is recommended to promote salicylate excretion in patients with:
- Severe neurologic impairment,
- Renal or respiratory insufficiency,
- Acidemia despite correction, or
- Extremely high serum salicylate levels.

CLINICAL NOTE

Therapeutic levels needed for the anti-inflammatory effects of salicylates range from 15 to 30 mg per dL (1.10-2.15 mmol per L).

CLINICAL PEARLS

1. Salicylates impair cellular respiration by uncoupling oxidative phosphorylation.
2. Salicylate toxicity can result from chronic or acute ingestion. Acute ingestion of >150 mg/kg can cause severe toxicity.
3. Chronic intoxication is seen less frequently and generally has a poorer outcome, because of a low index of suspicion and delay in proper treatment.
4. Diagnosis is clinical, supplemented by measurement of the anion gap, ABGs, and serum salicylate levels.
5. Treatment is with activated charcoal and alkaline diuresis or hemodialysis.

Chapter 11

Vitamins

LEARNING OBJECTIVES

To understand:

❖ Chemistry, metabolism, and functions, and the clinical implications of deficiencies or toxicities of water and fat-soluble vitamins

CASE STUDIES

CASE STUDY 1

Theme: Causes and Clinical Implications of Thiamine Deficiency

A 20-year-old female was brought to the emergency department with respiratory distress. She gave a history of fever from the previous few days. She was a known alcoholic, but used to take alcohol only during episodes of depression.

On examination, she was pale, malnourished, agitated, and acutely ill. She was in acute respiratory distress. Her pulse was 110/minute, there was marked tachycardia, and a systolic murmur was heard along the left sternal edge. Bilateral crepitations were felt in the lungs, neck veins were engorged, and liver was also enlarged, although nontender. Bilateral foot drop was also there.

What is the probable diagnosis?

What type of investigations should be carried out to confirm the diagnosis?

CASE DETAILS

The patient is most probably suffering from cardiac beriberi. The criteria for diagnosing cardiac beriberi are: (1) signs of heart failure, (2) signs of neuropathies, (3) history of alcoholism or poor nutritional history, (4) exclusion of other signs of heart failure, (5) low red cell transketolase activity, and (6) response by thiamine administration. The above said patient is a known alcoholic, malnourished, and has heart failure and bilateral foot drop. The probable diagnosis is thiamine deficiency, which can be confirmed by erythrocyte transketolase activity.

Thiamine deficiency (causing beriberi) is most common among people subsisting on white rice or highly refined carbohydrates in developing countries and among alcoholics. Symptoms include diffuse polyneuropathy, high-output heart failure, and Wernicke-Korsakoff syndrome. Thiamine is given to help diagnose and treat the deficiency.

BASIC CONCEPT

Thiamine

Thiamine (vitamin B_1) is widely available in the diet. Thiamine is involved in carbohydrate, fat, amino acid, glucose, and alcohol metabolism. It is essentially nontoxic. The body cannot produce it and can only store up to 30 mg of thiamine in its tissues. Thiamine is mostly concentrated in the skeletal muscles. Other organs where it is found are the brain, heart, liver, and kidneys. The half-life of thiamine is 9 to 18 days. It is excreted by the kidney.

PATHOPHYSIOLOGY OF THIAMINE DEFICIENCY (BERIBERI)

Deficiency causes degeneration of peripheral nerves, thalamus, mammillary bodies, and cerebellum. Cerebral blood flow is markedly reduced, and vascular resistance is increased.

The heart may become dilated; muscle fibers become swollen, fragmented, and vacuolized, with interstitial spaces dilated by fluid. Vasodilation occurs and can result in edema in the feet and legs. Arteriovenous shunting of blood increases. Eventually, high-output heart failure may occur.

Dry beriberi: Nervous system involvement is termed dry beriberi. The neurologic findings can be peripheral neuropathy characterized by symmetric impairment of sensory, motor, and reflex functions of the extremities, especially in the distal lower limbs. Another presentation of neurologic involvement is **Wernicke's encephalopathy**, in which an orderly sequence of symptoms occurs, including vomiting, horizontal nystagmus, palsies of the eye movements, fever, ataxia, and progressive mental impairment leading to **Korsakoff syndrome**.

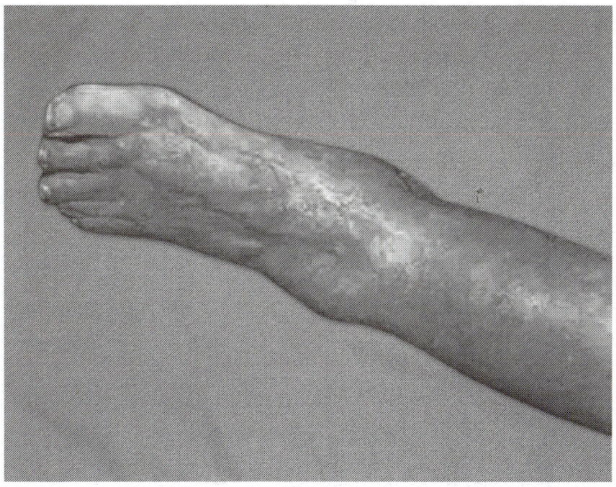

Fig. 11.1: Wet beriberi—edema of the lower extremity.

Wet beriberi is the term used for the cardiovascular involvement of thiamine deficiency. The chronic form of wet beriberi consists of three stages. In the first stage, peripheral vasodilation occurs, leading to a high cardiac output state. This leads to salt and water retention mediated through the renin–angiotensin–aldosterone system in the kidneys. As the vasodilation progresses, the kidneys detect a relative loss of volume and respond by conserving salt. With the salt retention, fluid is also absorbed into the circulatory system. The resulting fluid overload leads to edema of the dependent extremities **(Fig. 11.1)**.

By the time significant edema occurs, the heart has been exposed to a severely high workload in order to pump the required cardiac output needed to satisfy end-organ requirements. Parts of the heart muscle undergo overuse injury, which results in the physical symptoms of tachycardia, edema, and high arterial and venous pressures. These changes can lead to myocardial injury, expressed as chest pain.

Shoshin beriberi: A more rapid form of wet beriberi is termed acute fulminant cardiovascular beriberi, or Shoshin beriberi. The predominant injury is to the heart, and rapid deterioration follows the inability of the heart muscle to satisfy the body's demands because of its own injury. In this case, edema may not be present. Instead, cyanosis of the hands and feet, tachycardia, distended neck veins, restlessness, and anxiety occur.

Infantile beriberi occurs in infants (usually by age 3 to 4 weeks) who are breastfeed by thiamine-deficient mothers.

FREQUENCY

Beriberi is observed in developed nations in persons with alcoholism, people on fad diets, persons on long-term peritoneal dialysis without thiamine replacement, persons undergoing long-term starvation, or persons receiving intravenous fluids with high glucose concentration. No accurate statistics are available on the incidence of this condition.

CLINICAL MANIFESTATIONS

Early symptoms are nonspecific: Fatigue, irritability, poor memory, sleep disturbances, precordial pain, anorexia, and abdominal discomfort.

Dry beriberi refers to peripheral neurologic deficits due to thiamine deficiency. These deficits are bilateral and roughly symmetric, occurring in a stocking-glove distribution. They affect predominantly the lower extremities, beginning with paresthesias in the toes, burning in the feet (particularly severe at night), muscle cramps in the calves, pains in the legs, and plantar dysesthesias. Calf muscle tenderness, difficulty rising from a squatting position, and decreased vibratory sensation in the toes are early signs. Muscle wasting occurs. Continued deficiency worsens polyneuropathy, which can eventually affect the arms.

Wernicke-Korsakoff syndrome, which combines Wernicke's encephalopathy and Korsakoff's psychosis, occurs in some alcoholics, who do not consume foods fortified with thiamine. Wernicke's encephalopathy consists of psychomotor slowing or apathy, nystagmus, ataxia, ophthalmoplegia, impaired consciousness, and, if untreated, coma and death. It probably results from severe acute deficiency superimposed on chronic deficiency. Korsakoff psychosis consists of mental confusion, dysphonia, and confabulation with impaired memory of recent events. It probably results from chronic deficiency and may develop after repeated episodes of Wernicke's encephalopathy.

Cardiovascular (wet) beriberi is myocardial disease due to thiamine deficiency. The first effects are vasodilation, tachycardia, a wide pulse pressure, sweating, warm skin, and lactic acidosis. Later, heart failure develops, causing orthopnea and pulmonary and peripheral edema. Vasodilation can continue, sometimes resulting in shock.

Infantile beriberi: Heart failure (which may occur suddenly), aphonia, and absent deep tendon reflexes are characteristic.

Because thiamine is necessary for glucose metabolism, glucose infusions may precipitate or worsen symptoms of deficiency in thiamine-deficient people.

Causes

- **Lack of thiamine intake**
  - Diets consisting mainly of the following:
    - Food containing a high level of thiaminase, including milled rice, raw freshwater fish, raw shellfish, and ferns

- Food high in anti-thiamine factor, such as tea, coffee, and betel nuts
- Processed food with a content high in sulfite, which destroys thiamine
- Alcoholic state
- Starvation state

- **Increased consumption states**
  - Diets high in carbohydrate or saturated fat intake
  - Pregnancy
  - Hyperthyroidism
  - Lactation
  - Fever—severe infection
  - Increased physical exercise
- **Increased depletion**
  - Diarrhea
  - Diuretic therapies
  - Peritoneal dialysis
  - Hemodialysis
  - Hyperemesis gravidarum
- **Decreased absorption**
  - Chronic intestinal disease
  - Alcoholism
  - Malnutrition
  - Gastric bypass surgery
  - Malabsorption syndrome—celiac and tropical sprue
  - **Folate deficiency:** For example, in patients undergoing chemotherapy with high-dose methotrexate
    - Thiamine serves as a coenzyme (in the form of thiamine pyrophosphate) in a variety of metabolic processes. In these processes, thiamine pyrophosphate is regenerated via the donation of a proton from the reduced form of nicotinamide adenine dinucleotide (NADH).
    - Folic acid is essential to having enough dihydrofolate reductase to regenerate NADH from its oxidative form. This regeneration allows NADH to continue to be present to regenerate thiamine pyrophosphate without being consumed in the process.
    - If folic acid is deficient in cells, it causes an indirect thiamine deficiency, because thiamine is present, but cannot be activated.

LABORATORY STUDIES

Diagnosis is usually based on a favorable response to treatment with thiamine in a patient with symptoms or signs of deficiency. Similar bilateral lower extremity polyneuropathies due to other disorders (e.g., diabetes, alcoholism, vitamin B_{12} deficiency, heavy metal poisoning) do not respond to thiamine. Single-nerve neuritides (mononeuropathy, e.g., sciatica) and multiple mononeuropathy (mononeuritis multiplex) are unlikely to result from thiamine deficiency.

Electrolytes, including Mg, should be measured to exclude other causes. For confirmation in equivocal cases, erythrocyte transketolase activity and 24-hour urinary thiamine excretion may be measured.

Diagnosis of cardiovascular beriberi can be difficult if other disorders that cause heart failure are present. A therapeutic trial of thiamine can help.

TREATMENT

Supplemental thiamine, with dose based on clinical manifestations

For mild polyneuropathy, thiamine 10 to 20 mg once/day is given for 2 weeks. For moderate or advanced neuropathy, the dose is 20 to 30 mg/day; it should be continued for several weeks after symptoms disappear. For edema and congestion due to cardiovascular beriberi, thiamine 100 mg IV once/day is given for several days. Heart failure is also treated.

For Wernicke-Korsakoff syndrome, thiamine 50 to 100 mg IM or IV bid must usually be given for several days, followed by 10 to 20 mg once/day until a therapeutic response is obtained. Anaphylactic reactions to IV thiamin are rare. Symptoms of ophthalmoplegia may resolve in a day; improvement in patients with Korsakoff psychosis may take 1 to 3 months. Recovery from neurologic deficits is often incomplete in Wernicke-Korsakoff syndrome and in other forms of thiamine deficiency.

Because thiamine deficiency often occurs with other B vitamin deficiencies, multiple water-soluble vitamins are usually given for several weeks. Patients should continue to consume a nutritious diet, supplying one to two times the daily recommended intake (DRI) of vitamins; all alcohol intake should stop.

PROGNOSIS

The prognosis for beriberi is usually good, unless patients have established Korsakoff syndrome. When patients have progressed to this stage, the degree of damage is only minimally reversible.

CLINICAL NOTE

Because thiamine is necessary for glucose metabolism, glucose infusions may precipitate or worsen symptoms of deficiency in thiamine-deficient people.

CLINICAL PEARLS

1. Thiamine deficiency (causing beriberi) is most common among people subsisting on white rice or highly refined carbohydrates in developing countries and among alcoholics.
2. Symptoms include diffuse polyneuropathy, high-output heart failure, and Wernicke-Korsakoff syndrome.
3. Diagnosis is usually based on a favorable response to treatment with thiamine in a patient with symptoms or signs of deficiency.
4. For confirmation in equivocal cases, erythrocyte transketolase activity and 24-hours urinary thiamine excretion may be measured.
5. Because thiamine deficiency often occurs with other B vitamin deficiencies, multiple water-soluble vitamins are usually given for several weeks.

CASE STUDY 2

Theme: Thiamine—Chemistry, Metabolism, Coenzyme Role, and Clinical Implications of Thiamine Deficiency in Alcoholics

A 45-year-old male was brought to the emergency department after a family member found him extremely confused and disoriented. He had an unsteady gait and strange irregular eye movements. The patient had been a known heavy drinker from the past 6 years. There was no history of any known medical problem and he denied any other drug usage.

On examination, he was afebrile with a pulse of 90 beats per minute and a normal blood pressure of 110/80 mm Hg. Chest and abdominal examination were normal. He was extremely disoriented and agitated. Horizontal rapid eye movements on lateral gaze were noted bilaterally. His gait was very unsteady. The remainder of his examination was normal. The urine drug screen was negative and he had a positive blood alcohol level. Blood pyruvate and lactate levels were high.

What is the most likely diagnosis?

CASE DETAILS

The most likely diagnosis is Wernicke-Korsakoff syndrome (thiamine deficiency) often associated with chronic alcoholics. Thiamine deficiency is uncommon except in alcoholics as a result of nutritional deficiencies and malabsorption. The term Wernicke's encephalopathy is used to describe the clinical triad of confusion, ataxia, and nystagmus (or ophthalmoplegia). When persistent learning and memory deficits are present, the symptom complex is often called Wernicke-Korsakoff syndrome. Clinically, this term is best conceptualized as two distinct syndromes with acute/subacute confusional state and often reversible findings of Wernicke's encephalopathy versus persistent and irreversible findings of Korsakoff dementia.

BASIC CONCEPT

Thiamine

Thiamine, also known as vitamin B_1, is an important water-soluble vitamin which is active in the form of thiamine pyrophosphate and is required as a coenzyme in enzymatic reactions that involve the transfer of an aldehyde group.

Synthesis

Thiamine can be synthesized by plants and some microorganisms, but not usually by animals. Hence, human beings require thiamine from diet, though small amounts may be obtained from synthesis by intestinal bacteria.

Occurrence

Because of its importance in metabolic reactions, it is present in large amounts in skeletal muscle, heart, liver, kidney, and brain. It has a widespread distribution in foods, but there can be a substantial loss of thiamine during cooking above 100°C (212°F). Thiamine is absorbed in the intestine by both active transport mechanisms and passive diffusion. The active form of the coenzyme, thiamine pyrophosphate (thiamine diphosphate, TPP), is synthesized by an enzymatic transfer of a pyrophosphate group from ATP to thiamine **(Fig. 11.2)**.

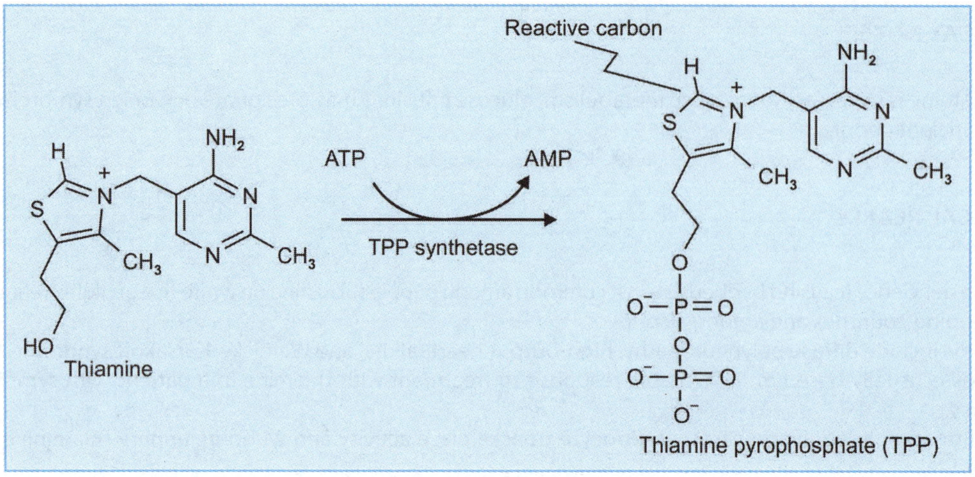

Fig. 11.2: Activation of thiamine-to-thiamine pyrophosphate.

Metabolic Role

Thiamine pyrophosphate is an essential cofactor for enzymes that catalyze the oxidative decarboxylation of α-keto acids to form an acylated coenzyme A (acyl CoA). These include pyruvate dehydrogenase, α-keto glutarate dehydrogenase, and branched-chain α-keto acid dehydrogenase. These three enzymes operate by a similar catalytic mechanism. Each of these enzymes is a multisubunit complex with three enzymatic activities that require the participation of several cofactors. The first activity (E1) is the dehydrogenase complex, which has TPP as the enzyme-bound cofactor. The carbanion form of TPP attacks the carbonyl carbon of the α-keto acid, releasing CO_2 and leaving a hydroxyalkyl-TPP intermediate. The hydroxyalkyl group reacts with the oxidized form of lipoamide, the prosthetic group of dihydrolipoyl transacetylase (E2), which is the second component of the complex. The resulting acyl lipoamide reacts with coenzyme A (CoASH) to form the product, acyl CoA, and leaving lipoamide in the fully reduced form. To regenerate the fully oxidized form of lipoamide for further rounds of the reaction, it interacts with the third component of the complex, dihydrolipoyl dehydrogenase (E3), which has covalently bound FAD. The FAD accepts the reducing equivalents from the reduced lipoamide to form $FADH_2$ and oxidized lipoamide. The reducing equivalents are then transferred to NAD^+ to form NADH, which is regenerated via the electron transport system with the production of ATP **(Fig. 11.3)**.

The E1 and E2 components are specific for each of the pyruvate dehydrogenase, α-keto glutarate dehydrogenase, and branched-chain α-keto acid dehydrogenase complexes. However, the E3 component is identical for all of the enzymes.

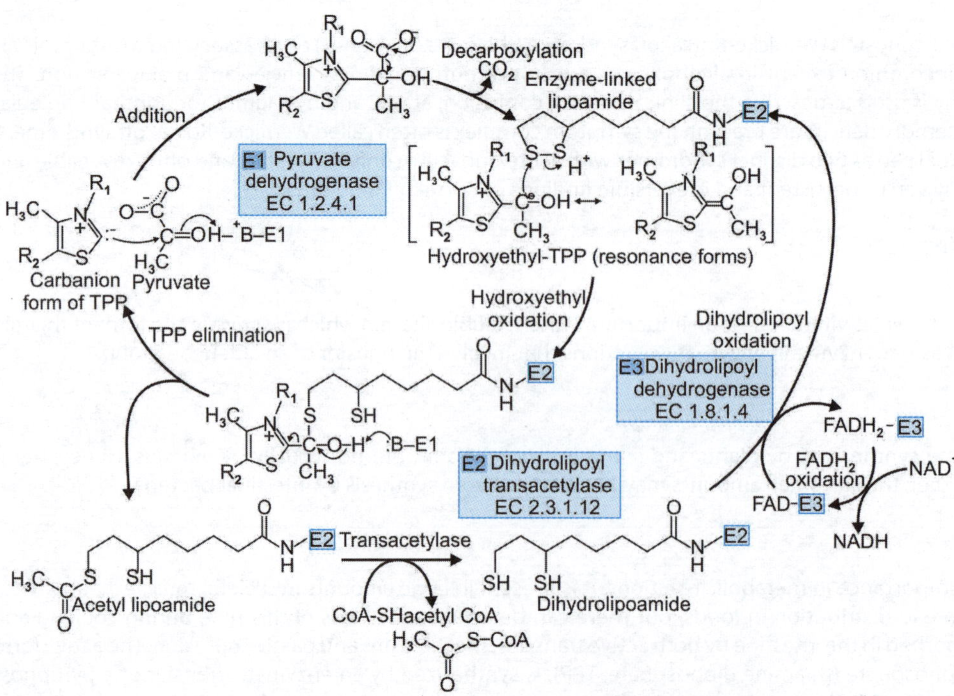

Fig. 11.3: Role of TPP in the conversion of pyruvate to acetyl CoA.

Thiamine pyrophosphate is also an important cofactor for the transketolase reactions in the pentose phosphate pathway of carbohydrate metabolism. These reactions are important in the reversible transformation of pentoses into the glycolytic intermediates fructose 6-phosphate and glyceraldehyde 3-phosphate. Again, it is the reactive carbon on the thiazole ring of TPP that reacts with a ketose phosphate (xylulose 5-phosphate) to cause the release of an aldose phosphate with two fewer carbons (glyceraldehyde 3-phosphate). The TPP-bound glycoaldehyde unit is then transferred to a different aldose phosphate (ribose 5-phosphate or erythrose 4-phosphate) to produce a ketose phosphate that has two carbons more (sedoheptulose 7-phosphate or fructose 6-phosphate) **(Fig. 11.4)**.

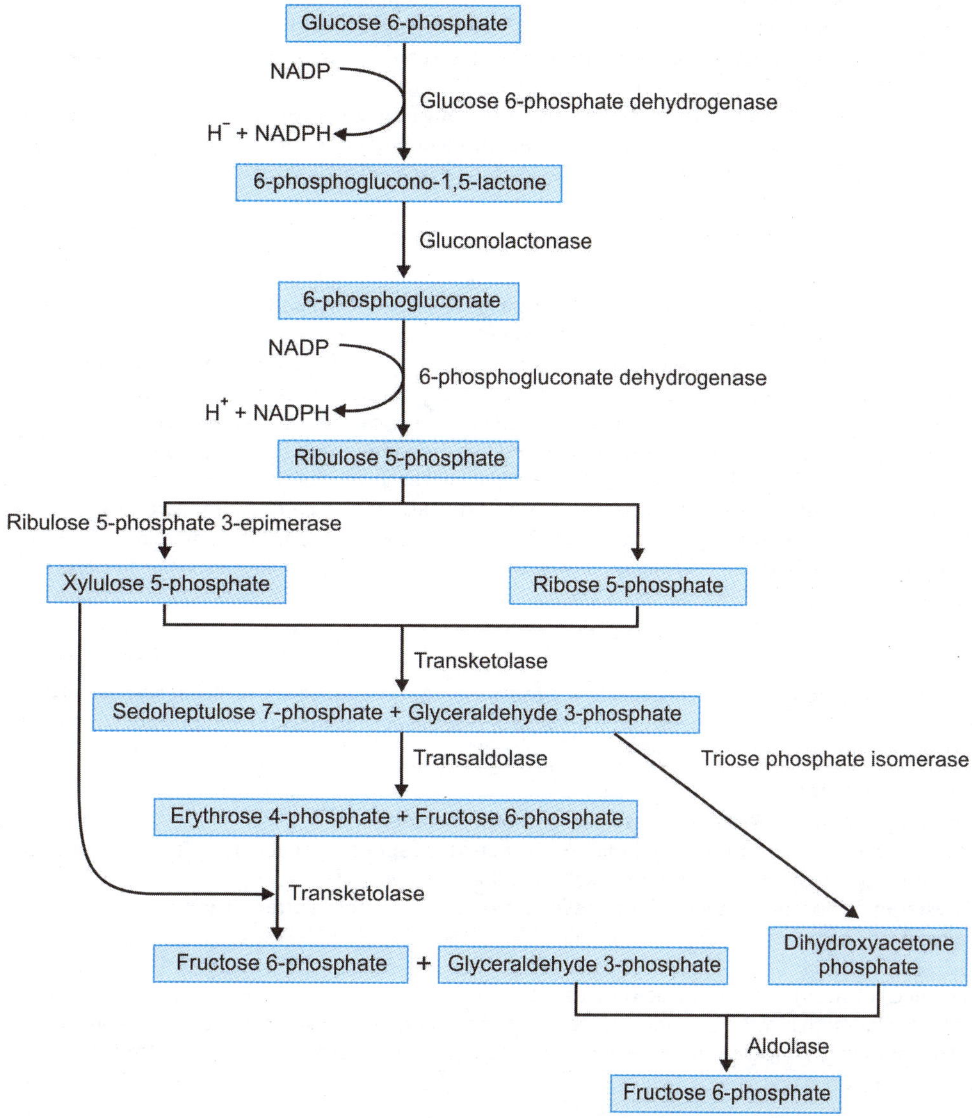

Fig. 11.4: HMP pathway. TPP is required as a coenzyme for the transketolase enzyme.

A deficiency in thiamine will decrease the efficiency of the enzymes for which TPP is required as a cofactor. Thus, the rate of conversion of pyruvate to acetyl-CoA and the flow of acetyl-CoA through the tricarboxylic acid cycle will be depressed as a result of the inefficiency of the TPP-requiring enzymes pyruvate dehydrogenase and α-keto glutarate dehydrogenase. The production of the reduced electron carrier, NADH, and the ATP produced from it via oxidative phosphorylation will be decreased as a consequence. Because nervous tissue and heart use at high rates ATP synthesized from the oxidation of NADH produced from pyruvate conversion to acetyl-CoA and from the TCA cycle, these tissues are most affected by a deficiency in thiamine. When deficient in thiamine, the brain can no longer efficiently metabolize pyruvate through the TCA cycle to produce ATP and thus must convert it to lactate to produce ATP. The main function of these enzymes in the brain is lipid (myelin sheath) and carbohydrate metabolism, production of amino acids, and production of glucose-derived neurotransmitters. Thiamine appears to have a role in axonal conduction particularly in acetyl cholinergic and serotoninergic neurons. A reduction in the function of these enzymes leads to diffuse impairment in the metabolism of glucose in key regions of the brain resulting in impaired cellular energy metabolism.

A deficiency in thiamine also adversely affects the flux of glucose metabolized by the pentose phosphate pathway. Transketolase activity requires the cofactor TPP to transfer the glycoaldehyde unit from a ketose to an aldose in the remodeling reactions of the pathway. When these reactions cannot proceed, precursor metabolites build up, and the flow through the pathway is decreased. This results in a decreased production of NADPH and decreased conversion of glucose to pentose, including ribose. This can lead to decreased regeneration of reduced glutathione and susceptibility to oxidative stress.

Thiamine turnover is rapid because of the ubiquitous presence of thiaminase enzymes that hydrolyze thiamine into its pyrimidine and thiazole components. Thus, symptoms of thiamine deficiency can appear within 2 weeks of a diet depleted in thiamine.

Thiamine is also required for the metabolism of tryptophan (as a coenzyme for tryptophan pyrrolase).

Deficiency affects the metabolism of tryptophan as well.

In Western societies, severe thiamine deficiency is most frequently found in alcoholics. Patients who chronically misuse alcohol are prone to thiamine deficiency arising from a number of factors including poor nutrition, poor absorption, and storage, as well as an increased breakdown of TPP and chronic liver diseases lead to decreased activation of thiamine pyrophosphate from thiamine.

WERNICKE'S-KORSAKOFF SYNDROME

PATHOPHYSIOLOGY

Heavy, long-term alcohol use is most commonly associated with Wernicke-Korsakoff syndrome. Within 2 to 3 weeks of decreased intake and thiamine depletion, areas of the brain with the highest thiamine content and turnover will demonstrate cellular impairment and injury. The main consequence of these metabolic changes is the loss of osmotic gradients across cell membranes. The earliest biochemical change is the decrease in α-keto glutarate-dehydrogenase activity in astrocytes.

Symptoms of Wernicke-Korsakoff syndrome are attributed to these focal areas of damage. Ocular motor signs are attributable to lesions in the brainstem affecting the abducens nuclei and eye movement centers in the pons and midbrain. These lesions are characterized by a lack of significant destruction to nerve cells, which accounts for the rapid improvement and degree of recovery observed with thiamine repletion. Ataxia is a manifestation of damage to the cerebellum, particularly the superior vermis. The amnestic component is related to damage in the diencephalon, including the medial thalamus, and connections with the medial temporal lobes and amygdala. The slow and incomplete recovery of memory deficits suggests that amnesia is related to irreversible structural damage.

MORTALITY/MORBIDITY

The mortality rate is up to 10 to 15% in severe cases. Since, the presentation is variable and often clinically missed, the exact mortality rate is difficult to estimate. Prognosis depends on the stage of disease at presentation and prompt treatment.

CLINICAL MANIFESTATIONS

Common signs and symptoms of Wernicke-Korsakoff syndrome include:

- Mental status changes—confusion, apathy, indifference, paucity of speech, hallucination, agitation and confabulation (patient fills in gaps of memory with data that can be recalled at that moment)
- Horizontal nystagmus, ophthalmoplegia (due to weakness of one or more extraocular muscles
- Visual impairment
- Ataxia
- Symptoms of alcohol withdrawal may also be present
- Cardiovascular dysfunction may be observed. Overt signs of beriberi heart disease are rare in patients with Wernicke-Korsakoff syndrome. The following symptoms may be observed and generally improve with administration of thiamine:
  - Postural hypotension
  - Tachycardia
  - Syncope
- Late-stage Wernicke-Korsakoff syndrome may result in stupor, coma, or even death.

CAUSES

- Chronic alcoholism
- Nutritional deficiency
- Persistent emesis
  - Hyper emesis gravidarum
  - Gastric malignancy
  - Intestinal obstruction

    - Bariatric surgery: Wernicke's encephalopathy can present as early as 2 weeks after surgery. Recovery typically occurs within 3–6 months of initiation of therapy, but may be incomplete if this syndrome is not recognized promptly and treated. The highest risk is in young women with vomiting.
- Systemic diseases
    - Malignancy
    - Disseminated tuberculosis
    - Acquired immunodeficiency syndrome (AIDS)
    - Uremia
- Starvation
    - Anorexia nervosa
    - Schizophrenia
    - Terminally-ill cancer patient
- Iatrogenic
    - Intravenous hyperalimentation
    - Refeeding after starvation
    - Chronic hemodialysis

LABORATORY STUDIES

- **Electrolytes:** Electrolyte studies are used to rule out an acute metabolic derangement causing mental confusion.
- **Serum thiamine levels:** Thiamine or the phosphorylated esters of thiamine in serum or blood can also be measured by high-performance liquid chromatography (HPLC) to detect deficiency.
- **Arterial blood gas:** To evaluate for hypoxemia, acidosis, or alkalosis.
- **Serum/urine toxic drug screen:** To rule out acute toxic ingestion. This is most helpful if results are available rapidly.
- **Liver-associated enzymes:** This may provide evidence of alcohol abuse or liver dysfunction.
- **Erythrocyte transketolase activity:** Thiamine deficiency is most frequently assessed by assaying erythrocyte transketolase activity in the presence and absence of added TPP. If the red blood cells have sufficient thiamine, the transketolase will be fully saturated with TPP, and no increase in activity will be observed when TPP is added to the assay system. An increase in transketolase activity indicates that the patient is thiamine deficient.

IMAGING STUDIES

- **CT brain scan:** Computed tomography (CT) scan can help in rapid assessment for hemorrhage, mass effect, edema, and large subacute stroke.
- **MRI of the brain:** Magnetic resonance imaging (MRI) demonstrates acute lesions of Wernicke-Korsakoff syndrome.

TREATMENT

Wernicke's encephalopathy is a medical emergency. Prompt recognition of the symptom complex and a high index of suspicion are crucial to ensure early treatment. Parenteral thiamine (100 mg) is the treatment of choice. Early treatment can rapidly reverse the ophthalmoplegia and improve ataxia/disequilibrium and early mental confusion, as well as prevent development of the amnestic state.

After the initial IV dose, continue daily doses of thiamine (100 mg) as IV, IM, or oral doses depending on patient's status. Supplementation of electrolytes, particularly magnesium and potassium (often low in people with alcoholism), may be required in addition to thiamine. Magnesium acts as a cofactor for many enzymes (e.g., transketolase for the conversion of thiamine-to-thiamine pyrophosphate) and, therefore, its deficiency may lead to refractory response to thiamine supplementation. In patients who are chronically malnourished, the remainder of the B vitamins should also be supplemented. Administration of intravenous glucose to patients, who are severely malnourished can exhaust their supply of thiamine and precipitate Wernicke-Korsakoff syndrome.

PROGNOSIS

Mortality may be secondary to infections and hepatic failure, but some deaths are directly attributable to irreversible defects of severe and prolonged thiamine deficiency (e.g., coma).

CLINICAL NOTE

Thiamine deficiency is most frequently assessed by assaying erythrocyte transketolase activity in the presence and absence of added TPP.

CLINICAL PEARLS

1. The term Wernicke's 's encephalopathy is used to describe the clinical triad of confusion, ataxia, and nystagmus (or ophthalmoplegia).When persistent learning and memory deficits are present, the symptom complex is often called Wernicke-Korsakoff syndrome.
2. Patients who chronically misuse alcohol are prone to thiamine deficiency due to poor nutrition, poor absorption, and storage, as well as an increased breakdown and decreased formation of TPP.
3. Thiamine deficiency is most frequently assessed by assaying erythrocyte transketolase activity in the presence and absence of added TPP.
4. Parenteral thiamine (100 mg) is the treatment of choice, followed by daily doses of thiamine (100 mg) as IV, IM, or oral doses depending on patient's status.
5. Early treatment can rapidly reverse the ophthalmoplegia improve ataxia and early mental confusion.

CASE STUDY 3

Theme: Chemistry, Metabolism, Coenzyme Role, and Clinical Implications of Vitamin B_2 Deficiency

A 45-year-old male, a known alcoholic from the previous 10 years reported to the physician for consultation. He complained of burning of eyes and a sore tongue. There was history of reduced appetite and mild abdominal discomfort.

The examination revealed cracks on the lips and in the corners of the mouth. The tongue was red, fissured, and inflamed. The hair was dull, skin was oily, and nails were split.

What is the probable cause for all these manifestations?

What type of investigations should be carried out to know the cause of the disease?

CASE DETAILS

The patient is most probably suffering from vitamin B_2 deficiency (Riboflavin deficiency).

Vitamin B_2 deficiency is frequent in chronic alcoholics. It can also occur in patients with chronic liver diseases, and in hospitalized patients who receive total parenteral nutrition (TPN) with inadequate riboflavin supplementation. Riboflavin is essential for healthy skin, nails, hair growth, and general good health, including regulating thyroid activity. Riboflavin supports energy production by aiding in the metabolism of fats, carbohydrates, and proteins. Characteristic symptoms of riboflavin deficiency include lesions of the skin, especially in the corners of the mouth, and a red, sore tongue. Assessment of riboflavin status can be done by erythrocyte glutathione reductase activity.

BASIC CONCEPT

Overview of Riboflavin Metabolism

Riboflavin, or vitamin B_2, was initially isolated from milk whey. Originally called lactochrome, it was also once known as vitamin G. Riboflavin is important for energy production, enzyme function, and normal fatty acid and amino acid synthesis and is necessary for the reproduction of glutathione, a free radical scavenger.

Riboflavin functions in several different enzyme systems. Two derivatives, riboflavin 5'phosphate [flavin mononucleotide (FMN)] and riboflavin 5'adenosine diphosphate [flavin adenine dinucleotide (FAD)], are the coenzymes that unite with specific apoenzyme proteins to form flavoprotein enzymes. Most of the flavin coenzyme systems help to regulate cellular metabolism.

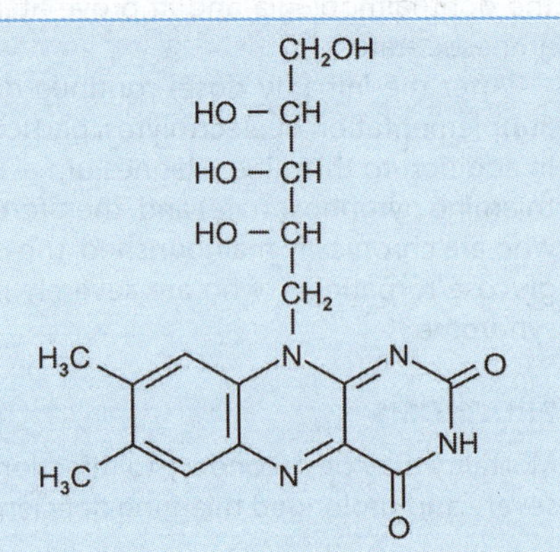

Fig. 11.5: Structure of riboflavin. It contains D-ribitol, isoalloxazine ring (flavin nucleus), one carbon is attached to the ninth position of isoalloxazine nucleus.

Functions

Flavin mononucleotide (FMN) and FAD function as coenzymes for a wide variety of oxidative enzymes and remain bound to the enzymes during the oxidation–reduction reactions. Flavins can act as oxidizing agents because of their ability to accept a pair of hydrogen atoms. Reduction of isoalloxazine ring **(Fig. 11.5)** (FAD, FMN oxidized form) yields the reduced forms of the flavoprotein ($FMNH_2$ and $FADH_2$).

Mechanism of action

Enzymes that contain flavin adenine dinucleotide (FAD) or flavin-mononucleotide (FMN) as prosthetic groups are known as flavoenzymes.

The functions of these flavoenzymes/flavoproteins are:

- Flavoproteins play very important roles in the electron transport chain.
- Decarboxylation of pyruvate and α-keto glutarate requires FAD besides other coenzymes.
- FAD is required as a coenzyme for monoamine oxidase and glutathione reductase.
- Fatty acyl CoA dehydrogenase requires FAD in fatty acid oxidation.
- Oxidative deamination of amino acids requires flavoproteins.
- FAD is required for the conversion of succinate to fumarate.
- Mitochondrial glycerol-3-p dehydrogenase requires FAD.
- FAD is required in the conversion of xanthine to uric acid.
- FAD is required by glycine oxidase enzyme.

FAD is a cofactor for methyltetrahydrofolate reductase and, therefore, modulates homocysteine metabolism.
The vitamin also plays a role in drug and steroid metabolism, including detoxification reactions.

RIBOFLAVIN DEFICIENCY

Water-soluble riboflavin is not stored in ample amounts; minute reserves are stored in the liver, kidneys, and heart. A constant supply is needed. Deficiency in this vitamin is usually part of a multiple-nutrient deficiency and does not occur in isolation.

Riboflavin, being water soluble is minimally stored in liver, kidneys, and heart. Hence, an optimum supply needs to be maintained. The isolated deficiency of riboflavin is rare; deficiency usually occurs as a component of multiple-nutrients deficiencies.

Nutritional deficiency

Riboflavin is abundantly found in milk, dairy products, cereals, meats, and dark green vegetables; hence, deficiency can occur as a result of dietary deficiency of these nutrients. Riboflavin is exceptionally light sensitive; milk stored in transparent containers can have photodegradation of riboflavin. The incidence of riboflavin deficiency has declined with the fortification of many foods including grains and cereals. Daily intake of breakfast cereals and milk is expected to maintain a sufficient supply of riboflavin.

Additional Risk Factors

a. Increased physiological demand as in pregnancy and lactation
b. Photodegradation, as in phototherapy for hyperbilirubinemia, especially in premature infants
c. Advanced age
d. Mental depression
e. Low socioeconomic status
f. Malabsorption as in sprue, malignancies, or alcoholism
g. Deficiency of riboflavin binding protein

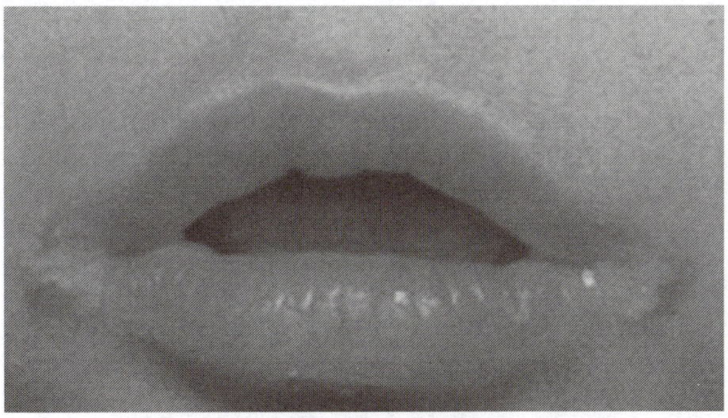

Fig. 11.6: Cheilosis.

CLINICAL MANIFESTATIONS

The isolated riboflavin deficiency is very rare; it is usually a component of multiple nutritional deficiencies. Therefore, multiple clinical manifestations are observed, such as:

- Cheilosis, or chapping and fissuring of the lips **(Fig. 11.6)**
- Glossitis—A sore, red, and fissured tongue **(Fig. 11.7)**
- Oily, scaly rashes on the skin, scalp, scrotum, vulva, and philtrum
- Red and itchy eyes
- Growth retardation in infants and children
- Night blindness
- Cataract
- Migraines
- Peripheral neuropathy
- Mild anemia (secondary to interference with iron absorption)
- Fatigue
- Deficiency can be associated with some developmental abnormalities, such as:
  - Cleft lip and palate deformities
  - Congenital heart defects.

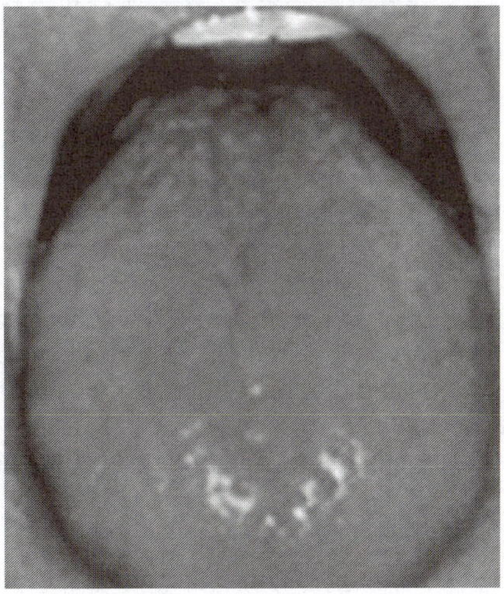

Fig. 11.7: Glossitis.

LABORATORY INVESTIGATIONS

- Measurement of RBC glutathione reductase activity may help in the detection of riboflavin deficiency. An increase in the stimulation of this enzymatic reaction confirms a low level of riboflavin.
- Riboflavin can cause false elevations of urinary catecholamines and false-positive urine urobilinogen reactions (Ehrlich test).
- Measurement of red blood cell or urinary riboflavin concentrations can also help in diagnosis.

TREATMENT

- Treatment for riboflavin deficiency consists of riboflavin replenishment, with care taken not to overlook coexisting B complex deficiencies.
- The recommended nutrient intake (RNI) of riboflavin is 0.6 mg/5000 kJ daily.
- The daily RNI ranges are 0.3 to 0.6 mg for infants, 0.7 to 1.1 mg for children, 1.1 to 1.4 mg for adolescents, and 1 to 1.6 mg for adults.
- Recommended increased requirements for pregnant and lactating women are as follows:
  - Additional 0.1 mg/day in the first trimester
  - Additional 0.3 mg/day in the second and third trimesters
  - Additional 0.4 mg/day during lactation
- Oral riboflavin doses of 1 to 4 mg daily are usually considered sufficient as a nutritional supplement in patients with normal gastrointestinal (GI) absorption. These doses should be present in the normal diet. Doses for deficiency treatment are slightly higher.
- Because the capacity of the GI tract to absorb riboflavin is limited (~20 mg if given in one oral dose), riboflavin toxicity has not been described.

CLINICAL NOTE

Riboflavin deficiency is almost always due to dietary deficiency.

CLINICAL PEARLS

1. Riboflavin is essential for healthy skin, nails, hair growth, and general good health, including regulating thyroid activity. Riboflavin supports energy production by aiding in the metabolism of fats, carbohydrates, and proteins.
2. Riboflavin deficiency is usually associated with other vitamin B complex deficiencies, and isolated deficiency is rare.
3. Measurement of RBC glutathione reductase activity may help in the detection of riboflavin deficiency.
4. Characteristic symptoms of riboflavin deficiency include lesions of the skin, especially in the corners of the mouth, and a red, sore tongue.
5. Oral riboflavin doses of 1 to 4 mg daily are usually considered sufficient as a nutritional supplement in patients with normal GI absorption.

CASE STUDY 4

Theme: Chemistry, metabolism, coenzyme role, and clinical implications of niacin deficiency and toxicity

A 60-year-old chronic smoker and alcoholic man suffering from odynophagia (painful swallowing), insomnia, epigastric discomfort, and recurrent diarrhea presented to the outpatient department. Clinical examination revealed memory disorientation, stomatitis, glossitis, esophagitis, and exfoliative dermatitis with some vesicles on erythematous bases on photo exposed sites.

Blood examinations showed leukocytosis and serological markers (elevated AST, ALT, and γGT) of heavy drinking. Chest X-ray and abdominal ultrasound showed emphysematous lungs and fatty liver; CT of the brain was normal. Treatment with nicotinamide 500 mg daily was initiated. The rash improved and upon re-examination after three weeks the dermatitis had resolved. Moreover, it was suggested that he restrict alcohol and smoking and increase consumption of other B complex vitamins and food sources of niacin.

What is the most likely diagnosis for this patient?

CASE DISCUSSION

Disoriented memory, diarrhea, and dermatitis are the signs of pellagra. The patient is a heavy drinker and smoker. Emphysematous lung is as a result of smoking and fatty liver is a consequence of chronic alcoholism. Chronic alcoholics are more prone to vitamin deficiencies.

The generalized signs of other vitamin deficiencies are also apparent in this patient, but pellagra is grossly apparent and since the rash improved and the dermatitis improved after niacin therapy, so there cannot be any other cause for the above said manifestations. The final clinical diagnosis is pulmonary emphysema with fatty liver and pellagra. The treatment is symptomatic, avoidance of alcohol, restriction of smoking, and supplementation with niacin and B complex vitamins.

OVERVIEW OF NIACIN METABOLISM

Niacin (nicotinic acid and nicotinamide) is also known as vitamin B_3. Both nicotinic acid **(Fig. 11.8)** and nicotinamide **(Fig. 11.9)** can serve as the dietary source of vitamin B_3. Niacin is a pyridine carboxylic acid that is converted into an amide in the body.

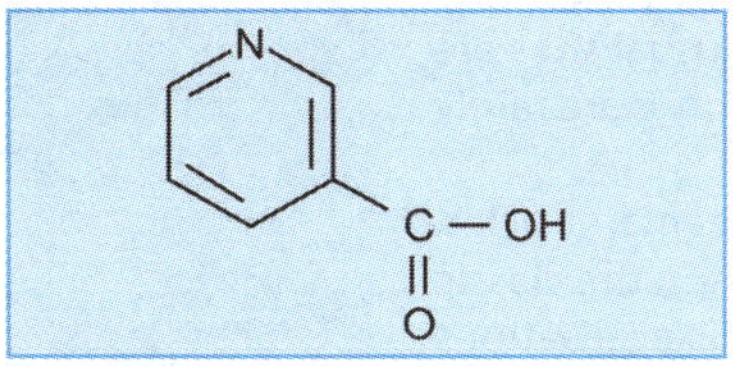

Fig. 11.8: Structure of nicotinic acid.

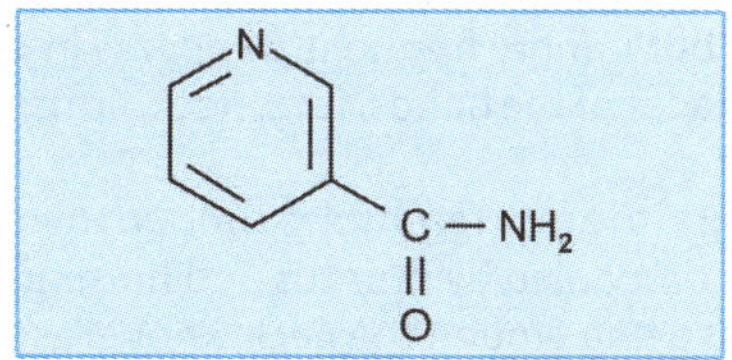

Fig. 11.9: Structure of nicotinamide.

Niacin is not a true vitamin in the strictest definition since it can be derived from the amino acid tryptophan. However, the ability to utilize tryptophan for niacin synthesis is inefficient (60 mg of tryptophan is required to synthesize 1 mg of niacin). Also, synthesis of niacin from tryptophan requires vitamins B_1, B_2, and B_6 which would be limiting in themselves on a marginal diet. The recommended daily requirement for niacin is 13 to 19 niacin equivalents (NE) per day for a normal adult. One NE is equivalent to 1 mg of free niacin. Nicotinic acid and nicotinamide are absorbed well from the stomach and small intestine. Niacin bioavailability is high from beans, milk, meat, and eggs; bioavailability from cereal grains is lower. Since flour is enriched with the "free" niacin (i.e., noncoenzyme form), bioavailability is excellent.

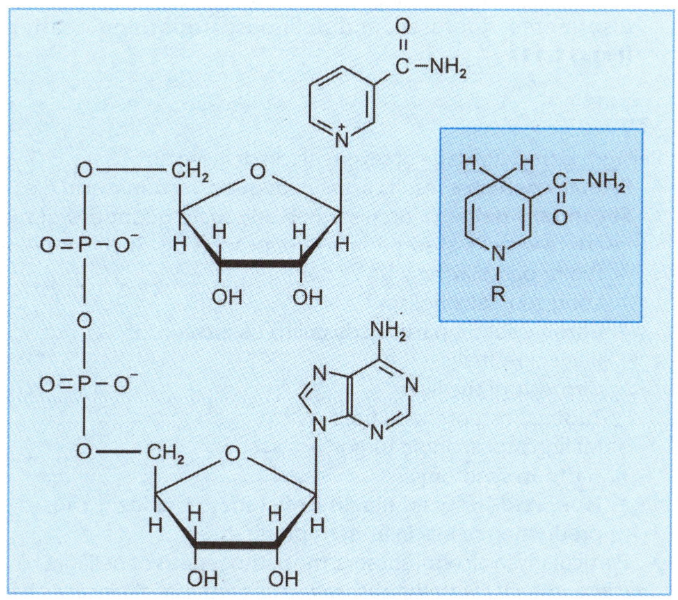

Fig. 11.10: Structure of NAD^+, NADP has extraphosphate attached to the ribose.

Niacin is required for adequate cellular function and metabolism as an essential component in coenzyme I [oxidized form of nicotinamide adenine dinucleotide (NAD)] and coenzyme II [reduced form of nicotinamide adenine dinucleotide phosphate (NADP) **Fig. 11.10**], which either donate or accept hydrogen ions in vital oxidation–reduction reactions. These compounds are important coenzymes for glycolysis, protein and amino acid metabolism, pyruvate metabolism, pentose biosynthesis, high-energy phosphate bond generation, glycerol metabolism, and fatty acid metabolism. In addition to its coenzyme role, NAD is the source of ADP-ribose for the ADP-ribosylation of proteins and poly-ADP-ribosylation of nucleoproteins involved in the DNA repair mechanism.

Pellagra

Pellagra is clinically manifested by the 4 D's: photosensitive dermatitis, diarrhea, dementia, and death. The full tetrad of symptoms is usually not well developed in infants and children. Pellagra is the most frequent clinical feature of nutritional deficiency in adults in rural populations in the third world, whose staple diet is niacin-deficient jawar or maize with inadequate animal protein, fruits, and vegetables.

Frequency

Although the exact incidence of pellagra in other countries is not known, pellagra occurs mainly in developing nations in which corn and corn products are the major food sources, if the corn is not especially treated. Pellagra also occurs in ethnic populations whose diets are deficient in niacin and/or tryptophan.

Mortality/Morbidity

Untreated pellagra results in death from multiorgan failure. The morbidity of pellagra is related to its effects on the organ systems involved.

Clinical Manifestations

- Dietary history, the three identifying factors (i.e., diarrhea, dermatitis, and dementia), localization, and seasonal appearance all contribute to the diagnosis.
- The early symptoms of pellagra include loss of appetite, generalized weakness, irritability, abdominal pain, and vomiting.
- Later symptoms are bright red glossitis, chronic or recurrent diarrhea (watery, but occasionally bloody), which leads to a state of malnutrition and cachexia.
- The characteristic skin rash is characterized by pigmentation and scaling, particularly involving the sun-exposed areas. Pellagra can affect any part of the body surface, but it more frequently appears in certain areas. The usual sites are the dorsal surfaces of the hands, face, neck, arms, and feet. The changes are rarely seen elsewhere.
- In acute pellagra, the rash resembles sunburn (with symmetric erythema, vesicles, and bullae accompanied by pruritus and burning). In advanced cases, the classic eruption forms a ring around the neck, known as "Casal's necklace." Exacerbations follow re-exposure to sunlight.
- As pellagra advances, neuropsychiatric symptoms, such as photophobia, asthenia, depression, hallucinations, memory loss, and psychosis begin. The patient becomes disoriented, confused, and delirious; stupor and death result if untreated **(Fig. 11.11)**.

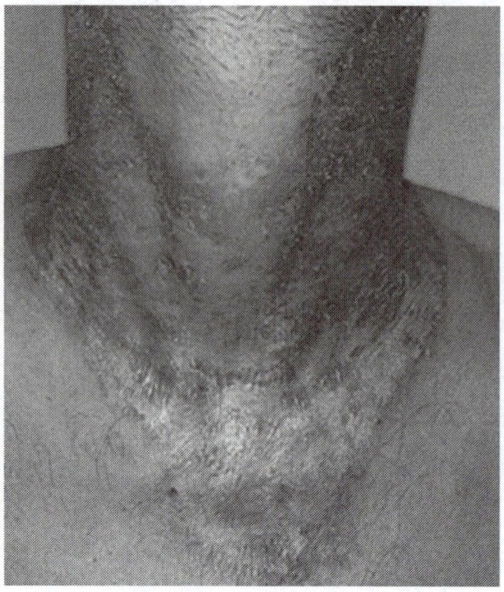

Fig. 11.11: Typical rash of niacin deficiency (casal necklace).

Causes

Pellagra is the late stage of severe niacin deficiency.

- **Primary pellagra** results from inadequate nicotinic acid (i.e., niacin) and/or tryptophan intake in the diet.
- **Secondary pellagra** occurs when adequate quantities of niacin are present in the diet, but other diseases or conditions interfere with its absorption and/or processing. Such conditions include the following:
  - Prolonged diarrhea
  - Long-term alcoholism
  - Chronic colitis, particularly colitis ulcerosa
  - Ileitis terminalis
  - Cirrhosis of the liver
  - Tuberculosis of the GI tract
  - Malignant carcinoid tumor
  - Hartnup syndrome
  - **Isoniazid-induced niacin deficiency:** Isoniazid causes a depletion of pyridoxal phosphate that is required for the production of niacin from tryptophan.

Particularly in alcohol abusers, the pathogenesis of pellagra has not been fully elucidated. It has not been determined if alcohol interferes directly with the absorption or synthesis of niacin as has been shown with thiamine. However, in developed countries, alcoholic pellagra encephalopathy (APE), which exhibits a disturbance of consciousness, has been reported decreased intake, malabsorption, reduced storage, and impaired utilization of niacin in a context of the increased metabolic needs in alcoholics are some of the main causes of pellagra in alcoholics. Finally, the high sun exposure in Mediterranean countries is an additional cause for the appearance of pellagra.

Laboratory Studies

- The therapeutic response to niacin in a patient with the typical symptoms and signs of pellagra establishes the diagnosis.
- Blood counts (anemia), findings of hypoproteinemia, higher levels of serum calcium and lower levels of serum potassium and phosphorus, liver function test results, and serum porphyrin levels can help in diagnosing pellagra.
- Low serum niacin, tryptophan, NAD, and NADP levels can reflect niacin deficiency and confirm the diagnosis of pellagra.
- Low urinary levels of N-methylnicotinamide and pyridone suggest niacin deficiency and support the diagnosis of pellagra. The combined excretion of *N*-methylnicotinamide and pyridone of less than 1.5 mg in 24 hours indicates severe niacin deficiency.

Treatment

Nicotinamide and Other Nutrients

Because multiple deficiencies are common, a balanced diet, including other B vitamins (particularly riboflavin and pyridoxine), is needed. Nicotinamide is usually used to treat deficiency, because nicotinamide, unlike nicotinic acid (the most common form of niacin), does not cause flushing, itching, burning, or tingling sensations. Nicotinamide is given in doses ranging from 40 mg/day to 250 mg/day PO in divided doses three to four times a day.

Niacin (nicotinic acid) in large amounts is sometimes used to lower LDL cholesterol and triglyceride levels and to increase HDL cholesterol levels.

Niacin Toxicity

Prostaglandin-mediated flushing due to binding of the vitamin to a G protein-coupled receptor has been observed at daily doses as low as 50 mg of niacin when taken as a supplement or as therapy for dyslipidemia. It may be more intense after alcohol ingestion, aerobic activity, sun exposure, and consumption of spicy foods. There is no evidence of toxicity from niacin derived from food sources. Flushing always starts in the face and may be accompanied by skin dryness, itching, paresthesias, and headache. Premedication with aspirin may alleviate these symptoms. Flushing is subject to tachyphylaxis and often improves with time. Nausea, vomiting, and abdominal pain also occur at similar doses of niacin. Hepatic toxicity is the most serious toxic reaction due to niacin and may present as jaundice with elevated aspartate aminotransferase (AST) and alanine aminotransferase (ALT) levels. A few cases of fulminant hepatitis requiring liver transplantation have been reported at doses of 3 to 9 g/day. Other toxic reactions include glucose intolerance, hyperuricemia, macular edema, and macular cysts. The upper limit for daily niacin intake has been set at 35 mg. However, this upper limit does not pertain to the therapeutic use of niacin.

Complications

- Dermatitis of pellagra can be distressing and disfiguring.
- Denudation of the vesiculated and blistered skin lesions can potentially become infected secondarily.
- Severe glossitis causes dysphagia.
- GI tract involvement leads to a malabsorptive state.
- Depression, anxiety, delusions, hallucinations, and coma are the neuropsychiatric complications observed in patients with pellagra.
- The malnourished state associated with pellagra results in death if untreated.

Prognosis

If pellagra is diagnosed and treated appropriately, the prognosis for recovery is excellent.

CLINICAL NOTE

Pellagra should be considered as a presumptive diagnosis in patients with chronic alcoholism, malnutrition, and amino acid imbalance in industrialized countries, even if they exhibit only neurological symptoms.

CLINICAL PEARLS

1. Pellagra is clinically manifested by the 4 D's: photosensitive dermatitis, diarrhea, dementia, and death.
2. Primary pellagra results from inadequate nicotinic acid (i.e., niacin) and/or tryptophan intake in the diet. Secondary pellagra occurs when adequate quantities of niacin are present in the diet, but other diseases or conditions interfere with its absorption and/or processing.
3. Diagnosis can be established by measurement of a decreased serum level of niacin, a low urinary level of N-methylnicotinamide and pyridone, and the improvement of cutaneous eruptions within 24 to 48 hours after oral niacin administration.
4. Nicotinamide is usually used to treat deficiency, because nicotinamide, unlike nicotinic acid (the most common form of niacin), does not cause flushing, itching, burning, or tingling sensations.
5. Niacin (nicotinic acid) in large amounts is sometimes used to lower LDL cholesterol and triglyceride levels and to increase HDL cholesterol levels.

CASE STUDY 5

Theme: Folic acid—Chemistry, Metabolism, Functions, and Clinical Implications of Folic Acid Deficiency

A 44-year-old man who had lost his job because of absenteeism presented to his physician complaining of loss of appetite, fatigue, muscle weakness, and emotional depression.

The physical examination revealed a somewhat enlarged liver that was firm and nodular, and there was a hint of jaundice in the sclerae and a hint of alcohol in his breath. The initial laboratory profile included a hematological analysis that showed that he had an anemia with enlarged red blood cells (macrocytic). A bone marrow aspirate confirmed the suspicion that he had a megaloblastic anemia because it showed a greater than normal number of red and white blood cell precursors, most of which were larger than normal. Further analyzes revealed that his serum folic acid level was1.2 ng/mL (normal 2.5 to 20), his serum B_{12} level was 253 pg/mL (normal 200 to 900), but his serum iron level was normal.

What is the cause of megaloblastic anemia in this patient?
What is its correlation with alcoholism?

CASE DETAILS

The megaloblastic anemias are a group of disorders characterized by the presence of distinctive morphologic appearances of the developing red cells in the bone marrow. The cause is usually deficiency of either cobalamin (vitamin B_{12}) or folate, but megaloblastic anemia may arise because of genetic or acquired abnormalities affecting the metabolism of these vitamins or because of defects in DNA synthesis not related to cobalamin or folate. Megaloblastic anemia in folate deficiency is identical to anemia resulting from vitamin B_{12} deficiency However, the serum vitamin B_{12} level is normal in this patient so that rules out vitamin B_{12} deficiency. Alcoholics in particular are at risk for folate deficiency because of impaired gastrointestinal absorption and poor nutrition. Folate is essential for many biochemical processes in the body, including DNA synthesis and red blood cell synthesis. Oral doses of 5 to 15 mg folic acid daily are satisfactory to treat the deficiency, as sufficient folate is absorbed from these extremely large doses even in patients with severe malabsorption. It is essential to exclude cobalamin deficiency before large doses of folic acid are given, and deficiency if present must be corrected, otherwise cobalamin neuropathy may develop, despite a response of the anemia of cobalamin deficiency to folate therapy.

BASIC CONCEPT

Overview of Folic Acid

Folic acid is the term commonly used for pteroylmonoglutamic acid. Folic acid is present in most fruits and vegetables (especially citrus fruits and green leafy vegetables) and daily requirements of 50 to 100 μg/day are usually met in the diet. Total body stores of folate are approximately 5000 μg, enough to supply requirements for 2 to 3 months.

By far the most common cause of folate deficiency is inadequate dietary intake. Alcoholics, anorectic patients, persons who do not eat fresh fruits and vegetables, and those who overcook their food are candidates for folate deficiency. Reduced folate absorption is rarely seen, since absorption occurs from the entire gastrointestinal tract. However, drugs such as phenytoin, trimethoprim-sulfamethoxazole, or sulfasalazine may interfere with folate absorption. Folic acid requirements are increased in pregnancy, hemolytic anemia, and exfoliative skin disease, and in these cases, the increased requirements (five to ten times normal) may not be met by a normal diet. Patients with increased folate requirements should receive supplementation with 1 mg/day of folic acid.

Biochemical functions

In its simplest form, folate consists of three connected chemical moieties: a pteridine ring (6-methylpterin), p-amino benzoic acid (PABA), and glutamate. In nature, folate is generally polyglutamated (decorated by two to seven additional glutamic acid residues) **(Fig. 11.12)**. Conjugases (γ-glutamyl carboxypeptidases) in the intestinal lumen cleave off extra glutamic acid residues, and folate is absorbed by the mucosa of the small intestine.

In cases of chronic alcoholism, folate deficiency may result from poor nutrition or from poor absorption of folate secondary to a conjugase deficiency. Once folate deficiency occurs, abnormal megaloblastic replication of epithelial mucosa can occur, which further impairs folate uptake. After absorption, folate is reduced to THF by dihydrofolate reductase. The majority of circulating folate is in the form of N5-methyl THF. Cells use specific transporters for THF uptake, and cellular machinery polyglutamates the folate to aid in cellular retention.

Folates (as the intracellular polyglutamate derivatives) act as coenzymes in the transfer of single-carbon units. Two of these reactions are involved in purine and one in pyrimidine synthesis necessary for DNA and RNA replication. Folate is also a coenzyme for methionine synthesis, in which methylcobalamin is also involved and in which THF is regenerated. THF is the acceptor of single carbon units newly entering the active pool via conversion of serine to glycine. Methionine, the other product of the methionine synthase reaction, is the precursor for s-adenosyl methionine (SAM), the universal methyl donor involved in >100 methyltransferase reactions.

Role of Folic Acid in Nucleotide Synthesis

Folate exists in a pool of interconvertible intermediates each carrying a one-carbon fragment, in several different oxidation states. Two different forms of folate are required for different aspects of nucleotide biosynthesis. N10-formyl THF provides the C-2 and C-8 carbons for the de novo synthesis of purine rings, and thus is critical for DNA metabolism. The methylene form, N5, N10-methylene THF, is required for the production of dTMP from dUMP. This reaction involves the transfer of a CH2 group and hydrogen from N5, N10-methylene THF. In this process, THF is oxidized to dihydrofolate (DHF) **(Fig. 11.12)**. For subsequent dTMP production, THF must be regenerated. THF is produced from DHF by the enzyme DHF reductase (DHFR) in a reaction requiring NADPH. DHFR is the target of methotrexate, an antifolate cancer chemotherapeutic, which by limiting the available pool of N5, N10-methylene

THF, inhibits DNA synthesis in rapidly dividing cancer cells. Methotrexate therapy can produce side effects resembling folate deficiency. (See details in methotrexate therapy.)

Additionally, bacterial DHFR is a target for antimicrobials.

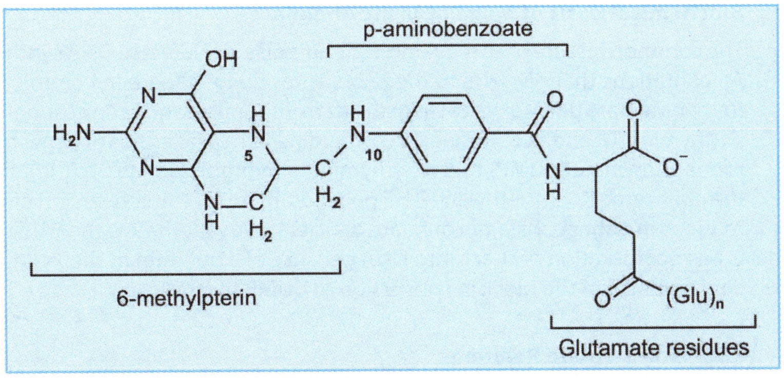

Fig. 11.12: Structure of tetrahydrofolate (active form of folic acid).

Role of Folic Acid in Transmethylation Reactions

Outside of DNA synthesis, folate plays a role in methylation metabolism. The major methyl donor is s-adenosyl methionine (SAM), which is required for many reactions. For example, SAM is needed for the production of norepinephrine from epinephrine and for DNA methylation, which can influence gene transcription. After methyl group transfer, SAM is converted to S-adenosyl homocysteine (SAH), which is hydrolyzed to homocysteine and adenosine. To restore the levels of methionine (an essential amino acid), homocysteine must be methylated. This reaction is dependent on N5-methyl THF and vitamin B_{12}. Methionine levels can be limiting, making the availability of N5-methyl THF for the conversion of homocysteine to methionine critical. Further, in the absence of B_{12}, THF can be trapped in the N5-methyl THF form and thus be removed from the THF pool. This is referred to as the "methyl trap," which can impact other areas of one-carbon metabolism, such as dTMP production.

Thus, methyl trap is the sequestering of tetrahydrofolate as N5-methyl THF because of decreased conversion of homocysteine to methionine as a result of a deficiency of methionine synthase or its cofactor, cobalamin (vitamin B_{12}) **(Fig. 11.13)**.

In summary, folate is a vitamin acquired from the diet that is essential for one-carbon metabolism. Inadequate folate levels inhibit DNA synthesis by limiting purine nucleotide and dTMP levels, which results in the abnormal cellular proliferation observed in megaloblastic anemia. Manifestations of folate deficiency thereafter, not surprisingly, would involve impairment of cell division, accumulation of possibly toxic metabolites, such as homocysteine, and impairment of methylation reactions involved in the regulation of gene expression, thus increasing neoplastic risks.

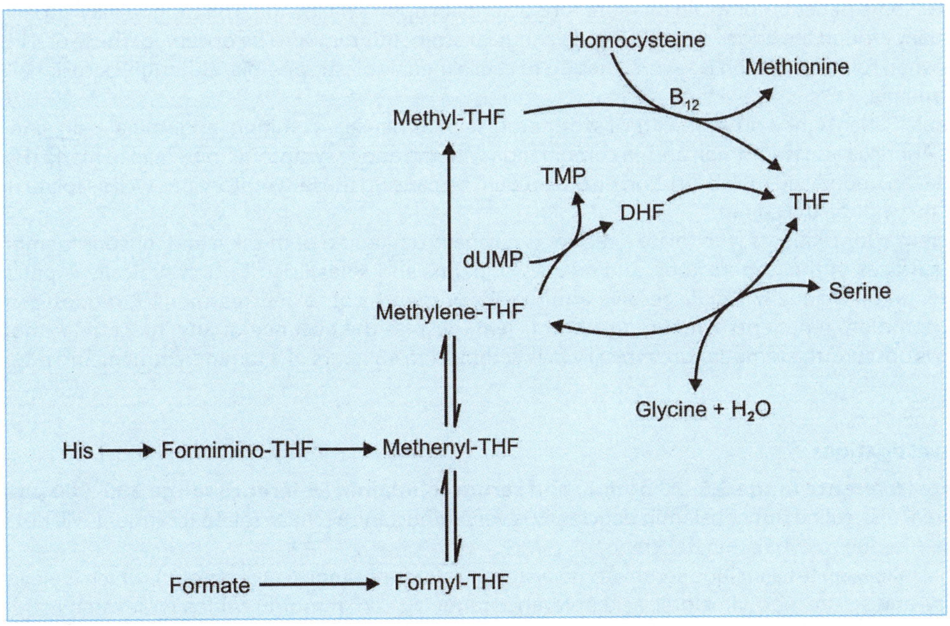

Fig. 11.13: One-carbon transfer reactions.

MEGALOBLASTIC ANEMIA DUE TO FOLATE DEFICIENCY

Incidence

The current standard of practice is that serum folate levels less than 3 ng/mL and a red blood cell (RBC) folate level less than 140 ng/mL put an individual at high-risk of folate deficiency. The RBC folate level generally indicates folate stored in the body, whereas the serum folate level tends to reflect acute changes in folate intake. The prevalence of folic acid deficiency has decreased since the United States and Canada introduced a mandatory folic acid food fortification program in November 1998. People with excessive alcohol intake and malnutrition are still at high-risk of folic acid deficiency.

Biochemical Basis of Megaloblastic Anemia

The common feature of all megaloblastic anemias is a defect in DNA synthesis that affects rapidly dividing cells in the bone marrow. All conditions that give rise to megaloblastic changes share in common a disparity in the rate of synthesis or availability of the four immediate precursors of DNA: the deoxyribonucleoside triphosphates (dNTPs): dA(adenine)TP and dG(guanine)TP (purines), dT(thymine)TP, and dC(cytosine)TP (pyrimidines). In deficiencies of either folate or cobalamin, there is failure to convert deoxyuridine monophosphate (dUMP) to deoxythymidine monophosphate (dTMP), the precursor of dTTP. This is because folate is needed as the coenzyme 5, 10-methylene-THF polyglutamate for the conversion of dUMP to dTMP; the availability of 5, 10-methylene-THF is reduced in either cobalamin or folate deficiency. An alternative theory for megaloblastic anemia in cobalamin or folate deficiency is misincorporation of Uracil into DNA because of a build-up of deoxyuridine triphosphate (dUTP) at the DNA replication fork as a consequence of the block in conversion of dUMP to dTMP.

Cobalamin–Folate Relations

Folate is required for many reactions in mammalian tissues. Only two reactions in the body are known to require cobalamin. Methylmalonyl CoA isomerization, which requires adenosyl cobalamin and the methylation of homocysteine to methionine, requires both methylcobalamin and both 5-methyltetrahydrofolate (5-MTHF). This reaction is the first step in the pathway by which 5-MTHF, which enters bone marrow and other cells from plasma, is converted into all the intracellular folate coenzymes. The coenzymes are all polyglutamated (the larger size-aiding retention in the cell), but the enzyme folate polyglutamate synthase can use only THF, not MTHF, as substrate. In cobalamin deficiency, MTHF accumulates in plasma, while intracellular folate concentrations fall due to the failure of formation of THF, the substrate on which folate polyglutamates are built. This has been termed THF starvation, or the methylfolate trap. This theory explains the abnormalities of folate metabolism that occur in cobalamin deficiency and also why the anemia of cobalamin deficiency will respond to folic acid in large doses.

CLINICAL MANIFESTATIONS

1. **History:** In folate deficiency, the patient's history is important because it may reveal the underlying disorder. Very often, a patient presents with a history of excessive alcohol intake with concurrent poor diet intake. Other times, patients may be pregnant or lactating; may take certain drugs, such as phenytoin, sulfonamides, or methotrexate; may have chronic hemolytic anemia; or may have underlying malabsorption.
2. **Oral lesions:** Some patients complain of a sore tongue or pain upon swallowing. The tongue may appear swollen, beefy, red, or shiny, usually around the edges and tips initially. Angular stomatitis may also be observed. These oral lesions typically occur at the time when folate depletion is severe enough to cause megaloblastic anemia, although, occasionally, lesions may occur before the anemia.
3. **GI symptoms:** Patients may present with GI symptoms, such as nausea, vomiting, abdominal pain, and diarrhea, especially after meals. Anorexia also is common and, in combination with the above symptoms, may lead to marked weight loss. However, be aware that an underlying malabsorption disorder could be causing these symptoms, as well as folate depletion. The lack of folate itself may not be the culprit.
4. **Hyperpigmentation:** Patients with folate deficiency may have darkening of the skin and mucous membranes, particularly at the dorsal surfaces of the fingers, toes, and creases of palms and soles. Distribution typically is patchy. Fortunately, the hyperpigmentation gradually should resolve after weeks or months of folate treatment. A modest temperature elevation (<102°F) is common in patients who are folate deficient, despite the absence of any infection. Although the underlying mechanism is obscure, the temperature typically falls within 24 to 48 hours of vitamin treatment and returns to normal within a few days.

Laboratory Investigations

- **Serum folate (reference range 2.5–20 ng/mL) and serum cobalamin (reference range 200–900 pg/mL)**
  - As the initial test, ruling out cobalamin deficiency is very important because folate treatment will not improve neurologic abnormalities due to cobalamin deficiency.
  - Additional follow-up tests include serum homocysteine (reference range 5–16 mmol/L), which is elevated in B_{12} and folate deficiency, and serum methylmalonic acid (reference range 70–270 mmol/L), which is elevated in B_{12} deficiency only.
  - Red blood cell folate levels (reference range >140 ng/mL) tend to reflect chronic folate status rather than acute changes in folate that are reflected in serum folate levels,
- **Hematological findings**
  - **Peripheral blood film:** Oval macrocytes, usually with considerable anisocytosis and poikilocytosis, are the main feature. The MCV is usually >100 fL unless a cause of microcytosis (e.g., iron deficiency or thalassemia trait) is present. Some of the neutrophils are hyper hypersegmented (more than five nuclear lobes). There may be leukopenia due to a reduction in granulocytes and lymphocytes, but this is usually $>1.5\times10^9$/L; the platelet count may be moderately reduced, rarely to $<40 \times 10^9$/L. The severity of all these changes parallels the degree of anemia. In the nonanemic patient, the presence of a few macrocytes and hypersegmented neutrophils in the peripheral blood may be the only indication of the underlying disorder **(Fig. 11.14)**.

- **Bone marrow:** Bone marrow morphology is characteristically abnormal. Marked erythroid hyperplasia is present as a response to defective red blood cell production (ineffective erythropoiesis). Megaloblastic changes in the erythroid series include abnormally large cell size and asynchronous maturation of the nucleus and cytoplasm, i.e., cytoplasmic maturation continues while impaired DNA synthesis causes retarded nuclear development. In the myeloid series, giant metamyelocytes are characteristically seen.
- **Chromosomes:** Bone marrow cells, transformed lymphocytes, and other proliferating cells in the body show a variety of changes including random breaks, reduced contraction, spreading of the centromere, and exaggeration of secondary chromosomal constrictions and over prominent satellites. Similar abnormalities may be produced by antimetabolite drugs (e.g., cytosine arabinoside, hydroxyurea, and methotrexate) that either interfere with DNA replication or folate metabolism and that also cause megaloblastic appearances.

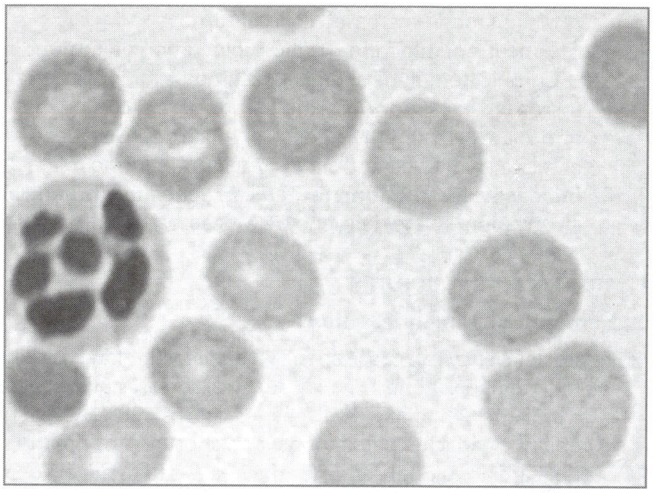

Fig. 11.14: Peripheral blood film in megaloblastic anemia. Macrocytes are observed and some of the red blood cells show ovalocytosis. A six-lobed polymorph nuclear leukocyte is present.

- **Ineffective hematopoiesis:** There is an accumulation of unconjugated bilirubin in plasma due to the death of nucleated red cells in the marrow (ineffective erythropoiesis). Other evidence for this includes raised urine urobilinogen, reduced haptoglobin and positive urine hemosiderin, and a raised serum lactate dehydrogenase. A weakly positive direct antiglobulin test due to complement can lead to a false diagnosis of autoimmune hemolytic anemia.

Causes of Folate Deficiency

The essential causes of folate deficiency are:

a. **Dietary deficiency:** Dietary deficiency of folate can be related to:
   - Chronic alcoholism (poor nutrition)
   - Psychiatric illness
   - Older adults (physical deformities, ill-fitting dentures, or depression)
   - Prolonged cooking (folate is heat labile)
   - Liver or kidney failure
   - Anorexia (loss of appetite due to any reason)

b. **Impaired absorption:** Various factors affecting folate absorption may be categorized as:
   - **Transporter deficiency:** Folate absorption across the intestinal cell membrane occurs mainly through a carrier-mediated active transport. Folate transporter is substrate and pH specific; saturable, and sodium dependent. Absorption of folate by passive diffusion does occur, but only to a minute extent. Therefore, deficiency of folate transporter or its metabolic inhibition due to any specific reason may cause folate deficiency.
   - **Small bowel resection or mesenteric vascular insufficiency**: A reduced absorptive area resulting from small bowel resection or mesenteric vascular insufficiency may cause folate deficiency.
   - **Villous atrophy:** Celiac disease, tropical sprue, and advancing age may cause folate deficiency due to atrophy of villi.
   - **Achlorhydria** by increasing gastric pH can impair folate absorption (pH dependence of folate transporter).
   - **Drugs**: Anticonvulsant drugs, such as Dilantin by inhibiting mucosal conjugase, decrease folate absorption.
   - **Zinc deficiency**: Zinc is a cofactor of the mucosal conjugase enzyme. Therefore, zinc deficiency may impair folate absorption.

c. **Impaired metabolism:** The following factors causing an inability to metabolize folate may result in folate deficiency:
   - **Antimetabolites:** Methotrexate and trimethoprim, acting as structural analogs of folate, competitively inhibit dihydrofolate reductase enzyme causing reduced bioavailability of folate.
   - **Reduced levels of metabolizing enzymes,** such as dihydrofolate reductase and methylene tetrahydrofolic acid (THFA) reductase are observed in hypothyroidism.
   - **Congenital deficiency or absence of metabolizing enzymes** may also decrease the bioavailability of folate.
   - **Chronic alcoholism**: Highly active alcohol dehydrogenase in chronic alcoholism, through binding with folate, may impair its utilization.

d. **Increased daily requirement**: Folate deficiency can occur due to increased folate demand in the following conditions:
   - Children—active growth
   - Pregnancy—rapid fetal growth and uterine enlargement
   - Lactation—folate uptake into breast milk

- Malignancy—increased cellular turnover
- Concurrent infection—rapid proliferation of immune cells (immunoproliferative response)
- Chronic hemolytic anemia—a stimulus for increased hematopoiesis

e. **Increased excretion/loss:** Increased folate excretion may occur as a result of vitamin B_{12} deficiency. B_{12} deficiency is known to trap folate in the methylated form, which deprives the tissues of the active form of folate (folate trap). As a result, large amounts of folate are filtered and are excreted out, causing folate deficiency concurrent to B_{12} deficiency.

f. **Increased destruction:** Free radicals generated through alcohol metabolism or cigarette smoking may cause increased folate inactivation. Folate deficiency is widespread in chronic alcoholics and cigarette smokers.

MORTALITY/MORBIDITY

Hematological Manifestations

Folate deficiency can cause anemia. The presentation typically consists of macrocytosis and hypersegmented polymorph nuclear leukocytes (PMNs). The anemia usually progresses over several months, and the patient typically does not express symptoms as such until the hematocrit level reaches less than 20%. At that point, symptoms, such as weakness, fatigue, difficulty concentrating, irritability, headache, palpitations, and shortness of breath can occur. Furthermore, heart failure can develop in light of high-output cardiac compensation for the decreased tissue oxygenation. Angina pectoris may occur in predisposed individuals due to increased cardiac work demand. Tachycardia, postural hypotension, and lactic acidosis are other common findings. Less commonly, neutropenia and thrombocytopenia will also occur, although it usually will not be as severe as the anemia. In rare cases, the absolute neutrophil count can drop below 1000/mL and the platelet count below 50,000/mL.

Elevated Serum Homocysteine and Atherosclerosis

Folate in the 5-methyl THFA form is a cosubstrate required by methionine synthase when it converts homocysteine to methionine. As a result, in the scenario of folate deficiency, homocysteine accumulates. Several recent clinical studies have indicated that mild-to-moderate hyperhomocysteinemia is highly associated with atherosclerotic vascular disease, such as coronary artery disease (CAD) and stroke. In this case, mild hyperhomocysteinemia is defined as a total plasma concentration of 15 to 25 mmol/L and moderate hyperhomocysteinemia is defined as 26 to 50 mmol/L.

Elevated homocysteine levels might act as an atherogenic factor by converting a stable plaque into an unstable, potentially occlusive, lesion. Homocysteine is believed to have atherogenic and prothrombotic properties via multiple mechanisms.

Pregnancy Complications

Possible pregnancy complications secondary to maternal folate status may include spontaneous abortion, abruption placentae, and congenital malformations (e.g., neural tube defect).

Although the exact mechanism is not understood, a relative folate shortage may exacerbate an underlying genetic predisposition to neural tube defects.

Effects on Carcinogens

Diminished folate status is associated with enhanced carcinogenesis.

Effects on Cognitive Function

Low folate and high homocysteine levels are a risk factor for cognitive decline in high-functioning older adults and high homocysteine level is an independent predictor of cognitive impairment among long-term stay geriatric patients.

Mechanistically speaking, current theory proposes that folate is essential for synthesis of S-adenosylmethionine, which is involved in numerous methylation reactions. This methylation process is central to the biochemical basis of proper neuropsychiatric functioning.

MEGALOBLASTIC ANEMIA: TREATMENT

Oral doses of 5 to 15 mg folic acid daily are satisfactory. The length of time therapy must be continued depending on the underlying disease. It is customary to continue therapy for about 4 months, when all folate-deficient red cells will have been eliminated and replaced by new folate-replete populations.

Cobalamin deficiency must be excluded and, if present, corrected, otherwise cobalamin neuropathy may develop, despite a response of the anemia of cobalamin deficiency to folate therapy. Long-term folic acid therapy is required when the underlying cause of the deficiency cannot be corrected and the deficiency is likely to recur. Where mild but chronic folate deficiency occurs, it is preferable to encourage improvement in the diet after correcting the deficiency with a short course of folic acid. In any patient receiving long-term folic acid therapy, it is important to measure the serum cobalamin level at regular (e.g., once yearly) intervals to exclude the coincidental development of cobalamin deficiency.

Prevention

- Patients whose folic acid deficiency is related to dietary factors should be counseled to include green vegetables and fruit in their diet.
- Prophylactic treatment of pregnant patients and patients with chronic hemolytic anemias can prevent folic acid deficiency due to the increased requirement for folate in these conditions.

CLINICAL NOTE

It is essential to exclude cobalamin deficiency before large doses of folic acid are given, and deficiency if present must be corrected, otherwise cobalamin neuropathy may develop, despite a response of the anemia of cobalamin deficiency to folate therapy.

CLINICAL PEARLS

1. The megaloblastic anemias are a group of disorders characterized by the presence of distinctive morphologic appearances of the developing red cells in the bone marrow.
2. The cause is usually deficiency of either cobalamin (vitamin B_{12}) or folate, but megaloblastic anemia may arise because of genetic or acquired abnormalities affecting the metabolism of these vitamins or because of defects in DNA synthesis not related to cobalamin or folate.
3. The common feature of all megaloblastic anemias is a defect in DNA synthesis that affects rapidly dividing cells in the bone marrow.
4. Folate deficiency can result from several possible causes, including inadequate ingestion, impaired absorption, impaired metabolism leading to inability to utilize folate that is absorbed, increased requirement, increased excretion, and increased destruction.
5. Oral doses of 5 to 15 mg folic acid daily are satisfactory to treat the deficiency.

CASE STUDY 6

Theme: Chemistry, Metabolism, Coenzyme role, and Clinical Implications of Deficiency of Vitamin B_{12}

A 45-year-old female presented to her primary care doctor with fatigue and tingling/numbness in her extremities (bilateral). The symptoms had been gradually getting worst over the past one year. Upon further questioning, she reported frequent episodes of diarrhea and weight loss. She was a total vegetarian and was also on a fad diet from the previous 2 months.

Examination revealed that she was moderately built but anemic, there was no icterus, and pulse and blood pressure were normal. Her tongue was beefy red, fissured and a neurologic examination revealed numbness in all extremities with decreased vibration senses. A peripheral blood film demonstrated megaloblastic anemia.

What is the cause of megaloblastic anemia in this patient?

CASE DETAILS

Most probably the patient is suffering from megaloblastic anemia due to cobalamin deficiency. The cause for this anemia is strict vegetarian dietary pattern and lack of cobalamin supplementation. Cobalamin deficiency can occur from a lack of intake (such as with complete vegetarians), absence of intrinsic factor (either inherited or from removal/damage to gastric mucosa), intestinal organisms, or ileal abnormalities (tropical sprue). Patients present with anemic symptoms, such as fatigue, weakness, palpitations, vertigo, and tachycardia. GI symptoms include sore, beefy-red tongue, weight loss, and diarrhea. Both folate and cobalamin deficiencies have similar anemic and GI symptoms. However, cobalamin deficiency can also present with numerous neurologic manifestations including: numbness, paresthesias, weakness, ataxia, abnormal reflexes, and diminished vibratory sensation. Treatment consists of identifying/treating the underlying cause of deficiency and replacement of cobalamin or folate.

MEGALOBLASTIC ANEMIAS

The megaloblastic anemias are a group of disorders characterized by the presence of distinctive morphological appearances of the developing red cells in the bone marrow. The cause is usually deficiency of either cobalamin (vitamin B_{12}) or folate, but megaloblastic anemia may arise because of genetic or acquired abnormalities affecting the metabolism of these vitamins or because of defects in DNA synthesis not related to cobalamin or folate.

Cobalamin

Cobalamin (vitamin B_{12}) exists in a number of different chemical forms. All have a cobalt atom at the center of a corrin ring. In nature, the vitamin is mainly in the 2-deoxyadenosyl (ado) form, which is located in mitochondria. It is the cofactor for the enzyme methylmalonyl CoA mutase. The other major natural cobalamin is methylcobalamin, the form in human plasma and in cell cytoplasm. It is the cofactor for methionine synthase. There are also minor amounts of hydroxocobalamin to which methyl- and adenosyl cobalamin are rapidly converted by exposure to light.

Cobalamin is somewhat analogous to heme in its structure having as its base a tetrapyrrole ring. Instead of iron as a metal cofactor for heme, cobalamin has cobalt in a coordination state of six with a benzimidazole group nitrogen coordinated to one axial position, the four equatorial positions coordinated by the nitrogens of the four pyrrole groups and the sixth position occupied by either a deoxyadenosine group, a methyl group **(Fig. 11.15)** or a CN– group in the commercially available form in vitamin tablets. Dietary cobalamin is absorbed in the Co^{3+} oxidation state and must be reduced by intracellular reductases to the Co^{+} form for use.

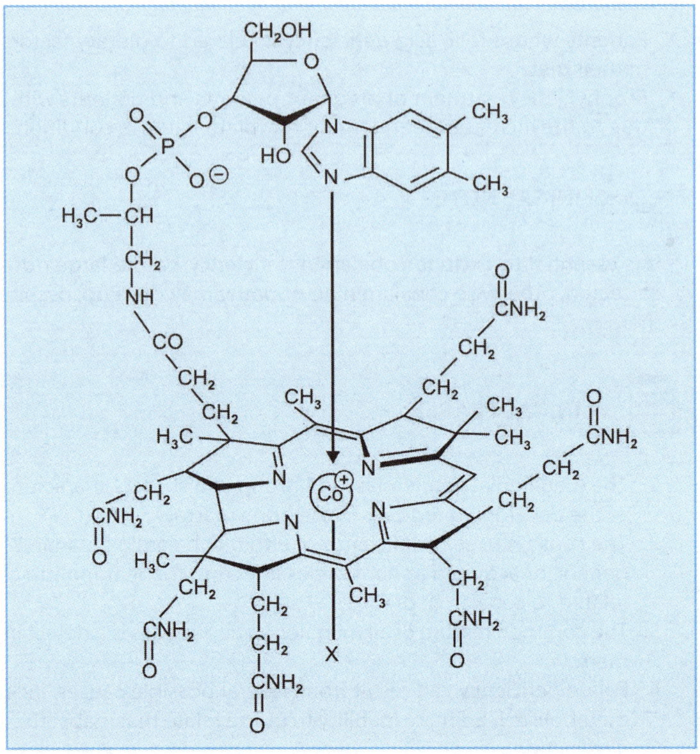

Fig. 11.15: Structure of cobalamin.

Dietary Sources and Requirements

Cobalamin is synthesized solely by microorganisms. Ruminants obtain cobalamin from the foregut, but the only source for humans is food of animal origin, e.g., meat, fish, and dairy products. Vegetables, fruits, and other foods of non-animal origin are free from cobalamin unless they are contaminated by bacteria. A normal Western diet contains between 5 µg and 30 µg of cobalamin daily. Adult daily losses (mainly in the urine and feces) are between 1 µg and 3 µg (~0.1% of body stores) and, as the body does not have the ability to degrade cobalamin, daily requirements are also about 1 to 3 µg. Body stores are of the order of 2 to 3 mg, sufficient for 3 to 4 years if supplies are completely cut off.

Absorption

Two mechanisms exist for cobalamin absorption. One is passive, occurring equally through buccal, duodenal, and ileal mucosa; it is rapid but extremely inefficient, <1% of an oral dose being absorbed by this process. The normal physiologic mechanism is active; it occurs through the ileum and is efficient for small (a few micrograms) oral doses of cobalamin and is mediated by gastric intrinsic factor (IF). Dietary cobalamin is released from protein complexes by enzymes in the stomach, duodenum, and jejunum; it combines rapidly with a salivary glycoprotein that belongs to the family of cobalamin-binding proteins known as haptocorrins (HCs). In the intestine, the haptocorrin is digested by pancreatic trypsin and the cobalamin transferred to IF.

Intrinsic factor (IF) is produced in the gastric parietal cells of the fundus and body of the stomach, and its secretion parallels that of hydrochloric acid. The IF-cobalamin complex passes to the ileum, where IF attaches to a specific receptor (cubulin) on the microvillus membrane of the enterocytes. Cubulin with its ligand IF-cobalamin complex is endocytosed. The cobalamin-IF complex enters the ileal cell where IF is destroyed. After a delay of about 6 hours, the cobalamin appears in portal blood attached to transcobalamine (TC) II. In the absence of the intrinsic factor, inadequate amounts of cobalamin are absorbed (the dietary requirement is approximately 200 ng/day) resulting in megaloblastic anemia. When the root cause of the resultant megaloblastic anemia is absence of or inadequate amounts of intrinsic factor, the condition is called pernicious anemia.

Between 0.5 µg and 5.0 µg of cobalamin enters the bile each day. This binds to IF, and a major portion of billiary cobalamin is normally reabsorbed together with cobalamin derived from sloughed intestinal cells. Because of the appreciable amount of cobalamin undergoing enterohepatic circulation, cobalamin deficiency develops more rapidly in individuals who malabsorb cobalamin than it does in vegans, in whom reabsorption of billiary cobalamin is intact.

Transportation and Storage of Cobalamin

Three plasma transport proteins have been identified. Transcobalamine I and III (differing only in carbohydrate structure) are secreted by white blood cells. Although approximately 90% of plasma vitamin B_{12} circulates bind to these proteins, only transcobalamine II is capable of transporting vitamin B_{12} into cells. The liver contains 2000 to 5000 µg of stored vitamin B_{12}. Since daily losses are

3 to 5 μg/day, the body usually has sufficient stores of vitamin B_{12} so that vitamin B_{12} deficiency develops more than 3 years after vitamin B_{12} absorption ceases.

Since vitamin B_{12} is present in all foods of animal origin, dietary vitamin B_{12} deficiency is extremely rare and is seen only in vegans—strict vegetarians who avoid all dairy products as well as meat and fish. Abdominal surgery may lead to vitamin B_{12} deficiency in several ways. Gastrectomy will eliminate that site of intrinsic factor production; blind loop syndrome will cause competition for vitamin B_{12} by bacterial overgrowth in the lumen of the intestine; and surgical resection of the ileum will eliminate the site of vitamin B_{12} absorption. Rare causes of vitamin B_{12} deficiency include fish tapeworm (Diphyllobothrium latum) infection, in which the parasite uses luminal vitamin B_{12}, pancreatic insufficiency (with failure to inactivate competing cobalamin-binding proteins), and severe Crohn's disease, causing sufficient destruction of the ileum to impair vitamin B_{12} absorption.

Metabolic Role of Cobalamin

1. Cobalamin plays a vital role in the catabolism of odd-chain fatty acids, threonine, methionine, and the branched-chain amino acids (leucine, isoleucine, and valine). The degradation of each of these compounds produces the same metabolite, propionyl-CoA.

Fate of Propionyl CoA

This activated three-carbon fatty acid enters the energy generating metabolic pathway at the level of the citric acid cycle as succinyl-CoA. The process requires three specialized enzymes. Propionyl-CoA carboxylase adds another carbon to propionyl-CoA to form D-methylmalonyl-CoA in a reaction which requires ATP and the CO2-binding cofactor biotin. A racemase converts the D-isomer of methylmalonyl-CoA to the L isomer. The last step is catalyzed by methylmalonyl-CoA mutase, a deoxyadenosylcobalamine requiring enzyme that moves the acyl-CoA group from the methylene carbon to the methyl carbon to form succinyl-CoA **(Fig. 11.16)**. In cases of cobalamin deficiency, this reaction is compromised and leads to an accumulation of methylmalonyl-CoA in serum, which has been suggested as a possible source of neurologic defects seen in cobalamin deficiency by decreasing lipid synthesis.

On the other hand, impaired biosynthesis of phosphatidylcholine due to decreased levels of methionine and S-adenosylmethionine (SAM) may play a role for the neurologic symptoms of cobalamin deficiency by compromising the repair of demyelination.

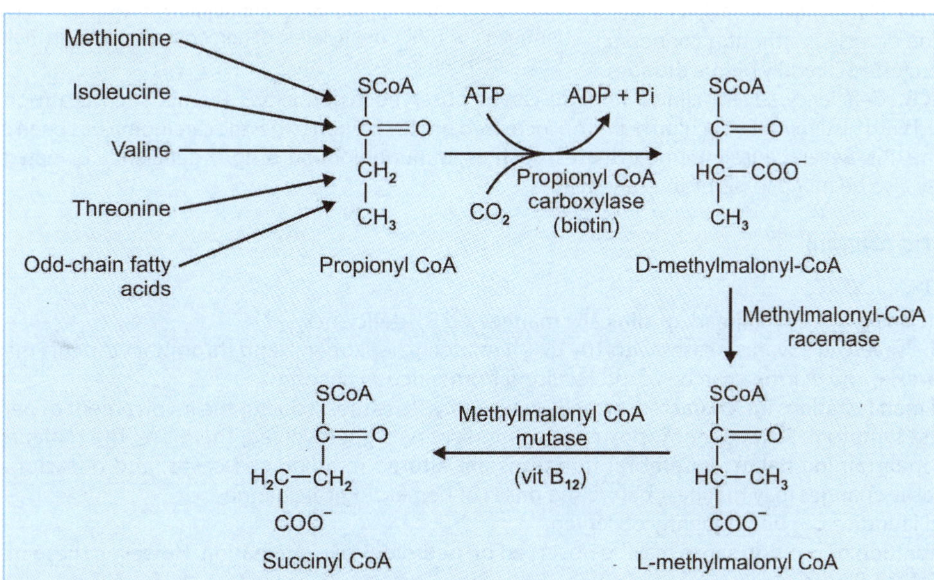

Fig. 11.16: Formation and fate of propionyl CoA.

2. **Role of cobalamin in DNA synthesis and the biochemical basis of megaloblastic anemia:** The cause of megaloblastic anemia seen in strict vegetarians is attributed to the effects of cobalamin deficiency on DNA synthesis, specifically the thymidylate synthetase reaction which converts dUMP → dTMP.
   Inadequate dTMP restricts DNA but not RNA synthesis leading to the appearance of large erythroid cells with small nuclei containing a high ratio of RNA to DNA. These cells are removed from the circulation, thus stimulating erythrogenesis and giving rise to anemia with an elevated presence of megaloblasts.
3. **Role of cobalamin in methionine metabolism:** Cobalamin is required for the conversion of homocysteine into methionine. Cobalamin must first undergo methyl transfer to form methyl cobalamin. It receives the methyl group from N5-methyltetrahydrofolate thus regenerating tetrahydrofolate to participate in other one-carbon transfers in purine metabolism

or pyrimidine remodeling. If there is a cobalamin deficiency, then the methionine synthase reaction cannot occur, N5-methyltetrahydrofolate accumulates, and the other C-1 donor forms of tetrahydrofolate cannot be formed. If N5, N10-methylenetetrahydrofolate, which is required for the methylation of dUMP to dTMP, cannot be formed, the thymidylate synthase reaction will be slowed and dTMP levels will drop **(Fig. 11.17).**

An added complication is that the thymidylate synthase reaction produces dihydrofolate unlike all the other C-1 pool reactions, which produce tetrahydrofolate. The dihydroform must be reduced to the tetrahydroform by dihydrofolate reductase, which can be inhibited by many drugs. Thus, in the absence of cobalamin methionine synthesis from homocysteine ceases allowing the "trapping" of the folate pool as N5-methyltetrahydrofolate, diminishing levels of N5, N10-methylenetetrahydrofolate, and impairing dTMP formation, and, therefore, DNA synthesis. Cells requiring regeneration due to turnover feel the brunt of this situation early and thus megaloblastic anemia is a result.

Causes of Vitamin B_{12} Deficiency

- Dietary deficiency (rare)
- Decreased production of intrinsic factor
- Pernicious anemia
- Gastrectomy
- Pancreatic insufficiency
- Fish tapeworm (rare)
- *Helicobacter pylori* infection
- Decreased ileal absorption of vitamin B_{12}
- Crohn's disease
- Surgical resection
- Transcobalamine II deficiency (rare)
- Competition for vitamin B_{12} in gut Blind loop syndrome.

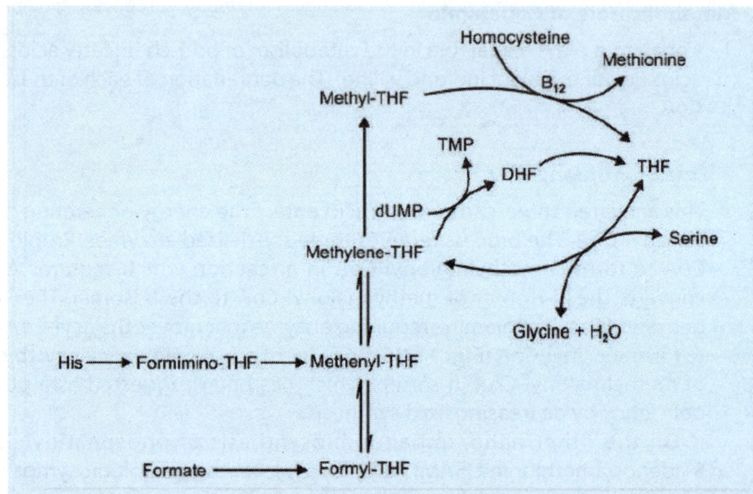

Fig. 11.17: Overlapping role of cobalamin and folic acid in DNA synthesis (through formation of TMP), methylation of homocysteine to form methionine, and the folate trap if cobalamin is deficient.

B_{12} deficiency

"Pernicious anemia" is the most common cause of B_{12} deficiency. The disease is although congenital, yet it is rarely manifested clinically before the age of 35 years. Besides B_{12} deficiency, several clinical findings can be observed in pernicious anemia, such as atrophic gastritis, which is usually associated with histamine-fast achlorhydria. An increased predisposition to gastric carcinoma has been observed in patients with atrophic gastritis. Several autoimmune diseases, such as immunoglobulin A (IgA) deficiency or polyglandular endocrine insufficiency may also be found in pernicious anemia.

MEGALOBLASTIC ANEMIA

Clinical Findings

- Megaloblastic anemia is the hallmark of clinically manifested B_{12} deficiency.
- Anemia can be severe in advances cases with 10–15% hematocrit; leukopenia and thrombocytopenia may also be observed.
- Glossitis, anorexia, and diarrhea can be found resulting from mucosal changes.
- Neurological manifestations are characteristic of B_{12} deficiency. Paresthesia due to the involvement of peripheral nerves may be the earliest symptom. Subsequently, posterior columns nerves get involved; therefore, the patients may present with difficulty in maintaining balance. Cerebral functions are altered in advanced cases, and occasionally, dementia and neuropsychiatric changes may manifest before the onset of hematological changes.
- Pallor or mild jaundice can be frequently observed.
- Decreased vibration or position sense may be observed on neurological examination. However, these may be normal in the initial phase of the illness.

Laboratory Findings

Anemia of varying severity can be observed in the megaloblastic state, which occasionally can be extremely severe.

- **MCV**: The MCV is usually higher than usual, ranging between 110 fL and 140 fL; however, normal MCV can also be observed, which might be due to coexistent thalassemia or iron deficiency anemia, and in certain conditions, no cause can be ascribed. This observation implies that patients with neurological manifestations having clinical signs suggestive of vitamin B_{12} deficiency should be evaluated despite a normal MCV and the absence of anemia.
- **The peripheral blood smear** is typically abnormal, with anisocytosis and poikilocytosis. Macro-ovalocytes and hypersegmented neutrophils are characteristically found with several other abnormal shaped cells (see blood smear). The reticulocyte count is decreased. Since vitamin B_{12} deficiency affects all hematopoietic cell lines, therefore, in extremely severe cases, the white blood cell count and the platelet count are reduced, and pancytopenia may be present.

- **Bone marrow morphology** is strikingly abnormal. Marked erythroid hyperplasia occurs in response to ineffective erythropoiesis. Megaloblastic changes in the erythroid series include abnormally large cell size and non-parallel maturation of the nucleus and cytoplasm, i.e., cytoplasmic maturation continues while DNA synthesis is impaired causing delayed nuclear development. In the myeloid series, giant metamyelocytes are typically observed.
- **Other laboratory findings** include high serum lactate dehydrogenase (LDH) and a moderately increased indirect serum bilirubin. These two findings are indicative of intramedullary destruction of maturing abnormal erythroid cells and are similar to those observed in peripheral hemolytic anemias.
- **Serum cobalamine level:** The diagnosis of vitamin B_{12} deficiency is confirmed by observing an abnormally low serum vitamin B_{12} (cobalamin) level. The average vitamin B_{12} level is >240 pg/mL, whereas in the majority of the patients with overt vitamin B_{12} deficiency, serum levels can be <170 pg/mL, and in symptomatic patients the levels <100 pg/mL may be found. The levels of 170–240 pg/mL are borderline. In conditions when the serum levels of vitamin B_{12} are marginal, the diagnosis can be confirmed by finding an elevated level of serum methylmalonic acid (>1000 nmol/L). However, high levels of serum methylmalonic acid can also be observed in renal insufficiency.
- **The Schilling test** is nowadays rarely used.
- **Essentials of Diagnosis are** macrocytic anemia, macro-ovalocytes and hypersegmented neutrophils on peripheral blood smear, and serum vitamin B_{12} level less than 100 pg/mL.

Differential Diagnosis

Vitamin B_{12} deficiency should be differentiated from folic acid deficiency, in which red blood cell folate is low while vitamin B_{12} levels are normal. The differentiation between vitamin B_{12} deficiency and myelodysplasia (the other common cause of macrocytic anemia with abnormal morphology) is based on the characteristic morphology of the cells and the low vitamin B_{12} level.

Treatment

The indications for initiating cobalamin therapy are well-diagnosed megaloblastic anemia or other hematological abnormalities or neuropathies due to B_{12} deficiency.

Patients with pernicious anemia are treated with parenteral therapy. Intramuscular injections of 100 μg of vitamin B_{12} are sufficient for each dose. Supplementation is usually given daily for the first week, weekly for the first month, and then monthly for life. It is a lifelong disorder, and if patients discontinue their monthly therapy, vitamin deficiency can recur. Oral cobalamin may be used instead of parenteral therapy and can provide similar results. The dose is 1000 μg/d and must be continued indefinitely.

Patients respond to therapy with an immediate improvement in their symptoms. Hypokalemia may complicate the first several days of treatment, mainly if the anemia is severe. Quick reticulocytosis occurs in 5–7 days, and the hematologic picture normalizes in two months. Central nervous system symptoms and signs are reversible if they are of relatively short duration (less than six months) but become permanent if treatment is not initiated immediately.

CLINICAL NOTE

Both folate and cobalamin deficiencies have similar anemic and GI symptoms. However, cobalamin deficiency can also present with numerous neurologic manifestations including: numbness, paresthesias, weakness, ataxia, abnormal reflexes, and diminished vibratory sensation.

CLINICAL PEARLS

1. The megaloblastic anemias are a group of disorders characterized by the presence of distinctive morphological appearances of the developing red cells in the bone marrow.
2. The cause is usually deficiency of either cobalamin (vitamin B_{12}) or folate, but megaloblastic anemia may arise because of genetic or acquired abnormalities affecting the metabolism of these vitamins or because of defects in DNA synthesis not related to cobalamin or folate.
3. Patients present with anemic symptoms, such as fatigue, weakness, palpitations, vertigo, and tachycardia. GI symptoms include sore, beefy-red tongue, weight loss, and diarrhea.
4. Essentials of diagnosis are macrocytic anemia. Macro-ovalocytes and hyper segmented neutrophils on peripheral blood smear and serum vitamin B_{12} level less than 100 pg/mL.
5. Intramuscular injections of 100 μg of vitamin B_{12} are adequate for each dose. Oral cobalamin may be used instead of parenteral therapy and can provide equivalent results. The dose is 1000 μg/day and must be continued indefinitely.

CASE STUDY 7

Theme: Differential Diagnosis of Megaloblastic Anemia

A 55-year-old female reported to the general physician with complaints of weight loss of 10 lbs, general ill health, weakness, generalized body aches, numbness and paresthesias in legs, reduced appetite, and abdominal discomfort from the previous six months. Past history did not reveal any medical illness.

On general examination, patient was pale with moderate jaundice, tongue was beefy red and fissured, and nails were brittle. Mild tachycardia was there but blood pressure was normal. She was hospitalized with a general diagnosis of moderate anemia, jaundice, and neurological symptoms. The laboratory investigations report was as follows:

CBC

WBC:	4.5 × 109/L	Differential:	
RBC:	2.50 × 1012/L	Lymphocyte %	36.0
HGB:	10.0 g/dL	Monocytes %	3.8
		Neutrophils %	59.4
MCV:	124.0 fL	Eosinophils %	1.0
MCH:	40.5 pg/dL	Basophils %	0.0
MCHC:	32.7 g/dL		
PLT:	155 × 109/L		

Peripheral smear: Macrocytes, anisocytosis, poikilocytosis, ovalocytes, basophilic stippling, occasional Howell-Jolly bodies, and moderate number of hyper segmented neutrophils.

B_{12}:	<50 pg/mL	(Low)
Folate:	10.3 ng/mL	(Normal)
Total bilirubin	2.5 mg/dL	(High)
AST:	35 U/mL	(Normal)
ALT:	30 U/mL	(Normal)

Examination of a bone marrow aspirate revealed an erythroblastic hyperplasia with megaloblastic norm oblasts.

Schilling test: Part I, before intrinsic factor: 1% (Normal is >7.5%)
Part II, after intrinsic factor: 8%

Based on the information obtained so far, what is the most likely diagnosis?

CASE DETAILS

There is a vitamin B_{12} deficiency. The patient was admitted with signs of a moderate hemolytic anemia and neurological symptoms. Her CBC shows that she has a macrocytic anemia. Her leukocyte and platelet counts are the lower end of the normal range, indicating a developing pancytopenia. The blood smear revealed hypersegmented neutrophils, ovalocytes, and Howell-Jolly bodies. Her bilirubin values support a diagnosis of hemolysis. On a differential diagnosis, neurological symptoms typically accompany B_{12} deficiency rather than a folate deficiency. Based on her serum vitamin B_{12} and folate results, she can definitively be diagnosed as having a megaloblastic anemia due to a vitamin B_{12} deficiency. There is no liver disease. Since the liver enzymes are normal, liver disease is ruled out as a source of jaundice or the macrocytic anemia. A common cause of vitamin B_{12} deficiency in a patient with no previous gastrointestinal history is pernicious anemia. The Schilling test can determine if the deficiency is due to the absence of intrinsic factor, or some malabsorption disorder. The Schilling test result in Part I showed less than 7% of the initially radioactively tagged radioactive dose of oral vitamin B_{12} in the urine 24 hours later. When the test was repeated with intrinsic factor, a greater amount of radioactive B_{12} was found in the urine 24 hours later. The diagnosis of PA is supported by the finding of intrinsic factor blocking antibodies in her blood. So the likely diagnosis for this patient is pernicious anemia.

BASIC CONCEPT

Pernicious Anemia

Pernicious anemia is a chronic illness caused by impaired absorption of vitamin B_{12} because of a lack of intrinsic factor (IF) in gastric secretions. Pernicious anemia occurs as a relatively common adult form of anemia that is associated with gastric atrophy and a loss of IF production and as a rare congenital autosomal recessive form in which IF production is lacking without gastric atrophy.

The disease was named pernicious anemia because it was fatal before treatment became available, first as liver therapy and, subsequently, as purified vitamin B_{12}. The term pernicious is no longer appropriate, but it is retained for historical reasons.

Pathophysiology

Dietary Cobalamin (Cbl) is acquired mostly from meat and milk and is absorbed in a series of steps, which require proteolytic release from foodstuffs and binding to a gastric protein secreted by parietal cells that is known as IF. Subsequently, recognition of the IF-Cbl complex by specialized ileal receptors must occur for internalization of the complex.

Classic pernicious anemia is caused by the failure of gastric parietal cells to produce sufficient IF to permit the absorption of adequate quantities of dietary vitamin B_{12}.

Pernicious anemia probably is an autoimmune disorder with a genetic predisposition. Pernicious anemia is more common than is expected in families of patients with pernicious anemia, and the disease is associated with human leukocyte antigen (HLA) Types A2, A3, and B7 and Type A blood group.

Antiparietal cell antibodies occur in 90% of patients with pernicious anemia, but in only 5% of healthy adults. Similarly, binding and blocking antibodies to IF are found in most patients with pernicious anemia. A greater association than anticipated exists between pernicious anemia and other autoimmune diseases, which include thyroid disorders, Type I diabetes mellitus, ulcerative colitis, Addison disease, infertility, and acquired agammaglobulinemia.

Other disorders that interfere with the absorption and metabolism of vitamin B_{12} can also produce cobalamin (Cbl) deficiency, with the development of a macrocytic anemia and neurological complications.

Cbl deficiency may result from dietary insufficiency of vitamin B_{12}; disorders of the stomach, small bowel, and pancreas; certain infections; and abnormalities of transport, metabolism, and utilization. Deficiency may be observed in strict vegetarians. Breastfed infants of vegetarian mothers are also affected. Severely affected infants of vegetarian mothers who do not have overt Cbl deficiency have been reported to be deficient. Meat and milk are the main source of dietary Cbl. Because body stores of Cbl usually exceed 1000 μg and the daily requirement is about 1 μg, strict adherence to a vegetarian diet for more than 5 years usually is required to produce findings of Cbl deficiency.

In adults, pernicious anemia is associated with severe gastric atrophy and achlorhydria, which are irreversible. Coexistent iron deficiency is common because achlorhydria prevents solubilization of dietary ferric iron from foodstuffs. Patients with pernicious anemia have a 2- to 3-fold increased incidence of gastric carcinoma.

MORTALITY/MORBIDITY

The disease is called pernicious anemia because it was fatal prior to the discovery that it was a nutritional disorder. Presently, patients on appropriate treatment have a normal lifespan.

CLINICAL MANIFESTATIONS

- The onset of pernicious anemia is generally slow and indistinct. The diagnostic triad of **weakness, sore tongue, and paresthesia may be observed but frequently is not the main symptom complex.** Patients usually seek medical intervention because of the clinical symptoms suggestive of cardiac, renal, genitourinary, gastrointestinal, infectious, psychiatric, or neurological disorders. The patients are anemic with macrocytic cellular indices.
- **General observations:** Weight loss of about 10–15 pounds is observed in approximately 50% of patients, which is most probably due to underlying anorexia in this disease.
- **Anemia:** The anemia is less distressing; however, tachycardia and increased cardiac output may develop with hematocrit less than 20%. In patients with preexisting heart disease, congestive heart failure and coronary insufficiency may occur.
- **Gastrointestinal findings:** About 50% of patients present with a **tender, smooth, and beefy red** tongue; the smooth tongue is due to the loss of papillae. Some patients may present with constipation or increased frequency of passage of semisolid stools. These findings can be due to megaloblastic alterations of the intestinal mucosal cells.
- Some vague gastrointestinal symptoms are typical, such as anorexia, taste alterations, nausea, vomiting, belching, and gaseous distension. Infrequently, patients present with severe abdominal pain, owing to underlying spinal cord pathology.
- **Neurological symptoms:** Neurological symptoms can be observed in the majority of the patients. These symptoms include generalized weakness, paresthesia, clumsiness, and an unsteady gait. The neurological symptoms occur because of the degeneration of myelin sheath, loss of nerve fibers in the dorsal and lateral columns of the spinal cord and cerebral cortex.
- **Genitourinary system**: Spinal cord damage causes retention of urine and impaired micturition. The predisposition to urinary tract infections is increased in such patients.
- Mild jaundice and low-grade fever are although common, but being mild, they may be left undiagnosed.
- Tachycardia accompanied by flow murmurs is frequently observed. Dyspnea, tachypnea, and symptoms suggestive of congestive heart failure may be present with severe anemia.
- Hepatomegaly associated with congestive heart failure can be observed.
- Mild splenomegaly can be found in about 20% of patients.

Causes

- **Hereditary**: A higher incidence of pernicious anemia in families is suggestive of hereditary nature of the disease.
- **Autoimmune destruction:** Patients with pernicious anemia report with an increased predisposition to autoimmune disorders indicating an immunological aspect of the disease.
- Children who develop cobalamin deficiency usually have a genetic disorder, and the cause of their cobalamin deficiency is distinct from the etiology observed in classic pernicious anemia.
- **Congenital pernicious anemia** presents with an absence of intrinsic factor without gastric atrophy.

- **Gastric disorders** which may cause B_{12} deficiency are gastrectomy, gastric stapling, and bypass procedures for obesity and extensive infiltrative disease of the gastric mucosa. Generally, these disorders accompany a decreased ability to mobilize dietary Cbl rather than malabsorption of Cbl. Thus, patients with these disorders may have a normal Schilling test.
- **Pancreatic disorders** can produce Cbl deficiency.
- **Hyperacidity**: Cbl deficiency is reported in the **Zollinger-Ellison syndrome**. The underlying mechanism is probably due to the acidic pH of the distal small intestine which does not allow efficient binding of Cbl-IF complex with the ileal receptors.
- **Disorders of the ileum** due to the loss of the ileal receptors for the Cbl-IF complex may cause Cbl deficiency. Therefore, post-surgical loss of the ileum or inflammatory diseases of the intestine, such as gluten-enteropathy, ulcerative colitis, and ileal lymphoma interfere with B_{12} absorption.
- **Congenital deficiency of the ileal** IF receptors and hereditary Transcobalamin I (TC I) deficiency produce B_{12} deficiency and are usually diagnosed early in life.
- **Drug-induced:** Many drugs such as nitrous oxide, cholestyramine, *para*-amino-salicylic acid, neomycin, metformin, phenformin, and colchicine, may affect B_{12} uptake in the ileum but may not cause symptomatic vitamin B_{12} deficiency as they are not prescribed long enough to exhaust body stores of Cbl.
- **Abnormalities in the intestinal lumen** can produce Cbl deficiency. Patients with blind intestinal loops, stricture, and large diverticula may develop bacterial overgrowth, which utilize dietary Cbl for their metabolic needs.
- **Worm infestations:** Infestation with *Diphyllobothrium latum* causes Cbl deficiency. Tapeworm infestation occurs from eating poorly cooked and infected lake fish. Since the parasites have a high requirement for Cbl, that might be the cause of B_{12} deficiency in such patients.

Laboratory Studies

Peripheral blood: The peripheral blood usually shows a macrocytic anemia with a mild leukopenia and thrombocytopenia. The mean cell volume (MCV) and mean cell hemoglobin (MCH) are increased, with a mean corpuscular hemoglobin concentration (MCHC) within the reference range. The leukopenia and thrombocytopenia usually parallel the severity of the anemia.

The peripheral smear shows oval macrocytes, hypersegmented granulocytes, and anisopoikilocytosis. In severe anemia, red blood cell inclusions may include Howell-Jolly bodies, Cabot rings, and punctate basophilia. The macrocytosis can be obscured by the coexistence of iron deficiency, thalassemia minor or inflammatory disease.

Serum: The indirect bilirubin may be elevated because pernicious anemia is a hemolytic disorder associated with increased turnover of bilirubin. The serum lactic dehydrogenase usually is markedly increased. Increased values for other red blood cells, enzymes, and serum iron saturation are also observed. The serum potassium, cholesterol, and skeletal alkaline phosphatase often are decreased.

Gastric secretions: Total gastric secretions are decreased to about 10% of the reference range. Most patients with pernicious anemia are achlorhydric, even with histamine stimulation. IF is either absent or markedly decreased.

Serum Cbl levels: The serum Cbl is low in patients with pernicious anemia; however, it may be within the reference range in certain patients with other forms of Cbl deficiency.

Schilling test: The Schilling test measures Cbl absorption by increasing urine radioactivity after an oral dose of radioactive Cbl. The test is useful in demonstrating that the anemia is caused by an absence of IF and is not secondary to other causes of Cbl deficiency. Likewise, it is helpful because it is used to identify patients with classic pernicious anemia, even after they have been treated with vitamin B_{12}.

Histologic Findings

The bone marrow biopsy and aspirate usually are hypercellular and show trilineage differentiation. Erythroid precursors are large and often oval.

TREATMENT

Supplemental Vitamin B_{12}

Vitamin B_{12} 1000 to 2000 μg per oral can be given once/day to patients who do not have severe deficiency or neurologic symptoms or signs. Large oral doses can be absorbed by mass action, even when intrinsic factor is absent. For more severe deficiency, vitamin B_{12} 1 mg IM is usually given one to four times/week for several weeks until hematologic abnormalities are corrected; then it is given once/month.

Although hematologic abnormalities are usually corrected within 6 weeks (reticulocyte count should improve within 1 week), resolution of neurologic symptoms may take much longer. Neurologic symptoms that persist for months or years become irreversible. In most elderly people with vitamin B_{12} deficiency and dementia, cognition does not improve after treatment. Vitamin B_{12} treatment must be continued for life unless the pathophysiological mechanism for the deficiency is corrected.

Infants of vegan mothers should receive supplemental vitamin B_{12} from birth.

Complications

- If patients are not treated early in the disease, neurological complications can become permanent.
- Severe anemia can cause congestive heart failure or precipitate coronary insufficiency.
- The incidence of gastric adenocarcinoma is 2- to 3-fold greater in patients with pernicious anemia than in the general population of the same age.

Prognosis

Early recognition and treatment of pernicious anemia provides a normal, and usually uncomplicated, lifespan. Delayed treatment permits progression of the anemia and neurological complications. The mental and neurological damage can become irreversible without therapy.

CLINICAL NOTE

The macrocytosis in pernicious anemia can be obscured by the coexistence of iron deficiency, thalassemia minor, or inflammatory disease.

CLINICAL PEARLS

1. Pernicious anemia is a chronic illness caused by impaired absorption of vitamin B_{12} because of a lack of intrinsic factor (IF) in gastric secretions.
2. Pernicious anemia probably is an autoimmune disorder with a genetic predisposition.
3. The onset of pernicious anemia usually is insidious and vague. The classic triad of weakness, sore tongue, and paresthesias may be elicited but usually is not the chief symptom complex.
4. The peripheral blood usually shows a macrocytic anemia with a mild leukopenia and thrombocytopenia.
5. Vitamin B_{12} 1000 to 2000 µg per oral can be given once/day to patients who do not have severe deficiency or neurologic symptoms or signs. Large oral doses can be absorbed by mass action, even when intrinsic factor is absent. For more severe deficiency, vitamin B_{12} 1 mg IM is usually given one to four times/week for several weeks until hematologic abnormalities are corrected; then it is given once/month.

CASE STUDY 8

Theme: Chemistry, Metabolism, Coenzyme Role, Functions, and Clinical Significance of Vitamin C

A 4-year-old boy was brought for consultation for hematuria, edema of lower extremities, as well as swollen right leg. He was the 12th born in a poor family, where one previous child died from malnutrition and dehydration in the period of infancy. The child was fed only with cow's milk and biscuits. No vaccination and antirickets prophylaxis were applied. From the period of 5 months, the boy manifested irritability, sweating, poor appetite, and cried when somebody touched him.

At admission, the baby was afebrile, pale, and malnourished; his hair was dry and cracked. The anthropometric measures showed high and weight on the third percentile. Clinical evaluation showed no organomegaly, no neurological signs, gingival bleeding was there, and only one tooth was present.

Laboratory findings were as follows:

Red blood cell count 3.5 million/mm^3
Hemoglobin (Hb) 7 g/dL
Hematocrit (Hct) 30%
Serum iron low
Liver functional tests were in the normal range.
Ultrasound of kidney was normal.

Doppler of blood vessels of both legs was normal which excluded thrombophlebitis. Swelling of the right leg indicated radiological investigation. Massive subperiostal hematoma on the right femur, dilated metaphyses, general osteoporosis, epiphysiolysis, and dislocation of the epiphysis had been present on the radiogram.

What is the probable diagnosis?

CASE DETAILS

Considering the osteoskeletal manifestation, malnutrition, anemia, irritability, and the anamnesis of poor nutrition, as well as the radiological findings, deficiency of vitamin C is concluded.

Vitamin C—An Overview

Vitamin C (ascorbic acid) plays a role in collagen, carnitine, hormone, and amino acid formation. It is essential for wound healing and facilitates recovery from burns. Vitamin C is also an antioxidant, supports immune function, and facilitates the absorption of iron.

Humans, other primates, and guinea pigs are unable to synthesize L-ascorbic acid (vitamin C); therefore, they require it in their diet. The enzyme, L-gluconolactone oxidase, which usually would catalyze the conversion of L-gulono-gamma-lactone to L-ascorbic acid, is defective due to a mutation or inborn error in carbohydrate metabolism.

Coenzyme Role of Vitamin C

Vitamin C is the coenzyme for two groups of hydroxylases.
Ascorbic acid has specific roles in the copper-containing hydroxylases and the a-ketoglutarate-linked iron-containing hydroxylases.

Copper-Containing Hydroxylases

- **Dopamine β-hydroxylase:** It is a copper-containing enzyme involved in the synthesis of the catecholamines, norepinephrine, and epinephrine, from tyrosine in the adrenal medulla and central nervous system. During hydroxylation, the Cu^{+} is oxidized to Cu^{2+}; reduction back to Cu^{+} specifically requires ascorbate, which is oxidized to monodehydroascorbate.
- A number of peptide hormones have a carboxyl terminal amide that is derived from a terminal glycine residue. This glycine is hydroxylated on the *a*-carbon by a copper-containing enzyme, peptidylglycine hydroxylase, which, again, requires ascorbate for reduction of Cu^{2+}.
- ***a*-ketoglutarate-linked iron-containing hydroxylases:** A number of iron-containing, ascorbate-requiring hydroxylases share a common reaction mechanism, in which hydroxylation of the substrate is linked to decarboxylation of *a* ketoglutarate. Many of these enzymes are involved in the modification of precursor proteins.
  - Proline and lysine hydroxylases are required for the postsynthetic modification of procollagen to collagen. Vitamin C is necessary for the triple-helix formation of collagen. Deficiency of vitamin C leads to impaired collagen synthesis, causing capillary fragility, poor wound healing, and bony abnormalities in affected adults and children.
  - Proline hydroxylase is also required in the formation of osteocalcin and the C1q component of complement.
  - Aspartate β-hydroxylase is required for the postsynthetic modification of the precursor of protein C, the vitamin K-dependent protease that hydrolyzes activated factor V in the blood-clotting cascade.
  - Trimethyllysine and γ-butyrobetaine hydroxylases are required for the synthesis of carnitine.

Other Functions

- Vitamin C is required as a redox agent, reducing metal ions in many enzymes and removing free radicals. In this capacity, it protects DNA, protein, and vessel walls from damage caused by free radicals.
- Although the clinical manifestations are unclear, vitamin C is also a cofactor in the metabolism of cholesterol and in the synthesis of carnitine, peptide hormones, corticosteroids, and aldosterone.
- It also enhances the absorption of iron from the small intestine. This may contribute to the anemia seen with vitamin C deficiency.
- It is a component of many drug-metabolizing enzyme systems, particularly the mixed-function oxidase systems.

Absorption and Dietary Sources

Almost complete absorption of vitamin C occurs if <100 mg is administered in a single dose; however, only 50% or less is absorbed at doses >1 g. Enhanced degradation and fecal and urinary excretion of vitamin C occur at higher intake levels.

Good dietary sources of vitamin C include citrus fruits, green vegetables (especially broccoli), tomatoes, and potatoes. Consumption of five servings of fruits and vegetables a day provides vitamin C in excess of the RDA, 90 mg/day for males and 75 mg/day for females. Smoking, hemodialysis, pregnancy, and stress (e.g., infection, trauma) appear to increase vitamin C requirements.

VITAMIN C (ASCORBIC ACID) DEFICIENCY—SCURVY

Incidence

The incidence of scurvy peaks in children aged 6 to 12 months who are fed a diet deficient in citrus fruits or vegetables. Incidence also peaks in elderly populations, who sometimes have "tea-and-toast" diets deficient in vitamin C. The predictors of plasma vitamin C levels at or below the depleted range include being male, having a low dietary intake of vitamin C, not taking vitamin supplements, and smoking.

Pathophysiology

Formation of intercellular cement substances in connective tissues, bones, and dentin is defective, resulting in weakened capillaries with subsequent hemorrhage and defects in bone and related structures.

Bone tissue formation becomes impaired, which, in children, causes bone lesions and poor bone growth. Fibrous tissue forms between the diaphysis and the epiphysis, and costochondral junctions enlarge. Densely calcified fragments of cartilage are embedded in the fibrous tissue. Subperiostal hemorrhages, sometimes due to small fractures, may occur in children or adults.

CLINICAL MANIFESTATIONS

- Early symptoms are malaise and lethargy **(Fig. 11.18)**.
- After 1 to 3 months, patients develop shortness of breath and bone pain. Myalgias may occur because of reduced carnitine production.
- Other symptoms include skin changes with roughness, easy bruising, and petechiae, gum disease, loosening of teeth, poor wound healing, and emotional changes.

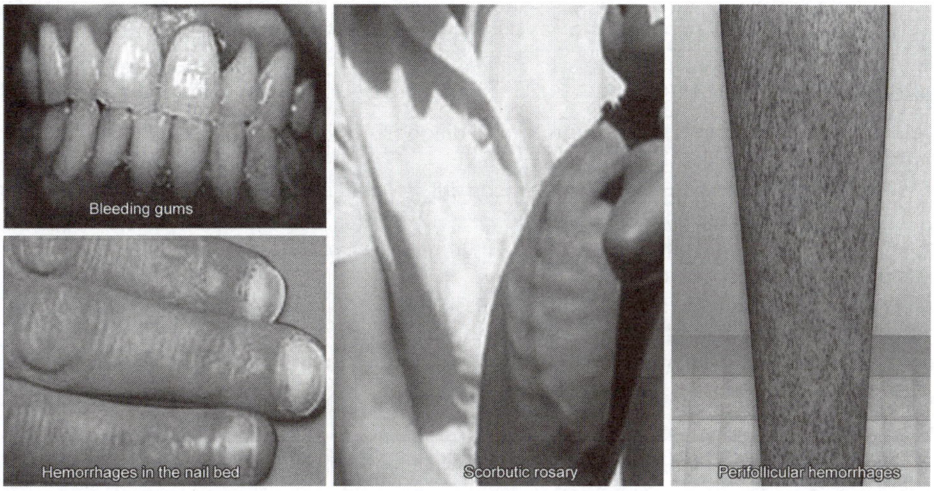

Fig. 11.18: Bleeding gums, hemorrhages, and scorbutic rosary: Clinical signs of vitamin C deficiency.

- Dry mouth and dry eyes similar to Sjögren syndrome may occur.
- In the late stages, jaundice, generalized edema, oliguria, neuropathy, fever, and convulsions can be seen.
- **Vital signs:** Hypotension may be observed late in the disease. This may be due to an inability of the resistance vessels to constrict in response to adrenergic stimuli.
- **Skin:** Perifollicular hyperkeratotic papules, perifollicular hemorrhages, purpura, and ecchymoses are seen most commonly on the legs and buttocks where hydrostatic pressure is the greatest. Poor wound healing and breakdown of old scars may be seen.
- **Nails:** Splinter hemorrhages may occur.
- **Head and neck:** Gum swelling, friability, bleeding, and infection with loose teeth; mucosal petechia; scleral icterus (late, probably secondary to hemolysis); and pale conjunctiva are seen. Conjunctival hemorrhage, flame-shaped hemorrhages, and cotton-wool spots may be seen. Bleeding into the periorbital area, eyelids, and retrobulbar space can also be seen. Alopecia may occur secondary to reduced disulfide bonding.
- **Chest and cardiovascular:** Scorbutic rosary (i.e., sternum sinks inward) may occur in children. High-output heart failure due to anemia can be observed. Bleeding into the myocardium and pericardial space has been reported.
- **Extremities:** Fractures, dislocations, and tenderness of bones are common in children. Bleeding into muscles and joints may be seen. Edema may occur late in the disease.
- **Gastrointestinal:** Loss of weight secondary to anorexia is common.

Causes

- Scurvy is caused by a dietary deficiency of vitamin C. The body's pool of vitamin C can be depleted in 1 to 3 months.
- Risk factors include the following:
  - Babies who are fed only cow's milk during the first year of life are at risk.
  - Alcoholism and conforming to food fads are risk factors.
  - Elderly individuals who eat a tea-and-toast diet are at risk. Retired people who live alone and those who eat primarily fast food face increased risk of deficiency.
  - Economically disadvantaged persons tend to not purchase foods high in vitamin C (e.g., green vegetables, citrus fruits), which results in them being at high risk.
  - More recently, vitamin C deficiency has been noted in refugees who are dependent on external suppliers for their food and have limited access to fresh fruits and vegetables.

- Cigarette smokers require increased intake of vitamin C because of lower vitamin C absorption and increased catabolism.
- Pregnant and lactating women and those with thyrotoxicosis require increased intake of vitamin C because of increased utilization.
- People with anorexia nervosa or anorexia from other diseases, such as AIDS or cancer are at increased risk of vitamin C deficiency.
- People with Type 1 diabetes have increased vitamin C requirements, as do those on hemodialysis and peritoneal dialysis.
- Because vitamin C is absorbed in the small intestine, people with disease of the small intestine, such as Crohn's, Whipple's, and celiac disease are at risk.
- Iron overload disorders may lead to renal vitamin C wasting.

Diagnosis

Diagnosis is usually made clinically in a patient who has skin or gingival signs and is at risk of vitamin C deficiency are normal.

Laboratory Investigations

- A plasma or leukocyte vitamin C level can confirm clinical diagnosis.
- Scurvy occurs at levels generally less than 0.1 mg/dL.
    - Symptoms occur at levels below 2.5 mg/L, which is considered deficiency.
    - Levels of 2.5 to 5 mg/L indicate depletion.
    - Levels can be low in patients who have tuberculosis, rheumatic fever, or other chronic illnesses; those who smoke cigarettes; and patients on oral contraceptive drugs.
- Capillary fragility can be checked by inflating a blood pressure cuff and looking for petechia on the forearm.
- Bleeding time, clotting time, and prothrombin time are normal.
- An Fe deficiency anemia is generally observed.

Imaging Studies

Skeletal X-rays can help diagnose childhood (but not adult) scurvy. Changes are most evident at the ends of long bones, particularly at the knee.

- Early changes resemble atrophy
- Loss of trabeculae results in a ground-glass appearance
- The cortex thins
- A line of calcified, irregular cartilage (white line of Fraenkel) may be visible at the metaphysis.
- A zone of rarefaction or a linear fracture proximal and parallel to the white line may be visible as only a triangular defect at the bone's lateral margin but is specific.
- The epiphysis may be compressed.
- Healing subperiosteal hemorrhages may elevate and calcify the periosteum.

Differential Diagnosis

In adults, scurvy must be differentiated from arthritis, hemorrhagic disorders, gingivitis, and protein-energy malnutrition. Hyperkeratotic hair follicles with surrounding hyperemia or hemorrhage are almost pathognomonic. Bleeding gums, conjunctival hemorrhages, most petechia, and ecchymoses are nonspecific.

Treatment

Patients should take ascorbic acid at 100 mg three to five times a day until total of 4 g is reached, and then they should decrease intake to 100 mg daily.

Alternately, ascorbic acid may be taken at 1 g/day for the first 3 to 5 days followed by 300 to 500 mg/day for a week. Then the recommended daily allowance is resumed.

- Divided doses are given because intestinal absorption is limited to 100 mg at one time.
- Parenteral doses are necessary in those with gastrointestinal malabsorption.

Diet

- Foods high in vitamin C include the following:
    - Citrus fruits, especially grapefruits and lemons
    - Vegetables, including broccoli, green peppers, tomatoes, potatoes, and cabbage.
- The recommended daily allowance for vitamin C varies. The current recommendation for adults is 120 mg daily, although a dose of 60 mg daily is all that is required to prevent scurvy. Some experts think the level should be as high as 200 mg daily to match the level present in five servings of fruits and vegetables daily, a diet shown to decrease cancer risk.

- Vitamin C supplementation has also been reported to be useful in Chédiak-Higashi syndrome and osteogenesis imperfecta. Diets high in vitamin C have been claimed to lower the incidence of certain cancers, particularly esophageal and gastric cancers. If proved, this effect may be due to the fact that vitamin C can prevent the conversion of nitrites and secondary amines to carcinogenic nitrosamines.

Toxicity

Taking >2 g of vitamin C in a single dose may result in abdominal pain, diarrhea, and nausea. Since vitamin C may be metabolized to oxalate, it is feared that chronic, high-dose vitamin C supplementation could result in an increased prevalence of kidney stones. Thus, it is reasonable to advise patients with a past history of kidney stones not to take large doses of vitamin C. There is also an unproven but possible risk that chronic high doses of vitamin C could promote iron overload in patients taking supplemental iron. High doses of vitamin C can induce hemolysis in patients with glucose-6-phosphate dehydrogenase deficiency, and doses >1 g/day can cause false-negative guaiac reactions as well as interfere with tests for urinary glucose.

CLINICAL NOTE

Vitamin C is required as a redox agent, reducing metal ions in many enzymes and removing free radicals.

CLINICAL PEARLS

1. Vitamin C deficiency can occur as part of general under nutrition, but severe deficiency (causing scurvy) is uncommon.
2. Symptoms include fatigue, depression, and connective tissue defects (e.g., gingivitis, petechiae, rash, internal bleeding, impaired wound healing). In infants and children, bone growth may be impaired.
3. Severe deficiency results in scurvy, a disorder characterized by hemorrhagic manifestations and abnormal osteoid and dentin formation.
4. Diagnosis is usually clinical.
5. Treatment consists of oral vitamin C.

CASE STUDY 9

Theme: Chemistry, Metabolism, Functions, and Clinical Significance of Vitamin A

A 2-year-old child presented with chronic cough and bronchitis, growth failure, and passage of light colored, foul smelling stools. Mother of the child reported that the child was finding it difficult to locate things in the dim light and during night time.

What could be the possible problem with this child?
What is the cause for these symptoms?
How this disease can be treated or prevented?

CASE DETAILS

The child is probably suffering from vitamin A deficiency.

The child has chronic cough, bronchitis, growth failure, and passage of light colored, foul smelling stools. All these symptoms are due to increased susceptibility to infections as a result of the keratinization of mucous membranes in the respiratory, GI, and urinary tracts. The thickened mucosa cracks easily and the risk for bacterial infections increases. During infection, the synthesis of retinol binding protein is reduced in response to infection since it is a negative "acute phase protein," that results in decreased circulatory concentration of the vitamin with further deterioration of the immune system. The diagnostic feature of vitamin A deficiency, i.e., night blindness, is also there in this child. So, it is clearly a case of vitamin A deficiency. The diagnosis can be confirmed by estimating serum retinol and retinol binding protein.

BASIC CONCEPT

Vitamin A

Vitamin A, in the strictest sense, refers to retinol **(Fig. 11.19)**. However, the oxidized metabolites, retinaldehyde and retinoic acid, are also biologically active compounds. The term retinoids includes all molecules (including synthetic molecules) that are chemically

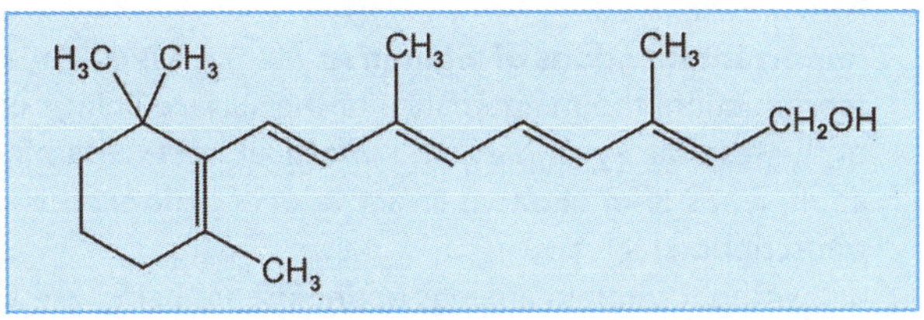

Fig. 11.19: Structure of vitamin A (retinol).

related to retinol. Retinaldehyde (11-cis) is the essential form of vitamin A that is required for normal vision, whereas retinoic acid is necessary for normal morphogenesis, growth, and cell differentiation. Retinoic acid does not function in vision and, in contrast to retinol, is not involved in reproduction. Vitamin A also plays a role in iron utilization, humoral immunity, T cell-mediated immunity, natural killer cell activity, and phagocytosis. Vitamin A is commercially available in esterified forms (e.g., acetate, palmitate) since it is more stable as an ester.

There are more than 600 carotenoids in nature, and approximately 50 of these can be metabolized to vitamin A. β-carotene is the most prevalent carotenoid in the food supply that has provitamin A activity. In humans, significant fractions of carotenoids are absorbed intact and are stored in liver and fat. The a-, β-, and γ-carotenes and cryptoxanthin are quantitatively the most important provitamin A carotenoids. Although it would appear that one molecule of β-carotene should yield two of retinol, this is not so in practice; 6 μg of β carotene is equivalent to 1 μg of preformed retinol. The total amount of vitamin A in foods is, therefore, expressed as micrograms of retinol equivalents.

Dietary Sources

Liver, fish, and eggs are excellent food sources for preformed vitamin A; vegetable sources of provitamin A carotenoids include dark green and deeply colored fruits and vegetables. Moderate cooking of vegetables enhances carotenoid release for uptake in the gut. Carotenoid absorption is also aided by some fat in a meal. Infants are particularly susceptible to vitamin A deficiency because neither breast nor cow's milk supplies enough vitamin A to prevent deficiency.

Metabolism

The liver contains approximately 90% of the vitamin A reserves and secretes vitamin A in the form of retinol, which is bound to retinol-binding protein. Once this has occurred, the retinol-binding protein complex interacts with a second protein, transthyretin. This trimolecular complex functions to prevent vitamin A from being filtered by the kidney glomerulus, to protect the body against the toxicity of retinol and to allow retinol to be taken up by specific cell-surface receptors that recognize retinol-binding protein. A certain amount of vitamin A enters peripheral cells even if it is not bound to retinol-binding protein. After retinol is internalized by the cell, it becomes bound to a series of cellular retinol-binding proteins, which function as sequestering and transporting agents as well as co-ligands for enzymatic reactions. Certain cells also contain retinoic acid-binding proteins, which have sequestering functions but also shuttle retinoic acid to the nucleus and enable its metabolism.

Retinoic acid has a role in the regulation of gene expression and tissue differentiation: Retinoic acid is a ligand for certain nuclear receptors that act as transcription factors. Two families of receptors (RAR and RXR receptors) are active in retinoid-mediated gene transcription. Retinoid receptors regulate transcription by binding as dimeric complexes to specific DNA sites, the retinoic acid response elements, in target genes. The receptors can either stimulate or repress gene expression in response to their ligands. RAR binds all-trans retinoic acid and 9-cis retinoic acid, whereas RXR binds only 9-cis retinoic acid.

The retinoid receptors play an important role in controlling cell proliferation and differentiation. Retinoic acid is useful in the treatment of cystic acne because it inhibits keratinization, decreases sebum secretion, and possibly alters the inflammatory reaction. RXRs dimerize with other nuclear receptors to function as coregulators of genes responsive to retinoids, thyroid hormone, and calcitriol.

Vitamin A has a function in vision: In the retina, retinaldehyde functions as the prosthetic group of the light-sensitive opsin proteins, forming rhodopsin (in rods) and iodopsin (in cones) **(Fig. 11.20)**. Any one cone cell contains only one type of opsin, and is sensitive to only one color. In the pigment epithelium of the retina, all-trans-retinol is isomerized to 11-cis-retinol and oxidized to 11-cis-retinaldehyde. This reacts with a lysine residue in opsin, forming the holoprotein rhodopsin. The absorption of light by rhodopsin causes isomerization of the retinaldehyde from 11-cis to all-trans, and a conformational change in opsin. This results in the release of retinaldehyde from the protein, and the initiation of a nerve impulse. The formation of the initial excited form of rhodopsin, bathorhodopsin, occurs within picoseconds of illumination. There is then a series of conformational changes leading to the formation of metarhodopsin II, which initiates a guanine nucleotide amplification cascade and then a nerve impulse. The final step is hydrolysis to release all-trans-retinaldehyde and opsin. The key to initiation of the visual cycle is the availability of 11-cis-retinaldehyde, and hence vitamin A. In deficiency, both the time taken to adapt to darkness and the ability to see in poor light are impaired.

Important functions of vitamin A: Vitamin A is essential for vision (especially dark adaptation), immune response, bone growth, reproduction, the maintenance of the surface linings of the eyes, epithelial cell growth and repair, and the epithelial integrity of the respiratory, urinary, and intestinal tracts. Vitamin A is also important for embryonic development and the regulation of adult genes. It functions as an activator of gene expression by retinoid alpha-receptor transcription factor and ligand-dependent transcription factor.

Synthetic vitamin analogs (retinoids) are being used increasingly in dermatology. The possible protective role of β-carotene, retinol, and retinoids against some epithelial cancers is under study. However, risk of certain cancers may be increased after β-carotene supplementation.

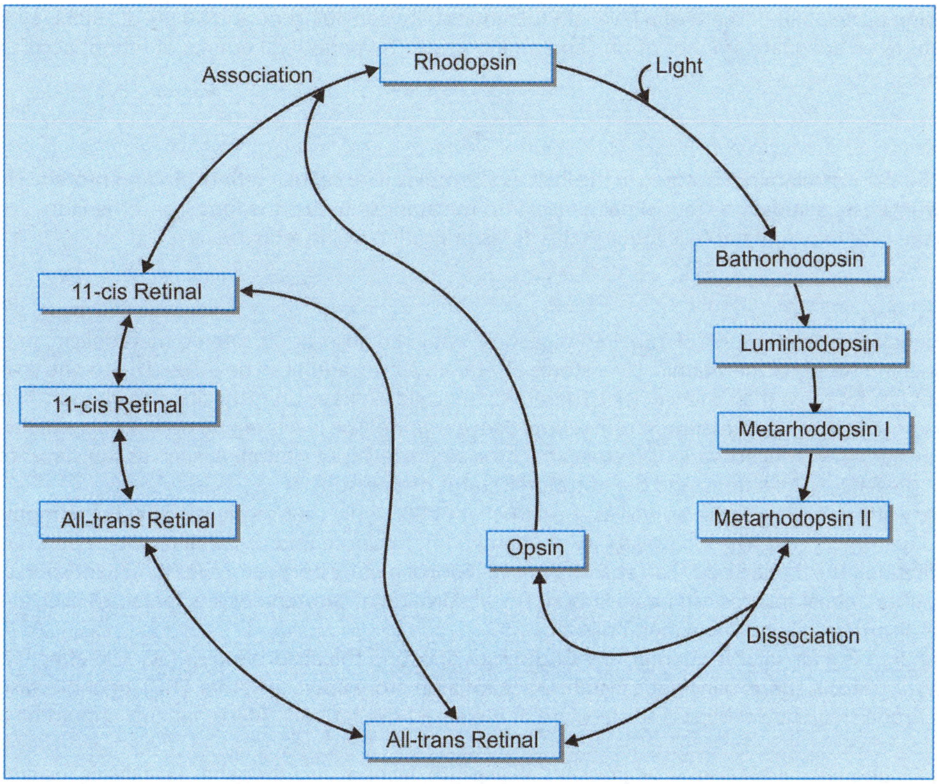

Fig. 11.20: Wald's visual cycle—Role of vitamin A in vision.

VITAMIN A DEFICIENCY

Vitamin A deficiency can result from inadequate intake, fat malabsorption, or liver disorders. Deficiency impairs immunity and hematopoiesis and causes skin rashes and typical ocular effects (e.g., xerophthalmia, night blindness). Diagnosis is based on typical ocular findings and low vitamin A levels. Treatment consists of vitamin A given orally or, if symptoms are severe or malabsorption is the cause, parenterally.

Etiology

Primary vitamin A deficiency is usually caused by prolonged dietary deprivation. It is endemic in areas, such as Southern and Eastern Asia, where rice, devoid of β-carotene, is the staple food. The risk is also increased in vegans, refugees, and persons with alcoholism, toddlers, and preschool children living below the poverty line. Xerophthalmia due to primary deficiency is a common cause of blindness among young children in developing countries.

Secondary vitamin A deficiency may be due to decreased bioavailability of provitamin A carotenoids or to interference with absorption, storage, or transport of vitamin A. Interference with absorption or storage is likely in sprue, cystic fibrosis, pancreatic insufficiency, duodenal bypass, chronic diarrhea, bile duct obstruction, giardiasis, and cirrhosis. Vitamin A deficiency is common in prolonged protein-energy malnutrition not only because the diet is deficient but also because vitamin A storage and transport is defective. In children with complicated measles, vitamin A can shorten the duration of the disorder and reduce the severity of symptoms and risk of death.

Pathophysiology

Digestion and Absorption

The protein-bound provitamin A is freed from their complexes in the stomach. As the retinol can be quickly and efficiently absorbed, therefore, the esters of vitamin A (retinyl esters) are hydrolyzed to retinol in the small intestine. The dietary carotenoids are first broken down into molecules of retinaldehyde, which are eventually reduced to retinol to be absorbed. The retinol is eventually esterified to retinyl esters in the intestinal mucosal cells.

Transportation

The transportation of the retinyl esters (of both retinoid and carotenoid origin) takes place as components of chylomicrons first in the lymphatics of the intestine, and then through blood to the liver. Vitamin A is transported in the blood bound to transthyretin and retinol binding protein (RBP). The serum level of RBP ranges between 40 μg/dL and 50 μg/dL. RBP is synthesized in the liver; the process requires an adequate amount of zinc and amino acids. The peripheral uptake of retinol occurs through a receptor-mediated process.

Storage

Approximately, 50–80% of vitamin A is stored in the liver as a complex with cellular retinol binding protein. The rest of the vitamin A is stored as retinyl esters (mostly as retinyl palmitate) into the adipose tissue, the lungs, and the kidneys. The mobilization of vitamin A from the liver to peripheral cells requires the de-esterification of the retinyl esters.

Vitamin A deficiency

Vitamin A deficiency occurs as a result of impaired digestion, impaired absorption, altered metabolism, or due to an imbalance between demand and supply of the vitamin. Liver stores of vitamin A in an adult can be utilized up to one year, whereas, in a child, the stores do not last for more than a few weeks. Therefore, the children have predisposition to vitamin A deficiency. The status of vitamin A can be assessed by estimating serum retinol concentration. The levels of RBP do not fall until the total body stores of vitamin A are considerably reduced. Various factors affect the serum levels of vitamin A, such as the status of the liver, the levels of zinc and iron, presence of infections, and the nutritional status of a person.

Zinc deficiency affects the synthesis as well as the turnover of RBP, which subsequently affects the mobilization of vitamin A from the liver to peripheral cells. The bioavailability of vitamin A from carotenoids is variable and depends upon the absorption and the yield of retinol. The human body can absorb only 40–60% of dietary beta carotene from plant sources. However, 80–90% of retinyl esters from animal sources can be absorbed. The absorption of carotenoids is affected by diet, availability of zinc and protein, and the disorders of lipoprotein metabolism.

Because vitamin A is a fat-soluble vitamin, any GI diseases affecting the absorption of fats also affect vitamin A absorption. Patients with cystic fibrosis, sprue, pancreatic insufficiency, inflammatory bowel disorder (IBD), or cholestasis, as well as persons who have undergone small-bowel bypass surgery, are at increased risk for VAD. These patients should be advised to consume vitamin A.

One factor affecting the metabolism of vitamin A is alcoholism. Alcohol dehydrogenase catalyzes the conversion of retinol to retinaldehyde, which is then oxidized to retinoic acid. The affinity of alcohol dehydrogenase to ethanol impedes the conversion of retinol to retinoic acid.

Increased requirements of vitamin A most commonly occur among sick children. The World Health Organization (WHO) and the United Nations International Children's Emergency Fund (UNICEF) have issued joint statements recommending that vitamin A be administered to all children, especially those younger than 2 years, who are diagnosed with measles. Coexistent VAD in young children increases the risk of death.

Pregnant women do not require increased vitamin A supplementation because of the possible risk of cranial neural crest defects and other malformations resulting from excessive use of vitamin A during pregnancy. The recommended daily allowance (RDA) of 800 μg for all adult females is also appropriate for pregnant women, because their stores of vitamin A meet the fetal accretion rate. The requirement for lactating women is 1300 μg in the first 6 months and 1200 μg in the second 6 months.

The RDAs of vitamin A for various age groups are as follows:

- Infants aged 1 year or younger—375 μg
- Children aged 1 to 3 years— 400 μg
- Children aged 4 to 6 years—500 μg
- Children aged 7 to 10 years—700 μg
- All males older than 10 years—1000 μg
- All females older than 10 years—800 μg

Frequency

An estimated 250 million children are at risk for vitamin deficiency syndromes. The most widely affected group includes up to 10 million malnourished children, who develop xerophthalmia and have an increased risk of complications and death from measles. Each year, 250,000 to 500,000 children become blind because of VAD.

CLINICAL MANIFESTATIONS

- **Bitot spots:** Areas of abnormal squamous cell proliferation and keratinization of the conjunctiva can be seen in young children with VAD.
- **Blindness due to retinal injury:** Vitamin A has a major role in phototransduction. VAD leads to a lack of visual pigments; this reduces the absorption of various wavelengths of light, resulting in blindness.
- **Poor adaptation to darkness (nyctalopia),** which can lead to night blindness, is an early symptom.
- **Xerophthalmia** results from keratinization of the conjunctiva **(Fig. 11.21)**.
- **Keratomalacia:** In advanced deficiency; the cornea becomes hazy and can develop erosions, which can lead to its destruction (keratomalacia).

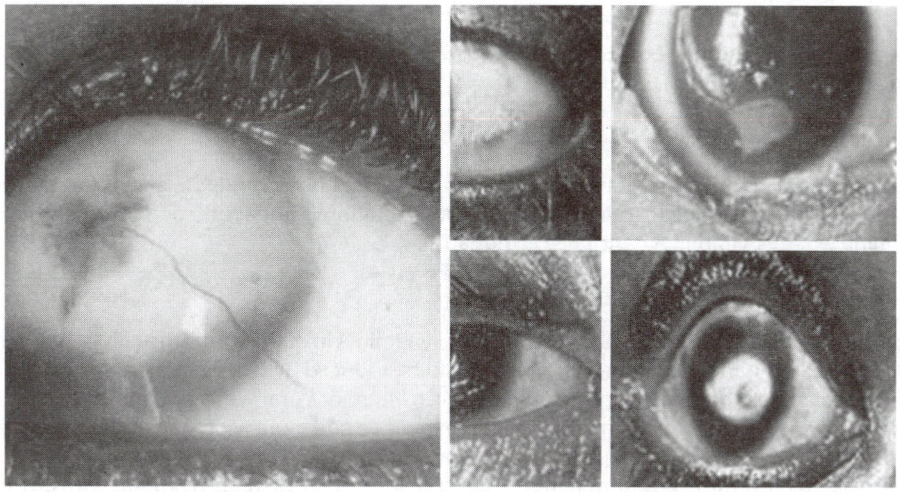

Fig. 11.21: Ophthalmological changes in vitamin A deficiency.

- Dry skin
- Dry hair
- Pruritus
- Broken fingernails
- Follicular hyperkeratosis (phrynoderma) secondary to blockage of hair follicles with plugs of keratin
- Excessive deposition of periosteal bone secondary to reduced osteoclastic activity
- Anemia
- Keratinization of mucous membranes in the respiratory, GI, and urinary tracts
- Drying, scaling, and follicular thickening of the skin and respiratory infections can result impairment of the humoral and cell-mediated immune system.
- **Increased susceptibility to infections:** Vitamin A also has an important role in differentiation of immune system cells, and even mild deficiency leads to increased susceptibility to infectious diseases. During infection, the synthesis of retinol binding protein is reduced in response to infection since it is a negative "acute phase protein," that results in decreased circulatory concentration of the vitamin with further deterioration of the immune system. Keratinization of the mucous membranes of respiratory tracts and urinary tract takes place, further increasing the susceptibility to infections.
- The younger the patient, the more severe are the effects of vitamin A deficiency.
- Growth retardation and infections are common among children.
- Mortality rate can exceed 50% in children with severe vitamin A deficiency.

Subclinical forms of VAD may not cause any symptoms, but the risk of developing respiratory and diarrheal infections is increased, the growth rate is decreased, and bone development is slowed. Patients may have a recent history of increased infections, infertility secondary to impaired spermatogenesis, or recent spontaneous abortion secondary to impaired embryonic development. The patient may also report increased fatigue, as a manifestation of VAD anemia.

LABORATORY INVESTIGATIONS

- **A serum retinol level:** Direct measure using high-performance liquid chromatography. Normal range is 28 to 86 µg/dL (1 to 3 µmol/L). However, levels decrease only after the deficiency is advanced because the liver contains large stores of vitamin A. Also, decreased levels may result from acute infection, which causes retinol-binding protein and transthyretin (also called prealbumin) levels to decrease transiently. A therapeutic trial of vitamin A may help confirm the diagnosis.
- A serum RBP study is easier to perform and less expensive than a serum retinol study, because RBP is a protein and can be detected by an immunologic assay. RBP is also a more stable compound than retinol with respect to light and temperature. However, RBP levels are less accurate, because they are affected by serum protein concentrations and because types of RBP cannot be differentiated.
- A zinc level is useful because zinc deficiency interferes with RBP production.
- An iron panel is useful because iron deficiency can affect the metabolism of vitamin A.
- Albumin levels are indirect measures of vitamin A levels.
- Obtain a complete blood count (CBC) with differential if anemia, infection, or sepsis is a possibility.
- An electrolyte evaluation and liver function studies should be performed to evaluate for nutritional and volume status.

Imaging Studies

In children, radiographic films of the long bones may be useful when an evaluation is being made for bone growth and for excessive deposition of periosteal bone.

Other Tests

Ocular findings suggest the diagnosis. Dark adaptation can be impaired in other disorders (e.g., zinc deficiency, retinitis pigmentosa, severe refractive errors, cataracts, diabetic retinopathy). If dark adaptation is impaired, rod scotometry and electroretinography are done to determine whether vitamin A deficiency is the cause.

TREATMENT

- Any stage of xerophthalmia should be treated with 60 mg of vitamin A in oily solution, usually contained in a soft-gel capsule. The same dose is repeated 1 and 14 days later. Doses should be reduced by half for patients 6 to 11 months of age.
- Mothers with night blindness or Bitot's spots should be given vitamin A orally, either 3 mg daily or 7.5 mg twice a week for 3 months. These regimens are efficacious, and they are less expensive and more widely available than injectable water-miscible vitamin A.
- A common approach to prevention is to supplement young children living in high-risk areas with 60 mg every 4 to 6 months, with a half-dose given to infants 6 to 11 months of age.
- One high-risk group, extremely low-birth-weight infants (<1000 g), is likely to be vitamin A-deficient and should be supplemented with 1500 μg (or RAE) of vitamin A, three times a week for 4 weeks. Severe measles in any society can lead to secondary vitamin A deficiency.
- Children hospitalized with measles should receive two 60 mg doses of vitamin A on two consecutive days.
- Vitamin A deficiency most often occurs in patients with malabsorptive diseases (e.g., celiac sprue, short-bowel syndrome), who have abnormal dark adaptation or symptoms of night blindness without other ocular changes.

Typically, such patients are treated for 1 month with 15 mg/day of a water-miscible preparation of vitamin A. This is followed by a lower maintenance dose with the exact amount determined by monitoring serum retinol.

- There are no specific deficiency signs or symptoms that result from carotenoid deficiency. It was postulated that β-carotene would be an effective chemopreventive agent for cancer because numerous epidemiologic studies had shown that diets high in β-carotene were associated with lower incidences of cancers of the respiratory and digestive systems. However, intervention studies in smokers found that treatment with high doses of β-carotene actually resulted in more lung cancers than did treatment with placebo.
- Non-provitamin A carotenoids, such as lutein and zeaxanthin, have been suggested to protect against macular degeneration. The non-provitamin A carotenoid lycopene has been proposed to protect against prostate cancer. However, the effectiveness of these agents has not been proven by intervention studies, and the mechanisms underlying these purported biologic actions are unknown.

Prevention

The diet should include dark green leafy vegetables, deep-or bright-colored fruits (e.g., papayas, oranges), carrots, and yellow vegetables (e.g., squash, pumpkin). Vitamin A–fortified milk and cereals, liver, egg yolks, and fish liver oils are helpful. Carotenoids are absorbed better when consumed with some dietary fat. If milk allergy is suspected in infants, they should be given adequate vitamin A in formula feedings. In developing countries, prophylactic supplements of vitamin A palmitate in oil 60,000 RAE (200,000 IU) po every 6 months are advised for all children between 1 and 5 years of age; infants <6 months can be given a one-time dose of 15,000 RAE (50,000 IU), and those aged 6 to 12 months can be given a one-time dose of 30,000 RAE (100,000 IU).

Vitamin A Toxicity

Vitamin A toxicity can be acute, which is usually an outcome of accidental ingestion of vitamin or chronic. Both the forms typically cause headache and exhibit signs of increased intracranial pressure. Acute toxicity often causes nausea and vomiting, whereas chronic toxicity is mostly characterized by dermatological changes, impairment of liver functions, and congenital disabilities (toxicity in pregnant women). The diagnosis is made clinically; except in infants with congenital disabilities, the dose adjustment ensures a complete recovery.

In children, acute vitamin A toxicity results from an accidental ingestion of > 300,000 IU or > 100,000 RAE. The acute toxicity has also been reported in adults, especially arctic explorers, who ingest polar or seal livers containing a very high content of vitamin A.

In older children and adults, chronic toxicity develops after a prolonged consumption of > 30,000 RAE (> 100,000 IU)/day. Birth defects have been reported in children of women on "isotretinoin" for the treatment of acne during pregnancy.

Excessive consumption of carotene does not cause vitamin A toxicity; however, it does cause carotenemia, which is usually asymptomatic, but may cause yellow discoloration of the skin (carotenodermia). Supplementation of β-carotene (not the dietary carotenoids) has been reported to increase the predisposition for cancer.

Clinical Manifestations

The symptoms are variable; the initial symptoms are headache and rash, which generally develop during acute or chronic toxicity. The signs of raised intracranial pressure are common in acute toxicity. Irritability, pain abdomen, nausea, vomiting, and drowsiness are commonly observed. Peeling of the skin is found in some patients.

The following symptoms characterize chronic toxicity:

Early signs and symptoms: Thickening of the hair, thinning of the eyebrows, rough and dry skin, cracked lips, and dry eyes.

Late signs and symptoms: Severe headache, generalized weakness, bone pains, easy fractures, cortical hyperostosis of bones, and pseudotumor cerebri. In children, anorexia, itching, pruritis, and failure to thrive are common; however, in extreme cases, hepatomegaly and splenomegaly may also be observed. In carotenodermia, deep yellow discoloration, especially on the palms and soles, is observed.

Diagnosis

- **Clinical evaluation**

  Diagnosis is clinical. Blood vitamin levels correlate poorly with toxicity. However, if clinical diagnosis is equivocal, laboratory testing may help. In vitamin A toxicity, fasting plasma retinol levels may increase from normal (28 to 86 µg/dL [1 to 3 µmol/L]) to > 100 µg/dL (> 3.49 µmol/L), sometimes to > 2000 µg/dL (> 69.8 µmol/L). Hypercalcemia is common.

  Differentiating vitamin A toxicity from other disorders may be difficult. Carotenodermia may also occur in severe hypothyroidism and anorexia nervosa, possibly because carotene is converted to vitamin A more slowly.

Prognosis

Complete recovery usually occurs if vitamin A ingestion stops. Symptoms and signs of chronic toxicity usually disappear within 1 to 4 weeks. However, birth defects in the fetus of a mother who has taken megadoses of vitamin A are not reversible.

Treatment

Vitamin A is stopped.

CLINICAL NOTE

In children with complicated measles, vitamin A can shorten the duration of the disorder and reduce the severity of symptoms and risk of death.

CLINICAL PEARLS

1. Vitamin A deficiency can result from inadequate intake, fat malabsorption, or liver disorders.
2. Deficiency impairs immunity and hematopoiesis and causes skin rashes and typical ocular effects (e.g., xerophthalmia, night blindness).
3. Diagnosis is based on typical ocular findings and low vitamin A levels.
4. Treatment consists of vitamin A given orally or, if symptoms are severe or malabsorption is the cause, parenterally.
5. Excessive intake can lead to toxicity since the vitamin is stored in the body. Symptoms of toxicity include anorexia, irritability, headache, peeling of skin, drowsiness, and vomiting. Bony exostosis and hepatomegaly are also seen.

CASE STUDY 10

Theme: Chemistry, Metabolism, Functions, and Clinical Significance of Vitamin D

A 3-year-old girl was brought for consultation. Significant past medical history included the following: She was an adopted child and was born to a mother who suffered from alcohol abuse. She was born prematurely (gestational age not available) with weight 2000 g and length 44 cm; furthermore, she had previously been diagnosed with encephalopathy and anemia; the adopted mother had her on vitamin supplements for 7 weeks. The mother stated that the child began walking at the age of 27 months.

She was seen by both orthopedics and pediatrics and her physical examination was as follows: She was well below the 5th percentile for both height and weight; there was delayed psychomotor and speech development, multiple rachitic deformities of the skeleton to include severe bowing of the tibias bilaterally (45 degrees), pigeon chest (pectus carinatum), and thickened/

widened wrists bilaterally and a Trendelenburg gait on the left side. Laboratory investigation report was as follows: Serum Ca: normal, PO_4^- low alkaline phosphatase: mildly increased and vitamin D low.

X-ray studies revealed—"cupping" of the distal radius and distal femur, widening of the epiphysis, and angular deformities.

What is the most probable diagnosis?

CASE DETAILS

The child is suffering from nutritional rickets. As the history reveals, the child was born prematurely and ever since birth she had been an ignored child. The mile stones were delayed. The nutritional deficiencies are grossly apparent from the low height and weight. The skeletal deformities are characteristic of rickets. The laboratory investigations and the X-ray findings also signify vitamin D deficiency.

Vitamin D deficiency leads to impaired intestinal absorption of calcium, resulting in decreased serum total and ionized calcium values. This hypocalcemia results in secondary hyperparathyroidism, a homeostatic response that initially maintains serum calcium levels at the expense of the skeleton. Due to the PTH-induced increase in bone turnover, alkaline phosphatase levels are often increased. In addition to increasing bone resorption, PTH decreases urinary calcium excretion, while promoting phosphaturia. This results in hypophosphatemia, which exacerbates the mineralization defect in the skeleton. In the long bones, laying down of uncalcified osteoid at the metaphases leads to spreading of those areas, producing knobby deformity, which is visualized on radiography as cupping and flaring of the metaphyses.

OVERVIEW OF VITAMIN D

Vitamin D is Really a Hormone

Vitamin D is not strictly a vitamin, since, it can be synthesized in the skin, and under most conditions, that is the major source of the vitamin. Only when sunlight exposure is inadequate is a dietary source required. Its main function is in the regulation of calcium absorption and homeostasis; most of its actions are mediated by way of nuclear receptors that regulate gene expression. Deficiency, leading to rickets in children and osteomalacia in adults, continues to be a problem in northern latitudes, where sunlight exposure is inadequate.

SYNTHESIS OF VITAMIN D

In response to ultraviolet radiation of the skin, a photochemical cleavage results in the formation of vitamin D from 7-dehydrocholesterol. Cutaneous production of vitamin D is decreased by melanin and high solar protection factor sunblocks, which effectively impair skin penetration of ultraviolet light. The increased use of sunblocks in North America and Western Europe and a reduction in the magnitude of solar exposure of the general population over the past several decades have led to an increased reliance on dietary sources of vitamin D. In the United States and Canada, these sources largely consist of fortified cereals and dairy products, in addition to fish oils and egg yolks. Vitamin D from plant sources is in the form of vitamin D_2, whereas that from animal sources is vitamin D_3. These two forms have equivalent biologic activity and are activated equally well by the vitamin D hydroxylases in humans. Vitamin D enters the circulation, whether absorbed from the intestine or synthesized cutaneously, bound to vitamin D-binding protein, an a-globulin synthesized in the liver. Vitamin D is subsequently 25-hydroxylated in the liver by cytochrome P450-like enzymes in the mitochondria and microsomes. The activity of this hydroxylase is not tightly regulated, and the resultant metabolite, 25-hydroxyvitamin D [25(OH)D], is the major circulating and storage form of vitamin D. Approximately 88% of 25(OH)D circulates bound to the vitamin D-binding protein, 0.03% is free, and the rest circulates bound to albumin. The half-life of 25(OH)D is approximately 2 to 3 weeks; however, it is dramatically shortened when vitamin D-binding protein levels are reduced, as can occur with increased urinary losses in the nephrotic syndrome.

The second hydroxylation, required for the formation of the mature hormone, occurs in the kidney. The 25-hydroxyvitamin D-1-hydroxylase is a tightly regulated cytochrome P450-like mixed function oxidase expressed in the proximal convoluted tubule cells of the kidney. PTH and hypophosphatemia are the major inducers of this microsomal enzyme, whereas calcium and the enzyme's product, 1, 25(OH)2D, repress it. The 25-hydroxyvitamin D-1-hydroxylase is also present in epidermal keratinocytes, but keratinocyte production of 1, 25(OH)2D is not thought to contribute to circulating levels of this hormone. In addition to being present in the trophoblastic layer of the placenta, the 1-hydroxylase is produced by macrophages associated with granulomata and lymphomas. In these latter pathologic states, the activity of the enzyme is induced by interferon and TNF-a but is not regulated by calcium or 1, 25(OH)2D; therefore, hypercalcemia, associated with elevated levels of 1,25 (OH)2D, may be observed.

The major pathway for inactivation of vitamin D metabolites is an additional hydroxylation step by the vitamin D 24-hydroxylase, an enzyme that is expressed in most tissues. 1, $25(OH)_2$ D is the major inducer of this enzyme; therefore, this hormone promotes its own inactivation, thereby limiting its biologic effects. Polar metabolites of 1,25(OH)2D are secreted into the bile and reabsorbed via the enterohepatic circulation. Impairment of this recirculation, seen with diseases of the terminal ileum, leads to accelerated losses of vitamin D metabolites.

Vitamin D Metabolism is Both Regulated by and Regulates Calcium Homeostasis

The main function of vitamin D is in the control of calcium homeostasis, and in turn, vitamin D metabolism is regulated by factors that respond to plasma concentrations of calcium and phosphate. Calcitriol acts to reduce its own synthesis by inducing the

24-hydroxylase and repressing the 1-hydroxylase in the kidney. The principal function of vitamin D is to maintain the plasma calcium concentration. Calcitriol achieves this in three ways: it increases intestinal absorption of calcium; it reduces excretion of calcium (by stimulating resorption in the distal renal tubules); and it mobilizes bone mineral. In addition, calcitriol is involved in insulin secretion, synthesis and secretion of parathyroid and thyroid hormones, inhibition of production of interleukin by activated T-lymphocytes and of immunoglobulin by activated B-lymphocytes, differentiation of monocyte precursor cells, and modulation of cell proliferation. In most of these actions, it acts like a steroid hormone, binding to nuclear receptors and enhancing gene expression, although it also has rapid effects on calcium transporters in the intestinal mucosa.

Vitamin D Deficiency Affects Children and Adults

In the vitamin D deficiency disease rickets, the bones of children are under mineralized as a result of poor absorption of calcium. Similar problems occur as a result of deficiency during the adolescent growth spurt. Osteomalacia in adults results from the demineralization of bone, especially in women who have little exposure to sunlight, often after several pregnancies. Although vitamin D is essential for prevention and treatment of osteomalacia in the elderly, there is little evidence that it is beneficial in treating osteoporosis.

Rickets

Rickets is a disease of growing bone that is unique to children and adolescents. It is caused by a failure of osteoid to calcify in a growing person. Failure of osteoid to calcify in adults is called osteomalacia. Vitamin D deficiency rickets occurs when the metabolites of vitamin D are deficient. Less commonly, a dietary deficiency of calcium or phosphorus may also produce rickets.

Pathophysiology

In the vitamin D deficiency state, hypocalcemia develops, which stimulates excess parathyroid hormone, which stimulates renal phosphorus loss, further reducing deposition of calcium in the bone. Excess parathyroid hormone also produces changes in the bone similar to those occurring in hyperparathyroidism. Early in the course of rickets, the calcium concentration in the serum decreases. After the parathyroid response, the calcium concentration usually returns to the reference range, though phosphorus levels remain low. Alkaline phosphatase, which is produced by overactive osteoblast cells, leaks to the extracellular fluids so that its concentration rises to anywhere from moderate elevation to very high levels.

Intestinal malabsorption of fat and diseases of the liver or kidney may produce the clinical and secondary biochemical picture of nutritional rickets. Anticonvulsant drugs (e.g., phenobarbital, phenytoin) accelerate metabolism of calcitriol, which may lead to insufficiency and rickets, particularly in children who are kept indoors in institutions.

Calcium and vitamin D intakes are low in infants who are fed vegan diets, particularly lacto vegans, and monitoring of their vitamin D status is essential.

Frequency

Although the prevalence of vitamin D deficiency varies, the third National Health and Nutrition Examination Survey (NHANES III) revealed that vitamin D deficiency is prevalent throughout the United States. Vitamin D deficiency rickets does not occur in formula-fed infants because formula and milk sold in the United States contains 400 IU of vitamin D per liter. Except in pediatric patients with chronic malabsorption syndromes or end-stage renal disease, nearly all cases of rickets occur in breastfeed infants who have dark skin and receive no vitamin D supplementation.

Causes of Vitamin D Deficiency

The clinical syndrome of vitamin D deficiency can be a result of (a) deficient production of vitamin D in the skin, (b) lack of dietary intake, (c) accelerated losses of vitamin D, (d) impaired vitamin D activation, or (e) resistance to the biologic effects of 1,25(OH)2D.

The elderly people are particularly at risk for vitamin D deficiency, since both the efficiency of vitamin D synthesis in the skin and the absorption of vitamin D from the intestine decline with age.

Similarly, intestinal malabsorption of dietary fats leads to vitamin D deficiency. This is further exacerbated in the presence of terminal ileal disease, which results in impaired enterohepatic circulation of vitamin D metabolites. In addition to intestinal diseases, accelerated inactivation of vitamin D metabolites can be seen with drugs that induce hepatic cytochrome P450 mixed function oxidases, such as barbiturates, phenytoin, and rifampin. Impaired 25-hydroxylation, associated with severe liver disease or isoniazid, is an infrequent cause of vitamin D deficiency. Impaired 1-hydroxylation is prevalent in the population with profound renal dysfunction and a decrease in functional renal mass. Thus, therapeutic interventions should be considered in patients whose creatinine clearance is <0.5 mL/sec (30 mL/minute).

Mutations in the renal-1-hydroxylase are the basis for the genetic disorder, pseudo-vitamin D-deficiency rickets. This autosomal recessive disorder presents with the syndrome of vitamin D deficiency in the first year of life. Patients present with growth retardation, rickets, and hypocalcemic seizures. Serum 1, 25(OH)2D levels are low, despite normal 25(OH)D levels and elevated parathyroid hormone (PTH) levels. Treatment with vitamin D metabolites that do not require 1-hydroxylation results in disease remission, although lifelong therapy is required.

A second autosomal recessive disorder, hereditary vitamin D-resistant rickets, a consequence of vitamin D receptor mutations, is a greater therapeutic challenge. These patients present in a similar fashion during the first year of life, but alopecia often accompanies the disorder, demonstrating a functional role of the VDR (vitamin D receptor) in postnatal hair regeneration. Serum levels of 1,25(OH)2D are dramatically elevated in these individuals, both because of increased production due to stimulation of 1-hydroxylase activity as a consequence of secondary hyperparathyroidism and because of impaired inactivation, since induction of the 24-hydroxylase by 1,25(OH)2D requires an intact VDR. Since the receptor mutation results in hormone resistance, daily calcium and phosphorus infusions may be required to bypass the defect in intestinal mineral ion absorption.

Occasionally, deficiency severe enough to cause maternal osteomalacia results in rickets with metaphyseal lesions in neonates.

Summary of Causes of Impaired Vitamin D Action

- Vitamin D deficiency
  - Impaired cutaneous production
  - Dietary absence
  - Malabsorption
- Accelerated loss of vitamin D
  - Impaired enterohepatic circulation
- Impaired 25-hydroxylation
  - Liver disease
  - Isoniazid
- Impaired 1-hydroxylation
  - Hypoparathyroidism
  - Renal failure
  - Ketoconazole
  - 1-Hydroxylase mutation
- X-linked hypophosphatemic rickets
- Target organ resistance
  - Vitamin D receptor mutation
  - Phenytoin

CLINICAL MANIFESTATIONS

- Generalized muscular hypotonia of an unknown mechanism is observed in most patients with clinical signs of rickets.
- Craniotabes manifests early in infants with vitamin D deficiency, although this feature may be normal in infants, especially for those born prematurely.
- If rickets occurs at a later age, thickening of the skull develops. This produces frontal bossing and delays the closure of the anterior fontanelle. In the long bones, laying down of uncalcified osteoid at the metaphases leads to spreading of those areas, producing knobby deformity, which is visualized on radiography as cupping and flaring of the metaphyses.
- Weight-bearing produces deformities, such as bowlegs and knock-knees.
- In the chest, knobby deformities result in the rachitic rosary along the costochondral junctions. The weakened ribs pulled by muscles also produce flaring over the diaphragm, which is known as Harrison groove. The sternum may be pulled into a pigeon-breast deformity.
- In more severe instances in children older than 2 years, vertebral softening leads to kyphoscoliosis. The ends of the long bones demonstrate that same knobby thickening **(Fig. 11.22)**. At the ankle, palpation of the tibial malleolus gives the impression of a double epiphysis (Marfan sign). Because the softened long bones may bend, they may fracture one side of the cortex (i.e., greenstick fracture).

Regardless of the cause, the clinical manifestations of vitamin D deficiency are largely a consequence of impaired intestinal calcium absorption. Mild-to-moderate vitamin D deficiency is asymptomatic, whereas long-standing vitamin D deficiency results in hypocalcemia accompanied by secondary hyperparathyroidism, impaired mineralization of the skeleton (osteopenia on X-ray or decreased bone mineral density), and proximal myopathy. In the absence of an intercurrent illness, the hypocalcemia associated with long-standing vitamin D deficiency rarely presents with acute symptoms of hypocalcemia, such as numbness, tingling, or seizures. However, the concurrent development of hypomagnesemia, which impairs parathyroid function, or the administration of potent bisphosphonates, which impair bone resorption, can lead to acute symptomatic hypocalcemia in vitamin D-deficient individuals.

Laboratory Investigations

- Early on in the course of rickets, the calcium (ionized fraction) is low; however, it is often within the reference range at the time of diagnosis as parathyroid hormone levels increase.
- Calcitriol levels maybe normal or elevated because of increased parathyroid activity. Because levels of serum 25(OH)D reflect body stores of vitamin D and correlate with symptoms and signs of vitamin D deficiency better than levels of other vitamin

D metabolites, 25(OH)D (D2+D3) measurement is generally considered the best way to diagnose deficiency. Goal 25(OH)D levels are 30 to 40 ng/mL (about 75–100 nmol/L); whether levels above this may be beneficial remains uncertain.

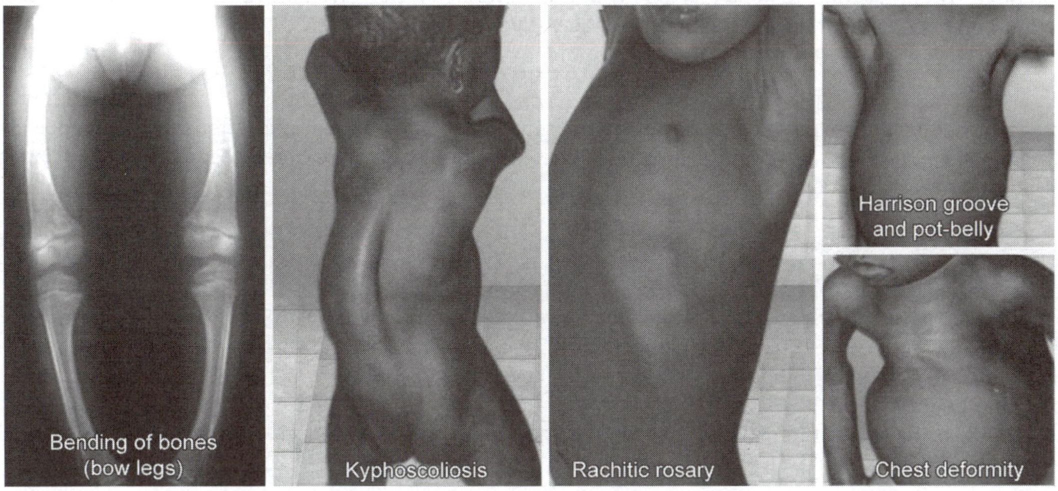

Fig. 11.22: Vitamin D deficiency manifestations.

- If the diagnosis is unclear, serum levels of 1,25(OH)2D and urinary Ca concentration can be measured. In severe deficiency, serum 1, 25(OH)2D is abnormally low, usually undetectable. Urinary Ca is low in all forms of the deficiency except those associated with acidosis.
- The phosphorus level is invariably low for age unless recent partial treatment or recent exposure to sunlight has occurred.
- Alkaline phosphatase levels are elevated.
- A generalized aminoaciduria occurs from the parathyroid activity; aminoaciduria does not occur in familial hypophosphatemia rickets (FHR).
- Parathyroid hormone (PTH) levels are also measured to confirm the diagnosis, because in vitamin D deficiency, PTH level is high.

Imaging Studies

Bone changes, seen on X-rays, precede clinical signs. In rickets, changes are most evident at the lower ends of the radius and ulna. The diaphyseal ends lose their sharp, clear outline; they are cup-shaped and show a spotty or fringy rarefaction. Later, because the ends of the radius and ulna have become noncalcified and radiolucent, the distance between them and the metacarpal bones appears increased. The bone matrix elsewhere also becomes more radiolucent. Characteristic deformities result from the bones bending at the cartilage–shaft junction because the shaft is weak. As healing begins, a thin white line of calcification appears at the epiphysis, becoming denser and thicker as calcification proceeds. Later, the bone matrix becomes calcified and opacified at the subperiosteal level.

Treatment

- Correction of Ca and P deficiencies
- Supplemental vitamin D.

  Ca deficiency (which is common) and P deficiency should be corrected. As long as Ca and P intake is adequate, adults with osteomalacia and children with uncomplicated rickets can be cured by giving vitamin D 40 µg (1600 IU) po once/day. Serum 25(OH)D and 1,25(OH)2D begin to increase within 1 or 2 days. Serum Ca and phosphate increase and serum alkaline phosphatase decreases within about 10 days. During the third week, enough Ca and P are deposited in bones to be visible on X-rays. After about 1 month, the dose can usually be reduced gradually to the usual maintenance level of 10 to 15 µg (400 to 600 IU) once/day. If tetany is present, vitamin D should be supplemented with IV Ca salts for up to 1 week. Because rickets and osteomalacia due to defective production of vitamin D metabolites are vitamin D-resistant, they do not respond to the doses usually effective for rickets due to inadequate intake. Endocrinologic evaluation is required because treatment depends on the specific defect. When 25(OH) D production is defective, vitamin D 50 µg (2000 IU) once/day increases serum levels and results in clinical improvement. Patients with kidney disorders often need 1, 25(OH)2D supplementation.

Vitamin D Toxicity

Usually, vitamin D toxicity results from taking excessive amounts. Marked hypercalcemia commonly causes symptoms. Diagnosis is typically based on elevated blood levels of 25(OH)D. Treatment consists of stopping vitamin D, restricting dietary Ca, restoring intravascular volume deficits, and, if toxicity is severe, giving corticosteroids or bisphosphonates.

Because synthesis of 1,25(OH)2D (the most active metabolite of vitamin D) is tightly regulated, vitamin D toxicity usually occurs only if excessive doses (prescription or megavitamin) are taken. Vitamin D 1000 μg (40,000 IU)/day produces toxicity within 1 to 4 months in infants. In adults, taking 1250 μg (50,000 IU)/day for several months can produce toxicity. Vitamin D toxicity can occur iatrogenically when hypoparathyroidism is treated too aggressively.

Symptoms

The main symptoms result from hypercalcemia. Anorexia, nausea, and vomiting can develop, often followed by polyuria, polydipsia, weakness, nervousness, pruritus, and eventually renal failure. Proteinuria, urinary casts, azotemia, and metastatic calcifications (particularly in the kidneys) can develop.

Diagnosis

- Hypercalcemia plus risk factors or elevated serum 25(OH)D levels

  A history of excessive vitamin D intake may be the only clue differentiating vitamin D toxicity from other causes of hypercalcemia. Elevated serum Ca levels of 12 to 16 mg/dL (3 to 4 mmol/L) are a constant finding when toxic symptoms occur. Serum 25(OH) D levels are usually elevated >150 ng/mL (>375 nmol/L). Levels of 1,25(OH)2D, which need not be measured to confirm the diagnosis, may be normal.

  Serum Ca should be measured often (weekly at first, then monthly) in all patients receiving large doses of vitamin D, particularly the potent 1,25(OH)2D.

Treatment

IV hydration plus corticosteroids or bisphosphonates.

After stopping vitamin D intake, hydration with IV normal saline and corticosteroids or bisphosphonates (which inhibit bone resorption) are used to reduce blood Ca levels.

Kidney damage or metastatic calcifications, if present, may be irreversible.

Prevention of Rickets

- Adequate ultraviolet light or 10 mcg (400 IU) PO daily of a vitamin D preparation and an adequate dietary supply of calcium and phosphorus prevent rickets.
- As little as 20 min/day of ultraviolet light to the face of a light-skinned baby is sufficient; however, significantly longer periods of exposure are necessary for children with increased skin pigmentation.

CLINICAL NOTE

Impaired 1-hydroxylation is prevalent in the population with profound renal dysfunction and a decrease in functional renal mass. Thus, therapeutic interventions should be considered in patients whose creatinine clearance is <0.5 mL/sec (30 mL/minute).

CLINICAL PEARLS

1. Vitamin D deficiency is a common cause of rickets and osteomalacia, but these disorders may also result from other conditions, such as various renal tubular disorders, familial hypophosphatemic (vitamin D-resistant) rickets, chronic metabolic acidosis, hypoparathyroidism (which reduces vitamin D absorption), inadequate dietary Ca, and disorders or drugs that impair the mineralization of bone matrix.
2. Vitamin D deficiency causes hypocalcemia, which stimulates production of PTH, causing hyperparathyroidism. Hyperparathyroidism increases absorption, bone mobilization, and renal conservation of Ca but increases excretion of phosphate. As a result, the serum level of Ca may be normal, but because of hypophosphatemia, bone mineralization is impaired.
3. In young infants, rickets causes softening of the entire skull (craniotabes). In older infants with rickets, sitting and crawling are delayed, as is fontanelle closure; there is bossing of the skull and costochondral thickening. Costochondral thickening can look like beadlike prominences along the lateral chest wall (rachitic rosary). In children 1 to 4 years, epiphyseal cartilage at the lower ends of the radius, ulna, tibia, and fibula enlarge; kyphoscoliosis develops, and walking is delayed. In older children and adolescents, walking is painful; in extreme cases, deformities, such as bowlegs and knock-knees develop.
4. Diagnosis may be suspected based on any of the following: A history of inadequate sunlight exposure or dietary intake, symptoms and signs of rickets, osteomalacia, or neonatal tetany and characteristic bone changes seen on X-ray.
5. Children with uncomplicated rickets can be cured by giving vitamin D 40 μg (1600 IU) po once/day. Vitamin D should always be repleted in conjunction with calcium supplementation since most, if not all, of the consequences of vitamin D deficiency are a result of impaired mineral ion homeostasis.

CASE STUDY 11

Theme: Chemistry, Metabolism, Functions, and Deficiency of Vitamin E

A 16-year-old female came with history of imbalance while walking, "weakness" in both lower limbs since 5 years, and slurring of speech since 3 years. There was no history of tingling or numbness in upper or lower limbs. She had difficulty in combing hair and buttoning clothes.

There was no history of exposure to heavy metals, or chronic ingestion of drugs.

She was born of second-degree consanguineous marriage but none of the family members had similar complaints.

Examination revealed averagely built and nourished female with normal vital signs. She had slurred speech and nystagmus. Cognition was normal. Fundoscopic evaluation was normal. There was no skin, hair, or skeletal system abnormality. Both the lower limbs had rigidity. Power was normal in both lower limbs as well as upper limbs but coordination was impaired. Finger nose finger and heel knee shin test were impaired indicating ataxia. Rhomberg's test revealed increased swaying on closing eyes. Her gait was ataxic. Vibration sense and joint position sense were impaired in the lower limbs. Bilateral knee and ankle reflexes were absent while other reflexes were normal.

Her investigations revealed the following:

Hemoglobin—98 g/L, white blood cell count—6.7 × 109/L (N: 60%, L: 38%, E: 02%, B: 00%, M: 00%).

Electrolytes, blood sugar, renal function test, and liver function tests were normal. MRI and CT brain were normal.

Thyroid function tests were normal. Serum vitamin E—11 µmol/L (N: 18–29 µmol/L). Serum lipid levels were normal:

Triglycerides 1.37 mmol/L, serum cholesterol 4.78 mmol/L, and LDL cholesterol 3.0 mmol/L.

Stool fat excretion was normal. There were no gastrointestinal abnormalities.

What is the most probable diagnosis?

CASE DETAILS

The patient is most probably suffering from vitamin E deficiency.

Vitamin E deficiency can result in ataxia with clinical presentation similar to Friedreich's ataxia—ataxia with isolated vitamin E deficiency. Vitamin E is one of the most important lipid-soluble antioxidant nutrients. Cystic fibrosis, chronic cholestatic liver disease, abetalipoproteinemia, short-bowel syndrome, isolated vitamin E deficiency syndrome, and other malabsorption syndromes all may cause varying degrees of vitamin E deficiency. Vitamin E replacement can influence outcome significantly; therefore, screening for vitamin E deficiency is beneficial for patients with ataxia of unknown cause.

BASIC CONCEPT

Vitamin E

Vitamin E is a collective name for all stereoisomers of tocopherols and tocotrienols **(Fig. 11.23)**. The most biologically active is α-tocopherol, but β-, γ-, and δ-tocopherols, four tocotrienols, and several stereoisomers may also have important biologic activity. Vitamin E acts as a chain-breaking antioxidant and is an efficient pyroxyl radical scavenger, which protects low-density lipoproteins (LDLs) and polyunsaturated fats in membranes from oxidation. A network of other antioxidants (e.g., vitamin C, glutathione) and enzymes maintains vitamin E in a reduced state.

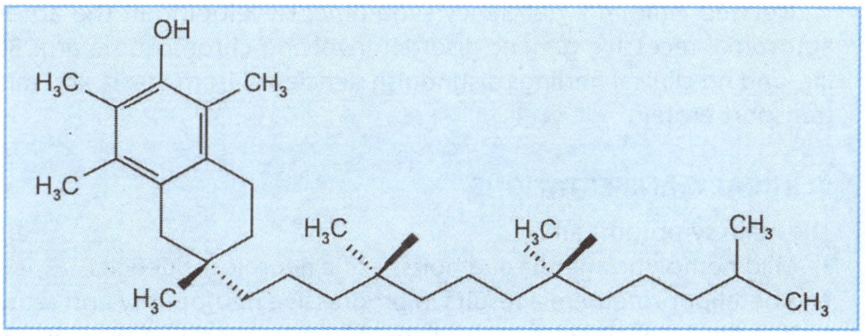

Fig. 11.23: Vitamin E (α-tocopherol).

Absorption and Metabolism

After absorption, vitamin E is taken up from chylomicrons by the liver, and a hepatic α-tocopherol transport protein mediates intracellular vitamin E transport and incorporation into very low-density lipoprotein (VLDL). The transport protein has particular affinity for the RRR isomeric form of α-tocopherol; thus, this natural isomer has the most biologic activity.

Requirement

Vitamin E is widely distributed in the food supply and is particularly high in sunflower oil, safflower oil, and wheat germ oil; γ tocotrienols are notably present in soybean and corn oils. Vitamin E is also found in meats, nuts, and cereal grains, and small amounts are present in fruits and vegetables. The RDA for vitamin E is 15 mg/day (34.9 µmol or 22.5 IU) for all adults. Diets high in polyunsaturated fats may necessitate a slightly higher requirement for vitamin E. Although the amount of vitamin E in many fortified foods and supplements is given in IU, current recommendations are to use mg.

Functions of Vitamin E

No unequivocal unique function for vitamin E has been defined.

- It acts as a lipid-soluble antioxidant in cell membranes, and is important in maintaining the fluidity of cell membranes.
- It also has a (relatively poorly defined) role in cell signaling.
- The main function of vitamin E is as a chain-breaking, free-radical trapping antioxidant in cell membranes and plasma lipoproteins by reacting with the lipid peroxide radicals formed by peroxidation of polyunsaturated fatty acids. The tocopheroxyl radical product is relatively unreactive, and ultimately forms nonradical compounds. Commonly, the tocopheroxyl radical is reduced back to tocopherol by reaction with vitamin C from plasma. The resultant monohydroascorbate radical then undergoes enzymic or nonenzymic reaction to yield ascorbate and dehydroascorbate, neither of which is a radical.
- The stability of the tocopheroxyl free radical means that it can penetrate further into cells and, potentially, propagate a chain reaction. Therefore, vitamin E may, like other antioxidants, also have pro-oxidant actions, especially at high concentrations. This may explain why, although studies have shown an association between high blood concentrations of vitamin E and lower incidence of atherosclerosis, but trials of high doses of vitamin E have been disappointing.
- Vitamin E also inhibits prostaglandin synthesis and the activities of protein kinase C and phospholipase A2.
- Vitamin E supplements do not protect against cardiovascular disorders; whether supplements can protect against Alzheimer's disease, tardive dyskinesia, and prostate cancer among smokers is controversial.

Vitamin E Deficiency

Dietary vitamin E deficiency is common in developing countries; deficiency among adults in developed countries is uncommon and usually due to fat malabsorption. The main symptoms are hemolytic anemia and neurologic deficits. Diagnosis is based on measuring the ratio of plasma α-tocopherol to total plasma lipids; a low ratio suggests vitamin E deficiency. Treatment consists of oral vitamin E, given in high doses if there are neurologic deficits or if deficiency results from malabsorption.

Vitamin E deficiency causes fragility of RBCs and degeneration of neurons, particularly peripheral axons and posterior column neurons.

Etiology

Absorption of vitamin E depends on normal pancreatic biliary function, biliary secretion, micelle formation, and penetration across intestinal membranes. Interference with any of these processes could result in a deficiency state.

In developing countries, the most common cause is inadequate intake of vitamin E. In developed countries, the most common causes are disorders that cause fat malabsorption, including abetalipoproteinemia (Bassen-Kornzweig syndrome, due to genetic absence of apolipoprotein B), chronic cholestatic hepatobiliary disease, pancreatitis, short bowel syndrome, and cystic fibrosis. Vitamin E deficiency is seen in only severe and prolonged malabsorptive diseases, such as celiac disease, or after small-intestinal resection. Children with cystic fibrosis or prolonged cholestasis may develop vitamin E deficiency characterized by areflexia and hemolytic anemia. Children with abetalipoproteinemia cannot absorb or transport vitamin E and become deficient quite rapidly.

Isolated vitamin E deficiency syndrome: Developing in the absence of fat malabsorption, this syndrome is caused by an autosomal-recessive genetic disorder involving chromosome arm 8q. Neurologic findings develop within the first decade of life, and no clinical findings distinguish deficiency from ataxia and movement disorders. It is due to a defect in the α-tocopherol transport protein.

CLINICAL MANIFESTATIONS

The main symptoms are:

- Mild hemolytic anemia and nonspecific neurologic deficits.
- Abetalipoproteinemia results in progressive neuropathy and retinopathy in the first two decades of life.
- Vitamin E deficiency may contribute to retinopathy of prematurity (also called retrolental fibroplasia) in premature infants and to some cases of intraventricular and subependymal hemorrhage in neonates.
- Affected premature neonates have muscle weakness.
- Vitamin E deficiency causes axonal degeneration of the large myelinated axons and results in posterior column and spinocerebellar symptoms. Peripheral neuropathy is initially characterized by areflexia, with progression to an ataxic gait, and by decreased vibration and position sensations.
- In adults with malabsorption, vitamin E deficiency very rarely causes spinocerebellar ataxia because adults have large vitamin E stores in adipose tissue.

Diagnosis

Low α-tocopherol level or low ratio of plasma α-tocopherol to plasma lipids without a history of inadequate intake or a predisposing condition, vitamin E deficiency is unlikely. Confirmation usually requires measuring the vitamin level. Measuring RBC hemolysis in response to peroxide can suggest the diagnosis, but is nonspecific. Hemolysis increases as vitamin E deficiency impairs RBC stability. Measuring the plasma α-tocopherol level is the most direct method of diagnosis. In adults, vitamin E deficiency is suggested if the α-tocopherol level is <5 μg/mL (<11.6 μmol/L). Because abnormal plasma lipid levels can affect vitamin E status, a low ratio of plasma α-tocopherol to plasma lipids (<0.8 mg/g total lipid) is the most accurate indicator in adults with hyperlipidemia. In children and adults with abetalipoproteinemia, plasma α-tocopherol levels are usually undetectable.

Prevention

Although premature neonates may require supplementation, human milk and commercial formulas have enough vitamin E for full-term neonates.

TREATMENT

Supplemental α-tocopherol

If malabsorption causes clinically evident deficiency, α-tocopherol 15 to 25 mg/kg po once/day should be given. However, larger doses given by injection are required to treat neuropathy during its early stages or to overcome the defect of absorption and transport in abetalipoproteinemia. Vitamin E in high doses may protect against oxygen-induced retrolental fibroplasia and bronchopulmonary dysplasia, as well as intraventricular hemorrhage of prematurity. Vitamin E has been suggested to increase sexual performance, to treat intermittent claudication, and to slow the aging process, but evidence for these properties is lacking. When given in combination with other antioxidants, vitamin E may help to prevent macular degeneration. High doses (60–800 mg/day) of vitamin E have been shown in controlled trials to improve parameters of immune function and to reduce colds, but intervention studies using vitamin E to prevent cardiovascular disease or cancer have not shown efficacy and, at doses > 400 mg/day, may even increase all-cause mortality.

Vitamin E Toxicity

Many adults take relatively large amounts of vitamin E (α-tocopherol 400 to 800 mg/day) for months to years without any apparent harm. Occasionally, muscle weakness, fatigue, nausea, and diarrhea occur. The most significant risk is bleeding. However, bleeding is uncommon unless the dose is >1000 mg/day or the patient takes oral coumarin or warfarin. Thus, the upper limit for adults aged ≥19 year is 1000 mg for any form of α-tocopherol. Recent analyzes of previous studies report that high vitamin E intakes may increase the risk of hemorrhagic stroke and premature death.

CLINICAL NOTE

In adults with malabsorption, vitamin E deficiency very rarely causes spinocerebellar ataxia because adults have large vitamin E stores in adipose tissue.

CLINICAL PEARLS

1. Absorption of vitamin E depends on normal pancreatic billiary function, billiary secretion, micelle formation, and penetration across intestinal membranes. Interference with any of these processes could result in a deficiency state.
2. The main symptoms are hemolytic anemia and neurologic deficits.
3. Diagnosis is based on measuring the ratio of plasma α-tocopherol to total plasma lipids; a low ratio suggests vitamin E deficiency.
4. Treatment consists of oral vitamin E, given in high doses if there are neurologic deficits or if deficiency results from malabsorption.
5. High dose >1000 mg/day of α-tocopherol can cause bleeding.

CASE STUDY 12

Theme: Chemistry, Metabolism, Functions, and Deficiency of Vitamin K

A term infant is born and does well with breastfeeding. Two days later, the mother calls frantically because baby is bleeding from the umbilical cord and nostrils.

What is the nature of the disease and how this can be treated?

BASIC CONCEPT

The child is suffering from vitamin K deficiency.

Hemorrhagic disease of newborn is caused by poor transfer of maternal vitamin K through placenta and by lack of intestinal bacteria in the infant for synthesis of vitamin K. The intestine is sterile at birth and becomes colonized over the first few weeks.

Vitamin K is required for the synthesis of blood clotting proteins. Vitamin K is the coenzyme for the carboxylation of the glutamate residues in the post-translational modifications of proteins to form the unusual amino acid γ-carboxyglutamic acid. γ-Carboxyglutamate chelates calcium ions, and so permits the binding of the blood clotting proteins to membranes.

Because of these factors, vitamin K is routinely administered to newborns. Deficiency of fat soluble vitamins A, E, D, and K can occur with intestinal malabsorption, but avid fetal uptake during pregnancy usually prevents infantile symptoms.

Overview of Vitamin K Metabolism

Vitamin K represents a group of lipophilic and hydrophobic vitamins. Three compounds have the biological activity of vitamin K phylloquinone, the normal dietary source, found in green vegetables; menaquinones, synthesized by intestinal bacteria, with differing lengths of side chain; and menadione and menadiol diacetate, synthetic compounds that can be metabolized to phylloquinone. Menaquinones are absorbed to some extent, but it is not clear to what extent they are biologically active as it is possible to induce signs of vitamin K deficiency simply by feeding a phylloquinone-deficient diet, without inhibiting intestinal bacterial action.

Vitamin K is the Coenzyme for Carboxylation of Glutamate in Postsynthetic Modification of Calcium-binding Proteins

Vitamin K-dependent proteins are a heterogeneous group, including clotting factor proteins and also proteins found in bone, lung, kidney, and placenta. Vitamin K is the cofactor for the carboxylation of glutamate residues in the postsynthetic modification of proteins to form the unusual amino acid γ-carboxyglutamate (Gla) **(Fig. 11.24)**. This is a critical step for the activity of vitamin K-dependent proteins for calcium binding and proper assembly to phospholipid membranes.

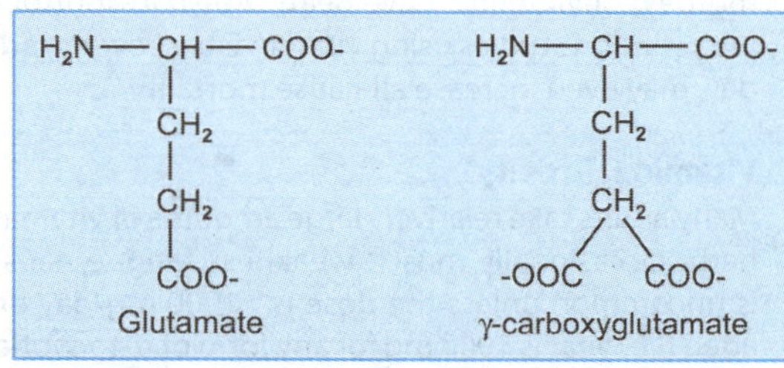

Fig. 11.24: Glutamate and γ-carboxyglutamate.

Initially, vitamin K hydroquinone is oxidized to the epoxide, which activates a glutamate residue in the protein substrate to a carbanion, which reacts nonenzymically with carbon dioxide to form γ-carboxyglutamate **(Fig. 11.25)**. Vitamin K epoxide is reduced to the quinone by a warfarin-sensitive reductase, and the quinone is reduced to the active hydroquinone by either the same warfarin-sensitive reductase or a warfarin-insensitive quinone reductase. In the presence of warfarin, vitamin K epoxide cannot be reduced, but accumulates and is excreted. If enough vitamin K (as the quinone) is provided in the diet, it can be reduced to the active hydroquinone by the warfarin-insensitive enzyme, and carboxylation can continue, with stoichiometric utilization of vitamin K and excretion of the epoxide. A high dose of vitamin K is the antidote to an overdose of warfarin. Prothrombin and several other proteins of the blood clotting system (factors VII, IX, and X, and proteins C and S) each contain 4 to 6 γ-carboxyglutamate residues.

γ-Carboxyglutamate chelates calcium ions, and so permits the binding of the blood clotting proteins to membranes. In vitamin K deficiency, or in the presence of warfarin, an abnormal precursor of prothrombin (preprothrombin) containing little or no γ-carboxyglutamate, and incapable of chelating calcium, is released into the circulation.

Vitamin K is also Important in Synthesis of Bone Calcium-Binding Proteins

Two proteins that contain γ-carboxyglutamate are present in bone, osteocalcin, and bone matrix Gla protein. Osteocalcin also contains hydroxyproline, so its synthesis is dependent on both vitamins K and C; in addition, its synthesis is induced by vitamin D. The release into the circulation of osteocalcin provides an index of vitamin D status.

Dietary Sources

Vitamin K is found in green leafy vegetables, such as kale and spinach, and appreciable amounts are also present in margarine and liver. Vitamin K is present in vegetable oils and is particularly rich in olive, canola, and soybean oils. The average daily intake by Americans is estimated to be approximately 100 µg/day.

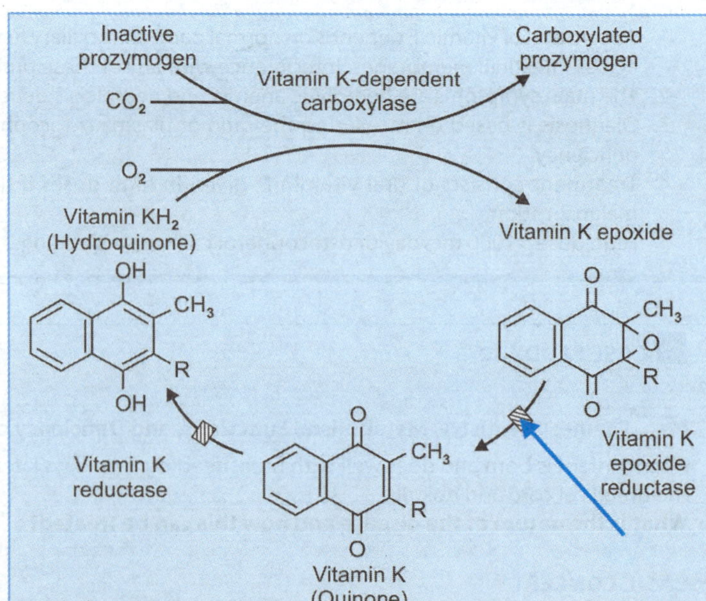

Fig. 11.25: Role of vitamin K in the gamma carboxylation of glutamate residues of various proteins. The arrow shows the site of action of warfarin.

DEFICIENCY OF VITAMIN K

Pathophysiology

Newborn infants are at risk of developing vitamin K deficiency, and this coagulation abnormality leads to serious bleeding. Transplacental transfer of vitamin K is very limited during pregnancy, and the storage of vitamin K in neonatal liver is also limited. This makes the newborn infant uniquely vulnerable to hemorrhagic disorders unless exogenous vitamin K is given for prevention of bleeding immediately after birth.

Once the infantile gut is colonized with bacterial flora, the microbial production of vitamin K results in a lower risk of infantile vitamin K deficiency bleeding. A gut-related microbial source of vitamin K is particularly important if dietary phylloquinone is restricted.

The most common sites of hemorrhage or bleeding are the umbilicus, mucous membrane, the GI tract, circumcision, and venipuncture sites. Hematomas frequently occur at the sites of trauma (i.e., large cephalohematomas, scalp bruising related to instrumentation used at delivery, and, rarely, intracranial hemorrhage). Neonatal mortality and long-term neurologic morbidity are severe consequences of vitamin K deficiency bleeding.

Breast milk is a poor source of vitamin K (breast milk levels are 1–4 µg/L). The recommended dietary intake of vitamin K is 1 µg/kg/day. Exclusively breastfeed infants have intestinal colonization with lactobacilli that do not synthesize vitamin K; thus, reduced production of menaquinones increases the neonatal risk of developing a hemorrhagic disorder if not supplemented with vitamin K. Formula-feed infants have higher fecal concentrations of vitamin K1 because of dietary intake and significant quantities of fecal menaquinones, reflecting the gut's microflora.

Preterm infants who are receiving total parenteral nutrition (TPN) are not at risk because they are receiving vitamin K via the multivitamin additive to the TPN. Special consideration is needed for very low-birth-weight infants whose intestinal tract bacterial flora is altered because of multiple courses of broad-spectrum antimicrobials. Once preterm infants are weaned off of TPN, they may develop vitamin K deficiency if they are exclusively fed breast milk.

Frequency

The routine intramuscular administration of vitamin K immediately after birth has made vitamin K deficiency bleeding an uncommon occurrence. The frequency of vitamin K deficiency bleeding varies from 0.25 to 1.7% in the first week of life in infants not receiving vitamin K prophylaxis. Late vitamin K deficiency bleeding (2–12 weeks after birth) appears to be reduced or prevented with parenteral administration of vitamin K at birth.

CLINICAL MANIFESTATIONS

- The main symptom is bleeding (hemorrhage)—into the skin (causing bruises), from the nose, from a wound, in the stomach, or in the intestine.
- Sometimes bleeding in the stomach causes vomiting with blood **(Fig. 11.26)**.
- Blood may be seen in the urine or stool. In newborns, life-threatening bleeding within or around the brain may occur.
- Having a liver disorder increases the risk of bleeding because proteins that help blood clot (clotting factors) are made in the liver.
- Vitamin K deficiency may also weaken bones.
- Most newborn infants are healthy upon examination, even if early onset bleeding is present; however, intracranial hemorrhage can occur during the delivery process and can lead to severe complications.
- Signs of intracranial hemorrhage include apnea with/without seizures and a shock, such as syndrome.
- Internal hemorrhage of organs other than the brain may be difficult to detect; however, if they are suspected, careful physical monitoring and serial imaging after birth are indicated.
- Soft tissue hemorrhage is easier to recognize, but sequential measurements of the bleeding into soft tissues or muscle are mandatory.

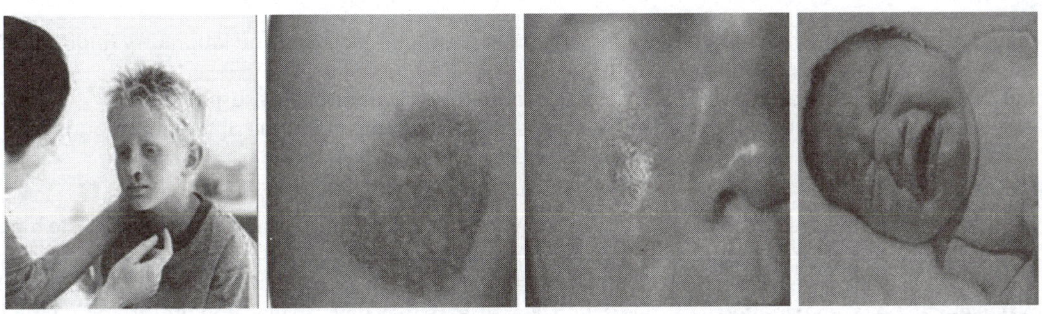

Fig. 11.26: A deficiency of vitamin K can lead to extreme bleeding, which can begin as a gum or nose discharge or bruising.

Causes

- Vitamin K deficiency in the newborn can be present for various reasons.
- Maternal medications that interfere with vitamin K stores or function (e.g., carbamazepine, phenytoin, barbiturates, some cephalosporins, rifampin, isoniazid, warfarin, or warfarin-like drugs) can result in vitamin K deficiency bleeding in the infant.
- In addition to breastfeeding, clinical states that are risk factors for late-onset vitamin K deficiency bleeding include:
  - Diarrhea
  - Hepatitis
  - Cystic fibrosis
  - Celiac disease
  - Alpha-1-antitrypsin deficiency
  - Short bowel syndrome
  - Intestinal bacterial overgrowth
  - Chronic exposure to broad spectrum antimicrobials.
- Vitamin K deficiency can result from lack of vitamin K in the diet. The amount of vitamin K in the diet is often limiting for the carboxylation reaction, and thus recycling of the vitamin K is essential to maintain normal levels of vitamin K-dependent proteins. In adults, low dietary intake alone is seldom reason for severe vitamin K deficiency but may become common in association with the use of broad-spectrum antibiotics.
- From disorders that impair fat absorption and that thus reduce the absorption of vitamin K. Disease or surgical interventions that affect the ability of the intestinal tract to absorb vitamin K, either through anatomic alterations or by changing the content of bile salts and pancreatic juices in the proximal small bowel, can result in significant reduction of vitamin K levels.
- Chronic liver diseases such as primary billiary cirrhosis also deplete vitamin K stores.
- Taking large amounts of mineral oil may reduce the absorption of vitamin K.
- Inherited deficiency of the functional activity of the enzymes involved in vitamin K metabolism results in bleeding disorders.

Laboratory Studies

- A prothrombin time (PT), activated partial thromboplastin time (aPTT), fibrinogen levels, and a platelet count should be included in the initial workup for vitamin K deficiency bleeding (VKDB) in a newborn. A thrombin clotting time (TCT) is optional.
  - A prolonged PT is usually the first laboratory test result to be abnormal in vitamin K deficiency bleeding due to reduction in prothrombin, FVII, FIX, and FX levels. FVII has the shortest half-life among these factors, which can prolong the PT before changes in the aPTT; however, no laboratory test result can confirm the diagnosis of vitamin K deficiency bleeding.
  - A direct blood measurement of vitamin K is not useful because levels normally are low in newborns.
  - Infants with vitamin K deficiency bleeding typically have a prolonged PT with platelet counts and fibrinogen levels within the normal range for newborns. Thrombocytopenia or a prolonged aPTT should prompt workup for other causes of bleeding during the neonatal period.
- The diagnosis of vitamin K deficiency bleeding is confirmed if administration of vitamin K halts the bleeding and reduces the PT value.

Imaging Studies

- Intracranial bleeding is rare and usually associated with other causes of bleeding, particularly thrombocytopenia; however, intracranial hemorrhage has been reported in vitamin K deficiency bleeding and can be fatal.
- Investigate any neurologic symptoms with imaging. MRI exposes the neonate to no radiation and is becoming the preferred way to study the brain because tissue damage can be better defined.

Other Tests

- A full coagulopathy workup and hematology consultation are required if clinical and laboratory findings are suggestive of non-vitamin K deficiency bleeding.
- A workup that includes functional tests and imaging is mandatory if liver disease is suspected.
- Hereditary defects in the coagulation system must always be considered among the differential diagnoses.

TREATMENT

A vitamin K injection in the muscle is recommended for all newborns to reduce the risk of bleeding within the brain after delivery. Otherwise, vitamin K is usually taken by mouth or given by injection under the skin. If a drug is the cause, the dose of the drug is adjusted or extra vitamin K is given. For patients with chronic malabsorption, 1 to 2 mg/day of vitamin K should be given orally, or 1 to 2 mg/week can be taken parenterally. Patients with liver disease may have an elevated prothrombin time because of liver cell destruction as well as vitamin K deficiency. If an elevated prothrombin time does not improve on vitamin K therapy, it can be deduced that it is not the result of vitamin K deficiency.

People who have vitamin K deficiency and a severe liver disorder may also need blood transfusions to replenish the clotting factors. A damaged liver may be unable to synthesize clotting factors even after vitamin K injections are given.

The reversal of excessive anticoagulant therapy with warfarin or warfarin-like drugs can be achieved by minimal doses of vitamin K (1 mg orally or by intravenous injection) for asymptomatic patients. This strategy can diminish the risk of bleeding while maintaining therapeutic anticoagulation for an underlying prothrombotic state.

Toxicity

Toxicity from dietary phylloquinone and menaquinones has not been described. High doses of vitamin K can impair the actions of oral anticoagulants.

Complications of Vitamin K Deficiency

- Intracranial hemorrhage is the primary serious complication of vitamin K deficiency bleeding.
- Complications of treatment include anaphylactoid, such as reactions during intravenous (IV) vitamin K administration, hyperbilirubinemia or hemolytic anemia after high doses of vitamin K, and hematomas at the site of injection, if administered IM.

Prevention

- Intramuscular (IM) vitamin K prophylaxis at birth is the standard of care in the United States.
- Commercial infant formulas in the United States contain supplemental vitamin K.
- These measures have served to make vitamin K deficiency bleeding a rarity. However, parental refusal of prophylaxis and an increasing frequency of breastfeeding may cause a resurgence of vitamin K deficiency bleeding in developed countries.

Prognosis

- In the absence of intracranial hemorrhage, the prognosis for vitamin K deficiency bleeding in an otherwise healthy infant is excellent.
- Prognosis after intracranial hemorrhage depends on the extent and location of the hemorrhage.
- Long-term sequelae of intracranial hemorrhage may include motor and intellectual deficits.

Vitamin K Antagonists

Warfarin

A water-soluble vitamin K antagonist initially developed as a rodenticide, warfarin, is the coumarin derivative **(Fig. 11.27)**. Like other vitamin K antagonists, warfarin interferes with the synthesis of the vitamin K-dependent clotting proteins, which include prothrombin (factor II) and factors VII, IX, and X. The synthesis of the vitamin K-dependent anticoagulant proteins, proteins C and S, is also reduced by vitamin K antagonists.

Mechanism of Action

Warfarin inhibits vitamin K epoxide reductase (VKOR), thereby blocking the γ-carboxylation process. This results in the synthesis of vitamin K-dependent clotting proteins that are only partially γ-carboxylated. Warfarin acts as an anticoagulant because these partially γ-carboxylated proteins have reduced or absent biologic activity.

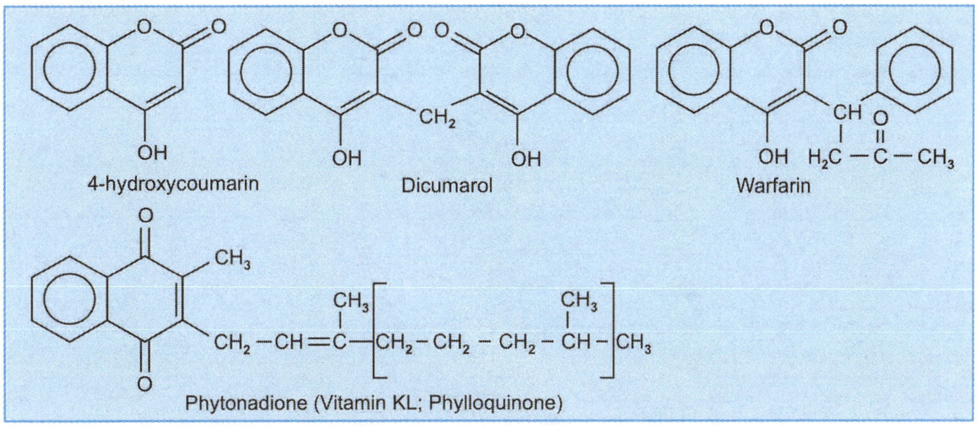

Fig. 11.27: Vitamin K antagonists, these are structural analogs of vitamin K.

The onset of action of warfarin is delayed until the newly synthesized clotting factors with reduced activity gradually replace their fully active counterparts.

The antithrombotic effect of warfarin depends on a reduction in the functional levels of factor X and prothrombin, clotting factors that have half-lives of 24 and 72 hours, respectively. Because of the delay in achieving an antithrombotic effect, initial treatment with warfarin is supported by concomitant administration of a rapidly acting parenteral anticoagulant, such as heparin, low-molecular-weight heparin (LMWH), or fondaparinux, in patients with established thrombosis or at high risk for thrombosis.

Like all anticoagulants, the major side effect of warfarin is bleeding. A rare complication is skin necrosis. Warfarin crosses the placenta and can cause fetal abnormalities. Treatment of pregnant women with warfarin can lead to fetal bone abnormalities (fetal warfarin syndrome). Consequently, warfarin should not be used during pregnancy.

In addition to genetic factors, the anticoagulant effect of warfarin is influenced by diet, drugs, and various disease states. Fluctuations in dietary vitamin K intake affect the activity of warfarin. A wide variety of drugs can alter absorption, clearance, or metabolism of warfarin.

Warfarin therapy is most often monitored using the prothrombin time, a test that is sensitive to reductions in the levels of prothrombin, factor VII, and factor X. The test is performed by adding thromboplastin, a reagent that contains tissue factor, phospholipid, and calcium, to citrated plasma and determining the time to clot formation.

Hydroxy coumarin **(Fig. 11.27)**, which was isolated from bacterial contaminants in the hay, interferes with vitamin K metabolism, thereby causing a syndrome similar to vitamin K deficiency.

Dicumarol **(Fig. 11.27)** is similar in action to warfarin; it causes inhibition of epoxide reductase enzyme and is given in the treatment of deep vein thrombosis. It is also an uncoupler of oxidative phosphorylation.

CLINICAL NOTE

In adults, low dietary intake alone is seldom reason for severe vitamin K deficiency but may become common in association with the use of broad-spectrum antibiotics.

CLINICAL PEARLS

1. Vitamin K is necessary for the synthesis of the clotting factors and thus for the normal clotting of blood. It is also needed for healthy bones and other tissues.
2. Newborns are prone to vitamin K deficiency because only small amounts of vitamin K cross the placenta and because, during the first few days after birth, their intestine does not contain bacteria to produce vitamin K.
3. Hemorrhagic disease is more likely in infants who are breastfeed or who have a disorder that impairs fat absorption or a liver disorder. Formulas for infants contain vitamin K.
4. The deficiency can cause hemorrhagic disease of the newborn, characterized by a tendency to bleed.
5. A prothrombin time (PT), activated partial thromboplastin time (aPTT), fibrinogen levels, and a platelet count should be included in the initial workup for vitamin K deficiency bleeding (VKDB) in a newborn.
6. A vitamin K injection is usually given to newborns to protect them from this disease.

Chapter 12

Minerals

LEARNING OBJECTIVES

To understand:

- ❖ Chemistry, metabolism, and functions of iron
- ❖ Clinical implications of iron deficiency and overload
- ❖ Calcium metabolism and homeostasis
- ❖ Clinical implications of hyper- and hypocalcemia
- ❖ Copper metabolism, functions, and clinical implications of copper deficiency and toxicity
- ❖ Zinc—metabolism, functions, and significance
- ❖ Selenium—functions, deficiency, and toxicity
- ❖ The sources of exposure, pathogenesis, clinical manifestations, laboratory diagnosis, and management of heavy metal toxicity

CASE STUDIES

CASE STUDY 1

Theme: Iron Metabolism, Function, and Iron Deficiency Anemia

An 18-year-old female reported to the physician for consultation. She complained of generalized weakness, lethargy, and inability to do the routine work from the previous few months. On further questioning, she revealed that she was having excessive bleeding during menstruation from the previous 6 months. She complained of breathlessness and palpitations while climbing stairs for her house. She also had experienced periods of lightheadedness, though not to the point of fainting. Other changes she had noticed were cramping in her legs, a desire to crunch on ice. There was no history of any fever, drug intake, or abdominal discomfort. Her appetite had also decreased and she was taking meals only once a day.

Upon examining, her physician found that she had tachycardia, pale gums, and nail beds, and her tongue was swollen. Given her history and the findings on her physical examination, the physician suspected that the patient was anemic and ordered a sample of her blood for examination. The results were as shown below:

Hb—8.0 g/dL Serum iron—32 μg/dL

What is the cause of anemia in this patient?
What are the possible complications in the untreated cases?

CASE DETAILS

The most likely diagnosis is iron deficiency anemia.

Generalized weakness, exercise intolerance, dyspnea, palpitations, history of blood loss during menstruation, tachycardia, and low Hb all are suggestive of iron deficiency anemia. Iron deficiency is the most prevalent single deficiency state on a worldwide basis. Iron deficiency is related in part to abnormal iron metabolism.

Overview of Iron Metabolism

The balance of iron in humans is tightly controlled and designed to conserve iron for reutilization. There is no regulated excretory pathway for iron, and the mechanisms by which iron is lost from the body are blood loss (via gastrointestinal bleeding, menses, or other forms of bleeding) and the loss of epithelial cells from the skin, gut, and genitourinary tract. Normally, the only route by which iron comes into the body is via absorption from food or from medicinal iron taken orally. Iron may also enter the body through red-cell transfusions or injection of iron complexes. The margin between the amount of iron available for absorption and the requirement for iron in growing infants and the adult female is narrow; this accounts for the great prevalence of iron deficiency worldwide—currently estimated at one-half billion people.

Iron Requirement

The amount of iron required from the diet to replace losses averages about 10% of body iron content a year in men and 15% in women of childbearing age. Dietary iron content is closely related to total caloric intake (approximately 6 mg of elemental iron per 1,000 calories). Iron bioavailability is affected by the nature of the foodstuff, with heme iron (e.g., red meat) being most readily absorbed. In the United States, the average iron intake in an adult male is 15 mg/day with 6% absorption; for the average female, the daily intake is 11 mg/day with 12% absorption. An individual with iron deficiency can increase iron absorption to about 20% of the iron present in a meat-containing diet but only 5–10% of the iron in a vegetarian diet. As a result, one-third of the female population in the United States has virtually no iron stores. Vegetarians are at an additional disadvantage because certain foodstuffs that include phytates and phosphates reduce iron absorption by about 50%. When ionizable iron salts are given together with food, the amount of iron absorbed is reduced. When the percentage of iron absorbed from individual food items is compared with the percentage for an equivalent amount of ferrous salt, iron in vegetables is only about one-twentieth as available, egg iron one-eighth, liver iron one-half, and heme iron one-half to two-thirds.

Infants, children, and adolescents may be unable to maintain normal iron balance because of the demands of body growth and lower dietary intake of iron. During the last two trimesters of pregnancy, daily iron requirements increase to 5–6 mg. That is the reason why iron supplements are strongly recommended for pregnant women in developed countries.

Iron absorption takes place largely in the proximal small intestine and is a carefully regulated process. For absorption, iron must be taken up by the luminal cell. That process is facilitated by the acidic contents of the stomach **(Fig. 12.1)**, which maintains the iron in solution. At the brush border of the absorptive cell, the ferric iron is converted to the ferrous form by a ferrireductase. Transport across the membrane is accomplished by divalent metal transporter 1 (DMT1, also known as Nramp2 or DCT-1). DMT1 is a general cation transporter. Once inside the gut cell, iron may be stored as ferritin or transported through the cell to be released at the basolateral surface to plasma transferrin through the membrane-embedded iron exporter, ferroportin. The function of ferroportin is negatively regulated by hepcidin, the principal iron regulatory hormone. In the process of release, iron interacts with another ferroxidase, hephaestin, which oxidizes the iron to the ferric form for transferrin binding. Hephaestin is similar to ceruloplasmin, the copper-carrying protein.

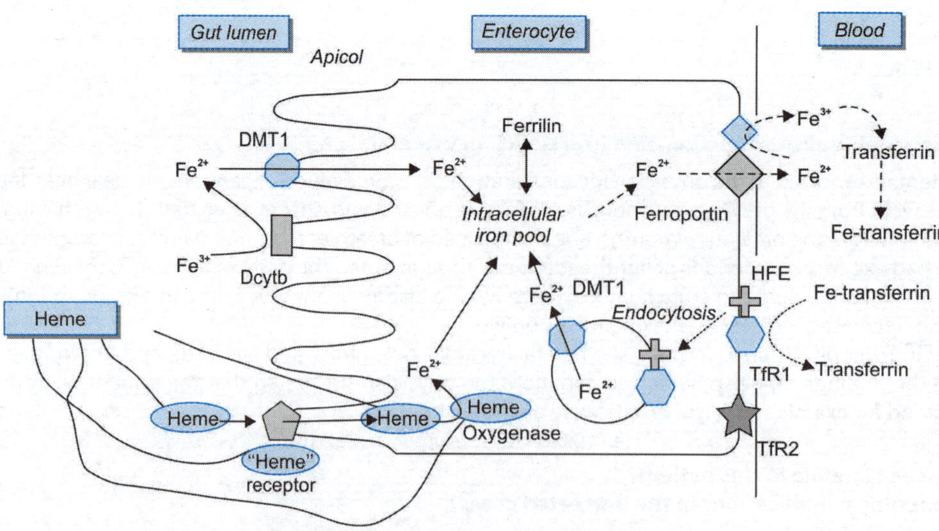

Fig. 12.1: Mechanism of iron absorption.

Iron absorption is influenced by a number of physiological states erythroid hyperplasia, for example, stimulates iron absorption, even in the face of normal or increased iron stores, and hepcidin levels are inappropriately low. The molecular mechanism underlying this relationship is not known. Thus, patients with anemias associated with high levels of ineffective erythropoiesis absorb excess amounts of dietary iron. Over time, this may lead to iron overload and tissue damage. In iron deficiency, hepcidin levels are low and iron is much more efficiently absorbed from a given diet; the contrary is true in states of secondary iron overload. The normal individual can reduce iron absorption in situations of excessive intake or medicinal iron intake; however, while the percentage of iron absorbed goes down, the absolute amount goes up. This accounts for the acute iron toxicity occasionally seen when children ingest large numbers of iron tablets. Under these circumstances, the amount of iron absorbed exceeds the transferrin-binding capacity of the plasma, resulting in free iron that affects critical organs, such as cardiac muscle cells.

Free Iron Toxicity

Iron is a critical element in the function of all cells, although the amount of iron required by individual tissues varies during development. At the same time, the body must protect itself from free iron, which is highly toxic because it participates in chemical reactions that generate free radicals, such as singlet O_2 or OH^-. In chemical reactions that generate free radicals, such as singlet O_2 or OH^-. Consequently, elaborate mechanisms have evolved that allow iron to be made available for physiological functions while at the same time conserving this element and handling it in such a way that toxicity is avoided.

Iron Transport

Iron absorbed from the diet or released from stores circulates in the plasma bound to *transferrin*, the iron transport protein. Transferrin is a bilobed glycoprotein with two iron-binding sites. Transferrin (Tf) is normally about one-third saturated with iron transferrin that carries iron, which exists in two forms—*monoferric* (one iron atom) or *diferric* (two iron atoms). The turnover (half-clearance time) of transferrin-bound iron is very rapid—typically 60–90 minutes. Because almost all of the iron transported by transferrin is delivered to the erythroid marrow, the clearance time of transferrin-bound iron from the circulation is affected most by the plasma iron level and the erythroid marrow activity. When erythropoiesis is markedly stimulated, the pool of erythroid cells requiring iron increases and the clearance time of iron from the circulation decreases. The half-clearance time of iron in the presence of iron deficiency is as short as 10–15 minutes. With suppression of erythropoiesis, the plasma iron level typically increases and the half-clearance time may be prolonged to several hours. Normally, the iron bound to transferrin turns over 10–20 times per day. Assuming a normal plasma iron level of 80–100 µg/dL, the amount of iron passing through the transferrin pool is 20–24 mg/day.

The iron-transferrin complex circulates in the plasma until it interacts with specific *transferrin receptors* on the surface of marrow erythroid cells. Diferric transferrin has the highest affinity for transferrin receptors; apotransferrin (transferrin not carrying iron) has very little affinity. While transferrin receptors are found on cells in many tissues within the body—and all cells at some time during development will display transferrin receptors—the cell having the greatest number of receptors (300,000–400,000/cell) is the developing erythroblast.

Utilization of Iron

Once the iron-bearing transferrin interacts with its receptor, the complex is internalized via clathrin-coated pits and transported to an acidic endosome, where the iron is released at the low pH. The iron is then made available for heme synthesis, while the transferrin-receptor complex is recycled to the surface of the cell, where the bulk of the transferrin is released back into circulation and the transferrin receptor reanchors into the cell membrane. At this point, a certain amount of the transferrin receptor protein may be released into circulation and can be measured as soluble transferrin receptor protein. Within the erythroid cell, iron in excess of the amount needed for hemoglobin synthesis binds to a storage protein, apoferritin, forming ferritin. This mechanism of iron exchange also takes place in other cells of the body expressing transferrin receptors, especially liver parenchymal cells where the iron can be incorporated into heme-containing enzymes or stored. The iron incorporated into hemoglobin subsequently enters the circulation as new red cells are released from the bone marrow. The iron is then part of the red cell mass and will not become available for reutilization until the red cell dies.

Conservation of Iron

In a normal individual, the average red cell lifespan is 120 days. Thus, 0.8–1.0% of red cells turn over each day. At the end of its lifespan, the red cell is recognized as senescent by the cells of the reticuloendothelial (RE) system, and the cell undergoes phagocytosis. Once within the RE cell, the hemoglobin from the ingested red cell is broken down, the globin and other proteins are returned to the amino acid pool, and the iron is shuttled back to the surface of the RE cell, where it is presented to circulating transferrin. It is the efficient and highly conserved recycling of iron from senescent red cells that supports steady state (and even mildly accelerated) erythropoiesis. Persistent errors in iron balance lead to either iron deficiency anemia or hemosiderosis. Both are disorders with potential adverse consequences.

Storage of Iron

Ferritin and hemosiderin are iron-containing compounds meant for storage of iron. Ferritin is a protein-bound, water-soluble, and mobilizable storage compound and is the major source of storage iron. Hemosiderin is a water-insoluble form that is less readily available for use. When the amount of total body iron is relatively low, storage iron consists predominately of ferritin. When iron stores are high, hemosiderin predominates. Unlike ferritin, hemosiderin stains with the Prussian blue stain (Pens reaction) and may be observed in tissues. Storage forms normally comprise approximately 30% of total body iron. Iron stores provide a source of iron when physiological demand is high, e.g., blood loss, pregnancy, and periods of rapid growth.

Metabolic Role of Iron

Iron is vital for all living organisms because it is essential for multiple metabolic processe, including oxygen transport, DNA synthesis, and electron transport.

The major role of iron in mammals is to carry O_2 as part of hemoglobin. O_2 is also bound by myoglobin in muscle. Iron is a critical element in iron-containing enzyme, including the cytochrome system in mitochondria. Without iron, cells lose their capacity for electron transport and energy metabolism. In erythroid cells, hemoglobin synthesis is impaired, resulting in anemia and reduced O_2 delivery to tissue.

Demand and Supply Imbalance

Since each milliliter of red cells contains 1 mg of elemental iron, the amount of iron needed to replace those red cells lost through senescence amounts to 16–20 mg/day (assuming an adult with a red cell mass of 2 L). Any additional iron required for daily red cell production comes from the diet. Normally, an adult male will need to absorb at least 1 mg of elemental iron daily to meet needs, while females in the childbearing years will need to absorb an average of 1.4 mg/day. However, to achieve a maximum proliferative erythroid marrow response to anemia, additional iron must be available. With markedly stimulated erythropoiesis, demands for iron are increased by as much as six- to eightfold. With extravascular hemolytic anemia, the rate of red cell destruction is increased, but the iron recovered from the red cells is efficiently reutilized for hemoglobin synthesis. In contrast, with intravascular hemolysis or blood loss anemia, the rate of red cell production is limited by the amount of iron that can be mobilized from stores. Typically, the rate of mobilization under these circumstances will not support red cell production >2.5 times normal. If the delivery of iron to the stimulated marrow is suboptimal, the marrow's proliferative response is blunted, and hemoglobin synthesis is impaired. The result is a hypoproliferative marrow accompanied by microcytic, hypochromic anemia.

Menstrual blood loss in women plays a major role in iron metabolism. The average monthly menstrual blood loss is approximately 50 mL, or about 0.7 mg/day. However, menstrual blood loss may be five times the average. To maintain adequate iron stores, women with heavy menstrual losses must absorb 3–4 mg of iron from the diet each day. This strains the upper limit of what may reasonably be absorbed, and women with menorrhagia of this degree will almost always become iron deficient without iron supplementation.

Pregnancy may also upset the iron balance, since requirements increase to 2–5 mg of iron per day during pregnancy and lactation. Normal dietary iron cannot supply these requirements, and medicinal iron is needed during pregnancy and lactation. Repeated pregnancy (especially with breastfeeding) may cause iron deficiency, if increased requirements are not met with supplemental medicinal iron. Decreased iron absorption can on very rare occasions cause iron deficiency and usually occurs after gastric surgery, though concomitant bleeding is frequent.

By far, the most important cause of iron deficiency anemia is blood loss, especially gastrointestinal blood loss. Chronic aspirin use may cause it even without a documented structural lesion. Iron deficiency demands a search for a source of gastrointestinal bleeding, if other sites of blood loss (menorrhagia, other uterine bleeding, and repeated blood donations) are excluded.

Chronic hemoglobinuria may lead to iron deficiency since iron is lost in the urine; traumatic hemolysis due to a prosthetic cardiac valve and other causes of intravascular hemolysis (e.g., paroxysmal nocturnal hemoglobinuria) should also be considered. Frequent blood donors may also be at risk for iron deficiency.

While blood loss or hemolysis places a demand on the iron supply, conditions associated with inflammation interfere with iron release from stores and can result in a rapid decrease in the serum iron level.

SUMMARY OF CAUSES OF IRON DEFICIENCY

Conditions that increase demand for iron, increase iron loss, or decrease iron intake or absorption can produce iron deficiency:

- **Increased demand for iron and/or hematopoiesis:**
  - Rapid growth in infancy or adolescence
  - Pregnancy
  - Erythropoietin therapy
- **Increased iron loss:**
  - Chronic blood loss
  - Menses
  - Acute blood loss
  - Blood donation
  - Phlebotomy as treatment for polycythemia vera.
- **Decreased iron intake or absorption:**
  - Inadequate diet
  - Malabsorption from disease (sprue, Crohn's disease)
  - Malabsorption from surgery (postgastrectomy)
  - Acute or chronic inflammation

IRON DEFICIENCY ANEMIA

Iron deficiency is defined as decreased total iron body content. Iron deficiency anemia occurs when iron deficiency is sufficiently severe to diminish erythropoiesis and cause the development of anemia. Iron deficiency is the most prevalent single deficiency state on a worldwide basis. It is important economically because it diminishes the capability of individuals who are affected to perform physical labor, and it diminishes both growth and learning in children.

Frequency

In countries where little meat is in the diet, iron deficiency anemia is 6–8 times more prevalent than in North America and Europe. This occurs despite consumption of a diet that contains an equivalent amount of total dietary iron because heme iron is absorbed better from the diet than nonheme iron. In certain geographic areas, intestinal parasites, particularly hookworm, worsen the iron deficiency because of blood loss from the gastrointestinal tract. Anemia is more profound among children and premenopausal women in these environs.

Mortality/Morbidity

Chronic iron deficiency anemia is seldom a direct cause of death; however, moderate or severe iron deficiency anemia can produce sufficient hypoxia to aggravate underlying pulmonary and cardiovascular disorders. In children, the growth rate may be slowed, and a decreased capability to learn is reported.

Clinical Manifestations

As a rule, the only symptoms of iron deficiency anemia are those of the anemia itself (easy fatigability, tachycardia, palpitations, and tachypnea on exertion). Severe deficiency causes skin and mucosal change, including a smooth tongue, brittle nails, and cheilosis. Dysphagia because of the formation of esophageal webs (Plummer–Vinson syndrome) also occurs. Many iron-deficient patients develop pica, craving for specific foods (ice chips, etc.) often not rich in iron.

Laboratory Findings

- **Complete blood count (CBC):**
  - This documents the severity of the anemia. In chronic iron deficiency anemia, the cellular indices show a microcytic and hypochromic erythropoiesis, i.e., both the mean corpuscular volume (MCV) and mean corpuscular hemoglobin concentration (MCHC) have values below the normal range for the laboratory performing the test. Reference range values for the MCV and MCHC are 83–97 fL and 32–36 g/dL, respectively.
  - Often, the platelet count is elevated (>450,000/µL), which normalizes after iron therapy.
  - The white blood cell (WBC) count is usually within reference ranges (4,500–11,000/µL).
  - If the CBC count is obtained after blood loss, the cellular indices do not enter the abnormal range until most of the erythrocytes produced before the bleed are destroyed at the end of their normal lifespan (120 days).
- **Peripheral smear:**
  - In the early stages, the MCV remains normal. Subsequently, the MCV falls and the blood smear shows hypochromic microcytic cells (blood smear; **Figure 12.2**). With further progression, anisocytosis (variations in red blood cell size) and poikilocytosis (variation in shape of red cells) develop. Severe iron deficiency will produce a bizarre peripheral blood smear, with severely hypochromic cells, target cells, hypochromic pencil-shaped cells, and occasionally small numbers of nucleated red blood cells **(Fig. 12.2)**. The platelet count is commonly increased.

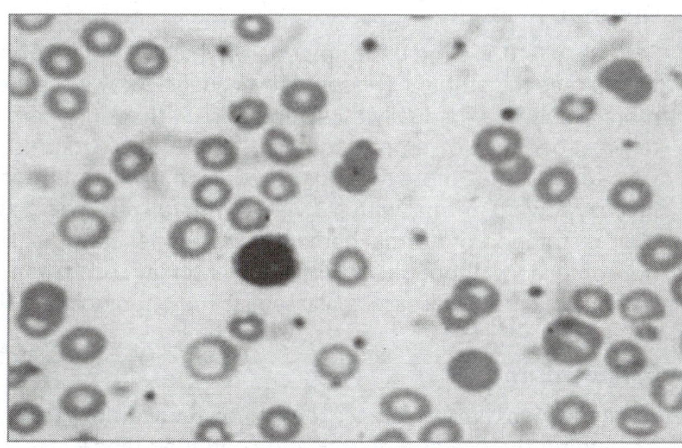

Fig. 12.2: Microcytic hypochromic cells in peripheral smear in a patient suffering from iron deficiency anemia.

  - Combined folate deficiency and iron deficiency are commonplace in areas of the world with little fresh produce and meat. The peripheral smear reveals a population of macrocytes mixed among the microcytic hypochromic cells. This combination can normalize the MCV.
- **Serum iron, total iron-binding capacity (TIBC), and serum ferritin:** Iron deficiency develops in stages. The first is depletion of iron stores. At this point, there is anemia and no change in red blood cell size. The serum ferritin will become abnormally low. A ferritin value <30 mcg/L is a highly reliable indicator of iron deficiency. The serum TIBC rises. After iron stores have been depleted, red blood cell formation will continue with deficient supplies of iron. Serum iron values decline to <30 mcg/dL and transferrin saturation to <15%. A low serum iron and ferritin with an elevated TIBC are diagnostic of iron deficiency. While a low serum ferritin is virtually diagnostic of iron deficiency, a normal serum ferritin can be seen in patients who are

deficient in iron and have coexistent diseases (hepatitis, anemia of chronic disorders). These test findings are useful in distinguishing iron deficiency anemia from other microcytic anemias.

- A bone marrow aspirate can be diagnostic of iron deficiency. Bone marrow biopsy for evaluation of iron stores is now rarely performed because of variation in its interpretation.
- Other laboratory tests are useful to establish the etiology of iron deficiency anemia and to exclude or establish a diagnosis of one of the other microcytic anemias.
  - Testing stool for the presence of hemoglobin is useful in establishing gastrointestinal bleeding as the etiology of iron deficiency anemia. Severe iron deficiency anemia can occur in patients with a persistent loss of <20 mL/day.
  - Hemoglobinuria and hemosiderinuria can be detected by laboratory testing. This documents iron deficiency to be due to renal loss of iron and incriminates intravascular hemolysis as the etiology.
  - Hemoglobin electrophoresis and measurement of hemoglobin A_2 and fetal hemoglobin are useful in establishing either beta-thalassemia or hemoglobin C or D as the etiology of the microcytic anemia. Unfortunately, simple tests do not exist for alpha-thalassemia in most laboratories, and it is a diagnosis of exclusion.
  - **Serum levels of transferrin receptor protein:** Because erythroid cells have the highest numbers of transferrin receptors on their surface of any cell in the body, and because transferrin receptor protein (TRP) is released by cells into the circulation, serum levels of TRP reflect the total erythroid marrow mass. Another condition in which TRP levels are elevated is absolute iron deficiency. Normal values are 4–9 µg/L determined by immunoassay. This laboratory test is becoming increasingly available an along with the serum ferritin, has been proposed to distinguish between iron deficiency and the anemia of chronic inflammation.

Differential Diagnosis

Other causes of microcytic anemia include anemia of chronic disease, thalassemia, and sideroblastic anemia. Anemia of chronic disease is characterized by normal or increased iron stores in the bone marrow and a normal or elevated ferritin level; the serum iron is low, often drastically so, and the TIBC is either normal or low. Thalassemia produces a greater degree of microcytosis for any given level of anemia than does iron deficiency. Red blood cell morphology on the peripheral smear is abnormal earlier in the course of thalassemia.

Treatment

The diagnosis of iron deficiency anemia can be made either by the laboratory demonstration an iron-deficient state or evaluating the response to a therapeutic trial of iron replacement.

Since the anemia itself is rarely life-threatening, the most important part of treatment is identification of the cause—especially a source of occult blood loss.

Oral Iron

Ferrous sulfate, 325 mg three times daily, which provides 180 mg of iron daily of which up to 10 mg is absorbed (though absorption may exceed this amount in cases of severe deficiency), is the preferred therapy. Compliance is improved by introducing the medicine more slowly in a gradually escalating dose with food. Alternatively, in cases of poor tolerance, one pill of ferrous sulfate can be taken at bed time on empty stomach. It is preferable to prescribe a lower dose of iron or to allow ingestion concurrent with food than to insist on a more rigorous schedule that will not be followed. An appropriate response is a return of the hematocrit level halfway toward normal within 3 weeks with full return to baseline after 2 months. Iron therapy should continue for 3–6 months after restoration of normal hematological values to replenish iron stores. Failure of response to iron therapy is usually due to noncompliance, although occasional patients may absorb iron poorly. Other reasons for failure to respond include incorrect diagnosis (anemia of chronic disease, thalassemia) and ongoing gastrointestinal blood loss that exceeds the rate of new erythropoiesis.

Parenteral Iron

The indications are intolerance to oral iron, refractoriness to oral iron, gastrointestinal disease (usually inflammatory bowel disease) precluding the use of oral iron, and continued blood loss that cannot be corrected. Because of the possibility of anaphylactic reactions, parenteral iron therapy should be used only in cases of persistent anemia after a reasonable course of oral therapy. Until recently, iron dextran had been the only form of parenteral iron available in the United States. Now, sodium ferric gluconate is available and has been shown to result in a lower incidence of severe anaphylaxis. To date, no deaths have been reported with the use of this preparation.

The dose (total 1.5–2 g) may be calculated by estimating the decrease in volume of red blood cell mass and then supplying 1 mg of iron for each milliliter of volume of red blood cells below normal. Approximately 1 g should then be added for storage iron. Total body iron ranges between 2 g and 4 g: Approximately 50 mg/kg in men and 35 mg/kg in women. Most (70–95%) of the iron is present in hemoglobin in circulating red blood cells. One milliliter of packed red blood cells (not whole blood) contains approximately 1 mg of iron. In men, red blood cell volume is approximately 30 mL/kg. A 70 kg man will therefore have approximately 2,100 mL of packed red blood cells and consequently 2,100 mg of iron in his circulating blood. In women, the red cell volume is about

27 mL/kg; a 50 kg woman will thus have 1,350 mg of iron circulating in her red blood cells. Thus, a woman whose hemoglobin is 9 g/dL would be treated with a total of 1,315 mg of parenteral iron, 315 mg for the increased red blood cell mass and 1,000 mg to provide iron stores. The entire dose may be given as an intravenous infusion over 4–6 hours. A test dose of a dilute solution is given first, and the patient should be observed during the entire infusion for anaphylaxis.

Red Cell Transfusion

Transfusion therapy is reserved for individuals who have symptoms of anemia, cardiovascular instability, continued and excessive blood loss from whatever source, and require immediate intervention. The management of these patients is less related to the iron deficiency than it is to the consequences of the severe anemia. Not only do transfusions correct the anemia acutely, but the transfused red cells provide a source of iron for reutilization, assuming they are not lost through continued bleeding. Transfusion therapy will stabilize the patient while other options are reviewed.

Prognosis

Iron deficiency anemia is an easily treated disorder with an excellent outcome; however, it may be caused by an underlying condition with a poor prognosis,, such as neoplasia. Similarly, the prognosis may be altered by a comorbid condition, such as coronary artery disease.

CLINICAL NOTE

The margin between the amount of iron available for absorption and the requirement for iron in growing infants and the adult female is narrow; this accounts for the great prevalence of iron deficiency worldwide—currently estimated at one-half billion people.

CLINICAL PEARLS

1. Iron deficiency anemia occurs when iron deficiency is sufficiently severe to diminish erythropoiesis and cause the development of anemia.
2. Symptoms of iron deficiency anemia are easy fatigability, tachycardia, palpitations, and tachypnea on exertion. Severe deficiency causes skin and mucosal change, including a smooth tongue, brittle nails, and cheilosis.
3. The diagnosis of iron deficiency anemia can be made either by the laboratory demonstration of an iron-deficient state or evaluating the response to a therapeutic trial of iron replacement.
4. CBC, peripheral blood smear, serum iron, ferritin, and serum total iron-binding capacity estimations are diagnostic of iron deficiency anemia.
5. Treatment of Fe deficiency anemia is based on treatment of the primary cause and iron supplementation orally, parenterally or by red cell transfusion depending upon the state of the patient.

CASE STUDY 2

Theme: Causes and Clinical Implications of Iron Overload

A 56-year-old Caucasian woman visited her family physician for her annual physical checkup. She stated that she was in generally good health but was experiencing some fatigue, mild depression, and mild-to-moderate joint pain from the previous several months. She was holding a full-time job as an accountant. Her medical history was significant only for hormone replacement therapy from the past 12 years. The patient stated that her consumption of alcohol was limited to one to two glasses of wine each week. She had been taking ibuprofen occasionally for joint pain but denied use of any other over-the-counter medication except daily vitamin tablets. Family history revealed that her father died 10 years ago of liver disease at age of 70. The patient was uncertain about the exact nature of her father's illness. Her mother was alive and was in good health. She also stated that she had two siblings—a brother and a sister who was recently diagnosed with diabetes.

Physical examination revealed a well-appearing female with normal vital signs. There was a mild hepatomegaly and joint tenderness. Laboratory studies were ordered on a fasting specimen and are as reported:

Laboratory data included—random blood glucose of 253 mg/dL, normal creatinine and electrolytes, aspartate aminotransferase (GOT) of 66 U/L (normal <44), alanine aminotransferase (ALT) of 133 U/L (normal <31 U/L), normal bilirubin and alkaline phosphatase levels, and negative hepatitis antigen screen.

Her iron level was 306 µg/dL (normal <155), with an iron-binding capacity of 315 µg/dL (normal <400), and percent saturation of 97% (normal <50%). Serum ferritin was 2,920 µg/L (normal <160). The polymerase chain restriction assay demonstrated homozygosity for the C282Y chromosome. Referral to the hepatology clinic resulted in a liver biopsy, which identified increased iron stores and early periportal fibrosis.

What is the probable diagnosis?

What is the basis for all the laboratory findings?

CASE DETAILS

The lady in question is most probably suffering from hemochromatosis. Hereditary hemochromatosis (HH) is a common inherited disorder of iron metabolism. This disease is usually diagnosed by elevated iron saturation, serum ferritin, a positive family history, hepatic abnormalities and cirrhosis, congestive heart failure, hypogonadism, arthritis, and *HFE* gene mutation (usually C282Y/C282Y) which is found in most cases.

The given patient has arthritis, a positive family history, raised transaminases, raised serum iron, iron-binding capacity, and high serum ferritin levels. PCR analysis also reveals the HFE gene mutation and the liver biopsy is revealing the increased iron stores. All these features are strongly in favor of hemochromatosis as a diagnosis.

BASIC CONCEPT

Hereditary hemochromatosis: Hereditary hemochromatosis (HH) is a fairly common disease in whites and is a result of iron deposition in hepatocytes, myocardial fibers, and other visceral cells. The classic tetrad of manifestations resulting from hemochromatosis consists of (1) cirrhosis, (2) diabetes mellitus, (3) hyperpigmentation of the skin **(Fig.12.3)**, and (4) cardiac failure. Clinical consequences also include hepatocellular carcinoma, impotence, and arthritis.

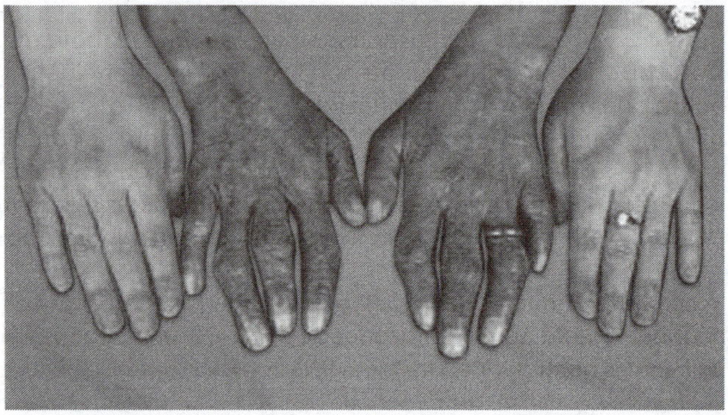

Fig. 12.3: Hyperpigmentation in hereditary hemochromatosis.

Biochemical Defect

The *hemochromatosis* gene is located on the long arm of chromosome 6 where it codes for a membrane protein, HFE, which is 343 amino acids in size. The exact mechanism of the role of HFE in iron metabolism is not completely understood. A popular hypothesis is that HFE, along with a second protein, beta-2 microglobulin (beta-2M), interacts with TfR on cell membranes. This interaction represses the affinity of Tf for the receptor, thus lowering the uptake of Tf into the cell. TfR have been found on the surface of a variety of cells, with the greatest concentration on the basolateral membrane of the intestine, hepatocytes, and erythrocyte precursors.

In HH, two mutations of the HFE gene have been described—*C282Y* and *H63D*. In the more prevalent *C282Y* mutation, there is a base substitution leading to a change in the amino acid in position 282 from cysteine (C) to tyrosine (Y).The loss of the sulfhydryl-containing amino acid disrupts the tertiary structure of HFE, so that it no longer binds to beta-2M. Beta-2M appears to act along with other proteins to chaperone the newly synthesized HFE out of the Golgi and to the cell surface where it can then bind to TfR. In the *C282Y* mutation, HFE remains in the Golgi, never making it to the cell surface. The result is that Tf binding to TfR is enhanced and excessive amounts of iron are absorbed in the small intestine, hepatocytes, and other tissues.

The second mutation, *H63D*, occurs when a histidine (H) residue in position 63 is replaced by an aspartic acid (D). The mechanism by which this mutation leads to increased iron uptake is less well understood when compared to the *C282Y* mutation. Unlike the *C282Y* mutation, the *H63D* mutation does not seem to affect the binding of beta-2M and intracellular trafficking, since detectable concentrations of the mutated protein are found on cell membranes. Some researchers speculate that the *H63D* mutation affects the binding of proteins involved in iron regulation and uptake at the cell surface.

A third *HFE* mutation, S65C, has also been described which appears to lead the mild to moderate hepatic iron overload without fibrosis in some cases.

Pathophysiology

Hemochromatosis is an autosomal recessive genetic disorder characterized by iron overload. Persons homozygous for mutations of the *hemochromatosis* gene, *HFE*, absorb 3–4 mg of dietary iron daily, a rate two to three times greater than normal. Normal storage sites become overloaded with iron, resulting in ferritin levels as much as ten times normal. With no mechanism to dispose of the excess, iron is deposited in the parenchymal cells of the liver, pancreas, pituitary, heart, synovium, and other tissues. Iron in excess of normal cellular ferritin stores contributes to the generation of free radicals and reactive oxygen intermediates that cause cell damage to organs and tissues. The amount of time needed for iron to increase in levels causing organ damage is variable and most likely partially dependent on gender and dietary factors. Blood loss through menstruation and pregnancy are thought to delay the onset of iron overload, and therefore symptoms, in women. Similarly, regular blood donation may confer some degree of protection. As levels of storage iron increase, clinical features of iron overload, including hepatic dysfunction or failure, diabetes, hypogonadism, arthritis, cardiomyopathy, hyperpigmentation and fatigue may become evident. Hyperpigmentation and fatigue may become evident. Symptomatic patients typically present in middle age between the ages of 30 and 60, although this is quite variable. Persons as young as 20 years of age may show clinical signs and symptoms of HH.

Frequency

Worldwide frequency of the *C282Y* and *H63D* mutations is found to be 1% and 8.1%, respectively. Marked disparity in the distribution of the C282Y mutation has been noted. Non-HFE–associated hereditary hemochromatosis was found in Mediterranean countries.

Diagnosis

Early identification of persons with HH is essential to prevent serious and irreversible complications associated with severe iron overload. Although rarely seen in clinical practice, the classic triad of skin hyperpigmentation (bronzing), type 2 diabetes, and hepatic cirrhosis has long been recognized as evidence of advanced iron overload.

HH is frequently discovered only during management of associated illness or routine health examinations. It has been estimated that only 10% of affected persons are actually being diagnosed at the present time.

Symptoms and Signs

Early symptoms are nonspecific (e.g., fatigue, arthralgias). Later clinical manifestations include arthropathy, hepatomegaly and evidence of hepatic insufficiency (late finding), skin pigmentation (combination of slate gray due to iron and brown due to melanin, sometimes resulting in bronze color), cardiac enlargement with or without heart failure or conduction defects, diabetes mellitus with its complications, and impotence in men. Interestingly, population studies have shown an increased prevalence of liver disease but not of diabetes, arthritis, or heart disease in C282Y homozygotes. Bleeding from esophageal varices may occur, and in patients in whom cirrhosis develops, there is a 15–20% frequency of hepatocellular carcinoma. Diagnosis of persons suspected of having iron overload depends on demonstrating excess iron in blood or tissues.

Laboratory Studies

- Serum iron concentration in patients with hereditary hemochromatosis is greater than 150 mcg/dL.
- Serum ferritin level is greater than 500 ng/mL.
- Transferrin saturation is usually >45%; however, transferrin saturation greater than 62% identifies hereditary hemochromatosis in 92% of patients. If transferrin saturation is greater than 45%, the presence of the *C282Y* or *H63D* mutation may be evaluated to confirm the diagnosis of hemochromatosis.
- Liver function test shows impairment in the liver functions with abnormally high transaminases and alkaline phosphatase levels.

Imaging Studies

- Radiographs demonstrate cardiomegaly and increased pulmonary vascular markings.
- Features of restrictive cardiomyopathy are visible on echocardiograms.

Other Tests

- Genetic tests for the *C282Y* and *H63D* mutations are widely available. Detection of hemochromatosis-associated mutations is conducted to confirm the diagnosis or to discover asymptomatic patients. Detection of homozygosity for the *C282Y* mutation or compound heterozygosity for the *C282Y/H63D* mutation definitely confirms the diagnosis of hereditary hemochromatosis.
- Supraventricular arrhythmias are often revealed on electrocardiograms.

Liver Biopsy

Liver biopsy, used to assess iron deposition in hepatic cells, has long been used to establish a diagnosis of HH. In addition, liver biopsy will determine the presence of cirrhosis, fibrosis, and other abnormalities. Results of liver biopsy are also useful in ruling out other causes of iron overload. The necessity for performing a liver biopsy for HH diagnosis is controversial, although it is considered a safe and minor procedure by most hepatologists. As with other invasive procedures, there are inherent risks.

Differential Diagnosis

HH must be differentiated from causes of secondary iron overload caused by hematological disorders or metabolic defects. Several types of anemia result in accumulation of excess iron including the thalassemia, sideroblastic anemias, and congenital dyserythropoietic anemias. Liver disease including alcoholic and nonalcoholic cirrhosis, and viral hepatitis are also the causes of iron overload and may result in increased TS levels. Other conditions associated with iron overload include rare defects of iron transport and porphyria cutanea tarda. Patients who undergo multiple transfusions and persons who overuse prescribed or over-the-counter iron supplements are also at risk for iron overload.

Patient history, liver biopsy, and/or biochemical and hematologic analyses may be needed to establish a diagnosis of conditions causing secondary iron overload. DNA tests for common mutations are very likely the most important diagnostic tool for identifying HH as the cause of iron overload. In some patients, both secondary causes and HH may be contributing to iron overload.

Treatment

1. Affected patients should avoid foods rich in iron (such as red meat), alcohol, vitamin C, raw shellfish, and supplemental iron.
2. Weekly phlebotomies of 1 or 2 units (250–500 mL) of blood (each containing about 250 mg of iron) are indicated in all symptomatic patients—those with a serum ferritin level of at least 1,000 mcg/L and those with an increased fasting iron saturation, and should be continued for up to 2–3 years to achieve depletion of iron stores.
3. The hematocrit and serum iron values should be monitored. When iron store depletion is achieved (iron saturation <50% and serum ferritin level <50 mcg/L), maintenance phlebotomies (every 2–4 months) are continued (although compliance has been reported to decrease with time).
4. The chelating agent, deferoxamine, is indicated for patients with hemochromatosis and anemia or in those with secondary iron overload due to thalassemia who cannot tolerate phlebotomies, treatment is painful and time-consuming.
5. An oral chelator, deferasirox—20 mg/kg once daily has been approved for treatment of iron overload due to blood transfusions.
6. Complications of hemochromatosis—arthropathy, diabetes, heart disease, portal hypertension, and hypopituitarism—also require treatment.
7. Liver transplantation for advanced cirrhosis associated with severe iron overload including hemochromatosis, has been reported to lead to survival rates that are lower than those for other types of liver disease because of cardiac complications and an increased risk of infections.

Prognosis

The major determinant of prognosis is the degree of organ damage from iron overload at the point of diagnosis. The presence of cirrhosis reduces life expectancy. Hemochromatosis patients with cirrhosis at the time of diagnosis are over five times more likely to die compared to hemochromatosis patients without cirrhosis.

CLINICAL NOTE

Although rarely seen in clinical practice, the classic triad of skin hyperpigmentation (bronzing), type 2 diabetes, and hepatic cirrhosis has long been recognized as evidence of advanced iron overload.

CLINICAL PEARLS

1. HH is a fairly common disease in whites and is a result of iron deposition in hepatocytes, myocardial fibers, and other visceral cells.
2. In HH, two mutations of the *HFE* gene have been described—*C282Y* and *H63D*.
3. Persons homozygous for mutations of the *hemochromatosis* gene, *HFE*, absorb 3–4 mg of dietary iron daily, a rate two to three times greater than normal. Normal storage sites become overloaded with iron, resulting in ferritin levels as much as ten times normal. With no mechanism to dispose of the excess, iron is deposited in the parenchymal cells of the liver, pancreas, pituitary, heart, synovium, and other tissues.
4. This disease is usually diagnosed by elevated iron saturation, serum ferritin, a positive family history, hepatic abnormalities and cirrhosis, congestive heart failure, hypogonadism, arthritis, and *HFE* gene mutation (usually *C282Y/C282Y*), which is found in most cases.
5. Weekly phlebotomies of 1 or 2 units (250–500 mL) of blood (each containing about 250 mg of iron) are indicated in all symptomatic patients—those with a serum ferritin level of at least 1,000 mcg/L and those with an increased fasting iron saturation, and should be continued for up to 2–3 years to achieve depletion of iron stores.

CASE STUDY 3

Theme: Asymptomatic Hypercalcemia

An asymptomatic 55-year-old woman on a routine physical examination was noted to have the following abnormalities in her biochemical profile:
Serum calcium = 11.3 mg/dL (normal: 8.4–10.2 mg/dL)
Serum phosphorous = 2.9 mg/dL (normal: 3.0–4.5 mg/dL)
Serum sodium = 140 mEq/L (normal: 135–147 mEq/L)
Serum potassium = 4.0 mEq/L (normal: 3.5–5.0 mEq/L)
Serum chloride = 106 mEq/L (normal: 95–105 mEq/L)
Serum bicarbonate = 20 mEq/L (normal: 22–28 mEq/L)

What is the differential diagnosis for hypercalcemia?
Is there a simple test that can help to differentiate the cause of her hypercalcemia?
What additional test should be ordered to confirm your diagnosis?

CASE DETAILS

Hypercalcemia in an ambulatory setting is most commonly due to primary hyperparathyroidism (HPTH), whereas in the hospital, it is most commonly secondary to malignancy with either metastasis to the bone marrow or the secretion of a parathormone-like peptide. Other diseases account for <25% of all cases of hypercalcemia; hence, the differential is primarily between HPTH and cancer-induced hypercalcemia. Since this patient is asymptomatic and ambulatory, primary HPTH is more likely. Parathormone (PTH) normally increases the distal reabsorption of calcium and inhibits the proximal reabsorption of phosphate. Hence, an excess of PTH secreted by a parathyroid adenoma (most common cause) will produce hypercalcemia and hypophosphatemia. The serum PTH level should be determined in this patient; it will be elevated in primary HPTH and depressed in any other cause of hypercalcemia.

CASE STUDY 4

Theme: Clinical Implications of Hypercalcemic Crisis

A 46-year-old woman stopped by airport police for erratic driving was sent by ambulance to the emergency department (ED) with an initial complaint of generalized confusion, which she stated started approximately 24 hours prior. She was at the airport to meet her daughter, who was due to arrive at 13:00, but the actual time she was detained by the officers was 20:30 (7½ hours after the pickup time). The daughter was contacted by phone and was able to provide a past medical history of alcohol abuse, depression, and hypertension. The patient was unable to recall her prescribed medications; she denied recent illicit drug or alcohol use or any allergies to medications. Her appearance was that of a clean, well-groomed individual.

She was extremely lethargic and fell asleep during her examination. Her initial vital signs were: Blood pressure 180/100 mm Hg, heart rate 77 beats per minute, respiratory rate of 18 breaths per minute, and a temperature of 97.8°F. Cardiac monitoring revealed sinus rhythm.

The patient's physical examination was essentially unremarkable with no focal motor or sensory deficits. Laboratory studies included the following: Comprehensive metabolic panel showed electrolyte derangements with hyponatremia, hypokalemia, and most importantly, hypercalcemia with an extremely elevated lipase level. The serum calcium level was 14.2 mg/dL, complete blood count was normal, cardiac enzymes and serum drug screen were all normal. BUN and creatinine were significantly high. Hormonal result revealed normal cortisol and TSH but high PTH [PTH-82.0 pg/mL (reference value-12–72pg/mL].

Bedside glucose reading was 115 mg/dL. No odors of acetone or alcohol were present and a serum alcohol was negative. In addition, an electrocardiograph (EKG), chest X-ray, and computed tomographic (CT) scan of the head were ordered. The EKG interpretation was normal sinus rhythm with nonspecific repolarization abnormality; the CT and chest X-ray were negative.

What is the probable diagnosis?

CASE DISCUSSION

The patient is suffering from hypercalcemic crisis.

The patient presented with a significant confused state of mind with drowsiness, lethargy, and hypertension. Based on the laboratory investigation report, she was found to be hyponatremic, hypokalemic, and most importantly, hypercalcemic. The clinical manifestations were vague, showing the effect on multiple organ systems. The altered mental status was due to severe hypercalcemia and associated electrolyte imbalance. The extremely elevated lipase level was as a result of acute pancreatitis probably secondary to hypercalcemia and/or her chronic alcoholism. The high BUN and creatinine were due to acute renal failure as a result of hypercalcemia. The PTH level was above normal, so hypercalcemia was likely to be PTH mediated.

Regulation of serum calcium within a range of 8.5–10.5 mg/dL, is tightly managed by two hormones—parathyroid hormone (PTH) and calcitriol. Several factors can affect the body's ability to maintain homeostasis. >90% of hypercalcemia is caused by primary hyperparathyroidism (HPT) or malignancy. Determining the etiology can be daunting during a hypercalcemic crisis due to the difficulty of obtaining an accurate history in the presence of the neurological dysfunction, which is common when calcium levels are greater than 12 mg/dL. Symptoms may also include muscle weakness, constipation, anorexia, nausea, vomiting, and abdominal pain. Other concurrent electrolyte abnormalities may coexist. Less common findings possibly seen in a hypercalcemic crisis when levels reach 15 mg/dL or more are pancreatitis, peptic ulcers, hypertension, and cardiac effects (bradycardia or shortened QT intervals). If left untreated, hypercalcemic crisis can eventually lead to renal failure and/or coma.

Treatment consists of rapid correction of hypercalcemia through intravenous hydration and loop diuretics, provided renal function is adequate. Several medications can also help to maintain calcium levels. However, if the patient is in renal failure, dialysis must be considered. Ultimately, the cause must be identified and treated.

HYPERCALCEMIA

Hypercalcemia is total serum Ca >12 mg/dL (3 mmol/L), or ionized Ca >6 mg/dL (1.5 mmol/L). The reference range of serum calcium levels is 8.7–10.4 mg/dL, with somewhat higher levels present in children. Approximately 40% of the calcium is bound to protein, primarily albumin, while 50% is ionized and is in physiologic active form. The remaining 10% is complexed to anions. Hypercalcemic crisis does not have an exact definition, although marked elevation of serum calcium, usually >14 mg/dL, is associated with acute signs and symptoms of hypercalcemia. Treatment of the elevated calcium level may resolve the crisis.

Causes

Plasma calcium is maintained within the reference range by a complex interplay of 3 major hormones—parathyroid hormone (PTH), 1,25-dihydroxyvitamin D (i.e., calcitriol), and calcitonin. These 3 hormones act primarily at bone, kidney, and small intestine sites to maintain appropriate calcium levels **(Fig. 12.4)**.

Calcium enters the body through the small intestine and eventually is excreted via the kidney. Bone can act as a storage depot. This entire system is controlled through a feedback loop; individual hormones respond as needed to increase or decrease the serum calcium concentration.

For hypercalcemia to develop, the normal calcium regulation system must be overwhelmed by an excess of PTH, calcitriol, some other serum factor that can mimic these hormones, or a huge calcium load.

Hypercalcemia is divided into PTH-mediated hypercalcemia (primary hyperparathyroidism) and nonPTH-mediated hypercalcemia.

PTH-mediated hypercalcemia is related to increased calcium absorption from the intestine. Primary hyperparathyroidism originally was the disease of "stones, bones, and abdominal groans". In most primary hyperparathyroidism cases, the calcium elevation is caused by increased intestinal calcium absorption. This is mediated by the PTH-induced calcitriol synthesis that enhances calcium absorption. The increase in serum calcium results in an increase in calcium filtration at the kidney. Because of PTH-mediated absorption of calcium at the distal tubule, less calcium is excreted than might be expected. In PTH-mediated hypercalcemia, bones do not play an active role because most of the PTH-mediated osteoclastic activity that breaks down bone is offset by hypercalcemic-induced bone deposition. Hypercalcemia of this disorder may remain mild for long periods because some parathyroid adenomas respond to the feedback generated by the elevated calcium levels. The cause of primary hyperparathyroidism may be solitary adenomas, multiple endocrine neoplasia, lithium therapy, or familial hypocalciuric hypercalcemia.

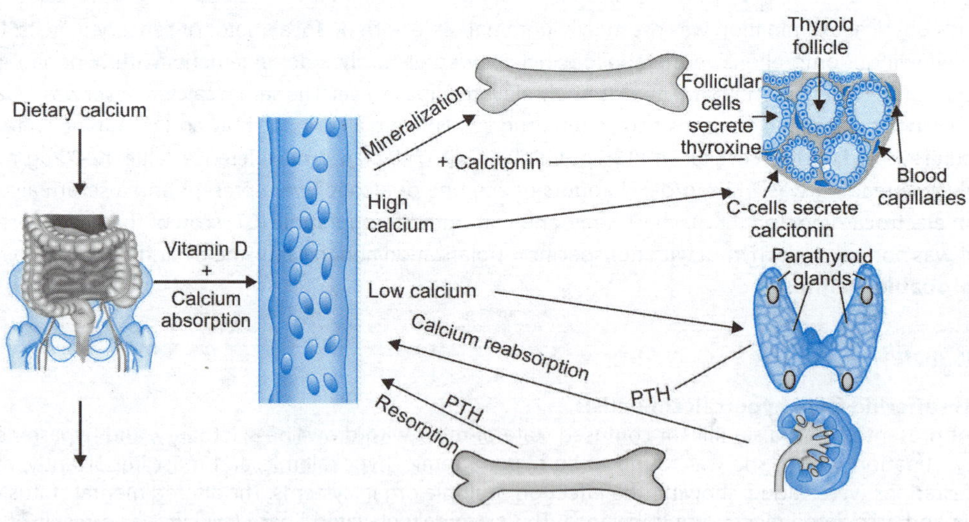

Fig. 12.4: The extracellular calcium concentrations are maintained within an exquisitely narrow range through a series of feedback mechanisms that involve parathyroid hormone (PTH) and the active vitamin D metabolite 1,25-dihydroxyvitamin D [1,25(OH)2D]. These feedback mechanisms are orchestrated by integrating signals between the parathyroid glands, kidney, intestine, and bone.

nonPTH-mediated hypercalcemia includes the following:

- **Hypercalcemia associated with malignancy:** Unlike PTH-mediated hypercalcemia, the elevation of calcium that results from malignancy generally worsens until therapy is provided. Hypercalcemia caused by malignancy is the result of increased osteoclastic activity within the bone. This results from one or both of the mechanisms that follow:
  - Extensive localized bone destruction may result from osteolytic metastasis of solid tumors. Evidence indicates that many malignant cells may release local osteoclastic activating factors.
  - Increased calcium levels resulting from malignancy caused by a PTH-related protein are a second mechanism. This protein is a humeral factor that acts on the skeleton to increase bone reabsorption; it acts on the kidney to decrease excretion of calcium. The gene that produces this protein is present in many malignant tissues.

- **Granulomatous disorders:** High levels of calcitriol may be found in patients with sarcoidosis and other granulomatous diseases. In these disorders, the increased level of calcitriol results from production within the macrophages, which constitute a large portion of some granulomas.
- **Iatrogenic:** In some cases, elevation of calcium is a known adverse effect of appropriate dosage. In other cases, large ingestions must be taken to induce the increase in calcium levels.

Other causes of hypercalcemia:

- **Neoplasms (nonparathyroid):** Metastasis to the bone from breast, multiple myeloma, and hematologic malignancies (breast cancer is one of the most common malignancies responsible for hypercalcemia)
- **Nonmetastatic (humoral-induced):** Ovary, kidney, lung, head and neck, esophagus, cervix, lymphoproliferative disease, multiple endocrine neoplasia, pheochromocytoma, and hepatoma
- **Pharmacological agents:** Thiazide, calcium carbonate (antacid), hypervitaminosis D, hypervitaminosis A, lithium, milk-alkali syndrome, and theophylline toxicity
- **Endocrinopathies (nonparathyroid):** Hyperthyroidism, adrenal insufficiency, and pheochromocytoma
- Familial hypocalciuric hypercalcemia
- **Tertiary hyperparathyroidism:** Postrenal transplant and initiation of chronic hemodialysis.
- **Miscellaneous:** Immobilization, hypophosphatasia, primary infantile hyperparathyroidism, AIDS, and advanced chronic liver disease.

Clinical Manifestations

- Mild hypercalcemia (up to 11–11.5 mg/dL) is usually asymptomatic and recognized only on routine calcium measurements.
- Some patients may complain of vague neuropsychiatric symptoms including trouble concentrating, personality changes, or depression.
- Other presenting symptoms may include peptic ulcer disease or nephrolithiasis, and fracture risk may be increased.
- More severe hypercalcemia (>12–13 mg/dL), particularly if it develops acutely, may result in lethargy, stupor, or coma, as well as gastrointestinal symptoms (nausea, anorexia, constipation, or pancreatitis).
- Hypercalcemia decreases renal concentrating ability which may cause polyuria and polydipsia.
- With long-standing hyperparathyroidism, patients may present with bone pain or pathological fractures.
- Finally, hypercalcemia can result in significant electrocardiographic changes including bradycardia, AV block, and short QT interval; changes in serum calcium can be monitored by following the QT interval.

Frequency

Hypercalcemia is a fairly common metabolic emergency. Between 20 and 40% of patients with cancer develop hypercalcemia at some point in their disease.

Primary hyperparathyroidism occurs in 25 per 100,000 persons in the general population and in 75 per 100,000 hospitalized patients. This condition is the most common cause of mild hypercalcemia which can be treated on an outpatient basis.

Laboratory Investigations

Serum Albumin Concentration

- The alterations in serum calcium levels can occur due to variations in the serum albumin levels. Therefore, during the diagnostic evaluation of hypo- or hypercalcemia, it is of profound importance to assess serum albumin levels. Out of the total, about 50% of the calcium is ionized, and the rest is bound chiefly to albumin. The direct estimations of ionized calcium are possible, but they are easily affected by the methods of sample collection. Therefore, the total calcium and albumin levels are estimated to correct for serum calcium concentration. In conditions of hypoalbuminemia (low serum albumin concentration), the exact calcium concentration is calculated by adding 0.2 mM (0.8 mg/dL) to the total calcium level for every reduction in serum albumin concentration of 1.0 g/dL below the reference value of 4.1 g/dL for albumin, and conversely the corrections are made for elevations in serum albumin concentrations.
- The attempts should be taken to determine the cause of hypercalcemia. Primary hyperparathyroidism and underlying malignancies are the two most common causes of hypercalcemia. A detailed history including previous use of drugs, any neck surgery, or symptoms suggestive of lymphoma or sarcoidosis can help in the differential diagnosis of hypercalcemia.
- After diagnosing true hypercalcemia, PTH levels are estimated using a two-site assay for the intact hormone. High PTH levels are usually associated with hypophosphatemia.
- As hypercalcemia is known to affect renal function, therefore, additionally, serum creatinine should be measured to assess the functional status of the kidney.
- In the presence of high calcium, low phosphorus, and high PTH (or "inappropriately normal") levels, the diagnosis of primary hyperparathyroidism is established. Patients with familial hypocalciuric hypercalcemia (FHH) can have similar findings. Therefore, the diagnosis of FHH should be ruled out, as the surgical intervention does not help these patients.

- A calcium/creatinine clearance ratio (calculated as urine calcium/serum calcium divided by urine creatinine/serum creatinine) of <0.01 suggests FHH, especially when there is a family history of mild, asymptomatic hypercalcemia. Ectopic PTH secretion is exceptionally uncommon.
- A low PTH level in the presence of hypercalcemia is inconsistent with parathyroid-mediated hypercalcemia; frequently, it is due to underlying malignancy.
- Serum calcitriol [1,25$(OH)_2$D] levels increase in granulomatous disorders. Therefore, clinical assessment in combination with laboratory testing can provide a background for the diagnosis of various disorders.

Imaging Studies

- No imaging studies definitively diagnose hypercalcemia.
- Consider hypercalcemia in patients with multiple nonspecific complaints and an associated lung mass.
- If laboratory evidence of primary hyperparathyroidism is present, CT scan of the head, MRI, ultrasound, or nuclear parathyroid scans may be helpful. Preoperative diagnostic imaging is essential in patients with previous neck surgery.

Hypercalcemia: Treatment

- No immediate treatment is required for the mild and symptomless hypercalcemia. The underlying cause guides the management of hypercalcemia. Irrespective of the cause, therapeutic intervention is necessary for the **profound symptomatic hypercalcemia.**
- The initial treatment of severe hypercalcemia starts with restoration of plasma volume since hypercalcemia inevitably causes dehydration. Therefore, 4–6 L of intravenous saline may be required over the first 24 hours because underlying comorbidities (e.g., congestive heart failure) may need the use of loop diuretics to increase sodium and calcium loss. However, loop diuretic therapy should not be commenced until the volume status has been revived to normal.
- In those conditions, when there is increased bone resorption,, such as in severe hyperparathyroidism or underlying malignancy, the drugs that prevent bone resorption should be considered. For example, zoledronic acid, pamidronate, and etidronate have been approved by the US Food and Drug Administration for the management of hypercalcemia of malignancy in adults. The onset of action might take place within 1–3 days but normalization of serum calcium levels are achieved in 60–90% of patients. Bisphosphonate infusions can be repeated in case relapse of hypercalcemia occurs.
- In rare instances, dialysis can be undertaken.
- Finally, as intravenous phosphate chelates calcium and lowers serum calcium levels, yet this therapy can be toxic since calcium–phosphate complexes may accumulate in tissues causing extensive organ damage.
- In patients with vitamin D-mediated hypercalcemia, glucocorticoids are preferred, as they lower vitamin D production. Intravenous hydrocortisone (100–300 mg daily) or oral prednisone (40–60 mg daily) for 3–7 days are used most often.
- Alternatively, drugs, such as ketoconazole, chloroquine, and hydroxychloroquine can also lower vitamin D production and are used frequently.
- Depending upon the state of the patient, the primary cause needs to be treated.

Prognosis

The prognosis depends upon the cause of hypercalcemia.

- Prognosis is worse in patients having malignancy with hypercalcemia.
- Prognosis is satisfactory, if the underlying cause is treatable, and treatment is started immediately.

CLINICAL NOTE

Although direct measurements of ionized calcium are possible, they are easily influenced by collection methods and other artifacts; thus, it is generally preferable to measure total calcium and albumin to "correct" the serum calcium.

CLINICAL PEARLS

1. Hypercalcemia is total serum Ca >12 mg/dL (3 mmol/L), or ionized Ca >6 mg/dL (1.5 mmol/L).
2. The most common cause is iatrogenic.
3. Gastrointestinal (GI) signs may occur (anorexia, vomiting, and constipation) and sometimes lethargy or seizures.
4. Mild, asymptomatic hypercalcemia does not require immediate therapy, and management should be dictated by the underlying diagnosis.
5. Treatment is IV saline plus furosemide and sometimes bisphosphonates.

CASE STUDY 5

Theme: Calcium Homeostasis and Clinical Implications of Hypocalcemia

A 14-year-old girl presented with muscle pain and cramps, stiffness, tingling of hands and feet, recurrent carpopedal spasms, and tetanic postures of both hands and feet since 2 months. She was born of third degree consanguineous marriage and was 2nd of 3 children with other siblings being normal. Her vegetarian diet contained no milk or milk products or vegetables.

On examination, she had no signs of rickets or short stature. Her blood pressure was normal. Her Trousseau's sign was positive. She had no skin pigmentation or oral thrush. Investigations showed hypocalcemia (serum calcium = 6.3 mg%) with hyperphosphatemia (serum phosphorus = 11.0 mg%) and elevated serum alkaline phosphatase (278 IU/L) with serum ionic calcium of 0.45 mmol/L. Her renal functions, blood gas analysis, hemogram, and urine calcium/creatinine were normal. Her serum parathyroid levels were low [10.1 pg/mL (normal = 12–72 pg/mL)] in spite of a low serum calcium. Her thyroid function tests were normal. Antimicrosomal antibody was elevated. She was treated with IV calcium, oral calcitriol, and calcium carbonate supplements.

What is the probable cause of hypocalcemia in this patient?

CASE DETAILS

The patient presents with muscle pain and cramps, stiffness, tingling of hands and feet with carpopedal spasms. Her Trousseau's sign is positive. Investigations reveal hypocalcemia with hyperphosphatemia. She is suspected to have hypocalcemic tetany, which could be due to hypoparathyroidism or chronic renal failure. Since the renal functions, blood gas analysis, hemogram, and urine calcium/creatinine are normal, so the possibility of renal failure as a cause is ruled out. Serum alkaline phosphatase is high, serum parathyroid levels are low, and antimicrosomal antibody is also elevated. Hypocalcemic tetany seems to be due to isolated autoimmune hypoparathyroidism. Hypoparathyroidism can occur due to aplasia or hypoplasia of parathyroid glands, parathyroid hormone gene mutations, autoimmune parathyroiditis, hemosiderosis, Wilson's disease, familial congenital variant with dysmorphic features or surgical removal or damage to the parathyroid glands during thyroidectomy.

Autoimmune hypoparathyroidism in the given patient is suggested by the finding of parathyroid antibodies. Autoimmune hypoparathyroidism is seen frequently in association with other autoimmune disorders. It is often seen as a part of polyglandular autoimmune disease type I (at least 2 of the following are required—autoimmune hypoparathyroidism, Addison's disease, and chronic mucocutaneous candidiasis). Since there are no clinical findings suggestive of either Addison's disease or chronic mucocutaneous candidiasis, so it is unlikely to be a part of polyglandular autoimmune disease type I. The likely diagnosis is isolated autoimmune hypoparathyroidism.

Overview of Calcium Metabolism

Calcium is required for the proper functioning of muscle contraction, nerve conduction, hormone release, and blood coagulation. In addition, proper Ca concentration is required for various other metabolic processes.

Maintenance of body Ca stores depends on:

- Dietary Ca intake
- Absorption of Ca from the GI tract
- Renal Ca excretion **(Fig. 12.4)**

In a balanced diet, roughly 1,000 mg of Ca is ingested each day and about another 200 mg/day is secreted into the GI tract in the bile and other GI secretions. Depending on the concentration of circulating vitamin D, particularly 1,25(OH)2D [1,25-dihydroxycholecalciferol, calcitriol, or active vitamin D, which is converted in the kidney from 25(OH)D, the inactive form], roughly 200–400 mg of Ca is absorbed from the intestine each day. The remaining 800–1,000 mg appears in the stool. Ca balance is maintained through renal Ca excretion averaging 200 mg/day.

Both extracellular and intracellular Ca concentrations are tightly regulated by bidirectional Ca transport across the plasma membrane of cells and intracellular organelles,, such as the endoplasmic reticulum, the sarcoplasmic reticulum of muscle cells, and the mitochondria. Cytosolic ionized Ca is maintained within the micromolar range (<1/1,000 of the serum concentration). Ionized Ca acts as an intracellular 2nd messenger; it is involved in skeletal muscle contraction, excitation–contraction coupling in cardiac and smooth muscle, and activation of protein kinases and enzyme phosphorylation. Ca is also involved in the action of other intracellular messengers,, such as cyclic adenosine monophosphate (cAMP) and inositol 1,4,5-triphosphate, and thus mediates the cellular response to numerous hormones including epinephrine, glucagon, ADH (vasopressin), secretin, and cholecystokinin. Parathyroid hormone (PTH) increases urinary cAMP.

Despite its important intracellular roles, roughly 99% of body Ca is in bone, mainly as hydroxyapatite crystals. Roughly 1% of bone Ca is freely exchangeable with the ECF and, therefore, is available for buffering changes in Ca balance.

Normal total serum Ca concentration ranges from 8.8–10.4 mg/dL (2.20–2.60 mmol/L). About 40% of the total blood Ca is bound to plasma proteins, primarily albumin. The remaining 60% includes ionized Ca plus Ca complexed with phosphate (PO_4) and citrate. Total Ca (i.e., protein-bound, complexed, and ionized Ca) is usually what is determined by clinical laboratory measurement. Ideally, the ionized or free Ca should be determined, because this is the physiologically active form of Ca in plasma; this direct determination of ionized calcium, because of its technical difficulty, is usually restricted to patients in whom significant alteration of protein binding of plasma Ca is suspected. Ionized Ca is generally assumed to be roughly 50% of the total serum Ca.

REGULATION OF CALCIUM METABOLISM

The metabolism of Ca and of PO_4 is intimately related. The regulation of both Ca and PO_4 balance is greatly influenced by concentrations of circulating PTH, vitamin D, and, to a lesser extent, calcitonin **(Fig. 12.4)**.

Carcinoma and inorganic PO_4 concentrations are also linked by their ability to chemically react to form $CaPO_4$. The product of concentrations of Ca and PO_4 (in mEq/L) is estimated to be 60 normally; when the product exceeds 70, precipitation of $CaPO_4$ crystals in soft tissue is much more likely. Calcification of vascular tissue accelerates arteriosclerotic vascular disease and may occur when the Ca × PO_4 product is even lower (>55), especially in patients with chronic kidney disease.

Parathormone is secreted by the parathyroid glands. It has several actions, but perhaps the most important is to defend against hypocalcemia. Parathyroid cells sense decreases in serum Ca and, in response release preformed PTH into the circulation **(Fig. 12.5)**. PTH increases serum Ca within minutes by increasing renal and intestinal absorption of Ca and by rapidly mobilizing Ca and PO_4 from bone (bone resorption). Renal Ca excretion generally parallels Na excretion and is influenced by many of the same factors that govern Na transport in the proximal tubule. However, PTH enhances distal tubular Ca reabsorption independently of Na. PTH also decreases renal PO_4 reabsorption and thus increases renal PO_4 losses. Renal PO_4 loss prevents the solubility product of Ca and PO_4 from being exceeded in plasma as Ca concentrations rise in response to PTH. PTH also increases serum Ca by stimulating conversion of vitamin D to its most active form, calcitriol. This form of vitamin D increases the percentage of dietary Ca absorbed by the intestine **(Fig. 12.5)**. Despite increased Ca absorption, long-term increases in PTH secretion generally result in further bone resorption by inhibiting osteoblastic function and promoting osteoclastic activity. PTH and vitamin D both function as important regulators of bone growth and bone remodeling.

Calcitonin is secreted by the thyroid parafollicular cells (C cells). Calcitonin tends to lower serum Ca concentration by enhancing cellular uptake, renal excretion, and bone formation. The effects of calcitonin on bone metabolism are much weaker than those of either PTH or vitamin D.

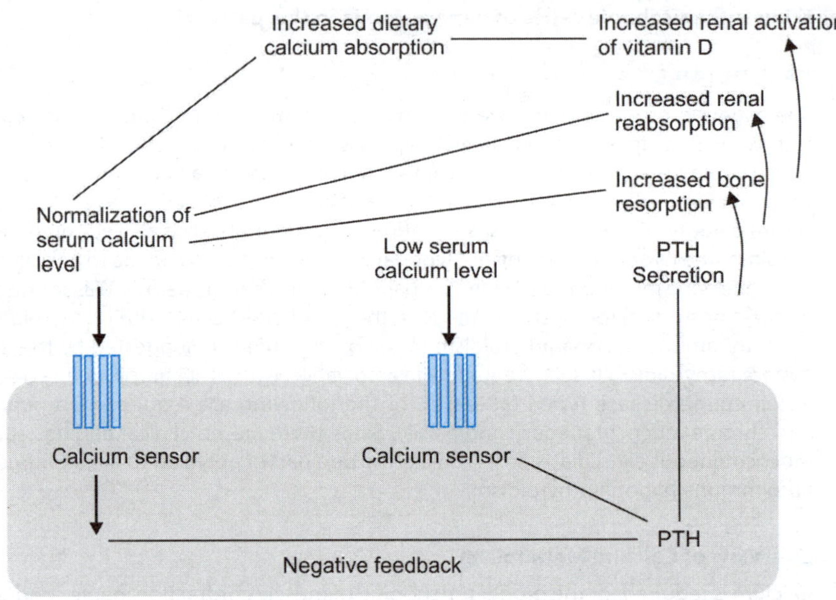

Fig. 12.5: A decrease in extracellular (ECF) calcium (Ca^{2+}) triggers an increase in PTH secretion (1) via activation of the calcium sensor receptor on parathyroid cells. PTH, in turn, results in increased tubular reabsorption of calcium by the kidney (2) and resorption of calcium from bone (2) and also stimulates renal 1,25(OH)2D production (3). 1,25(OH)2D, in turn, acts principally on the intestine to increase calcium absorption (4). Collectively, these homeostatic mechanisms serve to restore serum calcium levels to normal.

HYPOCALCEMIA

Causes

The causes of hypocalcemia include hypoalbuminemia, hypomagnesemia, hyperphosphatemia, multifactorial enhanced protein binding and anion chelation, medication effects, surgical effects, PTH deficiency or resistance, and vitamin D deficiency or resistance.

- Hypoalbuminemia is the most common cause of hypocalcemia and is due to cirrhosis, nephrosis, malnutrition, burns, chronic illness, and sepsis.
- Hypomagnesemia causes end-organ resistance to PTH and inhibits the hypocalcemic feedback loop through uncertain mechanisms. Causes of hypomagnesemia include pancreatitis, aminoglycoside treatment, amphotericin B, loop diuretics, alcoholism, and malnutrition.
- Hyperphosphatemia may be seen in critical illness and in patients who have ingested phosphate-containing enemas. Phosphate binds calcium avidly, causing acute hypocalcemia.
- Multifactorial causes are probably the most clinically relevant hypocalcemic emergencies in the ED and include the following:
  - Acute pancreatitis: Free fatty acids chelate calcium, causing saponification in the retroperitoneum.
  - Rhabdomyolysis: Increased phosphates from creatine phosphokinase (CPK) and other anions (i.e., lactate, bicarbonate) chelate calcium.

- Sepsis can cause hypocalcemia through many mechanisms.
- Toxic shock syndrome can cause hypocalcemia.
- High calcitonin levels cause low calcium.
- Malignancy: Osteoblastic metastases (e.g., breast cancer, prostate cancer) and tumor lysis syndrome may cause hypocalcemia (by differing mechanisms).
- Hepatic or renal insufficiency: Calciuresis, hypomagnesemia, hypoalbuminemia, and low active vitamin D levels may contribute to poor calcium homeostasis.
- Infiltrative disease: Sarcoidosis, tuberculosis, and hemochromatosis may infiltrate the parathyroids, causing dysfunction.

- **Enhanced protein binding and anion chelation:**
  - Protein binding is enhanced by elevated pH and free fatty acid release in high catecholamine states.
  - Anion chelation is seen in high-phosphate states (e.g., renal failure, rhabdomyolysis, mesenteric ischemia, oral administration of phosphate-containing enemas); high citrate states (e.g., massive blood transfusion, radiocontrast dyes); and high bicarbonate, lactate, and oxalate levels.
- **Medication effects:**
  - Proton pump inhibitors (PPIs) reduce gastric acid production resulting in reduced calcium absorption. An association with these medicines and an increased risk for hip fractures in elderly patients has been made due to decreased calcium absorption.
  - Selective serotonin inhibitors can have a calcium antagonistic effect on smooth muscle, particularly vascular endothelium.
  - Calcitonin and bisphosphonates cause chelation and end-organ inhibition.
  - Phenobarbital and phenytoin enhance vitamin D catabolism and decrease calcium resorption in the gut.
  - Ethylene glycol complexes with calcium.
  - Estrogen inhibits bone resorption.
  - Cimetidine decreases gastric pH, slowing fat breakdown, which is necessary to complex calcium for gut absorption.
  - Aluminum and alcohol suppress PTH.
  - Gadolinium-based contrast material can falsely lower serum calcium levels and should be considered, if levels are drawn shortly after magnetic resonance imaging.
- **Postsurgical effects:**
  - Parathyroid adenoma resection causes a transient hypocalcemia due to end-organ PTH resistance in the first postoperative day.
  - Vascular/parathyroid injury may occur during trauma or as an operative mishap.
  - Pancreatectomy prevents calcium absorption in the duodenum and the jejunum by eliminating necessary enzymes.
  - Small bowel syndrome causes hypocalcemia by reducing the surface available to absorb fatty acids and calcium.
- **PTH deficiency/resistance:**
  - Childhood/congenital causes are rare but include DiGeorge syndrome.
  - Idiopathic hypoparathyroidism interferes with calcium regulation.
  - Infiltrative diseases include Wilson's disease and metastatic cancer.
  - Pseudohypoparathyroidism is due to PTH resistance and has many forms, most notably Albright disease.
  - Renal failure can result in a variety of endocrine disorders, occasionally including hypocalcemia.
- **Vitamin D deficiency/resistance:**
  - Rickets may be due to lack of vitamin D or end-organ receptor resistance.
  - Hepatorenal disease: The liver and the kidney provide intermediary enzymes to form active 1,25$(OH)_2$D.

Incidence

The incidence of ionized hypocalcemia is difficult to quantify, but it has been reported to be 15–50% for ICU patients.

Mortality/Morbidity

Severe symptomatic hypocalcemia may result in cardiovascular collapse, hypotension unresponsive to fluids and vasopressors, and dysrhythmias. Neurological sequelae (e.g., tetany, seizures) may occur. Death is rare but has been reported. The disease causing hypocalcemia may have greater impact on morbidity than hypocalcemia itself.

Clinical Manifestations

Patients with hypocalcemia may be asymptomatic, if the decreases in serum calcium are relatively mild and chronic, or they may present with life-threatening complications. Moderate-to-severe hypocalcemia is associated with paresthesias, usually of the fingers, toes, and circumoral regions, and is caused by increased neuromuscular irritability. Chronic manifestations include cataracts, dry skin, coarse hair, brittle nails, psoriasis, chronic pruritus, and poor dentition. On physical examination, a Chvostek's sign (twitching of the circumoral muscles in response to gentle tapping of the facial nerve just anterior to the ear) may be elicited, although it is also present in ~10% of normal individuals. Carpal spasm may be induced by inflation of a blood pressure cuff to 20 mm Hg above the patient's systolic blood pressure for 3 minutes (Trousseau's sign). Severe hypocalcemia can induce seizures, carpopedal spasm, bronchospasm, laryngospasm, and prolongation of the QT interval. Acute hypocalcemia may lead to syncope, congestive heart failure (CHF), and angina due to the multiple cardiovascular effects.

Laboratory Investigations

Symptomatic patients with classic clinical findings of acute hypocalcemia require immediate resuscitation and evaluation. However, most cases of hypocalcemia are discovered by clinical suspicion and appropriate laboratory testing.

- **Calcium levels:**
  - A serum calcium level <8.5 mg/dL or an ionized calcium <1.0 mmol/L is considered hypocalcemia.
  - In respiratory alkalosis, total serum calcium is normal but ionized calcium is low.
  - Analysis for ionized level must be performed rapidly with whole blood to avoid changes in pH and anion chelation. Blood should be drawn in an unheparinized syringe for best results.
  - Falsely elevated calcium levels may be seen with elevated acetaminophen levels, alcohol, hydralazine, and hemolysis.
  - Falsely depressed levels can be seen with heparin, oxalate, citrate, or hyperbilirubinemia.
- Magnesium, phosphate, and other electrolyte levels should be obtained.
- Elevated BUN and creatinine levels may indicate renal dysfunction.
- Albumin, liver function studies, and coagulation parameters should be obtained to assess liver dysfunction and hypoalbuminemia.
- The PTH level (an antibody-mediated radioimmunoassay) should be checked as early as possible.
- Vitamin D levels should also be measured to know the cause of hypocalcemia.

Other Tests

Electrocardiogram (ECG) and electrocardiographic monitoring should be obtained to rule out dysrhythmias and a prolonged QT interval.

Hypocalcemia: Treatment

The approach to treatment depends on the severity of the hypocalcemia, the rapidity with which it develops, and the accompanying complications (e.g., seizures, laryngospasm).

Severe Symptomatic Hypocalcemia

In the presence of tetany, arrhythmias or seizures, calcium gluconate 10% (10–20 mL) administered intravenously over 10–15 minutes is indicated. Because of the short duration of action, calcium infusion is usually required. 10–15 mg of calcium per kilogram body weight, or six to eight 10 mL vials of 10% calcium gluconate (558–744 mg of calcium), are added to 1 L of D5W and infused over 4–6 hours. By monitoring the serum calcium level frequently (every 4–6 hours), the infusion rate is adjusted to maintain the serum calcium level at 7–8.5 mg/dL.

Asymptomatic Hypocalcemia

Oral calcium (1–2 g) and vitamin D preparations, including active vitamin D sterols, are used. Calcium carbonate is well tolerated and less expensive than many other calcium tablets. A check of urinary calcium excretion is recommended after the initiation of therapy because hypercalciuria (urine calcium excretion >200 mg/day or urine calcium/urine creatinine ratio >0.3) may impair kidney function in these patients. The low serum Ca^{2+} associated with low serum albumin concentration does not require replacement therapy. If serum Mg^{2+} is low, therapy must include replacement of magnesium, which by itself will usually correct hypocalcemia.

Prognosis

Prognosis is dependent on the etiology of hypocalcemia but is generally good.

CLINICAL NOTE

Hypocalcemia generally results from another disease process. Confirmation of the diagnosis for the diseases that caused hypocalcemia is important, so that the cause can be identified and managed early.

CLINICAL PEARLS

1. The causes of hypocalcemia include hypoalbuminemia, hypomagnesemia, hyperphosphatemia, multifactorial enhanced protein binding and anion chelation, medication effects, surgical effects, PTH deficiency or resistance, and vitamin D deficiency or resistance.
2. Moderate-to-severe hypocalcemia is associated with paresthesias, usually of the fingers, toes, and circumoral regions, and is caused by increased neuromuscular irritability.
3. On physical examination, a Chvostek's sign (twitching of the circumoral muscles in response to gentle tapping of the facial nerve just anterior to the ear) can be elicited and carpal spasm may be induced by inflation of a blood pressure cuff to 20 mm Hg above the patient's systolic blood pressure for 3 minutes (Trousseau's sign) in hypocalcemia.
4. Serum calcium, magnesium, electrolytes, vitamin D, PTH, BUN, and creatinine levels can be estimated for the diagnosis.
5. Severe symptomatic hypocalcemia requires calcium gluconate infusion while asymptomatic hypocalcemia requires oral calcium and vitamin D supplementation.

CASE STUDY 6

Theme: Neonatal Hypocalcemia

A 10-day-old boy was admitted with new-onset focal seizures. In the previous 6 days, his parents had noted the left-sided arm and leg twitching, right-sided head turning, and lip smacking. These episodes lasted for approximately 30 seconds, and their frequency had increased to seven times per hour before admission. There was no history of fever, trauma, sick contacts, or neonatal sepsis risk factors. The baby was breastfed and supplemented with formula. The pregnancy was unremarkable and the baby was born at term by an uncomplicated Cesarean section because of a previous Cesarean section. His birth weight was 4.1 kg (75–95th percentile). On admission, focal seizures, as described, were witnessed. He was afebrile with normal vital signs. He had no dysmorphic features and his physical examination was otherwise unremarkable.

Initial blood work showed normal renal function and electrolytes, with hypocalcemia [total calcium 1.80 mmol/L (normal: 1.96–2.66 mmol/L) and ionized calcium 0.82 mmol/L (normal: 1.14–1.29 mmol/L)] and hyperphosphatemia 3.30 mmol/L (normal: 1.62–3.10 mmol/L). His blood glucose level was within normal limits, 4.3 mmol/L.

The diagnosis was revealed after further maternal history and blood tests.

On further investigation, the mother was noted to have a diet low in calcium and she reported not taking any antenatal vitamin supplements. She also reported always wearing sunscreen when outdoors. The baby had not been started on vitamin D supplements.

Vitamin D deficiency in the infant was diagnosed on the basis of a low 25-hydroxyvitamin D level of 13 mmol/L (normal: 27–110 mmol/L), with a normal 1,25-hydroxyvitamin D level of 173 pmol/L (normal: 39–193 pmol/L).

A low 25-hydroxyvitamin D level indicates that vitamin D stores are low, while a normal 1,25-hydroxyvitamin D level confirms that the child is able to convert vitamin D to its active form. The infant's parathyroid hormone (PTH) level was appropriately elevated at 70 ng/L (normal: 10–65 ng/L). Urine calcium to creatinine ratio, head ultrasound, and electroencephalography were normal, there was no clinical or radiological evidence of rickets and there was no clinical or radiological evidence of rickets.

Maternal investigations demonstrated a normal calcium level of 2.27 mmol/L (normal: 2.19–2.60 mmol/L), 25-hydroxyvitamin D level of 16 nmol/L (normal: 17–95 nmol/L), and an elevated PTH level of 88 ng/L (normal: 10–65 ng/L). The baby was managed with an intravenous calcium gluconate infusion, oral calcium, vitamin D, and calcitriol (1,25-dihydroxyvitamin D). The seizures resolved within 48 hours of admission. The results of a full septic workup were negative.

What is the cause of hypocalcemia in this baby?

CASE DETAILS

The baby has symptomatic hypocalcemia due to maternal hypovitaminosis D. Hypocalcemia is a serum total Ca concentration < 8 mg/dL (<2 mmol/L) in term infants or <7 mg/dL (<0.75–1.10 mmol/L) in preterm infants depending on the method (type of electrode) used. The infant in the given case presented with symptomatic hypocalcemia at an unusually young age.

This is likely due to the profound degree of maternal hypovitaminosis D. She reported always wearing sunscreen outdoors. Sunscreen with a sun protection factor of 8 reduces cutaneous production of vitamin D by 98%. She did not supplement with vitamin D during pregnancy. Signs of hypocalcemia include hypotonia, apnea, and tetany. Treatment is IV or oral Ca supplementation.

NEONATAL HYPOCALCEMIA

Risk Factors for Neonatal Hypocalcemia

Symptomatic hypocalcemia without evidence of rickets may present in the early neonatal period. Risk factors for neonatal vitamin D deficiency secondary to maternal hypovitaminosis D include having a mother with dark skin, being born in the winter months, living at extremes of latitude, maternal diet low in vitamin D during pregnancy and lactation, and lack of maternal sun exposure.

Causes

Neonatal hypocalcemia may occur early (in the 1st 2 days of life) or late (>3 days); late-onset hypocalcemia is rare. Some infants with congenital hypoparathyroidism (e.g., from DiGeorge syndrome with agenesis or dysgenesis of the parathyroid glands) have both early and late (prolonged) hypocalcemia.

Risk factors for early hypocalcemia include prematurity, being small for gestational age, maternal diabetes, and perinatal asphyxia.

Normally, parathyroid hormone helps to maintain normal Ca levels when the constant infusion of ionized Ca across the placenta is interrupted at birth. A transient, relative hypoparathyroidism may cause hypocalcemia in preterm and some small for gestational age neonates, who have parathyroid glands that do not yet function adequately, and in infants of mothers with diabetes or hyperparathyroidism, because these women have higher-than-normal ionized Ca levels during pregnancy. Perinatal asphyxia may also increase serum calcitonin which inhibits Ca release from bone and results in hypocalcemia. In other neonates, the normal phosphaturic renal response to parathyroid hormone is absent; the elevated phosphate (PO_4) leads to hypocalcemia.

The cause of late-onset hypocalcemia is usually infant ingestion of cow's milk or formula preparations with too high a PO_4 load; elevated serum PO_4 leads to hypocalcemia. Clinical manifestations of neonatal hypocalcemia include:

- Jitteriness
- Muscle jerking
- Generalized or focal seizures
- Stridor (secondary to laryngospasm)
- Wheezing (secondary to bronchospasm)
- Vomiting (secondary to pylorospasm), and
- Prolonged QTc (QT interval corrected for rate) on electrocardiogram.

Laboratory Investigations

Initial investigations in the present scenario should include PTH, 25-hydroxyvitamin D, 1,25-dihydroxyvitamin D, and urine calcium to creatinine ratio. Other diagnostic investigations include renal function tests and plain X-rays (wrist or knee), looking for signs of rickets. Maternal calcium, 25-hydroxyvitamin D, and PTH levels should also be obtained.

Prevention

Vitamin D deficiency in infants and mothers is a re-emerging public health issue. There is no current consensus for maternal vitamin D requirements during pregnancy and lactation; however, 400 U/day is recommended for pregnant women.

Treatment

Early-onset hypocalcemia ordinarily resolves in a few days, and asymptomatic neonates with serum Ca levels >7 mg/dL (>1.75 mmol/L) or ionized Ca >3.5 mg/dL rarely require treatment. Those term infants with levels <7 mg/dL (<1.75 mmol/L) and preterm infants with Ca <6 mg/dL (<1.5 mmol/L) should be treated with 2 mL/kg of 10% Ca gluconate (200 mg/kg) by slow IV infusion over 30 minutes. Too rapid infusion can cause bradycardia, so heart rate should be monitored during the infusion. The IV site should also be watched closely because tissue infiltration by a Ca solution is irritating and may cause local tissue damage or necrosis.

After acute correction of hypocalcemia, Ca gluconate may be mixed in the maintenance IV infusion and given continuously. Starting with 400 mg/kg/day of Ca gluconate, the dose may be increased gradually to 800 mg/kg/day, if needed, to prevent a recurrence. When oral feedings are begun, the formula may be supplemented with the same daily dose of Ca gluconate, if needed, by adding the 10% Ca gluconate solution into the days formula. Supplementation is usually required for only a few days.

Treatment of late-onset hypocalcemia is addition of calcitriol or additional Ca to infant formula to provide a 4:1 molar ratio of Ca:PO_4 until normal Ca levels are maintained. Oral Ca preparations have a high sucrose content, which may lead to diarrhea in preterm infants.

CLINICAL NOTE

Ionized Ca is the more physiological measurement, because it obviates concerns about protein concentration and pH.

CLINICAL PEARLS

1. Hypocalcemia is a serum total Ca concentration <8 mg/dL (<2 mmol/L) in term infants or <7 mg/dL (<1.75 mmol/L) in preterm infants. It is also defined as an ionized Ca level <3.0–4.4 mg/dL (<0.75–1.10 mmol/L), depending on the method (type of electrode) used.
2. Signs include hypotonia, apnea, and tetany.
3. Risk factors for early hypocalcemia include prematurity, being small for gestational age, maternal diabetes, and perinatal asphyxia.
4. Diagnosis is done by measurement of serum total or ionized Ca; ionized Ca is the more physiological measurement, because it obviates concerns about protein concentration and pH. Prolongation of the corrected QT interval (QTc) on ECG also suggests hypocalcemia.
5. Treatment is IV or oral Ca supplementation.

CASE STUDY 7

Theme: Copper Metabolism and Clinical Implications of Copper Deficiency and Toxicity

A 15-year-old girl presented with abdominal pain and diarrhea for 3 days. She became jaundiced and a presumptive diagnosis of infective hepatitis was made, but serological tests were negative. She subsequently died of fulminant liver failure. At postmortem, her liver copper concentration was found to be grossly increased.
What is the probable diagnosis?
What kind of investigations should be carried out for her sister?

CASE DETAILS

High liver copper concentration indicates that the patient died of Wilson's disease, which is an autosomal recessive disorder caused by mutations in the *ATP7B* gene, a membrane-bound copper-transporting adenosine triphosphatase *(ATPase)*. Clinical manifestations are caused by copper toxicity and primarily involve the liver and the brain. Because effective treatment is available, it is important to make this diagnosis early. The patient's sister should be screened for Wilson's disease. Serum copper, ceruloplasmin, and urinary copper excretion may indicate, if she also has the disease. A liver biopsy may be indicated. DNA analysis can assist in the confirmation of diagnosis.

BASIC CONCEPT

Overview of Copper Metabolism

Copper is an essential trace element which is a component of many intracellular metalloenzymes, including cytochrome oxidase, tyrosinase, superoxide dismutase, lysyl oxidase, and dopamine β oxidase. Most of the copper in plasma is bound to ceruloplasmin.

About 50% of the average daily dietary copper of around 25 µmol (1.5 mg) is absorbed from the stomach and the small intestine. Absorbed copper is transported to the liver in portal blood bound to albumin and is exported to peripheral tissues mainly bound to ceruloplasmin and to a lesser extent to albumin.

Copper is present in all metabolically active tissues. The highest concentrations are found in liver and in kidney, with significant amount in cardiac and skeletal muscles and in bones. The liver contains 10% of the total body content of 1,200 µmol (80 mg). Excess copper is excreted in bile and then into gut, and the fecal copper output (12.5 µmol/24 hours) is the sum of the unabsorbed dietary copper and that re-excreted into the gut.

Copper Deficiency

Both children and adults can develop symptomatic copper deficiency. Premature infants are the most susceptible since copper stores in liver are laid down in the third trimester of pregnancy. In adults, copper deficiency is found in intestinal bypass surgeries or in patients who are on parenteral nutrition. Symptoms range from bone disease to iron-resistant microcytic hypochromic anemia.

Copper Toxicity

Copper toxicity is uncommon and is mostly due to administration of copper sulfate solutions. Oral copper sulfate may lead to gastric perforation. Serum copper may be greatly elevated. Copper is toxic to many organs, but renal tubular damage is more common and is of major concern. Treatment is by chelation with penicillamine.

WILSON'S DISEASE

The condition is characterized by excessive deposition of copper in the liver, brain, and other tissues. The major physiological aberration is excessive absorption of copper from the small intestine and decreased excretion of copper by the liver. Patients with Wilson's disease usually present with liver disease during the first decade of life or with neuropsychiatric illness during the third decade. The diagnosis is confirmed by measurement of serum ceruloplasmin, urinary copper excretion, and hepatic copper content, as well as the detection of Kayser–Fleischer rings.

Biochemical Defect

The genetic defect, localized to chromosome arm 13q, has been shown to affect the copper-transporting adenosine *ATPase* gene (*ATP7B*) in the liver. The *WD* gene product is a 1411 amino acid protein with highest levels of expression in the liver, kidneys, and placenta. The WD gene codes for P-type copper-transporting *ATPase*, now characterized as *ATP7B*. Many of the gene defects for *ATP7B* are small deletions, insertions, or missense mutations. Most patients carry different mutations on each of their 2 chromosomes. >200 different mutations have been identified, the most common of which is a change from a histidine to a glutamine (H1069Q).

Pathophysiology

In Wilson's disease, the processes of incorporation of copper into ceruloplasmin and excretion of excess copper into bile are impaired. The transport of copper by the copper-transporting P-type ATPase is defective secondary to one of several mutations in the *ATP7B* gene. The excess copper acts as a promoter of free radical formation and causes oxidation of lipids and proteins. Initially, the excess copper is stored in the liver and causes damage to the hepatocytes.

Defective copper incorporation into apoceruloplasmin leads to excess catabolism and low blood levels of ceruloplasmin. Serum copper levels are usually lower than normal because of low blood ceruloplasmin, which normally binds >90% of serum copper. As the disease progresses, nonceruloplasmin serum copper ("free" copper) levels increase, resulting in copper buildup in other parts of the body,, such as the brain leading to neurological and psychiatric disease.

Frequency

The frequency of Wilson's disease in most populations is about 1 in 30,000–40,000, and the frequency of carriers of *ATP7B* mutations is thus ~1%.

Mortality/Morbidity

Fulminant Wilson's disease leads to rapidly progressive liver failure, encephalopathy, coagulopathy, and eventually death if emergent liver transplantation is not performed. The fulminant presentation of Wilson's disease is more common in females than in males (4:1). Wilson's disease manifests as liver disease in children and adolescents, peaking at ages 10–13 years, and as neuropsychiatric illness in young adults aged 19–20 years.

Clinical Manifestations

Hepatic

Wilson's disease may present as hepatitis, cirrhosis, or as hepatic decompensation. An episode of hepatitis may occur, with elevated blood transaminase enzymes, with or without jaundice, and then spontaneously regresses. Hepatitis often reoccurs, and most of these patients eventually develop cirrhosis.

Hepatic decompensation is associated with elevated serum bilirubin, reduced serum albumin and coagulation factors, ascites, peripheral edema, and hepatic encephalopathy. In severe hepatic failure, hemolytic anemia may occur because large amounts of copper derived from hepatocellular necrosis are released into the bloodstream. The association of hemolysis and liver disease makes Wilson's disease a likely diagnosis.

Neurological

The neurological manifestations of Wilson's disease typically occur in patients in their early twenties, although the age of onset extends into the sixth decade of life. MRI and CT scans reveal damage in the basal ganglia and occasionally in the pons, medulla, thalamus, cerebellum, and subcortical areas. The three main movement disorders include: Dystonia, incoordination, and tremor. Dysarthria and dysphagia are common. In some patients, the clinical picture closely resembles that of Parkinson disease. Dystonia can involve any part of the body. Autonomic disturbances may include orthostatic hypotension and sweating abnormalities as well as bowel, bladder, and sexual dysfunction. Memory loss, migraine-type headaches, and seizures may occur. Patients have difficulties focusing on tasks, but cognition is not usually grossly impaired. Sensory abnormalities and muscular weakness are not features of the disease.

Psychiatric

A history of behavioral disturbances with onset in the 5 years before diagnosis, is present in half of patients with neurological disease. The features are diverse and may include loss of emotional control (temper tantrums, crying bouts), depression, hyperactivity, or loss of sexual inhibition.

Other Manifestations

Some female patients have repeated spontaneous abortions, and most become amenorrheic prior to diagnosis. Cholelithiasis and nephrolithiasis occur with increased frequencies. Some patients may have osteoarthritis, particularly of the knee. Microscopic hematuria is common, and increased urinary excretion of phosphates, amino acids, glucose, or urates may occur; however, a full-blown Fanconi syndrome is rare. Sunflower cataracts and Kayser–Fleischer rings (copper deposits in the outer rim of the cornea) may be seen. Electrocardiographic and other cardiac abnormalities have been reported but are not common.

Diagnosis

Laboratory Studies

- The presence of Kayser–Fleischer rings and ceruloplasmin levels of <20 mg/dL in a patient with neurological signs or symptoms suggest the diagnosis of Wilson's disease. If a patient is asymptomatic, exhibits isolated liver disease, and lacks corneal rings, the coexistence of a hepatic copper concentration of >250 mg/g of dry weight and a low serum ceruloplasmin level is sufficient to establish a diagnosis.
- **Serum ceruloplasmin:**
  - Serum ceruloplasmin levels are low in newborns and gradually rise within the first 2 years of life. Approximately 90% of all patients with Wilson's disease have ceruloplasmin levels of <20 mg/dL (reference range: 20–40 mg/dL).
  - Ceruloplasmin is an acute phase reactant and may be increased in response to hepatic inflammation, pregnancy, estrogen use, or infection.
  - Falsely low ceruloplasmin levels may be observed in any protein deficiency state including nephrotic syndrome, malabsorption, protein-losing enteropathy, and malnutrition. Ceruloplasmin levels may also be decreased in 10–20% of *WD* gene heterozygotes, who do not develop Wilson's disease and do not require treatment.
- **Urinary copper excretion:**
  - The urinary copper excretion rate is greater than 100 mg/day (reference range: <40 mg/day) in most patients with symptomatic Wilson's disease. The rate may also be elevated in other cholestatic liver diseases.
  - Both the sensitivity and the specificity of this test are suboptimal for use as a screening test; however, it may be useful to confirm the diagnosis and to evaluate the response to chelation therapy.
- **Hepatic copper concentration:**
  - This test is regarded as the criterion standard for diagnosis of Wilson's disease.
  - A liver biopsy with sufficient tissue reveals levels of >250 mcg/g of dry weight even in asymptomatic patients. Special collection vials are available to help avoid contamination.
  - A normal hepatic copper concentration (reference range: 15–55 mcg/g) effectively excludes the diagnosis of untreated Wilson's disease. An elevated hepatic copper concentration may be found in other chronic hepatic (mostly cholestatic) disorders.
- **Radiolabeled copper:** Radiolabeled copper testing directly assays hepatic copper metabolism.
- **Genetic diagnosis:** Linkage analysis has been used in family studies for presymptomatic testing; however, the multiplicity of mutations (>200 mutations of *ATP7B* have been identified) that requires screening in individuals without affected family members is large, making such analysis impractical.
- **Imaging studies:** CT and MRI of brain and abdomen can be carried out to confirm the diagnosis.
- **Kayser–Fleischer rings:** It can only be diagnosed definitively by an ophthalmologist using a slit lamp. They are present in >99% of patients with neurological/psychiatric forms of the disease and have been described very rarely in the absence of Wilson's disease **(Fig. 12.6)**. Kayser–Fleischer rings are present in only ~30–50% of patients diagnosed in the hepatic or presymptomatic state; thus, the absence of rings does not exclude the diagnosis.

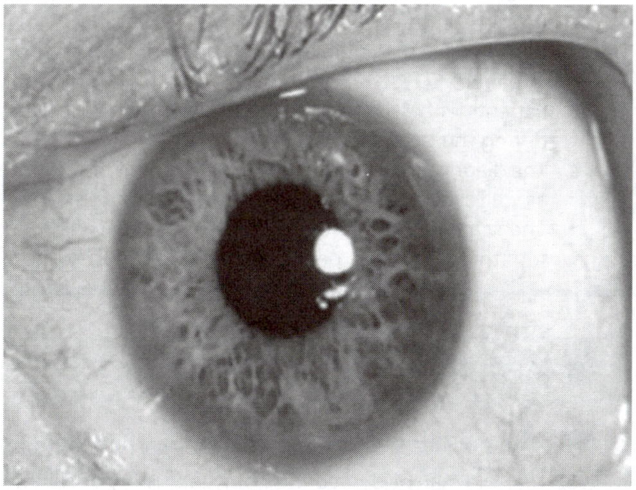

Fig. 12.6: Kayser–Fleischer ring in a patient suffering from Wilson's disease.

Treatment

Medication

The mainstay of therapy for Wilson's disease is pharmacological treatment with chelating agents.

Chelating agents bind excess copper. Ammonium tetrathiomolybdate is being used under the investigational new drug approval of the US Food and Drug Administration at the University of Michigan as an initial treatment for those who present with neurological or psychiatric manifestations. This drug works as both a chelating agent and an inhibitor of copper absorption from the GI tract.

Penicillamine was previously the primary anticopper treatment but now plays a minor role because of its toxicity and because it often worsens existing neurological disease, if used as initial therapy. If penicillamine is given, it should always be accompanied by 25 mg/day of pyridoxine. Trientine is a less toxic chelator and is supplanting penicillamine when a chelator is indicated.

For patients with hepatitis or cirrhosis, but without evidence of hepatic decompensation or neurological/psychiatric symptoms, zinc is the therapy of choice, although some advocate therapy with trientine. Zinc has proven efficacy in Wilson's disease and is essentially nontoxic. It produces a negative copper balance by blocking intestinal absorption of copper, and it induces hepatic metallothionein synthesis, which sequesters additional toxic copper. All presymptomatic patients should be treated prophylactically, since the disease is close to 100% penetrant. B_6 and dimercaprol can also be used as a part of the treatment.

Anticopper therapy must be given for life long. With treatment, liver function usually recovers after about a year, although residual liver damage is usually present. Neurological and psychiatric symptoms usually improve between 6 and 24 months of treatment.

Surgical Care

- The use of surgical decompression or transjugular intrahepatic shunting (TIPS) in the treatment of portal hypertension is reserved for individuals with recurrent or uncontrolled variceal bleeding that is unresponsive to standard conservative measures.
- Orthotopic liver transplantation is a potentially curative treatment of Wilson's disease.

Complications

The major complications in patients with untreated Wilson's disease are those associated with liver failure and a chronic, relentless course to cirrhosis, which is characterized by a progressive lassitude, fatigue, anorexia, jaundice, spider angiomas, splenomegaly, and ascites. Bleeding from varices, hepatic encephalopathy, hepatorenal syndrome, and coagulation abnormalities occur as liver failure ensues.

CLINICAL NOTE

The association of hemolysis and liver disease makes Wilson's disease a likely diagnosis.

CLINICAL PEARLS

1. Wilson's disease is an autosomal recessive disorder caused by mutations in the *ATP7B* gene, a membrane-bound copper transporting ATPase.
2. In this disease, the processes of incorporation of copper into ceruloplasmin and excretion of excess copper into bile are impaired.
3. Patients with Wilson's disease usually present with liver disease during the first decade of life or with neuropsychiatric illness during the third decade.
4. The diagnosis is confirmed by measurement of serum ceruloplasmin, urinary copper excretion, and hepatic copper content, as well as the detection of Kayser–Fleischer rings.
5. The mainstay of therapy for Wilson's disease is pharmacological treatment with chelating agents like—ammonium tetrathiomolybdate, penicillamine, zinc and trientine.

CASE STUDY 8

Theme: Zinc—Metabolism, Functions, and Significance

A 62-year-old man presented with a 4-week history of painful, scaly, and edematous palms and soles. The patient had a longstanding history of eczematous dermatitis of the soles, which never involved the palms in the past. The remainder of the skin examination including body folds and mucosa were normal. The patient's weight had been stable since significant weight loss from gastric bypass surgery 3 years prior.

The patient was initially treated with oral prednisone for 2 weeks without any improvement. There was no history of constitutional symptoms, joint pains, or diarrhea.

Laboratory investigation report:

- Normal erythrocyte sedimentation rate, complete blood count, and basic metabolic panel
- Serum zinc levels—68 µg/dL (low).

Serum zinc levels were below the normal limits and given the patient's history of gastric bypass and the clinical presentation, the patient was diagnosed with a nutritional deficiency. The patient was advised supplementation with zinc sulfate 220 mg/day with near resolution of his hand dermatitis occurred in just 6 days, further supporting the diagnosis. Although biotin and essential fatty acid deficiency were in the differential diagnosis, the rapid improvement of the patient's skin after only zinc supplementation suggested zinc deficiency to be the cause.

What is the metabolic role of zinc?

What are the causes and clinical implications of zinc deficiency?

CASE DETAILS

The patient is suffering from **acquired zinc (Zn) deficiency**. Zinc deficiency can be inherited in the form of acrodermatitis enteropathica or acquired by low nutritional intake, malabsorption (including bariatric surgery, celiac sprue), excessive loss of zinc (such as diarrhea secondary to viral, protozoal, and bacterial pathogens), chronic diseases (liver or renal disease, diabetes, malignancies, and sickle-cell disease), or a combination of these factors. Both the inherited and acquired forms can present with similar clinical features.

ZINC

Basic Concept

Zinc is an essential component of a large number (>300) of enzymes participating in the synthesis and degradation of carbohydrates, lipids, proteins, and nucleic acids as well as in the metabolism of other micronutrients. Zinc is present in all body tissues and fluids. The total body zinc content has been estimated to be 30 mmol (2 g). Skeletal muscle accounts for approximately 60% of the total body content and bone mass, with a zinc concentration of 1.5–3 mmol/g (100–200 mg/g), for approximately 30%.

Plasma zinc has a rapid turnover rate and it represents only about 0.l% of total body zinc content. Plasma zinc is complexed to organic ligands.

Sources of Zinc

Oysters, shellfish, red meats, liver, and egg yolks are rich sources of dietary zinc. Whole grains, nuts, legumes, and pumpkin seeds are relatively good plant sources.

Zinc from meat sources has a higher bioavailability due the presence of amino acids (such as glycine, histidine, lysine, methionine, and cysteine) that improve zinc absorption. Other compounds known to enhance zinc absorption include picolinic acid (secreted by the pancreas), vitamin B_6 (increases picolinic acid secretion), and citrate.

The zinc in whole grain products and other plant sources is less bioavailable because of their high content of phytic acid, a compound that inhibits zinc absorption, and fiber. In addition to fiber and phytates, minerals, such as calcium, iron, copper, and manganese have been shown to reduce zinc absorption by competing for transport across the brush border membrane.

Metabolism of Zinc

The dietary intake of zinc is around 10–15 mg/day. Zinc absorption is concentration dependent and occurs throughout the small intestine. Active transport of zinc into portal blood is mediated by metallothionein. Zinc competes with other metals for absorption, and absorption is greatly retarded by ingestion of fiber and phytates.

Zinc is lost from the body through the kidneys, skin, and intestine. The endogenous intestinal losses can vary from 7 mmol/day (0.5 mg/day) to >45 mmol/day (3 mg/day), depending on zinc intake. Urinary and skin losses are of the order of 7–10 mmol/day (0.5–0.7 mg/day) each and depend less on normal variations in zinc intake. Starvation and muscle catabolism increase zinc losses in urine. Strenuous exercise and elevated ambient temperatures can lead to losses by perspiration. The body has no zinc stores; in conditions of bone resorption and tissue catabolism, zinc is released and can be reutilized to some extent.

Zn-containing Enzymes

Zinc is an integral component of about 300 enzymes, within the enzymes, the role of zinc can be catalytic, cocatalytic, and structural **(Table 12.1)**:

a. **Catalytic function:** When the Zn^{2+} is directly involved in catalysis and its depletion causes loss of enzyme activity.
b. **Cocatalytic function:** In addition to zinc, 2 or more metals are needed for the catalytic action of the enzyme.
c. **Structural function:** Zinc is necessary to maintain tertiary structure and in some cases, the quaternary of the apoenzyme (metalloproteins involved in the regulation of gene expression: Zinc-fingers proteins).

TABLE 12.1: Zinc requiring enzymes.

Category	*Enzyme*	*Function*
a. Catalytic function	1. Carbonic anhydrase	Catalyzes the rapid interconversion of carbon dioxide and water to bicarbonate and protons and so is essential for respiration. A zinc prosthetic group in the enzyme is coordinated in three positions by histidine side chains. The fourth coordination position is occupied by water
	2. Alcohol dehydrogenases	Alcohol dehydrogenases are a group of dehydrogenase enzymes that occur in many organisms and facilitate the interconversion between alcohols and aldehydes or ketones with the reduction of nicotinamide adenine dinucleotide (NAD+ to NADH). They are dimeric proteins, with each subunit binding two Zn ions, only one of which is catalytically active.
	3. Carboxypeptidase	Carboxypeptidase is a protease that hydrolyzes the peptide bond of an amino acid residue at the carboxyl-terminal (C-terminal) end.
	4. Insulin protease or insulin-degrading enzyme	Insulin protease or insulin-degrading enzyme is a thiol zinc-metalloendopeptidase and is the major enzyme for the degradation of insulin. It regulates the level of insulin, amyloid β protein, and amyloid β precursor protein
b. Cocatalytic function	Superoxide dismutase	Superoxide dismutases are a class of enzymes that catalyze the dismutation of superoxide into oxygen and hydrogen peroxide. They act as antioxidant enzymes.
		In particular, SOD1 contains copper and zinc and its structure consists of two subunits of identical molecular weight joined by a disulfide bond. There are two Cu^{2+} and two Zn^{2+} atoms per molecule.
c. Structural function	Zinc finger	A zinc finger is a small protein structural motif that is characterized by the coordination of one or more zinc ions (Zn^{2+}) in order to stabilize the fold. Originally coined to describe the finger-like appearance of a *Xenopus laevis* transcription factor IIIA, the zinc finger name has now come to encompass a wide variety of differing protein structures. Zinc fingers coordinate zinc ions with a combination of cysteine and histidine residues. Zinc fingers are present among proteins that perform a wide range of cellular functions including replication and repair, transcription and translation, metabolism, proliferation, and apoptosis.

Other Functions of Zinc

1. It has a fundamental role in gene expression, cell growth, and cell replication.
2. It is required for insulin production, secretion, and the action of insulin.
3. Zinc stabilizes the molecular structure of cellular components and membranes and thus helps in the maintenance of cell and organ integrity.
4. Zinc is needed for the sense of taste and smell and helps to regulate appetite.
5. Zinc plays a central role in the immune system. Zinc affects multiple aspects of the immune system including both nonspecific and specific immunity.
6. It is required for wound healing.
7. Zinc is an essential component of gonadal hormones.
8. Zinc is required for the hair growth and maintenance of integrity of skin.
9. Zinc is essential for healthy brain development and function. Zinc status affects growth and maturation of neurons, synthesis of neurotransmitters, and the function of certain receptors.
10. Zinc is an essential cofactor for enzymes involved in the synthesis of bone matrix. Zinc deficiency has been implicated as a risk factor in the development of osteoporosis.
11. Regulatory role: Zinc finger proteins have been found to regulate gene expression by acting as transcription factors (binding to DNA and influencing the transcription of specific genes). Zinc also plays a role in cell signaling and has been found to influence hormone release and nerve impulse transmission. Zinc has been found to play a role in apoptosis (gene-directed cell death), a critical cellular regulatory process with implications for growth and development, as well as a number of chronic diseases.
12. Zinc supplementation has been studied as a possible treatment for the common cold, age-related macular degeneration, diabetes mellitus, and HIV/AIDS.

Recommended dietary allowance (RDA): The RDA for adult men and women is 11 mg/day and 8 mg/day of zinc, respectively.

Nutrient Interactions

Copper

Taking large quantities of zinc (50 mg/day or more) over a period of weeks can interfere with copper bioavailability. High intake of zinc induces the intestinal synthesis of a copper-binding protein called metallothionein. Metallothionein traps copper within intestinal cells and prevents its systemic absorption.

Iron

Supplemental (38–65 mg/day of elemental iron) but not dietary levels of iron may decrease zinc absorption. This interaction is of concern in the management of iron supplementation during pregnancy and lactation.

Calcium

Calcium in combination with phytic acid or phytate might affect zinc absorption.

Folate

The bioavailability of dietary folate is increased by the action of a zinc-dependent enzyme, suggesting a possible interaction between zinc and folic acid.

Vitamin A

Zinc and vitamin A interact in several ways. Zinc is a component of retinol-binding protein, a protein necessary for transporting vitamin A in the blood. Zinc is also required for the enzyme that converts retinol (vitamin A) to retinal. This latter form of vitamin A is necessary for the synthesis of rhodopsin that absorbs light and thus is involved in dark adaptation. Zinc deficiency is associated with decreased release of vitamin A from the liver, which may contribute to symptoms of night blindness that are seen with zinc deficiency.

Zinc Deficiency

a. **Acrodermatitis enteropathica (Fig. 12.7):** It is a genetic disorder resulting from the impaired uptake and transport of zinc. The symptoms of severe zinc deficiency include the slowing or cessation of growth and development, delayed sexual maturation, characteristic skin rashes, chronic and severe diarrhea, immune system deficiencies, impaired wound healing, diminished appetite, impaired taste sensation, night blindness, swelling and clouding of the corneas, and behavioral disturbances.
   Oral zinc therapy results in the complete remission of symptoms, though it must be maintained indefinitely in individuals with the genetic disorder.
b. **Acquired zinc deficiency (Fig. 12.8):** Although dietary zinc deficiency is unlikely to cause severe zinc deficiency in individuals without a genetic disorder; zinc malabsorption or conditions of increased zinc loss, such as severe burns or prolonged diarrhea may also result in severe zinc deficiency. Severe zinc deficiency has also been reported in individuals undergoing total parenteral nutrition without zinc, in those who abuse alcohol, and in those who are taking certain medications like penicillamine.

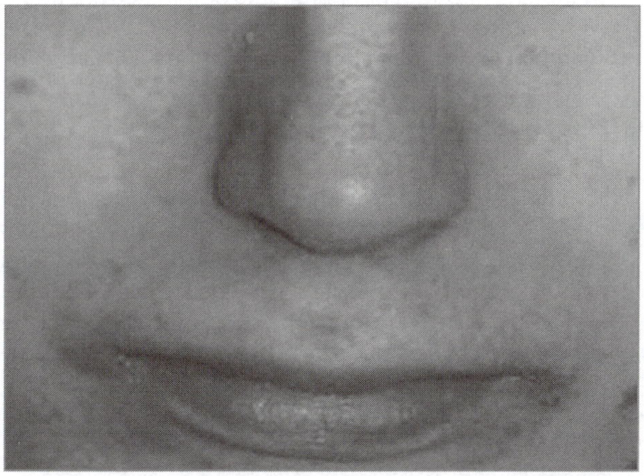

Fig. 12.7: Typical skin rash in acrodermatitis enteropathica.

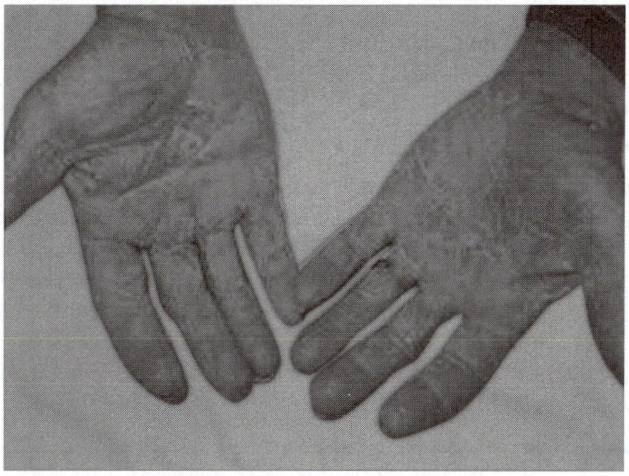

Fig. 12.8: Rashes in acquired zinc deficiency.

Risk Factors of Zinc Deficiency

- Premature and low-birth-weight infants
- Older breastfed infants and toddlers with inadequate intake of zinc-rich complementary foods
- Pregnant and lactating women
- Patients receiving total parenteral nutrition (intravenous feedings)
- Malnourished individuals including those with protein-energy malnutrition and anorexia nervosa

- Individuals with severe or persistent diarrhea
- Individuals with malabsorption syndromes including celiac disease and short bowel syndrome
- Individuals with inflammatory bowel disease including Crohn's disease and ulcerative colitis
- Alcoholics and those with alcoholic liver disease who have increased urinary zinc excretion and low liver zinc levels
- Individuals with chronic renal disease
- Individuals with sickle cell anemia
- Individuals who use medications that decrease intestinal zinc absorption, increase zinc excretion, or impair zinc utilization.
- Older adults (65 years and older)
- Strict vegetarians: The requirement for dietary zinc may be as much as 50% greater for strict vegetarians whose major food staples are grains and legumes, because high levels of phytic acid in these foods reduce zinc absorption.
- Patients who have undergone bariatric surgery are commonly at risk of developing nutritional deficiencies.

Laboratory Diagnosis

There is not a sensitive and specific biomarker to detect zinc deficiency in humans. Low plasma or serum zinc levels are typically used as a biomarker of zinc status but measuring blood concentration of zinc has a number of limitations including lack of sensitivity to detect marginal zinc deficiency, depression in response to inflammation, and diurnal variations. The repeated findings of a zinc concentration in a serum sample of <5 µmol/L are suggestive of impending zinc deficiency and require investigation. Unlike copper, serum zinc falls during the acute phase response to injury or infection.

Marginal zinc deficiency is best demonstrated by a positive clinical response to supplementation. Oral or intravenous zinc reverses the signs and symptoms of zinc deficiency within weeks.

Treatment

A number of zinc supplements are commercially available including zinc acetate, zinc gluconate, zinc picolinate, and zinc sulfate. Treatment for zinc deficiency should be initiated at 3 mg/kg/day of elemental zinc (50 mg of elemental zinc per 220 mg zinc sulfate). With treatment, prompt clinical improvement ensues, even before any significant changes in the serum zinc level may be observed. In addition to supplementation, any underlying cause for a nutritional deficiency should be investigated.

Zinc Toxicity

Acute zinc toxicity can occur as a result of the consumption of food or beverages contaminated with zinc released from galvanized containers. Signs of acute zinc toxicity are abdominal pain, diarrhea, nausea, and vomiting. Single doses of 225–450 mg of zinc usually induce vomiting. Milder gastrointestinal distress has been reported at doses of 50–150 mg/day of supplemental zinc. Metal fume fever can occur after the inhalation of zinc oxide fumes. Profuse sweating, weakness, and rapid breathing may develop within 8 hours of zinc oxide inhalation and persist 12–24 hours after exposure is terminated.

The long-term consumption of excessive zinc can cause copper deficiency. Total zinc intakes of 60 mg/day (50 mg supplemental and 10 mg dietary zinc) have been found to result in signs of copper deficiency.

CLINICAL NOTE

Zinc status affects growth and maturation of neurons, synthesis of neurotransmitters, and the function of certain receptors.

CLINICAL PEARLS

1. Zinc is an essential component of a large number (>300) of enzymes participating in the synthesis and degradation of carbohydrates, lipids, proteins, and nucleic acids.
2. Plasma zinc has a rapid turnover rate and it represents only about 0.l% of total body zinc content.
3. It has a fundamental role in gene expression, cell growth, and cell replication.
4. The requirement for dietary zinc may be as much as 50% greater for strict vegetarians whose major food staples are grains and legumes, because high levels of phytic acid in these foods reduce zinc absorption.
5. Zinc deficiency can be inherited in the form of acrodermatitis enteropathica or acquired by low nutritional intake, malabsorption (including bariatric surgery, celiac sprue), excessive loss of zinc (such as diarrhea secondary to viral, protozoal, and bacterial pathogens); chronic diseases (liver or renal disease, diabetes, malignancies, sickle-cell disease), or a combination of these factors.

CASE STUDY 9

Theme: Selenium—Functions, Deficiency, and Toxicity

In March, 2008, a chiropractor in Florida noted common symptoms of gastrointestinal illness and hair loss among several of his patients. In response to their symptoms, these patients had doubled the dose of a dietary supplement they had purchased at the chiropractic office. The patients subsequently noted worsening symptoms including nail discoloration. Two couples contacted the local health department, where investigators identified the common exposure and initiated an investigation. Active case finding was initiated by the local health department including contacting the chiropractor, who provided a list of patients to whom the dietary supplement had been sold. These patients were interviewed. Simultaneously, the US Food and Drug Administration (FDA) initiated an independent investigation as a result of similar complaints, at which time other agencies, including the poison control center and state health department, were notified. The dietary supplement was identified as the common exposure among all affected persons. The FDA subsequently tested the product and determined the selenium concentration to be 40,800 µg/1 oz, approximately 200 times the labeled concentration.

The misformulated liquid dietary supplement resulted in 201 cases of selenium poisoning, but the actual number of affected persons was likely greater.

What is the mechanism of selenium toxicity?
What are the sources of selenium exposure?

CASE DETAILS

Selenium is required for maintenance of health. It is obtained from food, and the RDA is 55 µg/day for persons 19 years or older, with a tolerable upper intake limit of 400 µg/day. The amount of selenium available in a diverse diet with meat, grains, vegetables, and nuts is typically sufficient to negate the necessity for supplementation. Selenium toxicity can occur with acute or chronic ingestion of excess selenium. Symptoms of selenium toxicity include nausea; vomiting; nail discoloration, brittleness, and loss; hair loss; fatigue; irritability; and foul breath odor (often described as "garlic breath").

BASIC CONCEPT

Selenium

Selenium is a trace element that is essential in small amounts, but like all essential elements, selenium can be toxic at high levels. Unlike plants, most animals—including humans—require selenium for the appropriate functioning of a number of selenium-dependent enzymes known as selenoproteins**.** Selenium is found in the environment in soil. Soils of certain areas in the Great Plains and western United States as well as other parts of the world have high concentrations of selenium, which are taken up by plants.

Functions of Selenium

Selenoproteins

Selenium exerts various biological functions mainly as part of the amino acid, selenocysteine, which is found in at least 25 selenocysteine-containing proteins (selenoproteins). During translation, the amino acid selenocysteine is incorporated into elongating proteins at very specific locations in the amino acid sequence in order to form functional selenoproteins. The insertion of selenocysteine is directed by the presence of a selenocysteine insertion sequence (SECIS) within selenoprotein mRNA **(Figs. 12.9A and B)**.

Figs. 12.9A and B: (A) Cysteine and (B) selenocysteine.

Some of the selenoproteins with an identified function include:

1. **Glutathione peroxidase:** Five selenium-containing glutathione peroxidases (GPx1-4 and GPx6) have been identified. GPx isoenzymes are all antioxidant enzymes that reduce potentially damaging reactive oxygen species (ROS), such as hydrogen peroxide and lipid hydroperoxides, to harmless products, such as water and alcohols by coupling their reduction with the oxidation of glutathione **(Fig. 12.10)**.

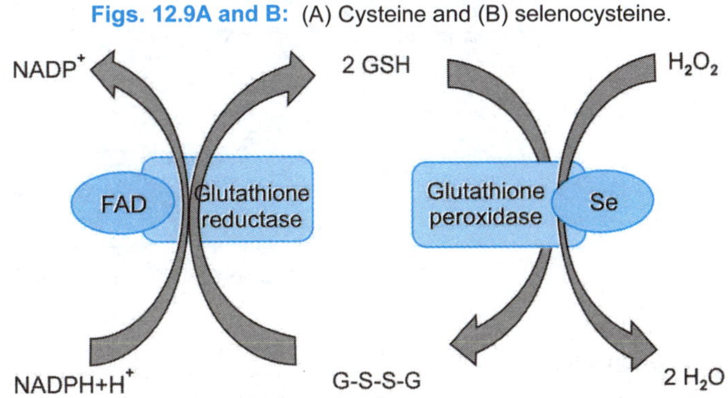

Fig. 12.10: Reduced glutathione is required for the activity of glutathione peroxidase, an antioxidant selenium-containing metalloenzyme enzyme that decomposes hydrogen peroxide to water.

2. **Thioredoxin reductases:** Thioredoxin reductases (TrxRs) are homodimeric enzymes, and each monomer contains FAD and NADPH-binding domains, and a selenocysteine-containing catalytic site. TrxRs catalyze the reduction of thioredoxin and serve as electron donors for the regeneration of small antioxidants, possibly recycling ascorbic acid (vitamin C), α-lipoic acid, α-tocopherol (vitamin E), and coenzyme Q10 from their oxidized forms. The protein thioredoxin, together with thioredoxin reductase (TrxR), NADPH, and FAD, constitutes the **thioredoxin antioxidant system** involved in the reduction of antioxidant enzymes [e.g., methionine sulfoxide reductases and ribonucleotide reductase **(Fig. 12.11)**] and of many oxidation/reduction (redox)-sensitive signaling proteins.
3. **Iodothyronine deiodinases (thyroid hormone deiodinases):** The thyroid gland releases very small amounts of biologically active thyroid hormone (triiodothyronine or T3) and larger amounts of an inactive form of thyroid hormone (T3 precursor: Thyroxine or T4) into the circulation. Most of the biologically active T3 in the circulation and inside cells is generated by the removal of one iodine atom from T4 in a reaction catalyzed by selenium-dependent iodothyronine deiodinase enzymes. Two different selenium-dependent iodothyronine deiodinases (DIOs type 1 and 2) can deiodinate T4, thus increasing circulating T3, while a third iodothyronine deiodinase (DIO type 3) can convert both T3 and T4 to inactive metabolites **(Fig. 12.12)**.

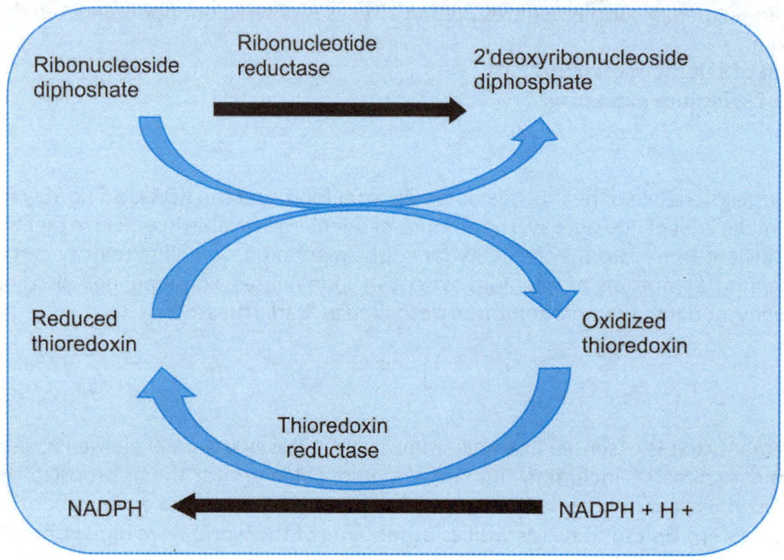

Fig. 12.11: The reaction catalyzed by ribonucleotide reductase; the enzyme complex requires reduced thioredoxin for its action.

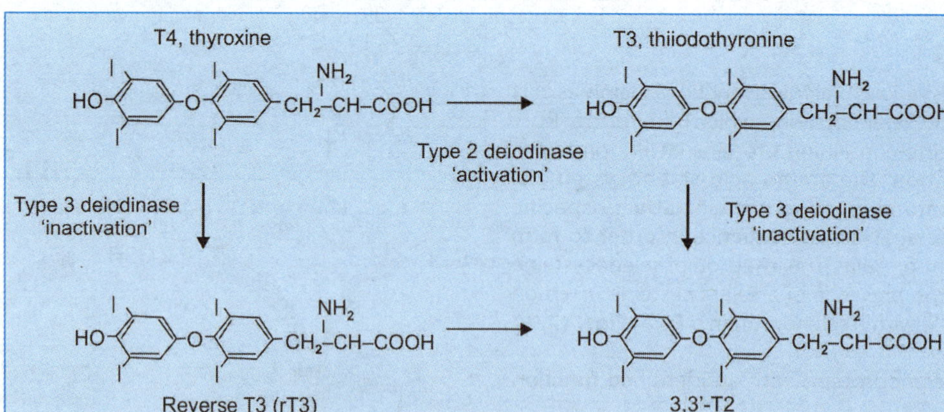

Fig. 12.12: Reaction catalyzed by selenium-dependent iodothyronine deiodinase.

Selenoprotein P

Selenoprotein P (SEPP1) is predominantly produced by the liver, a major storage site for selenium, and secreted in the plasma. SEPP1 also functions as an antioxidant that protects cells from oxidative damage by enabling full activity of thioredoxin reductases and glutathione peroxidases through adequate supply of selenium to extrahepatic tissues.

Methionine-R-sulfoxide reductase B1 (formerly selenoprotein R)

The methionine sulfoxide reduction system is involved in the protection against oxidative stress and is especially critical for the regeneration of proteins damaged by reactive oxygen species (ROS). ROS can oxidize methionine residues (methionine sulfoxides) within proteins and potentially impair their activities.

Selenoprotein W

Selenoprotein W (SEPW) is expressed in numerous tissues, with highest levels found in skeletal muscle and heart. SEPW contains a selenocysteine residue and a cysteine residue that binds to a glutathione molecule, suggesting a role in redox regulation. SEPW expression in the brain has been found to confer protection against oxidative stress-induced neuronal cell death.

At least 10 other selenoproteins exist, including one which is a component of the mitochondrial capsule of sperm cells, damage to which may account for the development of sperm abnormalities during selenium deficiency.

Selenium Deficiency

Insufficient selenium intake may negatively affect the activity of several selenium-responsive enzymes, including glutathione peroxidases, iodothyronine deiodinases, selenoprotein W, and methionine-R-sulfoxide reductase. Prolonged selenium deficiency may likely contribute to Keshan and Kashin–Beck diseases.

Risk factors of selenium deficiency

Selenium deficiency has been reported in:

- Chronically ill patients who were receiving total parenteral nutrition (TPN) without added selenium for prolonged periods of time.
- Following bariatric surgery
- Severe gastrointestinal conditions,, such as Crohn's disease
- Metabolic disorders, including phenylketonuria, homocystinuria, and maple syrup urine disease (if the treatment does not include supplementation with selenium).

Keshan Disease

Keshan disease is a fatal form of dilated cardiomyopathy that was first described in young women and children in a selenium-deficient region in China. The acute form of the disease is characterized by the sudden onset of cardiac insufficiency, while the chronic form results in moderate-to-severe heart enlargement with varying degrees of cardiac insufficiency.

Etiology

The incidence of Keshan disease is closely associated with very low dietary intakes of selenium and poor selenium nutritional status. Endemic in children aged 2–10 years and in women of childbearing age, this disease has a geographic distribution covering localities from northeast to southwest China. While selenium deficiency is a major etiological factor of Keshan disease, the seasonal and annual variation in disease occurrence suggested that other factors, especially an infectious agent, might be involved in addition to selenium deficiency. Coxsackievirus B3 is one virus type that has been isolated from Keshan patients, and animal studies have shown that this virus was capable of causing an inflammation of the heart (myocarditis) in selenium-deficient mice. Studies in mice also indicated that oxidative stress induced by selenium deficiency could result in changes in the viral genome,, such as to convert a relatively harmless strain of coxsackievirus B3 into a myocarditis-causing strain. Recent studies indicate that geochemical variables have an important influence on the distribution of Keshan disease. Acid soils high in organic matter and iron oxide content appear to be responsible for fixing selenium in forms which are poorly absorbed by staple crops which, in the instance of cereal grains, typically have a selenium content of <0.01 μg/g.

Clinical Manifestations

Typical manifestations are fatigue after even mild exercise, cardiac arrhythmia and palpitations, loss of appetite, cardiac insufficiency, cardiomegaly, and congestive heart failure.

Pathogenesis

Pathological changes include a multifocal myocardial necrosis and fibrosis. The coronary arteries are essentially unaffected. Ultrastructural studies show that membranous organelles,, such as mitochondria or sarcolemma, are affected earliest.

Prophylaxis

Once the disease is established, selenium is of little or no therapeutic value. Prophylaxis consisting of oral administration of selenium 3 months before the periods of highest anticipated risk is highly effective.

Kashin–Beck disease

A selenium-responsive bone and joint disease (osteoarthropathy) has been detected in children aged 5–13 years in China and less extensively in southeast Siberia. The disease is characterized by joint necrosis—epiphyseal degeneration of the arm and leg joints resulting in structural shortening of the fingers and long bones with consequent growth retardation and stunting. Although not identical to Keshan disease, Kashin–Beck disease also occurs in areas where the availability of soil selenium for crop growth is low. The selenium contents of hair and of whole blood are abnormally low and the blood content of glutathione peroxidase is reduced.

Recommended Dietary Allowance

Males and females—55 μg/day, the daily requirement increases in pregnancy and lactation. The Food and Nutrition Board (FNB) of the US Institute of Medicine set the tolerable upper intake level (UL) for selenium at 400 μg/day in adults based on the prevention of hair and nail brittleness and loss and early signs of chronic selenium toxicity. The UL of 400 μg/day for adults includes both selenium obtained from food and selenium from supplements.

Sources of Selenium

The richest food sources of selenium are organ meats and seafood, followed by muscle meats. Garlic, onion, and broccoli, wheat, other grains (including Brazil nuts), and soy are rich in selenomethionine and contain smaller amounts of selenocysteine and selenate.

Selenium supplements are available in several forms. Sodium selenite and sodium selenate are inorganic forms of selenium.

Selenium Toxicity

Although selenium is required for health, high doses of selenium can be toxic. Acute and fatal toxicities have occurred with accidental or suicidal ingestion of gram quantities of selenium. Chronic selenium toxicity (selenosis) may occur with smaller doses of selenium over long periods of time. The most frequently reported symptoms of selenosis are hair and nail brittleness and loss. Other symptoms may include gastrointestinal disturbances, skin rashes, a garlic breath odor, fatigue, irritability, and neurological disorders.

CLINICAL NOTE

The amount of selenium available in a diverse diet with meat, grains, vegetables, and nuts is typically sufficient to negate the necessity for supplementation.

CLINICAL PEARLS

1. Selenium is a trace element that is essential in small amounts, but like all essential elements, selenium can be toxic at high levels.
2. Selenium exerts various biological functions mainly as part of the amino acid, selenocysteine, which is found in at least 25 selenocysteine-containing proteins (selenoproteins).
3. Insufficient selenium intake may negatively affect the activity of several selenium-responsive enzymes, including glutathione peroxidases, iodothyronine deiodinases, selenoprotein W, and methionine-R-sulfoxide reductase.
4. Keshan disease is a fatal form of dilated cardiomyopathy that was first described in young women and children in a selenium-deficient region in China.
5. Kashin–Beck disease is characterized by joint necrosis—epiphyseal degeneration of the arm and leg joints resulting in structural shortening of the fingers and long bones with consequent growth retardation and stunting.

CASE STUDIES: HEAVY METAL TOXICITY

CASE STUDY 10

Theme: Lead Poisoning

A 16-year-old girl was admitted to medical OPD with severe abdominal pain, loss of appetite, nausea, and vomiting. The history revealed that the girl belonged to a family of potters, and that she also participated in the process of pottery and her father was diagnosed with lead poisoning 2 years ago. The patient's personal history underlined that approximately 1 year ago she presented with severe abdominal pain and was diagnosed with acute appendicitis for which she underwent appendectomy, but the pain persisted.

The clinical examination performed at the time of admission revealed: Jaundice, blue pigmentation of the nails, and painful abdomen at palpation. The blood pressure was 156/96 mm Hg.

Laboratory findings were:

Hemoglobin (Hb): 10.9 g/dL
Hematocrit (Hct): 31.6%
Mean corpuscular volume (MCV): 77.6 fL
Alanine aminotransferase (ALT): 158.9 U/L
Aspartate aminotransferase (AST): 63 U/L
Gamma-glutamyltransferase (GGT): 128 U/L
Conjugated hyperbilirubinemia [direct bilirubin (DB): 1.4 mg/dL]
Serum Na: 132 mmol/L
Serum K: 2.85 mmol/L
Blood lead level: 66.28 µg/dL
Urinary lead level: 419.7µg/L (normal <50 µg/L)
Delta-aminolevulinic acid: 7.66 mg/L (normal <4.5mg/L)

Abdominal ultrasound revealed a disappearance of the delimitation between the cortical and medullar parts in both kidneys.
Based on all these clinical and laboratory findings, the diagnosis of lead poisoning was established.

What are the causes of lead exposure?
What is the mechanism of lead toxicity?

CASE DETAILS

Lead poisoning representing a major health problem. It is a severe condition with potential multiorgan damage and even death, if lead is present in large amounts in the blood. A heavy metal lead has no physiological role in biological systems. It interferes with a number of body functions primarily affecting the central nervous, hematopoietic, hepatic, and renal system producing serious disorders. Acute toxicity is related to occupational exposure and is quite uncommon. Chronic toxicity on the other hand is much more common.

Sources of Exposure

Common sources of lead exposure include: paint chips, occupational exposure, glazed ceramics, herbal remedies (e.g., Ayurvedic medications), home remedies including antiperspirants, deodorants, jewelry, stored battery casings (or living near a battery smelter), lead-based gasoline, contaminated foods, cosmetics, foods in lead-containing cans, toys, home renovations, antique toys, or furniture. Major sources of exposure vary among and within countries; the major source of exposure in the United States remains old lead-based paint. As paint deteriorates, it chalks, flakes, and turns to dust. The dust can coat all surfaces, including children's hands. All of these forms of lead can be ingested. If heat is used to strip paint then lead vapor concentrations in the room can reach levels sufficient to cause lead poisoning via inhalation. The ways of contamination include ingestion, inhalation, prenatal exposure, and dermal exposure, but the most important and frequent ones are ingestion and inhalation.

Pathophysiology

The major mechanism of lead toxicity is due to increased generation of ROS and interference with generation of antioxidants. Lead inactivates glutathione by binding to GSHs sulfhydryl group, which causes GSH replenishment to become inefficient, thereby increasing oxidative stress. Lead also interferes with the activity of other antioxidant enzymes including superoxide dismutase and catalase. Lead entering the intravascular space binds quickly to red blood cells. Lead has a half-life of approximately 30 days in the blood, from where it diffuses into the soft tissues, including the kidneys, brain, liver, and bone marrow.

Lead then diffuses into bone and is stored there for a period that corresponds to a half-life of several decades. Increased bone turnover with pregnancy, menopause, lactation, or immobilization can increase blood lead levels. Estimations of blood lead levels are more useful for diagnosing acute lead poisoning, whereas the extent of past lead exposure can be estimated by determining the body burden of lead on the basis of results from the edetate (EDTA) calcium disodium ($CaNa_2$ EDTA) lead mobilization test. Lead is primarily excreted in urine and bile, but the elimination rate varies, depending on the tissue that absorbed the lead. The kidney excretes lead by means of glomerular filtration and tubular secretion. The effects of lead poisoning on the brain are manifold and include delayed or reversed development, permanent learning disabilities, seizures, coma, and even death. The long-term effect of lead exposure is maximal during the first 2 or 3 years of life, when the developing brain is in a critical formative stage.

Clinical Manifestations

The clinical presentation of lead poisoning includes the following:

Neurological Toxicity

Neurological symptoms include ataxia, stupor, coma, convulsions, hyperirritability, reduced IQ, shortened attention span, increased antisocial behavior, reduced educational attainment, and even death. In adults, chronic distal motor neuropathy (e.g., foot drop or wrist drop) may be seen with decreased reflexes and weakness of extensor muscles **(Fig. 12.13)**. Chronic lead exposure has been shown to cause optic neuritis and blindness.

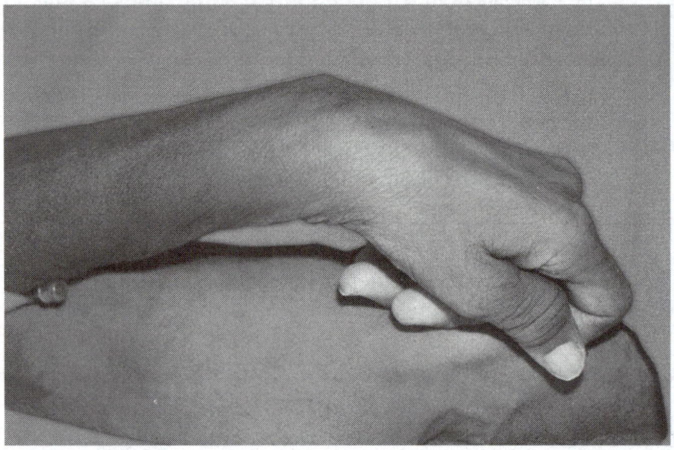

Fig. 12.13: Wrist drop in patient with lead poisoning.

Hematological Toxicity

Impairment of the hematological system may involve either disruption of heme synthesis or hemolysis, leading to anemia with its specific clinical signs, such as weakness and fatigue.

Renal Toxicity

The effects of lead on the renal system consist in proximal tubular function impairment leading to aminoaciduria, glycosuria, and hyperphosphaturia, interstitial nephritis in chronic exposure, and also impairment of calcium metabolism by interfering with activation of vitamin D, 1,2-dihydroxycholecalciferol.

Cardiovascular Toxicity

Lead exposure has been associated with the development of hypertension. The development of hypertension may be secondary to oxidative stress or an association with chronic nephropathy. Studies have also documented an association between lead toxicity and cardiovascular disease and stroke.

Reproductive Effects

In men, lead causes a reduction in libido, abnormal spermatogenesis, chromosomal damage, and infertility. Women experience an increase in the incidence of stillbirth, miscarriage, pregnancy-induced hypertension, and prematurity.

Gastrointestinal Effects

Patients may develop abdominal cramps, nausea, vomiting, and anorexia. Occasionally, some patients with acute poisoning can develop severe diarrhea and dehydration.

Dental Lines

Lead lines appearing on gingival tissue **(Fig. 12.14A)** are very unusual in children. Adults with poor dental hygiene may demonstrate this characteristic finding in any heavy metal poisoning. Lead can interfere with bone development, leading to the formation of lead lines at bone metaphyses. These lines represent periods of growth arrest, not lead toxicity per se **(Fig. 12.14B)**.

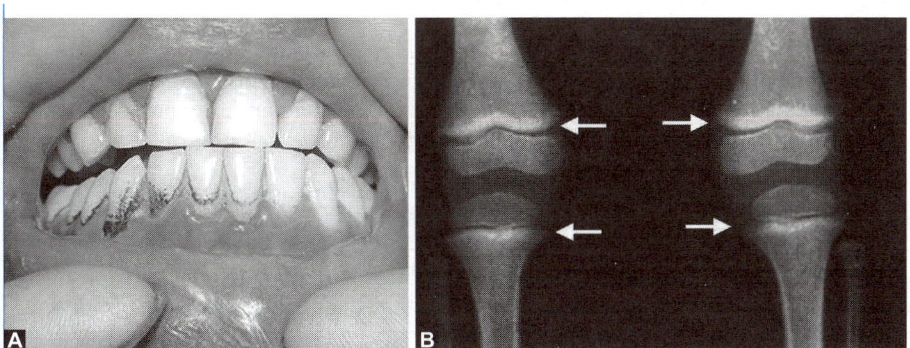

Figs. 12.14A and B: Lead lines in lead poisoning.

Laboratory Diagnosis

- **Blood lead level (BLL):** The diagnosis is established on the blood lead level, higher than 40µg/dL for occupational and 30µg/dL for nonoccupational exposure.
- **Free erythrocyte protoporphyrin (FEP) level:** Biochemical evidence of lead poisoning is by the finding of raised protoporphyrin levels in the erythrocytes due to the inhibition of the enzymes of heme biosynthetic pathway. Lead interferes with the enzyme ALA dehydratase and ferrochelatase (blocking the incorporation of iron into the protoporphyrin molecule) **(Fig. 12.15)**.
- A FEP level may be useful in demonstrating the degree of biological abnormalities that exist. FEP can also be used to help distinguish recent acute lead exposure from chronic exposure. If FEP is normal in the context of high blood lead levels, the exposure is more likely acute; if both are elevated, the exposure is more likely chronic.
- **Peripheral blood film:** Lead toxicity causes a hypochromic microcytic anemia and basophilic stippling of red blood cells **(Fig. 12.16)**. Hypochromia and microcytosis are typically seen in iron-deficiency anemia, which often coexists with lead toxicity. Assessing iron storage status (ferritin) in all cases of lead poisoning is important.

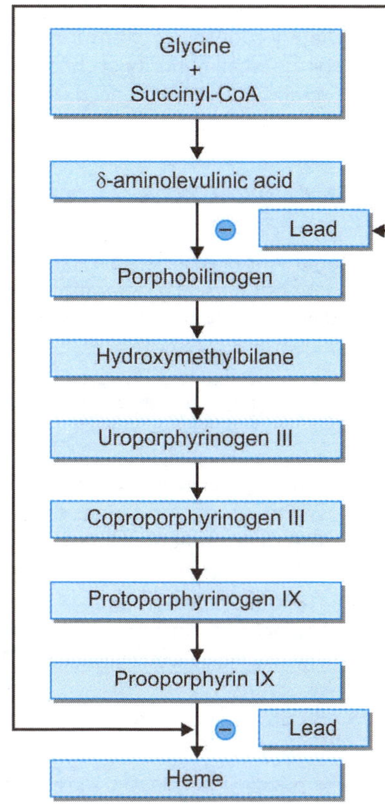

Fig. 12.15: Inhibition of enzymes of heme biosynthetic pathway in lead toxicity.

Radiography

In selected cases, abdominal radiographs may demonstrate lead-containing paint chips or other lead-containing objects. Radiographs of the long bones in growing children may reveal the characteristic lead lines **(Fig. 12.14B)**.

Neuroimaging

In general, neuroimaging [e.g., with magnetic resonance imaging (MRI) or computed tomography (CT)] does not play an important role in the diagnosis of lead poisoning. However, cerebral edema and microhemorrhages may be seen in patients presenting with acute encephalopathy on both CT and MRI. With chronic exposure to lead, patchy calcifications may be seen. Atrophy and white matter changes may be present with chronic exposures.

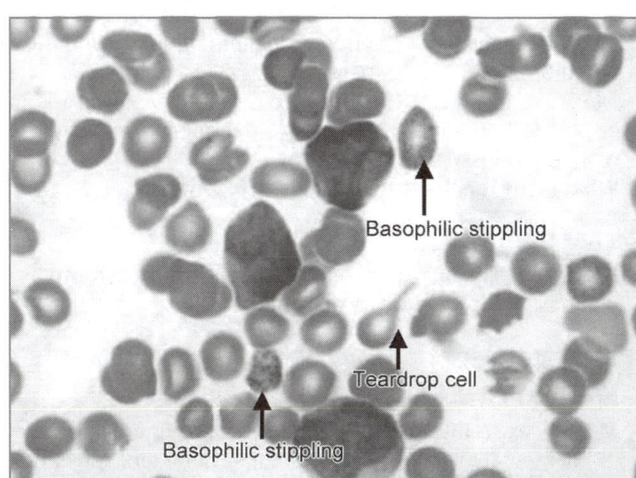

Fig. 12.16: Microcytic hypochromic anemia in lead toxicity. Lead may produce increased red blood cell (RBC) fragility and acute hemolytic anemia.

Treatment

Once lead is in bone, it is released slowly and is difficult to remove even with chelating agents. Because the cognitive/behavioral effects of lead may be irreversible, the main effort in treating lead poisoning is to prevent it from occurring and to prevent further ingestion by already poisoned children. The main components in the effort to eliminate lead poisoning are universally applicable to all children (and adults) and are as follows:

1. Identification and elimination of environmental sources of lead exposure

2. Behavioral modification to reduce nonnutritive hand-to-mouth activity
3. Dietary counseling to ensure sufficient intake of the essential elements—calcium and iron
4. For the small minority of children with more-severe lead poisoning, drug treatment is available that enhances lead excretion. Excretion can be enhanced using any of the chelating agents $NaCa_2$ EDTA, dimercaprol, or N-acetyl-penicillamine. Succimer is a water-soluble, oral chelating agent that is appropriate for use with BLLs higher than 45 µg/dL.

CLINICAL NOTE

Estimations of blood lead levels are more useful for diagnosing acute lead poisoning, whereas the extent of past lead exposure can be estimated by determining the body burden of lead on the basis of results from the edetate (EDTA) calcium disodium (CaNa2 EDTA) lead mobilization test.

CLINICAL PEARLS

1. Lead interferes with a number of body functions primarily affecting the central nervous, hematopoietic, hepatic, and renal system producing serious disorders.
2. The major mechanism of lead toxicity is due to increased generation of ROS and interference with generation of antioxidants.
3. The clinical presentation of lead poisoning involves nervous, hematologic, and renal systems impairment, but it can also lead to gastrointestinal disorders (anorexia, vomiting, constipation, and abdominal pain), hypertension, and infertility.
4. The diagnosis is established on the blood lead level, higher than 40µg/dL for occupational and 30µg/dL for nonoccupational exposure.
5. Because the cognitive/behavioral effects of lead may be irreversible, the main effort in treating lead poisoning is to prevent it from occurring and to prevent further ingestion by already poisoned children.

CASE STUDY 11

Theme: Mercury Poisoning

A 35-year-old woman presented to the emergency OPD with a 3-day history of abdominal pain, diarrhea, and fever. General physical examination of the patient revealed: BP—140/90 mm Hg; temperature—40°C; heart rate—110 beats/min and regular; respiration—16 breaths/min; O_2 saturation—94%. Nothing was remarkable on examination and routine laboratory tests.

The patient reported that 1 week ago, her daughter had brought mercury in the liquid form from the school and had put it on the heating stove. She was breastfeeding her 12-month-old daughter at that time. 24 hours after this event, her baby got fever and died before admission to the hospital, without any specific diagnosis. The autopsy report disclosed a suspected mercury poisoning, which might have led to cardiorespiratory collapse resulting in death of the infant.

Suspecting mercury poisoning in mother, blood was drawn and sent for mercury levels, which turned out to be 40 µg/dL (normal range: 0–10 µg/dL). As urinary mercury levels could not be tested in the city, symptomatic chelation treatment with N-acetylcysteine (NAC) was instituted with regard to presumptive diagnosis and history. In follow-up visit, the patient was asymptomatic without any clinical finding. Therefore, NAC treatment was terminated after 14 treatment days. The other children did not exhibit any manifestations of the disease.

What is the mechanism of mercury toxicity?

CASE DETAILS

History of exposure to mercury, gastrointestinal symptoms, and suspicious death of breastfed baby lead to the presumptive diagnosis of acute mercury poisoning.

BASIC CONCEPT

Mercury

Mercury exists in 3 forms: Elemental mercury, inorganic mercury salts, and organic mercury.

1. Elemental mercury is present in thermometers, sphygmomanometers, barometers, batteries, and some latex paints.
2. Inorganic mercury salts are found in pesticides, disinfectants, antiseptics, pigments, dry batteries, and explosives and as preservatives in some medicinal preparations.
3. Organic mercury in the diet, especially fish containing methyl mercury, is a major source of mercury exposure among the general population. Other sources of organic mercury exposure include through industries involved in chlorine and caustic

soda production, mining and metallurgy, electroplating, chemical and textile manufacturing, paper and pharmaceutical manufacturing, and leather tanning.

Mercury compounds in the environment are methylated to methyl mercury by soil and water microorganisms. Methyl mercury in the water rapidly accumulates in fish and other aquatic organisms, which are in turn consumed by humans.

Absorption

- Methyl mercury is the most avidly absorbed of the organic mercury compounds, with approximately 90% absorbed from the gastrointestinal tract.
- Inhaled elemental mercury vapor is 80% absorbed by the lungs and is distributed rapidly to the central nervous system because of its high lipid solubility. Elemental mercury liquid is poorly absorbed from the gastrointestinal tract, with <0.1% being absorbed. The half-life of elemental mercury in the tissues is approximately 60 days, most of the excretion occurring in the urine.
- Inorganic mercury salts are approximately 10% absorbed from the gastrointestinal tract and cross the blood–brain barrier to a lesser extent than elemental mercury.
- Mercuric salts are more soluble than mercurous salts and, therefore, produce greater toxicity. Elimination occurs primarily in the urine, with a half-life of approximately 40 days.

Pathophysiology

After absorption, mercury is distributed to all tissues, particularly the central nervous system and kidneys. Mercury reacts with sulfhydryl, phosphoryl, carboxyl, and amide groups, resulting in disruption of enzymes, transport mechanisms, membranes, and structural proteins. Widespread cellular dysfunction or necrosis results in the multiorgan toxicity characteristic of mercury poisoning.

Clinical Manifestations

Mercury poisoning may be acute or chronic and is related to exposure to elemental mercury vapors.

- Acute inhalation of elemental mercury vapor results in rapid onset of cough, dyspnea, chest pain, fever, chills, headaches, and visual disturbances.
- Gastrointestinal findings include metallic taste, salivation, nausea, vomiting, and diarrhea.
- Depending on the severity of the exposure, the illness may be self-limited or may progress to necrotizing bronchiolitis, interstitial pneumonitis, pulmonary edema, and death from respiratory failure.
- Younger children are more susceptible to pulmonary toxicity.
- Renal dysfunction and neurological disturbances (ataxia, persistent weakness, and emotional lability) may develop subacutely.

Acute ingestion of inorganic mercury salts (typically secondary to ingestion of a button battery) can manifest in a few hours as corrosive gastroenteritis, signified by metallic taste, oropharyngeal burns, nausea, hematemesis, severe abdominal pain, hematochezia, acute tubular necrosis, cardiovascular collapse, and death.

Chronic inorganic mercury intoxication produces the classic triad consisting of tremor, neuropsychiatric disturbances, and gingivitis.

Acrodynia, or pink disease, is a hypersensitivity reaction to mercury in children exposed to mercurous powders. The symptoms include:

- Generalized pain, paresthesias, and an acral (hands, feet) rash that may spread to involve the face **(Fig. 12.17)**.
- Anorexia, apathy, photophobia, and hypotonia.
- Irritability, tremors, diaphoresis, insomnia, hypertension, and tachycardia may be present.

The outcome is good after removal of the source of mercury exposure.

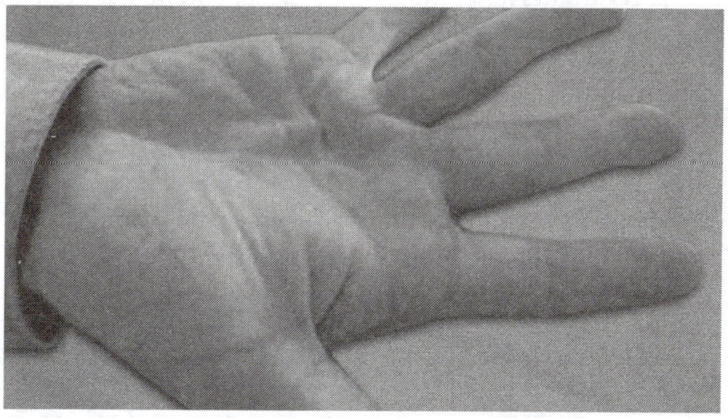

Fig. 12.17: Pink hands in mercury poisoning (pink disease).

Methyl mercury intoxication (also known as Minamata disease after the widespread mercury poisoning that occurred at Minamata Bay in Japan in people who had ingested contaminated fish**)** manifests as delayed neurotoxicity that appears after a latent period of weeks to months, and is characterized by:

- Ataxia, dysarthria, paresthesias, tremors, movement disorders, impairment of vision, hearing, smell, and taste
- Memory loss, progressive dementia, and death
- Infants exposed in utero are the most severely affected, with low birthweight, microcephaly, profound developmental delay, cerebral palsy, deafness, blindness, and seizures.
- Although there is significant residual morbidity from methyl mercury neurotoxicity; long-term follow-up of children can result in complete or partial resolution in most cases.

Laboratory Diagnosis

- The diagnosis of mercury intoxication is based on characteristic clinical findings, a history of exposure, and elevation of whole blood or urine mercury values, the last of which confirms the exposure.
- Thin layer and gas chromatographic techniques can be used to distinguish organic from inorganic mercury.
- Levels <10 µg/L in whole blood and <20 µg/L in a 24-hour urine specimen are considered normal. Although blood mercury levels may reflect acute exposure, they decrease as mercury redistributes into the tissues. Blood levels are used primarily in monitoring organic mercury poisonings.
- Urine mercury levels are most useful for identifying long-term exposures, except in the case of methyl mercury, which undergoes minimal urinary excretion.
- Hair analysis for mercury is not reliable because hair reflects both endogenous and exogenous mercury exposure (hair avidly binds mercury from the environment).
- Toenail: Toenail mercury has also been used as a measure of long-term mercury exposure, with mean levels of 0.25–0.45 mcg/g among Western samples. Toenail mercury has been correlated with fish and shellfish consumption.
- Abdominal radiographs may demonstrate ingested radiopaque mercury.
- Urinary markers of early nephrotoxicity include microalbuminuria, retinol-binding protein, β2-microglobulin, and N-acetyl-β-D-glycosaminidase.
- Early neurotoxicity may be detected with neuropsychiatric testing and nerve conduction studies, whereas severe central nervous system toxicity is apparent on CT or MRI.

Treatment

The principles of management include prompt removal from the source of poisoning, aggressive stabilization and supportive care, decontamination, and chelation therapy when appropriate.

Chelation for acute mercury poisoning is most effective when administered as soon as possible after the exposure. The efficacy of chelation in long-term exposures is reduced because heavy metal in the tissue compartment is relatively unexchangeable and some degree of irreversible toxicity has already occurred.

Dimercaprol, also known as 2,3-dimercaptopropanol or British anti-Lewisite (BAL), is the chelator of choice for a patient who cannot tolerate oral therapy, as often is true for critically ill patients and after ingestion of the corrosive inorganic arsenic and mercury salts. BAL is contraindicated for chelation of methyl mercury because BAL redistributes methyl mercury to the brain from other tissue sites, resulting in increased neurotoxicity.

D-Penicillamine is an orally administered chelator that can be considered for less-severe mercury poisoning. N-acetyl-D,L-penicillamine, an analog, is used with variable success in mercury poisoning. Oral chelating agents are used to replace the painful BAL injections when the patient is stable enough to tolerate oral therapy and prolonged chelation is necessary. **Succimer**, also known as 2,3-dimercaptosuccinic acid (DMSA), is an orally administered water-soluble derivative of BAL.

Patients with ingestion of elemental mercury require no follow-up unless there is an underlying disease that decreases the gastrointestinal transit time. Serial abdominal radiographs to document the progression of the metal are recommended. Acute inhalation of mercury fumes and ingestion of inorganic mercury require hospitalization to monitor the respiratory and gastrointestinal status, respectively.

Therapeutic abortion may be considered in pregnant patients, because of the teratogenic effect of mercury.

CLINICAL NOTE

Mercuric salts are more soluble than mercurous salts and, therefore, produce greater toxicity.

CLINICAL PEARLS

1. Mercury exists in 3 forms: Elemental mercury, inorganic mercury salts, and organic mercury.
2. Mercury reacts with sulfhydryl, phosphoryl, carboxyl, and amide groups, resulting in disruption of enzymes, transport mechanisms, membranes, and structural proteins.
3. Mercury poisoning may be acute or chronic and is related to exposure to elemental mercury vapors.
4. The diagnosis of mercury intoxication is based on characteristic clinical findings, a history of exposure, and elevation of whole blood or urine mercury values, the last of which confirms the exposure.
5. The principle of management includes prompt removal from the source of poisoning, aggressive stabilization and supportive care, decontamination, and chelation therapy when appropriate.

CASE STUDY 12

Theme: Arsenic Poisoning

A 35-year-old male is referred to a private clinic for evaluation. His symptoms began approximately 3 months ago, with the slow onset of numbness and tingling in his toes and fingertips, progressing slowly to involve the feet and hands in a symmetric "stocking-glove" fashion. In the past 2–3 weeks, the tingling has taken on a progressively painful, burning quality and he has noted weakness in gripping tools. The patient's medical history is remarkable for a flu-like illness approximately 4 months ago characterized by 3–4 days of fever, cough, diarrhea, and myalgias, which resolved spontaneously. Further questioning reveals the patient has been a carpenter since completing high school 17 years ago.

Neurological examination reveals diminished proprioception in the hands and feet, with a hyperesthetic response to pinprick sensation on the soles and slight bilateral muscular weakness in dorsiflexors of the toes and ankles.

Dermatologic examination reveals brown patches of hyperpigmentation, with scattered overlying pale spots in and around the axillae, groin, nipples, and neck. The palms and soles show multiple hyperkeratotic corn-like elevations 4–10 mm in diameter.

On initial laboratory evaluation, the CBC shows slight macrocytic anemia with hematocrit 35% (normal range: 40–52%), and MCV 111 fL (normal range: 80–100 fL). White blood cell count is 4.3 × 103/mm^3 (normal range: 3.9–11.7 × 103/mm^3); the differential reveals moderate elevation of eosinophils at 9% (normal range: 0–4%). Liver transaminases are slightly elevated. BUN, creatinine, and urinalysis are normal.

What might be the likely diagnosis?

CASE DETAILS

The patient is suffering from chronic arsenic poisoning. Peripheral neuropathy is a common complication of arsenic poisoning. The skin lesions occurring most frequently in arsenic-exposed humans are hyperpigmentation, hyperkeratosis, and skin cancer. Patchy hyperpigmentation, a pathologic hallmark of chronic exposure, may be found anywhere on the body, but occurs particularly on the eyelids, temples, axillae, neck, nipples, and groin. The classic appearance of the dark brown patches with scattered pale spots is sometimes described as "raindrops on a dusty road". In severe cases, the pigmentation extends broadly over the chest, back, and abdomen. Pigment changes have been observed in population chronically consuming drinking water containing 400 ppb or more arsenic.

BASIC CONCEPT

Arsenic

Arsenic is a metalloid that exists in 4 forms: Elemental arsenic, arsine gas, inorganic arsenic salts (pentavalent arsenate form or trivalent arsenite form), and organic arsenic compounds. Toxic manifestations are higher in the more soluble and higher-valence compounds. Arsine gas is the most toxic form of arsenic.

Sources of Arsenic Exposure (Table 12.2)

TABLE 12.2: Arsenic exposure.

S. No.	*Source*	*Examples*
1.	Natural sources	Arsenic-containing mineral ores Groundwater (especially near geothermal activity)
2.	Commercial products	Wood preservatives, pesticides, herbicides (weed killers, defoliants), fungicides, cotton desiccants, cattle and sheep dips, paints and pigments, leaded gasoline and fire salts (multicolored flame)
3.	Food products	Wine (grapes sprayed with arsenic-containing pesticides), tobacco (plants sprayed with arsenic-containing pesticides), and seafood
4.	Industrial processes	Purifying industrial gases, burning wood treated with arsenic preservatives, electronics manufacturing (microwave devices, lasers, light-emitting diodes, photoelectric cells, semiconductor devices), and hardening metal alloys, etc.
5.	Medicine	Fowler's solution, antiparasitic drugs (carbasone), veterinary pharmaceuticals, and some naturopathic remedies

Pharmacokinetics

Absorption

- Elemental arsenic is insoluble in water and bodily fluids and therefore, is insignificantly absorbed and nontoxic.
- Inhaled arsine gas is rapidly absorbed through the lungs.
- The inorganic arsenic salts are well absorbed through the gastrointestinal tract, lungs, and skin.
- The organic arsenic compounds are well absorbed through the gastrointestinal tract.

Transportation, Storage, and Excretion

After acute exposure, arsenic is initially bound to the protein portion of hemoglobin in the red blood cells (RBCs) and rapidly distributed to all tissues. Inorganic arsenic is methylated and is eliminated predominantly by the kidneys, with approximately 95% excreted in the urine and 5% excreted in the bile. Most of the arsenic is eliminated in the 1st few days, with the remainder slowly excreted over a period of several weeks. Arsenic concentrates in hair, nails, and skin. Measurement of the distance of **Mees' lines** (transverse white striae on the nail) from the nail bed can provide an estimate of time of exposure (nails grow at the rate of 0.4 mm/day) **(Fig. 12.18)**.

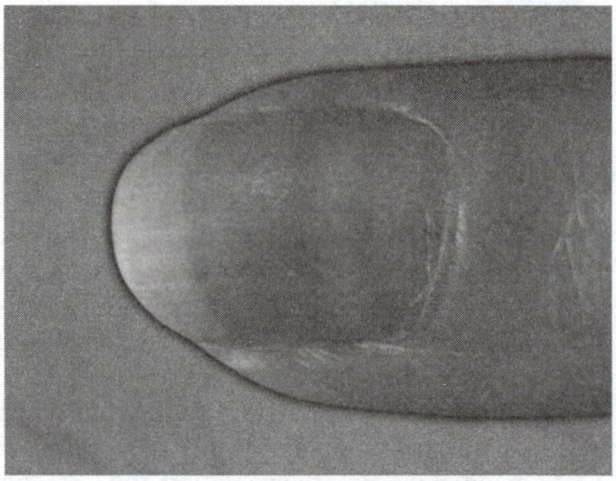

Fig. 12.18: Mees' lines in arsenic poisoning.

Pathophysiology

The absorbed arsine enters RBCs and is oxidized to arsenic dihydride and elemental arsenic. Complexing of these derivatives with red cell sulfhydryl groups results in cell membrane instability and massive hemolysis. The inorganic arsenic salts inhibit enzymatic processes vital to cellular metabolism. Trivalent arsenic binds to sulfhydryl groups, resulting in decreased production of ATP through the inhibition of pyruvate dehydrogenase, and α-ketoglutarate enzyme complexes. Pentavalent arsenic may be biotransformed to trivalent arsenic or substituted for phosphate in the glycolytic pathway, resulting in inhibition of the pathway and ATP production.

Clinical Manifestations

Acute Toxicity

- Inhalation causes no immediate symptoms.
- After a latent period of 2–24 hours, exposed individuals experience massive hemolysis, malaise, headache, weakness, dyspnea, nausea, vomiting, abdominal pain, hepatomegaly, pallor, jaundice, hemoglobinuria, and renal failure.
- Acute ingestion of arsenic produces gastrointestinal toxicity within minutes to hours and is manifested as nausea, vomiting, abdominal pain, and diarrhea.
- Hemorrhagic gastroenteritis with extensive fluid loss may result in hypovolemic shock.
- Cardiovascular toxicity includes QT interval prolongation, ventricular tachycardia, congestive cardiomyopathy, pulmonary edema, and cardiogenic shock.
- Acute neurologic toxicity includes delirium, seizures, cerebral edema, encephalopathy, and coma.
- Late sequelae include hematuria, proteinuria, and acute tubular necrosis.
- A delayed sensorimotor peripheral neuropathy may appear days to weeks after acute exposure, secondary to axonal degeneration.

Subacute toxicity is characterized by:

- Prolonged fatigue, malaise, weight loss, headache, chronic encephalopathy, peripheral sensorimotor neuropathy, leukopenia, anemia, thrombocytopenia, chronic cough, and gastroenteritis.
- Mees' lines in the nails become apparent 1–2 months after exposure in approximately 5% of patients.
- Dermatologic findings include alopecia, oral ulceration, peripheral edema, a pruritic macular rash, and desquamation.

Chronic Arsenic Toxicity

It causes significant morbidity in children resulting in skin lesions, lung disease, and defect in intellectual function.

- **Dermatologic lesions** include hyperpigmentation, hypopigmentation, hyperkeratoses (especially on the palms and soles) **(Fig. 12.19)**, squamous and basal cell carcinomas, and Bowen disease (cutaneous squamous cell carcinoma in situ).
- **Encephalopathy** and peripheral neuropathy may be present.
- Hepatomegaly, hypersplenism, noncirrhotic portal fibrosis, and portal hypertension occur.
- **Blackfoot disease** is an obliterative arterial disease of the lower extremities associated with chronic arsenic exposure that has been described in Taiwan.
- **Carcinogenicity** of chronic arsenic exposure is reflected in increased rates of cancers of the skin, lung, liver, bladder, and kidney as well as of angiosarcomas.

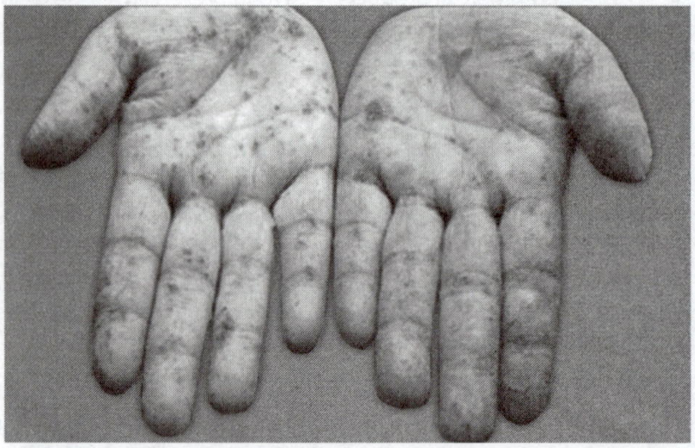

Fig. 12.19: Hyperkeratoses of the palms in arsenic poisoning.

Laboratory Findings

- The diagnosis of arsenic intoxication is based on characteristic clinical findings, a history of exposure, and elevated urinary arsenic values to confirm the exposure.
- **Urinalysis:** Concentrations greater than 50 µg/L in a 24-hour urine specimen are consistent with arsenic intoxication. Urinalysis may also show proteinuria, pyuria, and hematuria.
- **Blood arsenic levels** rarely are helpful because of their high variability and the rapid clearance of arsenic from the blood in acute poisonings.
- **Elevated arsenic values in the hair or nails** must be interpreted cautiously because of the possibility of external contamination.
- **Abdominal radiographs** may demonstrate ingested radiopaque arsenic.
- **Complete blood cell count** may show anemia, thrombocytopenia, and leukocytosis, followed by leukopenia, and basophilic stippling of RBCs.
- The serum concentrations of creatinine, bilirubin, and transaminases may be elevated.
- **Cerebrospinal fluid (CSF) examination** may show protein elevations.

Treatment

- **The principles of management** for arsenic and mercury intoxication include prompt removal from the source of poisoning, aggressive stabilization and supportive care, decontamination, and chelation therapy when appropriate.
- **Supportive care** for patients exposed to arsine gas requires close monitoring for signs of hemolysis including evaluation of the peripheral blood smear and urinalysis.
- **Acute ingestion** of inorganic arsenic salts results in hemorrhagic gastroenteritis, cardiovascular collapse, and multiorgan dysfunction. Fluid resuscitation, pressor agents, and transfusion of blood products may be required for management of cardiovascular instability. Severe respiratory distress, coma with loss of airway reflexes, intractable seizures, and respiratory paralysis are indications for intubation and mechanical ventilation.
- **Renal function** must be monitored carefully for signs of renal failure and the need for hemodialysis.
- **Gastrointestinal decontamination** after ingestion of the inorganic arsenic and mercury salts has not been well studied. Because of the corrosive effects of these compounds, induced emesis is not recommended, and endoscopy may be considered before gastric lavage. Arsenic and mercury are not well adsorbed to activated charcoal, but its use may be helpful, if coingestants are suspected. Whole-bowel irrigation is used to remove any radiopaque material remaining in the gastrointestinal tract.
- **Chelation therapy** is same as mercury toxicity.

CLINICAL NOTE

Acute ingestion of inorganic arsenic salts results in hemorrhagic gastroenteritis, cardiovascular collapse, and multiorgan dysfunction. Fluid resuscitation, pressor agents, and transfusion of blood products may be required for management of cardiovascular instability.

CLINICAL PEARLS

1. Arsenic is a metalloid that exists in 4 forms: elemental arsenic, arsine gas, inorganic arsenic salts (pentavalent arsenate form or trivalent arsenite form), and organic arsenic compounds.
2. After acute exposure, arsenic is initially bound to the protein portion of hemoglobin in the RBCs and rapidly distributed to all tissues.
3. After a latent period of 2–24 hours, exposed individuals experience massive hemolysis, malaise, headache, weakness, dyspnea, nausea, vomiting, abdominal pain, hepatomegaly, pallor, jaundice, hemoglobinuria, and renal failure.
4. The diagnosis of arsenic intoxication is based on characteristic clinical findings, a history of exposure, and elevated urinary arsenic values to confirm the exposure.
5. The principle of management for arsenic intoxication includes prompt removal from the source of poisoning, aggressive stabilization and supportive care, decontamination, and chelation therapy when appropriate.

Chapter 13

Heme Synthesis and Degradation

LEARNING OBJECTIVES

To understand:

- Steps of heme synthesis
- Clinical implications of impaired heme biosynthesis
- Steps of heme degradation and bilirubin synthesis
- Clinical implications of impaired bilirubin metabolism

CASE STUDIES

CASE STUDY 1

Theme: Bilirubin Metabolism and Differential Diagnosis of Jaundice

A 65-year-old male who was unwell from the previous few months came for consultation. Past history revealed that he was under a lot of mental stress and had developed loss of appetite, weakness, malaise, and nausea. He also reported that his eyes were dark yellow from the last few weeks, urine was also turning deep yellow but the stool color was pale. He had lost around 5 kg of weight since his last visit (2 months ago) when he was admitted in the same hospital for some abdominal problem. There was no history of any fever, drug intake, alcoholism, or any other problem.

On physical examination, the patient was found to be undernourished. Yellow discoloration of skin, sclera, and palate was observed.

The vital signs were normal. Liver was enlarged and tender. The laboratory investigation report was as follows:

Blood biochemistry:

- Total bilirubin: 10.2 mg%
- Indirect bilirubin: 1.5 mg%
- Direct bilirubin: 8.7 mg%
- Serum glutamate oxaloacetic transaminase (SGOT): 28 IU/L
- Serum glutamate-pyruvate transaminase (SGPT): 35 IU/L
- Serum alkaline phosphatase (ALP): 220 IU/L

Urine examination:

- Bile pigment: Positive
- Urobilinogen: Negative
- Bile salts: Positive

What is the probable diagnosis?

CASE DETAILS

The typical history, conjugated hyperbilirubinemia, normal level of transaminases, high ALP, and bilirubin in urine strongly signify that the patient is suffering from jaundice, which is most probably obstructive jaundice. The cause of obstruction seems to be malignancy, probably carcinoma head of the pancreas. The confirmation of the diagnosis can be done by ultrasound, computed tomography (CT) scan, or magnetic resonance cholangiopancreatography (MRCP).

JAUNDICE

Jaundice is a yellow discoloration of the skin, mucous membranes, and sclera caused by increased amounts of bilirubin in the blood. Jaundice is a sign of an underlying disease process.

BASIC CONCEPT

Formation and fate of bilirubin: Bilirubin is the end product of heme degradation. From 70 to 90% of bilirubin is derived from degradation of the hemoglobin of senescent red blood cells. Bilirubin produced in the periphery is transported to the liver within the plasma, where, due to its insolubility in aqueous solutions, it is tightly bound to albumin.

Under normal circumstances, bilirubin is removed from the circulation rapidly and efficiently by hepatocytes.

Transfer of bilirubin from blood to bile involves four distinct but interrelated steps:

1. **Hepatocellular uptake:** Uptake of bilirubin by the hepatocyte has carrier-mediated kinetics.
2. **Intracellular binding:** Within the hepatocyte, bilirubin is kept in solution by binding as a nonsubstrate ligand to several of the glutathione-S-transferases, formerly called ligandins.
3. **Conjugation:** Bilirubin is conjugated with one or two glucuronic acid moieties by a specific UDP-glucuronosyltransferase to form bilirubin mono- and diglucuronide, respectively**. Conjugation disrupts the internal hydrogen bonding that limits aqueous solubility of bilirubin, and the resulting glucuronide conjugates are highly soluble in water.** Conjugation is obligatory for excretion of bilirubin across the bile canalicular membrane into bile. The UDP-glucuronosyltransferases have been classified into gene families based on the degree of homology among the mRNAs for the various isoforms. Those that conjugate bilirubin and certain other substrates have been designated the UGT1 family. These are expressed from a single gene complex by alternative promoter usage. This gene complex contains multiple substrate-specific first exons, designated A1, A2, etc. each with its own promoter and each encoding the amino-terminal half of a specific isoform. Exon A1 and the four common exons, collectively designated the UGT1A1 gene, encode the physiologically critical enzyme bilirubin-UDP-glucuronosyltransferase (UGT1A1).
4. **Biliary excretion:** Bilirubin mono- and diglucuronides are excreted across the canalicular plasma membrane into the bile canaliculus by an ATP-dependent transport process mediated by a canalicular membrane protein called multidrug resistance-associated protein 2 (MRP2). Mutations of MRP2 result in the **Dubin–Johnson syndrome.**

Extrahepatic Aspects of Bilirubin Disposition

Bilirubin in the gut: Following secretion into bile, conjugated bilirubin reaches the duodenum and passes down the gastrointestinal tract without reabsorption by the intestinal mucosa. An appreciable fraction is converted by bacterial metabolism in the gut to the water-soluble colorless compound, urobilinogen. About 80–90% of these products are excreted in feces, either unchanged or oxidized to orange derivatives called urobilins. The remaining 10–20% of the urobilinogens are passively absorbed, enter the portal venous blood, and are re-excreted by the liver. A small fraction (usually <3 mg/dL) escapes hepatic uptake, filters across the renal glomerulus and is excreted in urine **(Fig. 13.1)**.

Unconjugated bilirubin ordinarily does not reach the gut except in neonates or, by ill-defined alternative pathways, in the presence of severe unconjugated hyperbilirubinemia [e.g., Crigler–Najjar syndrome type I (CNS-I)]. Unconjugated bilirubin that reaches the gut is partly reabsorbed, amplifying any underlying hyperbilirubinemia.

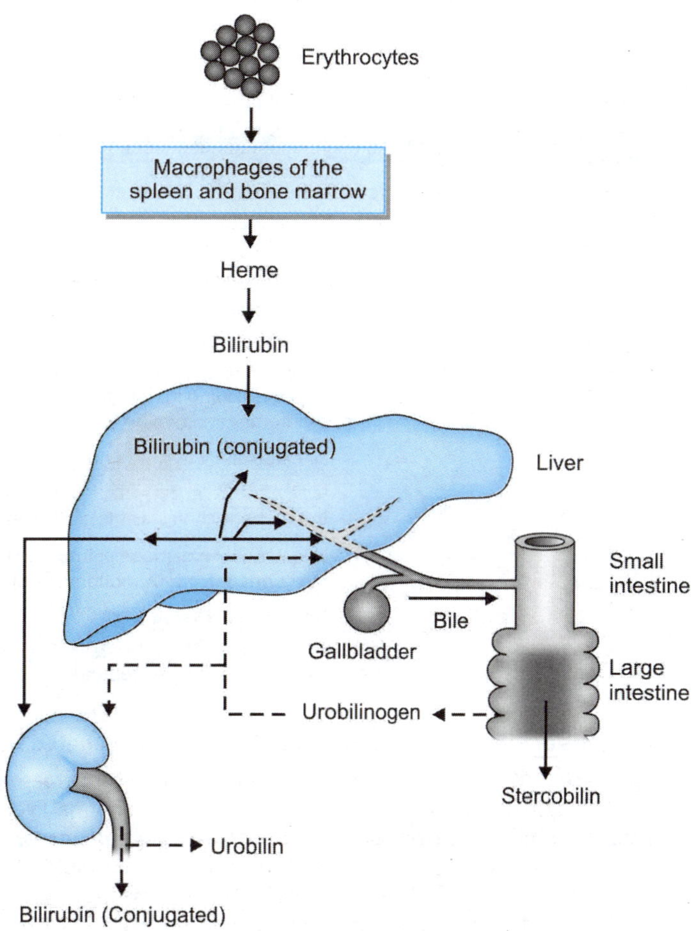

Fig. 13.1: Formation and fate of bilirubin.

Renal Excretion of Bilirubin Conjugates

Unconjugated bilirubin is not excreted in urine, as it is too tightly bound to albumin for effective glomerular filtration and there is no tubular mechanism for its renal secretion. In contrast, the bilirubin conjugates are readily filtered at the glomerulus and can appear in urine in disorders characterized by increased bilirubin conjugates in the circulation.

Biochemical Defect in Jaundice

Jaundice results from the accumulation of bilirubin. Hyperbilirubinemia may be due to abnormalities in the formation, transport, metabolism, and excretion of bilirubin. Total serum bilirubin is normally 0.2–1.2 mg/dL (mean levels are higher in men than women and higher in whites and Hispanics than blacks), and jaundice may not be recognizable until levels are about 3 mg/dL.

In the normal adult, the rate of systemic bilirubin production is equal to the rates of hepatic uptake, conjugation, and biliary excretion. Jaundice occurs (bilirubin levels may reach 30–40 mg/dL in severe disease) when the equilibrium between bilirubin production and clearance is disturbed by one or more of the following mechanisms: (1) excessive production of bilirubin, (2) reduced hepatic uptake, (3) impaired conjugation, (4) decreased hepatocellular excretion, and (5) impaired bile flow (both intrahepatic and extrahepatic). The first three mechanisms produce unconjugated hyperbilirubinemia, and the latter two produce predominantly conjugated hyperbilirubinemia. More than one mechanism may operate to produce jaundice, especially in hepatitis, which may produce unconjugated and conjugated hyperbilirubinemia. In general, however, one mechanism predominates, so that knowledge of the predominant form of plasma bilirubin is of value in evaluating possible causes of hyperbilirubinemia.

Classification of Jaundice

Jaundice can be classified in many ways:

Based on location of defect:

a. Prehepatic
b. Hepatic
c. Posthepatic

Based on type of hyperbilirubinemia:

a. Unconjugated hyperbilirubinemia
b. Conjugated hyperbilirubinemia
c. Mixed hyperbilirubinemia

The classification and different causes of jaundice are summarized in **Table 13.1**.

TABLE 13.1: Classification of jaundice based on type of hyperbilirubinemia.

Type of hyperbilirubinemia	*Location and cause*
Unconjugated hyperbilirubinemia (indirect-reacting bilirubin)	Increased bilirubin production (e.g., hemolytic anemia, hemolytic reactions, hematoma, pulmonary infarction) Impaired bilirubin uptake and storage (e.g., posthepatitis hyperbilirubinemia, Gilbert's syndrome, Crigler–Najjar syndrome, drug reactions)
Conjugated hyperbilirubinemia (predominant direct-reacting bilirubin)	**Hereditary cholestatic syndromes** Faulty excretion of bilirubin conjugates (e.g., Dubin–Johnson syndrome, Rotor's syndrome) or mutation in genes coding for bile salt transport proteins (e.g., progressive familial intrahepatic cholestasis syndromes and benign recurrent intrahepatic cholestasis)
	Hepatocellular dysfunction Biliary epithelial damage (e.g., hepatitis, hepatic cirrhosis) Intrahepatic cholestasis (e.g., certain drugs, biliary cirrhosis, sepsis, postoperative jaundice)
	Hepatocellular damage or intrahepatic cholestasis resulting from miscellaneous causes (e.g., spirochetal infections, infectious mononucleosis, cholangitis, sarcoidosis, lymphomas, industrial toxins)
	Biliary obstruction Choledocholithiasis, biliary atresia, carcinoma of biliary duct, sclerosing cholangitis, choledochal cyst, external pressure on common duct, pancreatitis, pancreatic neoplasms

Disorders of Bilirubin Metabolism Leading to Unconjugated Hyperbilirubinemia

Hemolysis: Increased destruction of erythrocytes leads to increased bilirubin turnover and unconjugated hyperbilirubinemia; the hyperbilirubinemia is usually modest in the presence of normal liver function. **In particular, the bone marrow is only capable of a sustained eight-fold increase in erythrocyte production in response to a hemolytic stress.** Therefore, hemolysis alone cannot result in a sustained hyperbilirubinemia of more than ~68 mol/L (4 mg/dL). Higher values imply concomitant hepatic dysfunction. When hemolysis is the only abnormality in an otherwise healthy individual, the result is a purely unconjugated hyperbilirubinemia, with the direct-reacting fraction as measured in a typical clinical laboratory being 15% of the total serum bilirubin. In the presence of systemic disease, which may include a degree of hepatic dysfunction, hemolysis may produce a component of conjugated hyperbilirubinemia in addition to an elevated unconjugated bilirubin concentration. Prolonged hemolysis may lead to the precipitation of bilirubin salts within the gallbladder or biliary tree, resulting in the formation of gallstones in which bilirubin, rather than cholesterol, is the major component. Such pigment stones may lead to acute or chronic cholecystitis, biliary obstruction, or any other biliary tract consequence of calculus disease.

Ineffective erythropoiesis: During erythroid maturation, small amounts of hemoglobin may be lost at the time of nuclear extrusion, and a fraction of developing erythroid cells is destroyed within the marrow. These processes normally account for a small proportion of bilirubin that is produced. **In various disorders—including thalassemia major, megaloblastic anemia due to folate or vitamin B_{12} deficiency, congenital erythropoietic porphyria, lead poisoning, and various congenital and acquired dyserythropoietic anemias—the fraction of total bilirubin production derived from ineffective erythropoiesis is increased, reaching as much as 70% of the total.** This may be sufficient to produce modest degrees of unconjugated hyperbilirubinemia.

Miscellaneous: Degradation of the hemoglobin of extravascular collections of erythrocytes, such as those seen in massive tissue infarctions or large hematomas, may lead transiently to unconjugated hyperbilirubinemia.

Decreased Hepatic Bilirubin Clearance

Decreased hepatic uptake: Decreased hepatic bilirubin uptake is believed to contribute to the unconjugated hyperbilirubinemia of Gilbert's syndrome (GS), although the molecular basis for this finding remains unclear. **Several drugs including flavaspidic acid, novobiocin, rifampin, and various cholecystography-contrast agents, have been reported to inhibit bilirubin uptake.** The resulting unconjugated hyperbilirubinemia resolves with cessation of the medication.

Impaired Conjugation

Physiological neonatal jaundice: Bilirubin produced by the fetus is cleared by the placenta and eliminated by the maternal liver. Immediately after birth, the neonatal liver must assume responsibility for bilirubin clearance and excretion. However, many hepatic physiological processes are incompletely developed at birth. Levels of UGT1A1 are low, and alternative excretory pathways allow passage of unconjugated bilirubin into the gut. Since the intestinal flora that convert bilirubin to urobilinogen are also undeveloped, an enterohepatic circulation of unconjugated bilirubin ensues. As a consequence, most neonates develop mild unconjugated hyperbilirubinemia between days 2 and days 5 after birth. Peak levels are typically <85–170 mol/L (5–10 mg/dL) and decline to normal adult concentrations within 2 weeks, as mechanisms required for bilirubin disposition mature. Prematurity, with more profound immaturity of hepatic function, or hemolysis, results in higher levels of unconjugated hyperbilirubinemia. **A rapidly rising unconjugated bilirubin concentration, or absolute levels >340 mol/L (20 mg/dL), puts the infant at risk for bilirubin encephalopathy, or kernicterus.** Under these circumstances, bilirubin crosses an immature blood–brain barrier and precipitates in the basal ganglia and other areas of the brain. The consequences range from appreciable neurological deficits to death. Treatment options include phototherapy, which converts bilirubin into water-soluble photoisomers that are excreted directly into bile and exchange transfusion **(Fig. 13.2)**. The canalicular mechanisms responsible for bilirubin excretion are also immature at birth, and their maturation may lag behind that of UGT1A1; this can lead to transient conjugated neonatal hyperbilirubinemia, especially in infants with hemolysis.

Acquired conjugation defects: A modest reduction in bilirubin-conjugating capacity may be observed in advanced hepatitis or cirrhosis. However, in this setting, conjugation is better preserved than other aspects of bilirubin disposition, such as canalicular excretion. Various drugs including pregnanediol, novobiocin, chloramphenicol, and gentamicin, may produce unconjugated hyperbilirubinemia by inhibiting UGT1A1 activity. Finally, **bilirubin conjugation may be inhibited by certain fatty acids that are present in breast milk but not serum of mothers whose infants have excessive neonatal hyperbilirubinemia (breast milk jaundice).** The pathogenesis of breast milk jaundice appears to differ from that of transient familial neonatal hyperbilirubinemia (Lucey–Driscoll syndrome), in which there is a UGT1A1 inhibitor in maternal serum.

Hereditary defects in bilirubin conjugation: Three familial disorders characterized by differing degrees of unconjugated hyperbilirubinemia have long been recognized. The defining clinical features of each are described below **(Table 13.2)**.

TABLE 13.2: Principal differential characteristics of Gilbert's and Crigler–Najjar syndromes.

	Crigler–Najjar syndrome		
Feature	*Type I*	*Type II*	*Gilbert's syndrome*
Total serum bilirubin (mg/dL)	[18–45 (usually >20)]	[6–25 (usually 20)]	Typically (4 mg/dL) in absence of fasting or hemolysis
Routine liver tests	Normal	Normal	Normal
Response to phenobarbital	None	Decreases bilirubin by >25%	Decreases bilirubin to normal
Kernicterus	Usual	Rare	No
Hepatic histology	Normal	Normal	Usually normal; increased lipofuscin pigment in some
Bile characteristics			
Color	Pale or colorless	Pigmented	Normal dark color
Bilirubin fractions	>90% unconjugated	Largest fraction (mean: 57%) monoconjugates	Normal dark color— mainly disconjugate monoconjugates are also increased (mean: 23%)
Bilirubin UDP-glucuronosyltransferase activity	Typically absent; traces in some patients	Markedly reduced: 0–10% of normal	Reduced: typically 10–33% of normal
Inheritance (all autosomal)	Recessive	Predominantly recessive	Promoter mutation: Recessive

Disorders of Bilirubin Metabolism Leading to Mixed or Predominantly Conjugated Hyperbilirubinemia

In hyperbilirubinemia due to acquired liver disease (e.g., acute hepatitis and common bile duct stone), there are usually elevations in the serum concentrations of both conjugated and unconjugated bilirubin. **Although, biliary tract obstruction or hepatocellular cholestatic injury may present on occasion with a predominantly conjugated hyperbilirubinemia, it is generally not possible to differentiate intrahepatic from extrahepatic causes of jaundice based upon the serum levels or relative proportions of unconjugated and conjugated bilirubin.** The major reason for determining the amounts of conjugated and unconjugated bilirubin in the serum is for the initial differentiation of hepatic parenchymal and obstructive disorders (mixed conjugated and unconjugated hyperbilirubinemia) from the inheritable and hemolytic disorders, discussed above, that are associated with unconjugated hyperbilirubinemia **(Table 13.3)**.

Liver Biochemical Tests

The following tests are undertaken for the differential diagnosis of jaundice **(Table 13.3)**.

TABLE 13.3: Liver biochemical tests—changes in three types of jaundice.

Tests	*Prehepatic jaundice*	*Hepatocellular jaundice*	*Uncomplicated obstructive jaundice*
Bilirubin			
Direct	—	Increased	Increased
Indirect	Increased	Increased	Increased
Urine bilirubin	None	Increased	Increased
Urine urobilinogen	Increased	Increased	Absent
Serum albumin/ total protein	Normal	Albumin decreased Total protein: 6.5–8.4 g/dL	Unchanged
Alkaline	Normal	Increased (+)	Increased (++++)
Phosphatase, prothrombin time	Normal	Prolonged if damage is severe and does not respond to parenteral vitamin K	Prolonged if obstruction marked, but responds to parenteral vitamin K
ALT, AST	Normal	Increased in hepatocellular damage, viral hepatitis	Minimally increased

(ALT: alanine aminotransferase; AST: aspartate aminotransferase)

Dubin–Johnson Syndrome

This benign and relatively rare disorder is characterized by low-grade, predominantly conjugated hyperbilirubinemia. **Total bilirubin concentrations are typically between 34 mol/L and 85 mol/L (2 mg/dL and 5 mg/dL) but on occasion can be in the normal range or as high as 340–430 mol/L (20–25 mg/dL) and can fluctuate widely in any given patient.** The degree of hyperbilirubinemia may be increased by intercurrent illness, oral contraceptive use, and pregnancy. As the hyperbilirubinemia is due to a predominant rise in conjugated bilirubin, bilirubinuria is characteristically present. Aside from elevated serum bilirubin levels, other routine laboratory tests are normal. Physical examination is usually normal except for jaundice, although an occasional patient may have hepatosplenomegaly.

Rotor Syndrome

This benign and autosomal recessive disorder is clinically similar to Dubin–Johnson syndrome (DJS), although it is seen even less frequently. **A major phenotypic difference is that the liver in patients with Rotor syndrome has no increased pigmentation and appears totally normal. The only abnormality in routine laboratory tests is an elevation of total serum bilirubin, due to a predominant rise in conjugated bilirubin. This is accompanied by bilirubinuria.** The pattern in Rotor syndrome resembles that of many acquired disorders of hepatobiliary function, in which coproporphyrin I, the major coproporphyrin isomer in bile, refluxes from the hepatocyte back into the circulation and is excreted in urine. Thus, total urinary coproporphyrin excretion is substantially increased in Rotor syndrome, in contrast to the normal levels seen in DJS.

Benign Recurrent Intrahepatic Cholestasis

This rare disorder is characterized by recurrent attacks of pruritus and jaundice. The typical episode begins with mild malaise and elevations in serum aminotransferase levels, followed rapidly by rises in alkaline phosphatase and conjugated bilirubin and onset of jaundice and itching. The first one or two episodes may be misdiagnosed as acute viral hepatitis. The cholestatic episodes, which may begin in childhood or adulthood, can vary in duration from several weeks to months, following which there is complete clinical and biochemical resolution. Intervals between attacks may vary from several months to years. Between episodes, physical examination is normal, as are serum levels of bile acids, bilirubin, transaminases, and alkaline phosphatase. The disorder is familial and has an autosomal recessive pattern of inheritance. **Benign recurrent intrahepatic cholestasis (BRIC) is considered a benign disorder in that it does not lead to cirrhosis or end-stage liver disease.** However, the episodes of jaundice and pruritus can be prolonged and debilitating, and some patients have undergone liver transplantation to relieve the intractable and disabling symptoms. Treatment during the cholestatic episodes is symptomatic; there is no specific treatment to prevent or shorten the occurrence of episodes.

Progressive Familial Intrahepatic Cholestasis

This name is applied to three phenotypically related syndromes. Progressive familial intrahepatic cholestasis (FIC) Type 1 (Byler disease) presents in early infancy as cholestasis that may be initially episodic. However, in contrast to BRIC, Byler disease progresses to malnutrition, growth retardation, and end-stage liver disease during childhood. Two other types of progressive FIC (Types 2 and 3) have been described. Although all three types of progressive FIC have similar clinical phenotypes, only Type 3 is associated with high serum levels of γ-glutamyl transferase activity. In contrast, activity of this enzyme is normal or only mildly elevated in symptomatic BRIC and progressive FIC Types 1 and 2.

Clinical Features

Unconjugated Hyperbilirubinemia

Stool and urine color are normal, and there is mild jaundice and indirect (unconjugated) hyperbilirubinemia with no bilirubin in the urine. Splenomegaly occurs in hemolytic disorders, except in sickle cell anemia.

Conjugated Hyperbilirubinemia

Hereditary cholestatic syndromes or intrahepatic cholestasis: The patient may be asymptomatic; cholestasis is often accompanied by pruritus, light-colored stools, and jaundice.

Hepatocellular Disease

Malaise, anorexia, low-grade fever, and right upper quadrant discomfort are frequent. Dark urine, jaundice, and, in women, amenorrhea occur. **An enlarged tender liver, vascular spiders, palmar erythema, ascites, gynecomastia, sparse body hair, fetor hepaticus, and asterixis may be present, depending** on the cause, severity, and chronicity of liver dysfunction.

Biliary Obstruction

There may be right upper quadrant pain, weight loss (suggesting carcinoma), jaundice, dark urine, and light-colored stools. Symptoms and signs may be intermittent, if caused by stone, carcinoma of the ampulla, or cholangiocarcinoma. Pain may be absent early in pancreatic cancer. Occult blood in the stools suggests cancer of the ampulla. Hepatomegaly and a palpable gallbladder (Courvoisier's sign) are characteristic, but neither specific nor sensitive, of a pancreatic head tumor. Fever and chills are more common in benign obstruction with associated cholangitis.

In newborns, as the bilirubin level rises, jaundice will typically progress from the head to the trunk, and then to the hands and feet. Additional signs and symptoms that may be seen in the newborn are—poor feeding, lethargy, changes in muscle tone, high-pitched crying, and seizures.

Diagnosis

The goal of testing is to determine the cause of the jaundice and to evaluate the severity of the underlying condition. The initial step is to obtain appropriate blood tests to determine if the patient has an isolated elevation of serum bilirubin. If so, is the bilirubin elevation due to an increased unconjugated or conjugated fraction? If the hyperbilirubinemia is accompanied by other liver test abnormalities **(Table 13.3)**, is the disorder hepatocellular or cholestatic? If cholestatic, is it intrahepatic or extrahepatic? All of these questions can be answered with a thoughtful history, physical examination, interpretation of laboratory and radiological tests and procedures.

Laboratory Studies

Measurement of serum bilirubin: The terms direct- and indirect-reacting bilirubin are based on the original **van den Bergh reaction**. This assay, or a variation of it, is still used in most clinical chemistry laboratories to determine the serum bilirubin level. In this assay, bilirubin is exposed to diazotized sulfanilic acid, splitting into two relatively stable dipyrrylmethene azopigments that absorb maximally at 540 nm, allowing for photometric analysis. **The direct fraction is that which reacts with diazotized sulfanilic acid in the absence of an accelerator substance, such as alcohol.** The direct fraction provides an approximate determination of the conjugated bilirubin in serum. **The total serum bilirubin is the amount that reacts after the addition of alcohol. The indirect fraction is the difference between the total and the direct bilirubin and provides an estimate of the unconjugated bilirubin in serum.**

With the van den Bergh method, the normal serum bilirubin concentration usually is 17 mol/L (<1 mg/dL). Up to 30%, or 5.1 mol/L (0.3 mg/dL), of the total may be direct-reacting (conjugated) bilirubin. Total serum bilirubin concentrations are between 3.4 mol/L and 15.4 mol/L (0.2 mg/dL and 0.9 mg/dL) in 95% of a normal population.

Measurement of urine bilirubin: Unconjugated bilirubin is always bound to albumin in the serum, is not filtered by the kidney, and is not found in the urine. Conjugated bilirubin is filtered at the glomerulus and the majority is reabsorbed by the proximal tubules; a small fraction is excreted in the urine. Any bilirubin found in the urine is conjugated bilirubin. The presence of bilirubinuria implies the presence of liver disease. A urine dipstick test (Ictotest) gives the same information as fractionation of the serum bilirubin. This test is very accurate. A false-negative test is possible in patients with prolonged cholestasis due to the predominance of conjugated bilirubin covalently bound to albumin.

Serum alanine and aspartate aminotransferase (ALT and AST) levels vary with age and correlate with body mass index. Elevated alkaline phosphatase levels are seen in cholestasis or infiltrative liver disease (such as tumor or granuloma). Alkaline phosphatase elevations of hepatic rather than bone, intestinal, or placental origin are confirmed by concomitant elevation of γ-glutamyl transpeptidase or 5′-nucleotidase levels. The differential diagnosis of any liver test elevation includes toxicity caused by drugs, herbal remedies, and toxins.

Liver Biopsy

Percutaneous liver biopsy is the definitive study for determining the cause and histologic severity of hepatocellular dysfunction or infiltrative liver disease. In patients with suspected metastatic disease or a hepatic mass, it is performed under ultrasound or CT guidance. Panels of blood tests (e.g., Fibrosure) and transient elastography (an ultrasonographic technique to measure liver stiffness) are under study to estimate the degree of liver fibrosis without the need for liver biopsy.

Imaging

Demonstration of dilated bile ducts by ultrasonography or CT scan indicates biliary obstruction (90–95% sensitivity). Ultrasonography, CT scan, and MRI may also demonstrate hepatomegaly, intrahepatic tumors, and portal hypertension. Magnetic resonance cholangiopancreatography (MRCP) is a sensitive and noninvasive method of detecting bile duct stones, strictures, and dilation; however, it is less reliable than endoscopic retrograde cholangiopancreatography (ERCP) for distinguishing malignant from benign strictures.

Treatment

The treatment is entirely dependent on the cause of the jaundice. In some cases, it will be curative, e.g., surgical removal of a gallstone blocking the common bile duct. Viral infections, e.g., hepatitis A may recover spontaneously. In other cases, treatment will modify the disease process and the jaundice will improve or disappear. Treatment may be purely symptomatic, e.g., drugs to relieve itching or palliative as in malignant disease. Some types of advanced liver disease causing jaundice may be treated by liver transplantation.

Phototherapy for Neonatal Jaundice

The goal of therapy is to lower the concentration of circulating bilirubin or keep it from increasing. Phototherapy achieves this by using light energy to change the shape and structure of bilirubin, converting it to molecules that can be excreted even when normal conjugation is deficient.

Phototherapy converts bilirubin to yellow photoisomers and colorless oxidation products that are less lipophilic than bilirubin and do not require hepatic conjugation for excretion. Photoisomers are excreted mainly in bile, and oxidation products predominantly in urine **(Fig. 13.2)**.

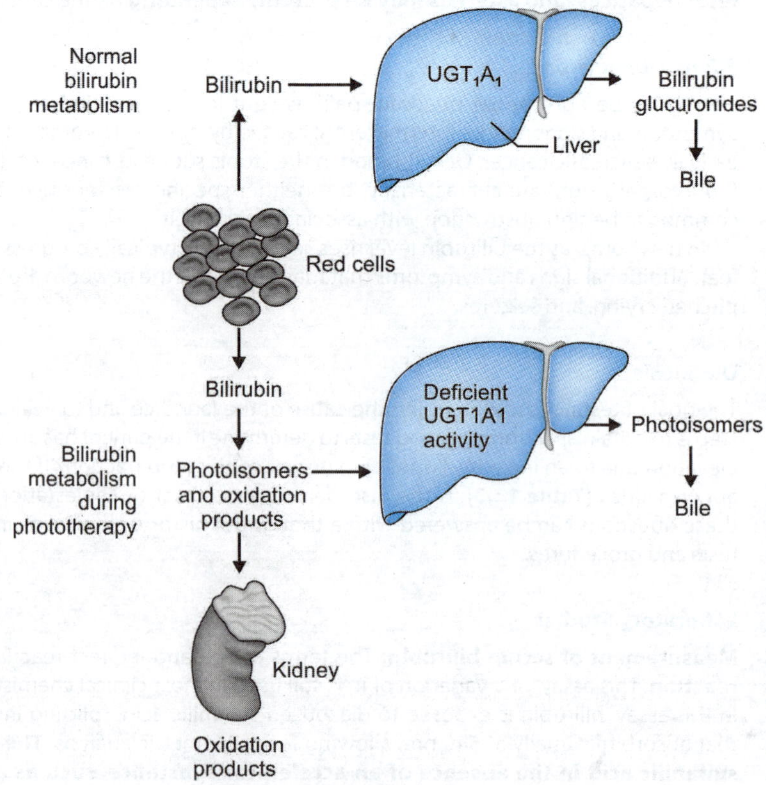

Fig. 13.2: Effect of phototherapy in jaundice.

Prognosis

It is fairly good in the treated cases, except in cases of malignant obstruction of common bile duct.

CLINICAL NOTE

The term "cholestasis" denotes retention of bile in the liver, and the term "cholestatic jaundice" is often used when conjugated hyperbilirubinemia results from impaired bile flow.

CLINICAL PEARLS

1. Jaundice results from the accumulation of bilirubin—a product of heme metabolism—in the body tissues. Hyperbilirubinemia may be due to abnormalities in the formation, transport, metabolism, and excretion of bilirubin.
2. Total serum bilirubin is normally 0.2–1.2 mg/dL (mean levels are higher in men than women and higher in whites and Hispanics than blacks), and jaundice may not be recognizable until levels are about 3 mg/dL.
3. The goal of testing is to determine the cause of the jaundice and to evaluate the severity of the underlying condition. Initial testing is usually focused on the liver.
4. The type of treatment is entirely dependent on the cause of the jaundice. In some cases, it will be curative, e.g., surgical removal of a gallstone blocking the common bile duct. Viral infections, e.g., hepatitis A, may recover spontaneously. In other cases, treatments will modify the disease process and the jaundice will improve or disappear.
5. Phototherapy converts bilirubin to yellow photoisomers and colorless oxidation products that are less lipophilic than bilirubin and do not require hepatic conjugation for excretion. Photoisomers are excreted mainly in bile, and oxidation products predominantly in urine.

CASE STUDY 2

Theme: Steps and Significance of Heme Synthesis

A 30-year-old woman had severe abdominal pain, nausea, vomiting, and diarrhea. Evaluations including upper and lower endoscopies did not establish any intestinal infection. She gradually improved and was discharged after 2 weeks. 2 years later, she was admitted to a psychiatric unit with acute mental changes and hallucinations, she had to be transferred to the emergency department due to abdominal pain, a grand mal seizure and hyponatremia.

Her pulse was 120 beats/min and BP was 174/114 mm Hg. She was disoriented but had no focal neurological signs. MRI showed subcortical abnormalities, and the spinal fluid was normal. After cholecystectomy for a distended gallbladder, she was discharged but she stayed with a family member in another city because her symptoms were worse and muscle weakness had developed. She was hospitalized and progressed to quadriparesis, respiratory failure, and aspiration pneumonia. Urinary porphobilinogen (PBG) was reported as 44 mg/24 hours (reference range 0–4).

What are the diagnosis and defect in this disease?
How is the diagnosis done and what is its prognosis?
What is the genetic basis of this disease?

CASE DISCUSSION

The patient is suffering from acute intermittent porphyria as is evident from the typical combination of abdominal pain, motor neuropathy, psychiatric symptoms and increased amounts of urinary porphyrins and their precursors. Acute intermittent porphyria (AIP) is a rare autosomal-dominant metabolic disorder affecting the production of heme. It is characterized by deficiency of enzyme porphobilinogen deaminase.

BASIC CONCEPT

Heme Synthesis

Heme biosynthesis involves eight enzymatic steps in the conversion of glycine and succinyl-CoA to heme **(Fig. 13.3)**. These eight enzymes are encoded by nine genes, as the first enzyme in the pathway, 5′-aminolevulinate synthase (ALA-synthase), has two genes that encode unique housekeeping (ALAS1) and erythroid-specific (ALAS2) isozymes. The first and last three enzymes in the pathway are located in the mitochondrion, whereas the other four are in the cytosol. Heme is required for a variety of hemoproteins, such as hemoglobin, myoglobin, respiratory cytochromes, and the cytochrome P450 enzymes (CYPs). **Hemoglobin synthesis in erythroid precursor cells accounts for approximately 85% of daily heme synthesis in humans. Hepatocytes account for**

most of the rest, primarily for synthesis of CYPs, which are especially abundant in the liver endoplasmic reticulum, and turn over more rapidly than many other hemoproteins, such as the mitochondrial respiratory cytochromes. As shown in **Figure 13.3**, pathway intermediates are the porphyrin precursors, ALA and PBG, and porphyrins (mostly in their reduced forms, known as porphyrinogens). At least in humans, these intermediates do not accumulate in significant amounts under normal conditions or have important physiological functions.

The first and rate-controlling step is the condensation of glycine and succinyl–coenzyme A (CoA) to form δ-aminolevulinic acid (ALA). The enzyme, ALA synthase, is activated by pyridoxal phosphate. In the liver, this rate-limiting enzyme can be induced by a variety of drugs, steroids, and other chemicals. The distinct nonerythroid (e.g., housekeeping) and erythroid-specific forms of ALA-synthase are encoded by separate genes located on chromosome 3p21.1 (ALAS1) and Xp11.2 (ALAS2), respectively. Defects in the erythroid gene ALAS2 cause X-linked sideroblastic anemia (XLSA).

The ALA formed is transported into the cytoplasm, where the second enzyme, ALA dehydratase (also known as porphobilinogen synthase), condenses two molecules of ALA to form the monopyrrole porphobilinogen. The third enzyme, porphobilinogen deaminase (also known as hydroxymethylbilane synthase), forms a linear tetrapyrrole, hydroxymethylbilane, which is normally rapidly converted, mainly to the cyclic intermediate uroporphyrinogen III, by the enzyme uroporphyrinogen III synthase (also known as uroporphyrinogen cosynthase). When uroporphyrinogen III synthase is deficient, as in congenital erythropoietic porphyria (Guenther's disease), hydroxymethylbilane rapidly undergoes nonenzymatic ring closure to form uroporphyrinogen I. The enzyme uroporphyrinogen decarboxylase carries out the stepwise decarboxylation of uroporphyrinogen I or III to form intermediates with 7-, 6-, 5-, and 4-carboxyl groups. Coproporphyrinogen is the common name for the 4-carboxyl–containing intermediate. Coproporphyrinogen III is transported back into mitochondria, where the enzyme coproporphyrinogen III oxidase carries out the stepwise oxidative decarboxylation of two of the remaining propionate β side chains, at positions 2 and 4 (on rings A and B, respectively), to vinyl groups, forming protoporphyrinogen IX. Next, the enzyme protoporphyrinogen oxidase carries out the oxidation of protoporphyrinogen IX to form protoporphyrin IX, after which the enzyme ferrochelatase (also called heme synthase) inserts ferrous iron into the protoporphyrin IX macrocycle to form the end product heme **(Fig. 13.3)**.

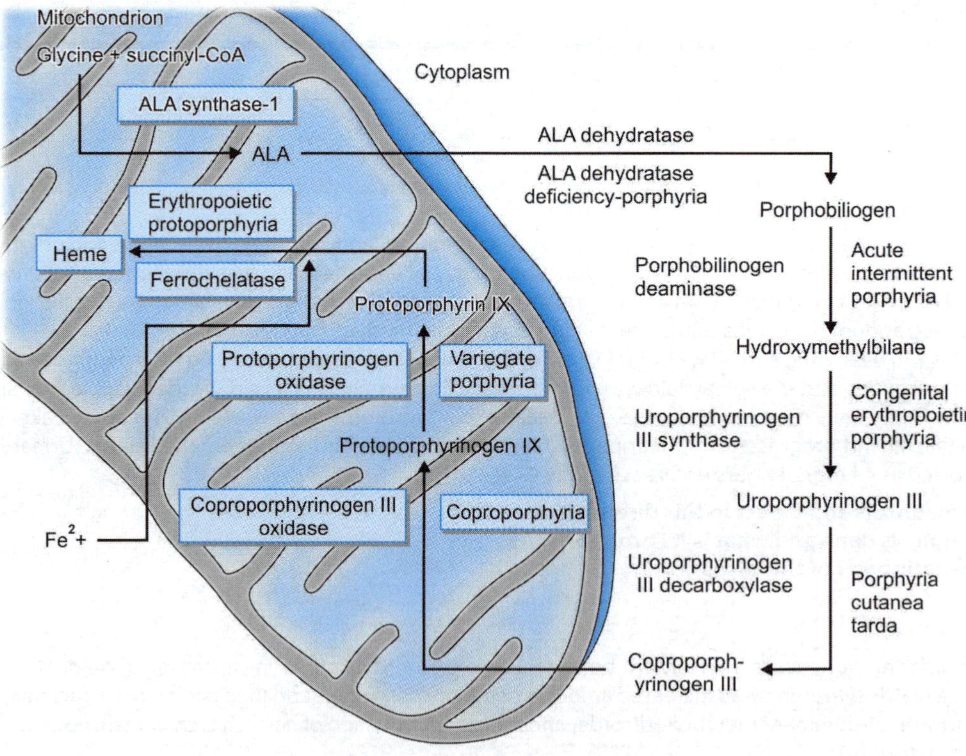

Fig. 13.3: Steps of heme synthesis.

Regulation of Heme Biosynthesis

Regulation of heme synthesis differs in the two major heme-forming tissues—the liver and erythron. In the liver, "free" heme regulates the synthesis and mitochondrial translocation of the housekeeping form of ALA synthase. Heme represses the synthesis of the ALA synthase mRNA and interferes with the transport of the enzyme from the cytosol into mitochondria. Hepatic ALA synthase is increased by many of the same chemicals that induce the cytochrome P450 enzymes in the endoplasmic reticulum of the liver. Because most of the heme in the liver is used for the synthesis of cytochrome P450 enzymes, hepatic ALA synthase and the cytochrome P450s are regulated in a coordinated fashion, and many drugs that induce hepatic ALA synthase also induce CYPs. The other hepatic heme biosynthetic enzymes are presumably expressed at constant levels, although their relative activities and kinetic properties differ. For example, normal individuals have high activities of ALA dehydratase but low activities of HMB synthase, the latter being the second rate-limiting step in the pathway.

In the erythron, novel regulatory mechanisms allow for the production of the very large amounts of heme needed for hemoglobin synthesis. The response to stimuli for hemoglobin synthesis occurs during cell differentiation, leading to an increase in cell number. **The erythroid-specific ALA synthase is expressed at higher levels than the housekeeping enzyme, and erythroid-specific control mechanisms regulate other pathway enzymes as well as iron transport into erythroid cells.**

PORPHYRIAS

The porphyrias are a group of rare metabolic disorders arising from reduced activity of any of the enzymes in the heme biosynthetic pathway. The disorders may be either acquired or inherited through a genetic defect in a gene encoding these enzymes. These deficiencies disrupt normal heme production and produce symptoms when increased heme is required. Porphyrin precursors, overproduced in response to synthetic pathway blockages, accumulate in the body and cause diverse pathological changes thereby becoming the basis for diagnostic tests. The diagnosis of acute porphyria can be confirmed by repeating the quantitation of urinary porphyrin during an acute episode and finding elevated levels (2–5 times of normal) of porphobilinogen.

Incidence

The prevalence of this condition is unknown, but probably it ranges from 1 in 500 to 50,000 worldwide. Certain types of porphyria are more common in specific populations, such as whites in South Africa and Scandinavians.

Classification

The porphyrias can be classified as either hepatic or erythropoietic, depending on whether the heme biosynthetic intermediates that accumulate and arise initially from the liver or developing erythrocytes, or as acute or cutaneous, based on their clinical manifestations. The porphyrias, their principal symptoms, and their major biochemical abnormalities are discussed in **Table 13.4**. Four of the five hepatic porphyrias—acute intermittent porphyria (AIP), hereditary coproporphyria (HCP), variegate porphyria (VP), and ALA dehydratase porphyria (ADP)—present during adult life with acute attacks of neurological manifestations and elevated levels of one or both of the porphyrin precursors, ALA and PBG, and are thus classified as acute porphyrias. The fifth hepatic disorder, porphyria cutanea tarda (PCT), presents with blistering skin lesions. HCP and VP also may have cutaneous manifestations similar to PCT.

The erythropoietic porphyrias—congenital erythropoietic porphyria (CEP) and erythropoietic protoporphyria (EPP)—are characterized by elevations of porphyrins in bone marrow and erythrocytes and present with cutaneous photosensitivity. **The skin lesions in CEP resemble PCT but are usually much more severe, whereas EPP causes a more immediate, painful, and nonblistering type of photosensitivity. EPP is the most common porphyria to cause symptoms before puberty.** Around 20% of EPP patients develop minor abnormalities of liver function, with up to about 5% developing hepatic complications that can become life-threatening.

Porphyrias are also classified based on the nature of the enzyme defect.

TABLE 13.4: Classification of porphyrias based on the enzyme defect.

Enzyme involved	*Type, class*	*Major signs and symptoms*	*Results of laboratory tests*
1. ALA synthase (erythroid form)	X-linked sideroblastic anemia (erythropoietic)	Anemia	Red cell counts and hemoglobin decreased
2. ALA dehydratase	ALA dehydratase deficiency (hepatic)	Abdominal pain, neuropsychiatric symptoms	Urinary ALA and coproporphyrin III increased
3. Uroporphyrinogen I synthase	Acute intermittent porphyria (hepatic)	Abdominal pain, neuropsychiatric symptoms	Urinary ALA and PBG increased
4. Uroporphyrinogen III synthase	Congenital erythropoietic (erythropoietic)	Photosensitivity	Urinary, fecal, and red cell uroporphyrins I increased
5. Uroporphyrinogen decarboxylase	Porphyria cutanea tarda (hepatic)	Photosensitivity	Urinary uroporphyrin I increased
6. Coproporphyrinogen oxidase	Hereditary coproporphyria (hepatic)	Photosensitivity, abdominal pain, neuropsychiatric symptoms	Urinary ALA, PBG, and coproporphyrin III and fecal coproporphyrin III increased
7. Protoporphyrinogen oxidase	Variegate porphyria (hepatic)	Photosensitivity, abdominal pain, neuropsychiatric symptoms	Urinary ALA, PBG, and coproporphyrin III and fecal protoporphyrin IX increased
8. Ferrochelatase	Protoporphyrin (erythropoietic)	Photosensitivity	Fecal and red cell protoporphyrin IX increased

Inheritance

Porphyria cutanea tarda (PCT) has both genetic and nongenetic causes. Mutations in the HFE gene (which also cause an iron overload disorder called hemochromatosis) increase the risk of developing porphyria cutanea tarda.

Most of the porphyrias are inherited. Inheritance patterns depend on the type of porphyria. Some forms of the condition are inherited in an autosomal dominant pattern, which means one copy of the altered gene is sufficient to cause the disorder. Other porphyrias are inherited in an autosomal recessive pattern which means two copies of the gene must be altered for a person to be affected by the condition.

Acute intermittent porphyria, variegate porphyria, and hereditary coproporphyria are inherited as autosomal dominant conditions with low penetrance. The homozygous forms are often associated with more florid and severe clinical features. Sequence analyses of the genes for all enzymes required for heme biosynthesis have revealed the porphyrias as highly heterogeneous, with multiple mutations underlying each type.

Porphyria cutanea tarda is usually an acquired disorder associated with liver disease and iron overload.

Typically, patients with the autosomal-dominant varieties present initially in adulthood, and those with homozygous variants present in early childhood. Symptomatic porphyria is thought to be more common in female than male patients with a female–male ratio of 5 to 1.

Hepatic Porphyrias

ALA-dehydratase–deficient porphyria

ADP is a rare autosomal recessive acute hepatic porphyria caused by a severe deficiency of ALA-dehydratase activity. The clinical presentation depends on the amount of residual ALA-dehydratase activity. Symptoms resemble those of AIP including abdominal pain and neuropathy. Infant with more severe disease manifests failure to thrive beginning at birth. Diagnosis is confirmed by significantly elevated levels of plasma and urinary ALA, urinary coproporphyrin III, and ALAD activity in erythrocytes <10% of normal.

The treatment of ADP acute attacks is similar to that of AIP.

Acute intermittent porphyria

Acute intermittent porphyria is inherited as an autosomal dominant, though it remains clinically silent in most patients who carry the trait. Clinical illness usually develops in women. Symptoms begin in the teens or 20s, but onset can begin after menopause in rare cases. The disorder is caused by partial deficiency of porphobilinogen deaminase activity, leading to increased excretion of aminolevulinic acid and porphobilinogen in the urine. The diagnosis may be elusive, if not specifically considered. The characteristic abdominal pain may be due to abnormalities in autonomic innervations in the gut. In contrast to other forms of porphyria, cutaneous photosensitivity is absent in acute intermittent porphyria. Attacks are precipitated by numerous factors including drugs and intercurrent infections. Hyponatremia may be seen, due in part to inappropriate release of antidiuretic hormone, though gastrointestinal loss of sodium in some patients may be a contributing factor.

Clinical Findings

Symptoms and signs: Patients show intermittent abdominal pain of varying severity; and in some instances, it may so simulate acute abdomen as to lead to exploratory laparotomy. Because the origin of the abdominal pain is neurologic, there is an absence of fever and leukocytosis. Complete recovery between attacks is usual. **Any part of the nervous system may be involved, with evidence for autonomic and peripheral neuropathy.** Peripheral neuropathy may be symmetric or asymmetric and mild or profound; in the latter instance, it can even lead to quadriplegia with respiratory paralysis. Other central nervous system manifestations include seizures, psychosis, and abnormalities of the basal ganglia. Hyponatremia may further cause or exacerbate central nervous system manifestations.

Laboratory findings: Often there is profound hyponatremia. The diagnosis can be confirmed by demonstrating an increased amount of porphobilinogen in the urine during an acute attack. Freshly voided urine is of normal color but may turn dark upon standing in light and air.

Prevention: Avoidance of factors known to precipitate attacks of acute intermittent porphyria—especially drugs can reduce morbidity. Starvation diets also cause attacks and so must be avoided.

Treatment: Treatment with a high-carbohydrate diet diminishes the number of attacks in some patients and is a reasonable empiric gesture considering its benignity. Acute attacks may be life-threatening and require prompt diagnosis, withdrawal of the inciting agent (if possible), and treatment with analgesics, intravenous glucose and hematin. A minimum of 300 g of carbohydrate per day should be provided orally or intravenously. Electrolyte balance requires close attention. Hematin therapy is still evolving and should be undertaken with full recognition of adverse consequences, especially phlebitis and coagulopathy. The intravenous dosage is up to 4 mg/kg once or twice daily. Liver transplantation may provide an option for patients with disease poorly controlled by medical therapy.

Porphyria Cutanea Tarda

It is the most common of the porphyrias, can be either sporadic (type 1) or familial (types 2 and 3), and can also develop after exposure to halogenated aromatic hydrocarbons. Hepatic URO-decarboxylase is deficient in all types of PCT, and for clinical symptoms to manifest, this enzyme deficiency must be substantial (~20% of normal activity or less).

Clinical Features

Blistering skin lesions that appear most commonly on the backs of the hands are the major clinical feature. These rupture and crust over, leaving areas of atrophy and scarring. Lesions may also occur on the forearms, face, legs, and feet. Occasionally, the skin over sun-exposed areas becomes severely thickened, with scarring and calcification that resembles systemic sclerosis. Neurological features are absent.

A number of susceptibility factors can be recognized clinically and can affect management. These include hepatitis C, HIV, excess alcohol, elevated iron levels, and estrogens. Excess alcohol is a long-recognized contributor, as is estrogen use in women. Multiple susceptibility factors that appear to act synergistically can be identified in the individual patient with PCT. Patients with PCT characteristically have chronic liver disease and sometimes cirrhosis and are at risk for hepatocellular carcinoma.

Diagnosis

Porphyrins are increased in the liver, plasma, urine, and stool. The urinary ALA level may be slightly increased, but the PBG level is normal. Urinary porphyrins consist mostly of uroporphyrin with lesser amounts of coproporphyrin. Plasma porphyrins are also increased. Isocoproporphyrins which are increased in feces and sometimes in plasma and urine are diagnostic for hepatic URO-decarboxylase deficiency.

Porphyria Cutanea Tarda: Treatment

Alcohol, estrogens, iron supplements, and, if possible, any drugs that may exacerbate the disease should be discontinued, but this step does not always lead to improvement. A complete response can almost always be achieved by the standard therapy, repeated phlebotomy, to reduce hepatic iron. A unit (450 mL) of blood can be removed every 1–2 weeks. **The aim is to gradually reduce excess hepatic iron until the serum ferritin reaches the lower limits of normal.** Because iron overload is not marked in most cases, remission may occur after only five or six phlebotomies; however, PCT patients with hemochromatosis may require more treatments to bring their iron levels down to the normal range.

An alternative when phlebotomy is contraindicated or poorly tolerated is a low-dose regimen of chloroquine or hydroxychloroquine, both of which complex with the excess porphyrins and promote their excretion. Small doses (e.g., 125 mg chloroquine phosphate twice weekly) should be given, because standard doses can induce transient, sometimes marked increases in photosensitivity and hepatocellular damage. Hepatic imaging can diagnose or exclude complicating hepatocellular carcinoma. Treatment of PCT in patients with end-stage renal disease is facilitated by administration of erythropoietin.

Hereditary Coproporphyria (HCP)

It is an autosomal dominant hepatic porphyria that results from the half-normal activity of COPRO-oxidase. The disease presents with acute attacks, as in AIP. Cutaneous photosensitivity also may occur, but much less commonly than in VP. HCP patients may have acute attacks and cutaneous photosensitivity together or separately. HCP is less common than AIP and VP.

Clinical Features

HCP is influenced by the same factors that cause attacks in AIP. The disease is latent before puberty, and symptoms which are virtually identical to those of AIP are more common in women. HCP is generally less severe than AIP. Blistering skin lesions are identical to PCT and VP.

Diagnosis

The COPRO III is markedly increased in the urine and feces in symptomatic disease and often persists, especially in feces, when there are no symptoms. Urinary ALA and PBG levels are increased (but less than in AIP) during acute attacks but may revert to normal more quickly than in AIP when symptoms resolve. Plasma porphyrins are usually normal or only slightly increased, but they may be higher in cases with skin lesions. The diagnosis of HCP is readily confirmed by increased fecal porphyrins consisting almost entirely of COPRO III, which distinguishes it from other porphyrias. An increase in the fecal COPRO III/COPRO I ratio is useful for detecting latent cases.

Although the diagnosis can be confirmed by measuring COPRO-oxidase activity, the assays for this mitochondrial enzyme are not widely available and require cells other than erythrocytes.

Hereditary Coproporphyria: Treatment

Neurological symptoms are treated as in AIP. Phlebotomy and chloroquine are ineffective when cutaneous lesions are present.

Variegate porphyria (VP)

It is an autosomal dominant hepatic porphyria that results from the deficient activity of PROTO-oxidase, the seventh enzyme in the heme pathway, and can present with neurological symptoms, photosensitivity, or both. VP is particularly common in South Africa, where 3 of every 1,000 whites have the disorder.

Clinical Features

VP can present with skin photosensitivity, acute neurovisceral crises, or both. **Acute attacks are identical to those in AIP and are precipitated by the same factors as AIP. Blistering skin manifestations are similar to those in PCT but are more difficult to treat and usually are of longer duration.** Homozygous VP is associated with photosensitivity, neurological symptoms, and developmental disturbances including growth retardation, in infancy or childhood.

Diagnosis

Urinary ALA and PBG levels are increased during acute attacks but may return to normal more quickly than in AIP. Increases in fecal protoporphyrin and COPRO III and in urinary COPRO III are more persistent. Plasma porphyrin levels also are increased, particularly when there are cutaneous lesions. VP can be distinguished rapidly from all other porphyrias by examining the fluorescence emission spectrum of porphyrins in plasma at neutral pH since VP has a unique fluorescence peak at neutral pH.

Assays of PROTO-oxidase activity in cultured fibroblasts or lymphocytes are not widely available.

Variegate Porphyria: Treatment

Acute attacks are treated as in AIP, and hemin should be started early in most cases. Other than avoiding sun exposure, there are a few effective measures for treating the skin lesions. β-carotene, phlebotomy, and chloroquine are not helpful.

Erythropoietic Porphyrias

In the erythropoietic porphyrias, excess porphyrins from bone marrow erythrocyte precursors are transported via the plasma to the skin and lead to cutaneous photosensitivity.

X-linked Sideroblastic Anemia

XLSA results from the deficient activity of the erythroid form of ALA-synthase and is associated with ineffective erythropoiesis, weakness, and pallor.

Clinical Features

Typically, males with XLSA develop refractory hemolytic anemia, pallor, and weakness during infancy. They have secondary hypersplenism, become iron overloaded, and can develop hemosiderosis. The severity depends on the level of residual erythroid ALA-synthase activity and on the responsiveness of the specific mutation to pyridoxal-5′-phosphate supplementation.

Diagnosis

Peripheral blood smear reveals a hypochromic, microcytic anemia with striking anisocytosis, poikilocytosis, and polychromasia; the leukocytes and platelets appear normal. Hemoglobin content is reduced, and the mean corpuscular volume and mean corpuscular hemoglobin concentration are decreased.

Bone marrow examination reveals hypercellularity with a left shift, megaloblastic erythropoiesis with an abnormal maturation. A variety of Prussian blue-staining sideroblasts are observed. Levels of urinary porphyrin precursors and of both urinary and fecal porphyrins are normal. The level of erythroid ALA synthase is decreased in bone marrow, but this enzyme is difficult to measure in the presence of the normal ALA synthase housekeeping enzyme. Definitive diagnosis requires the demonstration of mutations in the erythroid *ALAS* gene.

X-linked Sideroblastic Anemia: Treatment

The severe anemia may respond to pyridoxine supplementation. This cofactor is essential for ALA synthase activity, and mutations in the pyridoxine-binding site of the enzyme have been found in several responsive patients. Cofactor supplementation may make it possible to eliminate or reduce the frequency of transfusion. Unresponsive patients may be transfusion-dependent and require chelation therapy.

Congenital Erythropoietic Porphyria (CEP)

CEP, also known as Günther disease, is an autosomal recessive disorder. It is due to the markedly deficient, but not absent, activity of URO-synthase and the resultant accumulation of uroporphyrin I and coproporphyrin I isomers. CEP is associated with hemolytic anemia and cutaneous lesions.

Clinical Features

Severe cutaneous photosensitivity begins in early infancy. The skin over light-exposed areas is friable, and bullae and vesicles are prone to rupture and infection. Skin thickening, focal hypo- and hyperpigmentation, and hypertrichosis of the face and extremities are characteristic. Secondary infection of the cutaneous lesions can lead to disfigurement of the face and hands. Porphyrins are deposited in teeth and in bones. As a result, the teeth are reddish-brown and fluoresce on exposure to long-wave ultraviolet light called erythrodontia **(Fig. 13.4)**. Hemolysis is probably due to the marked increase in erythrocyte porphyrins and leads to splenomegaly. Adults with a milder form of the disease also have been described.

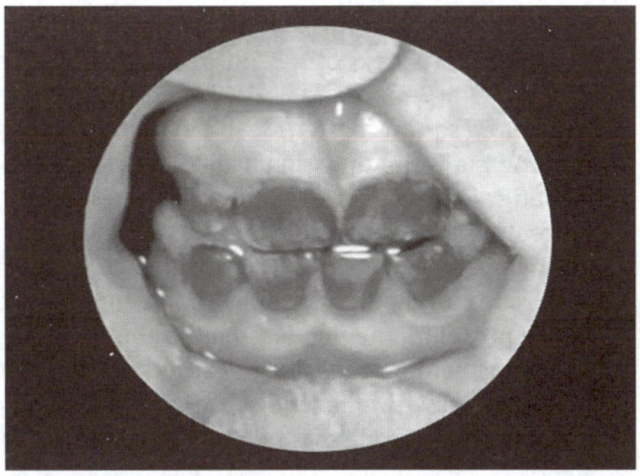

Fig. 13.4: Erythrodontia in congenital erythropoietic porphyria (the teeth are reddish-brown and fluoresce on exposure to long-wave ultraviolet light).

Diagnosis

Uroporphyrin and coproporphyrin (mostly type I isomers) accumulate in the bone marrow, erythrocytes, plasma, urine, and feces. The predominant porphyrin in feces is coproporphyrin I. The diagnosis of CEP can be confirmed by demonstration of markedly deficient URO-synthase activity and/or the identification of specific mutations in the *UROS* gene. The disease can be detected in utero by measuring porphyrins in amniotic fluid and URO-synthase activity in cultured amniotic cells or chorionic villi, or by the detection of the family's specific gene mutations.

Congenital Erythropoietic Porphyria: Treatment

Severe cases often require transfusions for anemia. Chronic transfusions of sufficient blood to suppress erythropoiesis are effective in reducing porphyrin production but results in iron overload. Splenectomy may reduce hemolysis and decrease transfusion requirements. Protection from sunlight and from minor skin trauma is important. β-carotene may be of some value. Complicating bacterial infections should be treated promptly. Recently, bone marrow and cord blood transplantation has proven effective in several transfusion-dependent children, providing the rationale for stem-cell gene therapy.

Erythropoietic Protoporphyria

Erythropoietic protoporphyria (EPP) is an inherited disorder resulting from the partial deficiency of ferrochelatase activity, the last enzyme in the heme biosynthetic pathway. EPP is the most common erythropoietic porphyria in children and, after PCT, the second most common porphyria in adults. EPP patients have ferrochelatase activities as low as 15–25% in lymphocytes and cultured fibroblasts. Protoporphyrin accumulates in bone marrow reticulocytes and then appears in plasma is taken-up in the liver and excreted in bile and feces. Protoporphyrin transported to the skin causes nonblistering photosensitivity.

Clinical Features

Skin photosensitivity, which differs from that in other porphyrias, usually begins in childhood and consists of pain, redness, and itching occurring within minutes of sunlight exposure. Photosensitivity is associated with substantial elevations in erythrocyte protoporphyrin and occurs only in patients with genotypes that result in ferrochelatase activities below ~35% of normal. Vesicular lesions are uncommon. Redness, swelling, burning, and itching can develop shortly after sun exposure and resemble angioedema. Symptoms may seem out of proportion to the visible skin lesions. Severe scarring is rare, as are pigment changes, friability, and hirsutism.

Although EPP is an erythropoietic porphyria, up to 20% of EPP patients may have minor abnormalities of liver function, and in about 5% of these patients, the accumulation of protoporphyrins causes chronic liver disease that can progress to liver failure and death. Protoporphyrin is insoluble and excess amounts form crystalline structures in liver cells and can decrease hepatic bile flow. Thus, rapidly progressive liver disease appears to be related to the cholestatic effects of protoporphyrins and is associated with increasing hepatic protoporphyrin levels due to impaired hepatobiliary excretion and increased photosensitivity.

Diagnosis

A substantial increase in erythrocyte protoporphyrin, which is predominantly free and not complexed with zinc, is the hallmark of this disease. Protoporphyrin levels are also variably increased in bone marrow, plasma, bile, and feces. Erythrocyte protoporphyrin concentrations are increased in other conditions, such as lead poisoning, iron deficiency, various hemolytic disorders, all homozygous forms of porphyria, and sometimes even in acute porphyrias. In all these conditions, however, in contrast to EPP, protoporphyrin is complexed with zinc. Therefore, after an increase in erythrocyte protoporphyrin is found in a suspected EPP patient, it is important to confirm the diagnosis by an assay that distinguishes free and zinc-complexed protoporphyrin. Erythrocytes in EPP also exhibit red fluorescence under a fluorescence microscopy at 620 nm. Urinary levels of porphyrins and porphyrin precursors are normal. Ferrochelatase activity in cultured lymphocytes or fibroblasts is decreased. DNA diagnosis by mutation analysis is recommended to detect the causative mutation.

Erythropoietic Protoporphyria: Treatment

Avoiding sunlight exposure and wearing clothes designed to provide protection for conditions with chronic photosensitivity are essential. Oral β-carotene (120–180 mg/dL) improves tolerance to sunlight in many patients. The dosage may need to be adjusted to maintain serum carotene levels in the recommended range of 10–15 mmol/L (600–800 mg/dL). Mild skin discoloration due to carotenemia is the only significant side effect. The beneficial effects of β-carotene may involve quenching of singlet oxygen or free radicals.

Treatment of hepatic complications, which may be accompanied by motor neuropathy, is difficult. Cholestyramine and other porphyrin absorbents, such as activated charcoal may interrupt the enterohepatic circulation of protoporphyrin and promote its fecal excretion, leading to some improvement. Splenectomy may be helpful when the disease is accompanied by hemolysis and significant splenomegaly. Plasmapheresis and intravenous hemin are sometimes beneficial.

Liver transplantation has been carried out in some EPP patients with severe liver complications and is often successful in the short-term. However, liver disease often recurs in the transplanted liver due to continued bone marrow production of excess protoporphyrin. Bone marrow transplantation is considered after the liver transplantation, if a suitable donor can be found.

Diagnosis of Porphyrias

The diagnosis of a specific type of porphyria can generally be established by consideration of the clinical and family history, the physical examination, and appropriate laboratory tests.

The biochemical distinction among the porphyrias resides with the measurement of porphyrins and their metabolites in urine and feces.

Porphyrin intermediates in the first half of the heme biosynthetic pathway (porphobilinogen, aminolevulinic acid, and uroporphyrins) are water soluble and fat insoluble. Thus, excessive excretions occur in urine, not stool. Terminal half porphyrin intermediates (coproporphyrin and protoporphyrin) are fat soluble and excreted through bile in the stool. Because coproporphyrin is water soluble as well, it may also be present.

Measuring the 24-hour urinary excretion of porphobilinogen and aminolevulinic acid during a symptomatic period is the most helpful method of determining whether a particular set of symptoms and signs is due to acute porphyria.

If levels of urine porphobilinogen or aminolevulinic acid or both are increased, diagnosis of an acute porphyria attack can be made. **When urine porphobilinogen is elevated more than 2–5 times its normal limits, an acute attack of acute intermittent porphyria, variegate porphyria, or hereditary coproporphyria should be suspected. During an acute attack, acute intermittent porphyria is distinguished from variegate porphyria or hereditary coproporphyria by normal or near-normal levels of fecal porphyrin.** Reduced activity of erythrocyte porphobilinogen deaminase further supports the diagnosis of acute intermittent porphyria.

Variegate porphyria and hereditary coproporphyria, like acute intermittent porphyria, have decreased porphobilinogen deaminase activity and resultant increased levels of urinary porphobilinogen during acute attacks. However, variegate porphyria is specifically distinguished by a deficiency of protoporphyrinogen oxidase, which leads to accumulation of both protoporphyrinogen and protoporphyrin in bile and feces. In variegate porphyria, the preponderant stool porphyrin is protoporphyrin with concentrations ranging from 3 times to 7 the normal value. Hereditary coproporphyria also has a distinct stool porphyrin pattern. Defective coproporphyrinogen oxidase leads to accumulation of coproporphyrin in both stool and urine. In hereditary coproporphyria, the concentration of stool coproporphyrinogen is at least 5 times normal.

A rapid and qualitative test for porphobilinogen in urine (the Hoesch or Watson–Schwartz test) is available in some laboratories. **An early diagnosis of an acute porphyria is more important than deciding which of the four types the patient has, since the immediate management is the same regardless of the type.**

Other Diagnostic Methods

Enzyme assays in erythrocytes or other cells or tissues are helpful in supporting the diagnosis but are best used to identify family members with latent disease.

The demonstration of decreased cellular enzyme activity proves the presence of the genetic defect but by itself is insufficient for implicating porphyria as the cause of a particular patient's symptoms.

Plasma peak fluorescence is used with fecal porphyrin quantification for diagnosis of variegate porphyria.

Treatment

Management strategies in acute episodes of porphyria are limited, and therapy is mainly supportive. Treatment mainstays include identifying and limiting possible precipitants, cessation or avoidance of porphyrogenic drugs, treatment of infections with safe drugs maintaining adequate intake of carbohydrates and fluids, and administering heme arginate.

Ingestion of large amounts of carbohydrates (glucose loading) or administration of hematin (a hydroxide of heme) may repress ALAS1, resulting in diminished production of harmful heme precursors.

Hematin: Most typically in the form of heme arginate is used.

The heme is taken up by hepatocytes, replenishes the regulatory heme pool, and downregulates ALA synthase 1, the rate-limiting enzyme in the heme biosynthetic pathway, with a resultant dramatic decline in porphyrin production. Within hours of heme administration, the overproduction and overexcretion of aminolevulinic acid and porphobilinogen are normalized.

Heme repletion may also improve 5-hydroxytryptophan and serotonin metabolism, which has been suggested to play a role in central nervous system disease. If given early, heme can prevent irreversible axonal death.

Within 2–4 days, most patients with acute porphyria show clinical improvement.

The antioxidant β-carotene is used to reduce the tissue damage from the exposure of the chemical reaction, which helps to reduce the symptoms of cutaneous porphyria.

Prevention

- Avoid sunlight
- Avoid fasting
- Avoid consumption of wine, beer, and alcoholic substances
- Avoid dehydration
- Avoid iron supplements and vitamins containing iron
- **High levels of lead can affect heme metabolism by combining with SH groups in enzymes, such as ferrochelatase and ALA dehydratase. This affects porphyrin metabolism.** Elevated levels of protoporphyrin are found in red blood cells, and elevated levels of ALA and of coproporphyrin are found in urine.
- ALA synthase is the key regulatory enzyme of the heme biosynthetic pathway in liver. A large number of drugs (e.g., barbiturates, griseofulvin) induce the enzyme. Most of these drugs do so by inducing cytochrome P450, which uses up heme and thus derepresses (induces) ALAS1. In patients with porphyria, increased activities of ALAS1 result in increased levels of potentially harmful heme precursors prior to the metabolic block. Thus, taking drugs that cause induction of cytochrome P450 (so-called microsomal inducers) can precipitate attacks of porphyria.

Prognosis

Normal lifespan is possible in many types of porphyrias. Limited treatments are available. Prognosis is not poor.

CLINICAL NOTE

An attack of acute intermittent porphyria may be precipitated by one of the "four Ms": Medication, menstruation, malnutrition, maladies.

CLINICAL PEARLS

1. The porphyrias are a group of rare metabolic disorders arising from reduced activity of any of the enzymes in the heme biosynthetic pathway.
2. The disorders may be either acquired or inherited through a genetic defect in a gene encoding these enzymes.
3. These deficiencies disrupt normal heme production, with symptoms prominent when increased heme is required.
4. Porphyrin precursors, overproduced in response to synthetic pathway blockages, accumulate in the body and cause diverse pathological changes thereby becoming the basis for diagnostic tests.
5. The diagnosis of acute porphyria can be confirmed by repeating the quantitation of urine porphyrin during an acute episode and finding elevated levels (2–5 times normal) of porphyrins in the urine.

Chapter 14

Hemoglobinopathies

LEARNING OBJECTIVES

To understand:
- Molecular basis,
- Clinical implications,
- Laboratory diagnosis, and
- Management of clinically important hemoglobinopathies

CASE STUDIES

CASE STUDY 1

Theme: Clinical Implications of Altered Hemoglobin Structure—Sickle Cell Disease (Qualitative Defect)

A 16-year-old African-American girl was admitted to the emergency room with complaints of fever and recurrent pain in her arms and legs.

Her laboratory tests revealed the following:

Hemoglobin	8.0 g/dL
Hematocrit	9.1%
Serum Iron	11 µg/dL
Serum albumin	4.4 g/dL

Blood smear showed target cells, poikilocytes, hypochromasia, sickle red cells, nucleated RBCs, and Howell-Jolly bodies.

Hb electrophoresis showed a slow moving band.

What could be the probable diagnosis?

CASE DISCUSSION

The patient is suffering from sickle cell disease.

Sickle cell disease (SCD) and its variants are genetic disorders of mutant hemoglobin (Hb).The most common form found in North America is homozygous HbS disease.

BASIC CONCEPT

The activity of a given protein is dependent on proper folding of its polypeptide chain to assume a defined three-dimensional structure. The importance of protein folding to molecular medicine is emphasized by the fact that many disease-causing mutations do not directly affect the active or ligand binding site of proteins, but instead cause local or global alterations in protein structure or disrupt the folding pathway such that the native protein fold is not achieved, or undesirable interactions with other proteins are promoted. The molecular defect that changes adult hemoglobin (HbA) to sickle hemoglobin (HbS), leading to sickle cell anemia, is a classic example of mutations that affect protein structure.

Normal hemoglobin has four subunits called globins. Adult hemoglobin has two α (α1 and α2) and two β (β1 and β2) globin chains. Each globin chain has an associated heme prosthetic group, which is the site of oxygen binding and release. All globin chains have similar primary sequences. The secondary structure of globin chains consists of approximately 75% α-helix. The similar primary sequence promotes a similar tertiary structure in all globins that is called the globin fold, which is compact and globular in overall conformation. The quaternary structure of HbA can be described as a dimer of α1 β1 and α2 β2 dimers. The αβ dimers move relative to one another during the binding and release of oxygen.

Hemoglobin must remain soluble at high concentrations within the red blood cell to support normal oxygen binding and release properties. This is made possible by a distribution of amino acid side chains in which hydrophobic residues are sequestered in the interior core of the folded globin subunits, while hydrophilic residues dominate the water-exposed surface of the globin fold. The disk-shaped heme prosthetic group is inserted into a hydrophobic pocket formed by the globin **(Fig. 14.1)**.

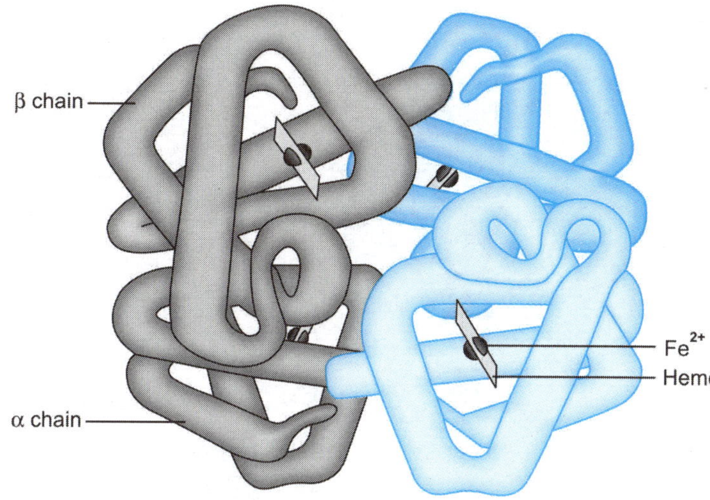

Fig. 14.1: Structure of HbA.

In sickle cell disease, also called as **sickle cell anemia**, a single nucleotide alteration (**point mutation**) in the β-globin gene of hemoglobin causes a change of thymine for adenine (GAG to GTG), at the sixth codon of the β-gene. This change encodes valine instead of glutamic acid in the sixth position on the β-globin molecule. The charge at this site is altered and allows for polymerization of hemoglobin under conditions of hypoxia. These properties are responsible for the profound clinical expressions of the sickling syndromes. The mutant β-globin chain is designated as βs, and the resulting hemoglobin is referred to as HbS.

SICKLE CELL DISEASE

Inheritance: It is a homozygous recessive disorder. It occurs in individuals who have inherited two abnormal genes (one from each parent) that code for the synthesis of β-chain of the Hb molecule. Heterozygotes have one normal and one sickle cell gene. The blood cells of these individuals contain both HbS and HbA. These individuals have sickle cell trait and they usually do not show the clinical symptoms and can have a normal life span.

Frequency: Sickle cell disease has been recognized in the malarial areas of the world. In malarial areas, there is a selective advantage to the heterozygote (HbAS). Individuals with sickle cell trait have lower levels of *Plasmodium falciparum* parasitemia, higher hemoglobin counts, and less severe reinfections than individuals with homozygous HbA. Sickling might protect a person from malaria by either of the following:

- Making it more difficult for the parasite to metabolize or to enter the sickled cell
- By accelerating sickling, parasitized cells are quickly removed.
- While children with sickle cell trait HbSA seem to have a milder form of falciparum malaria, those with homozygous HbS have a severe form that is associated with very high mortality rate.

Sickle cell disease is the most common in individuals of African descent, but is seen in Hispanics, Arabians, Indians, and whites. In the United States, the incidence is 1 in 625 live births to African-Americans.

Pathophysiology

The substitution of the nonpolar valine for a charged glutamate forms a protrusion on the β-globin that fits into a complementary site on the α-chain of another hemoglobin molecule in the cell. At low oxygen tension, HbS polymerizes inside the red blood cells (RBC), first forming a gel, then subsequently assembling into a network of fibrous polymers that stiffen and distort the cell, producing rigid misshapen erythrocytes—sickle-shaped erythrocytes **(Fig. 14.2)**. The life span of an erythrocyte homozygous for HbS is approximately 20 days compared to 120 days for a normal (RBC). The extent of sickling depends on the factors that increase the proportion of HbS in the deoxy state. These factors include decreased oxygen tension as a result of high altitude or flying in nonpressurized plane, increased pCO_2, decreased pH, and increased concentration of 2,3-bisphosphoglycerate. After recurrent episodes of sickling, membrane damage occurs and the cells are no longer capable of resuming the biconcave shape upon reoxygenation. Thus, they become irreversibly sickled cells (ISCs) **(Fig. 14.3)**. From 5% to 50% of RBCs permanently remain in the sickled shape. Such sickled cells frequently block the flow of blood in the narrow capillaries. The interruption in the supply of oxygen leads to tissue anoxia, causing pain and eventually death of cells (**infarction**) in the vicinity of blockage. Because of the disruption of the red cell membrane, the increased adhesiveness of sickle reticulocytes, and the increased leukocyte count, there is a thrombotic coagulopathy associated with sickle cell anemia that contributes to the severity of the disease.

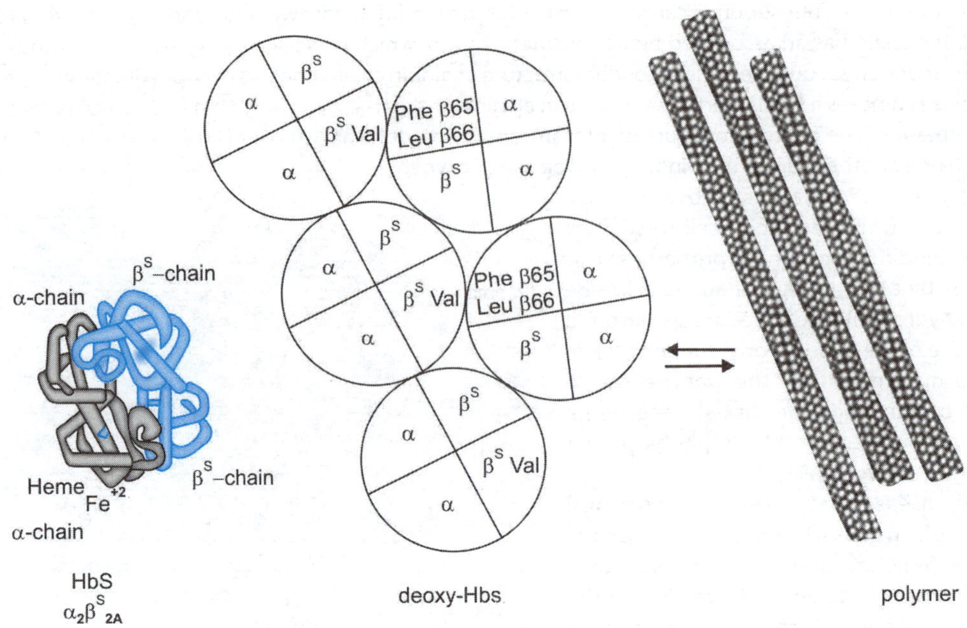

Fig. 14.2: Pathogenesis of sickle cell anemia.

Clinical Manifestations

The presenting symptoms of sickle cell disease (SCD) involve pain and anemia.

- SCD usually manifests early in childhood. For the first 6 months of life, infants are protected largely by elevated levels of HbF; soon thereafter, the condition becomes evident.
- During childhood and adolescence, the disease is associated with growth retardation, delayed sexual maturation, and being underweight.
- Anemia is universally present.
  - It is chronic and hemolytic in nature and usually very well tolerated.
  - Anemia may be complicated with megaloblastic changes secondary to folate deficiency. These result from increased RBC turnover and folate utilization.
  - A serious complication is the aplastic crisis
    - This is caused by infection with the parvovirus B-19 (B19V).The virus infects RBC progenitors in bone marrow, resulting in cessation of erythropoiesis.
    - Coupled with greatly shortened RBC lifespan, usually 10 to 20 days, a very rapid drop in Hb occurs.
    - The condition is self-limited, with bone marrow recovery occurring in 7 to 10 days, followed by brisk reticulocytosis.

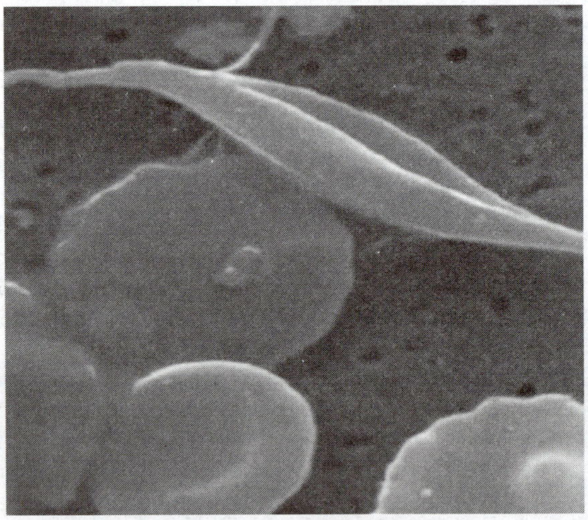

Fig. 14.3: Sickled red blood cells.

- The spleen enlarges in the latter part of the first year of life.
  - Occasionally, it undergoes a sudden very painful enlargement due to the pooling of large numbers of sickled cells. This phenomenon is known as splenic sequestration crisis.
  - The spleen undergoes repeated infarction, aided by low pH and low oxygen tension in the sinusoids and splenic cords.
  - Even while enlarged, its function is impaired.
    - Over time, the spleen becomes fibrotic and shrinks. This is, in fact, an autosplenectomy.
    - The nonfunctional spleen is a major contributor to the immune deficiency that exists in these individuals. Failure of opsonization and an inability to deal with infective encapsulated microorganisms, particularly *Streptococcus pneumoniae*, ensue.
- Pneumococcal infections are common in childhood.
  - During adult life, infections with Gram-negative organisms, especially *Salmonella*, predominate.
  - Of special concern is the frequent occurrence of *Salmonella* osteomyelitis in areas of bone weakened by infarction.
- Another problem occurring in infancy is hand-foot syndrome.

- This is a dactylitis presenting as painful swelling of the dorsum of the hand and foot.
- Cortical thinning and destruction of the metacarpal and metatarsal bones appear on radiographs 3–5 weeks after the swelling begins.
- Leukocytosis or erythema does not accompany the swelling.

- The most common clinical picture during adult life is vaso-occlusive crisis.
  - The crisis begins suddenly, sometimes as a consequence of infection or temperature change.
  - Severe deep pain is present in the extremities, involving long bones. The abdomen is affected with severe pain resembling acute abdomen. The face may also be involved. Pain may be accompanied by fever, malaise, and leukocytosis. The person in crisis is in extreme discomfort.
  - The crisis may last several hours to several days and terminate as abruptly as it began.
- Approximately half of the individuals with homozygous HbS disease experience vaso-occlusive crisis.
  - The frequency of crisis is extremely variable. Some have as many as six or more episodes annually, whereas others may have episodes only at great intervals or none at all.
  - Each individual typically has a consistent pattern for crisis frequency.
- Many individuals with HbS disease experience chronic low-level pain, mainly in bones and joints. Intermittent vaso-occlusive crisis may be superimposed, or chronic low-level pain may be the only expression of the disease.
- The acute chest syndrome consists of chest pain, fever, tachypnea, leukocytosis, and pulmonary infiltrates.
  - This is a medical emergency and must be treated immediately.
  - It probably begins with infarction of ribs, leading to chest splinting and atelectasis.
  - Fat embolism, resulting from bone marrow infarction, plays an important etiological role in the pathogenesis of this syndrome.
  - If not attended to promptly, it may lead to acute respiratory distress syndrome (ARDS).
- Central nervous system involvement is one of the most devastating aspects of SCD.
  - It is most prevalent in childhood and adolescence.
  - The most severe manifestation is stroke, resulting in varying degrees of neurological deficit. The stroke is mostly thrombotic, but it may also be hemorrhagic.
- The heart is involved due to chronic anemia and microinfarcts.
  - Hemolysis and blood transfusion lead to hemosiderin deposition in the myocardium.
  - Both ventricles and the left atrium are all dilated.
  - Usually, a systolic murmur is present, with wide radiation over the precordium.
- Chronic hemolysis with hyperbilirubinemia is associated with the formation of bile stones. Cholelithiasis may be asymptomatic or result in acute cholecystitis, requiring surgical intervention.
- Repeated infarction of joints, bones, and growth plates leads to aseptic necrosis, especially in weight-bearing areas, such as the femur. This complication is associated with chronic pain and disability and may require changes in employment and lifestyle.
- Blood in the pulmonary circulation is deoxygenated, resulting in a high degree of polymer formation.
  - The lungs develop areas of microinfarction. The resulting areas that lack oxygenation aggravate the sickling process.
  - Pulmonary hypertension may develop. This may be due in part to the depletion of nitric oxide. Various studies have found that more than 40% of adults with SCD have pulmonary hypertension that worsens with age.
- The kidneys lose concentrating capacity.
  - Isosthenuria results in a large loss of water, further contributing to dehydration in these patients. Renal failure may ensue, usually preceded by proteinuria.
  - Nephrotic syndrome is uncommon but may occur.
- Paraorbital facial infarction may result in ptosis.
  - Retinal vascular changes also occur.
  - A proliferative retinitis is common in HbSC disease and may lead to loss of vision.
- Leg ulcers are a chronic painful problem. They result from minor injury to the area around the malleoli. Because of relatively poor circulation, compounded by sickling and microinfarcts, healing is delayed and infection is established.
- Priapism is a serious complication and tends to occur repeatedly. When it is prolonged, it may lead to impotence.
- Pregnancy represents a special area of concern. The high rate of fetal loss is due to spontaneous abortion. Placenta previa and abruption are common due to hypoxia and placental infarction. At birth, the infant often is premature or has a low birth weight.

Laboratory Findings

1. A complete blood cell count usually reveals an increased reticulocytes count (5–15%).
2. Total leukocyte count (12,000–20,000/mm^3), upper limit of normal or greater.
3. Differential leukocyte count: normal or predominance of neutrophils.
4. Mean corpuscular volume (MCV): Normal (unless thalassemic hemoglobin is present).
5. Hb mild-to-moderate anemia (5–9 g/dL).

6. **Platelet count:** Normal to increased.
7. **Blood smear:** A diagnosis of sickle cell disease can be suspected by the examination of the peripheral blood film and that shows the presence of target cells, poikilocytes, hypochromasia, sickle red cells, nucleated RBCs, and Howell-Jolly bodies.
8. Sickling of the red blood cells on a blood film can be induced by the addition of sodium metabisulfite. The presence of sickle hemoglobin can also be demonstrated with the "sickle solubility test." A mixture of hemoglobin S (HbS) in a reducing solution (such as sodium dithionite) gives a turbid appearance, whereas normal Hb gives a clear solution **(Fig. 14.4)**.

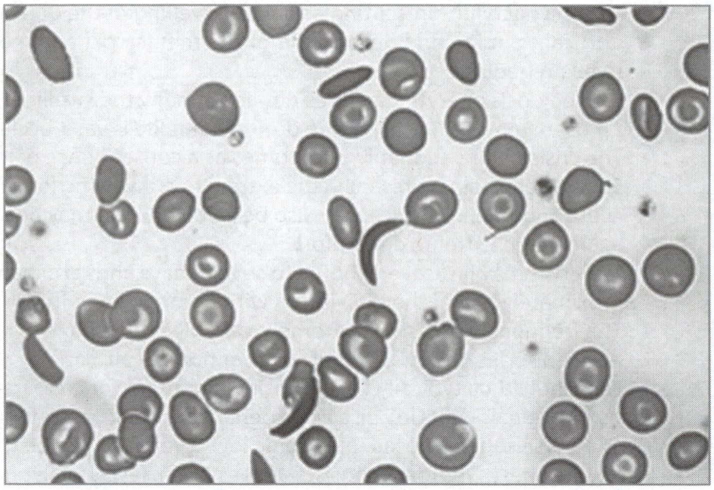

Fig. 14.4: Peripheral blood film in sickle cell disease, showing the presence of hypochromasia, sickle red cells, and nucleated RBCs.

9. **Hemoglobin electrophoresis:** The substitution of the nonpolar valine for the charged glutamic acid results in decreased mobility of the HbS in the electric field as compared to HbA. This altered mobility is due to the presence of less negative charge on the two β-globin chains, thus rendering HbS less negative than HbA. The diagnosis is confirmed by high-pressure liquid chromatography (HPLC).
10. Bone marrow is markedly hyperplastic with erythroid predominance.
11. Radiological studies may reveal characteristic bony findings of sickle cell disease in the vertebral bodies, mild expansion of the marrow cavities, osteoporosis, and possibly sclerosis of the long bones and femoral heads.
12. Liver function tests, as well as BUN, creatinine, and serum electrolytes are also required to be performed.

Treatment

Treatment strategies include the following seven goals: (1) management of vaso-occlusive crisis, (2) management of chronic pain syndromes, (3) management of the chronic hemolytic anemia, (4) prevention and treatment of infections, (5) management of the complications and the various organ damage syndromes associated with the disease, (6) prevention of stroke, and (7) detection and treatment of pulmonary hypertension.

- Vaso-occlusive crisis is treated with vigorous hydration and analgesics.
- Pain control is best achieved by the administration of opioids.
  - Morphine is the drug of choice. Morphine dosing has to be individualized.
  - Chronic pain is managed with long-acting oral morphine preparations and acetaminophen and nonsteroidal anti-inflammatory drugs (NSAIDs).
- Prevention of infection improves chances of survival in SCD.
  - Penicillin prophylaxis, commencing in infancy and continued until age 5 years or early teens, and the use of a pneumococcal vaccine at age 2 years with a booster dose at age 5 years greatly reduce the frequency of infections with *S. pneumoniae*.
  - In the adult patient, all infections must be treated promptly with broad-spectrum antibiotics until a causative organism is identified and therapy is tailored according to its antibiotic sensitivity.
- Allogeneic bone marrow transplantation (BMT) can cure the disease, but it is difficult to decide which patients should be offered BMT.
  - Many risks are associated with BMT, and the risk-to-benefit ratio must be assessed carefully.
  - With the advent of cord blood stem cell transplantation and with the development of less immunoablative conditioning regimens, perhaps BMT will gain wider acceptance and use.
  - The lack of availability of a matched donor may limit the utility of BMT.
- Although several attempts have been made to treat SCD with pharmacological agents over the years, the only drug currently approved by the US Food and Drug Administration (FDA) for the treatment of SCD is hydroxyurea.
- Effects of therapy with hydroxyurea
  - Hydroxyurea increases the production of HbF, which retards gelation and sickling. The Hb level rises, and the frequency and severity of vaso-occlusive crisis declines, sometimes being eliminated altogether. The reduction in the circulating leukocytes decreases the adherence of neutrophils to the vascular endothelium.
  - A decrease in chronic pain and the reticulocyte count occurs.
  - Hydroxyurea is a potentially leukemogenic and carcinogenic agent.
    - Potential complications referable to long-term use are not yet known.
    - Its use also requires frequent blood testing and monitoring, with special attention to development of leukopenia and/or thrombocytopenia.
- **Pharmacological advances**

- Oral glutamine therapy can be helpful to lower resting energy expenditure in growing children.
- Inhalation of nitric oxide has been successfully tried in the treatment of pulmonary hypertension.
- Locally acting GM-CSF has been reported to promote the healing of leg ulcers.
- Butyrate has been reported to decrease the vaso-occlusive crisis.
- Arginine has been used as a precursor of nitric oxide.

- **Treatment of anemia:** Anemia is generally less distressful.
  - Folate stores get depleted due to increased cellular turn-over. Therefore, supplementation of folic acid is helpful to raise Hb levels.
  - Any coexisting iron deficiency should be treated by iron supplementation, especially in premenopausal women.
  - Overall a balanced diet is essential.
  - A blood transfusion may be required in certain conditions, such as acute chest syndrome, stroke, pregnancy, aplastic crisis, and general anesthesia. The objective is to lower HbS concentration to less than 30%. However, repeated blood transfusions increase the risk of blood born infections and may cause iron overload and alloimmunization.
- **Surgical Treatment**
  Surgical treatment is restricted to treating complications of the disease.
  - Chronic leg ulcers are treated by skin grafting.
  - Avascular necrosis can be treated by hip replacement or alternative orthopedic procedures.
  - Cholecystectomy is recommended for the removal of gallstones, irrespective of the status that acute cholecystitis is coexistent or not.

Prevention

- **Screening for Hb S at birth:** This procedure allows early diagnosis and initiation of early treatment in the proven cases.
- **Prenatal diagnosis:** The procedures used in prenatal testing are sensitive and rapid. Prenatal testing is followed by genetic and psychological counseling.
- **Chorionic villus sampling:** This is a low-risk and safe procedure. DNA extracted from the chorionic villus biopsy at 8–12 weeks' gestation can be analyzed to detect the defect.
- **Amniocentesis:** DNA extracted from amniotic fluid cells can be analyzed at 16 weeks' gestation.
- **A DNA analysis of fetal cells:** Fetal cells can be isolated from maternal blood, and the DNA extracted from these calls can be used for DNA analysis.

Prognosis

Sickle cell anemia is a life-long disease; the quality of life and the prognosis can improve with early therapeutic interventions.

CLINICAL NOTE

The most common clinical picture during adult life is vaso-occlusive crisis.

CLINICAL PEARLS

1. The sickle cell disease, also called as sickle cell anemia, is due to a single nucleotide alteration (point mutation) in the β-globin gene of hemoglobin.
2. At low oxygen tension, HbS polymerizes inside the red blood cells, first forming a gel, then subsequently assembling into a network of fibrous polymers that stiffen and distort the cell, producing rigid misshapen erythrocytes-sickle-shaped erythrocytes.
3. Such sickled cells frequently block the flow of blood in the narrow capillaries. The interruption in the supply of oxygen leads to tissue anoxia, causing pain and eventually death of cells (infarction) in the vicinity of blockage.
4. A diagnosis of sickle cell disease can be suspected by the examination of the peripheral blood film and that shows the presence of target cells, poikilocytes, hypochromasia, sickle red cells, nucleated RBCs, and Howell-Jolly bodies.
5. Hydroxyurea increases the production of HbF, which retards gelations and sickling. The Hb level rises, and the frequency and severity of vaso-occlusive crisis declines.

CASE STUDY 2

Theme: Clinical Implications of Altered Hemoglobin Structure—Thalassemia (Quantitative Defect)

Adriana, a 7-year-old girl, was brought to the pediatrician for consultation by her parents. At the age of 3, she was in the 10th percentile for height and weight, pale, and her hemoglobin was 5.8 g/dL. Following further diagnostic studies, she was diagnosed with beta-thalassemia major. Over the course of the next 4 years, she was hospitalized every 1–2 months so that she could be transfused with packed red blood cells.

During a routine follow-up visit at the hematology clinic, Adriana's laboratory results were as follows:

Hemoglobin: 10 g/dL

Serum iron: 180 µg/dL

What is the defect in this disease?

What is the biochemical basis for the symptoms? What is the possible treatment for this defect?

CASE DISCUSSION

Thalassemias are a group of inherited microcytic, hemolytic anemias characterized by defective Hb synthesis. They are particularly common in people of Mediterranean, African, and Southeast Asian ancestry. Symptoms and signs result from anemia, hemolysis, splenomegaly, bone marrow hyperplasia, and iron overload (if there have been multiple transfusions. Diagnosis is based on genetic tests and quantitative Hb analysis. Treatment for severe forms may include transfusion, splenectomy, chelation, and stem cell transplantation.

Adriana in this case is experiencing anemia as indicated by her hemoglobin level of 10 g/dL; however, for children with beta-thalassemia, the goal of treatment is to maintain hemoglobin levels between 9 and 10 g/ dL. The more disturbing value is her total serum iron of 180 µg/dL. The normal level of serum iron for children is 50–175 µg/dL. This value indicates iron toxicity.

BASIC CONCEPT

THALASSEMIAS

The thalassemias are hereditary disorders characterized by reduction in the synthesis of globin chains (α or β). Reduced globin chain synthesis causes reduced hemoglobin synthesis and eventually causing hypochromic microcytic anemia because of defective hemoglobinization of red blood cells. Thalassemias can be considered among the hypoproliferative anemias, the hemolytic anemias, and the anemias related to abnormal hemoglobin, since all of these factors play a role in pathogenesis.

Normal adult hemoglobin is primarily hemoglobin A, which represents approximately 98% of circulating hemoglobin. Hemoglobin A is formed from a tetramer—two α chains and two β chains—and can be designated $\alpha_2\beta_2$. Two copies of the α-globin gene are located on chromosome 16, and there is no substitute for α-globin in the formation of hemoglobin. The β-globin gene resides on chromosome 11 adjacent to genes encoding the β-like globin chains, δ and γ. The tetramer of $\alpha_2\delta_2$ forms hemoglobin A_2, which normally comprises 1–2% of adult hemoglobin. The tetramer $\alpha_2\delta_2$ forms hemoglobin F, which is the major hemoglobin of fetal life but which comprises less than 1% of normal adult hemoglobin **(Fig. 14.5)**.

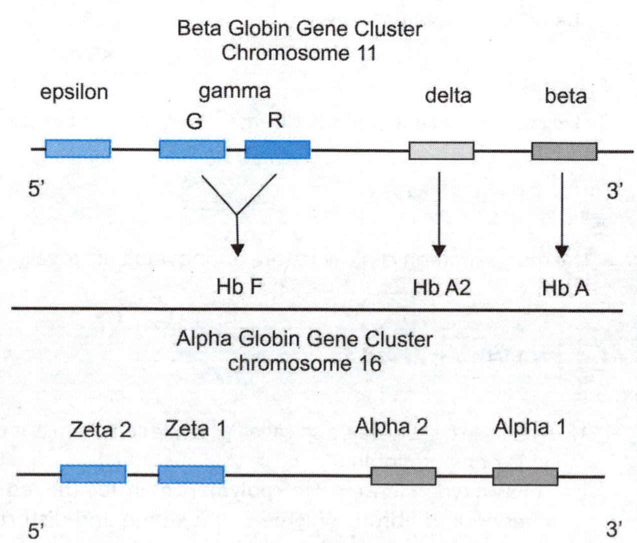

Fig. 14.5: Alpha and beta globin gene clusters.

Types of Thalassemia

Based on the defective chain, there are two main types:

i. Alpha thalassemia: Alpha thalassemia demonstrates problems with alpha globin chain production.
ii. Beta thalassemia: Beta thalassemia demonstrates problems with beta globin chain production.

Inheritance

Thalassemia is inherited in an autosomal recessive manner. The affected patients have a variable life span depending upon the severity of the disease.

Alpha Thalassemia

Alpha thalassemias primarily occur due to gene deletion causing impaired α-globin chain synthesis. The genes involved may be α-globin genes themselves (structural genes) or the regulatory genes, which regulate the expression of α-globin genes. As a consequence of impaired α-globin chain synthesis, the production of biologically functional hemoglobin is impaired.

Some mutational events such as point mutations or frameshift mutations may occur within or around the coding region of the α-globin gene cluster, and thus, may also impair the production of functional hemoglobin. These mutations can affect the RNA splicing or initiation of translation. Therefore, these events usually result in the synthesis of unstable α-chain variants.

From the genetic point of view, alpha thalassemias are highly heterogeneous; however, phenotypically alpha thalassemias can be explained based on the number of defective genes:

- **Alpha (0) thalassemia:** All the four α-globin genes are deleted; therefore, the affected patients fail to produce any of the functional hemoglobins, such as HbA, HbF, or HbA_2. This condition leads to the development of **hydrops fetalis, or Hb Bart,** a condition that is incompatible with life, the death of the fetus occurs in utero.
- **Alpha (+) thalassemia:** There is functional deletion of one of the four α-globin genes, hence, there is some α chain synthesis. The alpha (+) thalassemia can be subclassified into three general forms based on the number of gene deletions.
  - **A-Thalassemia** (**-α/α α**): It is identified by single α-globin gene deletion. However, three normal genes are inherited. These patients are denoted as a silent carrier of alpha thalassemia. This condition is also termed **alpha thalassemia minima, alpha thalassemia-2 trait, and heterozygosity for alpha (+) thalassemia minor.** There are no clinical manifestations, and the affected patients may exhibit normal hematological profile. Some may have a mild reduction in MCV and mean corpuscular hemoglobin (MCH).
  - **B-Inheritance of two normal alpha genes- (two genes' deletion):** There may be either heterozygosity for alpha (0) thalassemia (α α/--) or homozygosity for alpha (+) thalassemia (-α/-α), resulting in the development of **alpha thalassemia minor or alpha thalassemia-1 trait.** There are no significant clinical manifestations except for mild anemia and reduced mean corpuscular volume (MCV) and mean corpuscular hemoglobin (MCH).
  - **C-Inheritance of one normal alpha gene (-α/--)-(three genes deletions):** Since, there is only one functional alpha gene, therefore, this condition leads to the formation of hemoglobin H (tetramers of excess beta chains), based on that this type of alpha thalassemia is termed HbH disease. The patients present with moderate to severe degrees of hemolytic anemia (lifelong), moderate ineffective erythropoiesis, splenomegaly, and skeletal changes.

Other miscellaneous forms of alpha thalassemia are caused by translational defects, either premature or failed termination of translation. Some rare types of mutations cause thalassemia by inducing protein folding defects of normal globin chains **(Fig. 14.6)**.

Incidence

Alpha thalassemia is common in the malaria-endemic regions of the world. A protective effect from malaria by the presence of both single as well as double gene deletions has been reported by several studies. Although the anomalies affecting the α-globin genes have been reported worldwide, yet they are more common in people of Asian, African, and Mediterranean origin.

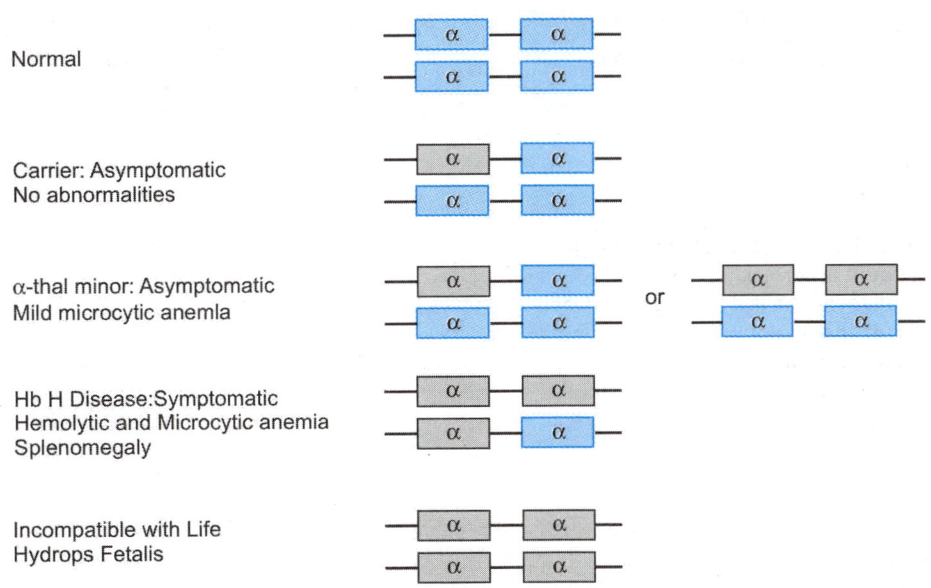

Fig. 14.6: Alpha thalassemia: Genetics and clinical manifestations.

Clinical Manifestations

Variations in the clinical courses and physical observations are identified in each of the four gene defects (**Table 14.1**). Furthermore, the clinical course of the disease can be altered by the collateral expression of beta chain hemoglobinopathies and beta-thalassemias.

- **Silent carrier/alpha-thalassemia-2 trait:** Patients are clinically asymptomatic. The silent carrier state gets manifested in children with HbH disease having both parents as carriers of these alleles.
- **Homozygous alpha (+) thalassemia:** The patients are clinically healthy. Although hemoglobin A2 concentration does not rise, elevations of hemoglobin F have been reported in this genotype.
- **Hemoglobin H disease:** The α-globin chain production is markedly reduced, resulting in the excess aggregation of beta globin chains as homotetrameric HbH. These unstable tetramers impair oxygen transportation (left-sided shift of oxygen dissociation curve). Additionally, this unstable hemoglobin precipitates and forms inclusion bodies within the red blood cells, resulting in chronic hemolytic anemia.
  - Symptoms are present at the time of birth; there may be anemia, neonatal jaundice, or even hydrops fetalis. Blood chemistry reveals indirect hyperbilirubinemia, high LDH levels, and low haptoglobin levels, all suggestive of hemolytic anemia. Hemolysis worsens when patients are exposed to oxidant drugs or infections.
  - Other complications include the following:
    - Hepatosplenomegaly
    - Chronic leg ulcers
    - Cholelithiasis
    - Aplastic or hypoplastic crises
    - Skeletal deformities such as marked frontal bossing (due to the expansion of bone marrow), prominent maxillae, delayed pneumatization of sinuses, box-like and convex ribs and long bones, shortened limbs due to premature closure of epiphyses, and the increased tendency of fractures due to bone fragility and osteopenia.
    - There may be compression fracture of the spine resulting in cord compression or other neurological deficits.
    - Besides these symptoms, there may be developmental and metabolic changes due to ineffective erythropoiesis.
    - Massive enlargement of the spleen may require splenectomy in the second or third decade of life.
    - Blood transfusions are also needed depending upon the severity of anemia—iron overload results as a consequence of repeated blood transfusions.
- **Hemoglobin Bart or hydrops fetalis (--/--):** There is no effective **α**-globin chain synthesis. The disease seems incompatible with life. The death of the fetus occurs in utero (hydrops fetalis). There is massive edema of the body resulting from high output cardiac failure secondary to extramedullary hematopoiesis and edematous friable placenta.

TABLE 14.1: Clinical course and hematological findings in each of the four genotypes of α-thalassemia.

Alphaglobin genes	*Syndrome*	*Hematocrit*	*MCV*
4	Normal	Normal	
3	Silent carrier	Normal	
2	Thalassemia minor	28–40%	60–75 fL
1	Hemoglobin H disease	22–32%	60–70 fL
0	Hydrops fetalis		

Laboratory Studies

- **Trait - α/α α**
  - Hemoglobin level is within the reference range.
  - Reticulocyte count is normal.
  - Mean corpuscular volume (MCV) ranges between 75 and 85 fL.
  - Mean corpuscular hemoglobin (MCH) is around 26 pg.
- **Alpha1 thalassemia minor**
  - Hemoglobin level is within the reference range.
  - Reticulocyte count is normal.
  - MCV is 65 to 75 fL.
  - MCH is around 22 pg.
- **Hemoglobin H disease**
  - Hemoglobin level is 7 to 10 g/dL.
  - Reticulocyte count is 5 to 10%.
  - MCV is 55 to 65 fL.
  - MCH is 20 pg.
  - The peripheral blood smear shows small misshapen red cells, hypochromia, microcytosis, and targeting.

- **Hydrops fetalis**
  - Hemoglobin is 4 to 10 g/dL.
  - MCV is 110 to 120 fL.
  - The peripheral blood smear shows severe anisopoikilocytosis, severe hypochromia, and nucleated red blood cells.
- Alpha thalassemia combined with sickle cell anemia causes a higher hemoglobin concentration and improved red blood cell survival.

Other Tests

- **Hemoglobin electrophoresis** separates hemoglobin into different types. Hemoglobin Bart is elevated at birth in patients with alpha thalassemia. In hemoglobin H disease, 20 to 40% of total hemoglobin is of hemoglobin Bart; however, in the silent carrier alpha thalassemia condition, the percentage is only 1 to 2% with low or normal amounts of hemoglobin A_2. Hemoglobin electrophoresis is generally not sufficiently sensitive to diagnose silent carrier alpha thalassemia.
- α to β synthetic ratios are altered in both alpha and beta thalassemias. Increasing ratios of β- to α-globin chains are observed in alpha-2 thalassemia, alpha-1 thalassemia, and hemoglobin H disease, respectively.
- Currently, **genetic testing** is used to establish the diagnosis in patients with a suggestive family history and or hematologic findings suggestive of alpha thalassemia.
  - Recombinant DNA technology can be diagnostic but is still a research tool
  - Gene mapping
  - Polymerase chain reaction (PCR)
  - Restriction endonucleases
  - Anti-L globin monoclonal antibodies

Procedures

Bone marrow aspiration and biopsy are not helpful in establishing the precise diagnosis and are not indicated unless other confounding problems exist.

Histologic Findings

Peripheral blood smear may reveal target cells, microcytosis, hypochromia, and anisopoikilocytosis **(Fig. 14.7)**. Most individuals with alpha-2 thalassemia (trait) have only mild microcytosis, which can be differentiated from other common causes of microcytosis based on serum iron and ferritin concentrations within the reference range.

Peripheral smear from a patient with hemoglobin H disease, showing target cells, microcytosis, hypochromia, and anisopoikilocytosis. Morphological abnormalities are similar to those observed in beta thalassemia. In alpha-2 thalassemia (silent trait), only mild microcytosis is observed.

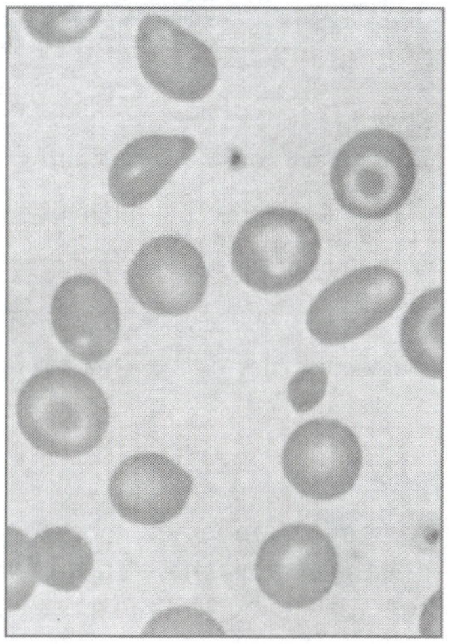

Fig. 14.7: Peripheral blood smear form a patient with hemoglobin H disease, showing target cells, microcytosis, hypochromia, and anisopoikilocytosis.

Treatment

Medical intervention

- Iron supplementation is not recommended as it causes iron overload and does not influence hematological indices or cell structure.
- Supplementation of folate is recommended to provide sufficient supply of the vitamin for increased demand resulting from the hemolytic process and higher bone marrow turnover rate.
- Immediate attention is to be given to treat infection, especially after splenectomy in children, and appropriate vaccines are administered to these individuals.
- A blood transfusion is to be used only if necessary.
- Iron chelation therapy to avoid iron overloading is recommended if chronic transfusion is needed (hemoglobin H disease).

Surgical Intervention

- Hemoglobin H disease
  - Splenectomy is performed if there are repeated transfusions.
  - Surgical or orthodontic corrections are undertaken to correct skeletal deformities of the skull and maxilla caused by erythroid hyperplasia.
- **Infrequently, allogeneic stem cell transplantation can be considered.**

Prognosis

- The prognosis is excellent for silent carriers.
- Because hydrops fetalis is incompatible with life, hemoglobin H (--/--) is the most serious syndrome.

- The overall survival for hemoglobin H disease is variable; however, it is generally good. Many patients survive into adulthood. However, some patients have a more complicated course and may not do as well.

β-thalassemias

β-thalassemias are usually caused by point mutations rather than deletions (**Table 14.2**). These mutations result in premature chain termination or in problems with transcription of RNA and ultimately result in reduced or absent β-globin chain synthesis. The molecular defects leading to β-thalassemia are numerous and heterogeneous. Defects that result in absent globin chain expression are termed β_0, whereas those causing reduced synthesis are termed β^+. The reduced β-globin chain synthesis in β-thalassemia results in a relative increase in the percentages of hemoglobins A_2 and F compared to hemoglobin A, as the β-like globins (δ and γ) substitute for the missing β chains. In the presence of reduced β chains, the excess α chains are unstable and precipitate, leading to damage of red blood cell membranes. This leads to intramedullary and peripheral hemolysis. The bone marrow becomes hyper plastic under the drive of anemia and ineffective erythropoiesis resulting from the intramedullary destruction of the developing erythroid cells. In cases of severe thalassemia, the marked expansion of the erythroid element in the bone marrow may cause severe bony deformities, osteopenia, and pathologic fractures.

Beta Thalassemia Syndromes

TABLE 14.2: Percentage of HbA1, HbA2 and HbF in different genotypes of beta thalassemia.

β-Globin genes		*Hb A_1*	*Hb A_2*	*HbF*
Normal	Homozygous β	97–99%	1–3%	<1%
Thalassemia major	Homozygous β^0	0%	4–10%	90–96%
Thalassemia major	Homozygous β^+	0–10%	4–10%	90–96%
Thalassemia intermedia	Homozygous β^+ (mild)	0–30%	0–10%	6–100%
Thalassemia minor	Heterozygous β^0	80–95%	4–8%	1–5%
Thalassemia minor	Heterozygous β^+	80–95%	4–8%	1–5%

Incidence

Thalassemia is among the most common genetic disorders worldwide.

The thalassemias have a distribution concomitant with areas where malaria is common. People with thalassemia minor are able to fight malaria better than those who do not have it—therefore, in parts of the world where malaria existed, thalassemia minor increased. This was of great value in the past since malaria was rampant and deadly. However, malaria is no longer a problem in many areas of the world, and thalassemia minor has no advantage to people in these areas. The beta thalassemias are seen primarily in the Mediterranean Sea area, Africa, and Southeast Asia. Due to global migration patterns, there has been an increase in the incidence of thalassemia in North America in the last 10 years.

Thalassemia has also been found in people of many ethnic backgrounds, so it cannot be called a Mediterranean disease. Other areas affected are the Middle East, India, Pakistan, and Southeast Asia.

Causes

Beta thalassemia is caused by a genetic mutation in the beta-globin gene; however, many additional factors influence the clinical manifestations of disease. The following factors are known to influence the clinical phenotype:

- Intracellular fetal Hb concentrations
  - The level of expression of fetal Hb (i.e., the expression level of the gamma-globin gene) determines, in part, the severity of the disease.
  - Patients with high fetal Hb have milder disease.
- Co-inheritance of alpha thalassemia
  - Patients with co-inheritance of alpha thalassemia have a milder clinical course because they have a less severe alpha–beta chain imbalance.
  - The coexistence of sickle cell trait and beta thalassemia is a major and symptomatic hemoglobinopathy with most of the symptoms and complications of sickle cell disease. Unlike sickle cell trait, in which most Hb-on-Hb electrophoresis is Hb A (AS), S is the dominant Hb (SA) and usually constitutes about 60% of the circulating Hb.

Clinical Findings

β-thalassemia

Affected children are normal at birth but after 6 months, when hemoglobin synthesis switches from hemoglobin F to hemoglobin A, develop severe anemia requiring transfusion. Numerous clinical problems ensue, including growth failure, bony deformities (abnormal facial structure, pathologic fractures), hepatosplenomegaly, and jaundice. The clinical course is modified significantly by transfusion therapy, but the transfusional iron overload (hemosiderosis) results in a clinical picture similar to hemochromatosis, with heart failure, cirrhosis, and endocrinopathies, usually after more than 100 units of red blood cells. These problems develop because of the body's inability to excrete the iron from transfused red cells. Before the application of allogeneic stem cell transplantation and the development of more effective forms of iron chelation, death from cardiac failure usually occurred between the ages of 20 and 30 years. This has been profoundly changed.

People with thalassemia major may also experience the following:

- Pallor
- Headaches
- Fatigue
- Shortness of breath
- An infant with thalassemia major appears normal at birth. If a child is well for the first five years of life, a diagnosis of thalassemia major is unlikely.
- Changes occur in the appearance of the face and head.
- The eyes appear slanted and the cheekbones become prominent.

The clinical manifestations are the direct result of the pathophysiologic process of thalassemia. Pallor is present because hemoglobin is a major factor in the normal skin color. Children with thalassemia are usually small for their age, reaching only the 5th percentile for growth. They experience recurrent severe anemia (hemoglobin 6 g/dL) and hepatosplenomegaly. The stress on the bone marrow causes the bones to thicken and becomes less flexible. This leads to pathological fractures and pain.

Thalassemia Intermedia

Patients homozygous for a milder form of β-thalassemia (allowing a higher rate of globin gene synthesis) have thalassemia intermedia. These patients have chronic hemolytic anemia but do not require transfusions except under periods of stress. They may also develop iron overload because of periodic transfusion. They survive into adult life, but with hepatosplenomegaly and bony deformities. Patients heterozygous for β-thalassemia have thalassemia minor and a clinically insignificant microcytic anemia.

Complications

Complications that may arise from regular blood transfusions include an overload of iron build-up in vital organs causing diabetes, liver disease, and heart failure. The spleen may become so enlarged or overactive that it has to be removed surgically.

The following are the complications possible:

- Anemia
- Leg ulcers
- Stillbirth—four gene deletions cause still birth
- Fractures
- Ineffective erythropoiesis
- Uric acid levels raised (plasma or serum)
- Hypersplenism
- Osteoporosis

Laboratory Findings

β-thalassemia Minor

As in β-thalassemia trait, these patients have a modest anemia with hematocrit between 28% and 40%. The MCV ranges from 55 to 75 fL, and the red blood cell count is normal or increased. The peripheral blood smear is mildly abnormal, with hypochromia, microcytosis, and target cells **(Fig. 14.8)**.

The reticulocyte count is normal or slightly elevated. Hemoglobin electrophoresis (using quantitative techniques) may show an elevation of hemoglobin A_2 to 4–8% and occasional elevations of hemoglobin F to 1–5%.

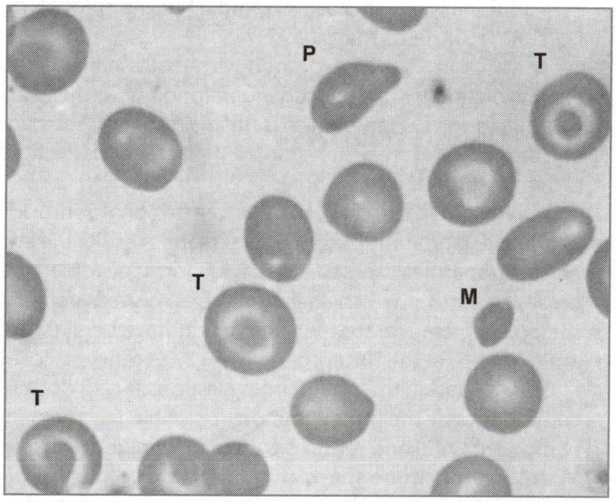

Fig. 14.8: Peripheral smear in beta-zero thalassemia minor showing microcytes (M), target cells (T), and poikilocytes.

β-thalassemia Major

β-thalassemia major produces severe anemia, and without transfusion, the hematocrit may fall to less than 10%. The peripheral blood smear is bizarre, showing severe poikilocytosis, hypochromia, microcytosis, target cells, basophilic stippling, and nucleated red blood cells. Little or no hemoglobin A is present. Variable amounts of hemoglobin A_2 are seen, and the major hemoglobin present is hemoglobin F **(Fig. 14.9)**.

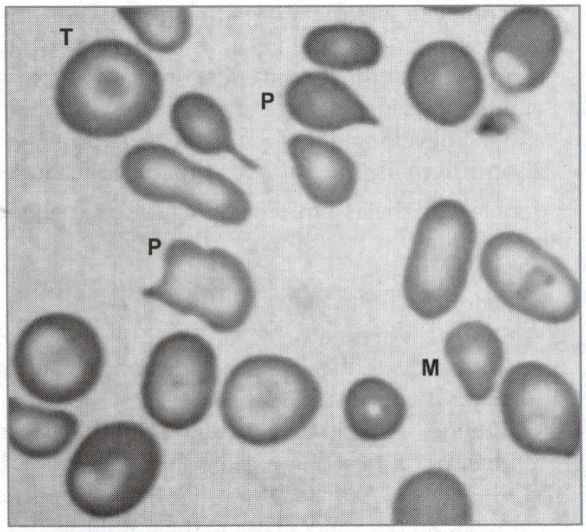

Fig. 14.9: Peripheral smear from a patient with beta-zero thalassemia major showing more marked microcytosis (M) and anisopoikilocytosis (P) than in thalassemia minor. Target cells (T) and hypochromia are prominent.

Imaging Studies

- The skeletal deformities in patients with thalassemia major include a widened bone marrow space, resulting in a decreased thickness of the bone cortex. These alterations are particularly striking in the skull, which may exhibit the typical **hair-on-end** appearance. Bone deformities can also be examined in the long bones, vertebrae, and pelvis.
- The evidence of extramedullary hematopoiesis and damage secondary to iron overload resulting from multiple transfusion therapy can be observed in the liver and biliary tract of patients with thalassemia major.
- Viral hepatitis resulting from repeated transfusions is another common finding which progresses to liver cirrhosis and portal hypertension. Gall stones can be visualized through gallbladder images.
- Iron overload and anemia can affect cardiac functions. The patients with thalassemia major can present with conduction system defects, decreased myocardial function, and fibrosis. Pericarditis can also develop in some patients.

Other tests

- Iron studies (iron, transferrin, and ferritin) are useful in excluding iron deficiency and the anemia of chronic disorders as the cause of the patient's anemia.
- Patients may require a bone marrow examination to exclude certain other causes of microcytic anemia.
- The Mentzer index is defined as mean corpuscular volume per red cell count. An index of less than 13 suggests that the patient has the thalassemia trait, and an index of more than 13 suggests that the patient has iron deficiency.
- Prenatal diagnosis is possible. Molecular diagnostic tests can precisely determine whether a mutation is present any time after approximately 8 weeks of gestation. The physician can establish the diagnosis in utero using DNA obtained from amniocentesis or by chorionic villus sampling. In most laboratories, the DNA is amplified using the polymerase chain reaction technique and then it is analyzed for the presence of the thalassemia mutation using a panel of oligonucleotide probes corresponding to known thalassemia mutations.

Treatment

Thalassemia trait: Normally, there are no treatments recommended. However, iron medication, if necessary. **Thalassemia major:** The primary treatment is regular blood transfusions, usually every four weeks. In addition to the blood transfusion, injections of Desferal to help the body flush out the extra iron created by the new blood.

Additionally, splenectomy (removal of the spleen), bone marrow transplants, and chelation therapy are being proposed as possible treatments for thalassemia.

The anemia that is associated with thalassemia may be severe and is accompanied by ineffective erythropoiesis, with bone expansion and extramedullary hematopoiesis in the liver, spleen, and other sites, such as paravertebral masses.

Transfusion therapy, which is the mainstay of treatment, allows for normal growth and development and suppresses ineffective erythropoiesis. Transfusion-transmitted infections (primarily hepatitis B and C) are an important cause of death in countries where proper testing is not available.

Iron overload results both from transfusional hemosiderosis and excess gastrointestinal iron absorption. Iron deposition in the heart, liver, and multiple endocrine glands results in severe damage to these organs, with variable endocrine organ failure. The endocrinopathies can be treated with hormone replacement. However, the most serious result of iron overload is life-threatening cardiotoxicity, for which chelation therapy is required. Thalassemia can be cured by bone marrow transplantation. Experimental therapies to ameliorate the anemia that have been or are currently under investigation include fetal hemoglobin modifiers and antioxidants. In the future, gene therapy or other molecular methods may be feasible.

Iron-chelation therapy is largely responsible for doubling the life expectancy of patients with thalassemia major. Deferoxamine continues to be the most common iron-chelating agent in use, but it has several limitations: the need for parenteral administration (which is painful and reduces compliance), side effects, and cost (which is prohibitive in underdeveloped countries).

Allogeneic bone marrow transplantation is the treatment of choice for β-thalassemia major. Children who have not yet experienced iron overload and chronic organ toxicity do well, with long-term survival in more than 80% of cases.

Additional treatments under development are experimental protocols to manipulate globin gene expression using gene therapy or using drugs that activate gamma-globin genes. Since fetal globin gene expression is associated with a milder phenotype, approaches to enhance intracellular Hb F levels (by activating gamma-globin gene expression) are under investigation. The two most widely studied drugs in this area are butyrates and hydroxyurea.

Gene-replacement therapy or gene therapy is being pursued by several research groups. Obstacles in gene therapy include inability to express high levels of the beta-globin gene in erythroid cells and inability to transduce hematopoietic pluripotent stem cells at high efficiency.

Prevention

Prenatal diagnosis is possible by analyzing DNA obtained via chorionic villi sampling at 8 to 10 weeks of gestation or by amniocentesis at 14 to 20 weeks of gestation. Since the genetic defects are quite variable, family genotyping usually must be completed for diagnostic linkage (segregation) analysis. With the anticipated availability of large-scale mutation screening by DNA chip technology, extensive pedigree analyses may be obviated. Genetic therapy strategies are currently in the early stages of development.

CLINICAL NOTE

The anemia that is associated with thalassemia may be severe and is accompanied by ineffective erythropoiesis, with bone expansion and extramedullary hematopoiesis in the liver, spleen, and other sites, such as paravertebral masses.

CLINICAL PEARLS

1. The thalassemias are hereditary disorders characterized by reduction in the synthesis of globin chains (α or β).
2. In the thalassemia patient, a point mutation or deletion of the genes that control globin chain production occurs. This leads to a decreased production of the corresponding globin chains and an abnormal hemoglobin ratio.
3. They are particularly common in people of Mediterranean, African, and Southeast Asian ancestry.
4. Symptoms and signs result from anemia, hemolysis, splenomegaly, bone marrow hyperplasia, and, if there have been multiple transfusions, iron overload.
5. Diagnosis is based on genetic tests and quantitative Hb analysis. Treatment for severe forms may include transfusion, splenectomy, chelation, and stem cell transplantation.

CASE STUDY 3

Theme: Clinical Implications of Altered Hemoglobin Methemoglobinemia (Qualitative Defect)

A 26-week-old baby was brought to the pediatric clinic because of increasing lethargy and cyanosis. The infant had been in good health at birth, and the mother attempted breastfeeding. Since the mother's milk flow had ceased, the family physician had recommended formula feeding. The child was unwell since then.

The blood sample was collected and a positive test for methemoglobin was obtained. A diagnosis of methemoglobinemia was made.

The baby was treated for two days. At the time of discharge, the child was alert and there was no cyanosis. The child was discharged with instructions to the mother concerning formula prepared with distilled water.

What is the cause for methemoglobinemia?

What type of treatment was given to the baby?

CASE DISCUSSION

Nitrites and nitrates, contaminants of water supply, are of particular concern in pediatrics because the infants consume a large amount of water. In rural areas, the well water is easily contaminated by the cattle feeding lots. Such well water might not harm an adult but can seriously compromise the health of a young child. The child in the given case suffered from methemoglobinemia due to the contamination of water only since the symptoms disappeared after formula feeding with distilled water. If the use of clean water in the baby' formula would not have eliminated the symptoms, then it could have been congenital methemoglobinemia.

METHEMOGLOBINEMIA

Biochemical Defect

The hemoglobin present in red blood cells is comprised of four globin chains, each associated with heme as a prosthetic group. Heme contains an iron molecule which in its reduced form (ferrous form) helps the acceptance of oxygen through sharing of an electron. Hemoglobin bound with oxygen is termed "oxyhemoglobin" **(Fig. 14.10)**. After unloading of oxygen, the iron molecule reverts to its original ferrous form. The acceptance and transportation of oxygen by hemoglobin are entirely dependent on the ferrous state of iron. Hemoglobin-containing iron in the ferric (Fe^{3+}) state is termed "methemoglobin."

As methemoglobin lacks electron to share with oxygen, it fails to accept and transport oxygen. As the red blood cells are regularly exposed to varying degrees of oxidative stress, under physiological conditions approximately 1% methemoglobin can be found in the normal blood.

The low concentration of methemoglobin is maintained through the following mechanisms:

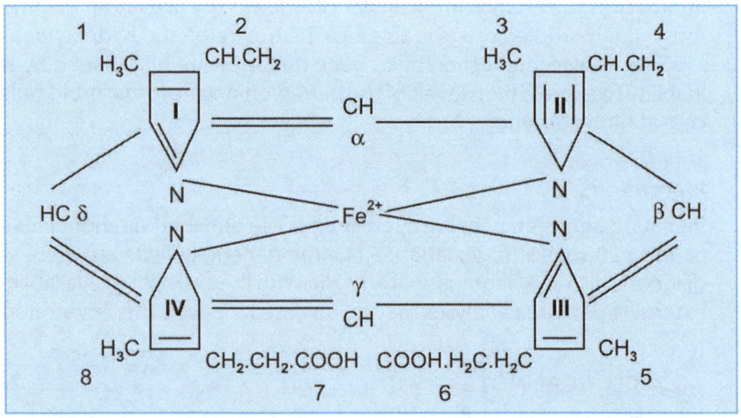

Fig. 14.10: The structure of heme showing Fe in the ferrous form.

1. **Through hexose-monophosphate shunt (HMP shunt) pathway:** This pathway helps to protect against the oxidants by generating NADPH that keeps glutathione in its reduced (the active) form. Reduced glutathione is essential for the activity of glutathione peroxidase, which is an antioxidant enzyme that helps to prevent the formation of methemoglobin.
2. **Through diaphorase I and diaphorase II:** These enzymes help in the reduction of methemoglobin. Diaphorase I and diaphorase II require nicotinamide adenine dinucleotide (NADH) and nicotinamide adenine dinucleotide phosphate (NADPH), respectively, for the reduction of methemoglobin to its usual ferrous state. In the physiological state, diaphorase II has a restricted ability to reduce hemoglobin. However, its activity can be increased to five times its normal action by the pharmacological drugs, such as methylene blue. Although methemoglobinemia is considered mainly an acquired disorder, some congenital cases have also been reported in the literature.

Pathophysiology

The oxidation of iron affects the oxygen-carrying capacity of hemoglobin. The delivery of oxygen to tissues is impaired (the oxygen–hemoglobin dissociation curve is shifted to the left), and a state of functional anemia is produced.

Organs with high oxygen demands (i.e., CNS, cardiovascular system) usually are the first systems to manifest toxicity. Oxygenated blood is red, deoxygenated blood is blue, and blood-containing methemoglobin is a dark reddish brown color. This dark hue imparts clinical cyanosis when methemoglobin levels are at 1.5 g/dL (approximately 10–15% methemoglobin concentration); however, a level of 5 g/dL of deoxygenated blood is required for similar effects. Therefore, when methemoglobin levels are relatively low, cyanosis may be observed without cardiopulmonary symptoms.

Methemoglobinemia may be passed down through families (inherited). Or, it may result from exposure to certain drugs, chemicals, or foods (acquired).

There are two forms of inherited methemoglobinemia. The first form is passed on by both parents. The parents usually do not have the condition themselves, but they carry the gene that causes the condition. It occurs when there is a problem with an enzyme called cytochrome b5 reductase.

There are two types of this form of methemoglobinemia:

- Type 1 (also called erythrocyte reductase deficiency) occurs when red blood cells lack the enzyme.
- Type 2 (also called generalized reductase deficiency) occurs when the enzyme does not work anywhere in the body.
  The second form of inherited methemoglobinemia, called hemoglobin M disease, is caused by defects in the hemoglobin molecule itself. Only one parent needs to pass on the abnormal gene in order for the child to inherit the disease.
- Acquired methemoglobinemia is more common than the inherited forms. It occurs after exposure to certain chemicals and drugs.
  The condition may also occur in infants who are very ill or who are fed too many vegetables containing nitrates (such as beets).

CLINICAL SYMPTOMS

Symptoms of Type 1 methemoglobinemia (erythrocyte reductase deficiency) include:

- Bluish coloring of skin.

Symptoms of Type 2 methemoglobinemia (generalized reductase deficiency) include:

- Developmental delay
- Failure to thrive
- Mental retardation
- Seizures

Symptoms of hemoglobin M disease include:

- Bluish coloring of the skin **(Fig. 14.11)**.

Symptoms of Acquired Methemoglobinemia

- Bluish coloring of the skin
- Headache
- Fatigue
- Shortness of breath
- Lack of energy
- Normal methemoglobin concentrations are 1 percent (range, 0–3%).
  - At concentrations of 3 to 15%, a slight discoloration (e.g., pale, gray, blue) of the skin may be present.
  - At fractions of 15 to 20%, the patient may be relatively asymptomatic, but cyanosis is likely to be present.
  - Signs and symptoms at fractions of 25 to 50% are as follows:
  - Headache
  - Dyspnea
  - Lightheadedness, even syncope
  - Weakness
  - Confusion
  - Palpitations, chest pain

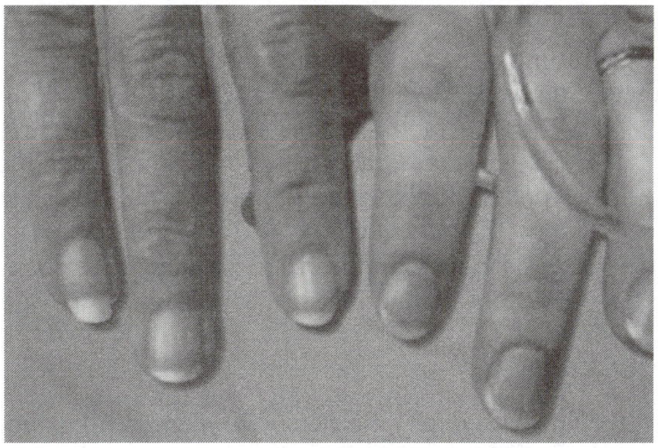

Fig. 14.11: Cyanosis in a patient with methemoglobinemia.

Signs and Symptoms at Fractions of 50 to 70%

- Cardiovascular
  - Abnormal cardiac rhythms
- CNS
  - Altered mental status
  - Delirium, seizures, coma
- Metabolic
  - Profound acidosis
- Discoloration of the skin and blood is the most striking physical finding.

Causes

- Compromised physiologic cellular defenses against oxidant stress occur in some patients, including the following:
  - Children younger than 4 months may have underdeveloped protective mechanisms (NADH methemoglobin reductase). Infections, especially GI infections, may cause a build-up of systemic oxidants by an overgrowth of gut bacteria.
  - **Congenital lack of protective cellular capabilities** includes those with the following:
    - Patients with NADH methemoglobin reductase (diaphorase I) deficiency may develop congenital methemoglobinemia.
    - Patients with hemoglobin M disease may have abnormal hemoglobin that is not amenable to reduction.
    - Patients with pyruvate kinase deficiency may have an impaired glycolytic pathway, which results in deficient NADH production.
    - Patients with G-6-PD deficiency may have impaired production of NADP in the hexose-monophosphate shunt.
- **Agents that inflict large oxidant stress** on patients include the following:
  - Pharmaceutical agents: Include local anesthetic agents (e.g., benzocaine, lidocaine), amyl nitrite, chloroquine, dapsone, nitrates, nitrites, nitroglycerin, nitroprusside, phenacetin, phenazopyridine, primaquine, quinones, and sulfonamides.
  - Environmental agents include the following: Aniline dyes, aromatic amines, combustion products, foods containing nitrates or nitrites (including well water), isobutyl nitrite, naphthalene, nitroaniline, nitrobenzen, nitrosobenzene, resorcinol, and silver nitrate.

Laboratory Diagnosis

- **Arterial blood gas:** Normal PaO_2 concentrations are usually found on analysis. Clinical cyanosis in the presence of normal arterial oxygen tensions is highly suggestive of methemoglobinemia ("saturation gap").
- **Imaging studies:** CT scanning of the head, when appropriate.
- **Other tests:** Adjunctive laboratory tests include determining lactate levels and serum electrolyte levels. These may be helpful in determining the degree of tissue hypoxia and end-organ dysfunction.
- The diagnosis of methemoglobinemia is confirmed by direct measurement of methemoglobin by a multiple wavelength co-oximeter. Newer multiwave length pulse oximeters can detect methemoglobinemia with an accuracy comparable to co-oximeters.

Treatment

- Administration of supplemental oxygen
- Removal of the offending oxidizing agent
- Methylene blue is the first-line antidotal agent. Methylene blue accelerates the enzymatic reduction of methemoglobin by NADP-methemoglobin reductase and also reduces to leukomethylene blue that, in turn, reduces methemoglobin
- Hyperbaric oxygen therapy or packed RBC exchange transfusions are alternative therapies for patients who are not candidates for methylene blue.
- Dermal decontamination (e.g., water rinse, soap scrub, water rinse again)
- GI decontamination (e.g., gastric lavage, activated charcoal administration).

Prognosis

People with Type 1 methemoglobinemia and hemoglobin M disease usually do well. Type 2 methemoglobinemia is much more serious, and usually causes death within the first few years of life.

People with acquired methemoglobinemia usually do very well once the drug, food, or chemical that caused the problem is identified and avoided.

For minor cases of methemoglobinemia, the prognosis is very favorable. In severe cases, prognosis is determined by the degree of anoxic end-organ damage.

Possible Complications

End-organ damage (e.g., myocardial infarction, seizure, coma, death).

CLINICAL NOTE

Methemoglobin absorbs light at wavelengths that also absorb deoxyhemoglobin and oxyhemoglobin. Thus, methemoglobin interferes with the colorimetric testing that is used to obtain the percentage of oxyhemoglobin to deoxyhemoglobin.

CLINICAL PEARLS

1. When hemoglobin loses an electron and becomes oxidized, it is converted to the ferric state (Fe^{3+}) or methemoglobin. Methemoglobin lacks the electron that is needed to form a bond with oxygen and, thus, is incapable of oxygen transport, because red blood cells are continuously exposed to various oxidant stresses.
2. This low level of methemoglobin is maintained by two important mechanisms. One protective mechanism against oxidizing agents is the hexose monophosphate shunt pathway within the erythrocyte. Through this pathway, oxidizing agents are reduced by glutathione prior to the formation of methemoglobin. The second and more important mechanism against methemoglobin formation uses two enzyme systems, diaphorase I and diaphorase II.
3. There are two types of this form of methemoglobinemia: Type 1 (also called erythrocyte reductase deficiency) occurs when red blood cells lack the enzyme. Type 2 (also called generalized reductase deficiency) occurs when the enzyme does not work anywhere in the body.
4. The diagnosis of methemoglobinemia is confirmed by the direct measurement of methemoglobin by a multiple wavelength co-oximeter.
5. Methylene blue is used to treat persons with severe methemoglobinemia. Intravenous ascorbic acid can also be used for the treatment.

Chapter 15

Hormones

LEARNING OBJECTIVES

To understand:
- Chemistry
- Mechanism of action
- Functions
- Clinical significance of hormones

CASE STUDIES

CASE STUDY 1

Theme: Biological and Clinical Significance of Growth Hormone

An 18-year-old diabetic student, who was 7 feet tall and a basketball player, had poorly controlled diabetes mellitus for 4 years. Despite following his diet and exercising regularly, he required more than 120 units of insulin each day. Because of the patient's extreme insulin resistance, the physician measured antibodies against insulin, but they were not present. A brain MRI scan revealed an enlarged pituitary gland. The patient was subsequently referred to a neuroendocrine clinical center for further evaluation of the pituitary mass.

On specific questioning, however, he admitted that his shoe size had increased and his ring, given by his mother, had also gone small for him. These changes were so subtle that he had not reported growth of hands or feet as a concern until he was prompted by questions focused on these changes. He denied snoring, mood change, or sweating.

The patient weighed 78.6 kg. His blood pressure was 130/80 mm Hg. Abnormal findings included minimal acne; proximal interphalangeal joint swelling bilaterally (most prominent in the third and fourth left digits) and he had puffy hands bilaterally. There was mild edema of his hands and distal lower extremities bilaterally. Classic acral or facial features of acromegaly were absent and the remainder of his physical examination was unremarkable. The results of the patient's laboratory investigations were remarkable for elevated insulin-like growth factor 1 (IGF-1) and mild hyperprolactinemia. The other neuroendocrine test results were normal.

What is the probable diagnosis?
How will you confirm the diagnosis?
What is the biochemical basis for all these clinical and laboratory findings?

CASE DISCUSSION

It is a case of acromegaly. Acromegaly results from excessive release of growth hormone that begins after epiphyseal closure and the cessation of long bone growth. Acral bone growth causes the characteristic facial changes (protruding jaw, enlarged nose, and the enlargement of the hands, feet and skull). Other findings include enlarged viscera, thickening of the skin, and a variety of metabolic problems including diabetes mellitus. Insulin resistance is a common finding in acromegaly as is evident in the given case.

BASIC CONCEP T

Growth Hormone

Growth hormone (GH) is the most abundant anterior pituitary hormone, and GH-secreting somatotrope cells constitute up to 50% of the total anterior pituitary cell population. The pituitary GH gene (hGH-N) produces two alternatively spliced products that give rise to 22-kDa GH (191 amino acids) and a less abundant 20-kDa GH molecule, with similar biological activity.

Secretion

Growth hormone (GH) secretion is controlled by complex hypothalamic and peripheral factors.

Growth hormone-releasing hormone (GHRH) is a 44-amino-acid hypothalamic peptide that stimulates GH synthesis and release. Ghrelin, an octanoylated gastric-derived peptide, as well as synthetic agonists of the GHRH receptor, induces GHRH and also directly stimulate GH release. Somatostatin [somatotropin-release inhibiting factor (SRIF)] is synthesized in the medial preoptic area of the hypothalamus and inhibits GH secretion. GHRH is secreted in discrete spikes that elicit GH pulses, whereas SRIF sets basal GH tone. SRIF is also expressed in many extrahypothalamic tissues, including the CNS, gastrointestinal tract, and pancreas, where it also acts to inhibit islet hormone secretion. IGF-1, the peripheral target hormone for GH, feeds back to inhibit GH; estrogen induces GH, whereas chronic glucocorticoid excess suppresses GH release.

Surface receptors on the somatotrope regulate GH synthesis and secretion. The GHRH receptor is a G protein-coupled receptor (GPCR) that signals through intracellular cyclic AMP pathway to stimulate somatotrope cell proliferation as well as GH production. Inactivating mutations of the GHRH receptor cause profound dwarfism. A distinct surface receptor for ghrelin, a gastric-derived GH secretagogue, is expressed in the hypothalamus and pituitary. Somatostatin binds to five distinct receptor subtypes (SSTR1 to SSTR5); SSTR2 and SSTR5 subtypes preferentially suppress GH (and TSH) secretion.

Growth hormone (GH) secretion is pulsatile, with highest peak levels occurring at night, generally correlating with sleep onset. GH secretory rates decline markedly with age, so that hormone levels in middle age are about 15% of pubertal levels. GH secretion is also reduced in obese individuals, though IGF-1 levels may not be suppressed, suggesting a change in the setpoint for feedback control. Elevated GH levels occur within an hour of deep sleep onset as well as after exercise, physical stress, trauma, and during sepsis. Integrated 24-hour GH secretion is higher in women and is also enhanced by estrogen replacement. GH secretion is profoundly influenced by nutritional factors. Increased GH pulse frequency and peak amplitudes occur with chronic malnutrition or prolonged fasting.

Action

The pattern of GH secretion may affect tissue responses. The 70-kDa peripheral GH receptor protein shares structural homology with the cytokine/hematopoietic superfamily. A fragment of the receptor extracellular domain generates a soluble GH-binding protein (GHBP) that interacts with GH in the circulation. The liver and cartilage contain the greatest number of GH receptors. GH binding to receptor dimers is followed by signaling through the JAK/STAT pathway. The activated STAT proteins translocate to the nucleus, where they modulate expression of GH-regulated target genes. GH analogs that bind to the receptor, but are incapable of mediating receptor signaling, are potent antagonists of GH action. A GH receptor antagonist (pegvisomant) has been approved for treatment of acromegaly.

Functions of growth hormone are:

- It induces protein synthesis and nitrogen retention.
- It impairs glucose tolerance by antagonizing insulin action.
- It stimulates lipolysis, leading to increased circulating fatty acid levels, reduced omental fat mass, and enhanced lean body mass.
- It promotes sodium, potassium, and water retention and elevates serum levels of inorganic phosphate.
- Linear bone growth occurs as a result of complex hormonal and growth factor actions, including those of IGF-1.
- Growth hormone stimulates epiphyseal prechondrocyte differentiation. These precursor cells produce IGF-1 locally and are also responsive to the growth factor.
- IGF-1 is what actually causes tissue growth in the body.

Insulin-like Growth Factors

Although GH exerts direct effects in target tissues, many of its physiological effects are mediated indirectly through IGF-1, a potent growth and differentiation factor. The liver is the major source of circulating IGF-1. In peripheral tissues, IGF-1 exerts local paracrine actions that appear to be both dependent on and independent of GH. Serum IGF-1 concentrations are profoundly affected by physiological factors. Levels increase during puberty, peak at 16 years, and subsequently decline by >80% during the aging process. IGF-1 concentrations are higher in women than in men. Because GH is the major determinant of hepatic IGF-1 synthesis, abnormalities of GH synthesis or action (e.g., pituitary failure, GHRH receptor defect, or GH receptor defect) reduce IGF-1 levels. Hypocaloric states are associated with GH resistance; IGF-1 levels are, therefore, low with cachexia, malnutrition, and sepsis. High levels of IGF-1, in turn, signal the pituitary to reduce GH production. In acromegaly, IGF-1 levels are invariably high and reflect a log-linear relationship with GH concentrations.

Chronic excess IGF-1 would presumably result in features of acromegaly.

ACROMEGALY

Acromegaly (from Greek akros "extreme" or "extremities" and megalos "large"—extremities enlargement) is a syndrome that results when the pituitary gland produces excess growth hormone (hGH) after epiphyseal plate closure at puberty. A number of disorders may increase the pituitary's GH output, although most commonly, it involves a growth hormone (GH) producing tumor called pituitary adenoma, derived from a distinct type of cell (somatotrophs).

Causes

Acromegaly is caused by prolonged overproduction of GH by the pituitary gland. Pituitary produces several important hormones that control body functions, such as growth and development, reproduction, and metabolism. GH is part of a cascade of hormones that, as the name implies, regulates the physical growth of the body. This cascade begins in hypothalamus. Normally, GHRH, somatostatin, GH, and IGF-1 levels in the body are tightly regulated by each other and by sleep, exercise, stress, food intake, and blood sugar levels. If the pituitary continues to make GH independent of the normal regulatory mechanisms, the level of IGF-1 continues to rise, leading to bone overgrowth and organ enlargement. High levels of IGF-1 also cause changes in glucose and lipid metabolism and can lead to diabetes, high blood pressure, and heart disease.

Pituitary Adenoma

In over 90% of acromegaly patients, the overproduction of growth hormones is caused by a benign tumor of the pituitary gland, called an adenoma. These tumors produce excess growth hormones and, as they expand, compress surrounding brain tissues,, such as the optic nerves. This expansion causes the headaches and visual disturbances that often accompany acromegaly. In addition, compression of the surrounding normal pituitary tissue can alter production of other hormones, leading to changes in menstruation and breast discharge in women and impotence in men because of reduced testosterone production.

There is a marked variation in rates of GH production and the aggressiveness of the tumor. Some adenomas grow slowly and symptoms of growth hormone excess are often not noticed for many years. In general, younger patients tend to have more aggressive tumors. These tumors may be locally invasive, particularly into the cavernous sinus. Less than 1% are malignant. Most are macroadenomas (over 1 cm in diameter).

Most pituitary tumors arise spontaneously and are not genetically inherited. Many pituitary tumors arise from a genetic alteration in a single pituitary cell, which leads to increased cell division and tumor formation. This genetic change, or mutation, is not present at birth, but is acquired during life. The mutation occurs in a gene that regulates the transmission of chemical signals within pituitary cells; it permanently switches on the signal the cell to divide and secrete growth hormones. The events within the cell that cause disordered pituitary cell growth and growth hormone oversecretion currently are the subject of intensive research.

Nonpituitary Tumors

Rarely, acromegaly is caused not by pituitary tumors, but by tumors of the pancreas, lungs, and other parts of the brain.

The disease may be associated with endocrine tumors of the parathyroids or pancreas (MEN 1). Acromegaly may also be seen in McCune–Albright syndrome and as part of Carney's syndrome (atrial myxoma, acoustic neuroma, lentigines, and adrenal hypercortisolism). These tumors also lead to excess GH, either because they produce GH themselves or, more frequently, because they produce GHRH that stimulates the pituitary to make GH.

Acromegaly is rarely caused by ectopic secretion of GHRH or GH secreted by a lymphoma, hypothalamic tumor, bronchial carcinoid, or pancreatic tumor. In patients with GHRH-producing nonpituitary tumors, the pituitary still may be enlarged and may be mistaken for a tumor. When these nonpituitary tumors are surgically removed, growth hormone (GH) levels fall and the symptoms of acromegaly improve.

Incidence

Small pituitary adenomas are common, affecting about 17% of the population. However, most of these tumors do not cause symptoms and rarely produce excess GH. Three to four out of every million people develop acromegaly each year and about 60 out of every million people suffer from the disease at any time. Because the clinical diagnosis of acromegaly is often missed, these numbers probably underestimate the frequency of the disease.

Clinical Manifestations

Acromegaly is most often diagnosed in middle-aged adults, although symptoms can appear at any age. Swelling of the hands and feet is often an early feature, with patients noticing a change in ring or shoe size, particularly shoe width **(Fig. 15.1)**. A doughy, moist handshake is characteristic.

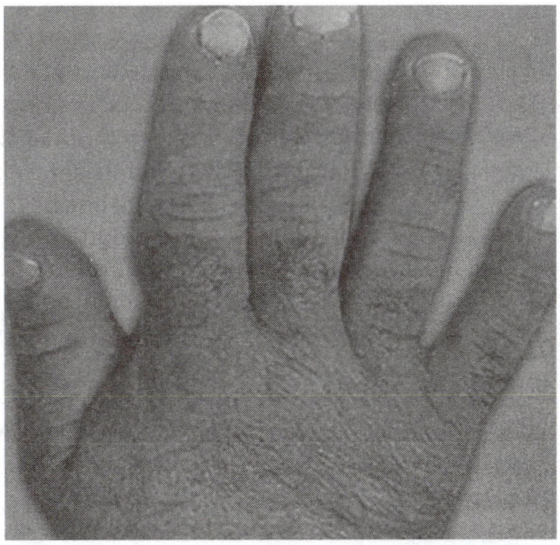

Fig. 15.1: Spade-shaped hand in acromegaly.

Gradually, bone changes alter the patient's facial features: the brow and lower jaw protrude, the nasal bone enlarges, and the teeth space out **(Fig. 15.2)**.

Other symptoms of acromegaly include **(Fig. 15.3)**:

- Joint aches, arthritis, carpal tunnel syndrome, and degenerative arthritis may occur. Overgrowth of vertebral bone can cause spinal stenosis.
- Thick, coarse, oily skin, skin tags, excessive sweating, and skin odor.
- Enlargement of lips, nose, and tongue (macroglossia), as does hypertrophy of pharyngeal, laryngeal tissue, and vocal cords; this causes a deep, coarse voice and sometimes makes intubation difficult.
- Obstructive sleep apnea may occur due to obstruction of the airways.
- Fatigue and weakness
- Headaches, impaired vision, temporal hemianopia may occur as a result of the optic chiasma being impinged by a suprasellar growth of the tumor.
- Abnormalities of the menstrual cycle and sometimes breast discharge in women.
- Erectile dysfunction in men and decreased libido. GH-secreting pituitary tumors usually cause some degree of hypogonadism, either by co-secretion of PRL or by direct pressure upon normal pituitary tissue.

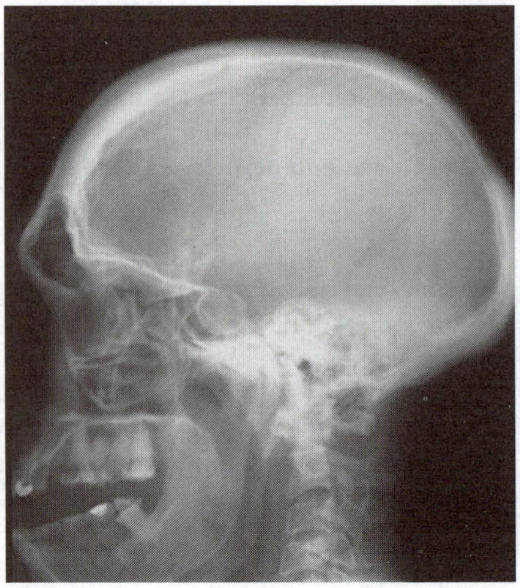

Fig. 15.2: Skull showing typical jaw shape.

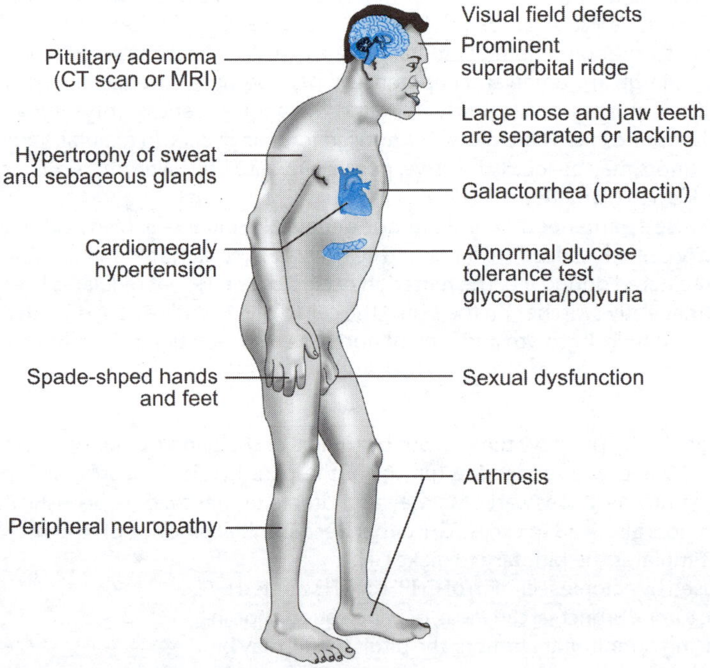

Fig. 15.3: Characteristics of acromegaly.

Routine Complications

- Diabetes mellitus [insulin resistance is usually present and frequently causes diabetes mellitus (30%)].
- Enlarged heart, hypertension, and heart failure. Hypertension (50%) and cardiomegaly are common. At diagnosis, about 10% of acromegalic patients have overt heart failure, with a dilated left ventricle and a reduced ejection fraction.
- Kidney failure
- Secondary hypothyroidism sometimes occurs; hypoadrenalism is unusual
- Carpal tunnel syndrome may cause thumb weakness and thenar atrophy. Arthritis of hips, knees, and spine can be troublesome. Cord compression may be seen.
- Visual field defects may be severe and progressive. Acute loss of vision or cranial nerve palsy may occur, if the tumor undergoes spontaneous hemorrhage and necrosis (pituitary apoplexy).
- Colon polyps are more likely to develop in patients with acromegaly.

Diagnosis

In suspected cases, the following tests are undertaken:

Blood tests:

1. **Estimation of GH levels:** A single measurement of an elevated blood GH level is not enough to diagnose acromegaly; because GH is secreted by the pituitary in impulses, or spurts, its concentration in the blood can vary widely from minute to minute. At a given moment, a person with acromegaly may have a normal GH level, whereas a GH level in a healthy person may even be five times higher.
2. **Oral glucose tolerance test:** More accurate information is obtained when GH is measured under conditions that normally suppress GH secretion. Often, the oral glucose tolerance test is used to diagnose acromegaly because drinking 75–100 g of glucose solution lowers blood GH levels to less than 1 nanogram per milliliter (ng/mL) in healthy people. In people with GH overproduction, this suppression does not occur. The oral glucose tolerance test is a highly reliable method for confirming a diagnosis of acromegaly.
3. **Estimation of IGF-1 levels:** IGF-1 levels can also be measured, which increase as GH levels go up, in people with suspected acromegaly. Because IGF-1 levels are much more stable than GH levels over the course of the day, they are often a more practical and reliable screening measure. Elevated IGF-1 levels almost always indicate acromegaly. However, a pregnant woman's IGF-1 levels are two to three times higher than normal. In addition, IGF-1 levels decline with age and may also be abnormally low in people with poorly controlled diabetes or liver or kidney disease.
4. **Other pituitary hormones** have to be assessed to address the secretory effects of the tumor as well as the mass effect of the tumor on the normal pituitary gland. They include serum free T4 and TSH (secondary hypothyroidism is common in acromegaly), gonadotropic hormones (FSH, LH), ACTH (adrenocorticotropic hormone), and prolactin.
5. **Miscellaneous tests:** Blood glucose (diabetes is common in acromegaly), liver enzymes and blood urea nitrogen (BUN) (hepatic or renal failure can misleadingly elevate GH), serum calcium (to screen for hyperparathyroidism), serum inorganic phosphorus (frequently elevated).
6. **Imaging:** After acromegaly has been diagnosed by measuring GH or IGF-1 levels, a magnetic resonance imaging (MRI) scan of the pituitary is used to locate and detect the size of the tumor causing GH overproduction. MRI is the most sensitive imaging technique, but computerized tomography (CT) scans can also be used.
7. If a head scan fails to detect a pituitary tumor, the physician should look for nonpituitary "ectopic" tumors in the chest, abdomen, or pelvis as the cause of excess GH. The presence of such tumors usually can be diagnosed by measuring GHRH in the blood and by a CT scan of possible tumor sites.

Rarely, a pituitary tumor secreting GH may be too tiny to detect even with a sensitive MRI scan.

Differential Diagnosis

Active acromegaly must be distinguished from familial coarse features, large hands and feet, and isolated prognathism and from inactive ("burned-out") acromegaly in which there has been a spontaneous remission due to infarction of the pituitary adenoma.

Misleadingly high serum GH levels can be caused by exercise or eating just prior to the test, acute illness or agitation, hepatic or renal failure, malnourishment, diabetes mellitus, or concurrent treatment with estrogens, beta-blockers, or clonidine. During normal adolescence, serum IGF-1 is usually elevated and GH may fail to be suppressed.

Treatment

Currently, treatment options include surgical removal of the tumor, medical therapy, and radiation therapy of the pituitary. Goals of treatment are to:

- Reduce excess hormone production to normal levels.
- Relieve the pressure that the growing pituitary tumor may be exerting on the surrounding brain areas.
- Preserve normal pituitary function or treat hormone deficiencies.
- Improve the symptoms of acromegaly.

Surgery

Surgery is the first option recommended for most people with acromegaly, as it is often a rapid and effective treatment. Surgery is most successful in patients with blood GH levels below 45 ng/mL before the operation and with pituitary tumors no larger than 10 millimeters (mm) in diameter. A possible complication of surgery is damage to the surrounding normal pituitary tissue, which requires lifelong use of pituitary hormone replacement. Even when surgery is successful and hormone levels return to normal, people with acromegaly must be carefully monitored for years for possible recurrence of the disease. More commonly, hormone levels improve, but do not return to normal. Additional treatment, usually medications, may be required.

Medical Therapy

Medical therapy is most often used, if surgery does not result in a cure and sometimes to shrink large tumors before surgery. Three medication groups are used to treat acromegaly.

1. **Somatostatin analogs** (SSAs) are the first medication group used to treat acromegaly. Octreotide and lanreotide are somatostatin analogs that are given by subcutaneous injection. They shut off GH production and are effective in lowering GH

and IGF-1 levels in 50–70% of patients. SSAs also reduce tumor size in around 0–50% of patients but only to a modest degree. Several studies have shown that SSAs are safe and effective for long-term treatment and in treating patients with acromegaly caused by nonpituitary tumors. Long-acting SSAs are given by intramuscular injection once a month. SSAs reduce the need for insulin and improve blood glucose control in some people with acromegaly who already have diabetes.

2. **GH receptor antagonists (GHRAs)**, which interfere with the action of GH, are the second group of medication. Pegvisomant is a GH receptor antagonist that blocks the effects of GH. Pegvisomant therapy produces symptomatic relief and normalizes serum IGF-1 levels in over 90% of patients. They do not, however, lower GH levels. Given once a day through injection, GHRAs are usually well-tolerated by patients. The long-term effects of these drugs on tumor growth are still under study. Side effects can include headaches, fatigue, and abnormal liver function.
3. **Dopamine agonists** make up the third medication group. These drugs are not as effective as the other medications at lowering GH or IGF-1 levels, and they normalize IGF-1 levels in only a minority of patients. Dopamine agonists are sometimes effective in patients who have mild degrees of excess GH and have both acromegaly and hyperprolactinemia—too much of the hormone prolactin. Cabergoline may be used first, since, it is an oral medication. Cabergoline therapy is most successful for tumors that secrete both PRL and GH but can also be effective for patients with normal serum PRL levels.

   Dopamine agonists can be used in combination with SSAs. Side effects can include nausea, headache, and lightheadedness.

Radiation Therapy

Radiation therapy is usually reserved for people who have some tumor remaining after surgery and do not respond to medications. These patients may be treated with stereotactic radiosurgery administered by gamma knife, heavy particle radiation, or adapted linear accelerator. Because radiation leads to a slow lowering of GH and IGF-1 levels, these patients often also receive medication to lower hormone levels. The full effect of this therapy may not occur for many years.

Follow-up

Acromegaly is a lifelong disease. Drug or radiation therapy typically goes on for several years. Even after successful therapy, levels of growth hormone and IGF-1 are required to be checked frequently.

Prognosis

Patients with acromegaly have increased morbidity and mortality from cardiovascular disorders and progressive acromegalic symptoms; those who are treated and have a glucose-suppressed serum GH level less than 2.5 ng/mL (radioimmunoassay) or under 1 ng/mL (immunofluorometric assay) and normal age-adjusted serum IGF-1 levels have reduced morbidity and mortality.

GIGANTISM

If excessive growth hormone production starts before the growth plates have closed (that is, in children), the condition produces gigantism. The long bones grow enormously. A person grows to unusually great stature, and the arms and legs lengthen. Puberty may be delayed, and the genitals may not develop fully.

CLINICAL NOTE

The oral glucose tolerance test is a highly reliable method for confirming a diagnosis of acromegaly.

CLINICAL PEARLS

1. Acromegaly is caused by prolonged overproduction of GH by the pituitary gland.
2. In over 90% of acromegaly patients, the overproduction of growth hormones is caused by a benign tumor of the pituitary gland, called an adenoma.
3. Swelling of the hands and feet is often an early feature; bone changes alter the patient's facial features. Arthritis, visual impairment, headaches, and menstrual abnormalities are other common manifestations.
4. Complications include hypopituitarism, hypertension, glucose intolerance or frank diabetes mellitus, cardiac enlargement, and cardiac failure.
5. Estimation of GH, IGF-1, oral glucose tolerance test, other hormones assays, liver and kidney function tests, and imaging can be undertaken to confirm the diagnosis.
6. Treatment involves surgery, medication, or radiation therapy.

CASE STUDY 2

Theme: Clinical Implications of Deficiencies of Adrenal Cortical Hormones

A 40-year-old male presented with vague symptoms of weakness, fatigue, and extreme lethargy from the previous few months. He reported that he had developed tanning of the skin all over the body. He was losing weight from the same duration despite a near normal appetite. There was some nausea and abdominal discomfort, due to which he sometimes avoided meals. History revealed that the patient fainted twice in the previous 2 months and each time his blood pressure was very low (as told to him by the emergency doctor). He avoided going out alone due to the fear of fainting again.

On general physical examination, pulse was 68 beats/min while BP was 100/60 mm Hg. Skin was bronze in color. No other abnormality was detected.

The attending physician suspected some hormonal disorder and sent blood sample for blood and urinary cortisol levels. Both the levels were low.

What is the probable diagnosis?
What is the underlying molecular disorder?
What is the biochemical basis for all the clinical manifestations?
What are the other confirmatory investigations for the diagnosis of this disease?

CASE DISCUSSION

The patient is suffering from **Addison's disease.**

The original description of Addison's disease—"general languor and debility, feebleness of the heart's action, irritability of the stomach, and a peculiar change of the color of the skin"—summarizes the dominant clinical features.

Addison's disease (also known as chronic adrenal insufficiency, hypocortisolism, or hypocorticism) is a rare endocrine disorder in which the adrenal glands do not produce enough steroid hormones (glucocorticoids and often mineralocorticoids). It may develop in children, adults, or some species of animals, and may occur as the result of many underlying causes.

The condition is named after Dr Thomas Addison, the British physician who first described the condition. The adjective "Addisonian" is used for features of the condition, as well as for patients with Addison's disease.

Role of Adrenal Cortical Hormones Cortisol

Cortisol belongs to a class of hormones called glucocorticoids, which affect almost every organ and tissue in the body. Cortisol's most important job is to help the body respond to stress. Among its many vital tasks, cortisol helps to:

- Maintain blood pressure and cardiovascular function
- Slow the immune system's inflammatory response
- Maintain levels of glucose in the blood
- Regulate the metabolism of proteins, carbohydrates, and fats
- The amount of cortisol produced by the adrenals is precisely balanced. Like many other hormones, cortisol is regulated by the brain's hypothalamus and the pituitary gland. **First, the hypothalamus releases a "trigger" hormone called corticotropin-releasing hormone (CRH) that signals the pituitary gland. The pituitary responds by sending out adrenocorticotropic hormone (ACTH), which in turn stimulates the adrenal glands. The adrenal glands respond by producing cortisol.** Completing the cycle, cortisol then signals back to both the pituitary and hypothalamus to decrease these trigger hormones **(Fig. 15.4)**.

The hypothalamus sends CRH to the pituitary, which responds by sending out ACTH. ACTH then causes the adrenals to release cortisol into the bloodstream.

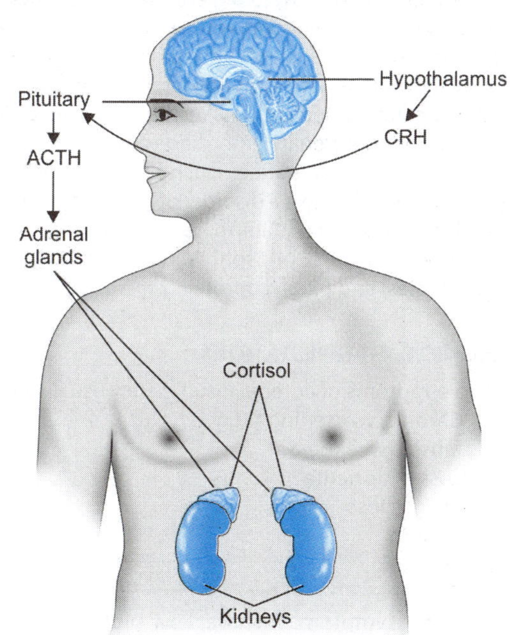

Fig. 15.4: Regulation of cortisol secretion by hypothalamus and pituitary gland.

Aldosterone

Aldosterone belongs to a class of hormones called mineralocorticoids, also produced by the adrenal glands. Aldosterone helps to maintain blood pressure and water and salt balance in the body by helping the kidneys to retain sodium and excrete potassium. When aldosterone production falls too low, the kidneys are not able to regulate water and salt balance, leading to a drop in both blood volume and blood pressure.

INCIDENCE

Addison's disease affects about 1–4 people per 100,000 in the US. It is found in patients of all ages and affects both males and females equally. Symptoms of insufficiency may not emerge until about 80–90% of the adrenal cortex has been destroyed.

ETIOLOGY AND PATHOGENESIS

Primary adrenal insufficiency: In US, about 70% of primary adrenal insufficiency is due to an autoimmune process. About 30% of the time, the adrenal damage is due to other causes, such as: tuberculosis, a common cause in areas of the world where tuberculosis is more prevalent; rarely, other lesions are encountered,, such as adrenoleukodystrophy, bilateral hemorrhage, tumor metastases, HIV, cytomegalovirus (CMV), amyloidosis, adrenomyeloneuropathy, familial adrenal insufficiency, or sarcoidosis. Rarely, it may be due to a genetic abnormality of the adrenal glands.

In early series, tuberculosis was responsible for 70–90% of cases, but the most frequent cause now is idiopathic atrophy, and an autoimmune mechanism is probably responsible. **Autoimmune destruction is probably secondary to cytotoxic T lymphocytes, although half of patients with idiopathic atrophy have circulating adrenal antibodies.** Specific adrenal antigens to which autoantibodies may be directed include 21-hydroxylase (CYP21A2) and side chain cleavage enzyme, but the significance of these antibodies in the pathogenesis of adrenal insufficiency is unknown. Some antibodies cause adrenal insufficiency by blocking the binding of ACTH to its receptors. Some patients also have antibodies to thyroid, parathyroid, and/or gonadal tissue.

Polyendocrine deficiency syndrome is classified into two separate forms—Type 1 and Type 2.

Type 1 is inherited and occurs in children. In addition to adrenal insufficiency, these children may have:

- Underactive parathyroid glands, which produce a hormone that regulates calcium and phosphorus balance in the body.
- Slow sexual development
- Pernicious anemia, a severe type of anemia
- Chronic *Candida* infections, a type of fungal infection
- Chronic active hepatitis, a liver disease.

Type 2, sometimes called Schmidt's syndrome, usually affects young adults and may include:

- An underactive thyroid gland, which produces hormones that regulate metabolism
- Slow sexual development
- Diabetes
- Vitiligo, a loss of pigment on areas of the skin.

Other causes: Medications, such as rifampin, phenytoin, ketoconazole, megestrol, and opiates may cause or potentiate adrenal insufficiency. Adrenal hemorrhage and infarction occur in patients on anticoagulants and in those with circulating anticoagulants and hypercoagulable states,, such as the antiphospholipid syndrome. [Antiphospholipid syndrome (APS or APLS) or antiphospholipid antibody syndrome is a disorder of coagulation that causes thrombosis in blood vessels, as well as pregnancy-related complications, such as miscarriage, stillbirth, preterm delivery, or severe preeclampsia. The syndrome occurs due to the production of autoimmune antibodies against phospholipid. In particular, the disease is characterized by antibodies against cardiolipin (anticardiolipin antibodies) and β2 glycoprotein.]

CLINICAL MANIFESTATIONS

The symptoms of adrenal insufficiency usually begin gradually. Characteristics of the disease are:

- Chronic, worsening fatigue
- Muscle weakness
- Loss of appetite
- Weight loss
- Nausea
- Vomiting
- Diarrhea
- Other symptoms include: Low blood pressure that falls further when standing, causing dizziness or fainting
- **Skin changes in Addison's disease, with areas of hyperpigmentation, or dark tanning, covering exposed and nonexposed parts of the body; this darkening of the skin is most visible on scars, skin folds, pressure points, such as the elbows, knees, knuckles and toes, lips, and mucous membranes (Fig. 15.5).**
- Addison's disease can cause irritability and depression. Because of salt loss, a craving for salty foods also is common.
- Hypoglycemia is more severe in children than in adults. In women, menstrual periods may become irregular or stop.

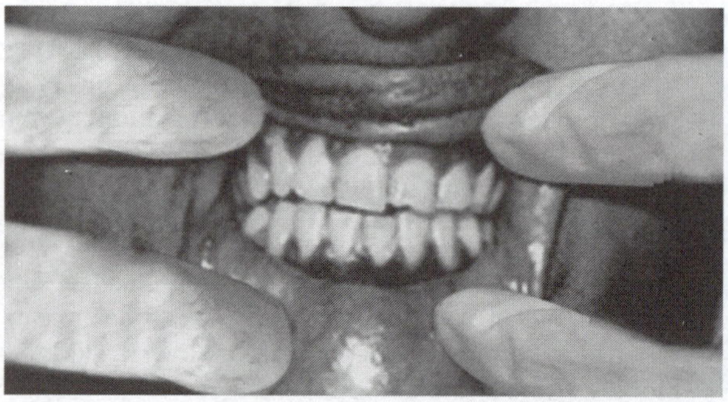

Fig. 15.5: Hyperpigmentation of mucous membranes.

- Because the symptoms progress slowly, they are usually ignored until a stressful event like an illness or an accident causes them to become worse. This is called an Addisonian crisis, or acute adrenal insufficiency. In most cases, symptoms are severe enough that patients seek medical treatment before a crisis occurs. However, in about 25% of patients, symptoms first appear during an Addisonian crisis.
- Symptoms of an Addisonian crisis include: sudden penetrating pain in the lower back, abdomen, or legs, severe vomiting and diarrhea, dehydration, low blood pressure, loss of consciousness; and if left untreated, an Addisonian crisis can be fatal.

DIAGNOSIS

In its early stages, adrenal insufficiency can be difficult to diagnose. A review of a patient's medical history based on the symptoms, especially the dark tanning of the skin, will lead a doctor to suspect Addison's disease.

1. **Laboratory investigations:** In the early phase of gradual adrenal destruction, there may be no demonstrable abnormalities in the routine laboratory parameters, but adrenal reserve is decreased—i.e., while basal steroid output may be normal, a subnormal increase occurs after stress.
2. **Adrenocorticotropic hormone (ACTH) stimulation test:** This is the most specific test for diagnosing Addison's disease. In this test, blood cortisol, urine cortisol, or both are measured before and after a synthetic form of ACTH is given by injection. In the so-called short, or rapid, ACTH test, measurement of cortisol in blood is repeated 30–60 minutes after an intravenous ACTH injection. The normal response after an injection of ACTH is a rise in blood and urine cortisol levels. Patients with either form of adrenal insufficiency respond poorly or do not respond at all.
3. **CRH stimulation test:** When the response to the short ACTH test is abnormal, a "long" CRH stimulation test is required to determine the cause of adrenal insufficiency. In this test, synthetic CRH is injected intravenously and blood cortisol is measured before and 30, 60, 90, and 120 minutes after the injection. Patients with primary adrenal insufficiency have high ACTHs but do not produce cortisol. Patients with secondary adrenal insufficiency have deficient cortisol responses but absent or delayed ACTH responses. Absent ACTH response points to the pituitary as the cause; a delayed ACTH response points to the hypothalamus as the cause.
4. **Estimation of serum electrolytes:** In more advanced stages of adrenal destruction, serum sodium, chloride, and bicarbonate levels are reduced, and the serum potassium level is elevated. The hyponatremia is due to both loss of sodium into the urine (due to aldosterone deficiency) and movement into the intracellular compartment. This extravascular sodium loss depletes ECFV and accentuates hypotension. Elevated plasma vasopressin and angiotensin II levels may contribute to the hyponatremia by impairing free water clearance. Hyperkalemia is due to a combination of aldosterone deficiency, impaired glomerular filtration, and acidosis. Basal levels of cortisol and aldosterone are subnormal and fail to increase following ACTH administration. Mild-to-moderate hypercalcemia occurs in 10–20% of patients for unclear reasons.
5. **Diagnosis during an emergency:** In patients suspected of having an Addisonian crisis, treatment is started with injections of salt, glucose-containing fluids, and glucocorticoids hormones immediately. Although a reliable diagnosis is not possible during crisis treatment, measurement of blood ACTH and cortisol during the crisis—before glucocorticoids are given—is enough to make a preliminary diagnosis. Low blood sodium, low blood glucose, and high blood potassium are also usually present at the time of an adrenal crisis. Once the crisis is controlled, an ACTH stimulation test can be performed to obtain the specific diagnosis.
6. **Other tests:** Once a diagnosis of primary adrenal insufficiency has been made, X-ray examinations of the abdomen may be taken to see if the adrenals have any signs of calcium deposits. Calcium deposits may indicate TB. A tuberculin skin test also may be used.

The electrocardiogram may show nonspecific changes, and the electroencephalogram exhibits a generalized reduction and slowing.

There may be a normocytic anemia, a relative lymphocytosis, and a moderate eosinophilia.

A magnetic resonance imaging (MRI) scan may also be used to produce a three-dimensional image of this region.

TREATMENT

All patients with adrenal insufficiency should receive specific hormone replacement. Replacement therapy should correct both glucocorticoids and mineralocorticoids deficiencies. Cortisol is replaced with a synthetic glucocorticoids, such as hydrocortisone, prednisone, or dexamethasone, taken orally once to three times each day, depending on which medication is chosen. If aldosterone is also deficient, it is replaced with oral doses of a mineralocorticoids, called fludrocortisone acetate (Florinef), taken once or twice a day. Because people with secondary adrenal insufficiency normally maintain aldosterone production, they do not require aldosterone replacement therapy. The doses of each medication are adjusted to meet the needs of the individual.

In female patients with adrenal insufficiency, androgen levels are also low. Thus, some physicians believe that daily replacement with 25–50 mg of DHEA PO may improve quality of life and bone mineral density.

During an Addisonian crisis, low blood pressure, low blood glucose, and high levels of potassium can be life-threatening. Standard therapy involves intravenous injections of glucocorticoids and large volumes of intravenous saline solution with dextrose. This treatment usually brings rapid improvement. When the patient can take fluids and medications by mouth, the amount of glucocorticoids is decreased until a maintenance dose is reached. If aldosterone is deficient, maintenance therapy also includes oral doses of fludrocortisone acetate.

Secondary Adrenal Insufficiency

Secondary adrenal insufficiency can be traced to a lack of ACTH. Without ACTH to stimulate the adrenal glands, the adrenals' production of cortisol drops. Aldosterone production is not usually affected.

A temporary form of secondary adrenal insufficiency may occur when a person who has been taking a synthetic glucocorticoids hormone, such as prednisone for a long time stops taking the medication, either abruptly or gradually. Glucocorticoids hormones, which are often used to treat inflammatory illnesses, such as rheumatoid arthritis, asthma, and ulcerative colitis, block the release of both CRH and ACTH. As a result, the adrenals may begin to atrophy—or shrink—from lack of ACTH stimulation and then fail to secrete sufficient levels of cortisol.

A person who stops taking a synthetic glucocorticoid hormone may have enough ACTH to function when healthy. However, when a person is under the stress of an illness, accident, or surgery, the person's body may not have enough ACTH to stimulate the adrenal glands to produce cortisol.

Another cause of secondary adrenal insufficiency is surgical removal of the noncancerous, ACTH-producing tumors of the pituitary gland that cause Cushing's disease. Cushing's disease is another disorder that leads to excess cortisol in the body. In this case, the source of ACTH is suddenly removed and replacement hormone must be taken until normal ACTH and cortisol production resumes.

Less commonly, adrenal insufficiency occurs when the pituitary gland either decreases in size or stops producing ACTH. These events can result from:

- Tumors or infections of the area
- Loss of blood flow to the pituitary
- Radiation for the treatment of pituitary tumors
- Surgical removal of parts of the hypothalamus
- Surgical removal of the pituitary gland

PROGNOSIS

Researchers are evaluating the use of another adrenal hormone, dehydroepiandrosterone, in improving the health-related quality of life in people with adrenal insufficiency. Scientists are also studying the occurrence of "relative" adrenal insufficiency—below normal production of adrenal hormones during critical illness—to further define this type of adrenal insufficiency, develop diagnostic tests, and identify the best treatment options.

CLINICAL NOTE

During an Addisonian crisis, low blood pressure, low blood glucose, and high levels of potassium can be life-threatening. Standard therapy involves intravenous injections of glucocorticoids and large volumes of intravenous saline solution with dextrose. This treatment usually brings rapid improvement.

CLINICAL PEARLS

1. Addison's disease (also known as chronic adrenal insufficiency, hypocortisolism, or hypocorticism) is a rare endocrine disorder in which the adrenal glands do not produce enough steroid hormones (glucocorticoids and often mineralocorticoids).
2. About 70% of primary adrenal insufficiency is due to an autoimmune process. About 30% of the time, the adrenal damage is due to other causes, such as tuberculosis, a common cause in areas of the world where tuberculosis is more prevalent; rarely, other lesions are encountered,, such as adrenoleukodystrophy, bilateral hemorrhage, tumor metastases, HIV, cytomegalovirus (CMV), amyloidosis, adrenomyeloneuropathy, familial adrenal insufficiency, or sarcoidosis. Rarely, it may be due to a genetic abnormality of the adrenal glands.
3. In its early stages, adrenal insufficiency can be difficult to diagnose. A review of a patient's medical history based on the symptoms, especially the dark tanning of the skin, will lead to suspicion of Addison's disease.
4. All patients with adrenal insufficiency should receive specific hormone replacement. Replacement therapy should correct both glucocorticoids and mineralocorticoids deficiencies.
5. Because people with secondary adrenal insufficiency normally maintain aldosterone production, they do not require aldosterone replacement therapy.

CASE STUDY 3

Theme: Clinical Implications of Hyperaldosteronism

A 44-year-old man was seen with a 3-year history of decreased energy, body aches, a sad mood, decreased concentration, and decreased interest in previously pleasurable activities, insomnia, and anxiousness. He had no past or family history of depression and substance abuse. He was diagnosed with hypertension and major depressive disorder. He was treated with antidepressants in consultation with a psychiatrist. He continued to have poorly controlled hypertension, depression, and hypokalemia despite using increasing doses of antihypertensive and antidepressants. He was referred to nephrology clinic.

Other than systolic and diastolic hypertension, his physical and neurological examinations were normal.

His serum sodium level was 129 mEq/L, and his potassium level was 2.1 mEq/L.

An examination of his arterial blood gas revealed metabolic alkalosis. Serum osmolality was 266 mOsmol/kg.

Urinary potassium was 40 mEq/L, while urine osmolality was 350 mOsmol/kg.

His plasma aldosterone-to-renin ratio was greater than 261 (aldosterone = 26.1 ng/dL, rennin <0.1 ng/mL).

What is the probable diagnosis?

What is the ideal treatment for this disease?

CASE DISCUSSION

The patient is suffering from Conn syndrome.

Hypertensions, hypokalemia, hypernatremia, high aldosterone-to-renin ratio are features of Conn syndrome.

Conn Syndrome

Conn syndrome is a disease of the adrenal glands involving excess production of aldosterone. Another name for the condition is primary hyperaldosteronism. In primary hyperaldosteronism, the cause for the excessive aldosterone production resides within the adrenal gland; in secondary aldosteronism, the stimulus is extra-adrenal.

BASIC CONCEPT

Aldosterone

Aldosterone is a steroid hormone (mineralocorticoid) produced by the outer section (zona glomerulosa) of the adrenal cortex in the adrenal gland, and acts on the distal tubules and collecting ducts of the kidney to cause the conservation of sodium, secretion of potassium, increased water retention, and increased blood pressure. The overall effect of aldosterone is to increase reabsorption of ions and water in the kidney. Aldosterone is part of the renin–angiotensin system. A measurement of aldosterone in blood may be termed as plasma aldosterone concentration (PAC), which may be compared to plasma renin activity (PRA) as a PAC/PRA ratio. Its activity is reduced in Addison's disease and increased in Conn syndrome.

Synthesis

The corticosteroids are synthesized from cholesterol within the adrenal cortex. Most steroidogenic reactions are catalyzed by enzymes of the Cytochrome P450 family. They are located within the mitochondria and require adrenodoxin as a cofactor (except 21-hydroxylase and 17α-hydroxylase) **(Fig. 15.6)**.

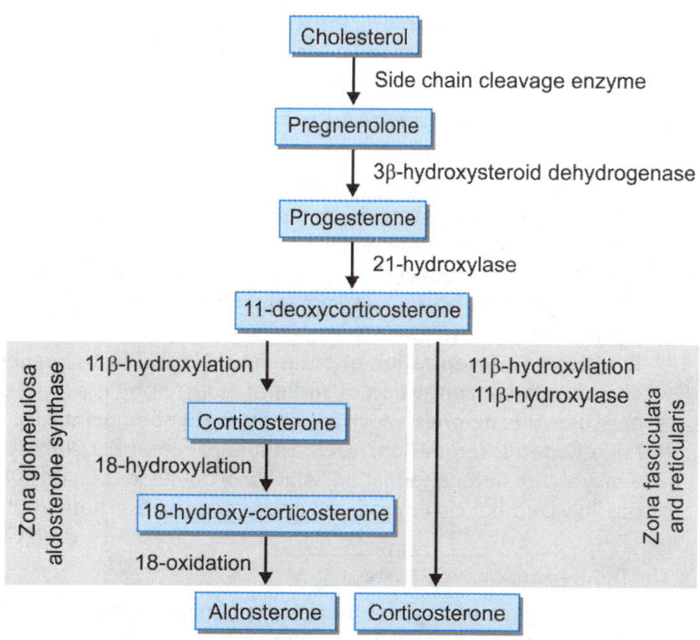

Fig. 15.6: Aldosterone and corticosterone synthesis.

Aldosterone and corticosterone share the first part of their biosynthetic pathway. The last part is either mediated by the aldosterone synthase (for aldosterone) or by the 11β-hydroxylase (for corticosterone). These enzymes are nearly identical (they share 11β-hydroxylation and 18-hydroxylation functions). But aldosterone synthase is also able to perform an 18-oxidation. Moreover, aldosterone synthase is found within the zona glomerulosa at the outer edge of the adrenal cortex; 11β-hydroxylase is found in the zona fasciculata and reticularis.

Functions

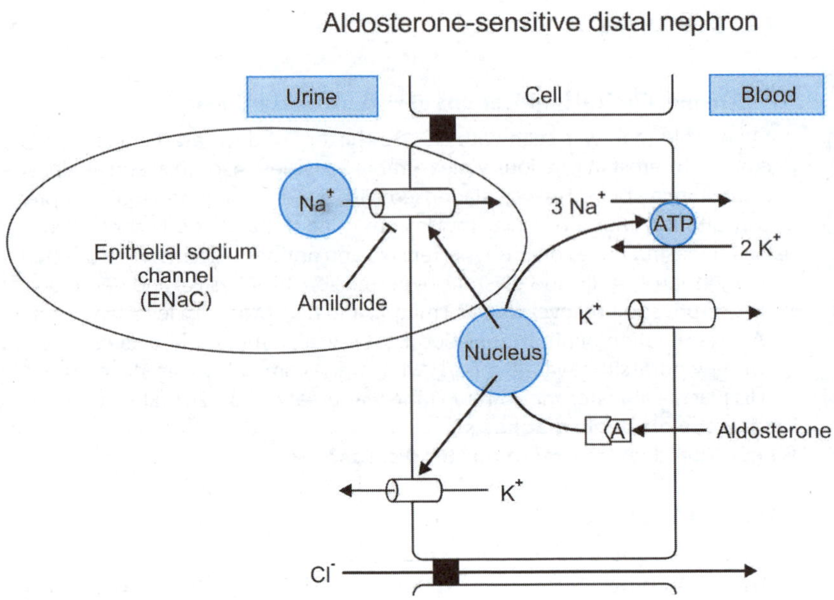

Fig. 15.7: Role of aldosterone in Na reabsorption.

Aldosterone is the primary of several endogenous members of the class of mineralocorticoids in human. Deoxycorticosterone is another important member of this class. At the late distal tubule and collecting duct, aldosterone has three main actions:

1. Acting on the mineralocorticoid receptors (MR) within the principal cells of the distal tubule and the collecting duct of the kidney nephron, it increases the permeability of the apical (luminal) membrane to potassium and sodium, hence **reabsorbing sodium (Na^+) ions and water into the blood, and secreting potassium (K^+) ions into the urine.** (Chlorine anions are also reabsorbed in conjunction with sodium cations to maintain the system's electrochemical balance) **(Fig. 15.7).**
2. Aldosterone **stimulates H^+ secretion** by intercalated cells in the collecting duct, regulating plasma bicarbonate (HCO_3^-) levels and its acid/base balance. A large proportion of Na^+ reabsorption results from an exchange reaction, in which H^+ ions are secreted and Na^+ is reabsorbed. Thus increased secretion of aldosterone promotes alkalosis due to loss of excessive H^+ ions.
3. Aldosterone has the same effect on the sweat glands, salivary glands, intestinal glands as on the renal tubules, greatly **reducing the loss of Na^+ and Cl^- in the glandular secretions.**

Aldosterone is responsible for the reabsorption of about 2% of filtered sodium in the kidneys, which is nearly equal to the entire sodium content in human blood under normal glomerular filtration rate (GFR).

Control of Aldosterone Release from the Adrenal Cortex

- The role of the renin-angiotensin system:
  Angiotensin is involved in regulating aldosterone secretion and is the core regulator. Angiotensin II acts synergistically with potassium, and the potassium feedback is virtually inoperative when no angiotensin II is present.
- The role of sympathetic nerves:
  The aldosterone production is also affected to one extent or another by nervous control, which integrates the inverse of carotid artery pressure, pain, posture, and probably emotion (anxiety, fear, and hostility) (including surgical stress). Pressure in the carotid artery decreases aldosterone.
- **The plasma concentration of potassium:** Aldosterone secretion is stimulated by the rise in serum potassium levels.
- **The plasma concentration of sodium:** Aldosterone is a function of the inverse of the sodium intake as sensed via osmotic pressure. Aldosterone is much increased at low sodium intakes.
- **Miscellaneous regulation:** ACTH, a pituitary peptide, also has some stimulating effect on aldosterone probably by stimulating deoxycorticosterone formation, which is a precursor of aldosterone. Aldosterone is increased by blood loss, pregnancy, and possibly by other circumstances, such as physical exertion, endotoxic shock, and burns.

The Renin–Angiotensin System

The renin–angiotensin system (RAS) or the renin–angiotensin–aldosterone system (RAAS) is a hormone system that regulates blood pressure and water (fluid) balance.

When blood volume is low, the kidneys secrete renin. Renin stimulates the production of angiotensin. Angiotensin causes blood vessels to constrict resulting in increased blood pressure. Angiotensin also stimulates the secretion of the hormone aldosterone from the adrenal cortex. Aldosterone causes the tubules of the kidneys to increase the reabsorption of sodium and water. This increases the volume of fluid in the body, which also increases blood pressure.

Activation of Renin–Angiotensin System

The system can be activated when there is a loss of blood volume or a drop in blood pressure (such as in hemorrhage).

1. A fall in sodium concentration, hypovolemia, and a fall in intracellular Ca^{++} stimulate release of renin from juxtaglomerular (JG) cells to the blood. Renin cleaves a zymogen, an inactive peptide, called angiotensinogen, converting it into angiotensin I **(Fig. 15.8)**.
2. Angiotensin I is then converted to angiotensin II by angiotensin-converting enzyme (ACE), which is found mainly in lung capillaries.
3. Angiotensin II is the major bioactive product of the renin–angiotensin system, binding to receptors on intraglomerular mesangial cells, causing these cells to contract along with the blood vessels surrounding them and causes the release of aldosterone from the zona glomerulosa in the adrenal cortex. Angiotensin II acts as an endocrine, autocrine/paracrine, and intracrine hormone.
4. By the activity of aminopeptidase, angiotensin II is converted to angiotensin III, which is less potent than angiotensin II.
5. Throughout the body, angiotensin II is a potent vasoconstrictor of arterioles.
6. Inhibitors of angiotensin-converting enzyme (ACE inhibitors) are often used to reduce the formation of the more potent angiotensin II. Captopril is an example of an ACE inhibitor.
7. Alternatively, angiotensin receptor blockers (ARBs) can be used to prevent angiotensin II from acting on angiotensin receptors. These drugs are one of the main ways to control hypertension, heart failure, kidney failure, and harmful effects of diabetes.

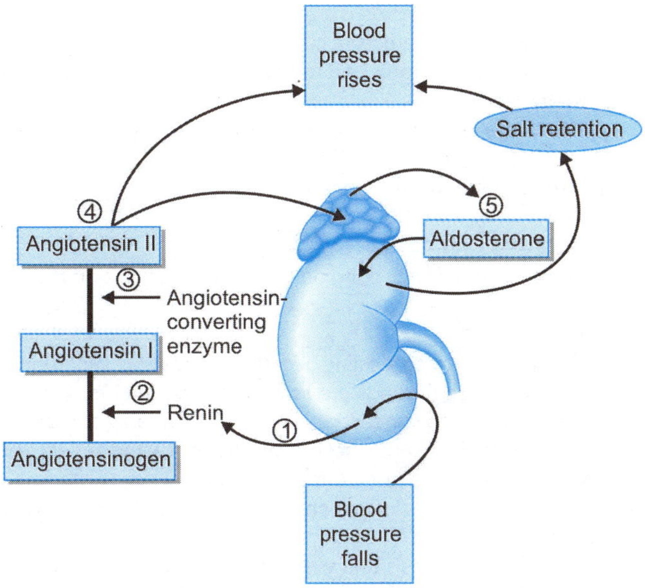

Fig. 15.8: Renin–angiotensin aldosterone system.

CONN SYNDROME

Pathogenesis

The excess secretion of the hormone aldosterone into the blood is from an abnormal adrenal gland or glands. Two types of abnormalities are seen: a benign tumor of one adrenal, called an adenoma or a general enlargement of both adrenals, called hyperplasia. In the original descriptions of excessive and inappropriate aldosterone production, the disease was the result of an aldosterone-producing adrenal adenoma (Conn syndrome). Most cases involve a unilateral adenoma, which is usually small and may occur on either side. Rarely, primary aldosteronism is due to an adrenal carcinoma.

In many patients with clinical and biochemical features of primary aldosteronism, a solitary adenoma is not found at surgery. Instead, these patients have bilateral cortical nodular hyperplasia. In the literature, this disease is also termed idiopathic hyperaldosteronism, and/or nodular hyperplasia. The cause is unknown.

Incidence

Conn syndrome is rare (one new case in a million people each year). However, when detailed investigations have been performed in patients with hypertension (high blood pressure), up to 10% may have this condition. Aldosteronism is twice as common in women as in men, usually occurs between the ages of 30 and 50. Although the prevalence of the tumor form of primary aldosteronism in the general hypertension population remains in the 1% range, the prevalence of the bilateral hyperplasia form has been reported to range as high as 10%, depending on the criteria used and the study population.

Clinical Manifestations

High blood pressure (hypertension) is the main, and often the only, symptom. Hypersecretion of aldosterone increases the renal distal tubular exchange of intratubular sodium for secreted potassium and hydrogen ions, with progressive depletion of body potassium and development of hypokalemia. Most patients have diastolic hypertension, which may be very severe, and headaches. The hypertension is probably due to the increased sodium reabsorption and extracellular volume expansion.

Potassium depletion is responsible for the muscle weakness and fatigue and is due to the effect of potassium depletion on the muscle cell membrane.

The polyuria results from impairment of urinary concentrating ability and is often associated with polydipsia. However, some individuals with mild disease, particularly most with the bilateral hyperplasia type, may have potassium levels in the low normal range and therefore have no symptoms associated with hypokalemia.

If potassium depletion is present, there may be electrocardiographic signs of hypokalemia including prominent U waves, cardiac arrhythmias, and premature contractions.

Electrocardiographic and roentgenographic signs of left ventricular enlargement are present which are, in part, secondary to the hypertension.

Structural damage to the cerebral circulation, retinal vasculature, and kidney occurs more frequently than would be predicted based on the level and duration of the hypertension. Proteinuria may occur in as many as 50% of patients with primary aldosteronism, and renal failure occurs in up to 15%.

Laboratory Diagnosis

Laboratory findings depend on both the duration and the severity of potassium depletion.

Urine Analysis

Urine pH is neutral to alkaline because of excessive secretion of ammonium and bicarbonate ions to compensate for the metabolic alkalosis. (These findings are infrequent in patients with bilateral hyperplasia.) An overnight concentration test often reveals impaired ability to concentrate the urine, probably secondary to the hypokalemia.

Hypokalemia may be severe (<3 mmol/L) and reflects body potassium depletion, in mild forms of primary aldosteronism, potassium levels may be normal.

Hypernatremia is infrequent but may be caused by sodium retention, concomitant water loss from polyuria, and resetting of the osmostat.

Metabolic alkalosis and elevation of serum bicarbonate are caused by hydrogen ion loss into the urine and migration into potassium-depleted cells. The alkalosis is perpetuated by potassium deficiency, which increases the capacity of the proximal convoluted tubule to reabsorb filtered bicarbonate.

If hypokalemia is severe, serum magnesium levels are also reduced.

The most rigorous method of diagnosis is to measure the blood levels of two hormones: aldosterone and renin (which plays a role in stimulating aldosterone production). In Conn syndrome, the aldosterone level is elevated and the renin level is low or undetectable.

The ratio of serum aldosterone to plasma renin activity is a very useful screening test. A high ratio (>30), when aldosterone is expressed as ng/dL and plasma renin activity as ng/mL per hour, strongly suggests autonomy of aldosterone secretion. Aldosterone levels need to be >500 pmol/L (>15 ng/dL) when salt intake is not restricted. Once hyposecretion of renin and failure of aldosterone secretion suppression are demonstrated, aldosterone-producing adenomas should be localized by abdominal CT scan, using a high-resolution scanner as many aldosteronomas of <1 cm in size can be localized.

If the CT scan is negative, percutaneous transfemoral bilateral adrenal vein catheterization with adrenal vein sampling may demonstrate a two- to three-fold increase in plasma aldosterone concentration on the involved side. In cases of hyperaldosteronism secondary to cortical nodular hyperplasia, no lateralization is found.

Clinical Diagnosis

The criteria for the diagnosis of primary aldosteronism are:

1. Diastolic hypertension without edema
2. Hyposecretion of renin (as judged by low plasma renin activity levels) that fails to increase appropriately during volume depletion (upright posture, sodium depletion).
3. Hypersecretion of aldosterone that does not suppress appropriately in response to volume expansion. Patients with primary aldosteronism characteristically do not have edema, since they exhibit an "escape" phenomenon from the sodium-retaining aspects of mineralocorticoids. Rarely, pretibial edema is present in patients with associated nephropathy and azotemia.

Escape Phenomenon

Although aldosterone has a potent effect in decreasing the rate of sodium ion excretion by the kidneys, the concentration of sodium in the extracellular fluid often rises only a few milliequivalents. The reason for this is that when sodium is reabsorbed by the tubules, there is simultaneous osmotic absorption of almost equivalent amounts of water.

Also, small increases in extracellular fluid sodium concentration stimulate thirst and increased water intake, if water is available. Therefore, the extracellular fluid volume increases almost as much as the retained sodium, but without much change in sodium concentration. An aldosterone-mediated increase in extracellular fluid volume lasting more than 1–2 days also leads to an increase in arterial pressure. The rise in arterial pressure then increases kidney excretion of both salt and water, called pressure natriuresis and pressure diuresis, respectively. This escape phenomenon is probably due to increased secretion of atrial natriuretic peptide (ANP). Because of increased excretion of Na^+ when the extracellular fluid (ECF) volume is expanded, mineralocorticoids do not produce edema in normal individuals and patients with hyperaldosteronism. However, escape may not occur in certain disease states and in these situations, continued expansion of ECF leads to edema.

Treatment

Primary aldosteronism due to an adenoma is usually treated by surgical excision of the adenoma.

However, dietary sodium restriction and the administration of an aldosterone antagonist—e.g., spironolactone—are effective in many cases. Hypertension and hypokalemia are usually controlled by doses of 25–100 mg of spironolactone every 8 hours. In some patients, medical management has been successful for years, but chronic therapy in men is usually limited by side effects of spironolactone, such as gynecomastia, decreased libido, and impotence. (Spironolactone is somewhat similar in chemical structure to the female sex hormone, estradiol, and therefore has some female hormone-like actions).

Eplerenone, a less potent but more specific MR antagonist with minimal, if any, antiandrogen effect is also useful in doses of 50–150 mg every 8 hours.

When idiopathic bilateral hyperplasia is suspected, surgery is indicated only when significant, symptomatic hypokalemia cannot be controlled with medical therapy, i.e., by spironolactone, Eplerenone, triamterene, or amiloride. Hypertension associated with idiopathic hyperplasia is usually not benefited by bilateral adrenalectomy.

` Without drug or surgical treatment, high blood pressure in many patients with Conn syndrome is difficult to control. Poorly controlled high blood pressure is associated with increased rates of stroke, heart disease, and kidney failure.

Prognosis

Treatment of Conn syndrome is usually successful. Many patients with a single adrenal adenoma will be able to stop drug treatment and will have normal blood pressures.

Nevertheless, many specialist centers will follow a patient with Conn syndrome for life. This is to monitor the rare possibility of growth of a second adenoma.

Patients with bilateral hyperplasia should have lifelong monitoring of effectiveness and side effects of drug treatment. Again, quality of life is generally good, although some patients may not be able to tolerate spironolactone treatment.

CLINICAL NOTE

A measurement of aldosterone in blood termed as plasma aldosterone concentration (PAC), compared to plasma renin activity (PRA) PAC/PRA ratio is reduced in Addison's disease and increased in Conn syndrome.

CLINICAL PEARLS

1. Conn syndrome is a disease of the adrenal glands involving excess production of aldosterone.
2. Hypertension, hypokalemia, and metabolic alkalosis are the hallmarks of Conn syndrome.
3. Edema is not seen despite excessive Na^+ reabsorption due to escape phenomenon.
4. The aldosterone level is elevated and the renin level is low or undetectable.
5. Treatment involves sodium restriction and the administration of spironolactone, Eplerenone, triamterene, or amiloride.
6. Surgery is indicated only when significant, symptomatic hypokalemia cannot be controlled with medical therapy.

CASE STUDY 4

Theme: Clinical Implications of Congenital Hypothyroidism

A 19-year-old male patient who allegedly had ceased to grow sometimes between 8 years and 12 years of age was brought for consultation. Although he completed his eighth grade, his intelligence was below normal. There was no family history of thyroid disease. Previous history revealed that as an infant, the patient slept much and cried little. The first teeth were markedly late in appearing, and were very irregular. His first loss of a deciduous tooth was at age 12 years and that was by surgical extraction because of extensive carious disease. The child walked at two and one-half years.

Physically, he was a short, stocky boy with a protuberant abdomen. His fingernails were soft, his skin was dry, and his speech was thick. He lacked pubic hair and had enlarged testicles.

Laboratory findings: Radioactive iodine uptake (RAIU) at 2, 6, and 24 hours was 2%; thyroid-stimulating hormone (TSH) was greater than 80 micrograms (μ) percent; 17-ketosteroid level was 4.5 milligrams (mg)/24 hours; thyroxine was 1.4 μg percent.

What is the probable diagnosis?

What is the possible defect?

What is the biochemical basis for these clinical manifestations?

CASE DETAILS

The patient is suffering from cretinism.

Cretinism (most likely from the Latin Christiānum, "Christian") is a condition of severely stunted physical and mental growth due to untreated congenital deficiency of thyroid hormones (hypothyroidism). The term cretin refers to a person so affected.

Causes

Congenital hypothyroidism can be endemic, genetic, or sporadic. It usually results from a congenital defect (e.g., absence of the thyroid, presence of only a rudimentary gland, and inability of the gland to produce thyroxine).

- Pituitary gland's failure to stimulate the thyroid
- Defective or abnormal formation of thyroid hormones
- **Incomplete development of the thyroid is the most common defect and occurs in about 1 out of every 3,000 births.**
- However, it can develop later if there is a lack of iodine in the diet, or if the thyroid is diseased or surgically removed.

Clinical Symptoms

Cretinism causes very serious retardation of physical and mental development; if the condition is left untreated, growth is stunted and the physical stature attained is that of a dwarf.

Poor length growth is apparent as early as the first year of life. Adult stature without treatment ranges from 1 meter to 1.6 meters, depending on severity, sex and other genetic factors. Bone maturation and puberty are severely delayed. Ovulation is impeded and infertility is common.

Neurological impairment may be mild, with reduced muscle tone and coordination, or so severe that the person cannot stand or walk. Cognitive impairment may also range from mild to so severe that the person is nonverbal and dependent on others for basic care. Thought and reflexes are slower.

Other signs may include thickened skin and a protruding abdomen.

Sporadic and genetic cretinism results from abnormal development or function of the fetal thyroid gland. This type of cretinism has been almost completely eliminated in developed countries by early diagnosis by newborn screening programs followed by lifelong treatment with thyroxine.

Endemic cretinism arises from a diet deficient in iodine and has affected far more people worldwide and continues to be a major public health problem in many countries. Iodine is an essential trace element, necessary primarily for the synthesis of thyroid hormones. Although it is found in many foods, it is not universally present in all soils in adequate amounts. The soils of many inland areas on all continents are iodine deficient, and plants and animals grown there are correspondingly deficient. Populations living in those areas without outside food sources are most at risk for iodine deficiency diseases. Iodine deficiency results in the impairments of varying degrees of physical and mental development. It also causes gradual enlargement of the thyroid gland, referred to as a goiter. It is being combatted in many countries by public health campaigns of iodine administration.

Laboratory Investigations

The diagnosis can be confirmed by radioactive iodine uptake, TSH, T_3, and T_4 assays. TSH is always high while T_3 and T_4 levels are low. Thyroid scan and the X-ray of the long bones can also be taken.

Treatment

Infants identified to be hypothyroid may be treated with either iodine, if they suffer from the earlier stages of endemic cretinism or thyroxine, if their thyroid gland is damaged, absent, or unable to produce the required amounts of thyroid hormone. Treatment at any time usually causes return of normal physical growth but after several weeks, mental retardation may already be permanent despite treatment. Frequent monitoring (every 2–3 weeks during the first months of life) is recommended to ensure that infants with congenital hypothyroidism remain within the high end of normal range, or euthyroid.

Endemic cretinism can be avoided if the mother eats foods with sufficient amounts of iodine. In some developed countries, endemic cretinism has been eliminated by correcting the iodine deficiency of expecting mothers as well as their children. However, several cases of hypothyroidism still appear every now and then. It is for this reason that many countries now screen newborns for hypothyroidism to recognize the full syndrome before it is too late.

CLINICAL NOTE

Incomplete development of the thyroid is the most common defect in cretinism and occurs in about 1 out of every 3,000 births.

CLINICAL PEARLS

1. Cretinism (most likely from the Latin Christiānum, "Christian") is a condition of severely stunted physical and mental growth due to untreated congenital deficiency of thyroid hormones (hypothyroidism). The term cretin refers to a person so affected.
2. Congenital hypothyroidism can be endemic, genetic, or sporadic. It usually results from a congenital defect (e.g., absence of the thyroid, presence of only a rudimentary gland, and inability of the gland to produce thyroxine).
3. However, it can develop later if there is a lack of iodine in the diet, or if the thyroid is diseased or surgically removed.
4. Cretinism causes very serious retardation of physical and mental development; if the condition is left untreated, growth is stunted and the physical stature attained is that of a dwarf.
5. The diagnosis can be confirmed by radioactive iodine uptake, TSH, T_3, and T_4 assays. TSH is always high while T_3 and T_4 levels are low. Thyroid scan and the X-ray of the long bones can also be taken.

CASE STUDY 5

Theme: Clinical Implications of Excess of Glucocorticoids

A 41-year-old female was admitted to the hospital with complaints of fatigue, weakness, lethargy, decreased concentration, and decreased memory over the last 18 months. She had also gained 40 lbs over the last 2 months with central distribution of fat and neck obesity.

Her physical examination was remarkable for Cushingoid appearance with body weight of 211 lbs, palmar erythema, and hirsutism.

Blood cortisol level was high. Her dexamethasone suppression test results were consistent with Cushing's disease.

What is Cushing's disease?
How does it differ from Cushing syndrome?
What are the clinical manifestations of this disease?
What is the defect in this disease?

CASE DETAILS

The term "Cushing's syndrome" is used to describe a condition resulting from long-term exposure of the body tissues to excessive glucocorticoids. The syndrome is most commonly caused by the therapeutic administration of exogenous glucocorticoids. The term "Cushing's disease" is reserved for Cushing's syndrome that is caused by excessive secretion of adrenocorticotropic hormone (ACTH) by a pituitary tumor, usually an adenoma.

Cushing's disease is responsible for roughly two-thirds of the cases of endogenous Cushing's syndrome. The remainders of the endogenous cases are caused by ectopic ACTH-secreting tumors and primary adrenal neoplasms.

BASIC CONCEPT

Normally, the production of cortisol follows a precise chain of events. First, the hypothalamus releases corticotropin-releasing hormone (CRH) for the pituitary gland. CRH causes the pituitary to secrete adrenocorticotropic hormone (ACTH), which stimulates the adrenal glands. The adrenals respond by releasing cortisol into the bloodstream.

Cortisol performs vital tasks in the body including helping to maintain blood pressure and cardiovascular functions, reducing the inflammatory response, balancing the effects of insulin, regulating the metabolism of proteins, carbohydrates, and fats. It is also excessively secreted in response to stress. When the amount of cortisol in the blood is adequate, the hypothalamus and pituitary release less CRH and ACTH. This process ensures that the amount of cortisol released by the adrenal glands is precisely balanced to meet the body's daily needs. However, under certain conditions, feedback regulation is lost and cortisol production can go awry.

Incidence

Cushing's disease occurs most frequently in women of reproductive age, but it can affect males and females of any age. An estimated 10–15 of every million people are affected each year.

Clinical Manifestations

Many of the signs and symptoms of Cushing's syndrome follow logically from the known action of glucocorticoids. Symptoms vary, but most people have:

- Upper body obesity, rounded face, increased fat around the neck, and thinning arms and legs. Children tend to be obese with slowed growth rates. Hypercortisolism promotes the deposition of adipose tissue in characteristic sites, notably the

upper face (producing the typical **"moon" facies**), the interscapular area (producing the **"buffalo hump"**), supraclavicular fat pads, and the mesenteric bed (producing **"truncal" obesity**). The reason for this peculiar distribution of adipose tissue is not known, but it is associated with insulin resistance and/or elevated insulin levels.
- Other symptoms appear in the skin, which becomes fragile and thin. It bruises easily and heals poorly. **Purplish pink stretch marks (striae)** may appear on the abdomen, thighs, buttocks, arms, and breasts. These are secondary to weakening and rupture of collagen fibers in the dermis **(Fig. 15.9)**.
- The bones are weakened, and routine activities may lead to backaches, rib and vertebral fractures. Catabolic responses in peripheral supportive tissue cause all these symptoms.
- Most people have severe fatigue, weak muscles, **high blood pressure, and high blood sugar.**
- Irritability, anxiety, and depression are common.
- Women usually have **excess hair growth** on the face, neck, chest, abdomen, and thighs. Menstrual periods may become irregular or stop. These symptoms are due to **increased levels of adrenal androgens**. Men have decreased fertility with diminished or absent libido.

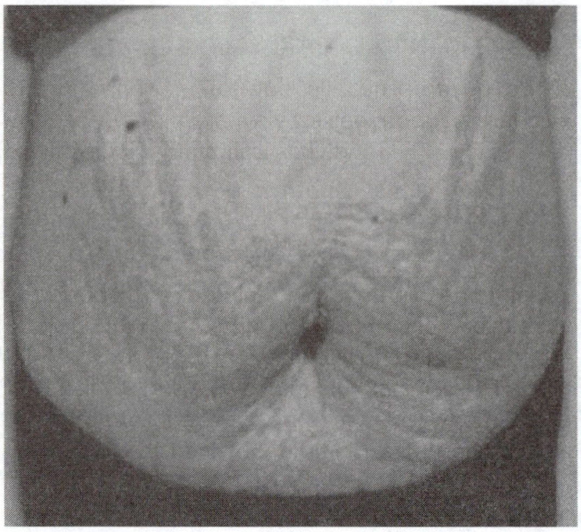

Fig. 15.9: Abdominal striae in Cushing's syndrome.

- Other common signs and symptoms include **increased thirst and urination**.
- Sometimes, other conditions have many of the same signs as Cushing's syndrome, even though people with these disorders do not have abnormally elevated cortisol levels. For example, polycystic ovary syndrome can cause menstrual disturbances, weight gain beginning in adolescence, excess hair growth, and impaired insulin action and diabetes. Metabolic syndrome—a combination of problems that includes excess weight around the waist, high blood pressure, abnormal levels of cholesterol and triglycerides in the blood, and insulin resistance—also mimics the symptoms of Cushing's syndrome.
- Another presentation or complication of Cushing's disease is opportunistic or bacterial infection. Immunosuppression resulting from corticosteroid excess is usually thought of as a cellular immune deficiency that increases the risk of opportunistic infections (*Cryptococcus neoformans*, *Candida* species, *Nocardia* species, and other organisms).

Etiology

The important causes of Cushing syndrome are as follows:
- Adrenal hyperplasia—secondary to pituitary ACTH overproduction
- Pituitary–hypothalamic dysfunction
- Pituitary ACTH-producing micro- or macroadenomas
- Secondary to ACTH or CRH-producing nonendocrine tumors (bronchogenic carcinoma, carcinoid of the thymus, pancreatic carcinoma, and bronchial adenoma)
- Adrenal macronodular hyperplasia
- Adrenal micronodular dysplasia
- Sporadic
- Familial
- Adrenal neoplasia: Adenoma or carcinoma
- Exogenous, iatrogenic causes, prolonged use of glucocorticoids, or ACTH.

Thus, excessive cortisol production may be ACTH dependent or it may be ACTH independent.

Diagnosis

Diagnosis is based on a review of a person's medical history, a physical examination, and laboratory tests. X-rays of the adrenal or pituitary glands can be useful in locating tumors. Easy bruising, typical striae, myopathy, and virilizing signs (although less frequent) are, if present, more suggestive of Cushing's syndrome.

Laboratory Tests to Diagnose Cushing's Syndrome

No single laboratory test is perfect and usually several are needed. The three most common tests used to diagnose Cushing's syndrome are the 24-hour urinary free cortisol test, measurement of midnight plasma cortisol or late-night salivary cortisol, and the low-dose dexamethasone suppression test. Another test, the dexamethasone–corticotropin-releasing hormone test, may be needed to distinguish Cushing's syndrome from other causes of excess cortisol.

1. **24-hour urinary free cortisol level:** In this test, a person's urine is collected over a 24-hour period and tested for cortisol. Levels higher than 50–100 micrograms a day for an adult suggest Cushing's syndrome.

2. **Midnight plasma cortisol and late-night salivary cortisol measurements:** The midnight plasma cortisol test measures cortisol concentrations in the blood. Cortisol production is normally suppressed at night, but in Cushing's syndrome, this suppression does not occur. If the cortisol level is more than 50 nanomoles per liter (nmol/L), Cushing's syndrome is suspected. Alternatively a late-night or bedtime saliva sample can be obtained, and tested to determine the cortisol level.
3. **Low-dose dexamethasone suppression test (LDDST):** In the LDDST, a low dose of dexamethasone, a synthetic glucocorticoids, is given every 6 hours for 2 days. Urine is collected before dexamethasone is administered and on each day of the test. Cortisol and other glucocorticoids signal the pituitary to release less ACTH, so the normal response after taking dexamethasone is a drop in blood and urine cortisol levels. If cortisol levels do not drop, Cushing's syndrome is suspected.
4. **Plasma ACTH level:** Measurement of plasma ACTH is useful in the diagnosis of ACTH-independent etiologies of the syndrome, since most adrenal tumors cause low or undetectable ACTH levels [<2 pmol/L (10 pg/mL)], while ACTH-secreting pituitary macroadenomas and ACTH-producing nonendocrine tumors usually result in elevated ACTH levels. Hence, the diagnosis can be confirmed by this test.
5. **Dexamethasone–corticotropin-releasing hormone (CRH) test:** Some patients have high cortisol levels, but do not develop the progressive effects of Cushing's syndrome,, such as muscle weakness, fractures, and thinning of the skin. These patients may have **pseudo-Cushing's syndrome**, a condition sometimes found in people who have depression or anxiety disorders, drink excess alcohol, have poorly controlled diabetes, or are severely obese. Pseudo-Cushing's does not have the same long-term effects on health as Cushing's syndrome and does not require treatment directed at the endocrine glands. The dexamethasone-CRH test rapidly distinguishes pseudo-Cushing's from mild cases of Cushing's. This test combines the LDDST and a CRH stimulation test. In the CRH stimulation test, an injection of CRH causes the pituitary to secrete ACTH. Pretreatment with dexamethasone prevents CRH from causing an increase in cortisol in patients with pseudo-Cushing's. Elevations of cortisol during this test suggest Cushing's syndrome.
6. **CRH stimulation test:** The CRH test, without pretreatment with dexamethasone, helps separate patients with pituitary adenomas from those with ectopic ACTH syndrome or adrenal tumors. As a result of the CRH injection, patients with pituitary adenomas usually experience a rise in blood levels of ACTH and cortisol because CRH acts directly on the pituitary. This response is rarely seen in people with ectopic ACTH syndrome and practically never in those with adrenal tumors.
7. **High-dose dexamethasone suppression test (HDDST):** The HDDST is the same as the LDDST, except it uses higher doses of dexamethasone. This test helps separate patients with excess production of ACTH due to pituitary adenomas from those with ectopic ACTH-producing tumors. High doses of dexamethasone usually suppress cortisol levels in patients with pituitary adenomas but not in those with ectopic ACTH-producing tumors.
8. **Radiological imaging—direct visualization of the endocrine glands:** Imaging tests reveal the size and shape of the pituitary and adrenal glands and help to determine if a tumor is present. The most common imaging tests are the computerized tomography (CT) scan and magnetic resonance imaging (MRI).

   Imaging procedures are used to find a tumor after a diagnosis has been made. Imaging is not used to make the diagnosis of Cushing's syndrome because benign tumors are commonly found in the pituitary and adrenal glands. These tumors, sometimes called incidentalomas, do not produce hormones in quantities that are harmful. They are not removed unless blood tests show they are a cause of symptoms or they are unusually large. Conversely, pituitary tumors may not be detectable by imaging in almost half of people who ultimately need pituitary surgery for Cushing's syndrome.
9. **Petrosal sinus sampling:** This test is not always required, but in many cases, it is the best way to distinguish pituitary from ectopic causes of Cushing's syndrome. Levels of ACTH in the petrosal sinuses are measured and compared with ACTH levels in a forearm vein. Higher levels of ACTH in the sinuses than in the forearm vein indicate a pituitary adenoma. Similar levels of ACTH in the petrosal sinuses and the forearm suggest ectopic ACTH syndrome.

Treatment

Treatment depends on the specific reason for excess cortisol and may include surgery, radiation, chemotherapy, or the use of cortisol-inhibiting drugs.

1. **Drug-induced Cushing's syndrome:** If the cause is long-term use of glucocorticoid hormones to treat another disorder, the dosage is gradually reduced to the lowest dose adequate for control of that disorder. Once control is established, the daily dose of glucocorticoid hormones may be doubled and given on alternate days to lessen side effects. In some cases, noncorticosteroid drugs can be prescribed.
2. **Pituitary adenomas:** Several therapies are available to treat the ACTH-secreting pituitary adenomas of Cushing's disease. The most widely used treatments are:
   a. **Surgical removal** of the tumor is also known as transsphenoidal adenomectomy. After curative pituitary surgery, the production of ACTH drops two levels below normal. This drop is natural and temporary, and patients are given a synthetic form of cortisol, such as hydrocortisone or prednisone to compensate. Most people can stop this replacement therapy in less than 1 or 2 years, but some must be on it for life.
   b. **Radiation therapy:** If transsphenoidal surgery fails or a patient is not a suitable candidate for surgery, radiation therapy is another possible treatment. Radiation to the pituitary gland is given over a 6-week period, with improvement occurring in 40–50% of adults and up to 85% of children. Another technique, called stereotactic radiosurgery or

gamma knife radiation, can be given in a single high-dose treatment. It may take several months or years before people feel better from radiation treatment alone.

c. **Combination therapy:** Combining radiation with cortisol-inhibiting drugs can help speed recovery. Drugs used alone or in combination to control the production of excess cortisol are ketoconazole, mitotane, aminoglutethimide, and metyrapone.

3. **Ectopic ACTH syndrome:** To cure the overproduction of cortisol caused by ectopic ACTH syndrome, all of the cancerous tissue that is secreting ACTH must be eliminated. The choice of cancer treatment—surgery, radiation, chemotherapy, immunotherapy, or a combination of these treatments—depends on the type of cancer. Because ACTH-secreting tumors may be small or widespread at the time of diagnosis, making them difficult to locate and treat directly, cortisol-inhibiting drugs are an important part of treatment. In some cases, if other treatments fail, surgical removal of the adrenal glands, called bilateral adrenalectomy, may replace drug therapy.
4. **Adrenal tumors:** Surgery is the mainstay of treatment for benign and cancerous tumors of the adrenal glands.
5. **Nodular adrenal hyperplasia:** Treatment of nodular adrenal hyperplasia usually requires surgical removal of both adrenal glands. Before surgery, medications that inhibit adrenal enzymes (ketoconazole, metyrapone, or aminoglutethimide) can lower cortisol levels.

After surgery, daily adrenal hormone replacement is usually necessary.

Removal of the adrenals in the absence of a known tumor is occasionally performed to eliminate the production of excess cortisol. In some occasions, this removes negative feedback from a previously occult pituitary adenoma, which starts growing rapidly and produces extreme levels of ACTH, leading to hyperpigmentation. This clinical situation is known as Nelson's syndrome.

Prognosis

The Cushing's syndrome prognosis varies depending on the cause of the disease; most cases of Cushing's syndrome can be cured. Many individuals with the hormonal disorder show significant improvement with Cushing's syndrome treatment, although some may find recovery complicated by various aspects of the causative illness. In addition, some kinds of tumors may return.

CLINICAL NOTE

Imaging is not used to make the diagnosis of Cushing's syndrome because benign tumors are commonly found in the pituitary and adrenal glands. Conversely, pituitary tumors may not be detectable by imaging in almost half of people who ultimately need pituitary surgery for Cushing's syndrome.

CLINICAL PEARLS

1. "Cushing's syndrome" is a condition resulting from long-term exposure of the body tissues to excessive glucocorticoids.
2. "Cushing's disease" is reserved for Cushing's syndrome that is caused by excessive secretion of adrenocorticotropic hormone (ACTH) by a pituitary tumor, usually an adenoma.
3. Easy bruising, typical striae, myopathy, and virilizing signs are suggestive of Cushing's syndrome.
4. Diagnosis is based on a review of a person's medical history, a physical examination, and laboratory tests. X-rays of the adrenal or pituitary glands can be useful in locating tumors.
5. The three most common tests used to diagnose Cushing's syndrome are—the 24-hour urinary free cortisol test, measurement of midnight plasma cortisol or late-night salivary cortisol, and the low-dose dexamethasone suppression test.
6. Treatment depends on the specific reason for excess cortisol and may include surgery, radiation, chemotherapy, or the use of cortisol-inhibiting drugs.

CASE STUDY 6

Theme: Clinical Implications of Antidiuretic Hormone (ADH) Deficiency

A 20-year-old girl noticed that she was waking up once, sometimes twice a night, by the need to go for urination. More recently, she had noticed that she needs to go during her school day much more frequently than before, sometimes as often as once every hour.

At first, she thought that her increased frequency of urination was due to the coffee she drank, but when she reduced her coffee consumption to one cup in the morning, she still needed to go for urination as earlier. In addition, she was buying bottled water too frequently, and she found herself never without a beverage in her hand or nearby. She also noticed that her urine seemed pale and colorless.

When she told her mother of her problem, her mother became very concerned and arranged for her to see the family physician.

Her physician found no abnormalities on physical examination. However, a blood chemistry profile revealed her plasma sodium level to be 149 mEq/L, plasma osmolarity was 308 mOsm/L, and her fasting plasma glucose was 85 mg/dL. An analysis of patient's urine showed a urine osmolarity of 200 mOsm/L. The urine sample was negative for the presence of glucose.

An extensive history revealed that no other member of the family had ever displayed similar symptoms.

She had no history of traumatic head injury and an MRI of her brain was normal.

Next, a 2-hour water deprivation test was performed on her. After 2 hours of not being able to drink water, the osmolarity of her plasma and urine was measured a second time, this time her urine osmolarity was unchanged; however, the osmolarity of her plasma increased to 315 mOsm/L.

What is the probable diagnosis?
Describe the mechanism by which normal fluid regulation in the body occurs.
Why there was no change in urinary osmolarity after fluid deprivation?

CASE DISCUSSION

The patient is suffering from diabetes insipidus. **Polyuria, polydipsia, high-plasma osmolarity, and low-urinary osmolarity are hallmarks of diabetes insipidus.** Diabetes insipidus is not the same as diabetes mellitus ("sugar" diabetes). Diabetes insipidus resembles diabetes mellitus because the symptoms of both diseases are increased urination and thirst. However, in every other respect, including the causes and treatment of the disorders, the diseases are completely unrelated. **Sometimes, diabetes insipidus is referred to as "water" diabetes to distinguish it from the more common diabetes mellitus or "sugar" diabetes.**

DIABETES INSIPIDUS

Diabetes insipidus (DI) is a condition characterized by excessive thirst and excretion of large amounts of severely diluted urine, with reduction of fluid intake having no effect on the latter. There are several different types of DI, each with a different cause. **The most common type is neurogenic DI, caused by a deficiency of arginine vasopressin (AVP), also known as antidiuretic hormone (ADH). The second common type of DI is nephrogenic diabetes insipidus, which is caused by an insensitivity of the kidneys to ADH.** It can also be an iatrogenic artifact of drug use.

Pathophysiology

Electrolyte and volume homeostasis is a complex mechanism that balances the body's requirements for blood pressure and the main electrolytes sodium and potassium. In general, electrolyte regulation precedes volume regulation. When the volume is severely depleted, however, the body will retain water at the expense of deranging electrolyte levels.

The regulation of urine production occurs in the hypothalamus, which produces ADH in the supraoptic and paraventricular nuclei. After synthesis, the hormone is transported in neurosecretory granules down the axon of the hypothalamic neuron to the posterior lobe of the pituitary gland where it is stored for later release. In addition, the hypothalamus regulates the sensation of thirst in the ventromedial nucleus by sensing increases in serum osmolarity and relaying this information to the cortex.

The main effector organ for fluid homeostasis is the kidney. **Antidiuretic hormone (ADH) acts by increasing water permeability in the collecting ducts and distal convoluted tubule, specifically it acts on proteins called aquaporins, which open to allow water into the collecting duct cells. This increase in permeability allows for reabsorption of water into the bloodstream, thus concentrating the urine.**

Signs and Symptoms

Excessive urination and extreme thirst are typical for diabetes insipidus (DI). **Symptoms of diabetes insipidus are quite similar to those of untreated diabetes mellitus, with the distinction that the urine does not contain glucose and there is no hyperglycemia.** Blurred vision is a rarity. Signs of dehydration may also appear in some individuals since the body cannot conserve much of the water it takes in.

The extreme urination continues throughout the day and the night. In children, DI can interfere with appetite, eating, weight gain, and growth as well. They may present with fever, vomiting, or diarrhea. Adults with untreated DI may remain healthy for decades as long as enough water is consumed to offset the urinary losses. However, there is a continuous risk of dehydration and loss of potassium.

Biochemical Defect

Diabetes insipidus is divided into four types, each of which has a different cause and must be treated differently.

1. **Central or neurogenic DI:** The most common type of DI is caused by a lack of vasopressin, a hormone that normally acts upon the kidney to reduce urine output by increasing the concentration of the urine. **This type of DI is usually due to the destruction of the "posterior" part of the pituitary gland where vasopressin is normally stored. Hence, it is commonly called pituitary DI.**

The posterior pituitary can be destroyed by a variety of underlying diseases including tumors, infections, head injuries, infiltrations, and various inheritable defects. The latter can be recognized by the onset of the DI in early childhood and a family history of parents, siblings, or other relatives with the same disorder. Nearly half the time, however, pituitary DI is "idiopathic" (that is, no cause can be found despite a thorough search including magnetic resonance imaging or MRI of the brain) and the underlying cause(s) is (are) still unknown. Pituitary DI is usually permanent and cannot be cured, but the signs and symptoms (i.e., constant thirst, drinking, and urination) can be largely or completely eliminated by treatment with various drugs including a modified from of vasopressin known as desmopressin or DDAVP. Because pituitary DI is sometimes associated with abnormalities in other pituitary hormones, tests and sometimes treatments for these other abnormalities are also needed.

2. **Gestagenic or gestational DI:** Occasionally, a lack of vasopressin can also develop during pregnancy, if the pituitary is slightly damaged and/or the placenta destroys the hormone too rapidly. **This second type of vasopressin deficiency is also treatable with DDAVP but, in this case, the deficiency and the DI often disappear 4–6 weeks after delivery at which time the DDAVP treatment can usually be stopped**. Often, however, the signs and symptoms of DI recur with subsequent pregnancies.
3. **Nephrogenic DI:** The third type of DI is caused by an inability of the kidneys to respond to the "antidiuretic effect" of normal amounts of vasopressin. The kidneys' ability to respond to ADH can be impaired by drugs—like lithium, for example—and by chronic disorders including polycystic kidney disease, sickle cell disease, kidney failure, partial blockage of the ureters, and inherited genetic disorders. **It cannot be treated with DDAVP and, depending on the cause, may/may not be curable by eliminating the offending drug or disease. The heritable form, for example, lasts for life and cannot be cured at present.** However, there are treatments that can partially relieve the signs and symptoms of nephrogenic DI.
4. **Dipsogenic DI:** The fourth form of DI occurs when vasopressin is suppressed by excessive intake of fluids. The latter is usually referred to as primary polydipsia and is most often caused by an abnormality in the part of the brain that regulates thirst. **This subtype is difficult to differentiate from pituitary DI particularly since the two disorders can result from many of the same brain diseases. The only sure way to tell them apart is to measure vasopressin during a stimulus, such as fluid deprivation or to observe the effects of DDAVP treatment**. In dipsogenic DI, DDAVP also eliminates the excessive urination but, unlike pituitary DI, it does not completely eliminate the increased thirst and fluid intake. Thus, it also results in water intoxication, a condition associated with symptoms, such as headache, loss of appetite, lethargy, and nausea and signs, such as an abnormally large decrease in the plasma sodium concentration (hyponatremia). Because of this and the current lack of a way to correct the underlying abnormality in thirst, dipsogenic DI cannot be treated at present, although the most troubling symptoms, nocturia, can be safely relieved by taking small doses of DDAVP at bedtime. The other subtype of primary polydipsia is due not to abnormal thirst but to psychosomatic causes and is often referred to as psychogenic polydipsia. It cannot be treated at present.

Diagnosis

Diagnosis is based on a series of tests, including urine analysis and a fluid deprivation test.

Urine analysis: The urine of a person with DI will be less concentrated.

A fluid deprivation test helps to determine whether DI is caused by one of the following:

- Excessive intake of fluid
- A defect in ADH production
- A defect in the kidneys' response to ADH.

This test measures changes in body weight, urine output, and urine composition when fluids are withheld. Sometimes measuring blood levels of ADH during this test is also necessary.

Desmopressin stimulation test: To distinguish between the main forms, desmopressin stimulation is also used; desmopressin can be taken by injection, a nasal spray, or a tablet. While taking desmopressin, a patient should drink fluids or water only when thirsty and not at other times, as this can lead to sudden fluid accumulation in the central nervous system. If desmopressin reduces urine output and increases osmolarity, the pituitary production of ADH is deficient, and the kidney responds normally. If the DI is due to renal pathology, desmopressin does not change either urine output or osmolarity.

In order to distinguish DI from other causes of excess urination, blood glucose levels, bicarbonate levels, and calcium levels need to be tested. Measurement of blood electrolytes can reveal a high sodium level (hypernatremia as dehydration develops).

In some patients, a magnetic resonance imaging (MRI) of the brain may be necessary as well.

Treatment

Central DI and gestational DI respond to desmopressin. Carbamazepine, an anticonvulsive medication, has also had some success in this type of DI. Gestational DI tends to abate on its own 4–6 weeks following labor, though some women may develop it again in subsequent pregnancies. In dipsogenic DI, desmopressin is not usually an option.

Desmopressin will be ineffective in nephrogenic DI. Instead, the diuretic hydrochlorothiazide (a thiazide diuretic) or indomethacin can improve nephrogenic diabetes insipidus. Thiazide diuretics are sometimes combined with amiloride to prevent hypokalemia. It seems paradoxical to treat an extreme diuresis with a diuretic but the thiazide diuretics will increase proximal tubule reabsorption of sodium and water and decrease distal delivery of fluid to the distal nephron thereby decreasing excretion rates. Again, adequate hydration is important for patients with DI, as they may become dehydrated easily.

CLINICAL NOTE

Adults with untreated DI may remain healthy for decades as long as enough water is consumed to offset the urinary losses. However, there is a continuous risk of dehydration and loss of potassium.

CLINICAL PEARLS

1. Diabetes insipidus (DI) is a condition characterized by excessive thirst and excretion of large amounts of severely diluted urine, with reduction of fluid intake having no effect on the latter.
2. There are several different types of DI, each with a different cause. The most common type is neurogenic DI, caused by a deficiency of arginine vasopressin (AVP), also known as antidiuretic hormone (ADH).
3. The second common type of DI is nephrogenic diabetes insipidus, which is caused by an insensitivity of the kidneys to ADH. It can also be an iatrogenic artifact of drug use.
4. Excessive urination and extreme thirst are typical for DI. Symptoms of diabetes insipidus are quite similar to those of untreated diabetes mellitus, with the distinction that the urine does not contain glucose and there is no hyperglycemia.
5. Diagnosis is based on a series of tests, including urine analysis and a fluid deprivation test.

CASE STUDY 7

Theme: Clinical Implications of Excess of Antidiuretic Hormone

A 56-year-old patient suffering from bronchial carcinoma (previously diagnosed 2 months back) was brought to the hospital with symptoms of headache, leg cramps, weakness, and generalized lethargy. The patient reported that he was having some weakness and lethargy from the last 1 month, but it had worsened from the previous 1 week and from that time only he was constantly having nausea, headache, and leg cramps. There was no fever, no history of any other apparent illness (except cough, sputum, breathlessness, etc., associated with bronchial carcinoma).

On general examination, the patient looked pale and confused. His pulse was 72 beats/min while BP was 100/60 mm Hg. There was no sign of edema or dehydration. The laboratory investigation reports revealed:

Blood glucose—78 mg/dL, blood urea—24 mg/dL, serum creatinine—0.8 mg/dL, serum sodium—126 mmol/L, and plasma osmolality was 258 mOsmol/kg.

Urinary sodium—45 mmol/L, urinary osmolality—350 mOsmol/kg and there was no sugar or protein present in urine.

The patient was diagnosed to be having syndrome of inappropriate antidiuretic hormone (SIADH).

What is SIADH? What are the possible causes of SIADH?
What is the cause of hyponatremia in this patient?
Is there any relation of bronchial carcinoma with SIADH?

CASE DETAILS

The syndrome of inappropriate antidiuretic hormone (SIADH) hypersecretion is a condition characterized by excessive release of antidiuretic hormone (ADH or vasopressin) from the posterior pituitary gland or another source. The result is hyponatremia, and sometimes fluid overload. This dilutional hyponatremia produces headache, nausea, vomiting, and confusion. Severe hyponatremia may cause convulsions or coma.

Hyponatremia, inappropriately elevated urine osmolality (>200 mOsm/kg), excessive urine sodium (UNa >30 mEq/L), and decreased serum osmolality are hallmarks of SIADH.

BASIC CONCEPT

The serum sodium concentration is regulated by the balance of water intake, renal filtration and reabsorption of sodium, and antidiuretic hormone (ADH)-mediated water conservation by the collecting duct.

Water balance is normally mediated by thirst, the secretion of antidiuretic hormone, the feedback mechanisms of the renin-angiotensin-aldosterone system, and renal handling of filtered sodium and water.

Disorders in any one of these components of sodium balance can result in hyponatremia.

Etiology and Pathogenesis

This disorder, commonly termed as the syndrome of inappropriate antidiuretic hormone secretion, is the most common cause of normovolemic hyponatremia and is due to the nonphysiological release of arginine vasopressin (AVP) from the posterior pituitary or an ectopic source.

Antidiuretic hormone (ADH) is secreted by supraoptic and paraventricular nuclei in the hypothalamus and transmitted via the neuronal axons to the posterior pituitary where it is stored. It is released when a decrease in the effective circulatory volume is sensed by vascular baroreceptors primarily located in the large arterial vessels. The key action of ADH in the kidney is to trigger the insertion of aquaporin-2 into the principal cells of the collecting duct. Aquaporins' selective permeability allows water reabsorption and consequently urine concentration. When water is ingested, it is taken up into the circulation and a reduction in plasma osmolality results, which is detected by osmoreceptors in the hypothalamus of the brain and these then switch off the release of ADH. The decreasing concentration of ADH effectively inhibits the aquaporins in the collecting ducts and distal convoluted tubules in the nephrons of the kidney. Hence, less water is reabsorbed, thereby increasing urine output, decreasing urine osmolality, and normalizing blood osmolality.

In SIADH, the release of ADH is not inhibited by a reduction in plasma osmolality when the individual ingests water and the osmolality of the plasma drops. As the main solute of plasma is sodium, this hypoosmolar state is usually detected as a low-sodium level on laboratory testing. **SIADH is therefore primarily a condition that results in the abnormal handling of water loading and not a problem with excessive solute loss. The key to the pathophysiology, signs, symptoms, and treatment of SIADH is to understand that the hyponatremia is a result of excess water and not a serum sodium deficiency.**

Two scenarios can occur in which vasopressin secretion will be not be correlated with the serum osmolality. First, a decrease in the effective circulatory volume may be falsely sensed by the large arterial baroreceptors in conditions, such as cirrhosis, nephrotic syndrome, and congestive heart failure. In these cases, the stimulus for ADH secretion overrides osmotic signals, which are conveying a hypoosmotic state. ADH secretion ensues despite hypoosmolality resulting in hyponatremia. In contrast to patients with SIADH, these patients appear hypervolemic.

Second, inappropriate ADH secretion occurs when there is dysregulation of cells secreting vasopressin or in the feedback mechanisms responsible for its release. A variety of ADH-secreting tumors both inside and outside the pituitary have been associated with SIADH, as well as certain CNS disorders, pulmonary disorders, and medications.

A mutation of the ADH receptor can make it more responsive to ADH and can result in the same clinical picture of hyponatremia, concentrated urine output, and decreased serum osmolality but with normal ADH secretion.

Causes of SIADH

Causes of syndrome of inappropriate antidiuretic hormone (SIADH) secretion vary widely. The syndrome was first described in patients with bronchogenic carcinoma. SIADH may be a marker for occult malignancy, such as head and neck cancers. SIADH may also be manifested in cases of hypothyroidism and is corrected when thyroid hormone is replaced.

Many therapeutic agents can induce **SIADH. Nonsteroidal anti-inflammatory drugs (NSAIDs) inhibit prostaglandin E2, which modulates vasopressin action and can result in decreased water excretion.** SIADH has been reported as an adverse effect of multiple psychotropic medications. While the exact mechanism of action is unknown, it has been proposed that serotonin and serotonergic medications cause increased ADH secretion via the 5-HT1C and 5-HT2 receptors.

The syndrome of inappropriate antidiuretic hormone (SIADH) should be differentiated from hospital-acquired hyponatremia often seen secondary to overzealous administration of hypotonic IV fluids.

Some of the causes of SIADH are listed below:

- **Central nervous system disease:** Tumor, trauma, infection, cerebrovascular accident, subarachnoid hemorrhage, Guillain-Barré syndrome, delirium tremens, and multiple sclerosis
- **Pulmonary disease:** Tumor, pneumonia, chronic obstructive pulmonary disease, lung abscess, tuberculosis, cystic fibrosis, and positive-pressure ventilation
- **Carcinoma:** Lung, pancreas, thymoma, ovary, and lymphoma
- **Drugs:** Exogenous vasopressin, nonsteroidal anti-inflammatory drugs, nicotine, diuretics, chlorpropamide, carbamazepine, tricyclic antidepressants, SSRIs (selective serotonin reuptake inhibitors), vincristine, thioridazine, cyclophosphamide, clofibrate, bromocriptine, haloperidol, thiothixene, exogenous oxytocin, MAOIs.
- **Surgery:** Postoperative
- Idiopathic

Classification of SIADH

The pattern of AVP secretion can be used to classify SIADH into four subtypes:

1. Erratic autonomous AVP secretion (ectopic production); lung cancer (especially small cell lung cancer, as well as other small-cell malignancies of other organs).
2. Normal regulation of AVP release around a lower osmolality set point or reset osmostat (cachexia, malnutrition).
3. Normal AVP response to hypertonicity with failure to suppress completely at low osmolality (incomplete pituitary stalk section).
4. Normal AVP secretion with increased sensitivity to its actions or secretion of some other antidiuretic factor (rare). Patients with the nephrogenic syndrome of inappropriate antidiuresis have clinical and laboratory features consistent with SIADH but undetectable levels of AVP. It is hypothesized that this disorder is due to gain of function mutations in the V2 receptor.

Clinical Features

In general, increased ADH causes water retention and extracellular fluid volume expansion without edema or hypertension, owing to natriuresis (retention of water and passing of sodium in urine). The water retention and sodium loss both cause hyponatremia, which is a key feature in SIADH. The clinical manifestations of hyponatremia are related to osmotic water shift leading to increased ICF volume, specifically brain cell swelling or cerebral edema. Therefore, the symptoms are primarily neurologic, and their severity is dependent on the rapidity of onset and absolute decrease in plasma Na^+ concentration. Patients may be asymptomatic or complain of nausea and malaise. As the plasma Na^+ concentration falls, the symptoms progress to include headache, lethargy, confusion, and obtundation. Stupor, seizures, and coma do not usually occur unless the plasma Na^+ concentration falls acutely below 120 mmol/L or decreases rapidly.

Laboratory Investigations

- **Serum:** Electrolytes, BUN, creatinine, glucose levels, and osmolality
  - Hyponatremia (sodium <135 mEq/L): Serum potassium and bicarbonate levels are normal in SIADH. Hypokalemia and metabolic alkalosis suggest diuretic therapy or vomiting.
  - BUN and serum uric acid levels tend to fall because of plasma dilution and increased excretion of nitrogenous products.
  - Low serum osmolality (<280 mOsm/kg)
  - Hyperkalemia and metabolic acidosis coexisting with hyponatremia suggest adrenal insufficiency.
  - Elevated glucose levels decrease the measured serum sodium levels by 1.6 mEq/L for every 100 mg/dL increase in glucose. This results from the osmotic effect of glucose drawing water into the intravascular space. The serum sodium level rises as hyperglycemia is corrected.
- **Urine:** Electrolytes and osmolality (specific gravity is nonspecific but sensitive)
  - Elevated urinary sodium level (>20 mmol/L). It would be preferable to check urine electrolytes at the same time as the serum electrolytes to determine the fractional excretion of sodium.
  - Urine osmolality generally >100 mOsm/L
- Plasma cortisol level may be obtained to exclude adrenal insufficiency.
- Pseudohyponatremia occurs with severe hyperlipidemia and with hypoproteinemia (levels >10 g/dL, as seen in multiple myeloma).

Imaging Studies

- Chest radiographs may reveal an underlying cause (e.g., pulmonary disease, lung carcinoma).
- CT scan of the head may be appropriate in selected cases.
  - CT scan may show evidence of cerebral edema (e.g., narrowing of the ventricles) or may identify a CNS disorder responsible for SIADH (e.g., brain tumor).
  - CT helps to rule out other potential causes of acute changes in neurologic status.

Other Tests

- Serum ADH levels
- Isolated hyponatremia has no consistent effect on ECG.

Treatment

Management of SIADH includes:

- Treating underlying causes when possible.
- Fluid restriction to 800–1,000 mL/day should be obtained to increase serum sodium.
- Intravenous saline: For very symptomatic patients (severe confusion, convulsions, or coma), hypertonic saline (5%) 200–300 mL IV in 3–4 hours should be given.
- **Drugs:**
  - Demeclocycline can be used in chronic situations when fluid restrictions are difficult to maintain; demeclocycline is the most potent inhibitor of AVP action.
  - **Conivaptan**—an antagonist of both V1A and V2 vasopressin receptors. Its indications are "treatment of euvolemic hyponatremia (e.g., the syndrome of inappropriate secretion of antidiuretic hormone, or in the setting of hypothyroidism, adrenal insufficiency, pulmonary disorders, etc.) in hospitalized patients".
  - **Tolvaptan**—an antagonist of the V2 vasopressin receptor (under trial and showed that it can raise the serum sodium by 5 mmol/L).

Avoid correction by more than 12 mEq/L/day.

The risk of correcting hyponatremia too rapidly is the development of the osmotic demyelination syndrome (ODS). This is a neurologic disorder characterized by flaccid paralysis, dysarthria, and dysphagia. The diagnosis is usually suspected clinically and can be confirmed by appropriate neuroimaging studies. There is no specific treatment for the disorder, which is associated with significant morbidity and mortality. Patients with chronic hyponatremia are most susceptible to the development of ODS, since their brain cell volume has returned to near normal as a result of the osmotic adaptive mechanisms described above. Therefore, administration of hypertonic saline to these individuals can cause sudden osmotic shrinkage of brain cells. In addition to rapid or overcorrection of hyponatremia, risk factors for ODS include prior cerebral anoxic injury, hypokalemia, and malnutrition, especially secondary to alcoholism. Water restriction in primary polydipsia and intravenous saline therapy in ECF volume-contracted patients may also lead to overly rapid correction of hyponatremia as a result of AVP suppression and a brisk water diuresis. This can be prevented by administration of water or use of an AVP analog to slow down the rate of free water excretion.

Prognosis

The fatality rate of patients with hyponatremia (sodium <130 mEq/L) is 60-fold compared to that of patients without documented hyponatremia, though the mortality is typically related to comorbid conditions rather than the hyponatremia itself.

The recent development of nonapeptide vasopressin antagonists has introduced a new selective treatment for euvolemic and hypervolemic hyponatremia.

CLINICAL NOTE

The risk of correcting hyponatremia too rapidly is the development of the osmotic demyelination syndrome (ODS), which is a neurologic disorder characterized by flaccid paralysis, dysarthria, and dysphagia.

CLINICAL PEARLS

1. The syndrome of inappropriate antidiuretic hormone secretion is the most common cause of normovolemic hyponatremia and is due to the nonphysiologic release of AVP from the posterior pituitary or an ectopic source.
2. Hyponatremia, inappropriately elevated urine osmolality (>200 mOsm/kg), excessive urine sodium (UNa >30 mEq/L), and decreased serum osmolality are hallmarks of SIADH.
3. The syndrome was first described in patients with bronchogenic carcinoma. SIADH may be a marker for occult malignancy, such as head and neck cancers. SIADH may also be manifested in cases of hypothyroidism, pulmonary, CNS diseases, or it may be drug induced.
4. The symptoms are primarily neurologic, and their severity is dependent on the rapidity of onset and absolute decrease in plasma Na^+ concentration.
5. Management of SIADH includes: treating underlying causes when possible, fluid restriction, intravenous saline—for very symptomatic patients (severe confusion, convulsions, or coma) hypertonic saline (5%) 200–300 mL IV in 3–4 hours should be given or drugs can be given to inhibit the effects of ADH.

CASE STUDY 8

Theme: Clinical Implications of Hyperthyroidism (Autoimmune Disease)

A 35-year-old female presented to the clinic for a routine health checkup. The patient reported that she felt tired, nervous, and anxious all the time with frequent palpitations. On further questioning, she reported that she had lost nearly 10 kg of weight in the past 3 months and was having diarrhea from the same duration. She had also noticed a change in hair texture, fingernail growth, and she frequently felt warm while others were cold or comfortable. She denied any history of depression or anxiety disorder, but she felt difficulty in falling asleep from the previous few weeks for which she was not taking any medications.

On examination, her heart rate was 110 beats per minute. She had a slight tremor and had increased reflexes in all extremities. A nontender thyroid enlargement was appreciated in the thyroid region. Her thyroid-stimulating hormone (TSH) level was low at 0.1 mIU/mL. The patient was told that she had an autoimmune antibody process.

What is the most likely diagnosis?
What is the biochemical mechanism for this disorder?

CASE DETAILS

The patient is suffering from **Graves' disease.** Graves' disease accounts for 60–80% of thyrotoxicosis. It is an autoimmune disease and most commonly affects thyroid, frequently causing it to enlarge to twice its size or more. **Thyroid becomes overactive with related hyperthyroid symptoms, such as increased heartbeat, muscle weakness, disturbed sleep, and irritability.** It can also affect the eyes, causing bulging eyes (exophthalmos). It affects other systems of the body, including the skin, heart, circulation, and nervous system.

GRAVES' DISEASE

It affects up to 2% of the female population, sometimes appears after childbirth. The disorder rarely begins before adolescence and typically occurs between 20 years and 50 years of age, but it also occurs in the elderly.

Pathophysiology

Graves' disease is an autoimmune disorder, in which antibodies are produced against the receptor for thyroid-stimulating hormone (TSH) (antibodies to thyroglobulin and to the thyroid hormones T3 and T4 may also be produced).

These antibodies cause hyperthyroidism because they bind to the TSH receptor and chronically stimulate it. The TSH receptor is expressed on the follicular cells of the thyroid gland and the result of chronic stimulation is an abnormally high production of T_3 and T_4.This, in turn, causes the clinical symptoms of hyperthyroidism, and the enlargement of the thyroid gland is visible as goiter.

The infiltrative exophthalmos that is frequently encountered has been explained by postulating that the thyroid gland and the extraocular muscles share a common antigen, which is recognized by the antibodies. Antibodies binding to the extraocular muscles would cause swelling behind the eyeball.

The "orange peel" skin has been explained by the infiltration of antibodies under the skin, causing an inflammatory reaction and subsequent fibrous plaques.

There are three types of autoantibodies to the TSH receptor currently recognized:

1. **Thyroid-stimulating immunoglobulins (TSI):** These antibodies (mainly IgG) act as LATS (long-acting thyroid stimulants), activating the cells in a longer and slower way than TSH, leading to an elevated production of thyroid hormone.
2. **Thyroid growth immunoglobulins (TGI):** These antibodies bind directly to the TSH receptor and have been implicated in the growth of thyroid follicles.
3. **Thyrotropin binding inhibiting immunoglobulins (TBII):** These antibodies inhibit the normal union of TSH with its receptor. Some will actually act as if TSH itself is binding to its receptor, thus inducing thyroid function. Other types may not stimulate the thyroid gland, but will prevent TSI and TSH from binding to and stimulating the receptor.

As in autoimmune hypothyroidism, a combination of environmental and genetic factors, including polymorphisms in HLA-DR, CTLA-4, and PTPN22 (a T cell regulatory gene), contributes to Graves' disease susceptibility. The concordance for Graves' disease in monozygotic twins is 20–30%, compared to <5% in dizygotic twins. **Indirect evidence suggests that stress is an important environmental factor, presumably operating through neuroendocrine effects on the immune system. Smoking is a minor risk factor for Graves' disease and a major risk factor for the development of ophthalmopathy. Sudden increases in iodine intake may precipitate Graves' disease, and there is a three-fold increase in the occurrence of Graves' disease in the postpartum period.**

Clinical Manifestations

The clinical presentation depends on the severity of thyrotoxicosis, the duration of disease, individual susceptibility to excess thyroid hormone, and the patient's age. In the elderly, features of thyrotoxicosis may be subtle or masked, and patients may present mainly with fatigue and weight loss, a condition known as apathetic thyrotoxicosis.

1. **Weight loss:** Thyrotoxicosis may cause unexplained weight loss, despite an enhanced appetite, due to the increased metabolic rate.
2. **Neurological manifestations:** The prominent features include hyperactivity, nervousness, and irritability, ultimately leading to a sense of easy fatigability in some patients. Insomnia and impaired concentration are common; apathetic thyrotoxicosis may be mistaken for depression in the elderly. Fine tremor is a frequent finding, best elicited by having patients stretch out their fingers while feeling the fingertips with the palm. Common neurological manifestations include hyperreflexia, muscle wasting, and proximal myopathy without fasciculation. Chorea is a rare feature. Thyrotoxicosis is sometimes associated with a form of hypokalemic periodic paralysis; this disorder is particularly common in Asian males with thyrotoxicosis.
3. **Cardiovascular manifestations:** The most common cardiovascular manifestation is sinus tachycardia, often associated with palpitations, occasionally caused by supraventricular tachycardia. The high-cardiac output produces a bounding pulse, widened pulse pressure, and an aortic systolic murmur and can lead to worsening of angina or heart failure in the elderly or those with preexisting heart disease. Atrial fibrillation is more common in patients >50 years. Treatment of the thyrotoxic state alone converts atrial fibrillation to normal sinus rhythm in about half of patients, suggesting the existence of an underlying cardiac problem in the remainder.
4. **Dermatological manifestations:** The skin is usually warm and moist, and the patient may complain of sweating and heat intolerance, particularly during warm weather. Palmar erythema, onycholysis, and, less commonly, pruritus, urticaria, and diffuse hyperpigmentation may be evident. Hair texture may become fine, and a diffuse alopecia occurs in up to 40% of patients, persisting for months after restoration of euthyroidism.

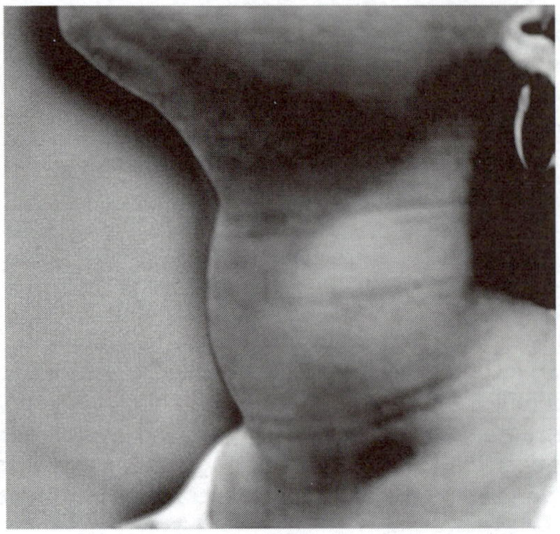

Fig. 15.10: Graves' disease (showing diffuse enlargement of thyroid gland).

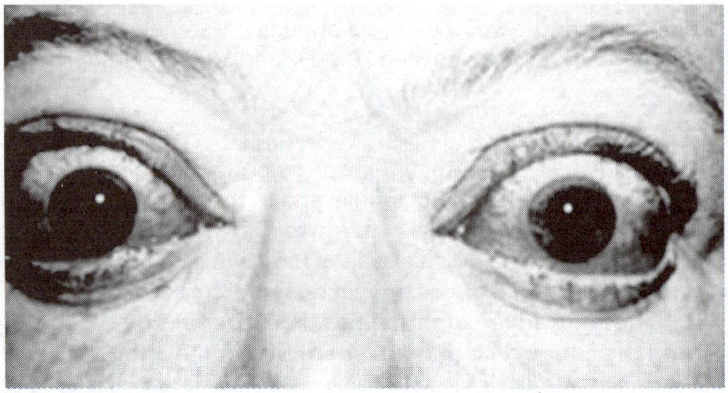

Fig. 15.11: Graves' ophthalmopathy.

5. **Gastrointestinal manifestations:** Gastrointestinal transit time is decreased, leading to increased stool frequency, often with diarrhea and occasionally mild steatorrhea.
6. **Menstrual irregularities:** Women frequently experience oligomenorrhea or amenorrhea; in men, there may be impaired sexual function and, rarely, gynecomastia.
7. **Effect on bones:** The direct effect of thyroid hormones on bone resorption leads to osteopenia in long-standing thyrotoxicosis; mild hypercalcemia occurs in up to 20% of patients, but hypercalciuria is more common. There is a small increase in fracture rate in patients with a previous history of thyrotoxicosis.
8. In Graves' disease, the thyroid is usually diffusely enlarged to two-to-three times its normal size. The consistency is firm. There may be a thrill or bruit due to the increased vascularity of the gland and the hyperdynamic circulation **(Fig. 15.10)**.
9. **Eye changes:** Lid retraction, causing a staring appearance, can occur in any form of thyrotoxicosis and is the result of sympathetic overactivity. However, Graves' disease is associated with specific eye signs that comprise **Graves' ophthalmopathy (Fig. 15.11)**. This condition is also called thyroid-associated ophthalmopathy, as it occurs in the absence of Graves' disease in 10% of patients. Most of these individuals have autoimmune hypothyroidism or thyroid antibodies. The onset of Graves' ophthalmopathy occurs within the year before or after the diagnosis of thyrotoxicosis in 75% of patients, but can sometimes precede or follow thyrotoxicosis by several years, accounting for some cases of euthyroid ophthalmopathy. **It is believed that fibroblasts in the orbital tissues may express the thyroid-stimulating hormone receptor (TSHr). This may explain why one autoantibody to the TSHr can cause disease in both the thyroid and the eyes.**
10. The two signs that are truly "diagnostic" of Graves' disease (i.e., not seen in other hyperthyroid conditions) are **exophthalmos and nonpitting edema**, over the anterior and lateral aspects of the lower leg, (hence, the term pretibial myxedema).

Laboratory Investigations

1. **T_3 and T_4 are elevated:** A sign of Graves' disease is hyperthyroidism, i.e., overproduction of the thyroid hormones T_3 and T_4. Normothyroidism is also seen, and occasionally also hypothyroidism, which may assist in causing goiter (though it is not the cause of the Graves' disease). Hyperthyroidism in Graves' disease is confirmed, as with any other cause of hyperthyroidism, by measuring elevated blood levels of free (unbound) T_3 and T_4.
2. Thyroid-stimulating hormone (TSH) is usually low in Graves' disease due to negative feedback from the elevated T_3 and T_4.
3. Protein-bound iodine is elevated.
4. **Radioactive iodine uptake test and thyroid scan:** Radioactive iodine uptake test measures the amount of iodine the thyroid collects from the bloodstream. High levels of iodine uptake can indicate Graves' disease. Nuclear imaging of Graves' disease is characterized by an enlarged gland and increased tracer uptake that is distributed homogeneously. Other causes of hyperthyroidism, such as nodules—small lumps in the gland—will show a different pattern of iodine distribution.
5. Thyroid-stimulating antibodies may also be detected serologically.
6. Biopsy to obtain histological testing is not normally required, but may be obtained if thyroidectomy is performed.

Treatment

The hyperthyroidism of Graves' disease is treated by reducing thyroid hormone synthesis, using antithyroid drugs, or reducing the amount of thyroid tissue with radioiodine (^{131}I) treatment or by thyroidectomy.

Antithyroid Drugs

The main antithyroid drugs are **carbimazole, methimazole, and propylthiouracil (PTU).** These drugs block the binding of iodine and coupling of iodotyrosines. The most dangerous side effect is agranulocytosis (1/250, more in PTU); this is an idiosyncratic reaction, which does not stop on cessation of drug. Others include granulocytopenia (dose dependent, which improves on cessation of the drug) and aplastic anemia. The most common side effects are rash and peripheral neuritis. These drugs cross the placenta and are also secreted in breast milk.

Radioiodine

Radioiodine (radioactive iodine-131) is suitable for most patients, although some prefer to use it mainly for older patients. Indications for radioiodine are failed medical therapy or surgery and where medical or surgical therapies are contraindicated. Hypothyroidism may be a complication of this therapy, but may be treated with thyroid hormones if it appears. Patients who receive the therapy must be monitored regularly. Contraindications to RAI are pregnancy (absolute), ophthalmopathy (relative; it can aggravate thyroid eye disease), solitary nodules. Disadvantages of this treatment are a high incidence of hypothyroidism (up to 80%) requiring eventual thyroid hormone supplementation in the form of a daily pill(s). The radioiodine treatment acts slowly (over months to years) to destroy the thyroid gland, and Graves' disease-associated hyperthyroidism is not cured in all persons by radioiodine, but has a relapse rate that depends on the dose of radioiodine which is administered.

Surgery

This modality is suitable for young patients and pregnant patients. Indications are a large goiter (especially when compressing the trachea), suspicious nodules or suspected cancer, and patients with ophthalmopathy. Subtotal or near-total thyroidectomy is an option for patients who relapse after antithyroid drugs and prefer this treatment to radioiodine.

Advantages are immediate cure and potential removal of carcinoma. Its risks are injury of the recurrent laryngeal nerve, hypoparathyroidism (due to removal of the parathyroid glands), hematoma (which can be life-threatening, if it compresses the trachea), and scarring.

Symptomatic Treatment

β-blockers (such as propranolol) may be used to inhibit the sympathetic nervous system symptoms of tachycardia and nausea until such time as antithyroid treatments start to take effect.

Treatment of Eye Disease

Mild cases are treated with lubricant eye drops or nonsteroidal anti-inflammatory drops. Severe cases, threatening vision (corneal exposure or optic nerve compression), are treated with steroids or orbital decompression. In all cases, cessation of smoking is essential.

Difficulty in closing eyes can be treated with lubricant gel at night, or with tape on the eyes to enable full, deep sleep.

Orbital decompression can be performed to enable bulging eyes to retreat back into the head. Bone is removed from the skull behind the eyes, and space is made for the muscles and fatty tissue to fall back into the skull.

Eyelid surgery can be performed on upper and/or lower eyelids to reverse the effects of Graves on the eyelids. Eyelid muscles can become tight with Graves, making it impossible to close eyes all the way. Eyelid surgery helps to reduce or eliminate dry eye symptoms.

Thyroid dermopathy does not usually require treatment but can cause cosmetic problems or interfere with the fit of shoes. Surgical removal is not indicated.

Graves' disease in children is usually managed with antithyroid drugs, often given as a prolonged course of the titration regimen. Surgery or radioiodine may be indicated for severe disease.

Complications of Graves' Disease

If left untreated, more serious complications could result, including birth defects in pregnancy and increased risk of a miscarriage.

Graves–Basedow disease is often accompanied by an increase in heart rate, which may lead to further heart complications including loss of the normal heart rhythm (atrial fibrillation), which may lead to stroke. If the eyes are proptotic (bulging) severely enough that the lids do not close completely at night, severe dryness will occur with a very high risk of a secondary corneal infection, which could lead to blindness. Pressure on the optic nerve behind the globe can lead to visual field defects and vision loss as well.

Thyrotoxic crisis, or thyroid storm, is rare and presents as a life-threatening exacerbation of hyperthyroidism, accompanied by fever, delirium, seizures, coma, vomiting, diarrhea, and jaundice. The mortality rate due to cardiac failure, arrhythmia, or hyperthermia is as high as 30%, even with treatment. Thyrotoxic crisis is usually precipitated by acute illness (e.g., stroke, infection, trauma, and diabetic ketoacidosis), surgery (especially on the thyroid), or radioiodine treatment of a patient with partially treated or untreated hyperthyroidism. Management requires intensive monitoring and supportive care, identification and treatment of the precipitating cause, and measures that reduce thyroid hormone synthesis.

CLINICAL NOTE

The two signs that are truly "diagnostic" of Graves' disease (i.e., not seen in other hyperthyroid conditions) are exophthalmos and nonpitting edema, over the anterior and lateral aspects of the lower leg, (hence, the term pretibial myxedema).

CLINICAL PEARLS

1. Graves' disease accounts for 60–80% of thyrotoxicosis.
2. It is an autoimmune disease and most commonly affects thyroid, frequently causing it to enlarge to twice its size or more.
3. Thyroid becomes overactive with related hyperthyroid symptoms, such as increased heartbeat, muscle weakness, disturbed sleep, and irritability. It can also affect the eyes, causing bulging eyes (exophthalmos).
4. It affects other systems of the body, including the skin, heart, circulation, and nervous system.
5. The hyperthyroidism of Graves' disease is treated by reducing thyroid hormone synthesis, using antithyroid drugs, or reducing the amount of thyroid tissue with radioiodine (^{131}I) treatment or by thyroidectomy.

CASE STUDY 9

Theme: Clinical Implications of Hypothyroidism (Autoimmune Disease)

A 51-year-old woman presented to her internist with complaints of swelling in the front of her neck. Upon history and physical examination, her physician noted that she had a weight gain, in the past year, of 28 pounds, had shortness of breath, and was easily fatigued. She indicated she had attributed these symptoms to getting older. In her family history, it was noted that her mother, aged 76, was living and had been taking thyroid medication for many years for reasons unknown to the patient.

The physician ordered a complete blood count, a basic metabolic panel, thyroid-stimulating hormone (TSH) assay, and a free thyroxine (fT4) assay. All results were in reference range except for an elevation in total cholesterol, TSH, and fT_4. Results are listed below:

Laboratory Results

Total Cholesterol: 278 mg/dL (6.9 mmol/L)

fT4: 0.5 (5.15 pmol/L)

TSH: 8.3 µIU/mL

Upon receipt of the laboratory reports of the elevated TSH and decreased fT_4, the physician requested TPOAb and TgAb testing. The results of the antibody testing indicated a markedly increased presence. With these laboratory findings and given the clinical symptoms, the physician diagnosed Hashimoto's thyroiditis. The patient was placed on L-thyroxine (levothyroxine) as a thyroid hormone replacement therapy to prevent further thyroid destruction.

What is Hashimoto thyroiditis?

What is the cause of thyroid destruction in this disease?

What is the genetic predisposition of this disease?

CASE DISCUSSION

Hashimoto's thyroiditis is an autoimmune disease in which the thyroid gland is gradually destroyed by a variety of cell and antibody-mediated immune processes. **Hashimoto's thyroiditis was first described by Dr Hakaru Hashimoto in 1912.** He described patients with chronic endocrine gland disorder of the thyroid as having struma lymphomatosa because of the diffuse infiltration of the gland with lymphocytes. The disease has been referred to as Hashimoto's thyroiditis or Hashimoto's disease since this original description. Other descriptions include chronic thyroiditis, lymphocytic thyroiditis, lymphadenoid goiter, and goitrous autoimmune thyroiditis.

Incidence

The mean annual incidence rate of autoimmune hypothyroidism is up to 4 per 1,000 women and 1 per 1,000 men. It is more common in certain populations,, such as the Japanese, probably because of genetic factors and chronic exposure to a high-iodine diet. The mean age at diagnosis is 60 years, and the prevalence of overt hypothyroidism increases with age. Subclinical hypothyroidism is found in 6–8% of women (10% over the age of 60) and 3% of men.

Inheritance

It is considered as an autoimmune disease and has demonstrated clustering in families as an apparently inherited dominant trait.

As with most autoimmune disorders, susceptibility to autoimmune hypothyroidism is determined by a combination of genetic and environmental factors, and the risk of either autoimmune hypothyroidism or Graves' disease is increased among siblings.

HLA-DR polymorphisms are the best documented genetic risk factors for autoimmune hypothyroidism, especially HLA-DR3, -DR4, and -DR5 in Caucasians. A weak association also exists between polymorphisms in CTLA-4, a T cell–regulatory gene, and autoimmune hypothyroidism. Both of these genetic associations are shared by other autoimmune diseases, which may explain the relationship between autoimmune hypothyroidism and other autoimmune diseases, especially Type 1 diabetes mellitus, Addison's disease, pernicious anemia, and vitiligo. HLA-DR and CTLA-4 polymorphisms account for approximately half of the genetic susceptibility to autoimmune hypothyroidism. The other contributory loci remain to be identified. A gene on chromosome 21 may be responsible for the association between autoimmune hypothyroidism and Down syndrome.

The female preponderance of thyroid autoimmunity is most likely due to sex steroid effects on the immune response, but an X chromosome-related genetic factor is also possible, which may account for the high frequency of autoimmune hypothyroidism in Turner syndrome.

Environmental susceptibility factors are poorly defined at present. **A high iodine intake may increase the risk of autoimmune hypothyroidism by immunologic effects or direct thyroid toxicity.** There is no convincing evidence for a role of infection except for the congenital rubella syndrome, in which there is a high frequency of autoimmune hypothyroidism. Viral thyroiditis does not induce subsequent autoimmune thyroid disease.

Pathology

The thyroid gland follicular cells enclose an amorphous colloid material composed of thyroglobulin. Thyroglobulin consists of the two hormones—triiodothyronine (T_3) and thyroxine (T_4). Regulation of the thyroid begins with thyrotropin-releasing hormone (TRH) secreted by the hypothalamus and acts on the pituitary gland to stimulate synthesis and release of TSH. It is TSH that binds to receptors in the thyroid gland to initiate the breakdown of thyroglobulin into free T_3 and T_4. TSH synthesis and release are regulated by a negative feedback mechanism by the level of free T_3 and T_4.

The exact mechanism for Hashimoto's thyroiditis is unknown, but it has been characterized by gradual thyroid failure because of an autoimmune destruction of the thyroid gland.

The disease is characterized by cellular and humoral responses, as demonstrated by serum antibodies to thyroid antigens and the lymphocytic infiltration of the gland. The thyroid autoantibodies present in patients include antithyroid peroxidase antibody (TPOAb), antithyroglobulin antibody (TgAb), and anti-TSH receptor autoantibodies (TSHRAb). **A high titer of at least 1 of the 3 antibodies has been found in 97% of patients with Hashimoto's thyroiditis.**

In Hashimoto's thyroiditis, the immunologic attack is aggressive and destructive. TgAbs are positive in about 60–80% of patients, and TPOAb in 95% of patients diagnosed with the disease. The positive titers for these antibodies are considered markers for the disease. TPOAb appears to be incapable of initiating the autoimmune process, but rather may be the consequence of the initial immune damage. As a result, antibodies to TPO may in fact be better indicators of active thyroid inflammation than TgAb. The circulating antibodies against components of the thyroid follicles act as thyroid blockers. Production of autoantibodies interferes with the process of TSH binding to receptors and the release of T_3 and T_4 from thyroglobulin. TgAbs are targeted against thyroglobulin. TSHRAbs in Hashimoto's disease bind to receptors and block the binding and function of TSH and are referred to as thyroxine-binding inhibitory immunoglobulins. TPOAbs bind with the microsomal antigens associated with the follicular cells lining the microsomal membrane. They are mainly IgG and fix complement and may be cytotoxic. This immune response progressively destroys the thyroid gland.

The thyroid lymphocytic infiltrate in autoimmune hypothyroidism is composed of activated CD^{4+} and CD^{8+} T cells, as well as B cells. Thyroid cell destruction is primarily mediated by the CD^{8+} cytotoxic T cells, which destroy their targets by either perforin-induced cell necrosis or granzyme B-induced apoptosis. In addition, local T cell production of cytokines,, such as tumor necrosis factor (TNF), IL-1, and interferon-α (IFN-α), may render thyroid cells more susceptible to apoptosis mediated by death receptors,, such as Fas, which are activated by their respective ligands on T cells. These cytokines also impair thyroid cell function directly and induce the expression of other proinflammatory molecules by the thyroid cells themselves,, such as cytokines, HLA class I and class II molecules, adhesion molecules, CD40, and nitric oxide. Administration of high concentrations of cytokines for therapeutic purposes (especially IFN-α) is associated with increased autoimmune thyroid disease, possibly through mechanisms similar to those in sporadic disease.

Progressive thyroid cell damage can change the apparent clinical picture from goitrous hypothyroidism to that of primary hypothyroidism and is considered to be the end stage of Hashimoto's thyroiditis.

Clinical Manifestations

Hashimoto's thyroiditis begins as a gradual enlargement of the thyroid gland followed by a usually slow development of hypothyroidism. Patients typically present with an enlarged thyroid resulting in diffuse goiter in the anterior region of the neck. The goiter is usually asymptomatic, but occasionally patients have difficulty in swallowing and a feeling of local pressure.

Hypothyroidism is a common late sequel of Hashimoto's thyroiditis and results in slowing of the metabolic processing of the body. The commonly encountered symptoms are as follows:

Dermatological changes: The skin is dry, and there is decreased sweating, thinning of the epidermis, and hyperkeratosis of the stratum corneum. Increased dermal glycosaminoglycan content traps water, giving rise to skin thickening without pitting (myxedema). Typical features include a puffy face with edematous eyelids and nonpitting pretibial edema. There is pallor, often with a yellow tinge to the skin due to carotene accumulation. Nail growth is retarded, and hair is dry, brittle, difficult to manage, and falls out easily.

In addition to diffuse alopecia, there is thinning of the outer third of the eyebrows, although this is not a specific sign of hypothyroidism.

Other common features include:

- Constipation and weight gain (despite a poor appetite): In contrast to popular perception, the weight gain is usually modest and due mainly to fluid retention in the myxedematous tissues.
- Libido is decreased in both sexes, and there may be oligomenorrhea or amenorrhea in long-standing disease, but menorrhagia is also common. Fertility is reduced and the incidence of miscarriage is increased. Prolactin levels are often modestly increased and may contribute to alterations in libido and fertility and cause galactorrhea.
- Myocardial contractility and pulse rate are reduced, leading to a reduced stroke volume and bradycardia. Increased peripheral resistance may be accompanied by hypertension, particularly diastolic.
- Blood flow is diverted from the skin, producing cool extremities.
- Pericardial effusions occur in up to 30% of patients but rarely compromise cardiac function. Fluid may also accumulate in other serous cavities and in the middle ear, giving rise to conductive deafness. Pulmonary function is generally normal, but dyspnea may be caused by pleural effusion, impaired respiratory muscle function, diminished ventilatory drive, or sleep apnea.
- Carpal tunnel and other entrapment syndromes are common, as is impairment of muscle function with stiffness, cramps, and pain. On examination, there may be slow relaxation of tendon reflexes and pseudomyotonia.
- Memory and concentration are impaired. Rare neurological problems include reversible cerebellar ataxia, dementia, psychosis, and myxedema coma.
- The hoarse voice and occasionally clumsy speech of hypothyroidism reflect fluid accumulation in the vocal cords and tongue.

The features described above are the consequence of thyroid hormone deficiency. However, autoimmune hypothyroidism may be associated with signs or symptoms of other autoimmune diseases, particularly vitiligo, pernicious anemia, Addison's disease, alopecia areata, and Type 1 diabetes mellitus.

Thyroid-associated ophthalmopathy, which usually occurs in Graves' disease, occurs in about 5% of patients with autoimmune hypothyroidism.

Autoimmune hypothyroidism is uncommon in children and usually presents with slow growth and delayed facial maturation. The appearance of permanent teeth is also delayed. Myopathy, with muscle swelling, is more common in children than in adults. In most cases, puberty is delayed, but precocious puberty sometimes occurs. There may be intellectual impairment, if the onset is before 3 years and the hormone deficiency is severe.

Diagnosis

The diagnosis is generally made from the clinical symptoms, but the confirmation is done by the laboratory investigations. Laboratory tests to determine thyroid function include:

- Free T_4 test (low)
- Serum TSH (high)
- T_3 (low or normal)
- Thyroid autoantibodies:
  - Antithyroid peroxidase antibody
  - Antithyroglobulin antibody

Imaging studies are generally not needed to diagnose Hashimoto's thyroiditis. This disease may also change the results of the following tests:

- Complete blood count
- Radioactive iodine uptake
- Serum prolactin
- Serum sodium
- If there is any doubt about the cause of a goiter associated with hypothyroidism, FNA biopsy can be used to confirm the presence of autoimmune thyroiditis.
- Other abnormal laboratory findings in hypothyroidism may include increased creatine phosphokinase, elevated cholesterol and triglycerides, and anemia (usually normocytic or macrocytic). Except when accompanied by iron deficiency, the anemia and other abnormalities gradually resolve with thyroxine replacement.

Increased levels of TSH are the first detectable abnormality seen in laboratory testing for correctly diagnosing hypothyroidism. This may occur even before the patient is symptomatic. As hypothyroidism progresses, the fT4 will decrease.

Recent methods for determining the thyroid status: Detection of the hormones requires sensitive analytical methods. The high sensitivity TSH (sTSH) assay is considered to be the first and best laboratory test for identification of thyroid abnormalities. The sTSH assay is extremely useful in the detection and confirmation of suspected primary hypothyroidism. sTSH has replaced the traditional monoclonal RIA technique for the hormone. Whereas the traditional RIA techniques measured an antigen–antibody complex, the 3rd-generation sTSH immunochemiluminometric assays (ICMA) use two or three separate monoclonal antibodies in the methodologies and provide a sensitivity of 0.01–0.02 mU/L. The requirement of binding to more than one site gives the sTSH its high specificity and sensitivity. The first antibody is in excess, bound to a solid phase support, and extracts the TSH molecule from the serum, and is usually specific for the beta subunit of the TSH molecule. The second antibody usually attaches to the alpha subunit of the TSH molecule.

Total T_4 (TT_4) assays detect both the T_4 bound to protein and the free, biologically active T_4. Although fT_4 is present as a very small fraction of TT_4 (approximately 0.02% of TT_4)8, fT_4 is the test of choice as an indicator of thyroid status.

The fT_4 determinations are most often performed using direct nonisotopic immunoassay, such as microparticle enzyme immunoassay (MEIA) and chemiluminescence.

The diagnosis of autoimmune thyroiditis may be confirmed by the detection of thyroid autoantibodies. TgAb and TPOAb are the most commonly detected thyroid autoantibodies. TPOAb assays are sensitive and specific and lend themselves to high-volume testing with RIA, ELISA, and, most recently, chemiluminescence. TgAb can be assayed by hemagglutination, RIA, ELISA, and ICMA.

Treatment

Hypothyroidism caused by Hashimoto's thyroiditis is treated with thyroid hormone replacement agents, such as levothyroxine. A tablet taken once a day generally keeps the thyroid hormone levels normal. In most cases, the treatment needs to be taken for the rest of the patient's life. In the event that hypothyroidism is caused by Hashimoto's thyroiditis, it is recommended that the TSH levels be kept as low as possible.

If there is no evidence of thyroid hormone deficiency, just regular observation is needed.

Prognosis

The outcome is usually very good. The disease stays stable for years. If it does slowly progress to thyroid hormone deficiency (hypothyroidism), it can be treated with thyroid replacement therapy.

Possible Complications

This condition can occur with other autoimmune disorders. In rare cases, thyroid cancer may develop.

CLINICAL NOTE

The traditional RIA techniques measured an antigen antibody complex, the 3rd-generation sTSH immunochemiluminometric assays (ICMA) use two or three separate monoclonal antibodies in the methodologies and provide a sensitivity of 0.01–0.02 mU/L.

CLINICAL PEARLS

1. Hashimoto's thyroiditis is an autoimmune disease in which the thyroid gland is gradually destroyed by a variety of cell and antibody-mediated immune processes.
2. The disease is characterized by cellular and humoral responses, as demonstrated by serum antibodies to thyroid antigens and the lymphocytic infiltration of the gland.
3. The diagnosis is generally made from the clinical symptoms, but the confirmation is done by the laboratory investigations.
4. Increased levels of TSH are the first detectable abnormality seen in laboratory. As hypothyroidism progresses, the fT4 will decrease. Thyroid autoantibodies, such as antithyroid peroxidase antibody and antithyroglobulin antibody, are also found.
5. Hypothyroidism caused by Hashimoto's thyroiditis is treated with thyroid hormone replacement agents, such as levothyroxine.

CASE STUDY 10

Theme: Clinical Implications of Hypothyroidism

A 65-year-old female presented to the clinic with complaints of lethargy, tiredness, and fatigue all the time. She had also noticed an increasing problem of constipation and gain in weight in the past 2 months, despite the fact that she had been too particular about her diet.

She was frequently feeling very cold when others were warm or comfortable. Her skin had become dry, and she had noticed a swelling sensation in her neck area.

On examination, she was afebrile with a pulse of 60 beats per minute. She was in no acute distress and appeared in good health. She had an enlarged, nontender thyroid noted on her neck. Her reflexes were diminished, and her skin was dry to touch.

What is the most likely diagnosis?

What laboratory test would you need to confirm the diagnosis?

What is the treatment of choice?

CASE DETAILS

The patient is suffering from hypothyroidism.

Hypothyroidism is the disease state caused by insufficient production of thyroid hormone by the thyroid gland.

There are many disorders that result in hypothyroidism. These disorders may directly or indirectly involve the thyroid gland. Because thyroid hormone affects growth, development, and many cellular processes, inadequate thyroid hormone has widespread consequences for the body.

Incidence

Hypothyroidism is a very common condition. It is estimated that 3–5% of the population has some form of hypothyroidism. The condition is more common in women than in men, and its incidence increases with age.

Causes

There are number of causes for hypothyroidism.

a. **Primary:** The defect is in thyroid itself
b. **Secondary (due to pituitary diseases):** Hypothyroidism occurs if the pituitary gland does not create enough thyroid-stimulating hormone (TSH) to induce the thyroid gland to produce enough thyroxine and triiodothyronine. Although not every case of secondary hypothyroidism has a clear-cut cause, it is usually caused by damage to the pituitary gland.
c. **Transient:** Hypothyroidism may occur transiently, the causes may be:
   1. Silent thyroiditis, including postpartum thyroiditis
   2. Subacute thyroiditis
   3. Withdrawal of thyroxine treatment in individuals with an intact thyroid
   4. After ^{131}I treatment or subtotal thyroidectomy for Graves' disease.

Clinical Manifestations

The symptoms of hypothyroidism are often subtle. They are not specific and are often attributed to aging. Patients with mild hypothyroidism may have no signs or symptoms. The symptoms generally become more obvious as the condition worsens and the majority of these complaints are related to a metabolic slowing of the body.

Common symptoms are listed below:

- Poor muscle tone (muscle hypotonia)
- Fatigue
- Cold intolerance, increased sensitivity to cold
- Depression
- Muscle cramps and joint pain
- Carpal tunnel syndrome
- Goiter
- Thin, brittle fingernails
- Thin, brittle hair
- Pallor
- Decreased sweating
- Dry, itchy skin
- Weight gain and water retention
- Bradycardia (low heart rate—less than 60 beats per minute)
- Constipation.

Late Symptoms

- Slow speech and a hoarse, breaking voice—deepening of the voice can also be noticed
- Dry puffy skin, especially on the face
- Thinning of the outer third of the eyebrows (sign of Hertoghe)
- Abnormal menstrual cycles
- Low basal body temperature.

Less Common Symptoms

- Impaired memory
- Impaired cognitive function (brain fog) and inattentiveness
- A slow heart rate with ECG changes including low-voltage signals. Diminished cardiac output and decreased contractility.
- Reactive (or postprandial) hypoglycemia
- Sluggish reflexes
- Hair loss
- Anemia caused by impaired hemoglobin synthesis (decreased EPO levels), impaired intestinal iron and folate absorption or B12 deficiency from pernicious anemia
- Difficulty swallowing
- Shortness of breath with a shallow and slow respiratory pattern
- Increased need for sleep
- Irritability and mood instability
- Yellowing of the skin due to impaired conversion of beta-carotene to vitamin A
- Impaired renal function with decreased GFR
- Elevated serum cholesterol
- Acute psychosis (myxedema madness) is a rare presentation of hypothyroidism
- Decreased libido due to impairment of testicular testosterone synthesis
- Decreased sense of taste and smell (anosmia)
- Puffy face, hands, and feet (late, less common symptoms)
- Gynecomastia

Laboratory Investigations

Following investigations are carried out to diagnose a case of hypothyroidism:

1. **TSH levels:** High levels of TSH indicate that the thyroid is not producing sufficient levels of thyroid hormone [mainly as thyroxine (T_4) and smaller amounts of triiodothyronine (T_3)]. This increase in TSH can actually precede the fall in thyroid hormones by months or years. If the decrease in thyroid hormone is actually due to a defect of the pituitary or hypothalamus, then the levels of TSH are abnormally low. This kind of thyroid disease is known as "secondary" or "tertiary" hypothyroidism. A special test, known as the TRH test, can help to distinguish, if the disease is caused by a defect in the pituitary or the hypothalamus.
2. **T_3 and T_4 levels:** Free triiodothyronine (fT_3), free levothyroxine (fT_4), total T_3 and total T_4 levels can be estimated. In early hypothyroidism, the level of thyroid hormones (T_3 and T_4) may be normal.
3. **Antithyroid antibodies**—for evidence of autoimmune diseases that may be damaging the thyroid gland.
4. **Serum cholesterol**—may be elevated in hypothyroidism.
5. **Prolactin**—as a widely available test of pituitary function.
6. **Thyroid scan:** A combination of the patient's clinical history, antibody screening (as mentioned above), and a thyroid scan can help to diagnose the precise underlying thyroid problem more clearly.
7. If a pituitary or hypothalamic cause is suspected, an MRI of the brain and other studies may be warranted.

Treatment

With the exception of certain conditions, the treatment of hypothyroidism requires lifelong therapy.

Thyroid replacement therapy: Hypothyroidism is treated with the levorotatory forms of thyroxine (L-T_4) and triiodothyronine (L-T_3). Both synthetic and animal-derived thyroid tablets are available. The most active thyroid hormone is actually T_3, but T_4 is preferred as a replacement. T_3 [liothyronine sodium (Cytomel)] is although available and there are certain indications for its use. However, for the majority of patients, a form of T_4 [levothyroxine sodium (Levoxyl, Synthroid)] is the preferred treatment. This is a more stable form of thyroid hormone and requires once a day dosing, whereas T_3 is much shorter acting and needs to be taken multiple times a day. In the overwhelming majority of patients, synthetic T_4 is readily and steadily converted to T_3 naturally in the bloodstream, and this conversion is appropriately regulated by the body's tissues.

- The average dose of T_4 replacement in adults is approximately 1.6 micrograms per kilogram per day.
- Children require larger doses.
- In young, healthy patients, the full amount of T_4 replacement hormone may be started initially.

In patients with pre-existing heart disease, this method of thyroid replacement may aggravate the underlying heart condition in about 20% of cases.

In older patients without known heart disease, starting with a full dose of thyroid replacement may result in uncovering heart disease, resulting in chest pain or a heart attack. For this reason, patients with a history of heart disease or those suspected of being at high-risk are started with 25 micrograms or less of replacement hormone, with a gradual increase in the dose at 6 weeks intervals.

Therapy for hypothyroidism is monitored at approximately 6 weeks intervals until stable. The goal is to maintain the TSH within normal limits. Once stable, the TSH can be checked yearly. Overtreating hypothyroidism with excessive thyroid medication is potentially harmful and can cause palpitations and poor blood pressure control and can also contribute to osteoporosis. Every effort should be made to keep the TSH within the normal range.

SUBCLINICAL HYPOTHYROIDISM

Subclinical hypothyroidism refers to a state in which patients do not exhibit the symptoms of hypothyroidism. These patients also have a normal amount of circulating thyroid hormone. The only abnormality is an increased TSH. This implies that the pituitary gland is working extra hard to maintain a normal circulating thyroid hormone level and that the thyroid gland requires extrastimulation by the pituitary to produce adequate hormones. The majority of these patients can be expected to progress to obvious hypothyroidism, especially if the TSH is above a certain level.

Such patients need treatment if they have a high serum cholesterol level. The abnormal cholesterol profile shows improvement with thyroid hormone replacement. If the cholesterol levels are normal, and the patient feels well, it is also reasonable to follow these patients without treatment and repeat the blood TSH and thyroid hormone levels in 4–6 months to see if more significant hypothyroidism is apparent.

CLINICAL NOTE

The increase in TSH can actually precede the fall in thyroid hormones by months or years. If the decrease in thyroid hormone is actually due to a defect of the pituitary or hypothalamus, then the levels of TSH are abnormally low. This kind of thyroid disease is known as "secondary" or "tertiary" hypothyroidism.

CLINICAL PEARLS

1. Hypothyroidism is the disease state caused by insufficient production of thyroid hormone by the thyroid gland.
2. There are many disorders that result in hypothyroidism. These disorders may directly or indirectly involve the thyroid gland. Because thyroid hormone affects growth, development, and many cellular processes; inadequate thyroid hormone has widespread consequences for the body.
3. Patients with mild hypothyroidism may have no signs or symptoms. The symptoms generally become more obvious as the condition worsens and the majority of these complaints are related to a metabolic slowing of the body.
4. High levels of TSH indicate that the thyroid is not producing sufficient levels of thyroid hormone [mainly as thyroxine (T_4) and smaller amounts of triiodothyronine (T_3)]. This increase in TSH can actually precede the fall in thyroid hormones by months or years. If the decrease in thyroid hormone is actually due to a defect of the pituitary or hypothalamus, then the levels of TSH are abnormally low.
5. Hypothyroidism is treated with the levorotatory forms of thyroxine (L-T_4) and triiodothyronine (L-T_3). Both synthetic and animal-derived thyroid tablets are available. The most active thyroid hormone is actually T_3, but T_4 is preferred as a replacement.

CASE STUDY 11

Theme: Clinical Implications of Hyperparathyroidism

A 45-year-old female reported to the emergency with severe pain in the left flank region, which was radiating towards lower leg and back. The patient was in acute distress and agony. History revealed that she frequently suffered from urinary tract infections and had several such episodes of pain. She further reported that she constantly felt weakness, fatigue, and bone pains from the previous few months. There was no history of fever and there was no personal or family history of medical problems.

Her physical examination was normal except for tenderness in the left renal region.

The attending physician ordered for complete blood count, electrolytes, and a complete urine analysis.

The laboratory investigation report revealed a normal complete blood count (CBC), and significantly elevated calcium level and low phosphorus level. Urine was cloudy and had plenty of pus cells. The patient was admitted and treated for renal colic.

What is the underlying cause for repeated episodes of renal colic?
What is the most likely diagnosis?
What is the relationship of bone pains and frequent urinary tract infections in this patient?
What is the cause for high serum calcium and low phosphorus level in this patient?

CASE DISCUSSION

The patient is suffering from hyperparathyroidism. Hypercalcemia, hypophosphatemia, recurrent urinary tract infections, renal stones, and bone pains, all signify the underlying hyperparathyroidism.

HYPERPARATHYROIDISM

Hyperparathyroidism is overactivity of the parathyroid glands resulting in excess production of parathyroid hormone (PTH). The parathyroid hormone regulates calcium and phosphate levels.

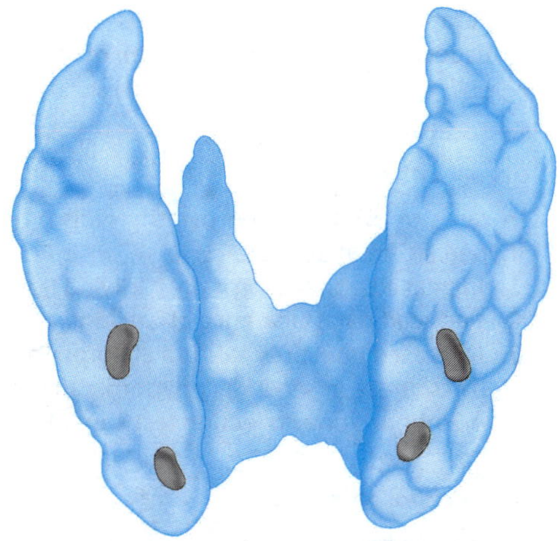

Fig. 15.12: Normal parathyroid glands.

Classification

Primary Hyperparathyroidism

Primary hyperparathyroidism results from a hyperfunction of the parathyroid glands themselves. There is oversecretion of PTH due to adenoma, hyperplasia or, rarely, carcinoma of the parathyroid glands **(Fig. 15.12)**.

Secondary Hyperparathyroidism

Secondary hyperparathyroidism is the reaction of the parathyroid glands to a hypocalcemia caused by something other than a parathyroid pathology, e.g., chronic renal failure or vitamin D deficiency.

Tertiary Hyperparathyroidism

Tertiary hyperparathyroidism results from hyperplasia of the parathyroid glands and a loss of response to serum calcium levels. This disorder is most often seen in patients with chronic renal failure. In cases of long-standing secondary hyperparathyroidism, the hypertrophied parathyroid glands can become autonomously functioning and continue to secrete parathyroid hormone (PTH) independent of whether the original stimuli to secrete PTH are still present.

In all cases, the raised PTH levels are harmful to bone, and treatment is often needed.

Clinical Manifestations

There are great variations in the manifestations:

- Patients may present with multiple signs and symptoms, including recurrent nephrolithiasis, peptic ulcers, mental changes, and, less frequently, extensive bone resorption.
- The manifestations may be subtle, and the disease may have a benign course for many years or a lifetime. This milder form of the disease is usually termed asymptomatic HPT.
- Rarely, hyperparathyroidism develops or worsens abruptly and causes severe complications,, such as marked dehydration and coma, so-called hypercalcemic parathyroid crisis.
- Manifestations of hyperparathyroidism involve primarily the kidneys and the skeletal system. Kidney involvement, due either to deposition of calcium in the renal parenchyma or to recurrent nephrolithiasis. Renal stones are usually composed of either calcium oxalate or calcium phosphate. In occasional patients, repeated episodes of nephrolithiasis or the formation of large calculi may lead to urinary tract obstruction, infection, and loss of renal function. Nephrocalcinosis may also cause decreased renal function and phosphate retention.
- The distinctive bone manifestation of hyperparathyroidism is osteitis fibrosa cystica. Histologically, the pathognomonic features are an increase in the giant multinucleated osteoclasts in scalloped areas on the surface of the bone and a replacement of the normal cellular and marrow elements by fibrous tissue.
- In symptomatic patients, dysfunctions of the CNS, peripheral nerve and muscle, gastrointestinal tract, and joints also occur.
- When present, neuromuscular manifestations may include proximal muscle weakness, easy fatigability, and atrophy of muscles and may be so striking as to suggest a primary neuromuscular disorder. The distinguishing feature is the complete regression of neuromuscular disease after surgical correction of the hyperparathyroidism.
- Gastrointestinal manifestations are sometimes subtle and include vague abdominal complaints and disorders of the stomach and pancreas. Again, cause and effect are unclear. In MEN-1 patients with hyperparathyroidism, duodenal ulcer may be the result of associated pancreatic tumors that secrete excessive quantities of gastrin (Zollinger–Ellison syndrome). Pancreatitis has been reported in association with hyperparathyroidism, but the incidence and the mechanism are not established.

Etiology

Parathyroid tumors are most often encountered as:

- Isolated adenomas without other endocrinopathies. A single abnormal gland is the cause in ~80% of patients; the abnormality in the gland is usually a benign neoplasm or adenoma and rarely a parathyroid carcinoma.
- They may also arise in hereditary syndromes,, such as **MEN syndromes (multiple endocrine neoplasia syndromes)**. MEN-1 (Wermer's syndrome) consists of hyperparathyroidism and tumors of the pituitary and pancreas, often associated with gastric hypersecretion and peptic ulcer disease (Zollinger–Ellison syndrome). MEN-2A is characterized by pheochromocytoma and medullary carcinoma of the thyroid, as well as hyperparathyroidism; MEN-2B has additional associated features, such as multiple neuromas but usually lacks hyperparathyroidism.

- Parathyroid tumors may also arise as secondary to underlying disease (excessive stimulation in secondary hyperparathyroidism, especially chronic renal failure), or after other forms of excessive stimulation,, such as lithium therapy.

Laboratory Tests

Serum Calcium

In cases of primary hyperparathyroidism or tertiary hyperparathyroidism, heightened PTH leads to increased serum calcium (hypercalcemia) due to:

1. Increased bone resorption, allowing flow of calcium from bone to blood.
2. Reduced renal clearance of calcium.
3. Increased intestinal calcium absorption.

By contrast, in secondary hyperparathyroidism, effectiveness of PTH is reduced.

A 24-hour urine collection test can help to determine how much calcium is being removed from the body.

Serum Phosphate

In primary hyperparathyroidism, serum phosphate levels are abnormally low as a result of decreased renal tubular phosphate reabsorption. However, this is only present in about 50% of cases. This contrasts with secondary hyperparathyroidism, in which serum phosphate levels are generally elevated because of renal disease.

Alkaline Phosphatase

Alkaline phosphatase levels are not elevated in all types of hyperparathyroidism.

Parathyroid immunoassay: The gold standard of diagnosis is the parathyroid immunoassay.

Bone density: Dual-energy X-ray absorptiometry (DEXA) of the spine provides reproducible quantitative estimates (within a few percent) of spinal bone density. Similarly, bone density in the extremities can be quantified by densitometry of the hip or of the distal radius. Cortical bone density is reduced while cancellous bone density, especially in the spine, is relatively preserved.

Bone X-rays and bone mineral density test can help to detect bone loss, fractures, or bone softening.
X-rays, ultrasound, or CT scans of the kidneys or urinary tract may show calcium deposits or a blockage.

Diagnosis

Once an elevated parathyroid hormone has been confirmed, goal of diagnosis is to determine whether the hyperparathyroidism is primary or secondary in origin by obtaining a serum calcium level. **In primary hyperparathyroidism, both PTH and serum calcium levels are high, while in secondary hyperparathyroidism PTH is high, but serum calcium level may be low or normal.**

Tertiary hyperparathyroidism has a high PTH and a high serum calcium concentration. It is differentiated from primary hyperparathyroidism by a history of chronic kidney failure and secondary hyperparathyroidism.

Treatment and Monitoring

Treatment depends upon the severity and cause of the condition. If there are mildly increased calcium levels due to primary hyperparathyroidism and no symptoms, just regular checkups are needed. If symptoms are present or calcium level is very high, surgery may be needed to remove the parathyroid gland that is overproducing the hormone. Treatment of secondary hyperparathyroidism depends on the underlying cause. Vitamin D and phosphorus supplementations can also be done. Magnesium deficiency impairs the secretion of PTH, and so hypomagnesemia should be corrected whenever detected.

Calcimimetics

A calcimimetics (cinacalcet) is a new type of drug for people with primary and secondary hyperparathyroidism on dialysis. It mimics the effect of calcium in tissues. This reduces PTH release from parathyroid glands, leading to lower calcium and phosphorus levels in blood. Calcimimetics control PTH release from parathyroid glands without increasing calcium and phosphorus levels. The most common side effects of calcimimetics are mild or moderate nausea and vomiting.

Prognosis

The outlook depends on the specific type of hyperparathyroidism.

Possible Complications

Complications may include:

- Increased risk of fractures
- Urinary tract infection due to kidney stones and blockage
- Peptic ulcer disease

- Pancreatitis
- Pseudogout

Surgery for hyperparathyroidism may lead to low blood calcium levels, which causes tingling and muscle twitching. This requires immediate treatment.

Prevention

Getting the proper amount of calcium in diet or through supplements may reduce risk of secondary hyperparathyroidism.

CLINICAL NOTE

Manifestations of hyperparathyroidism involve primarily the kidneys and the skeletal system. Kidney involvement is due to either deposition of calcium in the renal parenchyma or to recurrent nephrolithiasis.

CLINICAL PEARLS

1. Hyperparathyroidism is overactivity of the parathyroid glands resulting in excess production of parathyroid hormone (PTH).
2. Patients may present with multiple signs and symptoms, including recurrent nephrolithiasis, peptic ulcers, mental changes, and, less frequently, extensive bone resorption.
3. The distinctive bone manifestation of hyperparathyroidism is osteitis fibrosa cystica.
4. Parathyroid tumors are most often encountered as isolated adenomas without other endocrinopathies. They may also arise in hereditary syndromes,, such as multiple endocrine neoplasia (MEN) syndromes or they may arise secondary to underlying diseases.
5. Treatment depends upon the severity and cause of the condition. If there are mildly increased calcium levels and no symptoms, just regular checkups are needed. If symptoms are present or calcium level is very high, surgery may be needed to remove the parathyroid gland that is overproducing the hormone. Treatment of secondary hyperparathyroidism depends on the underlying cause. Vitamin D and phosphorus supplementations can also be done.

CASE STUDY 12

Theme: Clinical Implications of Hypoparathyroidism

A 36-year-old female diagnosed as hyperthyroid was on carbimazole. On stoppage of carbimazole, hyperthyroidism recurred and she was advised to have radioiodine treatment. Subsequently, she received ^{131}I. 2 months later, the patient developed severe carpopedal spasm and her plasma total calcium decreased to 6.4 mg/dL (normal range 8.5–10.5 mg/dL).

She was hospitalized for 4 days, her free T_3 was 1.4 pg/mL (normal range 1.4–4.2 pg/mL), free T_4 was 1.6 ng/dL (normal range 0.86–2.4 ng/dL), TSH was 1.0 mcU/mL (normal range 0.23–4.0 mcU/mL), and intact PTH was 1.00 pg/mL (normal range 12–72 pg/mL). She was immediately started on oral calcium and alfacalcidol; within 24 hours, the calcium rose to 7.2 mg/dL and plasma calcium was subsequently measured every 2 weeks. The patient received 1 μg of alfacalcidol and calcium lactate 10 g daily plus injection cholecalciferol 300,000 IU every 2 weeks. However, her calcium rose to only 7.7 mg/dL. The cholecalciferol dose was then increased to 600,000 units every 2 weeks and with this dose, the calcium level rose to 8.3 mg/dL.

What is the possible diagnosis?
What is the cause for hypocalcemia in this disease?

CASE DISCUSSION

The patient is suffering from hypoparathyroidism. Persistent hypoparathyroidism following ^{131}I treatment for hyperthyroidism is a rare, but recognized complication. Carpopedal spasm associated with low calcium level is a sign of hypoparathyroidism in this case. Calcium and vitamin D supplementation can restore the calcium level back to normal.

HYPOPARATHYROIDISM

Hypoparathyroidism is the state of decreased secretion or activity of parathyroid hormone (PTH). This leads to hypocalcemia and hyperphosphatemia.

Causes

Most people have 4 parathyroid glands, which make primary hypoparathyroidism uncommon. Hypocalcemia from hypoparathyroidism requires all 4 parathyroid glands to be affected.

- **Primary hypoparathyroidism** may be permanent or reversible. Permanent primary hypoparathyroidism may be congenital or acquired.
- **Iatrogenic:** The most common cause of primary hypoparathyroidism is excision of all parathyroid glands via surgery in the treatment of thyroid, laryngeal, or other neck malignancies. Patients with parathyroid hyperplasia, as observed in the multiple endocrine neoplasia (MEN) syndromes, are treated by surgical removal of the parathyroid glands. Repeated neck explorations for primary hyperparathyroidism due to parathyroid adenoma also may cause hypoparathyroidism.
- Extensive irradiation to the face, neck, or mediastinum may cause destruction of all 4 parathyroid glands with ensuing primary hypoparathyroidism and hypocalcemia.
- The **"hungry bone syndrome"** develops after a parathyroidectomy for hyperparathyroidism. The body has been accustomed to high levels of PTH, causing hypercalcemia. Much of this hypercalcemic effect is due to resorption of bone. When the parathyroid gland or glands responsible for the hypersecretion of PTH are removed, the PTH level in the blood drops suddenly, and the patient experiences transient hypoparathyroidism. The bone, which has been "starved" of calcium, avidly holds onto it under the influence of osteoblasts. Without PTH and with bone now using calcium to remineralize, the ECF ionized calcium level falls. Postoperatively, patients require aggressive treatment with calcium for several hours to several days. Eventually, the hypoparathyroid state resolves, and calcium homeostasis is reachieved.
- **Autoimmune polyglandular syndrome (also referred to as HAM syndrome)** includes primary hypoparathyroidism due to destruction of the parathyroid glands. On average, these patients develop primary hypoparathyroidism when aged 10 years.
- Autoimmune hypoparathyroidism may exist alone or in sporadic or familial forms. For patients with autoimmune primary hypoparathyroidism, the average age for development of hypocalcemia is aged 7 years, with a range of 6 months to 20 years.
- **Congenital:** Numerous conditions are there that result in congenital agenesis or hypoplasia and, therefore, can produce primary hypoparathyroidism with symptomatic hypocalcemia at birth or in the newborn period.
- Familial isolated hypoparathyroidism is a heterogeneous mixture of disorders.
- **Metal overload:** Hemochromatosis and thalassemia, both of which are associated with iron overload, may result in primary hypoparathyroidism.
- Wilson disease, with copper overload, also may cause primary hypoparathyroidism.
- Hypomagnesemia has been demonstrated to decrease PTH release. Correction of hypomagnesemia leads to correction of the primary hypoparathyroidism. Hypomagnesemia causes reversible functional primary hypoparathyroidism.
- **Neonatal:** The unborn baby of a mother with hypercalcemia has chronic suppression of parathyroid gland function. In the worst of circumstances, the parathyroid glands may become atrophic. At birth, the maternal calcium excess is gone, and newborns are at risk of hypocalcemia due to primary hypoparathyroidism. Clinically significant hypocalcemia may develop within the first 3 weeks of life, but may occur as late as 1 year after birth. The primary hypoparathyroidism in these patients is self-limiting.
- **Resistance to parathyroid hormone (pseudohypoparathyroidism):** This disease is very rare. Like hypoparathyroidism, this disease is characterized by hypocalcemia and hyperphosphatemia, but patients with pseudohypoparathyroidism have sufficient PTH, but the bones and kidneys become nonresponsive to PTH. They seem to have hypoparathyroidism, but actually they do not have; thus, the name pseudohypoparathyroidism.

Pathophysiology

The ionized calcium concentration in the extracellular fluid (ECF) remains nearly constant at a level of approximately 1 mm. Ionized calcium in the ECF is in equilibrium with ionized calcium in storage pools, such as bone, proteins in the circulation, and within the intracellular fluid. The intracellular fluid concentration of calcium is more than 10,000-fold lower than in the ECF. The maintenance of ionized calcium concentrations in both the intracellular and extracellular fluids is highly regulated and modulates the functions of bone, renal tubular cells, clotting factors, adhesion molecules, excitable tissues, and a myriad of intracellular processes. An extracellular calcium-sensing receptor has been isolated from parathyroid, kidney, and brain cells. In parathyroid cells, the extracellular calcium-sensing receptor regulates the secretion of PTH. A fall in ECF ionized calcium concentration leads to exocytosis of PTH.

1. **Effect of PTH on bones:** PTH has the overall effect of returning the ECF ionized calcium concentration to normal by its effects on the kidneys and the skeleton. PTH activates osteoclasts. Osteoclasts activation results in bone resorption and a release of ionized calcium into the ECF. Recent evidence suggests that small pulse doses of PTH activate osteoblasts, with ensuing bone deposition. The effect of PTH on osteoclasts seems more important than the effect on osteoblasts.
2. **Effect of PTH on kidneys:** PTH inhibits the proximal tubular transport of phosphate from the lumen to the interstitium. In conditions of primary PTH excess, hypophosphatemia tends to occur. Conversely, in hypoparathyroidism, the phosphate concentration in the plasma is normal or slightly elevated. PTH has a calcium-retaining effect on the distal tubule. The PTH-mediated calcium reabsorption is independent of any effects on sodium or water reabsorption. This effect of PTH is important in hypoparathyroidism because, in the absence of this distal tubular calcium reabsorption, the kidneys waste calcium. This depletes the ECF ionized calcium and increases the urinary calcium concentration.

3. **Concerted action with vitamin D (calcitriol):** PTH, through stimulation of renal 1-alpha-hydroxylase activity, helps in the activation of vitamin D. Calcitriol (1,25-dihydroxyvitamin D), the active vitamin D, promotes the absorption of dietary calcium. Therefore, calcitriol has a concerted action with PTH; both help in the maintenance of plasma calcium concentration. PTH deficiency causes impaired dietary calcium absorption, renal tubular reabsorption, bone resorption, and phosphaturic effect. Therefore, PTH deficiency eventually leads to hypocalcemia.

Clinical Manifestations

Hypocalcemia resulting from hypoparathyroidism exhibits a variety of symptoms. Besides neuromuscular irritability, which is the major outcome of hypocalcemia, the other clinical manifestations include:

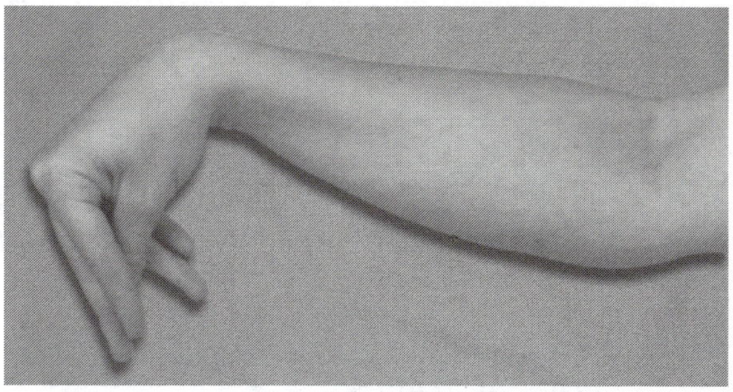

Fig. 15.13: Muscular spasm, a sign of hypocalcemia in hypoparathyroidism.

- **Psychological manifestations**—hyperirritability, tiredness, anxiety, depression, mood fluctuations, personality disorders, emotional instability, confusion, hallucinations, and psychosis.
- **Neurological manifestations**—paresthesia and convulsions
- **Electrolyte imbalance**—hypomagnesemia and hypokalemia
- **Acid-base imbalance**—alkalosis that worsens signs of hypocalcemia
- **Neuromuscular irritability**—muscular cramps, excessive sweating (diaphoresis), wheezing, breathlessness, hoarseness of voice, tetany, laryngospasm, and bronchospasm in severe cases
- The below-mentioned signs can elicit heightened neuromuscular irritability resulting from hypocalcemia:
  - **Chvostek's sign:** Facial twitching, chiefly around the mouth, is demonstrated by gently tapping the ipsilateral facial nerve just anterior to the ear.
  - **Trousseau sign (Fig. 15.13):** Carpal spasm is brought on by inflating a blood pressure cuff around the arm to pressure 20 mm Hg above occluding the radial pulse for 3–5 minutes.
- **Extrapyramidal choreoathetoid syndromes:** Hypocalcemia in patients with basal ganglia calcifications can lead to extrapyramidal choreoathetoid syndromes. Around 5% of patients with idiopathic hypoparathyroidism present with Parkinsonism, dystonia, hemiballismus, and oculogyric crises.
- **Neurological symptoms**, such as spastic paraplegia, ataxia, dysphagia, and dysarthria can be found in association with hypoparathyroidism-induced hypocalcemia.
- **Papilledema** may develop in severe hypocalcemia, which improves with treatment.
- **Chronic hypocalcemia** can be associated with ocular cataracts, abnormal dentition, dry, puffy, and rough skin.
- **Cardiovascular manifestations:** A prolongation of the QT interval is observed on ECG in severe hypocalcemia**.** Congestive heart failure can also develop.

Diagnosis

Diagnosis is by measurement of calcium, serum albumin, and PTH in blood. If necessary, measuring cAMP (cyclic AMP) in the urine after an intravenous dose of PTH can help in the distinction between hypoparathyroidism and other causes. Other tests include ECG for abnormal heart rhythms, and measurement of blood magnesium levels. CT scan of the brain in cases of hypoparathyroidism commonly reveals evidence of intracranial calcification.

Differential diagnoses are:

- Pseudohypoparathyroidism (normal PTH levels, but tissue insensitivity to the hormone, associated with mental retardation and skeletal deformities) and pseudopseudohypoparathyroidism
- Vitamin D deficiency or hereditary insensitivity to this vitamin (X-linked dominant)
- Malabsorption
- Kidney disease
- Medication: Steroids, diuretics, and some antiepileptics can also produce similar symptoms.

Treatment

1. **Medication:** Hypoparathyroidism requires lifelong treatment of oral supplements of calcium, vitamin D, in varying forms, and magnesium. These levels are checked regularly by blood tests. Acute symptomatic hypocalcemia, however, requires urgent correction with intravenous calcium.
2. **PTH:** It is not commercially available, but stage III clinical trials are underway for its use in osteoporosis. It soon may be available for patients with hypoparathyroidism.
3. **Surgical care:** Patients undergoing parathyroidectomy for parathyroid hyperplasia are at high risk of developing permanent primary hypoparathyroidism. Patients may be treated with an autotransplant of a segment of parathyroid gland to prevent hypoparathyroidism. If the autotransplantation fails, patients are treated as any other patient with hypoparathyroidism.

4. **Diet:** A diet rich in calcium content (i.e., emphasizing dairy products) is recommended for patients with primary hypoparathyroidism.

Complications

- Tetany can lead to a blocked airway, requiring a tracheostomy.
- Stunted growth, malformed teeth, and slow mental development can occur, if hypoparathyroidism develops in childhood.
- Overtreatment with vitamin D and calcium can cause hypercalcemia (high blood calcium) and sometimes interfere with kidney function.
- There is an increased risk of pernicious anemia, Addison's disease, cataract development, and Parkinson's disease.

CLINICAL NOTE

The most common cause of primary hypoparathyroidism is excision of parathyroid glands during surgery in the treatment of thyroid, laryngeal, or other neck malignancies.

CLINICAL PEARLS

1. Hypoparathyroidism is due to insufficient production of parathyroid hormone.
2. Causes of hypoparathyroidism include injury to the parathyroid glands, autoimmune disorder association, or congenital.
3. Symptoms of hypoparathyroidism include tingling fingers, toes, and lips, brittle nails, dry, coarse skin, dry hair, memory loss, headaches, severe muscle cramps, cataracts, malformed teeth, and convulsions.
4. Treatment of hypoparathyroidism is to restore the calcium and phosphorus to normal levels in the body.
5. Calcium and vitamin D are mainstay of treatment.

CASE STUDY 13

Theme: Clinical Implications of Excess Release of Catecholamines

A 45-year-old man with a 2 year history of refractory hypertension and symptoms of occasional "panic attacks" was referred to the hypertension clinic. The patient was apparently healthy but complained of sudden and unpredictable pounding headache with excessive sweating occurring off and on. He was a nonsmoker but used to take one vodka and tonic every night. His family history was positive for hypertension.

On examination, his blood pressure was 170/90 mm Hg in both arms and pulse was 72 beats/minute. His weight was 185 lbs. Fundoscopic examination revealed mild arteriolar narrowing (grade I).

He was taking beta blockers for treating hypertension. He tried many medications, but experienced side effects from majority of them.

Thyroid, chest, and abdominal examinations were normal; blood urea and serum creatinine were also normal.

Because of the patient's difficulty to control hypertension, the physician ordered 24 hours urine for vanillylmandelic acid (VMA), which was 8.0 mg% (normal <6 mg%).

What is the probable diagnosis?
What is the differential diagnosis?

CASE DETAILS

The patient is suffering from pheochromocytoma.

Pheochromocytoma

Pheochromocytomas and paragangliomas are catecholamine-producing tumors derived from the sympathetic or parasympathetic nervous system.

BASIC CONCEPT

Cells in the adrenal medulla synthesize and secrete epinephrine and norepinephrine. The ratio of these two catecholamines differs considerably among species: in humans, cats, and chickens, roughly 80, 60, and 30% of the catecholamine output is epinephrine.

Following release into blood, these hormones bind adrenergic receptors on target cells, where they induce essentially the same effects as direct sympathetic nervous stimulation.

Synthesis and Secretion of Catecholamines

Synthesis of catecholamines begins with the amino acid tyrosine, which is taken up by chromaffin cells in the medulla and converted to norepinephrine and epinephrine through the following steps **(Fig. 15.14)**:

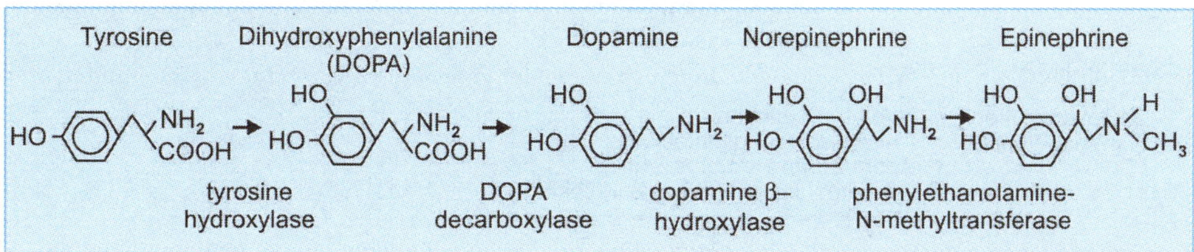

Fig. 15.14: Steps of formation of catecholamines from tyrosine.

Norepinephrine and epinephrine are stored in electron-dense granules, which also contain ATP and several neuropeptides. Secretion of these hormones is stimulated by acetylcholine release from preganglionic sympathetic fibers innervating the medulla. Many types of "stresses" stimulate such secretion, including exercise, hypoglycemia, and trauma. Following secretion into blood, the catecholamines bind loosely to and are carried in the circulation by albumin and perhaps other serum proteins.

Catecholamine Degradation

Catecholamines are degraded in the liver by two enzymes—COMT (catechol-O-methyltransferase) and MAO (monoamine oxidase) **(Fig. 15.15)**. By the action of COMT, epinephrine and norepinephrine are converted to metanephrine and normetanephrine, respectively. Both these products are further acted upon by MAO to form vanillylmandelic acid (VMA) and MOPG (3-methoxy-4-hydroxyphenylglycol) **(Fig. 15.16)**. These products are further excreted in urine. Epinephrine and norepinephrine can be acted upon directly also by MAO to form DOPG and DOMA. The excretory products are increased in pheochromocytoma and that forms the basis for the diagnostic test.

Adrenergic Receptors and Mechanism of Action

The physiological effects of epinephrine and norepinephrine are initiated by their binding to adrenergic receptors on the surface of target cells. These receptors are prototypical examples of seven-pass transmembrane proteins that are coupled to G proteins, which stimulate or inhibit intracellular signaling pathways.

Complex physiological responses result from adrenal medullary stimulation because there are multiple receptor types, which are differentially expressed in different tissues and cells. The alpha- and beta-adrenergic receptors and their subtypes were originally defined by differential binding of various agonists and antagonists and, more recently, by analysis of molecular clones.

Receptor	*Effectively binds*	*Effect of ligand binding*
Alpha-1	Epinephrine, norepinephrine	Increased free calcium
Alpha-2	Epinephrine, norepinephrine	Decreased cyclic AMP
Beta-1	Epinephrine, norepinephrine	Increased cyclic AMP
Beta-2	Epinephrine	Increased cyclic AMP

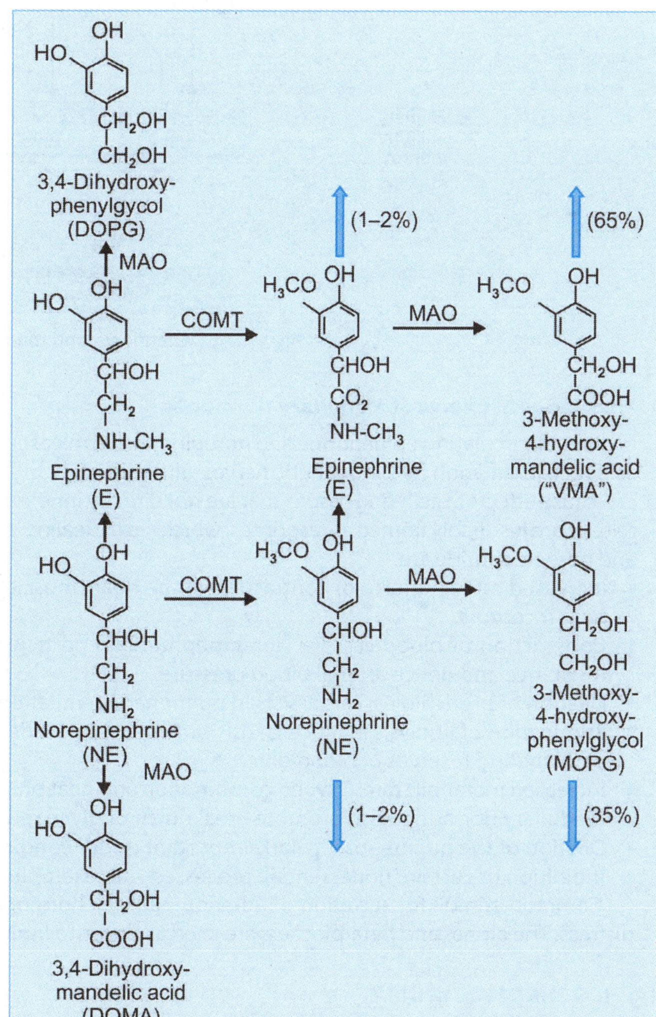

Fig. 15.15: Steps of degradation of catecholamines.

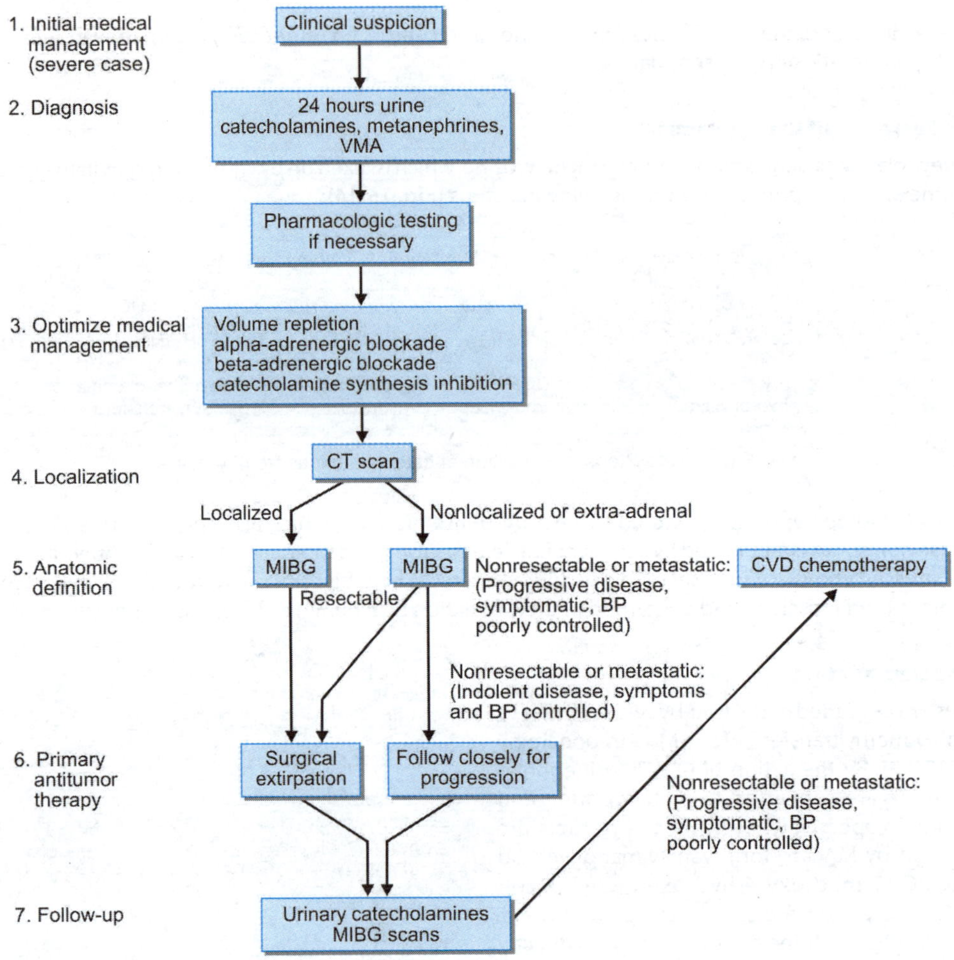

Fig. 15.16: Diagnosis and management of pheochromocytoma.

Physiological Effects of Medullary Hormones

In general, circulating epinephrine and norepinephrine released from the adrenal medulla have the same effects on target organs as direct stimulation by sympathetic nerves, although their effect is longer lasting. Additionally, of course, circulating hormones can cause effects in cells and tissues that are not directly innervated. The physiological consequences of medullary catecholamine release are justifiably framed as responses, which aid in dealing with stress. A listing of some major effects mediated by epinephrine and norepinephrine are:

- Increased rate and force of contraction of the heart muscle: This is predominantly an effect of epinephrine acting through beta receptors.
- Constriction of blood vessels: Norepinephrine, in particular, causes widespread vasoconstriction, resulting in increased resistance and hence arterial blood pressure.
- Dilation of bronchioles: This assists in pulmonary ventilation.
- Stimulation of lipolysis in fat cells: This provides fatty acids for energy production in many tissues and aids in conservation of dwindling reserves of blood glucose.
- Increased metabolic rate: Oxygen consumption and heat production increase throughout the body in response to epinephrine. Medullary hormones also promote breakdown of glycogen in skeletal muscle to provide glucose for energy production.
- Dilation of the pupils—particularly important under conditions of low ambient light.
- Inhibition of certain "nonessential" processes—an example is inhibition of gastrointestinal secretion and motor activity.

Common stimuli for secretion of adrenomedullary hormones include exercise, hypoglycemia, hemorrhage, and emotional distress. The alpha- and beta-blockers are used as drugs to inhibit the action of catecholamines.

PHEOCHROMOCYTOMA

Incidence

Pheochromocytoma is estimated to occur in 2–8 out of 1 million persons per year, and about 0.1% of hypertensive patients harbor a pheochromocytoma. The mean age at diagnosis is about 40 years, although the tumors can occur from early childhood until late in life. The "rule of tens" for pheochromocytomas states that about 10% are bilateral, 10% are extra-adrenal, and 10% are malignant. However, these percentages are higher in the inherited syndromes.

Inheritance

Up to 25% of pheochromocytomas may be familial. These tumors may arise sporadically or be inherited as features of multiple endocrine neoplasia Type 2 or several other pheochromocytoma-associated syndromes.

Etiology and Pathogenesis

Pheochromocytomas and paragangliomas are well-vascularized tumors that arise from cells derived from the sympathetic (e.g., adrenal medulla) or parasympathetic (e.g., carotid body, glomus vagale) paraganglia. The name pheochromocytoma reflects the black-colored staining caused by chromaffin oxidation of catecholamines. Although a variety of nomenclatures have been used to describe these tumors, most clinicians use the term pheochromocytoma to describe symptomatic catecholamine-producing tumors, including those located in extra-adrenal retroperitoneal, pelvic, and thoracic sites. The term paragangliomas is used to describe catecholamine-producing tumors in the head and neck, as well as tumors that arise from the parasympathetic nervous system, which may secrete little or no catecholamines. The etiology of most sporadic pheochromocytomas and paragangliomas is unknown.

Mutations of the genes VHL, RET, NF1, SDHB, and SDHD are all known to cause familial pheochromocytoma/extra-adrenal paragangliomas.

Pheochromocytoma is a tumor of the multiple endocrine neoplasia syndrome, Type IIA (also known as MEN-IIA) and Type IIB (MEN-IIB). The other component neoplasms of that syndrome include parathyroid adenomas, and medullary thyroid cancer. Mutations in the autosomal RET proto-oncogene drives these malignancies.

MEN-IIA also presents with hyperparathyroidism, while MEN-IIB also presents with mucosal neuroma.

Clinical Features

The clinical presentation is so variable that pheochromocytoma has been termed **"the great masquerader". Among the presenting symptoms, episodes of palpitations, headaches, and profuse sweating are typical and constitute a classic triad.** The presence of all the three symptoms, in association with hypertension, makes pheochromocytoma a likely diagnosis. On the other hand, a pheochromocytoma can be asymptomatic for years, and some tumors have grown to a considerable size before patients noted symptoms.

The signs and symptoms of a pheochromocytoma are those of sympathetic nervous system hyperactivity, including:

- Pain abdomen
- Pallor
- Nausea
- Weakness
- Tachycardia
- Hypertension, including paroxysmal (sporadic, episodic) high blood pressure, which sometimes can be more difficult to detect; another clue to the presence of pheochromocytoma is orthostatic hypotension (a fall in systolic blood pressure greater than 20 mm Hg or a fall in diastolic blood pressure greater than 10 mm Hg on making the patient stand).
- Palpitations
- Anxiety often resembling that of a panic attack
- Diaphoresis
- Headaches
- Polyurea
- Weight loss
- Localized amyloid deposits found microscopically
- Hypercalcemia
- Dilated cardiomyopathy
- Elevated blood glucose level [due primarily to catecholamine stimulation of lipolysis (breakdown of stored fat) leading to high levels of free fatty acids and the subsequent inhibition of glucose uptake by muscle cells. Further, stimulation of beta-adrenergic receptors leads to glycogenolysis and gluconeogenesis and thus elevation of blood glucose levels].
- A pheochromocytoma can also cause resistant arterial hypertension. A pheochromocytoma can be fatal, if it causes malignant hypertension, or severely high blood pressure. This hypertension is not well controlled with standard blood pressure medications.
- **Catecholamine crisis** can lead to heart failure, pulmonary edema, arrhythmias, and intracranial hemorrhage. During episodes of hormone release, which can occur at very divergent intervals, patients are anxious and pale, and they experience tachycardia and palpitations. These paroxysms generally last less than an hour and may be precipitated by surgery, positional changes, exercise, pregnancy, urination (particularly bladder pheochromocytoma), and various medications (e.g., tricyclic antidepressants, opiates, metoclopramide).

Diagnosis

The diagnosis is based on documentation of catecholamine excess by biochemical testing and localization of the tumor by imaging. Both are of equal importance, although measurement of catecholamines is traditionally the first step.

Biochemical Testing

Pheochromocytomas and paragangliomas synthesize and store catecholamines, which include norepinephrine (noradrenaline), epinephrine (adrenaline), and dopamine. Elevated plasma and urinary levels of catecholamines and the methylated metabolites, metanephrines, are the cornerstone for the diagnosis. The hormonal activity of tumors fluctuates, resulting in considerable variation in serial catecholamine measurements. Thus, there is some value in obtaining tests during or soon after a symptomatic crisis. On the other hand, most tumors continuously leak O-methylated metabolites, which are detected by metanephrines measurements.

Catecholamines and metanephrines can be measured using many different methods (e.g., high-performance liquid chromatography, enzyme-linked immunosorbent assay, and other immunoassays). In a clinical context suspicious for pheochromocytoma, when values are increased two to three times the upper limit of normal, a pheochromocytoma is highly likely, regardless of the assay used, assuming an appropriate clinical context.

1. **24-hour urinary tests for VMA,** metanephrines (total or fractionated), and catecholamines are widely available and commonly used for initial testing. Among these tests, the fractionated metanephrines and catecholamines are the most sensitive.
2. Plasma tests are more convenient and include measurements of catecholamines, metanephrines, and chromogranin A, a secretory product of endocrine cells. Plasma metanephrine measurements are most sensitive and are less susceptible to false-positive elevations from stress, including venipuncture.

   Care should be taken to rule out other causes of adrenergic (adrenalin-like) excess, such as hypoglycemia, stress, exercise, and drugs affecting the catecholamines, such as stimulants, methyldopa, dopamine agonists, or ganglion-blocking antihypertensives.

   The pattern of catecholamines can help in localizing the tumor, as epinephrine is virtually never increased in extra-adrenal pheochromocytomas.
3. **Pharmacologic tests,, such as the phentolamine test, the glucagon provocation test, and the clonidine suppression test, are of relatively low sensitivity and are rarely used.**

Diagnostic Imaging

A variety of methods have been used to localize pheochromocytomas and paragangliomas. CT and MRI are similar in sensitivity. CT should be performed with contrast. T2-weighted MRI with gadolinium contrast is optimal for detecting pheochromocytomas and is somewhat better than CT for imaging extra-adrenal pheochromocytomas and paragangliomas. About 5% of adrenal incidentalomas, usually detected by CT or MRI, prove to be pheochromocytomas after endocrinologic evaluation.

Tumors can also be localized using radioactive tracers including ^{131}I- or ^{123}I-metaiodobenzylguanidine (MIBG), ^{111}In-somatostatin analogs, or ^{18}F-dopa (or dopamine) positron-emission tomography (PET). Because these agents exhibit selective uptake in paragangliomas, nuclear imaging is particularly useful in the hereditary syndromes.

Differential Diagnosis

The differential diagnosis of pheochromocytoma includes:

- Anxiety disorders
- Paragangliomas
- Essential hypertension
- Hyperthyroidism
- Insulinoma
- Paroxysmal supraventricular tachycardia
- Renovascular hypertension
- Carcinoid
- When an asymptomatic adrenal mass is identified, likely diagnoses other than pheochromocytoma include a nonfunctioning adrenal adenoma, aldosteronomas, and cortisol-producing adenoma (Cushing's syndrome).

Treatment

Surgery

Surgical resection of the tumor is the treatment of first choice, either by open laparotomy or else laparoscopy. Given the complexity of preoperative management, and the potential for catastrophic intra- and postoperative complications, such surgery should be performed only at centers experienced in the management of this disorder. In addition to the surgical expertise that such centers can provide, they will also have the necessary endocrine and anesthesia resources. It may also be necessary to carry out adrenalectomy, a complete surgical removal of the affected adrenal gland(s).

Either surgical option requires prior treatment with the nonspecific and irreversible alpha-adrenoceptor blocker—phenoxybenzamine. Doing so permits the surgery to proceed while minimizing the likelihood of severe intraoperative hypertension (as might occur when the tumor is manipulated). Some authorities would recommend that a combined alpha-/beta-blocker, such as labetalol also be given in order to slow the heart rate. Regardless, a "pure" beta-blocker, such as atenolol must never be used in the presence of a pheochromocytoma due to the risk of such treatment leading to unopposed alpha agonism and, thus, severe and potentially refractory hypertension.

The patient with pheochromocytoma is invariably volume depleted. In other words, the chronically elevated adrenergic state characteristic of an untreated pheochromocytoma leads to near-total inhibition of renin–angiotensin activity, resulting in excessive fluid loss in the urine and thus reduced blood volume. Hence, once the pheochromocytoma has been resected, thereby removing the major source of circulating catecholamines, a situation arises where there is both very low sympathetic activity and volume depletion. This can result in profound hypotension. Therefore, it is usually advised to "salt load" pheochromocytoma patients before their surgery. This may consist of simple interventions, such as consumption of high salt food preoperatively, direct salt replacement or through the administration of intravenous saline solution.

Treatment of malignant pheochromocytoma or paragangliomas is challenging. Options include tumor mass reduction, alpha-blockers for symptoms, chemotherapy, and nuclear medicine radiotherapy.

Prognosis

Both malignant and benign pheochromocytomas can recur after surgery. The statistics vary from one study to the next but recurrence rates average around 10%. Therefore, long-term follow-up after surgery is very important.

CLINICAL NOTE

Among the presenting symptoms, episodes of palpitations, headaches, and profuse sweating are typical and constitute a classic triad.

CLINICAL PEARLS

1. Pheochromocytomas and paragangliomas are catecholamine-producing tumors derived from the sympathetic or parasympathetic nervous system.
2. Among the presenting symptoms, episodes of palpitations, headaches, and profuse sweating are typical and constitute a classic triad. The presence of all the three symptoms, in association with hypertension, makes pheochromocytoma a likely diagnosis.
3. Elevated plasma and urinary levels of catecholamines and the methylated metabolites, metanephrines, are the cornerstone for the diagnosis.
4. Complete tumor removal is the ultimate therapeutic goal.
5. Preoperative patient preparation is essential for safe surgery.

CASE STUDY 14

Theme: Causes, Clinical Implications, Diagnosis, and Treatment of Type 1 Diabetes Mellitus

A 10-year-old female presented to the clinic with an approximate 10 lb weight loss over the last few weeks, nausea, increased thirst, and urination. She denied abdominal pain. Her father was having Type 1 DM from the last 14 years and one cousin was also diagnosed with Type 1 DM at age of 18 months.

Physical examination revealed a thin, white female in no acute distress. Mucous membranes were dry. Rest of physical examination was normal. Laboratory studies revealed:

Random blood sugar	*411*	*(70–150 mg/dL)*
BUN	24	(7–20)
Sodium	129	(135–145)
Chloride	93	(96–110)
Potassium	5.4	(3.5–5.0)
Bicarbonate	23	(21–28)
pCO_2	23	(24–32)
Serum ketones	Positive	(Negative)
WBC	11,600	(5,000–10,000)

What is your diagnosis and plan for this patient?
What further testing is required to confirm your diagnosis?

CASE DETAILS

The patient is suffering from Type 1 diabetes mellitus with ketoacidosis. Age of the patient, family history, clinical symptoms, hyperglycemia, low sodium and bicarbonates, low pCO2 and the presence of ketones, all are suggestive of diagnosis of diabetes mellitus (Type1) with ketoacidosis.

DIABETES MELLITUS

Diabetes mellitus is a syndrome with disordered metabolism and inappropriate hyperglycemia due to either a deficiency of insulin secretion or to a combination of insulin resistance and inadequate insulin secretion to compensate. Type 1 diabetes is due to pancreatic islet B cell destruction predominantly by an autoimmune process, and these patients are prone to ketoacidosis. Type 2 diabetes is the more prevalent form and results from insulin resistance with a defect in compensatory insulin secretion.

BASIC CONCEPT

Insulin Biosynthesis, Secretion, and Action

Biosynthesis

Insulin is produced in the beta cells of the pancreatic islets. It is initially synthesized as a single-chain 86-amino-acid precursor polypeptide, preproinsulin. Subsequent proteolytic processing removes the amino terminal signal peptide, giving rise to proinsulin. Proinsulin is structurally related to insulin-like growth factors I and II, which bind weakly to the insulin receptor. Cleavage of an internal 31-residue fragment from proinsulin generates the C peptide and the A (21 amino acids) and B (30 amino acids) chains of insulin, which are connected by disulfide bonds. The mature insulin molecule and C peptide are stored together and cosecreted from secretory granules in the beta cells. Because the C peptide is cleared more slowly than insulin, it is a useful marker of insulin secretion and allows discrimination of endogenous and exogenous sources of insulin in the evaluation of hypoglycemia.

Secretion

Glucose is the key regulator of insulin secretion by the pancreatic beta cell, although amino acids, ketones, various nutrients, gastrointestinal peptides, and neurotransmitters also influence insulin secretion. Glucose levels >3.9 mmol/L (70 mg/dL) stimulate insulin synthesis, primarily by enhancing protein translation and processing. Glucose stimulation of insulin secretion begins with its transport into the beta cell by the GLUT2 glucose transporter. Glucose phosphorylation by glucokinase is the rate-limiting step that controls glucose-regulated insulin secretion. Further metabolism of glucose-6-phosphate via glycolysis generates ATP, which inhibits the activity of an ATP-sensitive K^+ channel. This channel consists of two separate proteins: one is the binding site for certain oral hypoglycemic (e.g., sulfonylureas, meglitinides), and the other is an inwardly rectifying K^+ channel protein. Inhibition of this K^+ channel induces beta cell membrane depolarization, which opens voltage-dependent calcium channels (leading to an influx of calcium), and stimulates insulin secretion **(Fig. 15.17)**.

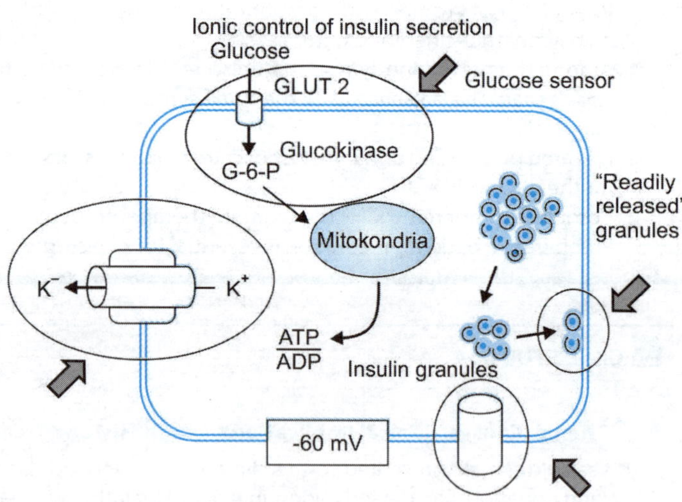

Fig. 15.17: Mechanism of secretion of insulin.

Insulin secretory profiles reveal a pulsatile pattern of hormone release, with small secretory bursts occurring about every 10 minutes, superimposed upon greater amplitude oscillations of about 80–150 minutes. Incretins are released from neuroendocrine cells of the gastrointestinal tract following food ingestion and amplify glucose-stimulated insulin secretion and suppress glucagon secretion. Glucagon-like peptide 1 (GLP-1), the most potent incretin, is released from L cells in the small intestine and that stimulates insulin secretion only when the blood glucose is above the fasting level. **Incretin analogs,, such as exenatide, are being used to enhance endogenous insulin secretion.**

Action

Once insulin is secreted into the portal venous system, ~50% is degraded by the liver. Unextracted insulin enters the systemic circulation where it binds to receptors in target sites. Insulin binding to its receptor stimulates intrinsic tyrosine kinase activity

(Fig. 15.18), leading to receptor autophosphorylation and the recruitment of intracellular signaling molecules,, such as insulin receptor substrates (IRS). IRS and other adaptor proteins initiate a complex cascade of phosphorylation and dephosphorylation reactions, resulting in the widespread metabolic and mitogenic effects of insulin. As an example, activation of the phosphatidylinositol-3′-kinase (Pi-3-kinase) pathway stimulates translocation of glucose transporters (e.g., GLUT4) to the cell surface, an event that is crucial for glucose uptake by skeletal muscle and fat. Activation of other insulin receptor signaling pathways induces glycogen synthesis, protein synthesis, lipogenesis, and regulation of various genes in insulin-responsive cells.

Glucose homeostasis reflects a balance between hepatic glucose production and peripheral glucose uptake and utilization. Insulin is the most important regulator of this metabolic equilibrium, but neural input, metabolic signals, and other hormones (e.g., glucagon) result in integrated control of glucose supply and utilization.

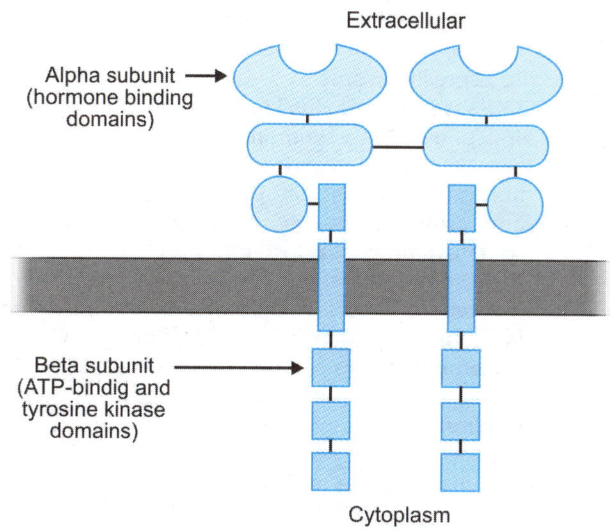

Fig. 15.18: Insulin receptor.

In the fasting state, low-insulin levels increase glucose production by promoting hepatic gluconeogenesis and glycogenolysis and reduce glucose uptake in insulin-sensitive tissues (skeletal muscle and fat), thereby promoting mobilization of stored precursors, such as amino acids and free fatty acids (lipolysis). Glucagon, secreted by pancreatic alpha cells when blood glucose or insulin levels are low, stimulates glycogenolysis and gluconeogenesis by the liver and renal medulla.

Postprandially, the glucose load elicits a rise in insulin and fall in glucagon, leading to a reversal of these processes. Insulin, an anabolic hormone, promotes the storage of carbohydrate and fat and protein synthesis. The major portion of postprandial glucose is utilized by skeletal muscle, an effect of insulin-stimulated glucose uptake. Other tissues, most notably the brain, utilize glucose in an insulin-independent fashion.

DIABETES MELLITUS

Classification

Several distinct types of DM exist and are caused by a complex interaction of genetics and environmental factors. Depending on the etiology of the DM, factors contributing to hyperglycemia include reduced insulin secretion, decreased glucose utilization, and increased glucose production.

Classification of Diabetes Mellitus

Diabetes mellitus (DM) is classified on the basis of the pathogenic process that leads to hyperglycemia, as opposed to earlier criteria, such as age of onset or type of therapy. The two broad categories of DM are designated Type 1 and Type 2. Both types of diabetes are preceded by a phase of abnormal glucose homeostasis as the pathogenic processes progresses.

Etiological Classification of Diabetes Mellitus

I. **Type 1 diabetes** (β-cell destruction, usually leading to absolute insulin deficiency).
   A. Immune-mediated
   B. Idiopathic
II. **Type 2 diabetes** (may range from predominantly insulin resistance with relative insulin deficiency to a predominantly insulin secretory defect with insulin resistance).
III. **Other specific types of diabetes:**
   A. Genetic defects of β-cell function characterized by mutations in:
      1. Hepatocyte nuclear transcription factor (HNF) 4 α (MODY 1)
      2. Glucokinase (MODY 2)
      3. HNF-1α (MODY 3)
      4. Insulin promoter factor-1 (IPF-1; MODY 4)
      5. HNF-1β (MODY 5)
      6. NEUROD1 (MODY 6)
      7. Mitochondrial DNA
      8. Subunits of ATP-sensitive potassium channel
      9. Proinsulin or insulin conversion.

B. Genetic defects in insulin action:
   1. Type A insulin resistance
   2. Leprechaunism
   3. Rabson–Mendenhall syndrome
   4. Lipodystrophy syndromes

C. Diseases of the exocrine pancreas—pancreatitis, pancreatectomy, neoplasia, cystic fibrosis, hemochromatosis, fibrocalculous pancreatopathy, mutations in carboxyl ester lipase.

D. Endocrinopathies—acromegaly, Cushing's syndrome, glucagonoma, pheochromocytoma, hyperthyroidism, somatostatinoma, aldosteronomas.

E. Drug- or chemical-induced—vacor, pentamidine, nicotinic acid, glucocorticoids, thyroid hormone, diazoxide, β-adrenergic agonists, thiazides, phenytoin, α-interferon, protease inhibitors, clozapine.

F. Infections—congenital rubella, cytomegalovirus, coxsackie.

G. Uncommon forms of immune-mediated diabetes—"Stiff-person" syndrome, anti-insulin receptor antibodies.

H. Other genetic syndromes sometimes associated with diabetes—Down's syndrome, Klinefelter's syndrome, Turner's syndrome, Wolfram's syndrome, Friedreich's ataxia, Huntington's chorea, Laurence–Moon–Biedl syndrome, myotonic dystrophy, porphyria, and Prader–Willi syndrome.

IV. **Gestational diabetes mellitus (GDM).**

(MODY—maturity onset of diabetes of the young)

Source: Adapted from American Diabetes Association, 2007.

The terms insulin-dependent diabetes mellitus (IDDM) and noninsulin-dependent diabetes mellitus (NIDDM) are obsolete. Since, many individuals with Type 2 DM eventually require insulin treatment for control of glycemia. Age is not a criterion in the classification system. Although Type 1 DM most commonly develops before the age of 30, an autoimmune beta cell destructive process can develop at any age. It is estimated that between 5% and 10% of individuals who develop DM after age of 30 have Type 1 DM. Likewise, Type 2 DM more typically develops with increasing age, but is now being diagnosed more frequently in children and young adults, particularly in obese adolescents.

Etiology of Type 1 Diabetes

The global incidence of Type 1 diabetes is increasing (approximately 3% each year). This form of diabetes is immune-mediated in over 90% of cases and idiopathic in less than 10%. The rate of pancreatic B cell destruction is quite variable, being rapid in some individuals and slow in others.

Immune-mediated type 1 diabetes mellitus: Approximately, one-third of the disease susceptibility is due to genes and two-thirds to environmental factors.

Genes that are related to the HLA locus contribute about 40% of the genetic risk. About 95% of patients with Type 1 diabetes possess either *HLA-DR3* or *HLA-DR4*. *HLA-DQ* genes are even more specific markers of Type 1 susceptibility, since a particular variety *(HLA-DQB10302)* is found in the DR4 patients with Type 1, while a "protective" gene *(HLA-DQB10602)* is often present in the DR4 controls. The other important gene that contributes to about 10% of the genetic risk is found at the 5'polymorphic region of the insulin gene. This polymorphic region affects the expression of the insulin gene in the thymus and results in depletion of insulin-specific T lymphocytes. In linkage studies, 16 other genetic regions of the human genome have been identified as being important to pathogenesis but less is known about them.

Children of diabetic parents are at increased lifetime risk for developing Type 1 diabetes. A child whose mother has Type 1 diabetes has a 3% risk of developing the disease and a 6% risk if the child's father has it. The risk in siblings is related to the number of HLA haplotypes that the sibling shares with the diabetic parent. If one haplotype is shared, the risk is 6% and if two haplotypes are shared, the risk increases to 12–25%. The highest risk is for identical twins, where the concordance rate is 25–50%.

Some patients with a milder expression of Type 1 diabetes mellitus initially retain enough B cell function to avoid ketosis, but as their B cell mass diminishes later in life, dependence on insulin therapy develops. Up to 15% of "Type 2" diabetic patients may actually have this mild form of Type 1 diabetes (latent autoimmune diabetes of adulthood; LADA).

Which environmental factor is responsible for the increased risk is not known. There have been a number of different hypotheses including infections with certain viruses (rubella, Coxsackie B_4) and consumption of cow's milk. None of these factors has so far been confirmed as the culprit.

Types of Autoantibodies (Immunological Markers)

1. **Islet cell cytoplasmic antibodies:** The primary antibodies found in 90% of Type 1 diabetics are against islet cell cytoplasmic proteins (termed ICCA, islet cell cytoplasmic antibodies). In nondiabetics, ICCA frequency is only 0.5–4%. The presence of ICCA is a highly accurate predictor of future development of IDDM. ICCA are not specific for the β-cells and recognize antigens in other cell types in the islet. However, the autoimmune attack appears to selectively destroy β-cells. Therefore, the antibodies may play a primary role in the destruction of islet cells. It is an equally likely possibility that the production of anti-islet antibodies occurs as a result of the destruction of β-cells. Whether a direct cause or an effect of islet cell destruction, the titer of the ICCA tends to decline over time.

2. **Islet cell surface antibodies:** Autoantibodies directed against cell-surface antigens (ICSA) have also been described in as many as 80% of Type 1 diabetics. Similar to ICCA, the titer of ICSA declines over time. Some patients with Type 2 diabetes have been identified that are ICSA positive.
3. **Specific antigenic targets of islet cells:** Antibodies to glutamic acid decarboxylase (GAD) have been identified in over 80% of patients newly diagnosed with IDDM. Like ICCA, anti-GAD antibodies decline over time in Type 1 diabetics. The presence of anti-GAD antibodies is a strong predictor of the future development of IDDM in high-risk populations. Anti-insulin antibodies (IAA) have been identified in IDDM patients and in relatives at risk to develop IDDM. These IAA are detectable even before the onset of insulin therapy in Type 1 diabetics. IAA are detectable in around 40% of young children with IDDM.

Idiopathic Type 1 Diabetes Mellitus

Less than 10% of subjects have no evidence of pancreatic B cell autoimmunity to explain their insulinopenia and ketoacidosis. This subgroup has been classified as "idiopathic Type 1 diabetes" and designated as "Type 1B". Although only a minority of patients with Type 1 diabetes fall into this group, most of these are of Asian or African origin. It was recently reported that about 4% of the West Africans with ketosis-prone diabetes are homozygous for a mutation in PAX-4 (Arg133Trp)—a gene that is essential for the development of pancreatic islets.

Pathophysiology of Type 1 Diabetes

Although other islet cell types [alpha cells (glucagon-producing), delta cells (somatostatin-producing), or PP cells (pancreatic polypeptide-producing)] are functionally and embryologically similar to beta cells and express most of the same proteins as beta cells, they are inexplicably spared from the autoimmune process.

Pathologically, the pancreatic islets are infiltrated with lymphocytes (in a process termed insulitis). After all beta cells are destroyed, the inflammatory process abates, the islets become atrophic, and most immunologic markers disappear. The precise mechanisms of beta cell death are not known but may involve formation of nitric oxide metabolites, apoptosis, and direct $CD8^+$ T cell cytotoxicity. The islet destruction is mediated by T lymphocytes rather than islet autoantibodies, as these antibodies do not generally react with the cell surface of islet cells.

The autoimmune destruction of pancreatic β-cells leads to a deficiency of insulin secretion. It is this loss of insulin secretion that leads to the metabolic derangements associated with IDDM. In addition to the loss of insulin secretion, the function of pancreatic α-cells is also abnormal. There is excessive secretion of glucagon in IDDM patients. Normally, hyperglycemia leads to reduced glucagon secretion. However, in patients with IDDM, glucagon secretion is not suppressed by hyperglycemia. The resultant inappropriately elevated glucagon levels exacerbate the metabolic defects due to insulin deficiency. The most pronounced example of this metabolic disruption is that patients with IDDM rapidly develop diabetic ketoacidosis in the absence of insulin administration. If somatostatin is administered to suppress glucagon secretion, there is a concomitant suppression in the rise of glucose and ketone bodies. Particularly problematic for long-term IDDM patients is an impaired ability to secrete glucagon in response to hypoglycemia. This leads to potentially fatal hypoglycemia in response to insulin treatment in these patients.

Although insulin deficiency is the primary defect in IDDM, in patients with poorly controlled IDDM, there is also a defect in the ability of target tissues to respond to the administration of insulin. There are multiple biochemical mechanisms that account for this impairment of tissues to respond to insulin. Deficiency in insulin leads to elevated levels of free fatty acids in the plasma as a result of uncontrolled lipolysis in adipose tissue. Free fatty acids suppress glucose metabolism in peripheral tissues, such as skeletal muscle. This impairs the action of insulin in these tissues, i.e., the promotion of glucose utilization. Additionally, insulin deficiency decreases the expression of a number of genes necessary for target tissues to respond normally to insulin, such as glucokinase in liver and the GLUT4 class of glucose transporters in adipose tissue. The major metabolic derangements, which result from insulin deficiency in IDDM, are impaired glucose, lipid, and protein metabolism.

Glucose metabolism: Uncontrolled IDDM leads to increased hepatic glucose output. First, liver glycogen stores are mobilized then hepatic gluconeogenesis is used to produce glucose. Insulin deficiency also impairs nonhepatic tissue utilization of glucose. In particular in adipose tissue and skeletal muscle, insulin stimulates glucose uptake. This is accomplished by insulin-mediated movement of glucose transporter proteins to the plasma membrane of these tissues. Reduced glucose uptake by peripheral tissues in turn leads to a reduced rate of glucose metabolism. In addition, the level of hepatic glucokinase is regulated by insulin. Therefore, a reduced rate of glucose phosphorylation in hepatocytes leads to increased delivery to the blood. Other enzymes involved in anabolic metabolism of glucose are affected by insulin (primarily through covalent modifications). The combination of increased hepatic glucose production and reduced peripheral tissues metabolism leads to elevated plasma glucose levels. When the capacity of the kidneys to absorb glucose is surpassed, glycosuria ensues. **Glucose is an osmotic diuretic and an increase in renal loss of glucose is accompanied by loss of water and electrolytes, termed polyuria. The result of the loss of water (and overall volume) leads to the activation of the thirst mechanism (polydipsia). The negative caloric balance, which results from the glucosuria and tissue catabolism leads to an increase in appetite and food intake (polyphagia).**

Lipid metabolism: One major role of insulin is to stimulate the storage of food energy following the consumption of a meal. This energy storage is in the form of glycogen in hepatocytes and skeletal muscle. Additionally, insulin stimulates hepatocytes to synthesize triglycerides and storage of triglycerides in adipose tissue. In opposition to increased adipocyte storage of triglycerides is insulin-mediated inhibition of lipolysis. In uncontrolled IDDM, there is a rapid mobilization of triglycerides leading to increased levels of plasma-free fatty acids. The free fatty acids are taken up by numerous tissues (however, not the brain) and metabolized to provide energy. Free fatty acids are also taken up by the liver.

Normally, the levels of malonyl-CoA are high in the presence of insulin. These high levels of malonyl-CoA inhibit carnitine palmitoyltransferase I, the enzyme required for the transport of fatty acyl-CoAs into the mitochondria where they are subject to oxidation for energy production. Thus, in the absence of insulin, malonyl-CoA levels fall and transport of fatty acyl-CoAs into the mitochondria increases. Mitochondrial oxidation of fatty acids generates acetyl-CoA, which can be further oxidized in the TCA cycle. However, in hepatocytes the majority of the acetyl-CoA is not oxidized by the TCA cycle, but is metabolized into the ketone bodies, acetoacetate and β-hydroxybutyrate. These ketone bodies leave the liver and are used for energy production by the brain, heart, and skeletal muscle. **In IDDM, the increased availability of free fatty acids and ketone bodies exacerbates the reduced utilization of glucose furthering the ensuing hyperglycemia.** Production of ketone bodies, in excess of the body's ability to utilize them, leads to ketoacidosis. In diabetics, this can be easily diagnosed by smelling the breath. **A spontaneous breakdown product of acetoacetate is acetone, which is volatilized by the lungs producing a distinctive odor.**

Normally, plasma triglycerides are acted upon by lipoprotein lipase (LPL), an enzyme on the surface of the endothelial cells lining the vessels. In particular, LPL activity allows fatty acids to be taken from circulating triglycerides for storage in adipocytes. **The activity of LPL requires insulin and, in its absence, a hypertriglyceridemia results.**

Protein metabolism: Insulin regulates the synthesis of many genes, either positively or negatively, that then affect overall metabolism. Insulin has a global effect on protein metabolism, increasing the rate of protein synthesis and decreasing the rate of protein degradation. Thus, insulin deficiency will lead to increased catabolism of protein. The increased rate of proteolysis leads to elevated concentrations in plasma amino acids. These amino acids serve as precursors for hepatic and renal gluconeogenesis. In liver, the increased gluconeogenesis further contributes to the hyperglycemia seen in IDDM.

SYMPTOMS AND SIGNS

Type 1 diabetes

1. **Polyuria:** Increased urination is a consequence of osmotic diuresis secondary to sustained hyperglycemia. This results in a loss of glucose as well as free water and electrolytes in the urine.
2. Thirst (polydipsia) is a consequence of the hyperosmolar state, as is blurred vision, which often develops as the lenses are exposed to hyperosmolar fluids.
3. Weight loss despite normal or increased appetite is a common feature of Type 1 when it develops subacutely. The weight loss is initially due to depletion of water, glycogen, and triglycerides; thereafter, reduced muscle mass occurs as amino acids are diverted to form glucose and ketone bodies.
4. Lowered plasma volume produces symptoms of postural hypotension. Total body potassium loss and the general catabolism of muscle protein contribute to the weakness.
5. Paresthesias may be present at the time of diagnosis, particularly when the onset is subacute. They reflect a temporary dysfunction of peripheral sensory nerves, which clears as insulin replacement restores glycemic levels closer to normal, suggesting neurotoxicity from sustained hyperglycemia. When absolute insulin deficiency is of acute onset, the above symptoms develop abruptly.
6. Ketoacidosis exacerbates the dehydration and hyperosmolality by producing anorexia and nausea and vomiting, interfering with oral fluid replacement. The patient's level of consciousness can vary depending on the degree of hyperosmolality. When insulin deficiency develops relatively slowly and sufficient water intake is maintained, patients remain relatively alert and physical findings may be minimal. When vomiting occurs in response to worsening ketoacidosis, dehydration progresses and compensatory mechanisms become inadequate to keep serum osmolality below 320–330 mOsm/L. Under these circumstances, stupor or even coma may occur. The fruity breath odor of acetone further suggests the diagnosis of diabetic ketoacidosis.
7. Hypotension in the recumbent position is a serious prognostic sign.
8. Loss of subcutaneous fat and muscle wasting are features of more slowly developing insulin deficiency. In occasional patients with slow, insidious onset of insulin deficiency, subcutaneous fat may be considerably depleted.

Laboratory Findings

Urinalysis

a. **Glycosuria:** Glycosuria allows for a good first-line screening test for diabetes mellitus. Normally, glucose does not appear in urine until the plasma glucose rises above 10 mmol/L or more. But in certain individuals due to low renal threshold, glucose may be present despite normal blood glucose levels. Conversely renal threshold increases with age so many diabetics may not have glycosuria despite high blood sugar levels.

   A specific and convenient method to detect glucosuria is the paper strip impregnated with glucose oxidase and a chromogen system (Clinistix, Diastix), which is sensitive to as little as 0.1% glucose in urine. Diastix can be directly applied to the urinary stream, and differing color responses of the indicator strip reflect glucose concentration.

   A normal renal threshold for glucose as well as reliable bladder emptying is essential for interpretation.

b. **Ketonuria:** Qualitative detection of ketone bodies can be accomplished by nitroprusside tests (Acetest or Ketostix). Although these tests do not detect beta-hydroxybutyric acid, which lacks a ketone group, the semiquantitative estimation of ketonuria thus obtained is nonetheless usually adequate for clinical purposes. Ketone bodies may be present in normal subject as a result of simple prolonged fasting.

c. **Microalbuminuria:** It may be defined as an albumin excretion rate intermediate between normality (2.5–25 mg/day) and macroalbuminuria (250 mg/day). The small increase in urinary albumin excretion is not detected by simple albumin stick tests and requires confirmation by careful quantization in a 24 hours urine specimen. The importance of microalbuminuria in the diabetic patient is that it is a signal of early reversible renal damage. Performing an albumin-to-creatinine ratio is probably easiest.

Unlike Type 1 diabetes mellitus, in which microalbuminuria is a good indicator of early kidney damage, microalbuminuria is a common finding (even at diagnosis) in Type 2 diabetes mellitus and is a risk factor for macrovascular (especially coronary heart) disease. It is a weaker predictor for future kidney disease in Type 2 diabetes mellitus.

Blood Testing Procedures

a. Glucose tolerance test

Methodology and normal fasting glucose: Plasma or serum from venous blood samples has the advantage over whole blood of providing values for glucose that are independent of hematocrit and that reflect the glucose concentration to which body tissues are exposed. For these reasons, and because plasma and serum are more readily measured on automated equipment, they are used in most laboratories. If serum is used or if plasma is collected from tubes that lack an agent to block glucose metabolism (such as fluoride), samples should be refrigerated and separated within 1 hour after collection. The glucose concentration is 10–15% higher in plasma or serum than in whole blood because structural components of blood cells are absent.

Fasting blood glucose: Fasting blood glucose is measured after an overnight fast of 10 hours. Fasting blood glucose estimation is better than random blood glucose. (1) FPG <5.6 mmol/L (100 mg/dL) is considered normal; (2) FPG = 5.6–6.9 mmol/L (100–125 mg/dL) is defined as IFG; and (3) FPG >7.0 mmol/L (126 mg/dL) warrants the diagnosis of DM.

Criteria for laboratory confirmation of diabetes mellitus: If the fasting plasma glucose level is 126 mg/dL or higher on more than one occasion, further evaluation of the patient with a glucose challenge is unnecessary. However, when fasting plasma glucose is less than 126 mg/dL in suspected cases, a standardized oral glucose tolerance test may be done.

75 g of glucose dissolved in 300 mL of water is given after an overnight fast to a person who has been receiving at least 150–200 g of carbohydrate daily for 3 days before the test. The data is interpreted in **Table 15.1**.

For proper evaluation of the test, the subjects should be normally active and free from acute illness. Medications that may impair glucose tolerance include diuretics, contraceptive drugs, glucocorticoids, niacin, and phenytoin should be avoided on that day.

Random blood glucose: Random is defined as without regard to time since the last meal. RBG measurement is required only during emergency. The current criteria for the diagnosis of DM emphasize that the FPG is the most reliable and convenient test for identifying DM in asymptomatic individuals. A random plasma glucose concentration >11.1 mmol/L (200 mg/dL) accompanied by classic symptoms of DM (polyuria, polydipsia, and weight loss) is sufficient for the diagnosis of DM.

TABLE 15.1: The Diabetes Expert Committee criteria for evaluating the standard oral glucose tolerance test.

Normal glucose tolerance		*Impaired glucose tolerance*	*Diabetes mellitus*
Fasting plasma glucose (mg/dL)	<110	110–125	>126
Two hours after glucose load	<140	140–199	>200

b. **Glycated hemoglobin (HbA1c) measurements:** Hemoglobin becomes glycated by ketoamine reactions between glucose and other sugars and the free amino groups on the alpha and beta chains. Only glycation of the N-terminal valine of the beta chain imparts sufficient negative charge to the hemoglobin molecule to allow separation by charge-dependent techniques. These charge-separated hemoglobins are collectively referred to as hemoglobin A1 (HbA1). The major form of HbA1 is hemoglobin A1c (HbA1c) where glucose is the carbohydrate. HbA1c comprises 4–6% of total hemoglobin A1. The remaining HbA1 species contain fructose 1,6-bisphosphate (HbA1a1), glucose-6-phosphate (HbA1a2), and unknown carbohydrate moiety (HbA1b). The hemoglobin A1c fraction is abnormally elevated in diabetic persons with chronic hyperglycemia.

Methods for measuring HbA1c include electrophoresis, cation-exchange chromatography, boronate affinity chromatography, and immunoassays. Office-based immunoassays using capillary blood give a result in about 9 minutes and this allows for immediate feedback to the patients regarding their glycemic control.

Since glycohemoglobins circulate within red blood cells whose lifespan lasts up to 120 days, they generally reflect the state of glycemia over the preceding 8–12 weeks, thereby providing an improved method of assessing diabetic control. Measurements should be made in patients with either type of diabetes mellitus at 3–4-month intervals, so that adjustments in therapy can be made.

In patients monitoring their own blood glucose levels, HbA1c values provide a valuable check on the accuracy of monitoring.

Use of HbA1c for screening is controversial. Sensitivity in detecting known diabetes cases by HbA1c measurements is only 85%, indicating that diabetes cannot be excluded by a normal value. On the other hand, elevated HbA1c assays are fairly specific (91%) in identifying the presence of diabetes.

The accuracy of HbA1c values can be affected by hemoglobin variants or derivatives; the effect depends on the specific hemoglobin variant or derivative and the specific assay used. Immunoassays that use an antibody to the glycated amino terminus of beta globin do not recognize the terminus of the gamma globin of hemoglobin F. Thus, in patients with high levels of hemoglobin F, immunoassays give falsely low values of HbA1c. Cation-exchange chromatography separates hemoglobin species by charge differences. Hemoglobin variants that coelute with HbA1c can lead to an overestimation of the HbA1c value. Chemically modified derivatives of hemoglobin, such as carbamoylation (in renal failure) or acetylation (high-dose aspirin therapy) can similarly coelute with HbA1c by some assay methods.

Any condition that shortens erythrocyte survival or decreases mean erythrocyte age (e.g., recovery from acute blood loss, hemolytic anemia) will falsely lower HbA1c irrespective of the assay method used. Alternative methods, such as fructosamine should be considered for these patients. Vitamins C and E are reported to falsely lower test results possibly by inhibiting glycation of hemoglobin.

c. **Serum fructosamine:** Serum fructosamine is formed by nonenzymatic glycosylation of serum proteins (predominantly albumin). Since serum albumin has a much shorter half-life than hemoglobin, serum fructosamine generally reflects the state of glycemic control for only the preceding 1–2 weeks. Reductions in serum albumin (e.g., nephrotic state or hepatic disease) will lower the serum fructosamine value. When abnormal hemoglobins or hemolytic states affect the interpretation of glycohemoglobins or when a narrower time frame is required,, such as for ascertaining glycemic control at the time of conception in a diabetic woman who has recently become pregnant, serum fructosamine assays offer some advantage. Normal values vary in relation to the serum albumin concentration and are 1.5–2.4 mmol/L when the serum albumin level is 5 g/dL.

d. **Self-monitoring of blood glucose:** Capillary blood glucose measurements performed by patients themselves, as outpatients, are extremely useful. In Type 1 patients, in whom "tight" metabolic control is attempted, they are indispensable. There are several paper strip (glucose oxidase, glucose dehydrogenase, or hexokinase) methods for measuring glucose on capillary blood samples. A reflectance photometer or an amperometric system is then used to measure the reaction that takes place on the reagent strip.

e. **Lipid profile:** Circulating lipoproteins are just as dependent on insulin as is the plasma glucose. In Type 1 diabetes, moderately deficient control of hyperglycemia is associated with only a slight elevation of LDL cholesterol and serum triglycerides and little if any change in HDL cholesterol. Once the hyperglycemia is corrected, lipoprotein levels are generally normal. However, in obese patients with Type 2 diabetes, a distinct "diabetic dyslipidemia" is characteristic of the insulin resistance syndrome. Its features are a high-serum triglyceride level (300–400 mg/dL), a low HDL cholesterol (less than 30 mg/dL), and a qualitative change in LDL particles, producing a smaller dense particle whose membrane carries supranormal amounts of free cholesterol. These smaller dense LDL particles are more susceptible to oxidation, which renders them more atherogenic. Since a low HDL cholesterol is a major feature predisposing to macrovascular disease, the term "dyslipidemia" has preempted the term "hyperlipidemia", which mainly denoted the elevated triglycerides. Measures designed to correct the obesity and hyperglycemia,, such as exercise, diet, and hypoglycemic therapy, are the treatment of choice for diabetic dyslipidemia, and in occasional patients in whom normal weight was achieved, all features of the lipoprotein abnormalities cleared.

f. **Additional tests:** In addition to the standard laboratory evaluation, the patient should be screened for DM-associated conditions (e.g., kidney, liver, and thyroid dysfunction). Individuals at high risk for cardiovascular disease should be screened for asymptomatic CAD by appropriate cardiac stress testing, when indicated.

The classification of the type of DM may be facilitated by laboratory assessments. Serum insulin or C-peptide measurements do not always distinguish Type 1 from Type 2 DM, but a low C-peptide level confirms a patient's need for insulin. Many individuals with new-onset Type 1 DM retain some C-peptide production.

Insulin levels generally are high early in the course of Type 2 diabetes mellitus and gradually wane over time. Stimulated C-peptide concentrations (after a standard meal challenge, such as sustacal or after glucagon) are somewhat preserved until late in the course of Type 2 diabetes mellitus. Absence of a C-peptide response to carbohydrate ingestion may indicate total beta cell failure.

Measurement of islet cell antibodies at the time of diabetes onset may be useful, if the type of DM is not clear based on the characteristics described above. Antibodies to insulin, islet cells, or glutamic acid decarboxylase (GAD) are absent in Type 2 diabetes mellitus.

Latent autoimmune diabetes of adults, or LADA, is a form of slow-onset Type 1 diabetes that occurs in middle-aged (usually white) adults. It can be differentiated from Type 2 diabetes by measuring anti-GAD65 antibodies. Such patients may respond to insulin secretagogue for a brief period (months).

DIFFERENTIAL DIAGNOSIS

Hyperglycemia Secondary to Other Causes

Secondary hyperglycemia has been associated with various disorders of insulin target tissues (liver, muscle, and adipose tissue). Other secondary causes of carbohydrate intolerance include endocrine disorders—often specific endocrine tumors—associated with excess production of growth hormone, glucocorticoids, catecholamines, glucagon, or somatostatin. With excess of glucocorticoids, catecholamines, or glucagon, increased hepatic output of glucose is a contributory factor; in the case of catecholamines, decreased insulin release is an additional factor in producing carbohydrate intolerance and, with excess somatostatin production, it is the major factor.

Secondary Causes of Hyperglycemia

A. Hyperglycemia due to tissue insensitivity to insulin

1. Hormonal tumors (acromegaly, Cushing's syndrome, glucagonoma, and pheochromocytoma)
2. Pharmacologic agents (corticosteroids, sympathomimetic drugs, and niacin)
3. Liver disease (cirrhosis and hemochromatosis)
4. Muscle disorders (myotonic dystrophy)
5. Adipose tissue disorders (lipodystrophy and truncal obesity)
6. Insulin receptor disorders (acanthosis nigricans syndromes and leprechaunism).

B. Hyperglycemia due to reduced insulin secretion

1. Hormonal tumors (somatostatinoma and pheochromocytoma)
2. Pancreatic disorders (pancreatitis, hemosiderosis, and hemochromatosis)
3. Pharmacologic agents (thiazide diuretics, phenytoin, and pentamidine).

A rare syndrome of extreme insulin resistance associated with acanthosis nigricans afflicts either young women with androgenic features as well as insulin receptor mutations or older people, mostly women, in whom a circulating immunoglobulin binds to insulin receptors and reduces their affinity to insulin.

Medications, such as diuretics, phenytoin, niacin, and high-dose corticosteroids can produce hyperglycemia that is reversible once the drugs are discontinued or when diuretic-induced hypokalemia is corrected. Chronic pancreatitis or subtotal pancreatectomy reduces the number of functioning B cells and can result in a metabolic derangement very similar to that of genetic Type 1 diabetes except that a concomitant reduction in pancreatic A cells may reduce glucagon secretion, so that relatively lower doses of insulin replacement are needed. Insulin-dependent diabetes is occasionally associated with Addison's disease and autoimmune thyroiditis (Schmidt's syndrome, or polyglandular failure syndrome). This occurs more commonly in women and represents an autoimmune disorder in which there are circulating antibodies to adrenocortical and thyroid tissue, thyroglobulin, and gastric parietal cells.

Nondiabetic Glycosuria

Nondiabetic glycosuria (renal glycosuria) is a benign asymptomatic condition wherein glucose appears in the urine despite a normal amount of glucose in the blood, either basally or during a glucose tolerance test. Its cause may vary from an autosomally transmitted genetic disorder to one associated with dysfunction of the proximal renal tubule (Fanconi syndrome, chronic renal failure), or it may merely be a consequence of the increased load of glucose presented to the tubules by the elevated glomerular filtration rate during pregnancy. **As many as 50% of pregnant women normally have demonstrable sugar in the urine, especially during the third and fourth months.** This sugar is practically always glucose except during the late weeks of pregnancy, when lactose may be present.

Management of Type 1 Diabetes Mellitus

The goals of therapy for Type 1 or Type 2 diabetes mellitus (DM) are to: (1) eliminate symptoms related to hyperglycemia, (2) reduce or eliminate the long-term microvascular and macrovascular complications of DM, and (3) allow the patient to achieve as normal a lifestyle as possible.

Because individuals with Type 1 DM partially or completely lack endogenous insulin production, administration of basal, exogenous insulin is essential for regulating glycogen breakdown, gluconeogenesis, lipolysis, and ketogenesis. Likewise, insulin replacement for meals should be appropriate for the carbohydrate intake and promote normal glucose utilization and storage.

Insulin Regimens

Two therapeutic regimens are currently in use, standard and intensive insulin treatment.

1. Standard treatment versus intensive treatment

   Standard treatment, which has its therapeutic goal, the clinical well-being of the patient, typically consists of one or two daily injections of insulin. Mean blood glucose obtained is typically in the 225–275 mg/dL range, with an HbA1c of 8–9% of the total hemoglobin. (The rate of formation of HbA1c is proportional to the average blood glucose concentration over the previous several months. Thus, HbA1c provides a measure of how well the treatment has normalized blood glucose in the diabetic over time.)

2. In contrast to standard therapy, intensive diabetes management has the goal of achieving euglycemia or near-normal glycemia. This approach requires multiple resources including thorough and continuing patient education, comprehensive recording of plasma glucose measurements and nutrition intake by the patient, and a variable insulin regimen that matches glucose intake and insulin dose. Insulin regimens usually include multiple-component insulin regimens, multiple daily injections (MDI), or insulin infusion devices. Mean blood glucose levels of 150 mg/dL can be achieved, with HbA1c 7% of the total hemoglobin. The patients on intensive therapy showed a 60% reduction in the long-term complications of diabetes-retinopathy, nephropathy, and neuropathy—compared with patients receiving standard care. This confirms that the complications of diabetes are related to an elevation of plasma glucose.

Insulin Preparations

Insulin is indicated for Type 1 diabetes as well as for Type 2 diabetic patients with insulinopenia whose hyperglycemia does not respond to diet therapy either alone or combined with other hypoglycemic drugs.

With the development of highly purified human insulin preparations, immunogenicity has been markedly reduced, thereby decreasing the incidence of therapeutic complications, such as insulin allergy, immune insulin resistance, and localized lipoatrophy at the injection site. However, the problem of achieving optimal insulin delivery remains unsolved with the present state of technology. It has not been possible to reproduce the physiologic patterns of intraportal insulin secretion with subcutaneous injections of short-acting or long-acting insulin preparations. Even so, with the help of appropriate modifications of diet and exercise and careful monitoring of capillary blood glucose levels at home, it has often been possible to achieve acceptable control of blood glucose by using various mixtures of short- and long-acting insulin injected at least twice daily or portable insulin infusion pumps.

Human insulin is produced by recombinant DNA techniques (biosynthetic human insulin) as Humulin (Eli Lilly) and as Novolin (Novo Nordisk). It is dispensed as either regular (R) or NPH (N) formulations. Five analogs of human insulin—three rapidly acting (insulin lispro, insulin aspart, and insulin glulisine) and two long-acting (insulin glargine and insulin detemir)—have been approved by the FDA for clinical use.

Insulin can be classified as short-acting or long-acting. The short-acting preparations are regular insulin and the rapidly acting insulin analogs. They are dispensed as clear solutions at neutral pH and contain small amounts of zinc to improve their stability and shelf life. The long-acting preparations are NPH insulin and the long-acting insulin analogs. NPH insulin is dispensed as a turbid suspension at neutral pH with protamine in phosphate buffer. The long-acting insulin analogs are also dispensed as clear solutions.

Mixed Insulin Preparations

Since intermediate insulin require several hours to reach adequate therapeutic levels, their use in patients with Type 1 diabetes requires supplements of regular or rapidly acting insulin analogs preprandially. For convenience, regular or rapidly acting insulin analogs and NPH insulin may be mixed together in the same syringe and injected subcutaneously in split dosage before breakfast and supper.

Summary of Bioavailability Characteristics of Insulin (Table 15.2)

Methods of Insulin Administration

1. **Insulin syringes and needles:** Plastic disposable syringes are available in 1-mL, 0.5-mL, and 0.3-mL sizes.
2. **Insulin pen injector devices:** Insulin pens eliminate the need for carrying insulin vials and syringes. Cartridges of insulin lispro, insulin aspart, insulin glargine, regular insulin, NPH insulin, and 70% NPH/30% regular insulin are available for reusable pens.

TABLE 15.2: Bioavailability characteristics of insulin.

Insulin preparations	*Onset of action*	*Peak action*	*Effective duration*
Insulin lispro, aspart, glulisine	5–15 minutes	1–1.5 hours	3–4 hours
Human regular	30–60 minutes	2 hours	6–8 hours
Human NPH	2–4 hours	6–7 hours	10–20 hours
Insulin glargine	1.5 hours	Flat	~24 hours
Insulin detemir	1 hour	Flat	17 hours

3. **Insulin pumps:** Insulin infusion pumps are used for subcutaneous delivery of insulin. These pumps are small (about the size of a pager) and very easy to program. They offer many features, including the ability to set a number of different basal rates throughout the 24 hours and to adjust the time over which bolus doses are given.
4. **Inhaled insulin:** A novel method for delivering a preprandial powdered form of insulin by inhalation (Exubera) has been approved by the FDA.

5. **Islet cell transplantation:** It is a minimally invasive procedure, wide application of this procedure for the treatment of Type 1 diabetes is limited by the dependence on multiple donors and the requirement for potent long-term immunotherapy.

A judicious balance of the size and frequency of meals with moderate regular exercise can often stabilize the insulin dosage in diabetics. A reasonable aim of therapy is to approach normal glycemic excursions without provoking severe or frequent hypoglycemia. What has been considered "acceptable" control includes blood glucose levels of 90–130 mg/dL before meals and after an overnight fast, and levels no higher than 180 mg/dL 1 hour after meals and 150 mg/dL 2 hours after meals. Glycohemoglobin levels should be no higher than 1% above the upper limit of the normal range.

Complications of Insulin Therapy

Hypoglycemia, insulin allergy, immune insulin resistance, and lipodystrophy at the injection site are some of the complications of insulin therapy.

Hypoglycemia in Type 1 Diabetes

One of the therapeutic goals of diabetes is to decrease blood glucose levels in an effort to minimize the development of the long-term complications of the disease. However, appropriate dosage is difficult to achieve in all patients, and hypoglycemia caused by excess insulin is the most common complication of insulin therapy, occurring in more than 90% of the patients. The frequency of hypoglycemic episodes, coma, and seizures is particularly high with intensive treatment regimens designed to achieve tight control of blood glucose. In normal individuals, hypoglycemia triggers a compensatory secretion of counter-regulatory hormones, most notably glucagon and epinephrine, which promote hepatic production of glucose. However, patients with Type 1 diabetes also develop a deficiency of glucagon secretion. This defect occurs early in the disease and is almost universally present 4 years after diagnosis. These patients thus rely on epinephrine secretion to prevent severe hypoglycemia. However, as the disease progresses, Type 1 diabetes patients show diabetic autonomic neuropathy and impaired ability to secrete epinephrine in response to hypoglycemia. The combined deficiency of glucagon and epinephrine secretion creates a condition sometimes called "hypoglycemia unawareness". Thus, patients with long-standing diabetes are particularly vulnerable to hypoglycemia. Hypoglycemia can also be caused by strenuous exercise. Exercise promotes glucose uptake into muscles and decreases the need for exogenous insulin. Patients should, therefore, check blood glucose levels before or after intensive exercise to prevent or abort hypoglycemia.

Around one-fourth of all patients who get Type 1 diabetes develop what is known as a "honeymoon" period within days or weeks of the onset of treatment. It is as if the patient has gone into remission and it can be confusing for the patient as it would appear that the condition has corrected itself. Some patients actually require no insulin during this phase and this may last for weeks or months. It is usually best to keep treating with insulin even if the requirements are negligible, to avoid possible insulin allergy upon re-exposure and also to maintain a treatment regimen and not give false hope to the patient.

Other Agents that Improve Glucose Control

The role of amylin, a 37-amino acid peptide cosecreted with insulin from pancreatic beta cells, in normal glucose homeostasis is uncertain. However, based on the rationale that patients who are insulin deficient are also amylin deficient, an analogue of amylin (pramlintide) was created and found to reduce postprandial glycemic excursions in Type 1 and Type 2 diabetic patients taking insulin.

Besides insulin therapy, lifelong dietary and lifestyle modifications are required to be done to achieve euglycemia.

Stem Cell Therapy

Stem cell therapy is one of the most promising treatments for the near future. It is expected that this kind of therapy can ameliorate or even reverse some diseases.

Complications of Type 1 Diabetes Mellitus

Out of all, diabetic ketoacidosis is the most common complication of Type 1 diabetes mellitus. Rest all complications are same as Type 2 diabetes mellitus. (See the details of complications in Type 2 diabetes mellitus.)

Prognosis

Prognosis of patients with Type 1 diabetes can be markedly improved by optimal care.

CLINICAL NOTE

Type 1 diabetes mellitus (DM) can be distinguished from Type 2 diabetes via a C-peptide assay, which measures endogenous insulin production.

CLINICAL PEARLS

1. Diabetes mellitus Type 1 (Type 1 diabetes, IDDM, or juvenile diabetes) is a form of diabetes mellitus that results from autoimmune destruction of insulin-producing beta cells of the pancreas.
2. The classical symptoms of Type 1 diabetes are polyuria, polydipsia, polyphagia, and weight loss.
3. Type 1 diabetes is fatal unless treated with insulin.
4. Injection is the most common method of administering insulin; insulin pumps and inhaled insulin have been available at various times.
5. Diabetic ketoacidosis is the most common complication of Type 1 DM.

CASE STUDY 15

Theme: Causes, Pathogenesis, Clinical Manifestations, Diagnosis, and Treatment of Type 2 Diabetes Mellitus

A 53-year-old African American presented to the physician for consultation about his health. He had been in good health until about 2 months ago when he started to feel weak and tired more rapidly than usual. On questioning, he admitted to getting up two or three times a night to urinate. He often felt thirsty and drank a glass of water each time.

His weight had been average throughout his high school, where he had been in the football team. After leaving school, he had gradually gained weight over the years. His appetite remained excellent but now he was losing weight and becoming weak.

The pain in his feet was worse at night and sometimes kept him awake. It was burning in character and sometimes his toes felt numb. The tingling and numbness in his fingers were causing him problems at his work as an auto mechanic because he frequently dropped small parts or had difficulty in making fine manual adjustments to engines. His vision was blurred at times, especially in the afternoon.

All other symptoms were negative. History revealed that his father died at age 69 from a massive stroke. His mother died at age 62 from end-stage kidney disease. She was found to have diabetes at age 48, and was on dialysis for 3 years before her death.

Physical examination:
Obese, weight 217 lbs, height 5'11"(BMI 30), pulse 76 beats/min, regular, and BP 142/78 mm Hg
Chest, abdomen, and genital examination—normal.

Laboratory tests:
Urinalysis: glucose 4^+, ketones and protein-negative
Random blood glucose: 456 mg/dL
Glycohemoglobin (HbA1c): 16.4%
Total cholesterol—243 mg/dL, HDL—20 mg/dL, and triglycerides—416 mg/dL.
What is the probable diagnosis?
What is the significance of all these investigations?

CASE DETAILS

The patient is suffering from diabetes mellitus Type 2.

Type 2 diabetes mellitus [formerly called noninsulin-dependent diabetes mellitus (NIDDM) or adult-onset diabetes mellitus] is a disorder that is characterized by high blood glucose in the context of insulin resistance and relative insulin deficiency. Circulating endogenous insulin is sufficient to prevent ketoacidosis but is inadequate to prevent hyperglycemia in the face of increased needs owing to tissue insensitivity (insulin resistance).

INCIDENCE

United States

In 2007, the estimated prevalence of diabetes in the United States was 7.8% (23.6 million people); almost one-third of cases were undiagnosed. More than 90% of cases of diabetes are Type 2 diabetes mellitus. With increasing obesity in the population, an older population, and an increase in the population of higher-risk minority groups, prevalence is increasing.

International

Type 2 diabetes mellitus is less common in non-Western countries where the diet contains fewer calories and caloric expenditure on a daily basis is higher. However, as people in these countries adopt Western lifestyles, weight gain and Type 2 diabetes mellitus are becoming virtually epidemic.

Age

While Type 2 diabetes mellitus traditionally has been thought to affect individuals older than 40 years, it is being recognized increasingly in younger persons, particularly in highly susceptible racial and ethnic groups and the obese. **In some areas, more Type 2 than Type 1 diabetes mellitus is being diagnosed in prepubertal children, teenagers, and young adults.**

Genetic Considerations

Genetic and environmental factors combine to cause both the insulin resistance and the beta cell loss. Most epidemiologic data indicate strong genetic influences, since in monozygotic twins over 40 years of age, concordance develops in over 70% of cases within a year whenever Type 2 diabetes develops in one twin. Individuals with a parent with Type 2 DM have an increased risk of diabetes; if both parents have Type 2 DM, the risk approaches 40%. Insulin resistance, as demonstrated by reduced glucose utilization in skeletal muscle, is present in many nondiabetic, first-degree relatives of individuals with Type 2 DM. **The disease is polygenic and multifactorial since in addition to genetic susceptibility, environmental factors (such as obesity, nutrition, and physical activity) modulate the phenotype.** Attempts to identify genes for Type 2 diabetics that cause the insulin resistance and the beta cell failure have as yet been unsuccessful, although linkage to a gene on chromosome 2 encoding a cysteine protease, Calpain-10, has been reported in a Mexican–American population. However, its association with other ethnic populations and any role it plays in the pathogenesis of Type 2 diabetes remain to be clarified. The mechanisms by which these genetic alterations increase the susceptibility to Type 2 diabetes are not clear.

Other Specific Types of Diabetes Mellitus

Maturity Onset Diabetes of the Young

This subgroup is a relatively rare monogenic disorder characterized by noninsulin-dependent diabetes with autosomal dominant inheritance and an age at onset of 25 years or younger. Patients are nonobese, and their hyperglycemia is due to impaired glucose-induced secretion of insulin. Six types of maturity onset diabetes of the young (MODY) have been described. Except for MODY 2, in which a glucokinase gene is defective, all other types involve mutations of a nuclear transcription factor that regulates islet gene expression.

Maturity onset diabetes of the young (MODY) 2 is quite mild, associated with only slight fasting hyperglycemia and few if any microvascular diabetic complications. It generally responds well to dietary modifications or low doses of oral hypoglycemic agents. MODY 3—the most common form—accounts for two-thirds of all MODY cases. The clinical course is similar to that of idiopathic Type 2 diabetes in terms of microangiopathy and failure to respond to oral agents with time.

Diabetes due to Mutant Insulin

This is a very rare subtype of nonobese Type 2 diabetes, with no more than ten families having been described. Since affected individuals were heterozygous and possessed one normal insulin gene, diabetes was mild, did not appear until middle age, and showed autosomal dominant genetic transmission. There is generally no evidence of clinical insulin resistance, and these patients respond well to standard therapy.

Diabetes due to Mutant Insulin Receptors

Defects in one of their insulin receptor genes have been found in more than 40 people with diabetes, and most have extreme insulin resistance associated with acanthosis nigricans. In very rare instances when both insulin receptor genes are abnormal, newborns present with a leprechaun-like phenotype and seldom live through infancy.

Diabetes Mellitus associated with a Mutation of Mitochondrial DNA

Since sperm do not contain mitochondria, only the mother transmits mitochondrial genes to her offspring. Diabetes due to a mutation of mitochondrial DNA that impairs the transfer of leucine or lysine into mitochondrial proteins has been described. Most patients have a mild form of diabetes that responds to oral hypoglycemic agents; some have a nonimmune form of Type 1 diabetes. Two-thirds of patients with this subtype of diabetes have a hearing loss, and a smaller proportion (15%) have a syndrome of myopathy, encephalopathy, lactic acidosis, and stroke-like episodes (MELAS).

Wolfram's Syndrome

Wolfram's syndrome is an autosomal recessive neurodegenerative disorder first evident in childhood. It consists of diabetes insipidus, diabetes mellitus, optic atrophy, and deafness, hence the acronym DIDMOAD. It is due to mutations in a gene named WFS1, which encodes a 100.3 kDa transmembrane protein localized in the endoplasmic reticulum. The function of the protein is not known. The diabetes mellitus, which is nonimmune and not linked to specific HLA antigens, usually presents in the first decade together with the optic atrophy. Cranial diabetes insipidus and sensorineural deafness develop during the second decade in 60–75% of patients. Ureterohydronephrosis, neurogenic bladder, cerebellar ataxia, peripheral neuropathy, and psychiatric illness develop later in many patients.

Transient or Permanent Neonatal Diabetes

Onset <6 months of age may be caused by several genetic mutations and requires treatment with insulin. Mutations in subunits of the ATP-sensitive potassium channel subunits are the major causes of permanent neonatal diabetes. Although these activating mutations impair glucose-stimulated insulin secretion, these individuals may respond to sulfonylureas and improve their glycemic control and can be treated with these agents. Homozygous glucokinase mutations cause a severe form of neonatal diabetes.

Insulin Resistance syndrome (Syndrome X; Metabolic Syndrome)

Twenty-five percent of the general nondiabetic obese population has insulin resistance of a magnitude similar to that seen in Type 2 diabetes. These insulin-resistant nondiabetic individuals are at much higher risk for developing Type 2 diabetes than insulin-sensitive persons. In addition to diabetes, these individuals have increased risk for elevated plasma triglycerides, lower high-density lipoproteins (HDLs), and higher blood pressure—a cluster of abnormalities termed syndrome X. These associations have now been expanded to include small, dense, low-density lipoprotein (LDL), hyperuricemia, abdominal obesity, prothrombotic state with increased levels of plasminogen activator inhibitor Type 1 (PAI-1), and proinflammatory state. These clusters of abnormalities significantly increase the risk of atherosclerotic disease.

Pathophysiology of Type 2 Diabetes Mellitus

Type 2 DM is characterized by impaired insulin secretion, insulin resistance, excessive hepatic glucose production, and abnormal fat metabolism. Obesity, particularly visceral or central (as evidenced by the hip-waist ratio), is very common in Type 2 DM. In the early stages of the disorder, glucose tolerance remains near-normal, despite insulin resistance, because the pancreatic beta cells compensate by increasing insulin output. As insulin resistance and compensatory hyperinsulinemia progress, the pancreatic islets in certain individuals are unable to sustain the hyperinsulinemia state. IGT, characterized by elevations in postprandial glucose, then develops. A further decline in insulin secretion and an increase in hepatic glucose production lead to overt diabetes with fasting hyperglycemia. Ultimately, beta cell failure may ensue.

Abnormal Muscle and Fat Metabolism

Insulin resistance, the decreased ability of insulin to act effectively on target tissues (especially muscle, liver, and fat), is a prominent feature of Type 2 DM and results from a combination of genetic susceptibility and obesity. Insulin resistance is relative, however, since supernormal levels of circulating insulin will normalize the plasma glucose. Insulin resistance impairs glucose utilization by insulin-sensitive tissues and increases hepatic glucose output; both effects contribute to the hyperglycemia. Increased hepatic glucose output predominantly accounts for increased fasting plasma glucose (FPG) levels, whereas decreased peripheral glucose usage results in postprandial hyperglycemia. In skeletal muscle, there is a greater impairment in glycogen formation than in glucose metabolism through glycolysis. Glucose metabolism in insulin-independent tissues is not altered in Type 2 DM.

The precise molecular mechanism leading to insulin resistance in Type 2 DM has not been elucidated. Insulin receptor levels and tyrosine kinase activity in skeletal muscle are reduced, but these alterations are most likely secondary to hyperinsulinemia and are not a primary defect. Therefore, "postreceptor" defects in insulin-regulated phosphorylation/dephosphorylation may play the predominant role in insulin resistance. For example, a PI-3-kinase signaling defect may reduce translocation of GLUT4 to the plasma membrane. Other abnormalities include the accumulation of lipid within skeletal myocytes, which may impair mitochondrial oxidative phosphorylation and reduce insulin-stimulated mitochondrial ATP production. Impaired fatty acid oxidation and lipid accumulation within skeletal myocytes may generate reactive oxygen species, such as lipid peroxides. Of note, not all insulin signal transduction pathways are resistant to the effects of insulin (e.g., those controlling cell growth and differentiation using the mitogenic-activated protein kinase pathway). Consequently, hyperinsulinemia may increase the insulin action through these pathways, potentially accelerating diabetes-related conditions, such as atherosclerosis.

The obesity accompanying Type 2 DM, particularly in a central or visceral location, is thought to be part of the pathogenic process. The increased adipocyte mass leads to increased levels of circulating free fatty acids and other fat cell products. For example, adipocytes secrete a number of biologic products (nonesterified free fatty acids, retinol-binding protein 4, leptin, TNF-α, resistin, and adiponectin). In addition to regulating body weight, appetite, and energy expenditure, adipokines also modulate insulin sensitivity. The increased production of free fatty acids and some adipokines may cause insulin resistance in skeletal muscle and liver. For example, free fatty acids impair glucose utilization in skeletal muscle, promote glucose production by the liver, and impair beta cell function. In contrast, the production by adipocytes of adiponectin, an insulin-sensitizing peptide, is reduced in obesity and this may contribute to hepatic insulin resistance. Adipocyte products and adipokines also produce an inflammatory state and may explain why markers of inflammation, such as interleukin-6 (IL-6) and C-reactive protein are often elevated in Type 2 DM.

Impaired Insulin Secretion

Insulin secretion and sensitivity are interrelated. In Type 2 DM, insulin secretion initially increases in response to insulin resistance to maintain normal glucose tolerance. Initially, the insulin secretory defect is mild and selectively involves glucose-stimulated insulin secretion. Eventually, the insulin secretory defect progresses to a state of grossly inadequate insulin secretion.

The reason(s) for the decline in insulin secretory capacity in Type 2 DM is unclear. The assumption is that a second genetic defect—superimposed upon insulin resistance—leads to beta cell failure. Islet amyloid polypeptide or amylin is cosecreted by the beta cell and forms the amyloid fibrillar deposit found in the islets of individuals with long-standing Type 2 DM. Whether such islet amyloid deposits are a primary or secondary event is not known. The metabolic environment of diabetes may also negatively impact islet function. For example, chronic hyperglycemia paradoxically impairs islet function ("glucose toxicity") and leads to a worsening of hyperglycemia. Improvement in glycemic control is often associated with improved islet function. In addition, elevation of free fatty acid levels ("lipotoxicity") and dietary fat may also worsen islet function. Beta cell mass is decreased in individuals with long-standing Type 2 diabetes.

Increased Hepatic Glucose and Lipid Production

In Type 2 DM, insulin resistance in the liver reflects the failure of hyperinsulinemia to suppress gluconeogenesis, which results in fasting hyperglycemia and decreased glycogen storage by the liver in the postprandial state. Increased hepatic glucose production occurs early in the course of diabetes, though likely after the onset of insulin secretory abnormalities and insulin resistance in skeletal muscle. As a result of insulin resistance in adipose tissue and obesity, free fatty acid (FFA) flux from adipocytes is increased, leading to increased lipid [very low-density lipoprotein (VLDL) and triglyceride] synthesis in hepatocytes. This lipid storage or steatosis in the liver may lead to nonalcoholic fatty liver disease and abnormal liver function tests. This is also responsible for the dyslipidemia found in Type 2 DM [elevated triglycerides, reduced high-density lipoprotein (HDL), and increased small dense low-density lipoprotein (LDL) particles].

Risk Factors for Type 2 Diabetes Mellitus

- Family history of diabetes (i.e., parent or sibling with Type 2 diabetes)
- Obesity (BMI >25 kg/m^2)
- Habitual physical inactivity
- Race/ethnicity (e.g., African American, Latino, Native American, Asian American, Pacific Islander)
- Previously identified IFG or IGT
- History of GDM or delivery of baby >4 kg (>9 lbs)
- Hypertension (blood pressure >140/90 mm Hg)
- HDL cholesterol level <35 mg/dL (0.90 mmol/L) and/or a triglyceride level >250 mg/dL (2.82 mmol/L)
- Polycystic ovary syndrome or acanthosis nigricans
- History of vascular disease.

Clinical Manifestations

1. While many patients with Type 2 diabetes present with increased urination and thirst, many others have an insidious onset of hyperglycemia and are asymptomatic initially. This is particularly true in obese patients, whose diabetes may be detected only after glycosuria or hyperglycemia is noted during routine laboratory studies.
2. Occasionally, Type 2 patients may present with evidence of neuropathic or cardiovascular complications because of occult disease present for some time prior to diagnosis.
3. Chronic skin infections are common. Generalized pruritus and symptoms of vaginitis are frequently the initial complaints of women. Diabetes should be suspected in women with chronic *Candida* vulvovaginitis as well as in those who have delivered large babies (>9 lbs, or 4.1 kg) or have had polyhydramnios, preeclampsia, or unexplained fetal losses.
4. Obese diabetics may have any variety of fat distribution; however, diabetes seems to be more often associated in both men and women with localization of fat deposits on the upper segment of the body (particularly the abdomen, chest, neck, and face) and relatively less fat on the appendages, which may be quite muscular. Standardized tables of waist-to-hip ratio indicate that ratios of "greater than 0.9" in men and "greater than 0.8" in women are associated with an increased risk of diabetes in obese subjects.
5. Mild hypertension is often present in obese diabetics.
6. Eruptive xanthomas on the flexor surface of the limbs and on the buttocks and lipemia retinalis due to hyperchylomicronemia can occur in patients with uncontrolled Type 2 diabetes who also have a familial form of hypertriglyceridemia.

Mortality/Morbidity

Diabetes mellitus is one of the leading causes of morbidity and mortality in the United States because of its role in the development of optic, renal, neuropathic, and cardiovascular disease. These complications, particularly cardiovascular disease (~50–75% of medical expenditures), are the major sources of expenses for patients with diabetes mellitus. Approximately two-thirds of people with diabetes die from heart disease or stroke. Men with diabetes face a twofold increased risk for coronary heart disease, and women have a threefold to fourfold increased risk. Diabetes mellitus is the leading cause of blindness in working-age adults in the United States; diabetic retinopathy accounts for 12,000–24,000 newly blind persons every year. Diabetes mellitus is the leading cause of end-stage renal disease (ESRD), accounting for 44% of new cases, according to the Centers for Disease Control and Prevention (CDC). Diabetes mellitus is the leading cause of nontraumatic lower limb amputations in the United States, with a 15- to 40-fold increase in risk over that of the nondiabetic population.

Laboratory Diagnosis

(Same as Type 1 Diabetes Mellitus).

Complications of Diabetes Mellitus

Acute Complications of DM

Diabetic ketoacidosis (DKA) and hyperglycemic hyperosmolar state (HHS) are acute complications of diabetes. DKA was formerly considered a hallmark of Type 1 DM, but it also occurs in individuals who lack immunologic features of Type 1 DM and who can subsequently be treated with oral glucose-lowering agents (these obese individuals with Type 2 DM are often of Hispanic or African American descent). HHS is primarily seen in individuals with Type 2 DM. Both disorders are associated with absolute or relative insulin deficiency, volume depletion, and acid-base abnormalities. DKA and HHS exist along a continuum of hyperglycemia, with or without ketosis. Both disorders are associated with potentially serious complications if not promptly diagnosed and treated.

1. **Diabetic ketoacidosis: (case study 16)**
2. **Hyperglycemic hyperosmolar state (HHS)**

Clinical Features

Hyperglycemic hyperosmolar state (HHS) occurs in elderly individuals with Type 2 DM, with a several week history of polyuria, weight loss, and diminished oral intake that culminates in mental confusion, lethargy, or coma. The physical examination reveals:

- Profound dehydration and hyperosmolality
- Hypotension, tachycardia, and altered mental status
- Nausea, vomiting, abdominal pain, and the Kussmaul respirations characteristic of DKA are absent.
- Hyperglycemic hyperosmolar state (HHS) is often precipitated by a serious, concurrent illness, such as myocardial infarction or stroke.
- Sepsis, pneumonia, and other serious infections are frequent precipitants and should be sought.

Pathophysiology

Relative insulin deficiency and inadequate fluid intake are the underlying causes of HHS. Insulin deficiency increases hepatic glucose production (through glycogenolysis and gluconeogenesis) and impairs glucose utilization in skeletal muscle. Hyperglycemia induces an osmotic diuresis that leads to intravascular volume depletion, which is exacerbated by inadequate fluid replacement. The absence of ketosis in HHS is not completely understood. Presumably, the insulin deficiency is only relative and less severe than in DKA. Lower levels of counterregulatory hormones and free fatty acids have been found in HHS than in DKA in some studies. It is also possible that the liver is less capable of ketone body synthesis or that the insulin/glucagon ratio does not favor ketogenesis.

Laboratory Abnormalities and Diagnosis

Most notable are the marked hyperglycemia [plasma glucose may be >55.5 mmol/L (1000 mg/dL)], hyperosmolality (>350 mOsmol/L), and prerenal azotemia. The measured serum sodium may be normal or slightly low despite the marked hyperglycemia. The corrected serum sodium is usually increased [add 1.6 mEq to measured sodium for each 5.6 mmol/L (100 mg/dL) rise in the serum glucose]. In contrast to DKA, acidosis and ketonemia are absent or mild. A small anion gap metabolic acidosis may be present secondary to increased lactic acid. Moderate ketonuria, if present, is secondary to starvation.

Treatment

In HHS, fluid losses and dehydration are usually more pronounced than in DKA due to the longer duration of the illness. The patient with HHS is usually older, more likely to have mental status changes, and more likely to have a life-threatening precipitating event with accompanying comorbidities. Even with proper treatment, HHS has a substantially higher mortality than DKA (up to 15% in some clinical series).

The rehydration in HHS should be slower to avoid neurological damage. Dilute (0.45%) saline has been used where the serum sodium level is above 160 mmol/L. However, recent data indicate that in most cases, the use of physiological (0.9%) saline is sufficient. The insulin dose requirements are usually lower than in DKA.

Lactic acidosis: Type 1 lactic acidosis occurs in hypoxic individuals and is due to an excessive production of lactate by peripheral tissues. Hypoxia is not a feature of lactic acidosis, which occurs due to impaired metabolism of lactate in the liver. Both are characterized by extreme metabolic acidosis. There is high-anion gap with low or absent ketones and high lactate levels.

Treatment

Large amount of intravenous sodium bicarbonate is needed to correct the acidosis. Alternatively, the patient may be dialyzed against a bicarbonate containing solution.

Chronic Complications of DM

Chronic complications can be divided into vascular and nonvascular complications.

The vascular complications of DM are further subdivided into microvascular (retinopathy, neuropathy, and nephropathy) and macrovascular complications [coronary artery disease (CAD), peripheral arterial disease (PAD), cerebrovascular disease]. Nonvascular complications include problems, such as gastroparesis, infections, and skin changes. Long-standing diabetes may be associated with hearing loss.

The risk of chronic complications increases as a function of the duration of hyperglycemia; they usually become apparent in the second decade of hyperglycemia. Since Type 2 DM often has a long asymptomatic period of hyperglycemia, many individuals with Type 2 DM have complications at the time of diagnosis.

Mechanisms of Complications

Following prominent theories, which are not mutually exclusive, have been proposed to explain how hyperglycemia might lead to the chronic complications of DM:

1. **Advanced glycosylation end products:** Increased intracellular glucose leads to the formation of advanced glycosylation end products (AGEs) via the nonenzymatic glycosylation of intra- and extracellular proteins. Nonenzymatic glycosylation results from the interaction of glucose with amino groups on proteins. AGEs have been shown to cross-link proteins (e.g., collagen, extracellular matrix proteins), accelerate atherosclerosis, promote glomerular dysfunction, reduce nitric oxide synthesis, induce endothelial dysfunction, and alter extracellular matrix composition and structure. The serum level of AGEs correlates with the level of glycemia, and these products accumulate as glomerular filtration rate declines.
2. **Sorbitol pathway:** Hyperglycemia increases glucose metabolism via the sorbitol pathway. Intracellular glucose is predominantly metabolized by phosphorylation and subsequent glycolysis, but when increased, some glucose is converted to sorbitol by the enzyme aldose reductase. Increased sorbitol concentration alters redox potential, increases cellular osmolality, generates reactive oxygen species, and likely leads to other types of cellular dysfunction.
3. **Activation of protein kinase C (PKC):** A third hypothesis proposes that hyperglycemia increases the formation of diacylglycerol leading to activation of protein kinase C (PKC). Among other actions, PKC alters the transcription of genes for fibronectin, Type IV collagen, contractile proteins, and extracellular matrix proteins in endothelial cells and neurons. Inhibitors of PKC are being studied in clinical trials.
4. **Hexosamine pathway:** A fourth theory proposes that hyperglycemia increases the flux through the hexosamine pathway, which generates fructose-6-phosphate, a substrate for O-linked glycosylation and proteoglycan production. The hexosamine pathway may alter function by glycosylation of proteins, such as endothelial nitric oxide synthase or by changes in gene expression of transforming growth factor β (TGF-β) or plasminogen activator inhibitor-1 (PAI-1).

   Growth factors appear to play an important role in DM-related complications, and their production is increased by most of these proposed pathways.
5. **Oxidative stress:** Hyperglycemia leads to increased production of reactive oxygen species or superoxide in the mitochondria; these compounds may activate all four of the pathways described above. Although hyperglycemia serves as the initial trigger for complications of diabetes, it is still unknown whether the same pathophysiological processes are operative in all complications or whether some pathways predominate in certain organs.

Vascular Complications

- **Microvascular complications**

  Ocular complications: Diabetes mellitus is the leading cause of blindness between the ages of 20 and 74 in the United States. Blindness is primarily the result of progressive diabetic retinopathy and clinically significant macular edema.

  Diabetic retinopathy: Diabetic retinopathy is classified into two stages: nonproliferative and proliferative. Nonproliferative diabetic retinopathy usually appears late in the first decade or early in the second decade of the disease and is marked by retinal vascular microaneurysms, blot hemorrhages, and cotton wool spots. Mild nonproliferative retinopathy progresses to more extensive disease, characterized by changes in venous vessel caliber, intraretinal microvascular abnormalities, and more numerous microaneurysms and hemorrhages.

  The appearance of neovascularization in response to retinal hypoxia is the hallmark of proliferative diabetic retinopathy. These newly formed vessels appear near the optic nerve and/or macula and rupture easily, leading to vitreous hemorrhage, fibrosis, and ultimately retinal detachment. Clinically significant macular edema can occur when only nonproliferative retinopathy is present.

  Duration of DM and degree of glycemic control are the best predictors of the development of retinopathy; hypertension is also a risk factor. Nonproliferative retinopathy is found in almost all individuals who have had DM for >20 years (25% incidence with 5 years, and 80% incidence with 15 years of Type 1 DM).

  Although there is genetic susceptibility for retinopathy, it confers less influence than either the duration of DM or the degree of glycemic control.

Treatment

The most effective therapy for diabetic retinopathy is prevention. Intensive glycemic and blood pressure control will delay the development or slow the progression of retinopathy in individuals with either Type 1 or Type 2 DM. Laser photocoagulation is very successful in preserving vision. Proliferative retinopathy is usually treated with panretinal laser photocoagulation, whereas macular edema is treated with focal laser photocoagulation.

- **Diabetic cataract:** Premature cataracts occur in diabetic patients and seem to correlate with both the duration of diabetes and the severity of chronic hyperglycemia. Nonenzymatic glycosylation of lens protein contributes to the premature occurrence of cataracts.
- **Glaucoma:** Glaucoma occurs in approximately 6% of persons with diabetes. It is responsive to the usual therapy for open-angle disease. Neovascularization of the iris in diabetics can predispose to closed-angle glaucoma, but this is relatively uncommon except after cataract extraction, when growth of new vessels has been known to progress rapidly, involving the angle of the iris and obstructing outflow.
- Renal complications
- **Diabetic nephropathy—See details in Chapter 21**
- **Diabetic neuropathy:** Diabetic neuropathy occurs in ~50% of individuals with long-standing Type 1 and Type 2 DM. It may manifest as polyneuropathy, mononeuropathy, and/or autonomic neuropathy. Both myelinated and unmyelinated nerve fibers are lost.
- **Polyneuropathy/mononeuropathy:** The most common form of diabetic neuropathy is distal symmetric polyneuropathy. It most frequently presents with distal sensory loss, but up to 50% of patients do not have symptoms of neuropathy. Loss of function appears in a stocking-glove pattern. Hyperesthesia, paresthesias, and dysesthesia also may occur. Symptoms may include a sensation of numbness, tingling, sharpness, or burning that begins in the feet and spreads proximally. Neuropathic pain develops in some of these individuals, occasionally preceded by improvement in their glycemic control. Pain typically involves the lower extremities, is usually present at rest, and worsens at night. Both an acute (lasting <12 months) and a chronic form of painful diabetic neuropathy have been described. As diabetic neuropathy progresses, the pain subsides and eventually disappears, but a sensory deficit in the lower extremities persists. Physical examination reveals sensory loss, loss of ankle reflexes, and abnormal position sense.

  Mononeuropathy (dysfunction of isolated cranial or peripheral nerves) is less common than polyneuropathy in DM and presents with pain and motor weakness in the distribution of a single nerve. A vascular etiology has been suggested, but the pathogenesis is unknown.
- **Autonomic neuropathy:** Individuals with long-standing Type 1 or 2 DM may develop signs of autonomic dysfunction involving the cholinergic, noradrenergic, and peptidergic (peptides, such as pancreatic polypeptide, substance P, etc.) systems. DM-related autonomic neuropathy can involve multiple systems, including the cardiovascular, gastrointestinal, genitourinary, and metabolic systems. Autonomic neuropathy may reduce counterregulatory hormone release, leading to an inability to sense hypoglycemia appropriately thereby subjecting the patient to the risk of severe hypoglycemia and complicating efforts to improve glycemic control. Anhidrosis of the feet can promote dry skin with cracking, which increases the risk of foot ulcers.

  Diabetic nerve damage can affect the nerves that are important for penile erection, causing erectile dysfunction. Erectile dysfunction can also be caused by poor blood flow to the penis rom diabetic blood vessel disease.

  Diabetic neuropathy can also affect nerves to the stomach and intestines, causing nausea, weight loss, diarrhea, and other symptoms of gastroparesis (delayed emptying of food contents from the stomach into the intestines, due to ineffective contraction of the stomach muscles).

Diabetic Neuropathy: Treatment

Despite advances in the understanding of the metabolic causes of neuropathy, treatments aimed at interrupting these pathological processes have been limited. Thus, with the exception of tight glucose control, treatments are for reducing pain and other symptoms.

Options for pain control include tricyclic antidepressants (TCAs), serotonin reuptake inhibitors (SSRIs), and antiepileptic drugs (AEDs).

Prognosis

The mechanisms of diabetic neuropathy are poorly understood. At present, treatment alleviates pain and can control some associated symptoms, but the process is generally progressive.

As a complication, there is an increased risk of injury to the feet because of loss of sensation. Small infections can progress to ulceration and this may require amputation.

Diabetic gangrene

The incidence of gangrene of the feet in diabetics is 30 times more than that in age-matched controls. The factors responsible for its development, in addition to peripheral vascular disease, are small vessel disease, peripheral neuropathy with loss of both pain sensation and neurogenic inflammatory responses, and secondary infection.

The peripheral sensory neuropathy interferes with normal protective mechanisms and allows the patient to sustain major or repeated minor trauma to the foot, often without knowledge of the injury. Motor and sensory neuropathy lead to abnormal foot muscle mechanics and to structural changes in the foot (hammer toe, claw toe deformity, prominent metatarsal heads, and charcot joint). Autonomic neuropathy results in anhidrosis and altered superficial blood flow in the foot, which promote drying of the skin and fissure formation. PAD and poor wound healing impede resolution of minor breaks in the skin, allowing them to enlarge and to become infected.

Approximately 15% of individuals with DM develop a foot ulcer (great toe or MTP areas are most common), and a significant subset will ultimately undergo amputation (14–24% risk with that ulcer or subsequent ulceration). Risk factors for foot ulcers or amputation include: male sex, diabetes >10 years' duration, peripheral neuropathy, abnormal structure of foot (bony abnormalities, callus, and thickened nails), peripheral arterial disease, and smoking, history of previous ulcer or amputation, and poor glycemic control.

Treatment

The optimal therapy for foot ulcers and amputations is prevention through identification of high-risk patients, education of the patient, and institution of measures to prevent ulceration. Despite preventive measures, foot ulceration and infection are common and represent a serious problem. Due to the multifactorial pathogenesis of lower extremity ulcers, management of these lesions is multidisciplinary.

Agents that reduce peripheral blood flow, such as tobacco and propranolol should be avoided. Control of other risk factors, such as hypertension is essential. Cholesterol-lowering agents are useful as adjunctive therapy when early ischemic signs are detected and when dyslipidemia is present. Patients should be advised to seek immediate medical care, if a diabetic foot ulcer develops. Improvement in peripheral blood flow with endarterectomy and bypass operations is possible in certain patients.

- **Skin and mucous membrane complications:** Chronic pyogenic infections of the skin may occur, especially in poorly controlled diabetic patients. Eruptive xanthomas can result from hypertriglyceridemia, associated with poor glycemic control. An unusual lesion termed necrobiosis lipoidica diabeticorum is usually located over the anterior surfaces of the legs or the dorsal surfaces of the ankles. They are oval or irregularly shaped plaques with demarcated borders and a glistening yellow surface and occur in women two to four times more frequently than in men.

Fungal infections are also very common in diabetics. Candidal infection can produce erythema and edema of intertriginous areas below the breasts, in the axillas, and between the fingers. It causes vulvovaginitis in most chronically uncontrolled diabetic women with persistent glucosuria and is a frequent cause of pruritus.

While antifungal creams containing miconazole or clotrimazole offer immediate relief of vulvovaginitis, recurrence is frequent unless glucosuria is reduced.

Large vessel diseases (Macrovascular complications)

Atherosclerosis and its effects produce the large vessel diseases.

a. Involvement of the coronary vessels can produce myocardial infarction.
b. Involvement of cerebral vessels can produce "stroke".
c. Peripheral vascular disease—atherosclerosis is markedly accelerated in the larger arteries. It is often diffused, with localized enhancement in certain areas of turbulent blood flow,, such as at the bifurcation of the aorta or other large vessels. Clinical manifestations of peripheral vascular disease include ischemia of the lower extremities, impotence, and intestinal angina.

Management of Type 2 Diabetes Mellitus

The goals of therapy for Type 2 DM are similar to those in Type 1. While glycemic control tends to dominate the management of Type 1 DM, the care of individuals with Type 2 DM must also include attention to the treatment of conditions associated with Type 2 DM (obesity, hypertension, dyslipidemia, and cardiovascular disease) and detection/management of DM-related complications. DM-specific complications may be present in up to 20–50% of individuals with newly diagnosed Type 2 DM. Reduction in cardiovascular risk is of paramount importance as this is the leading cause of mortality in these individuals.

a. **Weight reduction:** Treatment is directed toward achieving weight reduction, and prescribing a diet is only one means to this end. Behavior modification to achieve adherence to the diet—as well as increased physical activity to expend energy—is also required.
b. **Hypoglycemic agents:** If the patient is not able to achieve target glycemic control with weight management and exercise then pharmacologic therapy is indicated.

   Based on their mechanisms of action, glucose-lowering agents are subdivided into agents that increase insulin secretion, reduce glucose production, increase insulin sensitivity, and enhance GLP-1 action. Glucose-lowering agents (with the exception of α-glucosidase inhibitors and an amylin analog) are ineffective in Type 1 DM and should not be used for glucose management of severely ill individuals with Type 2 DM. Insulin is sometimes the initial glucose-lowering agent.

   1. **Insulin secretagogues:** Insulin secretagogues stimulate insulin secretion by interacting with the ATP-sensitive potassium channel on the beta cells. These drugs are most effective in individuals with Type 2 DM of relatively recent onset (<5 years), who have residual endogenous insulin production. Various examples of insulin secretagogues are as follows:

      a. Sulfonylurea—first generation
         Chlorpropamide
         Tolazamide
         Tolbutamide

b. Sulfonylurea—second generation
Glimepiride
Glipizide
Glipizide (extended release)
Glyburide
Glyburide (micronized)

c. Nonsulfonylureas
Repaglinide
Nateglinide
Insulin secretagogues are generally well tolerated. All of these agents, however, have the potential to cause profound and persistent hypoglycemia, especially in elderly individuals. Hypoglycemia is usually related to delayed meals, increased physical activity, alcohol intake, or renal insufficiency.

2. **Biguanides:** Metformin is the representative of this class of agents. It reduces hepatic glucose production through an undefined mechanism and improves peripheral glucose utilization slightly metformin reduces fasting plasma glucose and insulin levels, improves the lipid profile, and promotes modest weight loss.
The major toxicity of metformin, lactic acidosis, can be prevented by careful patient selection.
3. **α-glucosidase inhibitors:** α-glucosidase inhibitors (acarbose and miglitol) reduce postprandial hyperglycemia by delaying glucose absorption; they do not affect glucose utilization or insulin secretion. Postprandial hyperglycemia, secondary to impaired hepatic and peripheral glucose disposal, contributes significantly to the hyperglycemic state in Type 2 DM. These drugs, taken just before each meal, reduce glucose absorption by inhibiting the enzyme that cleaves oligosaccharides into simple sugars in the intestinal lumen. Therapy should be initiated at a low dose (25 mg of acarbose or miglitol) with the evening meal and may be increased to a maximal dose over weeks to months (50–100 mg for acarbose or 50 mg for miglitol with each meal). The major side effects (diarrhea, flatulence, and abdominal distention) are related to increased delivery of oligosaccharides to the large bowel and can be reduced somewhat by gradual upward dose titration. α-glucosidase inhibitors may increase levels of sulfonylureas and increase the incidence of hypoglycemia.
4. **Thiazolidinediones:** Thiazolidinediones reduce insulin resistance. These drugs bind to the PPAR-γ (peroxisome proliferator-activated receptor-γ) nuclear receptor. The PPAR-γ receptor is found at highest levels in adipocytes but is expressed at lower levels in many other tissues. Agonists of this receptor regulate a large number of genes, promote adipocyte differentiation, reduce hepatic fat accumulation, and appear to reduce insulin resistance indirectly by enhancing fatty acid storage and possibly by increasing adiponectin levels. Thiazolidinediones promote a redistribution of fat from central to peripheral locations. Circulating insulin levels decrease with use of the thiazolidinediones, indicating a reduction in insulin resistance. Rosiglitazone and pioglitazone belong to this category.
5. **Insulin therapy in Type 2 DM:** Insulin should be considered as the initial therapy in Type 2 DM, particularly in lean individuals or those with severe weight loss, in individuals with underlying renal or hepatic disease that precludes oral glucose-lowering agents, or in individuals who are hospitalized or acutely ill. Insulin therapy is ultimately required by a substantial number of individuals with Type 2 DM because of the progressive nature of the disorder and the relative insulin deficiency that develops in patients with long-standing diabetes.

CLINICAL NOTE

Glucose-lowering agents (with the exception of α-glucosidase inhibitors and an amylin analog) are ineffective in Type 1 DM and should not be used for glucose management of severely ill individuals with Type 2 DM. Insulin is sometimes the initial glucose-lowering agent.

CLINICAL PEARLS

1. Type 2 DM is characterized by impaired insulin secretion, insulin resistance, excessive hepatic glucose production, and abnormal fat metabolism.
2. While many patients with Type 2 diabetes present with increased urination and thirst, many others have an insidious onset of hyperglycemia and are asymptomatic initially.
3. Diabetic ketoacidosis (DKA) and hyperglycemic hyperosmolar state (HHS) are acute complications of diabetes. DKA was formerly considered a hallmark of Type 1 DM, but it also occurs in individuals who lack immunologic features of Type 1 DM and who can subsequently be treated with oral glucose-lowering agents.
4. Chronic complications are micro- and macrovascular complications involved in small and large blood vessels, respectively.
5. The care of individuals with Type 2 DM must also include attention to the treatment of conditions associated with Type 2 DM (obesity, hypertension, dyslipidemia, and cardiovascular disease) and detection/management of DM-related complications.

CASE STUDY 16

Theme: Biochemical Basis and Clinical Implications of Diabetic Ketoacidosis

A 22-year-old diabetic comes to the accident and emergency department. She gives a 2-day history of vomiting and abdominal pain. She is drowsy and her breathing is deep and rapid. There is distinctive smell from her breath.

What is the most likely diagnosis?
Which bedside test would you do to help you to confirm the diagnosis?
Which laboratory test would you request?

BASIC CONCEPT

The patient is suffering from **diabetic ketoacidosis.**

Diabetic ketoacidosis (DKA) is a state of inadequate insulin levels resulting in high blood sugar and accumulation of organic acids and ketones in the blood. It is a potentially life-threatening complication in patients with diabetes mellitus. It happens predominantly in Type 1 diabetes mellitus, but it can also occur in Type 2 diabetes mellitus under certain circumstances.

Cause

Diabetic ketoacidosis (DKA) most frequently occurs in known diabetics. **It may also be the first presentation in patients who had not previously been diagnosed as diabetics.** There is often a particular underlying problem that has led to the DKA episode. This may be intercurrent illness (pneumonia, influenza, gastroenteritis, and a urinary tract infection), pregnancy, inadequate insulin administration (e.g., defective insulin pen device), myocardial infarction (heart attack), stroke, or the use of cocaine. Young patients with recurrent episodes of DKA may have an underlying eating disorder, or may be using insufficient insulin for fear that it will cause weight gain. In 5% of cases, no cause for the DKA episode is found **(Fig. 15.19)**.

Diabetic ketoacidosis may occur in those previously known to have diabetes mellitus Type 2 or in those who on further investigations turn out to have features of Type 2 diabetes (e.g., obesity, strong family history); this is more common in African, African American, and Hispanic people. Their condition is then labeled "ketosis-prone Type 2 diabetes".

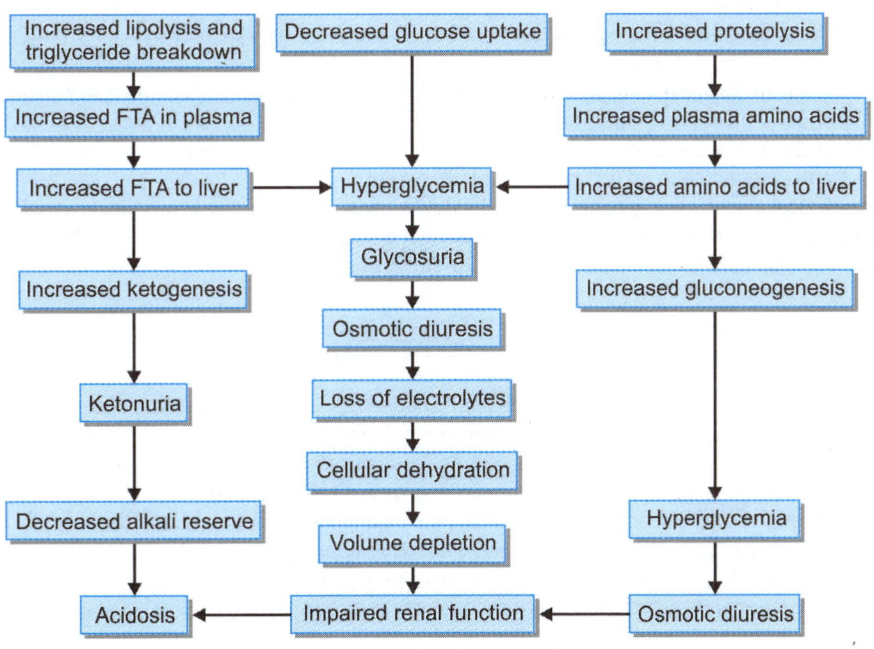

Fig. 15.19: Causes and consequences of diabetic ketoacidosis (DKA).

Pathophysiology

Diabetic ketoacidosis (DKA) results from relative or absolute insulin deficiency combined with counter-regulatory hormone excess (glucagon, catecholamines, cortisol, and growth hormone). **The decreased ratio of insulin to glucagon promotes gluconeogenesis, glycogenolysis, and ketone body formation in the liver, as well as increases in substrate delivery from fat and muscle (free fatty acids, amino acids) to the liver.**

The combination of insulin deficiency and hyperglycemia reduces the hepatic level of fructose 2,6 bisphosphate, which alters the activity of phosphofructokinase and fructose 1,6-bisphosphatase. Glucagon excess decreases the activity of pyruvate kinase, whereas insulin deficiency increases the activity of phosphoenolpyruvate carboxykinase. These changes shift the handling of pyruvate toward glucose synthesis and away from glycolysis. The increased levels of glucagon and catecholamines in the face of low insulin levels promote glycogenolysis. Insulin deficiency also reduces levels of the GLUT4 glucose transporter, which impairs glucose uptake into skeletal muscle and fat and reduces intracellular glucose metabolism.

Normally, the free fatty acids released by adipolysis are converted to triglycerides or VLDL in the liver. However, in DKA, hyperglucagonemia alters hepatic metabolism to favor ketone body formation, through activation of the enzyme carnitine palmitoyltransferase I. This enzyme is crucial for regulating fatty acid transport into the mitochondria, where beta oxidation and conversion to ketone bodies occur.

The ketone bodies, however, have a low pH and, therefore, turn the blood acidic (metabolic acidosis). The body initially buffers this with the bicarbonate buffering system, but this is quickly overwhelmed and other mechanisms to compensate for the acidosis,, such as hyperventilation to lower the blood carbon dioxide levels. This hyperventilation, in its extreme form, may be observed as Kussmaul respiration. Ketones, too, participate in osmotic diuresis and lead to further electrolyte losses. As a result of the above mechanisms, the average adult DKA patient has a total body water shortage of about 6 liters (or 100 mL/kg), in addition to substantial shortages in sodium, potassium, chloride, phosphate, magnesium, and calcium. Glucose levels usually exceed 13.8 mmol/L or 250 mg/dL.

Increased lactic acid production also contributes to the acidosis. The increased free fatty acids increase triglyceride and VLDL production. VLDL clearance is also reduced because the activity of insulin-sensitive lipoprotein lipase in muscle and fat is decreased. Most commonly, DKA is precipitated by increased insulin requirements, as might occur during a concurrent illness. Occasionally, complete omission of insulin by the patient with Type 1 DM precipitates DKA.

CLINICAL MANIFESTATIONS

The symptoms of an episode of diabetic ketoacidosis usually evolve over the period of about 24 hours. Predominant symptoms are nausea and vomiting, pronounced thirst, excessive urine production, and abdominal pain that may be severe. Hyperglycemia is always present. In severe DKA, breathing becomes labored and of a deep, gasping character (a state referred to as **"Kussmaul respiration"**). The abdomen may be tender to the point that an acute abdomen may be suspected,, such as acute pancreatitis, appendicitis, or gastrointestinal perforation. Coffee ground vomiting (vomiting of altered blood) occurs in a minority of patients; this tends to originate from erosions of the esophagus. In severe DKA, there may be confusion, lethargy, stupor, or even coma (a marked decrease in the level of consciousness).

On physical examination, there is usually clinical evidence of dehydration,, such as a dry mouth and decreased skin turgor. If the dehydration is profound enough to cause a decrease in the circulating blood volume, tachycardia (a fast heart rate), and low blood pressure may be observed. Often, a "ketotic" odor is present, which is often described as "fruity". If Kussmaul respiration is present, this is reflected in an increased respiratory rate.

Small children with DKA are relatively prone to cerebral edema (swelling of the brain tissue), which may cause headache, coma, loss of the pupillary light reflex, and progress to death. It occurs in 0.7–1.0% of children with DKA, and has been described in young adults, but is overall very rare in adults. It carries 20–50% mortality.

DIAGNOSIS

Investigations

Diabetic ketoacidosis (DKA) may be diagnosed when the combination of hyperglycemia (high blood sugars), ketones on urinalysis, and acidosis are demonstrated. Arterial blood gas measurement is usually performed to demonstrate the acidosis; this requires taking a blood sample from an artery. In addition to the above, blood samples are usually taken to measure urea and creatinine (measures of kidney function, which may be impaired in DKA as a result of dehydration) and electrolytes. Furthermore, markers of infection (complete blood count, C-reactive protein) and acute pancreatitis (amylase and lipase) may be measured. Given the need to exclude infection, chest radiography, and urinalysis are usually performed.

If cerebral edema is suspected because of confusion, recurrent vomiting, or other symptoms, computed tomography may be performed to assess its severity and to exclude other causes, such as stroke.

Management

The main aims in the treatment of diabetic ketoacidosis are replacing the lost fluids and electrolytes, while suppressing the high blood sugars and ketone production with insulin.

Fluid replacement: The amount of fluid depends on the estimated degree of dehydration. If dehydration is so severe, rapid infusion of saline is recommended to restore circulating volume.

Insulin is usually given continuously.

Potassium levels can fluctuate severely during the treatment of DKA, because insulin decreases potassium levels in the blood by redistributing it into cells. Serum potassium levels are initially often mildly raised even though total body potassium is depleted.

Hypokalemia often follows treatment. This increases the risk of irregularities in the heart rate. Therefore, continuous observation of the heart rate is recommended, as well as repeated measurement of the potassium levels and addition of potassium to the intravenous fluids once levels fall below 5.3 mmol/L. If potassium levels fall below 3.3 mmol/L, insulin administration may need to be interrupted to allow correction of the hypokalemia.

Bicarbonate

Sodium bicarbonate solution is administered to rapidly improve the acid levels in the blood.
Cerebral edema: Administration of fluids is slowed; intravenous mannitol and hypertonic saline (3%) are used.

Prognosis

With appropriate therapy, the mortality of DKA is low (<5%) and is related more to the underlying or precipitating event,, such as infection or myocardial infarction. The major nonmetabolic complication of DKA therapy is cerebral edema, which most often develops in children as DKA is resolving. The etiology of and optimal therapy for cerebral edema are not well-established, but overreplacement of free water should be avoided. The other known complications of DKA therapy are—hypoglycemia, hypokalemia, and hypophosphatemia.

Venous thrombosis, upper gastrointestinal bleeding, and acute respiratory distress syndrome occasionally complicate DKA.

Prevention of DKA

Following treatment, the physician and patient should review the sequence of events that led to DKA to prevent future recurrences. Foremost is patient education about the symptoms of DKA, its precipitating factors, and the management of diabetes during a concurrent illness. During illness or when oral intake is compromised, patients should:

1. Frequently measure the capillary blood glucose
2. Measure urinary ketones when the serum glucose >16.5 mmol/L (300 mg/dL)
3. Drink fluids to maintain hydration
4. Continue or increase insulin
5. Seek medical attention, if dehydration, persistent vomiting, or uncontrolled hyperglycemia develops. Using these strategies, early DKA can be prevented or detected and treated appropriately on an outpatient basis.

DIABETIC KETOACIDOSIS IN PREGNANCY

Diabetic ketoacidosis (DKA) in pregnancy is of special concern. It tends to occur at lower plasma glucose levels and more rapidly than in nonpregnant patients and usually occurs in the second and third trimesters because of increasing insulin resistance. Fetal mortality rates have previously been reported as high as 30% rising to over 60% in DKA with coma. However, with improvements in diabetic care, the figure for fetal loss has been reported as low as 9% in some countries. Prevention, early recognition, and aggressive management are vitally important to minimize fetal mortality.

CLINICAL NOTE

Despite apparently normal serum potassium levels, all patients with DKA have whole body depletion of potassium levels, which may be very severe.

CLINICAL PEARLS

1. DKA is a potentially life-threatening complication of diabetes mellitus.
2. Initial assessment must involve a rapid assessment of airway, breathing and circulation, and obtaining sufficient intravenous access.
3. The diagnosis of DKA requires a blood sugar of >14.0 mmol/L, positive urinary or plasma ketones, an arterial pH of <7.3, and serum bicarbonate of <18 mmol/L.
4. The basic principles of DKA management include rapid restoration of adequate circulation and perfusion with isotonic intravenous fluids, gradual rehydration and restoration of depleted electrolytes, insulin to reverse ketosis and hyperglycemia and regular monitoring of clinical signs and laboratory tests to detect and treat complications.
5. Acute cerebral edema is a potential complication possibly due to excessive fluid therapy or too rapid a fall in blood glucose.

CASE STUDY 17

Theme: Biochemical Basis and Clinical Implications of "Metabolic Syndrome"

A 64-year-old man is presented to his family doctor with complaints of frequent episodes of dizziness and of numbness in his legs.

During a routine history and physical examination, the doctor finds that the patient leads a sedentary lifestyle, is obese (body mass index of 32), and has hypertension (blood pressure of 200/120 mm Hg).

The patient is asked to return to the clinic a week later in the fasting state, during which time a blood specimen is obtained, and a glucose tolerance test is performed. Humoral analysis reveals fasting hyperglycemia, hyperinsulinemia, dyslipidemia, and glucose intolerance.

What is the probable diagnosis?
What other investigations should be carried out to confirm the diagnosis?
What is the possible treatment for this disease?

CASE DETAILS

The patient is suffering from "insulin resistance syndrome".

METABOLIC SYNDROME

Background

Metabolic syndrome also referred to as Syndrome X or insulin resistance syndrome consists of a number of metabolic risk factors that increase the risk for atherosclerotic cardiovascular disease (CVD) and other cardiovascular complications, such as cardiac arrhythmias, heart failure, and thrombotic events.

There are key components to the metabolic syndrome, which include hypertension, dyslipidemia, insulin resistance, chronic inflammation, impaired fibrinolysis, procoagulation, and most telling central obesity.

Incidence

A quarter of the world's adults are considered to have the metabolic syndrome. It is estimated that 47 million people in the United States have this multifactorial syndrome. Metabolic syndrome is generally observed with increased age, but may present in children and adolescents as well. Although a genetic predisposition exists in the development of metabolic syndrome, acquired causes also seem to play a role.

Diagnostic Criteria

In an effort to clinically identify patients with insulin resistance, various organizations have developed diagnostic criteria. The most commonly used criteria in the United States are those of the National Cholesterol Education Program/Adult Treatment Panel III (NCEP/ATP III).

- NCEP/ATP III criteria for the diagnosis of the metabolic syndrome include the following (diagnosis is made when 3 or more are present):
  - Waist circumference of more than 102 cm in men or more than 88 cm in women
  - Fasting triglyceride level of 150 mg/dL or higher
  - Blood pressure level of 130/85 mm Hg or higher
  - High-density lipoprotein cholesterol (HDL-C) level of less than 40 mg/dL in men or less than 50 mg/dL in women
  - Fasting glucose level of 110 mg/dL or higher [which has been changed to 100 mg/dL to reflect revised criteria for impaired fasting glucose (IFG)].

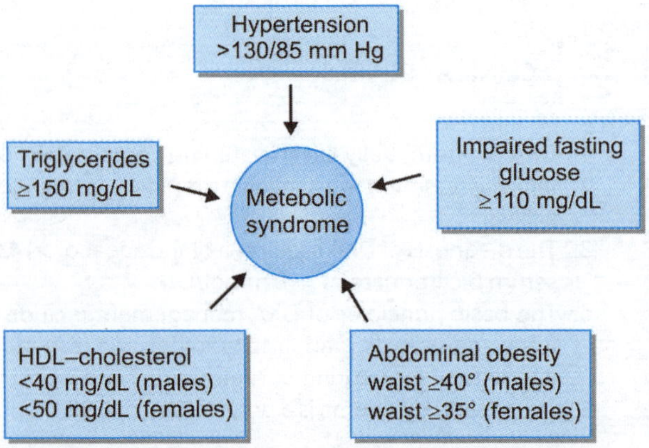

Fig. 15.20: Metabolic syndrome is associated with hypertension, dyslipidemia, obesity, and impaired glucose tolerance.

Pathophysiology

Metabolic syndrome is multifactorial—a combination of both metabolic and underlying risk factors is involved **(Fig. 15.20)**.

According to the National Cholesterol Education Program (NCEP) Adult Treatment Panel III (ATP III) report, there are six major components of metabolic syndrome relating to the development of CVD:

1. Abdominal obesity
2. Atherogenic dyslipidemia

3. Elevated blood pressure
4. Insulin resistance (with/without the presence of glucose intolerance)
5. Proinflammatory state, and
6. Prothrombotic state

1. **Abdominal obesity:** Abdominal obesity is assessed by waist circumference. Waist circumference is an important component of the most recent and frequently applied diagnostic criteria for the metabolic syndrome. However, measuring waist circumference does not reliably distinguish between a large waist due to increases in subcutaneous adipose tissue versus visceral fat; this distinction requires CT or MRI. With increases in visceral adipose tissue, adipose tissue-derived FFAs are directed to the liver. On the other hand, increases in abdominal subcutaneous fat release lipolysis products into the systemic circulation and avoid more direct effects on hepatic metabolism. **Relative increases in visceral versus subcutaneous adipose tissue with increasing waist circumference in Asians and Asian Indians may explain the greater prevalence of the syndrome in these populations compared to African American men in whom subcutaneous fat predominates.** Obesity in general is associated with a higher CVD risk and contributes to elevated blood pressure, elevated LDL-C levels, decreased HDL-C levels, and hyperglycemia. Increased waist circumference can, therefore, explain all the components of the metabolic syndrome.
2. **Atherogenic dyslipidemia:** Atherogenic dyslipidemia is defined as an increase in serum triglycerides, presence of small LDL-C particles, and a low HDL-C level. In general, FFA flux to the liver is associated with increased production of apoB-containing, triglyceride-rich very low-density lipoproteins (VLDLs). The effect of insulin on this process is complex, but hypertriglyceridemia is an excellent marker of the insulin-resistant condition.

   The other major lipoprotein disturbance in the metabolic syndrome is a reduction in HDL cholesterol. This reduction is a consequence of changes in HDL composition and metabolism. In the presence of hypertriglyceridemia, a decrease in the cholesterol content of HDL is a consequence of reduced cholesteryl ester content of the lipoprotein core in combination with cholesteryl ester transfer protein-mediated alterations in triglyceride making the particle small and dense. This change in lipoprotein composition also results in an increased clearance of HDL from the circulation. The relationships of these changes in HDL to insulin resistance are likely indirect, occurring in concert with the changes in triglyceride-rich lipoprotein metabolism. In addition to HDL, LDLs are also modified in composition. With fasting serum triglycerides >2.0 mM (~180 mg/dL), there is almost always a predominance of small dense LDLs. Small dense LDLs are thought to be more atherogenic. They may be toxic to the endothelium, and they are able to transit through the endothelial basement membrane and adhere to glycosaminoglycans. They also have increased susceptibility to oxidation and are selectively bound to scavenger receptors on monocyte-derived macrophages. Subjects with increased small dense LDL particles and hypertriglyceridemia also have increased cholesterol content of both VLDL1 and VLDL2 subfractions. This relatively cholesterol-rich VLDL particle may also contribute to the atherogenic risk in patients with metabolic syndrome.
3. **Hypertension:** The relationship between insulin resistance and hypertension is well-established. Under normal physiologic conditions, insulin is a vasodilator with secondary effects on sodium reabsorption in the kidney. However, in the setting of insulin resistance, the vasodilatory effect of insulin is lost, but the renal effect on sodium reabsorption is preserved. Sodium reabsorption is increased in Caucasians with the metabolic syndrome, but not in Africans or Asians. Insulin also increases the activity of the sympathetic nervous system, an effect that may also be preserved in the setting of the insulin resistance. Finally, insulin resistance is characterized by pathway-specific impairment in phosphatidylinositol 3-kinase signaling. In the endothelium, this may cause an imbalance between the production of nitric oxide and secretion of endothelin-1, leading to decreased blood flow. Hence by all means, insulin resistance results in hypertension.
4. **Insulin resistance:** It is a state in which less-than-anticipated biological effects are observed with a given amount of insulin. Alternatively, it may be defined as the state when the requirement of insulin, to achieve glycemic control and prevent ketosis, exceeds 200 or more units per day. Insulin resistance can be inherited or acquired. The inherited insulin resistance can be due to mutations involving the insulin receptor, glucose transporter, or signaling proteins. The causes of acquired insulin resistance include lack of physical exercise, unhealthy diet, drugs, hyperglycemia, advancing age, and high level of serum free fatty acids. The causes of insulin-resistant states can be categorized as follows:
   - **Prereceptor:**
     - Defective insulin (mutations)
     - Antibodies against insulin (anti-insulin antibodies)
   - **Receptor:**
     - Reduced number of receptors
     - Decreased binding of insulin
     - Defective insulin receptor (mutations)
     - Insulin receptor-blocking antibodies
   - **Post-receptor:**
     - Faulty signal transduction
     - Defective GLUT4
   - **Combinations of defects:** Some combinations of defects are frequently observed. For example, obesity is a significant cause of insulin resistance. It may be associated with post-receptor abnormality and a reduced number of insulin receptors.

- **Other conditions that are categorized as receptor or post-receptor insulin-resistant states:**
  - Leprechaunism
  - Lipodystrophy
  - Ataxia-telangiectasia
  - Werner syndrome
  - Rabson–Mendenhall syndrome
  - Pineal hypertrophic syndrome
- **Aging:** A decreased production of GLUT-4 with advancing age may cause insulin resistance.
- **Increased production of insulin antagonists:** Several disorders are associated with increased production of insulin antagonists, for example, Cushing syndrome, acromegaly, and conditions of stress, such as trauma, surgery, diabetes ketoacidosis, severe infection, uremia, and liver cirrhosis.
- **Drug-induced:** Drugs associated with insulin resistance syndrome include glucocorticoids, cyclosporine, niacin, and protease inhibitors.
- **Human immunodeficiency virus (HIV):** Protease inhibitor and nucleoside analogs have been reported to cause the development of insulin resistance.
- **Insulin treatment:**
  - The patients on insulin treatment almost always have low titer IgG anti-insulin antibody levels. Infrequently, the antibodies cause considerable prereceptor insulin resistance.
  - Increased inactivation of insulin at the site of subcutaneous injection site has also been implicated.

Glucose Intolerance

- The defects in insulin action lead to impaired suppression of glucose production by the liver and kidney and reduced glucose uptake and metabolism in insulin-sensitive tissues, i.e., muscle and adipose tissue. To compensate for defects in insulin action, insulin secretion and/or clearance must be modified to sustain euglycemia. Ultimately, this compensatory mechanism fails, usually because of defects in insulin secretion, resulting in progress from IFG and/or IGT to DM. Type 2 diabetes is characterized by increased hepatic glucose output, increased peripheral resistance to insulin action (due to receptor and postreceptor defects), and impaired insulin secretion. In skeletal muscle, various abnormalities, including defective glucose transport, may cause insulin resistance. Glucose transporter 4 (GLUT4) is the main insulin-responsive transporter.

5. **A prothrombotic state is characterized by abnormalities, specifically elevations, in procoagulant factors, antifibrinolytic factors, platelet alterations, and endothelial dysfunction.** Insulin resistance, the compensatory hyperinsulinemia, and other components are associated with increased risk of cardiovascular disease; endothelial dysfunction is a prominent feature of insulin resistance syndrome. An additional role of insulin resistance in the overall cardiac pathology associated with the metabolic syndrome relates to the normal role of insulin in platelet function. In platelets, insulin action leads to an increase in endothelial nitric oxide synthase (eNOS) activity that is due to its phosphorylation by AMPK. Activation of NO production in platelets leads to a decrease in thrombin-induced aggregation, thereby, limiting the procoagulant effects of platelet activation. This response of platelets to insulin function clearly indicates why disruption in insulin action is a major contributing factor in the development of the metabolic syndrome.
6. **A proinflammatory state is characterized by elevations of circulating inflammatory molecules, such as C-reactive protein (CRP), tumor necrosis factor-alpha, plasma resistin, interleukin (IL)-6, and IL-18.** CRP is a general marker of inflammation that has been linked to CVD in patients with metabolic syndrome. Adiponectin is an anti-inflammatory cytokine produced exclusively by adipocytes. Adiponectin enhances insulin sensitivity and inhibits many steps in the inflammatory process. In the liver, adiponectin inhibits the expression of gluconeogenic enzymes and the rate of glucose production. In muscle, adiponectin increases glucose transport and enhances fatty acid oxidation, partially due to activation of AMP kinase. Adiponectin is reduced in the metabolic syndrome. The relative contribution of adiponectin deficiency versus overabundance of the proinflammatory cytokines remains unclear.

These adipokines promote vascular dysfunction and atherogenesis either indirectly though metabolic risk factors or by direct action on the arterial wall.

Clinical Manifestations

The metabolic syndrome is typically unassociated with symptoms. On physical examination, waist circumference may be expanded and blood pressure elevated. The presence of one or either of these signs should alert the clinician to search for other biochemical abnormalities that may be associated with the metabolic syndrome. Less frequently, lipoatrophy or acanthosis nigricans is found on examination. Because these physical findings are typically associated with severe insulin resistance, other components of the metabolic syndrome should be expected.

Associated Diseases

1. **Cardiovascular disease:** The relative risk for new-onset CVD in patients with the metabolic syndrome, in the absence of diabetes, averages between 1.5- and threefold. Patients with metabolic syndrome are also at increased risk for peripheral vascular disease.

2. **Type 2 diabetes:** Overall, the risk for Type 2 diabetes in patients with the metabolic syndrome is increased three- to fivefold.
   Other associated conditions
   In addition to the features specifically associated with metabolic syndrome, insulin resistance is accompanied by other metabolic alterations. These included increases in apoB and C III, uric acid, prothrombotic factors (fibrinogen, plasminogen activator inhibitor 1), serum viscosity, asymmetric dimethylarginine, homocysteine, white blood cell count, proinflammatory cytokines, CRP, microalbuminuria, nonalcoholic fatty liver disease (NAFLD) and/or nonalcoholic steatohepatitis (NASH), polycystic ovarian disease (PCOS), and obstructive sleep apnea (OSA).
3. **Nonalcoholic fatty liver disease:** Fatty liver is relatively common. However, in NASH, both triglyceride accumulation and inflammation coexist. As the prevalence of overweight/obesity and the metabolic syndrome increases, NASH may become one of the more frequent causes of end-stage liver disease and hepatocellular carcinoma.
4. **Hyperuricemia:** Hyperuricemia reflects defects in insulin action on the renal tubular reabsorption of uric acid.
5. **Microalbuminuria:** Microalbuminuria may also be caused by altered endothelial pathophysiology in the insulin-resistant state.
6. **Polycystic ovary syndrome:** Polycystic ovary syndrome (PCOS) is highly associated with the metabolic syndrome, with a prevalence between 40% and 50%. Women with PCOS are 2 to 4 times more likely to have the metabolic syndrome compared to women without polycystic ovary syndrome (PCOS).
7. **Obstructive sleep apnea:** Obstructive sleep apnea (OSA) is commonly associated with obesity, hypertension, increased circulating cytokines, IGT, and insulin resistance. Continuous positive airway pressure (CPAP) treatment in OSA patients improves insulin sensitivity.

Diagnosis

The diagnosis of the metabolic syndrome relies on satisfying the criteria using tools at the bedside and in the laboratory. A person suspected of having this syndrome should have a thorough history taken especially with regard to family history and presence of other cardiovascular risk factors.

An examination should include:

- Recording the body weight
- Calculating the BMI
- Measurement of the waist circumference in inches
- Calculating the hip-waist ratio
- Measurement of the subcutaneous fat at 4 sites—biceps, triceps, subscapular, and suprailiac
- Blood pressure measurement

Laboratory Tests

1. Fasting lipids and glucose estimations are needed to determine, if the metabolic syndrome is present.
2. The measurement of additional biomarkers associated with insulin resistance must be individualized. Such tests might include apoB, high-sensitivity CRP, fibrinogen, uric acid, urinary microalbumin, and liver function tests.
3. A sleep study should be performed, if symptoms of OSA are present.
4. If PCOS is suspected based on clinical features and anovulation, testosterone, luteinizing hormone, and follicle-stimulating hormone should be measured

Treatment of Metabolic Syndrome

Treating the insulin resistance: While there is no drug treatment that directly treats the underlying insulin resistance in metabolic syndrome, there is, in fact, a way to reverse insulin resistance—diet and exercise. Those with metabolic syndrome should make every attempt to reduce their body weight to within 20% of their "ideal" body weight (calculated for age and height) and incorporate aerobic exercise (at least 20 minutes) into their daily lifestyle. With vigorous efforts to reduce weight and increase exercise, metabolic syndrome can be reversed and the risk for cardiovascular complications can be substantially improved. Several drug classes [biguanides, thiazolidinediones (TZDs)] increase insulin sensitivity. If insulin resistance is the primary pathophysiologic mechanism for the metabolic syndrome, then representative drugs in these classes should reduce its prevalence. Both metformin and TZDs enhance insulin action in the liver and suppress endogenous glucose production. TZDs, but not metformin, also improve insulin-mediated glucose uptake in muscle and adipose tissue. Benefits of both drugs have also been seen in patients with nonalcoholic fatty liver disease (NAFLD) and polycystic ovary syndrome (PCOS), and they have been shown to reduce markers of inflammation and small dense LDL. In general, the beneficial effects of TZDs appear superior to those of metformin.

Treating lipid abnormalities: While the lipid abnormalities seen with metabolic syndrome (low HDL, high LDL, and high triglycerides) respond nicely to weight loss and exercise, drug therapy is often required. Treatment should be aimed primarily at reducing LDL levels according to specific recommendations. Once reduced LDL targets are reached, efforts at reducing triglyceride levels and raising HDL levels should be made. Successful drug treatment usually requires treatment with a statin, a fibrate drug, or a combination of a statin with either niacin or a fibrate.

Treating the prothrombotic state: Patients with metabolic syndrome also exhibit a prothrombotic state due to the abnormalities in coagulation factors, which are not routinely measured in clinical practice.

Patients with metabolic syndrome should generally be placed on daily aspirin therapy to help in preventing such clotting events.

Treating the hypertension: High blood pressure is present in more than half the people with metabolic syndrome and, in the setting of insulin resistance, high blood pressure is especially important as a risk factor. Adequate blood pressure treatment in these individuals can substantially improve their outcome. Since underlying endothelial dysfunction is an important factor in such patients, drugs that improve hypertension and also the endothelial dysfunction are preferred, e.g., ACE inhibitors and angiotensin receptor blockers. Other antihypertensive, which lack this second property, like thiazide diuretics, beta-blockers, and calcium channel blockers should be reserved for second- and third-line therapies.

Treatment of impaired fasting glucose: In patients with the metabolic syndrome and Type 2 diabetes, aggressive glycemic control may favorably modify fasting triglycerides and/or HDL cholesterol. In those patients with IFG without a diagnosis of diabetes, a lifestyle intervention that includes weight reduction, dietary fat restriction, and increased physical activity has been shown to reduce the incidence of Type 2 diabetes. Metformin has also been shown to reduce the incidence of diabetes, although the effect was less than that seen with lifestyle intervention.

Lifestyle modifications: Management of metabolic syndrome is highly dependent on the control of all of the contributing factors. This includes both underlying risk factors as well as metabolic risk factors. Lifestyle modifications should be implemented immediately for all patients diagnosed with metabolic syndrome. Lifestyle modification includes weight reduction, increased physical activity, and nutritional therapy. Additional risk assessments should be performed in patients to assure appropriate goals of therapy throughout the course of the syndrome.

The key to preventing and metabolic syndrome, however, remains diet and exercise. Any person with a strong family history of metabolic syndrome or Type 2 diabetes should be especially careful to maintain a healthy lifestyle.

CLINICAL NOTE

The primary goal of clinical management of the metabolic syndrome is to reduce the risk for cardiovascular disease and Type 2 diabetes.

CLINICAL PEARLS

1. Insulin resistance is a generalized metabolic disorder, in which the body cannot use insulin efficiently.
2. People with the metabolic syndrome are at increased risk of coronary heart disease and other diseases related to plaque buildups in artery walls (e.g., stroke and peripheral vascular disease) and Type 2 diabetes.
3. Hypertension, dyslipidemia, polycystic ovarian syndrome, fatty liver disease, prediabetes, sleep and breathing disorder, certain cancers, and cognitive impairment are many of the presentations of the syndrome.
4. Lifestyle modification is the most important part of the management of people with the syndrome. Lately, medications have been recommended when lifestyle modification is not enough or when it fails.

CASE STUDY 18

Theme: Clinical Implications of Excess Release of Insulin (Insulinoma)

An 82-year-old woman presented to her primary care physician with a 10-year history of episodic confusion and somnolence. The episodes occurred about twice a year, typically in the morning, just after waking. They lasted minutes and were relieved when she ate her breakfast or had juice. Over the 8–10 months before presentation, the patient noted that the episodes were increasing in frequency as well as occurring throughout the day.

When the patient presented to her doctor with the above complaints, and was waiting for checkout, she developed confusion, immediately a capillary blood glucose test was performed, and she was noted to have a plasma glucose level of 28 mg/dL. She was given juice and her symptoms resolved after a few moments.

The patient was subsequently admitted to the hospital for further follow-up.

On examination, she was found to be a well-nourished woman in no apparent distress. She had mild hypertension. Her physical and neurological examinations were unremarkable. Her admission laboratory value of glucose level was 36 mg/dL. She was completely asymptomatic upon presentation and was thus placed on a fasting protocol.

The fasting protocol was continued until she became symptomatic. The subsequent laboratory results were consistent with the suspected diagnosis of an insulin secreting tumor. To localize the tumor, an abdominal CT with contrast was undertaken, which revealed an enhancing mass in the pancreatic head suggestive of an insulinoma.

What are the clinical signs and symptoms of insulinoma?
How is the diagnosis of insulinoma made?
What are the treatment options for insulinoma?

CASE DISCUSSION

Insulinoma

Insulinomas are almost always islet cell tumors of the pancreas and occur as single or multiple tumors. They are typically benign, although malignant tumors have been reported as well. Beta cells secrete insulin in response to increases in blood glucose. The resulting increase in insulin acts to lower blood glucose back to normal levels at which point further secretion of insulin is stopped. In contrast, the secretion of insulin by insulinomas is not properly regulated by glucose and the tumors will continue to secrete insulin causing glucose levels to fall further than normal. As a result, patients present with symptoms of low blood glucose (hypoglycemia), which are improved by eating.

Incidence

Insulinomas are rare neuroendocrine tumors with an incidence estimated at 1 to 4 new cases per million persons per year. Insulinoma is one of the most common types of tumor arising from the islets of Langerhans cells. Estimates of malignancy range from 5% to 30%. Over 99% of insulinomas originate in the pancreas, with rare cases from ectopic pancreatic tissue. About 5% of cases are associated with tumors of the parathyroid glands and the pituitary (multiple endocrine neoplasia Type 1) and are more likely to be multiple and malignant. Most insulinomas are small, less than 2 cm.

Clinical Manifestations

Insulinomas present with the neuroglycopenic and sympathoadrenal symptoms induced by hypoglycemia. These include recurrent headache, lethargy, diplopia, and blurred vision, particularly with exercise or fasting. Severe hypoglycemia may result in seizures, coma, and permanent neurological damage. Symptoms resulting from the catecholaminergic response to hypoglycemia (i.e., tremulousness, palpitations, tachycardia, sweating, hunger, anxiety, and nausea) are not as common. Sudden weight gain (the patient can become massively obese) is sometimes seen. Confusion is typical of insulinoma.

Interestingly, some patients have none of the sympathoadrenal symptoms. This phenomenon is known as "hypoglycemia unawareness" and occurs because the set point for catecholamine secretion in response to hypoglycemia is lowered.

Misdiagnosis of insulinoma is common. Patients with a psychiatric, seizure, or other neurological disorder can be misdiagnosed before the true diagnosis of insulinoma is made.

Diagnosis

The diagnosis of insulinoma is suspected in a patient with symptomatic fasting hypoglycemia. The conditions of Whipple's triad need to be met for the diagnosis of "true hypoglycemia" to be made:

1. Symptoms and signs of hypoglycemia
2. Concomitant plasma glucose level of 45 mg/dL (2.5 mmol/L) or less
3. Reversibility of symptoms with administration of glucose

Blood Tests

The following blood tests are needed to diagnose insulinoma:

- Glucose
- Insulin
- C-peptide

If available, a proinsulin level might be useful as well. Other blood tests may help to rule out other conditions, which can cause hypoglycemia.

Suppression Tests

Normally, endogenous insulin production is suppressed in the setting of hypoglycemia. A 72-hour fast, usually supervised in a hospital setting, can be done to see if insulin levels fail to suppress, which is a strong indicator of the presence of an insulin-secreting tumor.

During the test, the patient may have calorie-free and caffeine-free liquids. Capillary blood glucose is measured every 4 hours using a reflectance meter, until values <60 mg/dL (3.3 mmol/L) are obtained. Then, the frequency of blood glucose measurement is increased to every hour until values are <49 mg/dL (2.7 mmol/L). At that point, or when the patient has symptoms of hypoglycemia, a blood test is drawn for serum glucose, insulin, proinsulin, and C-peptide levels. The fast is stopped at that point, and the hypoglycemia treated with intravenous dextrose or calorie-containing food or drink.

Diagnostic Imaging

The insulinoma might be localized by noninvasive means, using ultrasound, CT scan, or by MRI techniques. An Indium-111 pentetreotide scan is more sensitive than ultrasound, CT, or MRI for detection of somatostatin receptor positive tumors.

Sometimes, angiography with percutaneous transhepatic pancreatic vein catheterization to sample the blood for insulin levels is required. Calcium can be injected into selected arteries to stimulate insulin release from various parts of the pancreas, which can be measured by sampling blood from their respective veins. The use of calcium stimulation improves the specificity of this test.

Diagnosis of insulinoma is established by demonstrating inappropriately high serum levels of endogenous insulin in the setting of hypoglycemia.

A serum insulin concentration of ≥6 μU/mL, when the serum glucose concentration is <45 mg/dL, indicates inappropriate secretion of insulin, consistent with insulinoma.

Treatment

The definitive management is surgical removal of the insulinoma. This may involve removing part of the pancreas as well (Whipple procedure and distal pancreatectomy).

Medications, such as diazoxide and somatostatin can be used to block the release of insulin for patients who are not surgical candidates or who otherwise have inoperable tumors.

Streptozotocin is used in islet cell carcinomas, which produce excessive insulin. Combination chemotherapy is used: doxorubicin + streptozotocin, or fluorouracil + streptozotocin in patients where doxorubicin is contraindicated.

In metastasizing tumors with intrahepatic growth, hepatic arterial occlusion or embolization can be used.

Prognosis

Most patients with benign insulinomas can be cured with surgery. Persistent or recurrent hypoglycemia after surgery tends to occur in patients with multiple tumors. About 2% of patients develop diabetes mellitus after their surgery.

CLINICAL NOTE

The conditions of Whipple's triad need to be met for the diagnosis of "true hypoglycemia" are—symptoms and signs of hypoglycemia, concomitant plasma glucose level of 45 mg/dL (2.5 mmol/L) or less, and reversibility of symptoms with administration of glucose.

CLINICAL PEARLS

1. Insulinomas are islet cell tumors of the pancreas and occur as single or multiple tumors.
2. Insulinomas present with the neuroglycopenic and sympathoadrenal symptoms induced by hypoglycemia.
3. A serum insulin concentration of ≥6 μU/mL, when the serum glucose concentration is <45 mg/dL, indicates inappropriate secretion of insulin, consistent with insulinoma.
4. The insulinoma might be localized by noninvasive means, using ultrasound, CT scan, or by MRI techniques.
5. The definitive management is surgical removal of the insulinoma. This may involve removing part of the pancreas as well (Whipple procedure and distal pancreatectomy).

CASE STUDY 19

Theme: Causes and Clinical Implications of Rebound Hypoglycemia

A 46-year-old male presented to the physician for follow-up of his diabetes. He was a known diabetic since the age of 10 and had been on insulin therapy. He complained of feeling very restless and diaphoretic around midnight. The physician advised him to observe the blood glucose level at the time of onset of symptoms. The patient on his next visit reported that the blood sugar was in the range of 40 mg/dL, which was very low. He, however, noted that his morning fasting blood sugar was high without taking any carbohydrates.

What is the probable diagnosis for such like symptoms?

What are the biochemical processes that govern the response to the night-time hypoglycemia?

CASE DETAILS

The patient is experiencing "Somogyi effect", also called "rebound hyperglycemia".

SOMOGYI EFFECT

The Somogyi effect is a pattern of undetected hypoglycemia (blood glucose values of less than 70) followed by hyperglycemia (blood glucose levels of more than 200). Typically, this happens in the middle of the night, but can also occur when too much insulin is circulating in the system.

Cause

The cause of Somogyi effect is said to be "man-made"—that is, the result of hyperfunctioning of insulin or oral hypoglycemic drugs at the wrong time. When the blood glucose level falls below normal, the body responds by releasing glucagon as well as the stress hormones epinephrine and cortisol. Glucagon facilitates release of glucose from the liver by glycogenolysis that raises the blood glucose immediately, and the stress hormones that cause insulin resistance for several hours, sustaining the elevated blood glucose. The physiological mechanisms driving the rebound are defensive. Sometimes, a person with diabetes will experience the Somogyi rebound when awake and notice symptoms of the initial low blood sugar or symptoms of the rebound. **At night, waking with a night sweat (perhaps combined with a rapid heart rate) is a symptom of the adrenaline and rebound hyperglycemia.**

CLINICAL MANIFESTATIONS

Symptoms include headache, nightmares, and night sweats.

Diagnosis

The diagnosis is established by measuring a 2 am glucose level, and when confirmed, then the bedtime insulin dose is needed to be decreased. The danger is that if nighttime blood glucose levels are not measured, the physician may interpret the patient as having hyperglycemia and require even higher doses of insulin. This would be exactly the wrong treatment, since the hypoglycemia is leading to counter-regulatory hormone reaction, and a very low sugar level causes the high sugar level in the morning.

Another disorder similar to the Somogyi effect is known as the dawn phenomenon. Although most diabetics are affected by this disorder, it seems to occur more often in pubescent adolescents. Adolescents' blood sugar is affected adversely by their body releasing counter-regulatory hormones. These counter-regulatory hormones (growth hormone, cortisol, and catecholamines) cause the glucose level to rise. For people with diabetes who do not have enough circulating insulin to keep this increase of glucose under control, the end result is a high glucose reading in the morning.

For pregnant women, the dawn phenomenon is even more exaggerated due to additional hormones released in the night produce precipitously high blood sugar levels. It is thought that the growth hormone has some impact in relation to the production of counter-regulatory hormones. Correction of the dawn phenomenon requires an increase in insulin coverage prior to bedtime.

CLINICAL NOTE

If nighttime blood glucose levels are not measured in Somogyi effect, the physician may interpret the patient as having hyperglycemia and require even higher doses of insulin. This would be exactly the wrong treatment.

CLINICAL PEARLS

1. The Somogyi effect is a pattern of undetected hypoglycemia (blood glucose values of less than 70) followed by hyperglycemia (blood glucose levels of more than 200).
2. Typically, this happens in the middle of the night, but can also occur when too much insulin is circulating in the system.
3. The physiological mechanisms driving the rebound are defensive.
4. When the blood glucose level falls below normal, the body responds by releasing glucagon as well as the stress hormones epinephrine and cortisol. Glucagon facilitates release of glucose from the liver by glycogenolysis that raises the blood glucose immediately, and the stress hormones that cause insulin resistance for several hours, sustaining the elevated blood glucose.
5. When confirmed, then the bedtime insulin dose is needed to be decreased.

Chapter 16

Detoxification

LEARNING OBJECTIVES

To understand:

- General mechanism of detoxification of drugs
- Mechanism of detoxification of acetaminophen
- Mechanism of entoxification
- Biochemical basis and management of ethylene glycol poisoning
- Mechanism and management of isoniazid toxicity.

CASE STUDIES

CASE STUDY 1

Theme: Phase 1 and 2 Reactions of Detoxification

An 18-year-old medical student was brought to the emergency department after being found in the dormitory room floor nauseated, having excessive vomiting, and complaining of severe abdominal pain. Her friends were concerned when she did not show up for an anatomy final at the local medical college. The patient had been under a lot of stress with finals, a breakup with a boyfriend, and trying to pay the college fee due to poor financial condition of the parents. In the dormitory room, one of her friends noticed an empty bottle of Tylenol (acetaminophen) near the bed with numerous pills lying on the ground near that girl.

On arrival to the emergency department, the patient was found to be in moderate distress and having excessive vomiting. The patient was quickly assessed and blood sample was sent for laboratory investigations. Patient had a hypokalemia noted on electrolytes and elevated liver enzymes. Her white blood cell count was normal. Her urine drug screen was negative and her acetaminophen blood level was above 200 μg/mL. The attending physician prescribed N-acetylcysteine to the patient.

What is the possible toxicity in this patient?

What is the biochemical mechanism whereby the N-acetylcysteine would help in this condition?

CASE DETAILS

The patient is having acetaminophen toxicity. The patient has described all the initial signs of a deliberate overdose of acetaminophen. Acetaminophen poisoning can cause gastroenteritis within hours and hepatotoxicity 1–3 days after ingestion. Severity of hepatotoxicity after a single acute overdose is predicted by serum acetaminophen levels. Treatment is with N-acetylcysteine to prevent or minimize hepatotoxicity.

BASIC CONCEPT

Acetaminophen Toxicity

Acetaminophen is contained in >100 products sold over-the-counter. Products include many children's preparations in liquid, tablet, and capsule form and many cough and cold preparations. Many prescription drugs also contain acetaminophen. Consequently, acetaminophen overdose is common.

Pathophysiology

After absorption, it is **metabolized mainly by glucuronidation and sulfation**, with a small fraction metabolized via the P450 mixed-function oxidase system to a highly toxic reactive intermediate N-acetyl-benzoquinone imine (NABQI) **(Fig. 16.1)**. This toxic intermediate is normally detoxified by cellular glutathione. With acute acetaminophen overdose (>140 mg/kg, or 7 g in an average adult), hepatocellular glutathione is rapidly depleted and the reactive intermediates attack other cell proteins, causing necrosis and possibly damage to other organs (e.g., kidneys, pancreas). **Patients with enhanced P450 activity,, such as chronic alcoholics and patients taking INH, are at increased risk of developing hepatotoxicity**. Hepatic toxicity may also occur after chronic accidental overuse of acetaminophen, e.g., as a result of taking two or three acetaminophen-containing products concurrently or intentionally exceeding the recommended maximum dose of 4 g/day.

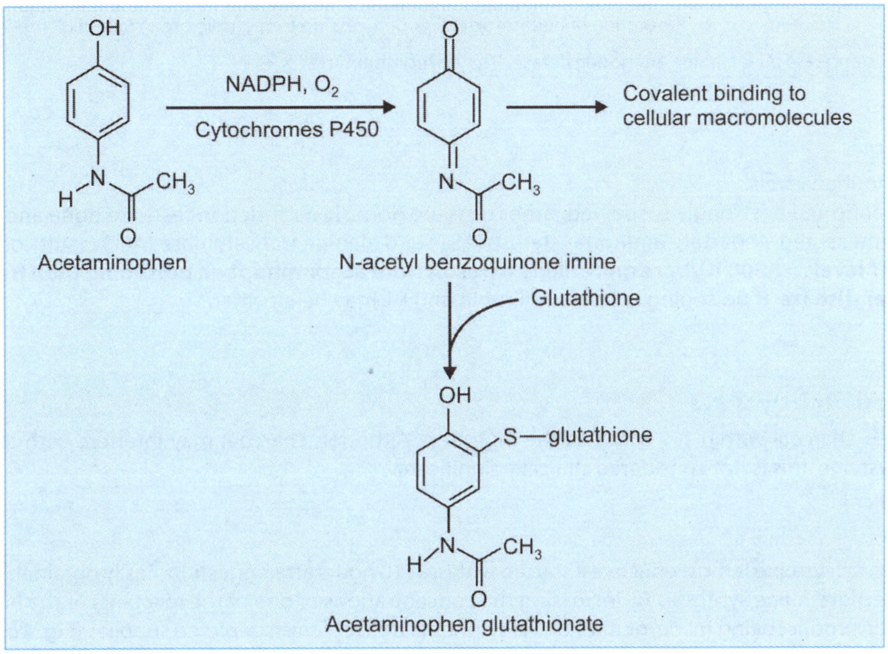

Fig. 16.1: Detoxification of acetaminophen.

Theoretically, **alcoholic liver disease or undernutrition could increase risk of toxicity because hepatic enzyme preconditioning may increase formation of NABQI and because undernutrition (also common among alcoholics) reduces hepatic glutathione stores**. This includes deficiencies of any of the enzymes involved in the synthesis of glutathione or that keep glutathione in its reduced state as well as any other fee radical generating process that consumes glutathione. However, whether the risk is actually increased is unclear. **Acute alcohol ingestion may be protective because hepatic P450 enzymes preferentially metabolize ethanol and thus cannot produce toxic NABQI.**

Clinical Findings

Shortly after ingestion, patients may have nausea or vomiting, but there are usually no other signs of toxicity until 24–48 hours after ingestion, when hepatic aminotransferase levels begin to increase. With severe poisoning, fulminant hepatic necrosis may occur, resulting in jaundice, hepatic encephalopathy, renal failure, and death. Rarely, massive ingestion (e.g., serum levels over 500–1,000 mg/L) can cause early onset of acute coma, hypotension, and metabolic acidosis unrelated to hepatic injury.

Acute Acetaminophen Toxicity

The diagnosis after acute overdose is based on measurement of the serum acetaminophen level. Symptoms which occur in 4 stages include anorexia, nausea, vomiting, and right upper quadrant abdominal pain. Renal failure and pancreatitis may occur, occasionally without liver failure. After >5 days, hepatotoxicity resolves or progresses to multiple organ failure which can be fatal **(Table 16.1)**.

Chronic Acetaminophen Poisoning

Chronic excessive use or repeated overdoses cause hepatotoxicity in a few patients. Usually, chronic overdose is not an attempt at self-injury but instead results from taking inappropriately high doses to treat pain. Symptoms may be absent or may include any of those that occur with acute overdose.

TABLE 16.1: Stages of acute acetaminophen poisoning.

Stages	*Time post ingestion*	*Description*
I	0–24 hours	Anorexia, nausea, and vomiting
II	24–72 hours	Right upper quadrant abdominal pain (common)
		AST, ALT, and, if poisoning is severe, bilirubin and PT sometimes elevated
III	72–96 hours	Vomiting and symptoms of liver failure
		Peaking of AST, ALT, bilirubin, and PT
		Sometimes renal failure and pancreatitis
IV	>5 days	Resolution of hepatotoxicity or progression to multiple organ failure (sometimes fatal)

AST: aspartate aminotranferase ;ALT: alanine aminotransferase; PT: prothrombin time

Laboratory Diagnosis

- Serum acetaminophen levels.
- If poisoning is confirmed or strongly suspected, other tests are done. Liver function tests are done and, in suspected severe poisoning, PT is measured. Aspartate aminotransferase (AST) and alanine transaminase (ALT) result correlate with the stage of poisoning. **AST levels >1,000 IU/L are more likely to result from acetaminophen poisoning than from chronic hepatitis or alcoholic liver disease**. If poisoning is severe, bilirubin and PT may be elevated.

Treatment

Emergency and Supportive Measures

Administer activated charcoal within 1–2 hours of the ingestion. Although charcoal may interfere with absorption of the oral antidote N-acetylcysteine, this is not considered clinically significant.

Specific Treatment

Treatment with *N*-acetylcysteine is most effective if started within 8–10 hours after ingestion. Easily obtainable and readily soluble, it serves to facilitate glutathione synthesis by increasing the concentrations of one of the reactants of the first synthetic step. The committed dipeptide product being made, glutathione is synthesized to replenish depleted supplies **(Fig. 16.2)**. **N-acetylcysteine seems most effective when given <10 hours after ingestion of acetaminophen but is recommended within the first 35 hours after ingestion.**

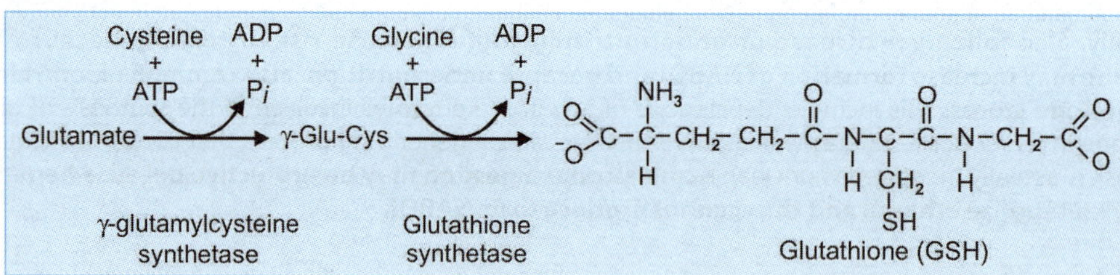

Fig. 16.2: Steps of glutathione synthesis.

Prognosis

With appropriate treatment, mortality is uncommon.

Poor prognostic indicators at 24–48 hours postingestion include all of the following:

- pH <7.3 after adequate resuscitation
- Serum creatinine >2.6
- Hepatic encephalopathy grade III (confusion and somnolence) or grade IV (stupor and coma)
- Hypoglycemia
- Thrombocytopenia

CLINICAL NOTE

Acute alcohol ingestion may be protective in acetaminophen toxicity because hepatic P450 enzymes preferentially metabolize ethanol and thus cannot produce toxic N-acetyl-benzoquinone imine.

CLINICAL PEARLS

1. Acetaminophen poisoning can cause gastroenteritis within hours and hepatotoxicity 1–3 days after ingestion.
2. It is metabolized mainly by glucuronidation and sulfation, with a small fraction metabolized via the P450 mixed-function oxidase system to a highly toxic reactive intermediate N-acetyl-p-benzoquinone imine. This toxic intermediate is normally detoxified by cellular glutathione. With acute acetaminophen overdose (>140 mg/kg, or 7 g in an average adult), hepatocellular glutathione is rapidly depleted and the reactive intermediates attack other cell proteins, causing necrosis and possibly damage to other organs (e.g., kidneys, pancreas).
3. Alcoholic liver disease or undernutrition can increase risk of toxicity.
4. Severity of hepatotoxicity after a single acute overdose is predicted by serum acetaminophen levels.
5. Treatment is with N-acetylcysteine to prevent or minimize hepatotoxicity.

CASE STUDY 2

Theme: Entoxification of Xenobiotics

A 3-year-old girl was brought into the emergency room. She was cold and clammy and was breathing rapidly. She was obviously confused and lethargic. Her mother indicated that she had accidentally ingested automobile antifreeze while playing in the garage.

Following gastrointestinal lavage and activated charcoal administration, a nasogastric tube for ethanol was administered.

What is the problem with the child, how will ethanol help in relieving the symptoms?

CASE DETAILS

This is a case of ethylene glycol poisoning.

BASIC CONCEPT

Ethylene Glycol Poisoning

Ethylene glycol is the major ingredient of almost all radiator fluid products. It is used to increase the boiling point and decrease the freezing point of radiator fluid, which circulates through the automotive radiator. These changes to the boiling and freezing points result from the colligative properties of the solute (they depend on the number of particles in the solution). Hence, ethylene glycol is added to prevent the radiator from overheating or freezing, depending on the season.

Pathophysiology

Ethylene Glycol Toxicity

The metabolic products of toxic alcohols are more harmful than the parent compounds. For example, ethylene glycol, the parent alcohol is comparatively a nontoxic compound; it may cause some changes in the mental state. However, its extreme toxicity characterizes the metabolic product of ethylene glycol.

Metabolism of Ethylene Glycol

Ethylene glycol is first metabolized to glycolaldehyde by alcohol dehydrogenase, which then is metabolized to glycolic acid (GA) through interaction with aldehyde dehydrogenase. These reactions are similar to the metabolic reactions of ethanol and methanol. *[Ethanol and methanol both are metabolized by alcohol* ***(Fig. 16.3)*** *dehydrogenase (ADH) pathway which is present in the liver and gastric mucosa and by the mixed-function oxidase (cytochrome P450) system found in the liver. The mixed-function oxidase component is more inducible than alcohol dehydrogenase]*.

Accidental ingestion of ethylene glycol in toxic concentrations causes a marked acidosis, the cause of which can be attributed to excess glycolic acid in the circulation. The patients might develop hyperventilation resulting as compensation to acidosis. The glycolic acid can further be converted to glyoxylic acid, which may be metabolized to highly toxic oxalate or relatively nontoxic metabolites of glutamate or α-ketoadipic acid. The oxalate formed in high concentrations may lead to the formation of calcium oxalate crystals, which accumulate in the blood and other tissues or precipitate in the renal cortex causing reduced glomerular filtration and renal insufficiency. The excess formation of calcium oxalate may also deplete calcium reserves, causing hypocalcemia.

The alcohol dehydrogenase-catalyzed step is the rate-limiting step of ethylene glycol metabolism. As ethanol is the true substrate of alcohol dehydrogenase, therefore, the affinity of alcohol dehydrogenase is more for ethanol than ethylene glycol. In fact, the presence of ethanol may even inhibit the metabolism of ethylene glycol.

Reactions

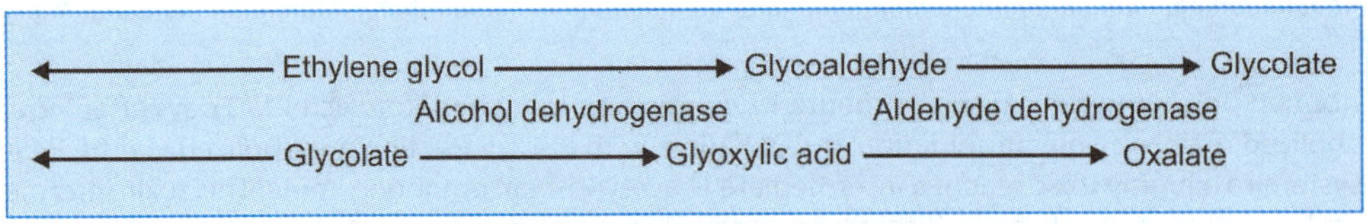

Fig. 16.3: Metabolism of ethylene glycol.

Clinical Manifestations

Shortly after ingestion of either of these agents, patients usually appear "drunk." The serum osmolality (measured with the freezing point device) is usually increased, but acidosis is often absent early. After several hours, metabolism to toxic organic acids leads to a **severe anion gap metabolic acidosis, tachypnea, confusion, convulsions, and coma. Ethylene glycol often produces oxalate crystalluria and renal failure**.

Causes

Causes of ethylene glycol poisoning include the following:
- Suicide attempts
- Accidental ingestions (mainly observed in children)
- Workplace beverage-container mix-ups.

Laboratory Investigations

- Serum ethylene glycol concentrations may be measured.
- **Serum osmolality:** Ethylene glycol exposure level is often estimated through measurement of the serum osmolality. This estimate is obtained by sampling a set of electrolyte levels (e.g., BUN, creatinine, and glucose) and calculating the expected osmolality in the patient's serum. A serum osmolality is then measured and the difference between the measured and calculated osmolality (**the osmolal gap**) is determined. Several formulas are effective for calculating the osmolality from serum electrolytes and other solutes.
- Serum electrolyte levels are also useful later in the course of intoxication because they can reveal the presence of **anion gap acidosis**. This information may be important when determining the need for dialysis and other interventions. The goal of therapy, however, is to treat the patient before acidosis develops.
- Additional laboratory tests that should be obtained in symptomatic patients include the following:
  - Serum calcium level determination is recommended
  - Arterial blood gas determination is recommended
  - **Urinalysis:** Urine may reveal the presence of calcium oxalate crystals, a sign usually observed late in the process of intoxication. **Oxalate crystals typically have the shape of a folded envelope.**

Treatment

Emergency and Supportive Measures

For patients presenting within 30–60 minutes after ingestion, the stomach is emptied by gastric lavage. **Charcoal is not very effective but should be administered if other poisons or drugs have also been ingested.**

Specific Treatment

Patients with significant toxicity (manifested by severe metabolic acidosis, altered mental status, and markedly elevated osmolar gap) should undergo hemodialysis as soon as possible to remove the parent compound and the toxic metabolites. Treatment with folic acid, thiamine, and pyridoxine may enhance the breakdown of toxic metabolites.

Ethanol blocks metabolism of the parent compounds by competing for the enzyme alcohol dehydrogenase. The desired serum ethanol concentration is 100 mg/day. Fomepizole (4-methylpyrazole, antizol) blocks alcohol dehydrogenase and can be used instead of ethanol.

CLINICAL NOTE

Treatment with folic acid, thiamine, and pyridoxine may enhance the breakdown of toxic metabolites in ethylene glycol poisoning.

CLINICAL PEARLS

1. Ethylene glycol is a relatively nontoxic compound before it is metabolized. The metabolites cause the distinctive toxicity associated with this compound.
2. Ethylene glycol is metabolized by alcohol dehydrogenase to form glycolaldehyde. Through interaction with aldehyde dehydrogenase, ethylene glycol is then metabolized to GA. This glycolate is then transformed into glyoxylic acid. At this point, the molecule may be transformed into the highly toxic oxalate or the safer glutamate or α-ketoadipic acid metabolites.
3. Causes of ethylene glycol poisoning include suicide attempts or accidental ingestions.
4. After several hours, metabolism to toxic organic acids leads to a severe anion gap metabolic acidosis, tachypnea, confusion, convulsions, and coma. Ethylene glycol often produces oxalate crystalluria and renal failure.
5. Ethanol blocks metabolism of the parent compounds by competing for the enzyme alcohol dehydrogenase, it is effective in treating the toxicity. Patients with significant toxicity should undergo hemodialysis as soon as possible to remove the parent compound and the toxic metabolites.

CASE STUDY 3

Theme: Isoniazid-induced Pyridoxal-phosphate Deficiency

A 4-year-old child with history of accidental ingestion of 13 tablets of isoniazid (INH) was brought to the emergency room, with generalized tonic-clonic seizures which were refractory to diazepam, phenytoin, and phenobarbitone. There was no previous history of such like seizures. There was no history of any medical illness.

There was no apparent abnormality detected except for seizures. Given in gram per gram amounts of the isoniazid ingested, intravenous pyridoxine (vitamin B_6) ultimately terminated the seizure activity.

What is the cause of seizures in this child? What is the line of treatment for this toxicity?

CASE DETAILS

The child is suffering from isoniazid toxicity. The toxic manifestations are due to deficiency of pyridoxine. **Isoniazid inhibits brain pyridoxal-5-phosphate, the active form of pyridoxine, resulting in decrease in the brain level of gamma-aminobutyric acid causing decrease in seizure threshold**.

BASIC CONCEPT

Isoniazid Toxicity

INH is an antibacterial drug used mainly in the treatment and prevention of tuberculosis. It may cause hepatitis with long-term use, especially in alcoholic patients and elderly persons. It produces acute toxic effects by inhibiting the brain pyridoxal-5-phosphate, resulting in lowered brain *gamma*-aminobutyric acid (GABA) levels. Acute ingestion of as little as 1.5–2 g of INH can cause toxicity and severe poisoning is likely to occur after ingestion of more than 80–100 mg/kg.

Pathophysiology

Isoniazid binds to pyridoxal-5-phosphate, the active form of pyridoxine (vitamin B6), to form INH-pyridoxal hydrazones. Pyridoxal-5-phosphate is a cofactor for glutamic acid decarboxylase and GABA transaminase in the GABA synthetic pathway. **The INH overdose results in decreased pyridoxal-5-phosphate, decreased GABA synthesis, increased cerebral excitability, and seizures. Co-ingestion of ethanol potentiates toxicity by enhancing degradation of phosphorylated pyridoxine**.

Toxic effects of INH also result from inhibition of lactate dehydrogenase, an enzyme that converts lactate to pyruvate and from inhibition of cytochrome P450. The INH undergoes N-acetylation in the liver to a variety of products that include acetylhydrazine, a potent hepatotoxin. These metabolites are excreted in the urine. With long-term administration at therapeutic doses, INH can cause clinically significant liver injury in 1% of patients and elevated liver enzyme levels in 10–20% of patients.

Clinical Manifestations

Symptoms are usually observed within 45 minutes of acute overdose but may be delayed up to 2 hours, when peak absorption occurs.

- Nausea
- Vomiting
- Dizziness

- Light sensitivity
- Seizures may occur abruptly and are often generalized and tonic-clonic, but focal seizures have been described
- The clinical triad of acute neurotoxicity consists of seizures (refractory to standard anticonvulsants), metabolic acidosis, and coma; it is usually observed in ingestions of more than 200 mg/kg
- Hyperpyrexia
- Hypotension
- Tachycardia
- Urinary retention
- Ataxia, slurred speech, stupor, and hyperreflexia.

Adverse effects from long-term ingestion include the following:

- **Peripheral neuritis:** Uncommon in healthy individuals but more common in persons with diabetes, those with alcoholism, and malnourished elderly individuals.
- **Hepatitis:** Increased risk with concomitant use of carbamazepine, phenobarbital, rifampin, and alcohol abuse.

Laboratory Investigations

- **No correlation exists between serum isoniazid (INH) levels and severity of acute intoxication. Laboratory** studies generally are not helpful in diagnosis of acute INH toxicity but may identify complications
- Elevated anion gap metabolic acidosis (caused by lactic acid)
- Hypokalemia
- Hyperglycemia
- Ketonemia
- Transient elevation of liver enzyme levels
- Leukocytosis
- Positive DIC panel
- Glycosuria
- Ketonuria

Laboratory abnormalities observed with INH therapy include the following:

- Elevated liver enzyme levels: **Patients with pretreatment AST levels above the upper limit of normal are predisposed to developing hepatotoxicity.**
- Granulocytopenia or agranulocytosis
- Eosinophilia
- Thrombocytopenia
- Anemia

Treatment

Emergency and Supportive Measures

Seizures may require higher than usual doses of benzodiazepines (e.g., lorazepam 3–5 mg intravenously) or administration of pyridoxine as an antidote.

Administer activated charcoal. **Do induce emesis, because of the risk of abrupt onset of seizures.**

Specific Treatment

Pyridoxine (vitâmin B_6) is a specific antagonist of the acute toxic effects of INH and is usually successful in controlling convulsions that do not respond to benzodiazepines. Give 5 g intravenously over 1–2 minutes, or if the amount ingested is known, give a gram-for-gram equivalent amount of pyridoxine. Patients taking INH are usually given 25–50 mg of pyridoxine orally daily to help prevent neuropathy.

Complications

Complications of isoniazid toxicity include the following:

- Aspiration
- Pneumonia
- Hypotension
- Cardiorespiratory arrest

Prognosis

- The prognosis is largely dependent on early identification and correction of complications.
- Advanced age, underlying seizure disorder, severe metabolic acidosis, and decreased renal function are associated with a poor prognosis.

CLINICAL NOTE

The clinical triad of acute neurotoxicity consists of seizures (refractory to standard anticonvulsants), metabolic acidosis, and coma; it is usually observed in ingestions of more than 200 mg/kg.

CLINICAL PEARLS

1. The INH is an antibacterial drug used mainly in the treatment and prevention of tuberculosis.
2. It produces acute toxic effects by inhibiting pyridoxal-5-phosphate, resulting in lowered brain GABA levels.
3. The clinical triad of acute neurotoxicity consists of seizures (refractory to standard anticonvulsants), metabolic acidosis, and coma; it is usually observed in ingestions of more than 200 mg/kg.
4. Elevated anion gap metabolic acidosis, hypokalemia and hyperglycemia, transient elevation of liver enzyme levels, leukocytosis, positive DIC panel, glycosuria, and ketonuria are observed in INH toxicity.
5. Pyridoxine (vitamin B_6) is a specific antagonist of the acute toxic effects of INH and is usually successful in controlling convulsions that do not respond to benzodiazepines. Give 5 g intravenously over 1–2 minutes, or if the amount ingested is known, give a gram-for-gram equivalent amount of pyridoxine.

Chapter 17

Diet and Nutrition

LEARNING OBJECTIVES

To understand:
- ❖ Causes, pathogenesis, and management of malnutrition
- ❖ Causes, pathogenesis, and management of obesity
- ❖ Biochemical deviations in starvation
- ❖ Chemistry and significance of dietary fiber.

CASE STUDIES

CASE STUDY 1

Theme: Protein-energy Malnutrition—Causes and Consequences

An 8-month-old girl was brought to the clinic because of excessive exhaustion and fatigue. On further questioning of the mother, she reported that she was previously breastfeeding but had to stop to return to work. To feed all of her other children, she had to dilute her formula with water to make the formula last longer for the entire family. On examination, the child was irritable, had starved appearance, weight was much below for height, mid-arm muscle circumference was 12 cm, and triceps thickness was 2 mm. The creatinine-height index (the 24-hour urinary creatinine excretion compared with normal values based on height) was low but serum albumin was normal.
What is the probable diagnosis?

CASE DETAILS

The child is suffering from **nutritional marasmus**. Marasmus is a state in which virtually all available body fat stores are exhausted due to starvation.

The given patient has starved appearance diagnostic of marasmus. The low body weight, diminished skinfold thickness, and reduced arm muscle circumference reflect the loss of fat reserves and the catabolism of proteins throughout the body. The low creatinine-height index also reflects the loss of muscle mass while the normal serum albumin differentiates it from kwashiorkor, which is primarily due to protein deficiency.

PROTEIN-ENERGY MALNUTRITION

The World Health Organization (WHO) defines malnutrition as "the cellular imbalance between the supply of nutrients and energy and the body's demand for them to ensure growth, maintenance, and specific functions". The term protein-energy malnutrition (PEM) applies to a group of related disorders that include marasmus, kwashiorkor, and intermediate states of marasmus-kwashiorkor. **The term marasmus is derived from the Greek word *marasmos*, which means withering or wasting. Marasmus involves inadequate intake of protein and calories and is characterized by emaciation. The term kwashiorkor is taken from the Ga language of Ghana and means "the sickness of the weaning". Kwashiorkor is due to inadequate intake of proteins and is characterized by edema.**

Incidence

Nearly 30% of humans currently experience one or more of the multiple forms of malnutrition. Close to 50 million children younger than 5 years have PEM and half of the children who die younger than 5 years are undernourished. Approximately 80% of these malnourished children live in Asia, 15% in Africa, and 5% in Latin America.

Classification and Etiology of Malnutrition

The term primary malnutrition refers to malnutrition resulting from inadequate food intake and secondary malnutrition refers to malnutrition resulting from increased nutrient needs, decreased nutrient absorption, and/or increased nutrient losses. Although both primary and secondary malnutrition occur in developing as well as developed countries, **primary malnutrition accounts for the major percentage of malnourished children in developing countries, whereas secondary malnutrition accounts for a higher percentage in developed countries**.

The PEM, whether primary or secondary, is graded as mild, moderate, or severe. Grade is determined by calculating weight as a percentage of expected weight for length or height using international standards (normal, 90–110%; mild PEM, 85–90%; moderate, 75–85%; and severe, <75%).

Primary PEM: Worldwide, primary protein-energy malnutrition (PEM) occurs mostly in children and the elderly who lack access to nutrients; although a common cause in the elderly is depression. Protein-energy undernutrition (PEU) can also result from fasting or anorexia nervosa. Child or elder abuse may be a cause.

Secondary PEM: This type most commonly results from the following:

- **Disorders that affect GI function:** These disorders can interfere with digestion (e.g., pancreatic insufficiency), absorption (e.g., enteritis, enteropathy), or lymphatic transport of nutrients (e.g., retroperitoneal fibrosis, Milroy's disease).
- **Wasting disorders:** In wasting disorders (e.g., AIDS, cancer) and renal failure, catabolism causes cytokine excess, resulting in undernutrition via anorexia and cachexia (wasting of muscle and fat). End-stage heart failure can cause cardiac cachexia, a severe form of undernutrition; mortality rate is particularly high. Factors contributing to cardiac cachexia may include passive hepatic congestion (causing anorexia), edema of the intestinal tract (impairing absorption), and, in advanced disease, increased O_2 requirement due to anaerobic metabolism. Wasting disorders can decrease appetite or impair metabolism of nutrients.
- **Conditions that increase metabolic demands:** These conditions include infections, hyperthyroidism, pheochromocytoma, other endocrine disorders, burns, trauma, surgery, and other critical illnesses.

Previously the most severe forms of PEM, marasmus, and kwashiorkor were considered distinct disorders. **Marasmus was thought to result primarily from inadequate energy intake, whereas kwashiorkor was thought to result primarily from inadequate protein intake. Currently, a third disorder, marasmic kwashiorkor, which has features of both disorders, is recognized.** The three conditions have distinct clinical and metabolic features, but they also have a number of overlapping features. For example, a low plasma protein concentration, often thought to be a manifestation of kwashiorkor, is common in children with both clinical marasmus and clinical kwashiorkor.

In recognition of the overlapping features of these two clinically distinct conditions, the terms currently preferred are edematous (kwashiorkor) and nonedematous (marasmus) PEM.

Nonedematous marasmus (also called the dry form of PEM) causes weight loss and depletion of fat and muscle. In developing countries, marasmus is the most common form of PEM in children.

Causes of Marasmus

The underlying causes of this spectrum of conditions are quite similar. Among these are:

- **Social and economic factors**, such as poverty and ignorance, frequently, malnutrition appears during weaning, especially if weaning is suboptimal, as can occur with a low-variety diet, or if weaning foods are introduced only in children older than 8–10 months.
- Social factors, such as food taboos.
- **Infections:** Associated infections often trigger, aggravate, or combine with marasmus. Infectious diseases more frequently associated with protein-energy malnutrition are gastroenteritis, respiratory infections, measles, and pertussis. HIV also plays an increasingly significant role in some countries.
- **Biologic factors**, such as maternal malnutrition and inadequate intakes of breast milk and other foods, as well as children of young or inexperienced mothers, twins, or female infants can be at a higher risk in some parts of the world.
- **Environmental factors**, such as overcrowded and unsanitary living conditions.

Causes of Kwashiorkor

Kwashiorkor (also called the wet, swollen, or edematous form) is associated with:

- **Premature abandonment of breastfeeding** which typically occurs when a younger sibling is born, displacing the older child from the breast. So, children with kwashiorkor tend to be older than those with marasmus.
- Kwashiorkor may also result from **an acute illness, often gastroenteritis** or another infection (probably secondary to cytokine release) in a child who already has PEM.

- A diet that is more deficient in protein than energy may be more likely to cause kwashiorkor than marasmus. Less common than marasmus, kwashiorkor tends to be confined to specific parts of the world,, such as rural Africa, the Caribbean, and the Pacific islands. In these areas, staple foods (e.g., yams, cassavas, sweet potatoes, and green bananas) are low in protein and high in carbohydrates.
- **In kwashiorkor, cell membranes leak, causing extravasation of intravascular fluid and proteins, resulting in peripheral edema**.

Starvation is a complete lack of nutrients. It occasionally occurs when food is available (as in fasting or anorexia nervosa) but usually occurs because food is unavailable (e.g., during famine or wilderness exposure).

Clinical Manifestations in PEM

Signs and symptoms of marasmus vary with the importance and duration of the energy deficit, age at onset, associated infections (e.g., GI infections), and associated nutritional deficiencies (e.g., iron deficiency, iodine deficiency).

Nonedematous PEM (Marasmus) (Fig. 17.1)

- Initially there is failure to gain weight and irritability, followed by weight loss and listlessness until emaciation results.
- The skin loses turgor and becomes wrinkled and loose as subcutaneous fat disappears. Loss of fat from the sucking pads of the cheeks may occur late and the infant's face may retain a relatively normal appearance, compared with the rest of the body, eventually becoming shrunken and wizened.
- The abdomen may be distended or flat with the intestinal pattern readily visible.
- There is muscle atrophy and resultant hypotonia. The most perceptible and frequent clinical feature in marasmus is the loss of muscle mass and subcutaneous fat mass. Some muscle groups,, such as buttocks and upper limb muscles are more frequently affected than others.
- The temperature is usually subnormal and the pulse is slow.
- Infants are usually constipated but may develop a starvation diarrhea with frequent small stools containing mucus.
- Anorexia is frequent and interferes with renutrition.

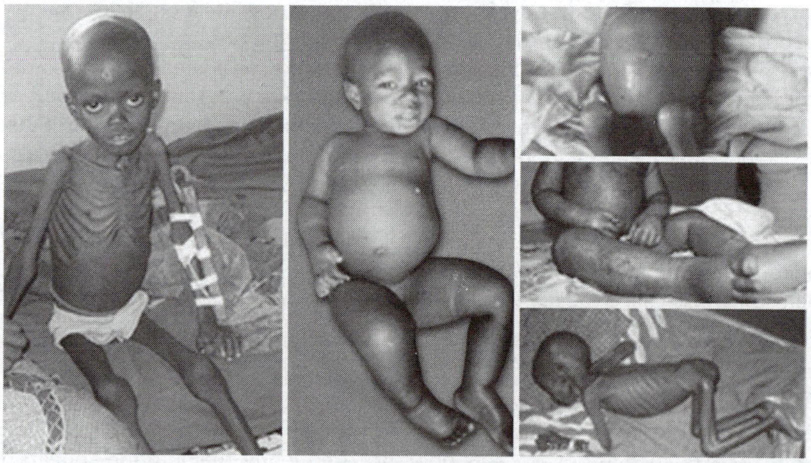

Fig. 17.1: Edematous (kwashiorkor) versus nonedematous (marasmus) protein-energy malnutrition.

Edematous PEM (Kwashiorkor) (Fig. 17.1)

- **Initially:** It may present as vague manifestations that include lethargy, apathy, or irritability.
- **Well-advanced:**
    - There is inadequate growth
    - Lack of stamina
    - Loss of muscle tissue
    - Increased susceptibility to infections
    - Vomiting
    - Diarrhea
    - Anorexia
    - Flabby subcutaneous tissues
    - Edema: **The edema usually develops early and may mask the failure to gain weight**, but the liver may enlarge early or late. The edema is often present in internal organs before it is recognized in the face and limbs.

- Dermatitis is common with darkening of the skin in irritated areas but not in areas exposed to sunlight, in contrast to pellagra.
- Depigmentation may occur after desquamation in these areas, or it may be generalized.
- The hair is sparse and thin and, in dark-haired children, may become streaky red or gray. Alternating episodes of undernutrition and adequate nutrition may cause the hair to have a dramatic "striped flag" appearance.
- The texture is coarse in chronic disease.
- Affected children may be apathetic, but become irritable when held.
- Eventually, there is stupor, coma, and death.

Marasmic kwashiorkor PEM: It is a mixed form of PEM and manifests as edema occurring in children who may or may not have other signs of kwashiorkor.

Clinical features of PEM in older children and adults are basically similar to those in young children, but skin and hair signs are less evident.

Pathophysiology

Malnutrition affects virtually every organ system. Dietary protein is needed to provide amino acids for synthesis of body proteins and other compounds that have various functional roles. Energy is essential for all biochemical and physiologic functions in the body. Furthermore, micronutrients are essential in many metabolic functions in the body as components and cofactors in enzymatic processes.

Weight loss: Many of the manifestations of PEM represent adaptive responses to inadequate energy and/or protein intakes. In the face of inadequate intakes, activity and energy expenditure decrease. However, despite this adaptive response, fat stores are mobilized to meet the ongoing, albeit lower, energy requirement. Once these stores are depleted, protein catabolism must provide the ongoing substrates for maintaining basal metabolism. Visceral organs and muscle are broken down and there is decrease in body weight. Loss of organ weight is greatest in the liver and intestine, intermediate in the heart and kidneys, and least in the nervous system.

Immunodeficiency: In addition to the impairment of physical growth and of cognitive and other physiologic functions, immune response changes occur early in the course of significant malnutrition in a child. Loss of delayed hypersensitivity, fewer T lymphocytes, impaired lymphocyte response, impaired phagocytosis secondary to decreased complement and certain cytokines, and decreased secretory immunoglobulin A (IgA) are some changes that may occur. These immune changes predispose children to severe and chronic infections, which further compromises nutrition causing anorexia, decreased nutrient absorption, increased metabolic needs, and direct nutrient losses. Bacterial infections (e.g., pneumonia, gastroenteritis, otitis media, UTIs, and sepsis) are common in both forms of PEM. Infections result in release of cytokines which produce anorexia, worsen muscle wasting, and cause a marked decrease in serum albumin levels.

Neurological changes: There are changes in the developing brain including a slowed rate of growth of the brain, lower brain weight, thinner cerebral cortex, decreased number of neurons, and insufficient myelinization.

Fatty degeneration and other effects: Other pathologic changes include fatty degeneration of the liver and heart, atrophy of the small bowel, and decreased intravascular volume leading to secondary hyperaldosteronism.

Laboratory Investigations

- The most helpful laboratory studies in assessing malnutrition in a child are hematological studies and laboratory studies evaluating protein status.
  - **Hematological studies** should include a complete blood cell (CBC) count with red blood cell (RBC) indices and a peripheral smear. This could also help exclude anemias from nutritional deficiencies, such as iron, folate, and vitamin B_{12} deficiencies.
  - **Measures of protein nutritional status** include serum albumin, retinol-binding protein, prealbumin, transferrin, creatinine, and BUN levels. Retinol-binding protein, prealbumin, and transferrin determinations are much better short-term indicators of protein status than albumin. However, in the field, a better measure of long-term malnutrition is serum albumin because of its longer half-life.
- **Additional diagnostic evaluation to find out the cause**:
  - In children who have a history of inadequate food intake and signs/symptoms of malnutrition, focus on identifying the cause of malnutrition. Perform laboratory studies based on information from a complete history and physical examination.
  - Initial diagnostic laboratory studies include **CBC count, sedimentation rate, serum electrolytes, and urinalysis and culture. Levels of blood glucose, electrolytes (especially K^+, occasionally Na^+), phosphate, Ca^+, and $Mg^·$ are usually low. BUN is often low unless renal failure is present. Metabolic acidosis may be present**.
  - **Stool specimens** should be obtained if the child has a history of abnormal stools. Stool cultures should be obtained and checked for ova and parasites, if diarrhea is severe or does not resolve with treatment.
  - Additional studies may focus on thyroid functions or sweat chloride tests. Children with suspected liver disease should have triglyceride and vitamin levels obtained.

- Blood cultures, tuberculin testing, and a chest X-ray are used to diagnose occult infections because people with PEM may have a muted response to infections.

Treatment

Mild-to-moderate PEM

A balanced diet can be recommended for the treatment of mild-to-moderate PEM and short-standing starvation. In conditions where solid food cannot be digested, liquid food (preferably lactose-free) can be supplemented. Oral feeding can worsen pre-existing diarrhea. In case of persistence of diarrhea, which is suggestive of lactose intolerance, yogurt-based rather than milk-based formulas are recommended. Vitamin supplementations are needed in all the circumstances.

Severe PEM

The patients with severe PEM or prolonged starvation require hospitalization. The fluid and electrolyte balance are restored. First, the existing infections are controlled and later the oral or nasogastric (NG) tube feeding is started. Parenteral nutrition is reserved for cases with severe malabsorption. Prophylactically, micronutrients are recommended about twice the recommended daily allowance (RDA) until full recovery.

Children

Underlying defect needs to be treated. Since the oral feeding can worsen diarrhea, therefore, the children are kept on oral or IV rehydration therapy first until diarrhea resolves. Oral feeds are given (6–12 times/day), but to avoid volume overload, the feed is given in small amounts, not exceeding >100 mL. Milk-based formulas with extra supplements are offered in progressively increasing quantities during the first week; after that, the full amount of 175 kcal/kg and 4 g of protein/kg may be given. Micronutrients, twice the RDA, are given and after 4 weeks, the whole milk and solid foods are started. The balanced diet should provide energy from 16% proteins, 50% fats, and 34% carbohydrates.

Adults

Underlying disorders should be treated.

Correction of PEM in adults generally resembles that in children; feedings are often limited to small amounts.

Treatment of institutionalized elderly patients with PEM requires multiple interventions:

- Feeding assistance
- Changes in diet (e.g., use of food enhancers and caloric supplements between meals)
- Treatment of depression and other underlying disorders.

Complications of treatment

Treatment of PEM can cause complications (refeeding syndrome) including fluid overload, electrolyte deficits, hyperglycemia, cardiac arrhythmias, and diarrhea. Diarrhea is usually mild and resolves; however, diarrhea in patients with severe PEM occasionally causes severe dehydration or death.

Because PEM can impair cardiac and renal function, hydration can cause intravascular volume overload. Treatment decreases extracellular K^+ and Mg^+. Depletion of K^+ or Mg^+ may cause arrhythmias. **Carbohydrate metabolism that occurs during treatment stimulates insulin release, which drives phosphate into cells. Hypophosphatemia can cause muscle weakness, paresthesias, seizures, coma, and arrhythmias.** Because phosphate levels can change rapidly during parenteral feeding, levels should be measured regularly.

During treatment, endogenous insulin may become ineffective leading to hyperglycemia. Dehydration and hyperosmolality can result. Fatal ventricular arrhythmias can develop, possibly caused by a prolonged QT interval.

Prognosis

Children: In children, mortality varies from 5 to 40%. Mortality rates are lower in children with mild PEM and those given intensive care. Death in the first days of treatment is usually due to electrolyte deficits, sepsis, hypothermia, or heart failure. Impaired consciousness, jaundice, petechiae, hyponatremia, and persistent diarrhea are ominous signs. Resolution of apathy, edema, and anorexia is a favorable sign. **Recovery is more rapid in kwashiorkor than in marasmus.**

Long-term effects of PEU in children are not fully documented. Some children develop chronic malabsorption and pancreatic insufficiency. In very young children, mild mental retardation may develop and persist until at least school age. Permanent cognitive impairment may occur, depending on the duration, severity, and age at onset of PEU.

Adults: In adults, PEU can result in morbidity and mortality (e.g., progressive weight loss increases mortality rate for elderly patients in nursing homes). In elderly patients, PEU increases the risk of morbidity and mortality due to surgery, infections, or other disorders. Except when organ failure occurs, treatment is uniformly successful.

CLINICAL NOTE

Alternating episodes of undernutrition and adequate nutrition may cause the hair to have a dramatic "striped flag" appearance in kwashiorkor.

CLINICAL PEARLS

1. The term PEM applies to a group of related disorders that include marasmus, kwashiorkor, and intermediate states of marasmus-kwashiorkor.
2. Marasmus results primarily from inadequate energy intake, kwashiorkor results primarily from inadequate protein intake, whereas marasmic kwashiorkor has features of both disorders.
3. Many of the manifestations of PEM represent adaptive responses to inadequate energy and/or protein intakes.
4. The most helpful laboratory studies in assessing malnutrition in a child are hematological studies and laboratory studies evaluating protein status.
5. Mild or moderate PEM including brief starvation, can be treated by providing a balanced diet, preferably orally. Severe PEM or prolonged starvation requires treatment in a hospital with a controlled diet.

CASE STUDY 2

Theme: Obesity—Causes and Consequences

A 16-year-old boy came for consultation to the physician. He complained of being lethargic most of the times and had practically no physical activity. He had been sleeping and eating excessively from the previous few months. On further questioning, he reported that his father was diabetic, hypertensive, and also very obese. His uncle and grandmother were also obese. His mother was average built. There was no present or past history of any medical illness.

On examination, the boy was overweight (90 kg), had truncal obesity, and pulse and blood pressure (BP) were normal. Chest was clear and no abnormality was detected on abdominal examination. Fasting blood sugar and thyroid profile were normal. Serum total cholesterol and triglycerides were high. Yellowish spots (xanthomas) were present on the exposed parts. The physician instructed the boy to reschedule the diet and to increase the physical activity. A diagnosis of obesity was made and a diet chart was given to the patient along with a drug orlistat to be taken after meals.

What is the cause of obesity in this boy?
What are the risk factors associated with obesity?
How can these risk factors be detected by simple biochemical investigations?
What is the mechanism of action of orlistat? Is it safe to give orlistat to any patient?

CASE DETAILS

OBESITY

Obesity is a state of excess adipose tissue mass. Physical examination is usually sufficient to detect excess body fat. The quantitative evaluation of obesity is performed by calculating the BMI.

The body mass index (BMI) closely correlates with excess adipose tissue. It is calculated by dividing measured body weight in kilogram by the height in meter square.

Classifications and Definitions of Obesity

Although several classifications and definitions for degrees of obesity are accepted, the most widely accepted is the World Health Organization (WHO) criteria based on BMI.

Under this convention for adults:

- Grade 1 overweight (commonly and simply called overweight) is a BMI of 25–29.9 kg/m^2
- Grade 2 overweight (commonly called obesity) is a BMI of 30–39.9 kg/m^2
- Grade 3 overweight (commonly called severe or morbid obesity) is a BMI greater than or equal to 40 kg/m^2

The surgical literature often uses a different classification to recognize particularly severe obesity. In this setting:

- **Severe obesity** a BMI greater than 40 kg/m^2 is described as severe obesity
- **Morbid obesity** a BMI of 40–50 kg/m^2 is termed morbid obesity, and
- **Super obese** a BMI greater than 50 kg/m^2 is termed superobese.

The definition of obesity in children involves BMIs greater than the 85th (commonly used to define overweight) or the 95th (commonly used to define obesity) percentile, respectively, for age-matched and sex-matched control subjects. Factors other than total weight, however, are also important. Upper body obesity (excess fat around the waist and flank) is a greater health hazard than lower body obesity (fat in the thighs and buttocks). **Obese patients with increased abdominal circumference (>102 cm in men and 88 cm in women) or with high waist-hip ratios (>1.0 in men and >0.85 in women) have a greater risk of diabetes mellitus, stroke, coronary artery disease, and early death than equally obese patients with lower ratios.** Further differentiation of the location of excess fat suggests that visceral fat within the abdominal cavity is more hazardous to health than subcutaneous fat around the abdomen.

Etiology of Obesity

Obesity is a heterogeneous group of disorders. The pathogenesis of obesity is far more complex than the simple paradigm of an imbalance between energy intake and energy output. There is a strong influence of genetic factors on an individual's body weight. Obesity is the outcome of interplay between the genetic and environmental factors.

1. **Energy balance: Physiologic regulation of energy balance**—body weight is regulated by both endocrine and neural components that ultimately influence the effector arms of energy intake and expenditure. This complex regulatory system is necessary because even small imbalances between energy intake and expenditure will ultimately have large effects on body weight. Alterations in stable weight by forced overfeeding or food deprivation induce physiologic changes that resist these perturbations: As with weight loss, appetite increases and energy expenditure falls; with overfeeding, appetite falls and energy expenditure increases. This latter compensatory mechanism frequently fails, however, permitting obesity to develop when food is abundant and physical activity is limited. A major regulator of these adaptive responses is the adipocyte-derived hormone leptin which acts through brain circuits (predominantly in the hypothalamus) to influence appetite, energy expenditure, and neuroendocrine function.
   a. **Energy input:** Appetite is influenced by many factors that are integrated by the brain, most importantly within the hypothalamus. Signals that impinge on the hypothalamic center include neural afferents, hormones and metabolites.
      - **Neural afferents:** Vagal inputs are particularly important, bringing information from viscera,, such as gut distention.
      - **Hormonal signals:** It includes leptin, insulin, cortisol, and gut peptides. Among the latter are ghrelin, which is made in the stomach and stimulates feeding, and peptide YY (PYY) and cholecystokinin, which are made in the small intestine and signal to the brain through direct action on hypothalamic control centers and/or via the vagus nerve.
      - **Metabolites** including glucose, can influence appetite, as seen by the effect of hypoglycemia to induce hunger; however, glucose is not normally a major regulator of appetite.

        These diverse hormonal, metabolic, and neural signals act by influencing the expression and release of various hypothalamic peptides [e.g., neuropeptide Y (NPY), agouti-related peptide (AgRP), α-melanocyte-stimulating hormone (α-MSH), and melanin-concentrating hormone (MCH)] that are integrated with serotonergic, catecholaminergic, endocannabinoid, and opioid signaling pathways.
      - Psychological and cultural factors also play a role in the final expression of appetite.

   b. **Energy expenditure:** It includes the following components: (1) resting or basal metabolic rate; (2) the energy cost of metabolizing and storing food; (3) the thermic effect of exercise; and (4) adaptive thermogenesis, which varies in response to chronic caloric intake (rising with increased intake). Basal metabolic rate accounts for ~ 70% of daily energy expenditure, whereas active physical activity contributes 5–10%.

      Adaptive thermogenesis occurs in brown adipose tissue (BAT) which plays an important role in energy metabolism in many mammals. **In contrast to white adipose tissue, which is used to store energy in the form of lipids, BAT expends stored energy as heat. A mitochondrial uncoupling protein-1 (UCP-1) in BAT dissipates the hydrogen ion gradient in the oxidative respiration chain and releases energy as heat.** The metabolic activity of BAT is increased by a central action of leptin, acting through the sympathetic nervous system, which heavily innervates this tissue.

      There is continued interest in the concept of a body weight "set point." This idea is supported by physiologic mechanisms centered around a sensing system in adipose tissue that reflects fat stores and a receptor, or "adipostat," that is in the hypothalamic centers. When fat stores are depleted, the adipostat signal is low and the hypothalamus responds by stimulating hunger and decreasing energy expenditure to conserve energy. Conversely, when fat stores are abundant, the signal is increased and the hypothalamus responds by decreasing hunger and increasing energy expenditure. The recent discovery of the *ob* gene and its product leptin and the *db* gene, whose product is the leptin receptor, provides important elements of a molecular basis for this physiologic concept.
2. **The adipocyte and adipose tissue:** Adipose tissue is composed of the lipid-storing adipose cell and a stromal/vascular compartment in which cells including preadipocytes and macrophages reside. Adipose mass increases by enlargement of adipose cells through lipid deposition as well as by an increase in the number of adipocytes. Obese adipose tissue is also characterized by increased numbers of infiltrating macrophages.

   Endocrinal role of adipose tissue: Although the adipocyte has generally been regarded as a storage depot for fat, it is also an endocrine cell that releases numerous molecules in a regulated fashion. These include the energy balance-regulating hormone:
   - Leptin
   - Cytokines, such as tumor necrosis factor (TNF) and interleukin (IL)-6
   - Complement factors, such as factor D (also known as adipsin)

- Prothrombotic agents, such as plasminogen activator inhibitor I
- A component of the blood pressure regulating system, angiotensinogen
- Adiponectin, an abundant adipose-derived protein whose levels are reduced in obesity, enhances insulin sensitivity and lipid oxidation and it has vascular protective effects
- Resistin and retinol-binding protein 4 (RBP4), their levels are increased in obesity, may induce insulin resistance. These factors and others are not yet identified, play a role in the physiology of lipid homeostasis, insulin sensitivity, blood pressure control, coagulation, and vascular health and are likely to contribute to obesity-related pathologies.

3. **Role of genes versus environment:** Obesity is commonly seen in families and the heritability of body weight is similar to that for height. Inheritance is usually not Mendelian, however, and it is difficult to distinguish the role of genes and environmental factors. Adopted children are more closely resemble to their biologic than adoptive parents with respect to obesity, providing strong support for genetic influences. Likewise, identical twins have very similar BMIs whether reared together or apart and their BMIs are much more strongly correlated than those of dizygotic twins. These genetic effects appear to relate to both energy intake and expenditure. Whatever the role of genes, it is clear that the environment plays a key role in obesity; genes influence the susceptibility to obesity in response to specific diets and availability of nutrition.

   Cultural factors are also important—these relate to both availability and composition of the diet and to changes in the level of physical activity. It appears that high-fat diets may promote obesity, especially when combined with diets rich in simple (as opposed to complex) carbohydrates.

   Leptin: The product of the *ob* gene is the peptide leptin, a name derived from the Greek root *leptos*, meaning thin. Leptin is secreted predominantly in the adipose cells and, to a lesser extent, in the placenta, skeletal muscle, and stomach fundus in rats. It acts primarily through the hypothalamus. Leptin has a myriad of functions in carbohydrate, bone, and reproductive metabolism that are still being unraveled, but its role in body weight regulation is the main reason it came to prominence. Its level of production provides an index of adipose energy stores. The major role of leptin in body-weight regulation is to signal satiety to the hypothalamus and, thus, reduce dietary intake and fat storage while modulating energy expenditure and carbohydrate metabolism to prevent further weight gain.

   Unlike the Ob/Ob mouse model in which this peptide was first characterized, most humans who are obese are not leptin deficient but rather leptin resistant. Therefore, they have elevated circulating levels of leptin.

Mutations in Various Genes

Leptin gene: Several families with morbid, early-onset obesity caused by inactivating mutations in either leptin or the leptin receptor have been described, thus demonstrating the biologic relevance of leptin in humans. The obesity in these individuals begins shortly after birth, is severe, and is accompanied by neuroendocrine abnormalities. The most prominent of these is hypogonadotropic hypogonadism, which is reversed by leptin replacement.

Mutations in *POMC* gene: Mutations in the gene encoding proopiomelanocortin (POMC) cause severe obesity through failure to synthesize α-MSH, a key neuropeptide that inhibits appetite in the hypothalamus. The absence of POMC also causes secondary adrenal insufficiency due to absence of adrenocorticotropic hormone (ACTH) as well as pale skin and red hair due to absence of α-MSH.

Proenzyme convertase-1 mutations: Proenzyme convertase-1 (PC-1) mutations are thought to cause obesity by preventing synthesis of α-MSH from its precursor peptide, POMC.

Melanocortin receptor mutations: α-MSH binds to the melanocortin-4 receptor (MC4R), a key hypothalamic receptor that inhibits eating. Heterozygous loss-of-function mutations of this receptor account for as much as 5% of severe obesity.

The *tub* gene mutations: The *tub* gene encodes a hypothalamic peptide of unknown function; mutation of this gene causes late-onset obesity.

The *fat* gene mutations: The *fat* gene encodes carboxypeptidase E, a peptide-processing enzyme; mutation of this gene is thought to cause obesity by disrupting production of one or more neuropeptides.

Secondary causes of obesity:

- Hypothyroidism
- Cushing syndrome
- Insulinoma
- Hypothalamic obesity
- Polycystic ovarian syndrome
- Genetic syndromes, such as Prader–Willi, Laurence–Moon–Biedl, Alström–Cohen, Carpenter, and Frohlich's syndrome
- Growth hormone deficiency
- Pregnancy
- Hypogonadism
- Pseudohypoparathyroidism
- Drug-induced [e.g., phenothiazines, sodium valproate, carbamazepine, tricyclic antidepressants, lithium, glucocorticoids, megestrol acetate, thiazolidinediones, sulfonylureas, insulin, adrenergic antagonists, and serotonin antagonists (especially cyproheptadine)]

- Eating disorders (especially binge-eating disorder, bulimia nervosa, and night-eating disorder)
- Smoking cessation
- Tube feeding-induced

Prevalence

The prevalence of obesity worldwide is increasing particularly in the developed nations of the Northern hemisphere,, such as the United States, Canada, and most countries of Europe. Conservative estimates suggest that as many as 250 million people (approximately 7% of the estimated current world population) are obese. Two to three times more people than this are probably overweight.

Age

The prevalence and age distribution of obesity have substantially changed in the last 2–3 decades.

- Although the prevalence has remained at 30–50% of the adult population in the United States, the prevalence in children has increased to 15–25%.
- As evidenced in secular trends, children and particularly adolescents who are obese have a high probability of growing to be adults who are obese; hence, the bimodal distribution of obesity portends a large-scale obesity epidemic in the next few decades.

Comorbidities Associated with Obesity

The following comorbidities are associated with obesity:

- **Cardiovascular:** Essential hypertension, coronary artery disease, left ventricular hypertrophy, cor pulmonale, obesity-associated cardiomyopathy, accelerated atherosclerosis, and pulmonary hypertension of obesity
- **CNS:** Stroke, idiopathic intracranial hypertension, and meralgia paresthetica
- **GI:** Gallbladder disease (cholecystitis, cholelithiasis), nonalcoholic steatohepatitis (NASH), fatty liver infiltration, and reflux esophagitis
- **Respiratory:** Obstructive sleep apnea, obesity hypoventilation syndrome (Pickwickian syndrome), increased predisposition to respiratory infections, and increased incidence of bronchial asthma
- **Malignant:** Association with endometrial, prostate, gallbladder, breast, colon, and, possibly, lung cancer
- **Psychologic:** Social stigmatization, depression
- **Orthopedic:** Osteoarthritis, coxa vara, slipped capital femoral epiphyses, and chronic lumbago
- **Metabolic:** Insulin resistance, hyperinsulinemia, type 2 diabetes mellitus, and dyslipidemia (characterized by high total cholesterol, high triglycerides, normal or elevated low-density lipoprotein, and low high-density lipoprotein)
- **Reproductive:** Anovulation, early puberty, infertility, hyperandrogenism and polycystic ovaries in women, and hypogonadotropic hypogonadism in men
- **Obstetric and perinatal:** Pregnancy-related hypertension, fetal macrosomia, and pelvic dystocia
- **Surgical:** Increased surgical risk and postoperative complications including wound infection, deep venous thrombosis, pulmonary embolism, and postoperative pneumonia
- **Pelvic:** Stress incontinence
- **Cutaneous:** Intertrigo (bacterial and/or fungal), acanthosis nigricans, hirsutism, increased risk for cellulitis, and carbuncles
- **Extremity:** Venous varicosities, lower extremity venous, and/or lymphatic edema
- **Miscellaneous:** Reduced mobility, difficulty in maintaining personal hygiene.

Medical Evaluation of the Obese Patient

Historical information: It should be obtained about age at onset, recent weight changes, family history of obesity, occupational history, eating and exercise behavior, cigarette and alcohol use, previous weight loss experience, and psychosocial factors including assessment for depression and eating disorders. Particular attention should be directed at use of laxatives, diuretics, hormones, nutritional supplements, and over-the-counter medications.

Physical examination: It should assess the degree and distribution of body fat, overall nutritional status, and signs of secondary causes of obesity.

Less than 1% of obese patients have an identifiable secondary, nonpsychiatric cause of obesity. Hypothyroidism and Cushing's syndrome are important examples that can usually be diagnosed by physical examination in patients with unexplained recent weight gain., such patients require further endocrinologic evaluation, including serum thyroid-stimulating hormone (TSH) determination and dexamethasone suppression testing. All obese patients should be assessed for medical consequences of their obesity by screening for the metabolic syndrome. Blood pressure, waist circumference, fasting glucose, low-density lipoprotein (LDL) and high density lipoprotein (HDL) cholesterol, and triglycerides should be measured.

Treatment

Most successful programs employ a multidisciplinary approach to weight loss, with hypocaloric diets, behavior modification to change eating behavior, aerobic exercise, and social support. Emphasis must be on maintenance of weight loss.

Dietary Instructions

A low-fat, high-complex carbohydrate and a high-fiber diet is recommended. This is achieved by emphasizing intake of a wide variety of predominantly "unprocessed" foods. Special attention is usually paid to limiting foods that provide large amounts of calories without other nutrients, i.e., fat, sucrose, and alcohol. There is no special advantage to diets that restrict carbohydrates, advocate relatively larger amounts of protein or fats, or recommend ingestion of foods one at a time. Long-term changes in eating behavior are required to maintain weight loss.

Behavior modification programs are available to which patients can be referred. Patients can be taught to plan menus and exercise sessions and to record their actual behavior. Patients can be taught to recognize "eating cues" (emotional, situational, etc.) and how to avoid or control them. Regular self-monitoring of weight is also associated with improved long-term weight maintenance.

Exercise offers a number of advantages to patients trying to lose weight and keep it off. Aerobic exercise directly increases the daily energy expenditure and is particularly useful for long-term weight maintenance. Exercise will also preserve lean body mass and partially prevent the decrease in basal energy expenditure (BEE) seen with semistarvation. When compared with no treatment, exercise alone results in small amounts of weight loss. Exercise plus diet results in greater weight loss than diet alone. A greater intensity of exercise is associated with a greater amount of weight loss. **Up to 1 hour of moderate exercise per day is associated with long-term weight maintenance in individuals who have successfully lost weight**.

Social support is essential for a successful weight loss program. Continued close contact with clinicians and involvement of the family and peer group are useful techniques for reinforcing behavioral change and preventing social isolation.

Patients with severe obesity may require more aggressive treatment regimens. Very-low-calorie diets (<800 kcal/day) result in rapid weight loss and marked initial improvement in obesity-related metabolic complications. Patients are commonly maintained on, such programs for 4–6 months and lose an average of 2 lb per week. Average weight loss is approximately 15% of initial weight. Side effects, such as fatigue, orthostatic hypotension, cold intolerance, fluid and electrolyte disorders are observed in proportion to the degree of calorie reduction and require regular supervision by a physician. Other less common complications include gout, gallbladder disease, and cardiac arrhythmias.

Medications

Several medications remain available for treatment of obesity. Older catecholaminergic medications (e.g., phentermine, diethylpropion, and mazindol) are approved for short-term use only and have limited utility. Two newer medications are approved for weight loss—sibutramine and orlistat. **Sibutramine blocks uptake of both serotonin and norepinephrine in the central nervous system. Orlistat reduces fat absorption in the gastrointestinal tract**.

Sibutramine, typically at doses of 10 mg/day, side effects include dry mouth, anorexia, constipation, insomnia, and dizziness. In some patients (<5%), sibutramine may substantially increase blood pressure.

Orlistat is the first approved medication for obesity that works in the gastrointestinal tract rather than the central nervous system. By inhibiting intestinal lipase, orlistat reduces fat absorption. As expected, orlistat may result in diarrhea, gas, and cramping and perhaps also reduced absorption of fat-soluble vitamins. The recommended dose of orlistat is 120 mg three times daily with meals. Despite FDA approval of sibutramine and orlistat and NIH guidelines supporting their use, long-term clinical benefits have not been demonstrated.

Bariatric surgery is an increasingly prevalent treatment option for patients with severe obesity. In the United States, gastric operations are considered the procedures of choice. Most popular is the Roux-en-Y gastric bypass (RYGB). In most centers, the operation can be done laparoscopically. The RYGB typically results in substantial amounts of weight loss—close to 50% of initial body weight in some studies. Complications occur in up to 40% of persons undergoing RYGB surgery and include peritonitis due to anastomotic leak, abdominal wall hernias, staple line disruption, gallstones, neuropathy, marginal ulcers, stomal stenosis, wound infections, thromboembolic disease, gastrointestinal symptoms, and nutritional deficiencies including iron, vitamin B_{12}, folate, calcium, and vitamin D.

Prognosis

For a person with a BMI of 25–28.9 kg/m^2, the relative risk for coronary heart disease is 1.72. This risk progressively increases with an increasing BMI.

- Overall, obesity is estimated to increase the cardiovascular mortality rate fourfold and the cancer-related mortality rate twofold.
- As a group, people who are severely obese have a six- to 12-fold increase in the all-cause mortality rate.

CLINICAL NOTE

Visceral fat within the abdominal cavity is more hazardous to health than subcutaneous fat around the abdomen.

CLINICAL PEARLS

1. Obesity is a state of excess adipose tissue mass. The BMI closely correlates with excess adipose tissue. It is calculated by dividing measured body weight in kilogram by the height in meter square.
2. The pathogenesis of obesity is far more complex than the simple paradigm of an imbalance between energy intake and energy output. Obesity is the outcome of interplay between the genetic and environmental factors.
3. The major role of leptin in body-weight regulation is to signal satiety to the hypothalamus and thus, reduce dietary intake and fat storage while modulating energy expenditure and carbohydrate metabolism to prevent further weight gain.
4. Obese people have a greater risk of diabetes mellitus, stroke, coronary artery disease, and early death than the normal nonobese individuals.
5. The treatment of obesity is based on inducing weight loss by hypocaloric diets, behavior modification to change eating behavior, aerobic exercise, and social support. The emphasis is laid on maintenance of reduced body weight.

CASE STUDY 3

Theme: Biochemistry of Starvation

A 25-year-old women living alone became severely depressed after the termination of her engagement. 2 months later, she was brought to the emergency room by a friend because of weakness and lethargy. She appeared thin and pale. Questioning revealed that she had not eaten for several weeks.

Analysis of a plasma sample indicated elevated levels of alanine, acetoacetate, β-hydroxybutyrate, and blood urea nitrogen (BUN). However, her plasma glucose concentration was within normal limits. She was hospitalized, given intravenous feeding and antidepressant medications, and subsequently shifted to a 1,800 cal (7,500 kJ) diet. Her recovery was uneventful.

How was the patient obtaining energy during the time when she was not eating?
How was the patient able to maintain her plasma glucose within normal limits even though she was not eating?
What does the elevation in plasma alanine indicate?
Why is BUN elevated?
What is indicated by the fact that the plasma acetoacetate and β-hydroxybutyrate levels are elevated?

CASE DISCUSSION

It is a case of starvation. The high alanine levels signify the catabolic state. Alanine in excessive amount is released from the muscles and to be taken to the liver to serve as a substrate for glucose production. Acetoacetate and β-hydroxybutyrate are ketone bodies, which serve as alternative fuel during starvation. High BUN signifies protein degradation; the carbon skeleton of amino acids is utilized for glucose production while amino group is converted to urea.

Starvation

Prolonged fasting may result from an inability to obtain food, from the desire to lose weight rapidly, or in clinical situations in which an individual cannot eat because of trauma, surgery, neoplasms, burns, etc. **In the absence of food, the plasma levels of glucose, amino acids, and triacylglycerols fall, triggering a decline in insulin secretion and an increase in glucagon release. The decreased insulin to glucagon ratio and the decreased availability of circulating substrates, make this period of nutritional deprivation a catabolic state, characterized by degradation of glycogen, triacylglycerol, and protein**. This sets into motion an exchange of substrates between liver, adipose tissue, muscle, and brain that is guided by two priorities: (i) the need to maintain glucose level to sustain the energy metabolism of brain, red blood cells, and other glucose requiring cells, and (ii) to supply energy to other tissues by mobilizing fatty acids from adipose tissues and converting them to ketone bodies to supply energy to other cells of the body.

Fuel Stores

A typical well-nourished 70 kg man has fuel reserves totaling about 161,000 kcal (670,000 kJ). The energy need for a 24-hour period ranges from about 1,600 kcal (6,700 kJ) to 6,000 kcal (25,000 kJ), depending on the extent of activity. Thus, stored fuels suffice to meet caloric needs in starvation for 1–3 months. However, the carbohydrate reserves are exhausted in only a day.

Energy Supply during Starvation

During starvation, the energy needs are fulfilled by three types of fuels—glucose, fatty acids, and ketone bodies.

a. **Glucose supply during starvation (gluconeogenesis):** Energy needs of brain and RBCs under starvation conditions, the blood-glucose level must be maintained above 2.2 mM (40 mg/dL). The first priority of metabolism in starvation is to provide sufficient glucose to the brain and other tissues (such as red blood cells) that are absolutely dependent on this fuel. However, precursors of glucose are not abundant. Most energy is stored in the fatty acyl moieties of triacylglycerols. **Fatty acids cannot be converted into glucose, because acetyl-CoA cannot be transformed into pyruvate.** The glycerol moiety of triacylglycerol can be converted into glucose, but only a limited amount is available. The only other potential source of glucose is amino acids derived from the breakdown of proteins. However, proteins are not stored and so any breakdown will necessitate a loss of function.

   Thus, the second priority of metabolism in starvation is to preserve protein, which is accomplished by shifting the fuel being used from glucose to fatty acids and ketone bodies.

b. **Fatty acid oxidation:** Energy need of liver the low blood-sugar level leads to decreased secretion of insulin and increased secretion of glucagon. Glucagon stimulates the mobilization of triacylglycerols in adipose tissue and gluconeogenesis in the liver. **The liver obtains energy for its own needs by oxidizing fatty acids released from adipose tissue.** The concentrations of acetyl-CoA and citrate consequently increase, which switches off glycolysis.

   Energy need of muscles: The uptake of glucose by muscle is markedly diminished because of the low insulin level, whereas fatty acids enter freely. Consequently, **muscle shifts almost entirely from glucose to fatty acids for fuel.** The beta-oxidation of fatty acids by muscle halts the conversion of pyruvate into acetyl-CoA because acetyl-CoA stimulates the phosphorylation of the pyruvate dehydrogenase complex which renders it inactive. Most of the pyruvate is transaminated to alanine at the expense of amino acids arising from breakdown of "labile" protein reserves synthesized in the fed state. The alanine, lactate, and much of the keto acids resulting from this transamination are exported from muscle and taken up by the liver, where the alanine is transaminated to yield pyruvate. The resultant amino acids are largely exported back to muscle to provide amino groups for formation of more alanine, while the pyruvate is a major substrate for gluconeogenesis in the liver **(Fig. 17.2)**.

   In adipose tissue, the decrease in insulin and increase in glucagon result in inhibition of lipogenesis, inactivation of lipoprotein lipase, and activation of intracellular hormone-sensitive lipase. This leads to release from adipose tissue of increased amounts of glycerol (which is a substrate for gluconeogenesis in the liver) and free fatty acids which are used by liver, heart, and skeletal muscle as their preferred metabolic fuel, therefore sparing glucose. **Glycerol derived from the cleavage of triacylglycerols is another raw material for the synthesis of glucose by the liver.**

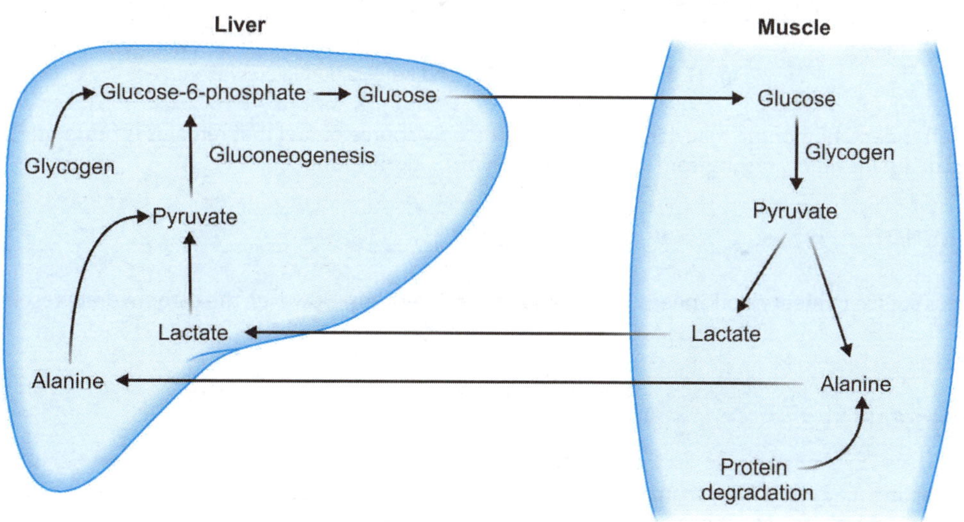

Fig. 17.2: Glucose-alanine and Cori's cycle.

   Loss of muscle mass: During starvation, degraded proteins are not replenished and serve as carbon sources for glucose synthesis. Initial sources of protein are those that turn over rapidly,, such as proteins of the intestinal epithelium and the secretions of the pancreas. Proteolysis of muscle protein provides some of three-carbon precursors of glucose. The nitrogen part of the amino acids is converted to urea (BUN).

c. **Ketosis:** Energy need of peripheral tissues after about 3 days of starvation, the liver forms large amounts of acetoacetate and β-hydroxybutyrate. Their synthesis from acetyl-CoA increases markedly because the citric acid cycle is unable to oxidize all the acetyl units generated by the degradation of fatty acids. **Gluconeogenesis depletes the supply of oxaloacetate which is essential for the entry of acetyl-CoA into the citric acid cycle. Consequently, the liver produces large quantities of ketone**

bodies which are released into the blood. At this time, the brain begins to consume appreciable amounts of acetoacetate in place of glucose. After 3 days of starvation, about a third of the energy needs of the brain are met by ketone bodies. The heart also uses ketone bodies as fuel. After several weeks of starvation, ketone bodies become the major fuel of the brain. Acetoacetate is activated by the transfer of CoA from succinyl-CoA to give acetoacetyl-CoA. Cleavage by thiolase then yields two molecules of acetyl-CoA which enters the citric acid cycle **(Fig. 17.3)**.

In essence, ketone bodies are equivalents of fatty acids that can pass through the blood–brain barrier. Only 40 g of glucose is then needed per day for the brain, compared with about 120 g in the first day of starvation. The effective conversion of fatty acids into ketone bodies by the liver and their use by the brain markedly diminishes the need for glucose. Hence, less muscle is degraded in the first days of starvation. The breakdown of 20 g of muscle daily compared with 75 g early in starvation is most important for survival.

A person's survival time is mainly determined by the size of the triacylglycerol depot.

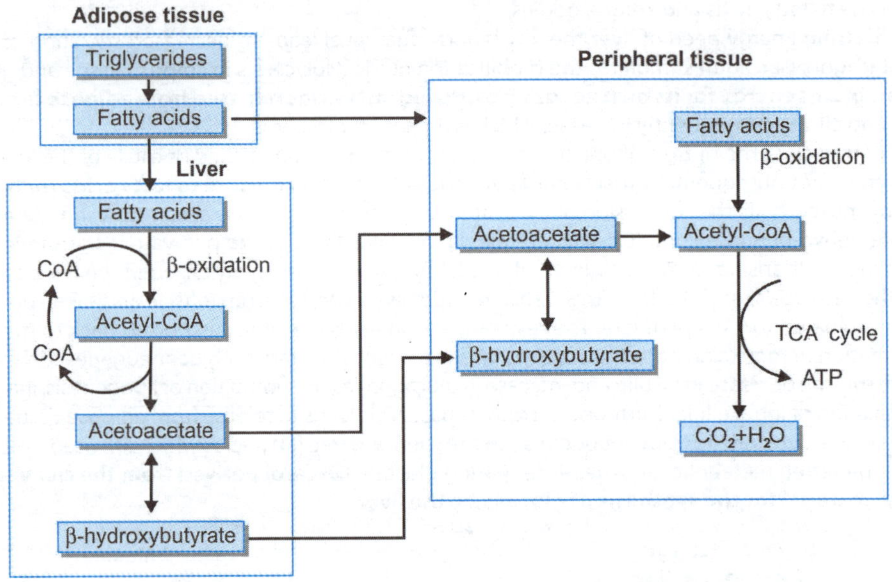

Fig. 17.3: Fatty acid oxidation and ketosis during starvation.

What happens after depletion of the triacylglycerol stores? The only source of fuel that remains is proteins. Protein degradation accelerates and death inevitably results from a loss of heart, liver, or kidney function.

CLINICAL NOTE

The stored fuels suffice to meet caloric needs in starvation for 1–3 months. However, the carbohydrate reserves are exhausted in only a day.

CLINICAL PEARLS

1. Prolonged fasting may result from an inability to obtain food, from the desire to lose weight rapidly, or in clinical situations in which an individual cannot eat because of trauma, surgery, neoplasms, burns, etc.
2. The decreased insulin to glucagon ratio and the decreased availability of circulating substrates, make this period of nutritional deprivation a catabolic state, characterized by degradation of glycogen, triacylglycerol, and protein.
3. In adipose tissue, the decrease in insulin and increase in glucagon result in inhibition of lipogenesis, inactivation of lipoprotein lipase, and activation of intracellular hormone-sensitive lipase. This leads to release from adipose tissue of increased amounts of glycerol (which is a substrate for gluconeogenesis in the liver) and free fatty acids, which are used by liver, heart, and skeletal muscle as their preferred metabolic fuel, therefore sparing glucose.
4. The alanine, lactate, and much of the keto acids resulting from this transamination are exported from muscle and taken up by the liver, where the alanine is transaminated to yield pyruvate.
5. The effective conversion of fatty acids into ketone bodies by the liver and their use by the brain markedly diminishes the need for glucose. Hence, less muscle is degraded in the first days of starvation. The breakdown of 20 g of muscle daily compared with 75 g early in starvation is most important for survival.

CASE STUDY 4

Theme: Biological and Clinical Significance of Dietary Fiber

A 36-year-old female presented to the clinic with complaints of alternating diarrhea and constipation. She reported some abdominal discomfort and bloating that were relieved with her bowel movement. She stated that her episodes were worse in times of stress. She denied any blood in her diarrhea. She denied any weight loss or anorexia. There was no history of fever or any drug intake.

Her physical examination was well within normal limits. She was prescribed a cellulose-containing dietary supplement which her doctor said would increase the bulk of her stools.

What is the most likely diagnosis?

What is the biochemical mechanism of the dietary supplement's effects on the intestines?

CASE DETAILS

The patient is most probably suffering from "irritable bowel syndrome".

IRRITABLE BOWEL SYNDROME

Background

Irritable bowel syndrome (IBS) is a chronic gastrointestinal disorder of unknown cause. Common symptoms include abdominal cramping or pain, bloating and flatulence, and altered bowel habits. **Irritable bowel syndrome has been called spastic colon, functional bowel disease, and mucous colitis**. However, IBS is not a true "colitis." The term colitis refers to a separate condition known as inflammatory bowel disease (IBD).

Irritable bowel syndrome is not contagious, inherited, or cancerous. However, IBS often disrupts daily living activities.

Causes

- The cause of irritable bowel syndrome is currently unknown. **The IBS is thought to result from interplay of abnormal gastrointestinal (GI) tract movements, increased awareness of normal bodily functions, and a change in the nervous system communication between the brain and the GI tract**. Abnormal movements of the colon, whether too fast or too slow, are seen in some, but not all, people who have IBS.
- Irritable bowel syndrome can also develop after episodes of gastroenteritis.
- It has been suggested that IBS is caused by dietary allergies or food sensitivities, but this has never been proven.
- Symptoms of irritable bowel syndrome may worsen during periods of stress or menses, but these factors are unlikely to be the cause that leads to development of IBS.
- Altered GI motility, visceral hyperalgesia, disturbance of brain-gut interaction, abnormal central processing, autonomic and hormonal events, genetic and environmental factors, and psychosocial disturbances are all variably involved, depending on the individual.

Clinical Manifestations

Irritable bowel syndrome affects each person differently. The hallmark of IBS is abdominal discomfort or pain. The following symptoms are also common:

- Abdominal cramping and pain that are relieved after bowel movements
- Alternating periods of diarrhea and constipation
- Change in the stool frequency or consistency
- Flatulence
- Passing mucus from the rectum
- Bloating
- Abdominal distension

The following are not symptoms or characteristics of IBS:

- Blood in stools or urine
- Vomiting (rare, though may occasionally accompany nausea)
- Pain or diarrhea that interrupts sleep
- Fever
- Weight loss

Diagnosis

IBS can be a very difficult diagnosis to make. The IBS is called a diagnosis of exclusion; this is done by performing tests to rule out other problems. A combination of history, physical examination, and selected tests are used to help diagnose irritable bowel syndrome. No single blood test or X-ray study confirms a diagnosis of IBS.

Ruling out parasitic infections, lactose intolerance, small intestinal bacterial overgrowth, and celiac disease are recommended for all patients before a diagnosis of irritable bowel syndrome is made. In patients over 50 years old, it is recommended that they undergo a screening colonoscopy.

Management

Reassurance and careful explanation of the functional nature of the disorder and of how to avoid obvious food precipitants are important first steps in patient counseling and dietary change. The following steps are undertaken to treat a patient of IBS:

1. **Stool-bulking agents:** High-fiber diets and bulking agents,, such as bran or hydrophilic colloid, are frequently used in treating IBS. Studies suggest that dietary fiber has multiple effects on colonic physiology. The water-holding action of fibers may contribute to increased stool bulk because of the ability of fiber to increase fecal output of bacteria. Fiber also speeds up colonic transit in most persons.
2. **Antispasmodics:** It has been observed that anticholinergic drugs may provide temporary relief for symptoms, such as painful cramps related to intestinal spasm.
3. **Antidiarrheal agents:** Peripherally acting opiate-based agents are the initial therapy of choice for IBS.
4. **Antidepressant drugs:** In addition to their mood-elevating effects, antidepressant medications have several physiologic effects that suggest they may be beneficial in IBS.
5. **Serotonin receptor agonist and antagonists:** Serotonin receptor antagonists have been evaluated as therapies for IBS-D. Serotonin acting on 5-HT3 receptors enhances the sensitivity of afferent neurons projecting from the gut. In humans, a 5-HT3 receptor antagonist, such as alosetron reduces perception of painful visceral stimulation in IBS. It also induces rectal relaxation, increases rectal compliance, and delays colonic transit.
6. **Chloride channel activators:** Lubiprostone is a bicyclic fatty acid that stimulates chloride channels in the apical membrane of intestinal epithelial cells. Chloride secretion induces passive movement of sodium and water into the bowel lumen and improves bowel function. The major side effects are nausea and diarrhea. Lubiprostone is a new class of compounds for treatment of chronic constipation with or without IBS.

ROLE OF DIETARY FIBERS

Dietary fiber is indigestible part of plant foods that makes stool soft and thus enables smooth bowel movements, prevents constipation, hemorrhoids, and diverticulosis.

It consists of all of the components of the cell walls of plants that are not broken down by the body's digestive enzymes.

Dietary Fiber and Total Fiber

Dietary fiber, as noted on the "Nutrition Facts Label" of commercial foods, is fiber originally present in the food. Total fiber consists of dietary fiber and added fiber—substances that are added to original food to increase their fiber content or to change their physical properties. Pectin, for example, is added to jam to give it a gel form.

Dietary fiber can be grouped into two main categories, those that are soluble and those that are insoluble in water.

Soluble Fiber: Soluble fiber (viscous fiber) partly dissolves in water and forms gel with it. Foods rich in soluble fiber include beans and other legumes (peas, soy, and lentils), oats, barley, citrus fruits (oranges, grapefruit), psyllium husk, and flax seed. Substances found in soluble fiber are gum, pectin, some hemicelluloses, mucilage, and storage polysaccharides (starch and glycogen).

Beneficial effects of soluble fiber:

- Soluble fiber may prevent both diarrhea and constipation. It absorbs water from the gut and thus makes stool soft, but not bulky.
- Soluble fiber may help in weight loss. It slows down the speed of the passage of food through the gut thus giving a feeling of fullness.
- Soluble fiber may help to prevent and treat diabetes type 2. It slows down absorption of glucose from the intestine into the blood thus preventing high spikes of glucose in the blood after a meal.
- Soluble fiber may lower total and LDL cholesterol and thus helps to prevent ischemic heart disease and stroke. It binds bile acids in the bowel and removes them from the body and thus reduces their absorption into the blood. Lost bile acids are replaced by synthesis from blood cholesterol. This is one theory about how soluble fiber lowers blood cholesterol levels.
- Soluble fiber may prevent bile salt diarrhea after a gallbladder removal.

Unwanted effects of soluble fiber:

Soluble fiber, if ingested in excess may cause:

- Abdominal bloating and flatulence
- Dehydration, if ingested without water
- Pectin may reduce absorption of cholesterol-lowering drugs, like lovastatin.

Soluble Fiber Supplements: Examples of soluble fiber supplements:

- Metamucil (psyllium—ispaghula)
- Citrucel (methylcellulose)
- Benefiber (wheat dextrin)
- Fiber choice (inulin)
- Pectin

The soluble fibers, such as pectin and true plant gums are mucilaginous and are digestible.

Pectins are predominantly polygalacturonic acids with varying amounts of other hexose or pentose residues. True plant gums are complex polysaccharides composed of primarily arabinose, fucose, galactose, mannose, rhamnose, and xylose. The gums are soluble in water and are digestible by the enzymes in the intestinal tract. Both pectins and gums are mucilaginous; they absorb water to form viscous gels in the stomach that decrease the rate of gastric emptying. The mucilaginous nature of the soluble fibers, pectins, and gums tends to decrease the rate at which carbohydrates are digested and absorbed, thus decreasing both the rise in blood glucose levels and the ensuing increase in insulin concentration.

Insoluble Fiber: Insoluble fiber cannot be dissolved in water. Foods rich in insoluble fiber include whole wheat and other whole grains and most dark green leafy vegetables, such as cabbage and cauliflower. Substances found in insoluble fiber include cellulose, hemicellulose, and lignin.

Beneficial effects of insoluble fiber: Insoluble fiber may help to prevent constipation, hemorrhoids, and diverticulosis. It binds water and thus makes stool soft and bulky; it also speeds up the passage of food through the intestine.

Unwanted effects of insoluble fiber:

- Ingesting foods with insoluble fiber containing sulfur (garlic, onions) may result in excessive gas.
- Insoluble fiber eaten on an empty stomach may aggravate symptoms of irritable bowel syndrome.
- Insoluble fiber ingested without water may result in severe constipation or even intestinal obstruction.
- Certain types of insoluble fiber may trigger diarrhea in sensitive people.
- Excessive ingestion of supplements containing insoluble fiber, especially in small children, may reduce absorption of calcium, magnesium, iron, copper, and zinc.

Substances found in insoluble fibers are as follows:

1. **Cellulose** is a major structural component of plant cell walls. Cellulose is a long, linear polymer of glucose (β-D-glucopyranose) units that are joined by β (1 → 4) glycosidic bonds. Cellulose molecules have an extended, rigid structure that is stabilized by interchain hydrogen bonds **(Fig. 17.4)**.
   Starch, the plant storage polysaccharide, which is also a polymer of glucose, differs in its structure in that the glucose monomer units are joined by α (1 → 4) glycosidic bonds. Starch is composed of two types of polymers, amylose, which has a nonbranched helical structure and amylopectin, which is branched with α (1 → 6) glycosidic bonds joining the branches to the main polymer chain **(Fig. 17.5)**. Although starch is easily digested by salivary and pancreatic amylase and the disaccharidases present on the brush border of intestinal mucosal cells, cellulose cannot be hydrolyzed. The β (1 → 4) glycosidic bonds of the cellulose chain cannot be cleaved by the amylases present in the digestive tract.

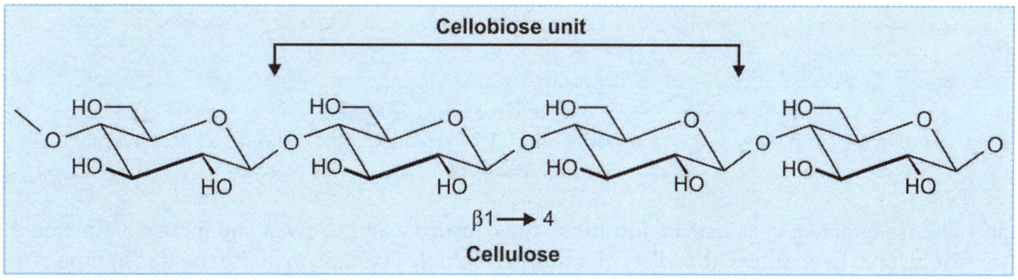

Fig. 17.4: Molecular structure of cellulose indicating the repeating disaccharide unit, cellobiose.

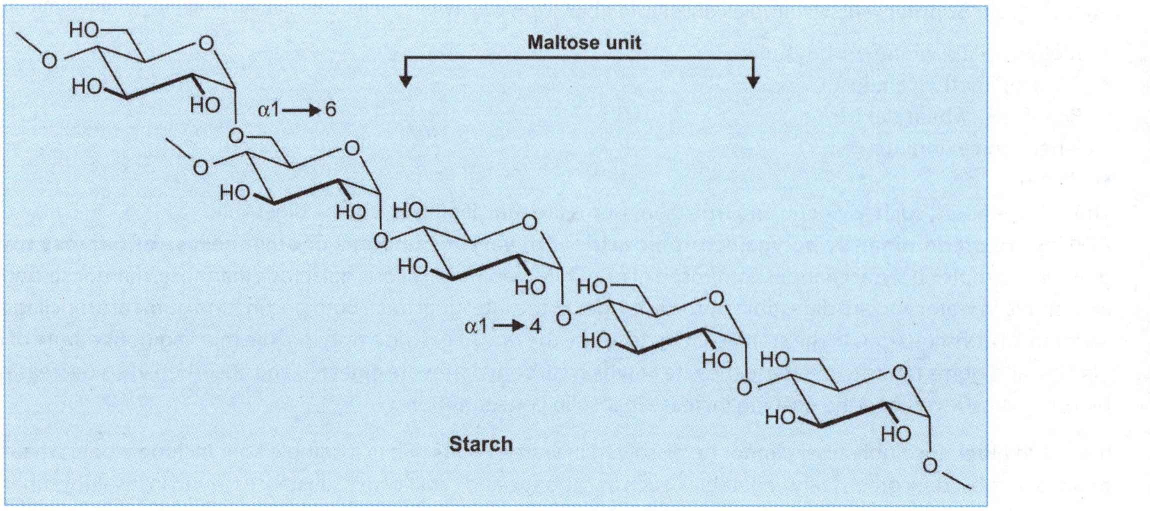

Fig. 17.5: Molecular structure of starch indicating the repeating disaccharide unit, maltose, as well as the α-1,6-glycosidic bond present in the branch points of amylopectin.

2. **Hemicelluloses** are also polysaccharides that are structural components of plant cell walls. However, unlike what their name implies, they are unrelated to cellulose. They are polymers that are made up of a variety of sugar monomers that include glucose, galactose, mannose, arabinose, and xylose, as well as acidic forms of these monosaccharides. Xylose is the monosaccharide that is most abundant. Hemicelluloses have a random, amorphous structure that is suitable for their location in the plant cell wall matrix. Depending on their molecular structure, hemicelluloses are partially digestible.
3. **Lignins** are formed by the irreversible dehydration of sugars that result in aromatic structures. The remaining alcohol or phenol OH groups can react with each other and with aldehyde and ketone groups to form polymers **(Fig. 17.6)**. These polymers cannot be broken down by the digestive enzymes and like cellulose and the indigestible portion of hemicelluloses, form the stool bulk.

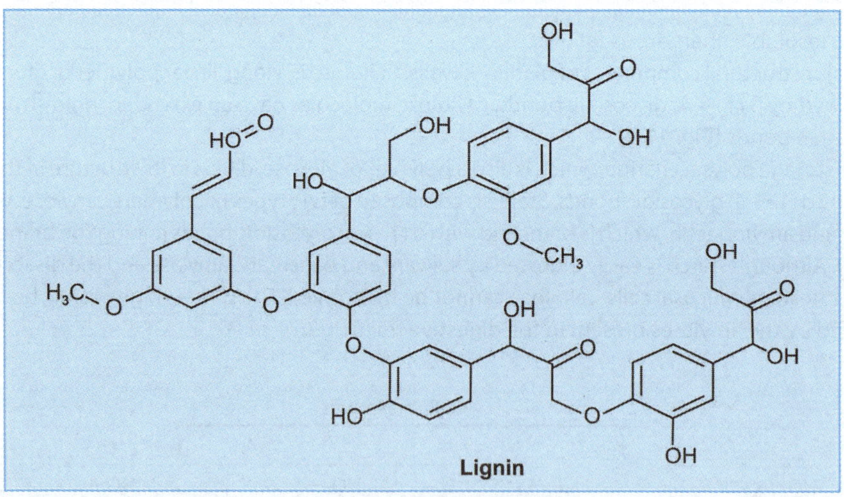

Fig. 17.6: A lignin molecule in an early stage of condensation. The aromatic rings are a result of irreversible dehydration of sugar residues.

Although cellulose and hemicellulose are insoluble, they absorb water to swell and increase the stool bulk. This results in larger, softer stools. It has been shown that diets plentiful in insoluble fiber also increase the transit time of food in the digestive tract and decrease intracolonic pressure. Lignins, in addition to increasing stool bulk, also bind organic molecules, such as cholesterol and many potential carcinogens.

CLINICAL NOTE

The hallmark of IBS is abdominal discomfort or pain that is relieved after bowel movement.

CLINICAL PEARLS

1. IBS is thought to result from interplay of abnormal GI tract movements, increased awareness of normal bodily functions, and a change in the nervous system communication between the brain and the GI tract.
2. Ruling out parasitic infections, lactose intolerance, small intestinal bacterial overgrowth, and celiac disease are recommended for all patients before a diagnosis of irritable bowel syndrome is made.
3. High-fiber diets and bulking agents,, such as bran or hydrophilic colloid, are frequently used in treating IBS.
4. Dietary fiber is indigestible part of plant foods that makes stool soft and thus enables smooth bowel movements, prevents constipation, hemorrhoids, and diverticulosis.
5. Soluble fiber may lower total and LDL cholesterol and thus helps to prevent ischemic heart disease and stroke.

Chapter 18

HIV Infection/Acquired Immunodeficiency Syndrome

LEARNING OBJECTIVES

To understand:

- ❖ Structural characteristics of HIV
- ❖ Modes of transmission
- ❖ Pathogenesis
- ❖ Clinical implications
- ❖ Laboratory diagnosis
- ❖ Management of HIV infection

CASE STUDIES

CASE STUDY

Theme: Human Immunodeficiency virus infection—causes and consequences.

A 29-year-old officer presented to emergency department with complaints of chills and breathing difficulty. He was a heroin abuser who was admitted in the same hospital 7 years ago because of drug overdosage. He had lost 10 kg of body weight since his last clinical visit.

On examination, he had multiple enlarged lymph nodes. Several red nodules were present on the skin of chest and arms. His body temperature was 40°C, BP was 170/50 mm Hg, and respiration was shallow with a respiratory rate of 40 breaths per minute. The chest radiograph showed diffuse pneumonia.

Sputum smear revealed numerous pneumocystis organisms while skin biopsy revealed Kaposi's sarcoma.

What is your presumptive diagnosis for this patient?
What are the different types of investigations required for confirmation of diagnosis?
What is the biochemical basis for the clinical manifestations in this patient?

CASE DISCUSSION

Patient is suffering from acquired immunodeficiency syndrome (AIDS). Intravenous drug usage seems to be the major causative factor. Patient's immune system has collapsed to the extent of loss of resistance to ordinary viral, fungal, and protozoal infections, which otherwise could have been controlled easily.

Acquired Immunodeficiency Syndrome

Acquired immunodeficiency syndrome, or AIDS, is a collection of symptoms due to underlying infections and malignancies resulting from specific damage to immune system caused by human immunodeficiency virus (HIV).

Incidence

Human immunodeficiency virus continues to be a major global public health issue. In 2016, an estimated 36.7 million people were living with HIV (including 1.8 million children)—with a global HIV prevalence of 0.8% among adults. Around 30% of these same people are not aware that they have the virus.

Since the start of the epidemic, an estimated 78 million people have become infected with HIV and 35 million people have died of AIDS-related illnesses. In 2016, 1 million people died of AIDS-related illnesses.

The vast majority of people living with HIV are located in low- and middle-income countries, with an estimated 25.5 million living in sub-Saharan Africa.

The first indication of this new syndrome came in 1981 in homosexual drug addict males; they had two things in common—*Pneumocystis* pneumonia and Kaposi's sarcoma. Both these are markers of collapsed immune system, the affected patients appeared to have lost their immune competence, rendering them vulnerable to overwhelming and fatal infections with relatively a virulent microorganisms, as well as to lymphoid and other malignancies. This condition was given the name acquired immunodeficiency syndrome (AIDS).

In 1986, the International Committee on Virus Nomenclature decided on the generic name of the causative virus as the human immunodeficiency virus.

Human Immunodeficiency Virus

Human immunodeficiency virus (HIV), the etiological agent of AIDS, belongs to *Lentivirus* subgroup of the Retroviridae family. This family of viruses is known for latency, persistent viremia, infection of the nervous system, and weak host immune responses. HIV has high affinity for CD4 T lymphocytes and monocytes. HIV binds to CD4 cells and becomes internalized. The virus replicates itself by generating a deoxyribonucleic acid (DNA) copy by reverse transcriptase. Viral DNA becomes incorporated into the host DNA, enabling further replication. Besides HIV, the related animal immunodeficiency viruses are also assigned to this group.

Structural Characteristics of HIV

- Human immunodeficiency virus (HIV) is a spherical enveloped virus of about 90–120 nm in diameter **(Fig. 18.1)**. There is a lipoprotein envelop, which consists of lipids derived from the host cell membrane and glycoproteins, which are viral coded. The major virus-coded envelop proteins are the projecting knob,, such as spikes on the surface and the anchoring transmembrane pedicles. The spikes, gp120, constitute the major surface component of the virus, which binds to the cell CD4 receptors on susceptible host cells. These specific receptors, known as cluster of differentiation 4 (CD4), are present on certain cells in the body, the cells possessing these receptors are called CD4$^+$ cells and these are T helper cells, B lymphocytes, macrophages, monocytes, and dendritic cells. Transmembrane pedicles gp41 cause cell-to-cell fusion.

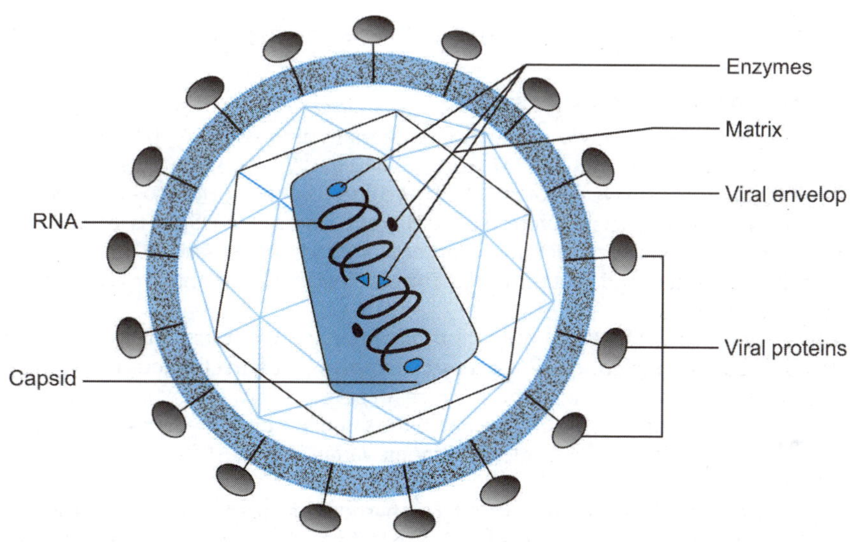

Fig. 18.1: Structure of human immunodeficiency virus (HIV). A cross-sectional schematic diagram of HIV virion, showing lipid bilayer in the form of viral envelop, nucleocapsid core, which includes a layer of a protein called p17 and an inner layer of a protein called p24. The HIV genome consists of two copies of the single-stranded ribonucleic acid (RNA), which are associated with two molecules of reverse transcriptase p64, protease p10, and integrase p32. The outer viral proteins are gp120 and gp41.

- Interior to the envelope is an outer icosahedral nuclear capsid shell and an inner cone-shaped core containing ribonucleoproteins. The enzymes integrase p32, protease p10, reverse transcriptase p55/66, and 2 copies of single-stranded genomic ribonucleic acid (RNA) are present inside the core. (The proteins and glycoproteins are indicated by their mass expressed as kilo-Daltons.) The reverse transcriptase enzyme is characteristic feature of retroviruses. When the virus infects a cell, the viral RNA is transcribed by the enzyme first into single-stranded deoxyribonucleic acid (DNA) and then into double-stranded DNA (provirus), which is integrated into the host cell chromosome. The provirus can remain latent for long period though it influences the host cell functions. At times in response to viral promoters, the provirus initiates viral replication by directing the synthesis of viral RNA and other components.

Genome of HIV

There are two types of genes analyzed **(Fig. 18.2)**:

a. **Structural genes encode for products, which participate in formation of functional structure of virus.**
   1. *gag* gene—encodes for core and shell of virus. The gene product is a precursor protein p55, which is cleaved into p17, p24, and p15. The p24 antigen (major core antigen) can be detected in serum during the early stages of infection till the appearance of the antibodies.

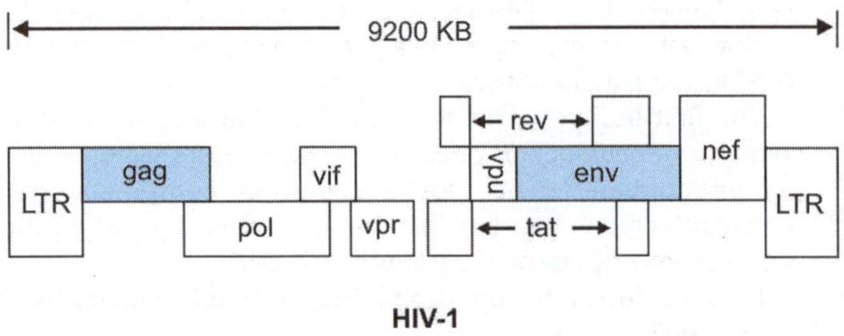

Fig. 18.2: Genome of human immunodeficiency virus (HIV).

   2. *pol* gene—encodes for the polymerase reverse transcriptase and other viral enzymes, such as protease and integrase. It is expressed as a precursor protein, which is cleaved into components like p64, which has reverse transcriptase and RNAse activity, p51 which has only reverse transcriptase activity, p10 is a protease that cleaves gag precursor and p32 is an integrase.
   3. *env* gene—determines the synthesis of envelop glycoprotein gp160, which is cleaved into gp120 and gp41. Glycosylation occurs after cleavage. The antibodies to gp120 are the first to appear after HIV infection and are present in circulation till the terminal stage of infection.

b. **Nonstructural and regulatory genes:**
   1. *vif* (viral infectivity factor gene) influences infectivity of viral particles.
   2. *vpr*—stimulates promoter region of the virus.
   3. *vpu* (only in HIV-1) and *vpx* (only in HIV-2) enhance maturation and release of progeny virus from cells. Detection of the type specific sequences *vpu* and *vpx* is useful in distinguishing between infection by HIV Types 1 and 2.
   4. *tat* (transactivating gene)—(2 copies) having stimulatory effect on synthesis of all viral proteins.
   5. *rev* (regulator of viral genes)—(2 copies) required for expression of structural genes.
   6. *nef* (negative factor gene) downregulates viral replication. It may be responsible for the regulation of latent state of virus.
   7. LTR (long terminal repeat)—sequences flanking on both sides giving promoter, enhancer, and integration signals.

Antigenic Variations in Human Immunodeficiency Virus

Based on molecular and antigenic differences, two types of human immunodeficiency virus (HIV) have been recognized. The original isolates of HIV and the related strains present all over the world belong to HIV Type 1. The HIV strains, first isolated from West Africa, which react with HIV Type 1 antiserum very weakly or not at all have been termed as HIV Type 2. It has 40% genetic similarity and is more closely related to simian immunodeficiency virus than to HIV-1. It can cause AIDS but is less pathogenic and is less common. It infects mainly monkeys and other similar species and is largely confined to West Africa, though isolations have been reported from some other areas, including Western and Southern India. The envelop antigens of the two types are different though their core peptides show some cross-reactivity.

Human immunodeficiency virus (HIV) is a highly mutable virus and exhibits frequent antigenic variations as well as differences in other features, such as nucleotide sequences, cell tropism, growth characteristics, and cytopathology. Not only are there differences between isolates of HIV from different races or persons, but also between sequential isolates from the same person, and even between those obtained from different sites of the same person at the same time. This great variability is believed to be due to error-prone nature of reverse transcription. Antigenic variation is most frequent in respect of the envelop proteins, but is also seen with other antigens.

HIV-1 strains have been classified into at least ten subtypes based on sequence analysis of their *gag* and *env* genes. These subtypes have been designated as A to J and constitute the Group M (for major), which cause the large majority of HIV-1 infections worldwide. A few HIV-1 strains isolated from West Africa do not fall within the major group and have been designated as group O (for outlier). Some later isolates of HIV-1 distinct from M and O groups have been called Group N (for new).

HIV subtypes show a geographical distribution.

- A—Worldwide
- B—America and Europe
- C—Asia, India, and China

The common subtypes in Africa are A, C, and D, while in Asia, the common subtypes are E, C, and B. Subtype E is the most common in Thailand.

Modes of Transmission

Human immunodeficiency virus (HIV) is transmitted when the virus enters the body, usually by injecting infected cells or semen. There are several possible ways in which the virus can enter.

- **Sexual contact:** In 75% cases, transmission is by sexual contact. Most commonly, HIV infection is spread by having sex with an infected partner. The virus can enter the body through the lining of the vagina, vulva, penis, rectum, or mouth during sex. People who already have a sexually transmitted disease,, such as syphilis, genital herpes, chlamydial infection, gonorrhea, or bacterial vaginitis, are more likely to acquire HIV infection during sex with an infected partner.
- **Parenteral:** In 15% cases, it is by blood transfusion or blood product transfusion. Blood products are now tested to minimize this risk. Sharing of unsterilized needles or syringes in drug addicts contaminated with blood from an infected person can also spread virus. HIV can be spread in healthcare settings through accidental needle sticks or contact with contaminated fluids. HIV can also spread through organ transplantation. If tissues or organs from an infected person are transplanted, the recipient may acquire HIV. Donors are now tested for HIV to minimize this risk.
- **From mother to child:** Women can transmit HIV to their babies during pregnancy or birth, when infected maternal cells enter the baby's circulation. Thirty percent of children born to infected mothers have the acquired infection unless virus is treated by antiviral drugs before pregnancy. In nursing mothers, transmission can occur through breast milk.

Mortality/Morbidity

The course of HIV infection is characterized primarily by latency. Unfortunately, profound immune suppression eventually develops and the illness appears to be almost uniformly lethal.

Progression from HIV infection to AIDS occurs 8–10 years after infection without antiretroviral treatment. In the recent past, most patients would not survive more than 1–2 years following diagnosis of AIDS. However, since the introduction of highly active antiretroviral therapy (HAART) and prophylaxis against opportunistic pathogens, death rates from AIDS have declined significantly. An HIV-positive patient older than 50 years with a nearly undetectable viral load and a CD4 count more than 350 now has less than 5% chance of dying or progressing to full-blown AIDS within 3 years.

Sex: In the United States, most HIV infections still occur in men via homosexual contact (72% of total cases). However, the frequency of infection in women is increasing. In the United States, fewer than 27% of all HIV cases are in women, whereas worldwide an estimated 50% of all HIV patients are women.

Age: Most AIDS cases occur in adults aged 25–49 years (70% of cases). Adolescents and young adults (aged 13–24 years) represent 25% of new cases. Young children represent less than 1% of AIDS cases in the United States. Internationally, children younger than 15 years are estimated to account for close to 10% of all HIV cases.

Pathogenesis: Infection is transmitted when virus enters the blood or tissues of a person and comes into contact with a suitable host cell, principally the CD4 lymphocytes. The virus may infect any cell bearing the CD4 antigen on the surface. Primarily, these are the $CD4^+$ helper T lymphocytes **(Fig. 18.3)**. Some other immune cells possessing CD4 antigens are also susceptible to infection, like B lymphocytes, monocytes, and macrophages including specialized macrophages, such as alveolar macrophages in the lungs and Langerhans cells in the dermis. Glial cells and microglial cells are also susceptible. Follicular dendritic cells from tonsils can be infected by HIV without the involvement of CD4. The steps of viral entry into the host cell are as follows:

1. **Attachment of virus into the host cell:** Specific binding of the virus to the CD4 receptors is by the envelop glycoprotein gp120.
2. **Cell-to-cell fusion:** For infection to take place, the cell fusion is essential. This is brought about by the transmembrane glycoprotein gp41. HIV-1 utilizes two major co-receptors along with CD4 to bind to, fuse with, and enter target cells; these co-receptors are CCR5 and CXCR4, which are also receptors for certain endogenous chemokines. Strains of HIV that utilize CCR5 as a co-receptor are referred to as macrophage tropic viruses. Strains of HIV that utilize CXCR4 are referred to as T cell-tropic viruses. Many virus strains are dual tropic in that they utilize both CCR5 and CXCR4. The natural chemokine ligands for the major HIV co-receptors can readily block entry of HIV. The mechanism of inhibition of viral entry is a steric inhibition of binding that is not dependent on signal transduction. The transmitting virus is almost invariably macrophage tropic virus that predominates during the early stages of HIV disease. In ~40% of HIV-infected individuals, there is a transition to a predominantly T cell-tropic virus that is associated with a relatively rapid progression of disease. However, at least 60% of infected individuals progress in their disease while maintaining predominance of macrophage tropic virus.

   The infected CD4 cells express a high level of gp120 on their surface. The gp120 on the surface of infected cells leads to fusion of these cells with CD4 protein of uninfected neighboring cells with formation of **multinucleated syncytial cells**. The lysis of fused cells finally occurs resulting in depletion of large number of uninfected cells from the circulation.
3. **Uncoating of the viral envelope and entry of nuclear capsid core into the cell:** After fusion of virus with the host cell membrane, HIV genome is uncoated and internalized into cell. Viral RNA is released into the core cytoplasm.
4. **Viral transcription:** Viral reverse transcriptase mediates transcription of its RNA; RNA–DNA hybrid is formed. Original RNA strand is degraded by ribonuclease H, followed by synthesis of second strand of DNA to yield double strand HIV-DNA.
5. **Integration into the host DNA as provirus:** The double-stranded DNA is integrated into the genome of the infected host cell through the action of the viral integrase enzyme, causing a latent infection.

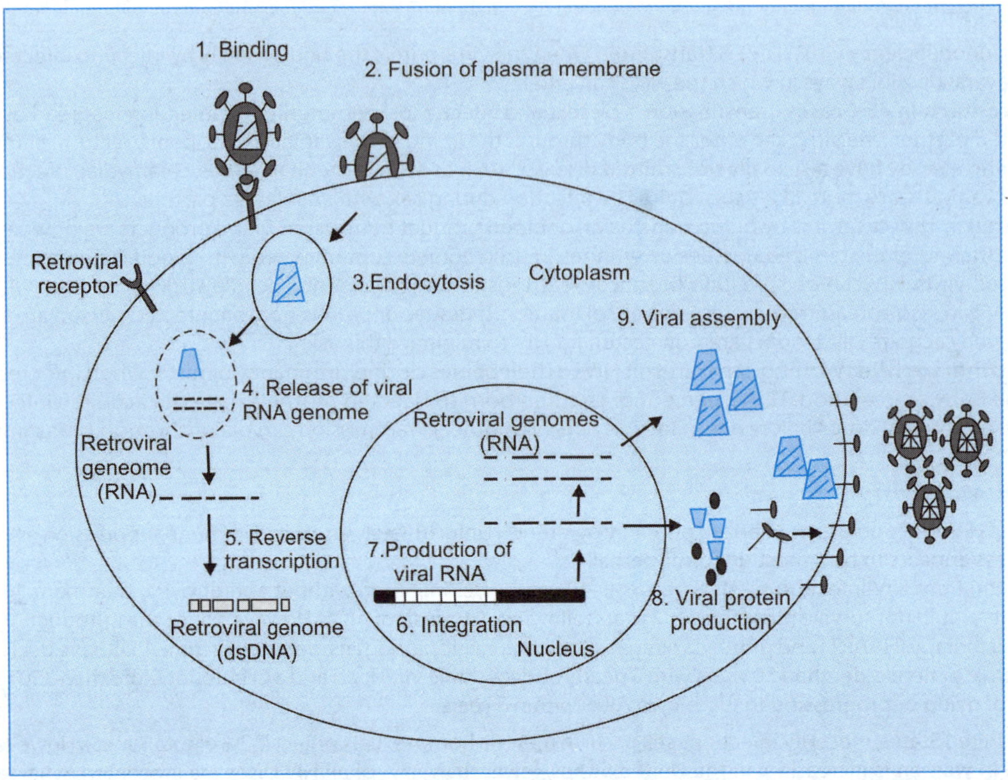

Fig. 18.3: Life cycle of human immunodeficiency virus (HIV) (integration and excision of viral genome).

6. **Fate of provirus:** From time to time, lytic infection is initiated releasing progeny virions, which infect other cells. The long and variable incubation period of HIV is because of the latency. In an infected individual, the virus can be isolated from the blood, lymphocytes, cell-free plasma, semen, cervical secretions, saliva, urine, and breast milk.
7. **Transcription back into RNA:** The viral DNA is transcribed into RNA and multiple copies of viral RNA are produced. There are only nine genes in HIV–RNA and these codes for the production of structural proteins, accessory proteins, and enzymes essential for the virus's replicative cycle.
8. **Virion assembly:** With the help of viral protease, the new virions are assembled into the polypeptide sequences needed for HIV virion formation and infectivity.
9. **Cell lysis:** The infected cell is made to burst open, presumably by the action of cellular proteins.

Causes of Immunodeficiency

The primary pathogenic mechanism in HIV infection is the damage caused to the CD4$^+$ T lymphocytes: The T4 cells decrease in numbers and the T4:T8 cell ratio is reversed. The infected cells do not release cytokines. This has a marked damping effect in the cell-mediated immune response. Though the major damage is to cellular immunity, the humoral mechanisms are also affected. AIDS patients are unable to respond to new antigens.

There is polyclonal activation of B lymphocytes leading to hypergammaglobulinemia. These are nonspecific antibodies and are irrelevant to antigens.

Monocyte-macrophage system is also affected apparently due to the lack of the activating factors by the T4 lymphocytes. The activity of NK cells and Tc (Tcytotoxic) cells are also affected. The clinical manifestations are due to failure of the immune responses. This renders the patient susceptible to life-threatening opportunistic infections and malignancies. The exceptions to this may be the neurological lesions seen in AIDS. Dementia and other degenerative neurological lesions seen in AIDS are due to direct toxic effects of HIV on the central nervous system.

Clinical Manifestations

AIDS is only the last stage in the wide spectrum of clinical features in HIV infection. The Center for Disease Control (USA) has classified the clinical course of HIV infection under various groups **(Fig. 18.4)**:

1. Group I: Acute HIV infection
2. Group II: Asymptomatic or latent infection

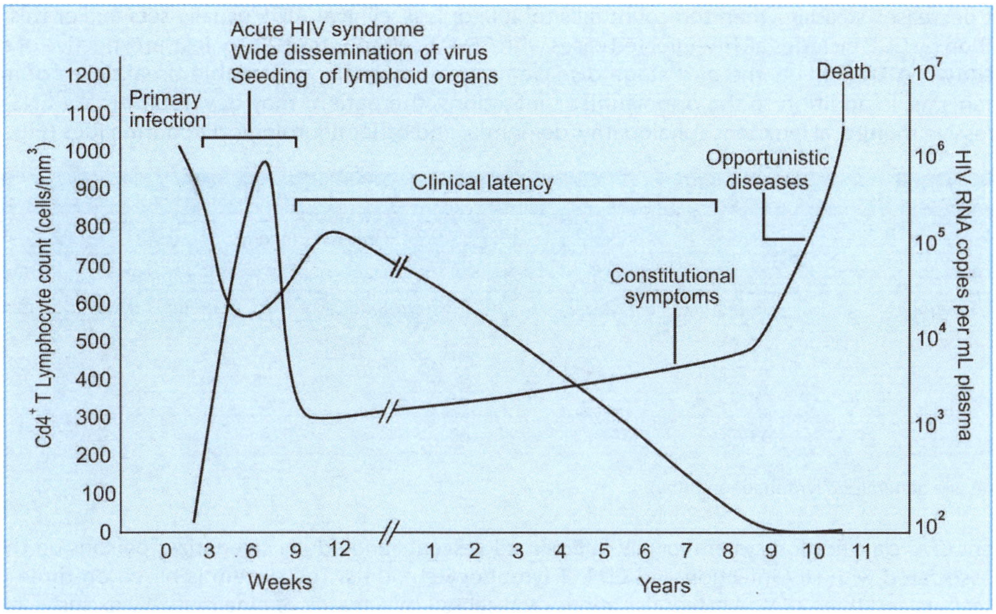

Fig. 18.4: Disease progression through different phases in HIV-infected cases. CD4 count comes down while the viral count goes high with the passage of time.

3. Group III: Persistent generalized lymphadenopathy (PGL)
4. Group IV:
   - Subgroup A: Constitutional diseases
   - Subgroup B: Neurological diseases
   - Subgroup C: Secondary infectious diseases
   - Subgroup D: Secondary cancers
   - Subgroup E: Other conditions

1. **Group I—acute HIV infection:** Many people do not develop symptoms after they first get infected with HIV. Others have a flu-like illness with fever, sore throat, headache, tiredness, skin rashes, and enlarged lymph nodes in the neck within several days to weeks after exposure to virus. These symptoms usually disappear of their own within a few weeks. The test for HIV antibodies appears negative while HIV antigenemia (p24 antigen) and viral nucleic acids can be demonstrated at the beginning of the phase. This phase is also called window period or phase of seroconversion.
2. **Group II—asymptomatic or latent infection:** All persons infected with HIV, pass through a phase of symptomless infection (clinical latency), which may last up to several years. The progression of disease varies widely among individuals. This state may last from a few months to more than 10 years. During this period, the virus continues to multiply actively and infects and kills the cells of the immune system. The virus destroys the CD4 cells that are the primary infection fighters.

   Even though the person has no symptoms, he or she is contagious and can pass HIV to others through the routes listed above. The patients show positive antibody tests during this phase. The infection progresses in course of time through various stages, CD4 lymphocytopenia, minor opportunistic infections, persistent generalized lymphadenopathy, AIDS-related complex, ultimately terminating in full-blown AIDS. The median time between primary HIV infection and development of AIDS has been stated as approximately 10 years. About 5–10% of the infected appear to escape clinical AIDS for 15 years or more. They have been "long-term survivors" or "long-term nonprogressors". The mechanism for, such long-time survivors is not exactly known, though many viral and host determinants are responsible.

   During this period, the host mounts an immune response against the virus, both humoral and cellular, which can only limit the viral load, but can not clear it completely. A chronic persistent infection with varying degree of multiplication is the result.
3. **Group III—persistent generalized lymphadenopathy (PGL):** This has been defined by presence of enlarged lymph nodes, at least 1 cm in diameter, in two or more noncontiguous extrainguinal sites, that persist for at least 3 months, in the absence of any current illness or medication that may cause lymphadenopathy. These are diagnostic of HIV when blood tests are positive for antibodies.
4. **Group IV:** This group includes patients with considerable immunodeficiency suffering from various constitutional symptoms of minor opportunistic infections. The patients present with weight loss—of more than 10% of body weight, persistent fever, diarrhea, generalized fatigue, and signs of other opportunistic infections may be apparent. The opportunistic infections are oral candidiasis, herpes zoster, salmonellosis or tuberculosis, and hairy cell leukoplakia **(Table 18.1)**. The patients are usually severely ill and many of them progress to AIDS in a few months. The CD4 cell

count decreases steadily when the count falls to 200, or less, clinical AIDS usually sets in. For this reason, the case definition by CDC includes all HIV-infected cases with $CD4^{+}$ T cell counts of 200 or less, irrespective of clinical condition.

5. **Full-blown AIDS:** This is the end-stage disease representing the irreversible breakdown of immune defense mechanisms. In addition to the opportunistic infections, the patient may develop primary CNS lymphomas and progressive multifocal leukoencephalopathy, dementia, and other neurological abnormalities **(Fig. 18.4)**.

TABLE 18.1: Revised classification system for HIV infection and expanded AIDS surveillance case definition for adolescents and adults.

	Clinical Categories		
CD4+ T Cell Categories	*A Asymptomatic, Acute (Primary) HIV or PGL*	*B Symptomatic, Not A or C Conditions*	*C AIDS-indicator Conditions*
>500/L	A1	B1	C1
200–499/L	A2	B2	C2
<200/L	A3	B3	C3

(PGL: progressive generalized lymphadenopathy)

The current CDC classification system for HIV-infected adolescents and adults categorizes persons on the basis of clinical conditions associated with HIV infection and $CD4^{+}$ T lymphocyte counts. The system is based on three ranges of $CD4^{+}$ T lymphocyte counts and three clinical categories and is represented by a matrix of nine mutually exclusive categories (see the details above). Using this system, any HIV-infected individual with a $CD4^{+}$ T cell count of <200/L has AIDS by definition, regardless of the presence of symptoms or opportunistic diseases. Once individuals have had a clinical condition in category B, their disease classification cannot be reverted back to category A, even if the condition resolves; the same holds true for category C in relation to category B.

Clinical Categories of HIV Infection

Category A: It consists of one or more of the conditions listed below in an adolescent or adult (>13 years) with documented HIV infection. Conditions listed in categories B and C must not have occurred.

- Asymptomatic HIV infection
- **Persistent generalized lymphadenopathy**
- **Acute (primary) HIV infection with accompanying illness or history of acute HIV infection.**

Category B: It consists of symptomatic conditions in an HIV-infected adolescent or adult that are not included among conditions listed in clinical category C and that meet at least one of the following criteria: (1) the conditions are attributed to HIV infection or are indicative of a defect in cell-mediated immunity; or (2) the conditions are considered by physicians to have a clinical course or to require management that is complicated by HIV infection. Examples include, but are not limited to the following:

- Bacillary angiomatosis
- Candidiasis, oropharyngeal (thrush)
- Candidiasis, vulvovaginal, persistent, frequent, or poorly responsive to therapy
- Cervical dysplasia (moderate or severe)/cervical carcinoma *in situ*
- Constitutional symptoms,, such as fever (38.5°C) or diarrhea lasting >1 month
- Hairy leukoplakia, oral
- Herpes zoster (shingles), involving at least two distinct episodes or more than one dermatome
- Idiopathic thrombocytopenic purpura
- Listeriosis
- Pelvic inflammatory disease, particularly, if complicated by tubo-ovarian abscess
- Peripheral neuropathy

Category C: Conditions listed in the AIDS surveillance case definition:

- Candidiasis of bronchi, trachea, or lungs
- Candidiasis, esophageal
- Cervical cancer, invasive
- Coccidioidomycosis, disseminated or extrapulmonary
- Cryptococcosis, extrapulmonary
- Cryptosporidiosis, chronic intestinal (>1 month's duration)
- Cytomegalovirus disease (other than liver, spleen, or nodes)
- Cytomegalovirus retinitis (with loss of vision)
- Encephalopathy, HIV-related
- Herpes simplex: chronic ulcer(s) (>1 month's duration); or bronchitis, pneumonia, or esophagitis

- Histoplasmosis, disseminated or extrapulmonary
- Kaposi's sarcoma **(Fig. 18.5)**
- Lymphoma, Burkitt's (or equivalent term)
- Lymphoma, primary, of brain
- *Mycobacterium avium* complex or *Mycobacterium kansasii*, disseminated or extrapulmonary
- *Mycobacterium tuberculosis*, any site (pulmonary or extrapulmonary)
- *Mycobacterium*, other species or unidentified species, disseminated or extrapulmonary
- *Pneumocystis jiroveci* pneumonia
- Pneumonia, recurrent
- Progressive multifocal leukoencephalopathy
- *Salmonella* septicemia, recurrent
- Toxoplasmosis of brain
- Wasting syndrome due to HIV

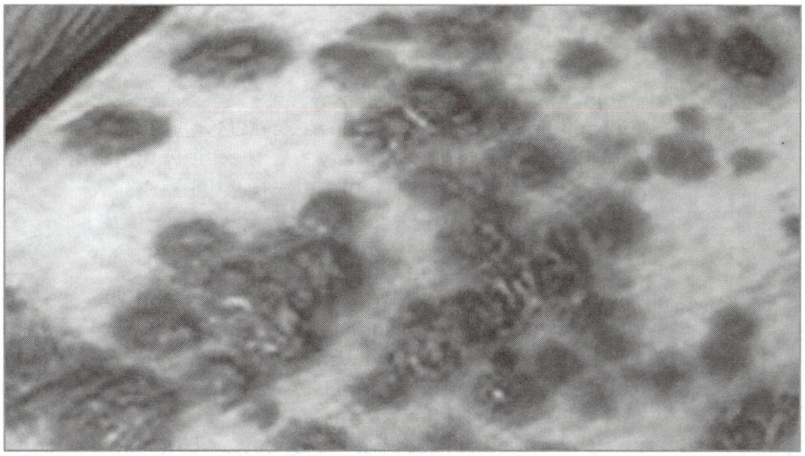

Fig. 18.5: Kaposi's sarcoma—it is an indolent, multifocal nonmetastasizing mucosal or cutaneous tumor probably of endothelial origin, represented in the form of purple spots in the skin.

Laboratory Diagnosis of HIV Infection

1. Laboratory procedures for the diagnosis of HIV infection include tests for immunodeficiency as well as specific tests for HIV.
   - **Nonspecific tests:** The following tests help to establish the immunodeficiency in HIV infection.
   - **Total leukocyte and lymphocyte count:** To demonstrate leukopenia and lymphopenia. The lymphocytic count is usually below 2,000/mm^3
   - **T cell subset assays:** Absolute CD4$^+$ cell count is less than 200/L. T4:T8 ratio is reversed. The decrease in CD4 is the hallmark for AIDS.
   - **Platelet count:** It shows thrombocytopenia.
   - IgA and IgG levels are raised.
   - **Diminished cell-mediated immunity as indicated by skin tests**
   - **Lymph node biopsy shows profound abnormalities.**
2. **Specific tests for HIV infection:** These include demonstration of HIV antigen, antibodies. Viral nucleic acids or other components and isolation of virus.
   i. **Detection of antigen:** Following a contact, as by blood transfusion, the viral antigen may be detectable in blood after about 2 weeks. The major core antigen p24 is the earliest virus marker to appear in blood. IgM antibodies appear in about 4–6 weeks, to be followed by IgG antibodies.
   If the infecting dose is small, as following a needle stick injury, the process may be considerably delayed. The appearance of p24 antigenemia and viremia, followed by IgM antibody response, coincides with the acute or seroconversion illness. Afterwards, free p24 antigen disappears from circulation and remains absent during the long asymptomatic phase to reappear only when severe clinical disease sets in. However, antibody bound p24 antigen continues to be demonstrable, after dissociation.
   The p24 capture ELISA assay, which uses anti-p24 antibody as the solid phase can be used for this. This test is positive in about 30% of the infected persons. In the first few weeks after infection and in the terminal phase, the test is uniformly positive. This test along with HIV ELISA is currently used for screening blood donors.
   ii. **Detection of antibodies:** Demonstration of antibodies is the simplest and most widely employed technique for the diagnosis of HIV infection. However, it takes 2–8 weeks to months for the antibodies to appear in circulation and during that period, the person may be highly infectious. Once antibodies appear they increase in titer for the next several months. IgM antibodies disappear in 8–10 weeks, while IgG antibodies remain throughout. When immunodeficiency becomes severe following clinical AIDS, some components of anti-p24 may disappear. There are two types of serological tests:

   Screening tests and supplemental tests.

   A. Screening tests include:
   a. ELISA
   b. Rapid tests:
      - Dot-blot assay
      - Particle agglutination tests
      - HIV spot and comb test
      - Fluorimetric microparticle technologies
   c. Simple tests—based on ELISA principle

B. Supplemental tests:
- ◊ Western blot test
- ◊ Indirect immunofluorescence test
- ◊ Radioimmunoprecipitation assay
- ◊ Enzyme-linked immunosorbent assay (ELISA) is the most frequently used method for screening of blood samples for HIV antibody. The sensitivity and specificity of the presently available commercial systems approaches 100% but false-positive and false-negative reactions occur.
- ◊ First generation—whole viral lysates
- ◊ Second generation—recombinant antigen
- ◊ Third generation—synthetic peptide
- ◊ Fourth generation—antigen + antibody (simultaneous detection of HIV antigen and antibody)—HIV duo antibody can be detected in a majority of individuals within 6–12 weeks after infection using the earlier generation of assays. But it can be detected within 3–4 weeks when using the newer third-generation ELISA. Due to their ability to detect p24 antigen, the fourth-generation ELISA will be of value in detecting early infection. The window period can be shortened to 2 weeks using p24-antigen assay.

Other test systems available include line immunoassay (LIA), immunofluorescence, Western blots, and radioimmunoprecipitation assay (RIPA). These are *supplemental or confirmatory assays.*

Western blotting: Western blots are regarded as the gold standard and seropositivity is diagnosed when antibodies against, both the env and the gag proteins are detected. The sensitivity of the test systems is currently being improved by the use of recombinant antigens.

Rapid tests: These are tests that can yield results in <30 minutes. The results are read by naked eye.

Rapid HIV assays have proven particularly useful for testing pregnant women in labor who have not received prenatal care. These are also helpful in detecting HIV-2 infection, which cannot be detected by ELISA.

3. **Demonstration of viral nucleic acid:** This can be accomplished by probes or by PCR techniques. The latter may be useful because of its extremely high sensitivity. Although standard tests that measure antibody response to the HIV virus have become increasingly sensitive, cases of HIV are occasionally missed because individuals can have negative antibody tests during the early stages of infection. Also, a few people with long-term HIV infection may have false-negative antibody tests or may be chronic carriers who are clinically asymptomatic. The NAAT (nucleic acid amplification test) helps to avoid these problems, as it amplifies the HIV viral RNA and detects viral genes instead of viral antibodies or antigens.

   PCR: In this, the target HIV–RNA or proviral DNA is amplified enzymatically in vitro by chemical reaction. It is an extremely sensitive assay because a single copy of proviral DNA can be amplified. Qualitative PCR is **useful** for diagnostic purposes.

   Three different techniques namely RT-PCR, nucleic acid sequence-based amplification (NASBA), and branched-DNA (b-DNA) assay have been employed to develop commercial kits.
4. **Virus isolation:** Virus isolation is accomplished by the cocultivation of the patient's lymphocytes with fresh peripheral blood cells of healthy donors or with suitable culture lines, such as T-lymphomas. The presence of the virus can be confirmed by reverse transcriptase assays, serological tests, or by changes in growth pattern of the indicator cells. However, virus isolation is tedious and time consuming (weeks) and is successful in only 70–90% of cases. Therefore, virus isolation is mainly used for the characterization of the virus.
5. **Alternative to classical tests:**
   a. Oral fluid (saliva) HIV tests
   b. Urine tests

Treatment

Virtually all treatment for HIV infection and AIDS today focuses on arresting the progression of the disease within the body as measured by T cell counts and tests for viral load. At present, a reasonable course of action is to initiate ARV therapy in anyone with the acute HIV syndrome; all pregnant women; patients with symptomatic disease; and patients with asymptomatic disease with $CD4^+$ T cell counts <350/L. In addition, one may wish to administer a 6-week course of therapy to uninfected individuals immediately following a high-risk exposure to HIV.

There are two principal approaches to treatment:

a. **Immunotherapy:** Immunotherapy is transfusion-based treatment designed to replace lost immunoglobulins needed to fight HIV infection (passive immunotherapy), to provide cellular factors, such as interleukins (IL-2) or to introduce selected or altered immune cells to attack cells harboring the virus (adoptive immunotherapy). The results of trials using this latter approach, however, have been inconclusive, and no group has yet shown a survival benefit.

b. **Anti-HIV drug treatment:** Treatment with anti-HIV drugs attempts to reduce viral load by blocking new infection in the host cell. The drugs are used to target two major enzymes of HIV, which are needed for the infection cycle: reverse transcriptase and protease.

   1. **Reverse transcriptase inhibitors:** Reverse transcriptase inhibitors act at the preintegration stage before the viral RNA has been converted to DNA and enter the host cell nucleus to integrate into the cell chromosome. These drugs block the reverse transcription of viral RNA into viral DNA. There are two types of reverse transcriptase inhibitors, both

of which accomplish the same objective: nucleoside and nucleotide analogs, and non-nucleoside reverse transcriptase inhibitors.

i. **Nucleoside analogs**, which constitute the most effective family of antiretroviral drugs, operate by mimicking nucleic acids normally incorporated into viral DNA. They interfere with reverse transcriptase and thus prevent infection. Nucleoside analogs can be placed in two groups, those replacing thymidine,, such as AZT and d4T, which protect activated T cells from infection, and nonthymidine analogs, such as ddl and 3TC, which protect resting T cells. Nucleotide analogs have the same action but are based around a different sugar.
   Despite their similarities in structure and action, nucleoside analogs have differing impacts on disease progression, viral burden, and the development of resistant virus. In addition, some must be activated within the infected cell before they become effective.
ii. **Non-nucleoside reverse transcriptase inhibitors** directly inhibit reverse transcription and, unlike nucleoside analogs, do not have to go through chemical changes in the infected cell before beginning their action. The two main non-nucleoside reverse transcriptase inhibitors are nevirapine, which can show toxicity and early resistance problems, and delavirdine, with which there is less clinical experience as yet.

2. **Protease inhibitors:** Protease inhibitors block HIV replication after integration. These drugs inhibit the function of the protease by acting as analogs for the peptide and non-peptide protease substrates needed to process the "gag-pol" polypeptide into proteins. As a result, no infectious virus can be manufactured.
   Since protease inhibitors act after integration, they can obstruct infectious HIV production in both acutely and chronically infected T cells and macrophages **(Fig. 18.6)**. (In contrast, reverse transcriptase inhibitors can only inhibit the acute infection of cells). Importantly, neither protease inhibitors nor reverse transcriptase inhibitors directly attack the cells in the body that are infected with the virus. These cellular reservoirs are the preferred source of resistant viruses. Protease inhibitors have also been shown to be less toxic than nucleoside analogs. So far only a few have been licensed for use, including saquinavir, ritonavir, indinavir, and, more recently, nelfinavir, although others are expected.
3. **Combination treatment:** Because reverse transcriptase inhibitors and protease inhibitors address different stages of viral replication, using both families of drugs in combination has been shown to be moreeffective than monotherapy in impeding the spread of HIV in the body and reducing viral loads. Although the optimum combination of anti-HIV drugs is as yet unknown, AZT, 3TC, and a protease inhibitor are usually the first drugs given. This combination of two reverse transcriptase inhibitors, one of which is a thymidine analog, and a protease inhibitor, blocks infection both before and after integration and in both activated and resting T cells. The aim of anti-HIV therapy has now shifted from simply delaying the progression of disease to finding a permanent cure. This combinational therapy is termed as highly active antiretroviral therapy (HAART).
   The current consensus is that one should give a potent combination of agents, HAART right from the start when treatment is indicated.
4. **The future:** In addition to the positive results shown by combination therapy trials, a number of developments may hold promise for the near future. These include genetically engineered killer T cells, which attack HIV before it reproduces, and research into genetically deactivating the CXCR4 and CCR5 T cell co-receptors, which are a path for HIV entry into cells.

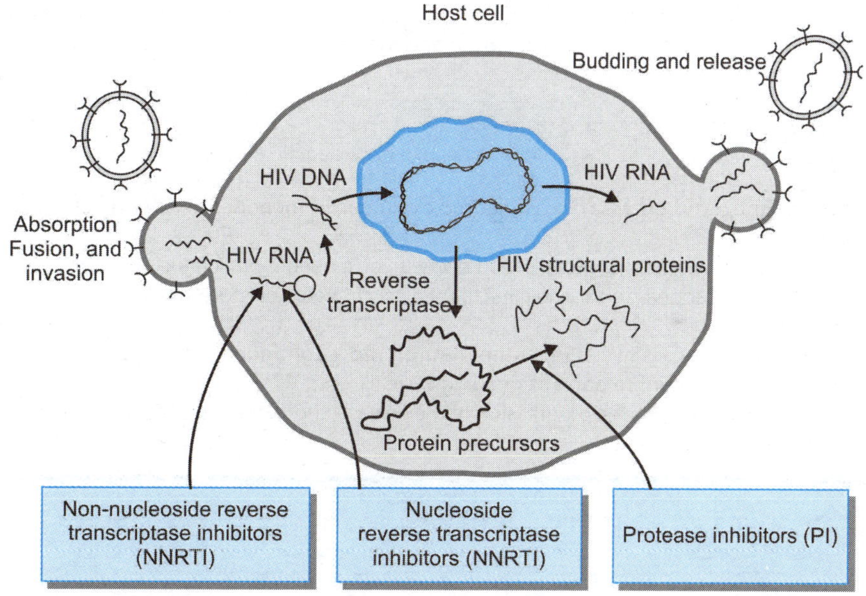

Fig. 18.6: Mechanism of action of different drugs used for the treatment of HIV infection.

Prevention

The risk of contracting HIV increases with the number of sexual partners. A change in the lifestyle would obviously reduce the risk.

The HIV-infected mothers are not recommended to have children at present and pregnancy itself would appear to be a risk factor for seropositive mothers. A recent clinical trial demonstrated the efficacy of AZT in preventing transmission of HIV from the mother to the fetus.

The spread of HIV through blood transfusion had virtually been eliminated since the introduction of blood donor screening in many countries. Blood products, such as factor VIII now undergo routine treatment, which appears to inactivate any HIV present effectively.

Development of Vaccine

An effective vaccine against HIV would have to elicit protection against both free virus and virus-infected cells. HIV-neutralizing antibodies do not prevent the progression of the disease. Individuals with high-neutralizing antibody titers, however, seem to have a longer disease-free interval. Cellular immune response may be important for protection and may take place through Tc cells, NK cells, and ADCC mechanisms. The role of these mechanisms in the protection against HIV infection and their relevance for anti-HIV vaccination are still unclear.

Another obstacle to the development of an effective HIV vaccine may be the high genetic variability of HIV, which resides mainly in the *env* gene. In certain regions of the envelope gene, the variability may be as high as 50%. However, conserved regions exist in the gp120 and the gp41 region, which can be recognized by HIV sera and neutralizing antibodies can be induced with peptides representing these regions. The main types of approaches to an AIDS vaccine are as follows:

1. Live attenuated virus
2. Inactivated virus
3. Live recombinant viruses
4. Synthetic peptides
5. Recombinant DNA products (gp120 and gp160)
6. Native envelope and/or core proteins
7. Anti-idiotype antibodies
8. Passive immunization

To date, the best hope lies in an inactivated vaccine.

Despite progress in dealing directly with HIV, however, the virus, by impairing the immune system, exposes the infected person to a range of opportunistic viral, bacterial, and parasitic infections and malignancies. It is these which are the actual cause of death in most patients with AIDS and, notwithstanding the success of anti-HIV drug treatment in reducing viral load, it is still unclear whether HIV-induced damage to the immune system can be reversed. New strains of HIV undetectable by current screening methods and resistant to the best antiretroviral drugs currently available have also now been discovered.

CLINICAL NOTE

The combination of two reverse transcriptase inhibitors and a protease inhibitor, termed as highly active antiretroviral therapy (HAART), blocks infection both before and after integration and in both activated and resting T cells.

CLINICAL PEARLS

1. Acquired immunodeficiency syndrome is a disease caused by human immunodeficiency virus and is characterized by marked immunosuppression.
2. The mode of transmission is by sexual contact, blood transfusions, needle prick injury, or from mother to child.
3. About 5–10% of the infected appear to escape clinical AIDS for 15 years or more. They have been "long-term survivors" or "long-term nonprogressors".
4. Enzyme-linked immunosorbent assay (ELISA) is the method most commonly employed for the screening purpose and Western blotting is used for the confirmation of the diagnosis.
5. Treatment is imparted simply to check the progression of the disease, there is no cure of AIDS and there is no vaccine available for prophylaxis of this disease.

Chapter 19

Acid-Base Balance and Imbalance

LEARNING OBJECTIVES

To understand:

- Significance of maintenance of plasma pH
- Mechanism of action of blood buffers
- Role of lungs in the maintenance of plasma pH
- Role of kidney in the maintenance of plasma pH
- Causes and clinical implications of acid-base imbalance.

CASE STUDIES

CASE STUDY

Theme: Regulation of Plasma pH in Normal Health

BASIC CONCEPT

An acid is a substance that can donate hydrogen ions (H^+) and a base is a substance that can accept H^+ ions, regardless of the substance's charge.

$$H_2CO_3 \text{ (acid)} \rightarrow H^+ + HCO_3^- \text{ (base)}$$

Strong acids are those that are completely ionized in body fluids and weak acids are those that are incompletely ionized in body fluids.

$$HCl \rightarrow H^+ + Cl^-$$

Hydrochloric acid (HCl) is considered as a strong acid because it is present only in a completely ionized form in the body, whereas H_2CO_3 is a weak acid because it is ionized incompletely and at equilibrium, all 3 reactants are present in body fluids.

The law of mass action states that the velocity of a reaction is proportional to the product of the reactant concentrations.

$$H_2CO_3 \text{ (acid)} \rightarrow H^+ + HCO_3^- \text{ (base)}$$

On the basis of this law, the addition of H^+ or bicarbonate (HCO_3^-) drives this reaction to the left.

In body fluids, the concentration of hydrogen ions (H^+) is maintained within very narrow limits, with the normal physiologic concentration being 40 nEq/L. The concentration of HCO_3^- (24 mEq/L) is 600,000 times that of (H^+). The tight regulation of (H^+) at this low concentration is crucial for normal cellular activities.

Maintenance of pH: It is important for proper physiological functioning of cells and tissues. Any changes in pH can alter enzyme activity, cellular uptake, incorporation and use of minerals and metabolites, uptake and release of oxygen, and the formation of biological structural components. Normal plasma pH = 7.40 (± 0.05). The pH range that is compatible with life is from 6.8 to 7.8. The body can comfortably tolerate a shift in pH of about 0.04. Most cells of the body have a pH = 7.0, but RBCs boast a pH of 7.2. The pH of the body affects its acid-base balance and the pH of blood has the greatest effect. The most common sources for pH disturbances are the body's production of organic acids (acetic, acetoacetate, propionic, butyric, lactic, etc.) which are the major sources of hydrogen ion.

Under normal conditions, acids and to a lesser extent, bases are being added constantly to the extracellular fluid compartment but still a physiologic (H^+) of 40 nEq/L is maintained and the following three processes must take place:

1. Buffering by extracellular and intracellular buffers
2. Alveolar ventilation, which controls $PaCO_2$
3. Renal H^+ excretion, which controls plasma (HCO_3^-).

BUFFERS

Buffers are weak acids or bases that are able to minimize changes in pH by taking up or releasing H^+. Phosphate is an example of an effective buffer, as in the following reaction:

$$HPO_4^{2-} + (H^+) \leftrightarrow H_2PO_4$$

Upon addition of an H^+ to extracellular fluids, the monohydrogen phosphate binds H^+ to form dihydrogen phosphate, minimizing the change in pH. Similarly, when (H^+) is decreased, the reaction is shifted to the left. Thus, buffers work as a first line of defense to blunt the changes in pH that would otherwise result from the constant daily addition of acids and bases to body fluids. With the constant pouring of H^+, the concentration of the monohydrogen phosphate will ultimately diminish and the pH will start falling.

The major buffer system of the body:

1. HCO_3^-/H_2CO_3 buffering system, HCO_3^-/CO_2 (bicarbonate/carbon dioxide)
2. HPO_4^{2-}/H_2PO_4 (phosphate)
3. Organic phosphate esters
4. Proteins

Proteins with side chains that contain more carboxyl-terminal groups than amino-terminal groups promote an acidic environment. Proteins with side chains that contain more amino-terminal groups than carboxyl-terminal groups promote an alkaline environment. Proteins with side chains containing equal numbers of amino and carboxyl side groups are neutral, not affecting the pH.

HCO_3^-/H_2CO_3 BUFFERING SYSTEM

In the extracellular fluid (ECF), bicarbonate buffer is the most important buffer.
Its function is illustrated by the following reactions:

$$H_2O + CO_2 \rightarrow H_2CO_3 \rightarrow H^+ + HCO_3^-$$

When an acid load (H^+) is added to the body fluids, it results in consumption of HCO_3^- by the added H^+. Carbonic acid, thus formed, in turn, forms water and CO_2. Carbon dioxide concentration is maintained within a narrow range via the respiratory drive, which eliminates accumulating CO_2. The kidneys regenerate the HCO_3^- consumed during this reaction.

Put simply, whereas simple buffers rapidly become ineffective as the association of the hydrogen ion and the weak anion of the weak acid reaches equilibrium, the bicarbonate system keeps working because the carbonic acid is removed as CO_2. The limit to the effectiveness of the bicarbonate system is the initial concentration of bicarbonate. The acid-base status of the patient is assessed by the bicarbonate concentration in the plasma. The association of hydrogen ion with bicarbonate occurs rapidly but the dissociation of H_2CO_3 to CO_2 and H_2O is slow. This process is accelerated by the enzyme carbonic anhydrase, which is present in the erythrocytes and in the kidney whenever this reaction is needed. Buffering at the expense of bicarbonate effectively removes hydrogen ions from ECF. Carbon dioxide is removed from the lungs and water assimilates in the ECF without producing any change in pH. The ECF contains a large amount of bicarbonate to the extent of 24 mmol/L; when the H^+ concentration increases, the bicarbonate concentration comes down since it is used up during the process of buffering.

This reaction continues to move to the left as long as CO_2 is constantly eliminated or until HCO_3^- is significantly depleted, making less HCO_3^- available to bind H^+. Since HCO_3^- and $PaCO_2$ can be managed independently (kidneys and lungs, respectively) that makes this a very effective buffering system. One of the major factors that make this system very effective is the ability to control $PaCO_2$ by changes in ventilation. As can be noted from this reaction, increased carbon dioxide (CO_2) concentration drives the reaction to the right, whereas a decrease in CO_2 concentration drives it to the left.

Assessing acid-base status: An indication of the acid-base status of the patient can be determined by measuring the components of the bicarbonate system. In chemical terms, the bicarbonate buffer system can be considered in the same way as any other chemical dissociation.

The Henderson–Hasselbalch equation describes the relationship between blood pH and the components of the H_2CO_3 buffering system.

$$pH = 6.1 + \log (HCO_3^-/H_2CO_3)$$

Bicarbonate (HCO_3^-) is in equilibrium with the metabolic components.

- Bicarbonate production in the kidney
- Acid production from endogenous or exogenous sources.

Carbonic acid (H_2CO_3) is in equilibrium with the respiratory component, as shown by the below equation:

$$H_2CO_3 = pCO_2 \text{ (mm Hg)} \times 0.03$$

Note that changes in pH or (H^+) are a result of relative changes in the ratio of $PaCO_2$ to (HCO_3^-) rather than to absolute change in either one. In other words, if both $PaCO_2$ and (HCO_3^-) change in the same direction, the ratio stays the same and the pH or (H^+) remains relatively stable. To diminish the alteration in pH that occurs when either HCO_3^- or $PaCO_2$ changes, the body, within certain limits, changes the other variable in the same direction.

Role of hemoglobin as a buffer: The buffering capacity of Hb is due to the presence of "imidazole" nitrogen group of histidine. Oxygenated Hb is a stronger acid than deoxygenated Hb. Acidity of the medium favors delivery of oxygen to the tissues. Alkalinity of the medium favors oxygenation of Hb. Sequence of events that occur in lungs and tissues are as follows:

- In the lungs: The formation of oxygenated hemoglobin from deoxygenated hemoglobin must release H^+, which will react with HCO_3^- to form H_2CO^3. Due to the low CO_2 tension in the lungs. H_2CO_3 dissociates to form CO_2 and H_2O.CO_2 is then eliminated in the expired air **(Fig. 19.1)**.
- **In the tissues:** Oxygenated Hb dissociates to give O_2 to the tissues and the deoxygenated Hb (reduced Hb) is formed. At the same time, CO_2 produced as a result of metabolism is hydrated to for H_2CO_3, which ionizes to form H^+ and HCO_3^-. Deoxygenated Hb acts as anion and accepts H^+ to form acid reduced Hb (**Fig. 19.2**).

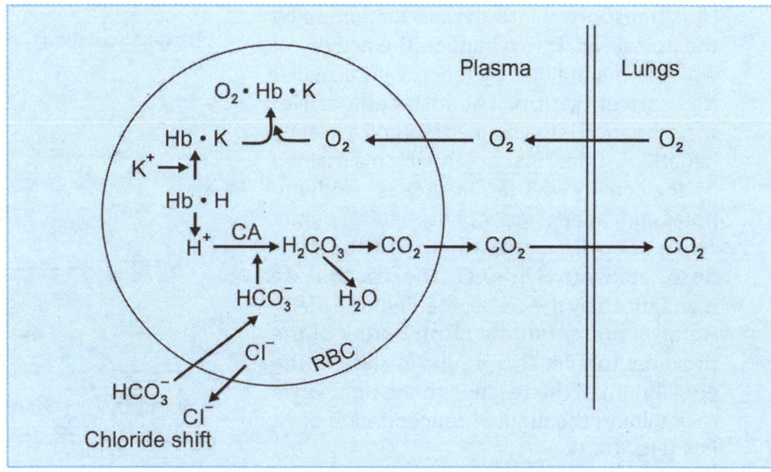

Fig. 19.1: Role of hemoglobin (Hb) as a buffer in the lungs.

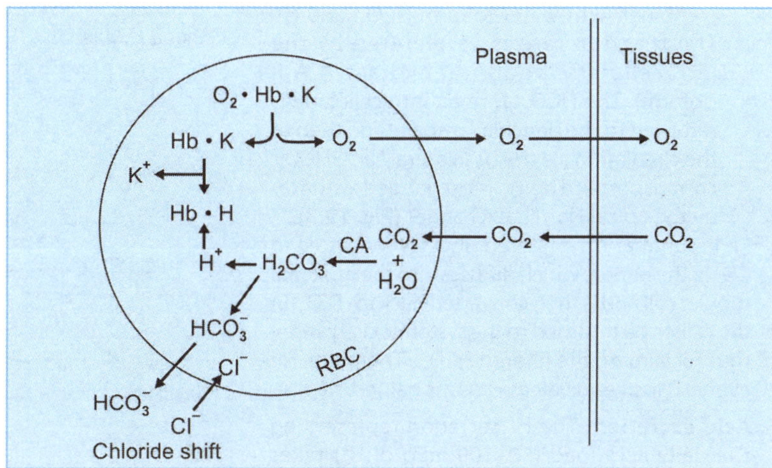

Fig. 19.2: Role of hemoglobin (Hb) as a buffer in the tissues.

Renal acid handling: Volatile (e.g., carbonic) and nonvolatile (e.g., sulfuric, phosphoric) acids are added continuously to the body fluids. Approximately, 15,000 mmol of CO_2 (carbonic acid) is produced daily from the metabolism of dietary carbohydrates and fats which is eventually eliminated through the lungs. Respiratory acidosis results from the failure to remove CO_2.

The nonvolatile acids (H_2SO_4 and H_3PO_4) are produced from the metabolism of sulfur-containing amino acids, sulfur-containing vitamins, sulfolipids, phosphoprotein, nucleoprotein, and phospholipids. These nonvolatile acids are first neutralized by the HCO_3^-/H_2CO_3 system:

$$H_2SO_4 + 2NaHCO_3 \rightarrow Na_2SO_4 + 2H_2CO_3 \rightarrow 2H_2O + 2CO_2$$

The strong acid is neutralized by the two molecules of HCO_3^- producing a weak acid (H_2CO_3) that resists the change in pH. The composition of the bicarbonate buffer is maintained by the involvement of the lungs and kidney. The CO_2 thus produced is excreted through the lungs and the bicarbonates that are consumed are replaced by the kidney. This neutralization process impedes progressive HCO_3^- loss and hinders the development of metabolic acidosis (mainly by secretion of H^+ in the collecting duct). Bicarbonate content is also maintained by the metabolism of amino acids, such as glutamate and aspartate that produce citrate and lactate, which are subsequently converted to HCO_3^-.

Approximately, 50–100 mEq of H^+ are contributed by diet each day. To maintain the normal pH, the kidney performs the following functions: (i) reabsorbs almost all the filtered bicarbonates and (ii) eliminates the daily H^+ load. Any loss of HCO_3^- is equal to the gain of an equimolar amount of H^+ and the loss of H^+ is equal to the addition of an equimolar amount of HCO_3^-.

HCO_3^- reabsorption

Approximately, 4,300 mEq of HCO_3^- is filtered daily in a healthy individual, with a glomerular ultrafiltrate of 180 L and serum HCO_3^- concentration of 24 mEq/L. All of the filtered bicarbonates are reabsorbed back; approximately 90% of the filtered HCO_3^- is reabsorbed back in the proximal tubule and the rest is reabsorbed in the thick ascending limb and the medullary collecting duct. The mechanism of bicarbonate reabsorption is as follows (shown in **Fig. 19.3**):

1. H^+ in the tubular lumen combines with filtered HCO_3^- in the following reaction:

$$HCO_3^- + H^+ \rightarrow H_2CO_3 \rightarrow H_2O + CO_2$$

H^+ is transported into the tubular lumen by the apical Na^+/H^+ exchanger, the activity of which is maintained by the low intracellular Na^+ concentration. The intracellular Na^+ concentration is maintained low and a relative negative intracellular potential is maintained by the activity of $3Na^+/2K^+$-ATPase (sodium-potassium adenosine triphosphatase) pump.

2. The carbonic acid, thus, produced is dissociated into $H_2O + CO_2$. The reaction rate is enhanced by the carbonic anhydrase (CA IV isoform) present in the brush border of the proximal tubule. This results in shifting the equilibrium of the reaction to the right while maintaining the luminal concentration of H^+ low **(Fig. 19.3)**.
3. CO_2 diffuses into the proximal tubular cell through the aquaporin-1 water channel and combines with water to form HCO_3^- and H^+. The reaction rate is accelerated by the intracellular carbonic anhydrase (CA II isoform). The HCO_3^- formed intracellularly is returned to the pericellular space and then to the circulation via the basolateral $Na^+/3HCO_3^-$ cotransporter. The H^+ is exchanged with Na^+ by the apical Na^+/H^+ exchanger **(Fig. 19.3)**.

In summary, the filtered HCO_3^- is converted to CO_2 in the lumen, which diffuses into the proximal tubular cell and is then converted back to HCO_3^- in the cell, to be returned to the systemic circulation, thus reclaiming the filtered HCO_3^-. Therefore, for every H^+ lost, equivalent HCO_3^- is gained.

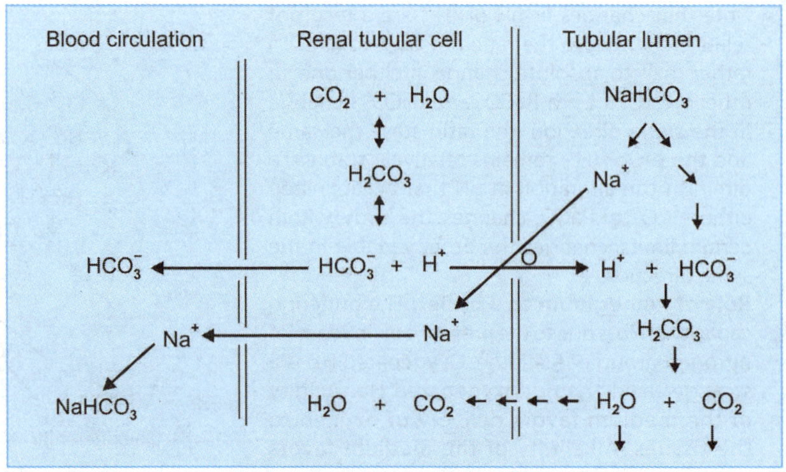

Fig. 19.3: Mechanism of reabsorption of HCO_3^-.

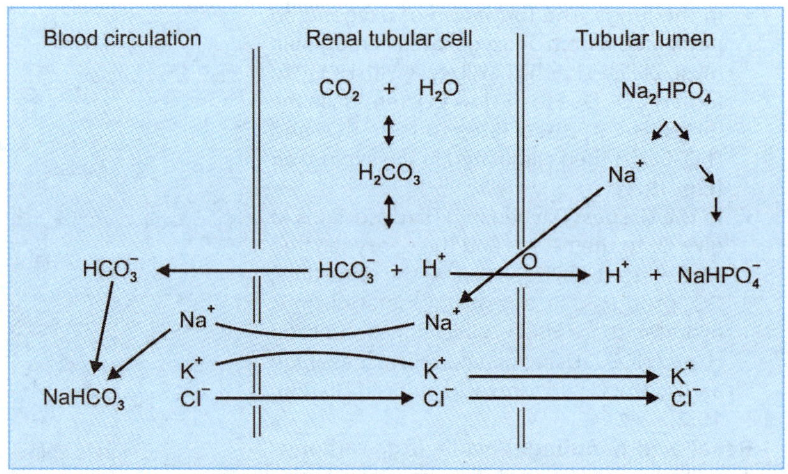

Fig. 19.4: Figure showing the buffering of secreted H^+ by HPO_4^{2-}.

Acid excretion: The H^+ secretion representing the daily acid load (50–100 mEq of H^+) takes place through the A-type intercalated cells of the collecting duct. H^+ enters the tubular lumen through either of the two apical proton pumps, H^+-ATPase or H^+/K^+-ATPase. The H^+ secretion in these segments is affected by Na^+ reabsorption in the adjacent principal cells of the collecting duct and the intracellular HCO_3^- is transported to the systemic circulation through the basolateral Cl^-/HCO_3^- exchanger.

More than 99.9% of the H^+ load is excreted in the bound form buffered by the weak bases,, such as NH_3 or phosphate. Hydrogen ions can be discharged as free ions, but at the least attainable urine pH of 5.0 that would require excretion of 5,000–10,000 L of urine per day. Urine pH cannot fall below 5.0 since the gradient against which H^+-ATPase pumps protons (intracellular pH 7.5 to luminal pH 5) becomes too steep. A highly acidified urine, despite a volume of 3 L, contains only 30 µEq of free H^+.

Titratable acidity: The amount of H^+ secreted by the renal tubular cell which is buffered by filtered weak acids is called titratable acidosis. Phosphate as HPO_4^{2-} is the primary buffer in this system, but other urine buffers include uric acid and creatinine.

$$H_2PO_4 \rightarrow H^+ + HPO_4^{2-}$$

The availability of phosphate filtered is limited and relatively fixed; therefore, only a small fraction of the secreted H+ can be buffered by HPO_4^{2-} **(Fig. 19.4)**.

Ammonia: Ammonia is a more significant urine-buffering system for secreted H^+ than phosphate. The buffering by ammonia (NH_3) occurs through the following reaction:

$$NH_3 + H^+ \rightarrow NH_4^+$$

Ammonia is produced in the proximal tubule from the amino acid glutamine by the action of glutaminase and the rate of this reaction is enhanced by an acid load and by hypokalemia. Ammonia is converted to ammonium (NH_4^+) by intracellular H^+ and is secreted into the proximal tubular lumen by the apical Na^+/H^+ (NH_4^+) antiporter. It can be secreted as such also and can later combine with H^+ in the lumen to form NH_4^+.

NH_4^+ is trapped in the lumen and excreted as the NH_4Cl salt and every H^+ ion buffered is an HCO_3^- gained to the systemic circulation. The kidneys can adjust the amount of NH_3 synthesized to meet demand, making this a robust system to buffer secreted H^+ in the urine **(Fig. 19.5)**.

NORMAL ACID-BASE HOMEOSTASIS AND ROLE OF LUNGS

Systemic arterial pH is maintained between 7.35 and 7.45 by extracellular and intracellular chemical buffering together with respiratory and renal regulatory mechanisms. The control of arterial CO_2 tension ($PaCO_2$) by the central nervous system and respiratory systems and the control of the plasma bicarbonate by the kidneys stabilize the arterial pH by excretion or retention of acid or alkali. The metabolic and respiratory components that regulate systemic pH are described by the Henderson–Hasselbalch equation:

$$pH = 6.1 + \log \frac{HCO_3^-}{PCO_2 \times .00301}$$

Under most circumstances, CO_2 production and excretion are matched and the usual steady-state $PaCO_2$ is maintained at 40 mm Hg. Underexcretion of CO_2 produces hypercapnia and overexcretion causes hypocapnia. Nevertheless, production and excretion are again matched at a new steady-state $PaCO_2$. Therefore, the $PaCO_2$ is regulated primarily by neural respiratory factors and is not subject to regulation by the rate of CO_2 production. Hypercapnia is usually the result of hypoventilation rather than of increased CO_2 production. Increases or decreases in $PaCO_2$ represent derangements of neural respiratory control or are due to compensatory changes in response to a primary alteration in the plasma (HCO_3^-).

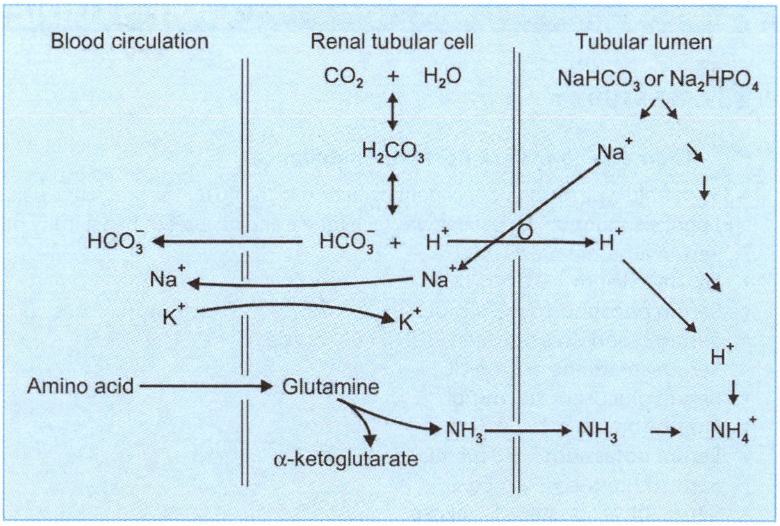

Fig. 19.5: Figure showing ammonia mechanism. Glutamine is first converted to glutamate and then to alpha-ketoglutarate.

Pathological aspect

There are two types of acid-base disorders: Respiratory and metabolic. Primary respiratory disorders affect blood acidity by causing changes in pCO_2 and primary metabolic disorders are caused by disturbances in the HCO_3^- concentration. The primary disturbances are usually accompanied by compensatory changes; however, even though these changes attenuate a pH shift from the normal value (7.40), they do not fully compensate for the primary acid-base disorders even if the disorders are chronic. Therefore, if the pH is <7.40, the primary process is acidosis (either respiratory or metabolic). If the pH is higher than 7.40, the primary process is either respiratory or metabolic alkalosis. The presence of one disorder with its appropriate compensatory change is a simple disorder. The presence of more than one simple disorder (not compensatory) is a mixed disorder. Double or triple disorders can coexist but not quadruple ones, because simultaneous respiratory acidosis and alkalosis are not possible. Primary respiratory disturbances (primary changes in $PaCO_2$) invoke compensatory metabolic responses [secondary changes in (HCO_3^-)] and primary metabolic disturbances elicit predictable compensatory respiratory responses. Metabolic acidosis due to an increase in endogenous acids (e.g., ketoacidosis) lowers extracellular fluid (HCO_3^-) and decreases extracellular pH. This stimulates the medullary chemoreceptors to increase ventilation and to return the ratio of (HCO_3^-) to $PaCO_2$ and thus pH, toward normal, although not to normal. The degree of respiratory compensation expected in a simple form of metabolic acidosis can be predicted from the relationship: $PaCO_2 = [1.5 \times (HCO_3^-)] + 8 \pm 2$, i.e., the $PaCO_2$ is expected to decrease 1.25 mm Hg for each mmol/L decrease in (HCO_3^-). Thus, a patient with metabolic acidosis and (HCO_3^-) of 12 mmol/L would be expected to have a $PaCO_2$ between 24 and 28 mm Hg. Values for $PaCO_2$ <24 mm Hg or >28 mm Hg define a mixed disturbance (metabolic acidosis and respiratory alkalosis or metabolic alkalosis and respiratory acidosis, respectively).

Mixed Acid-base Disorders

Mixed acid-base disorders—defined as independently coexisting disorders, not merely compensatory responses—are often seen in patients in critical care units and can lead to dangerous extremes of pH. A patient with diabetic ketoacidosis (metabolic acidosis) may develop an independent respiratory problem leading to respiratory acidosis or alkalosis. Patients with underlying pulmonary disease may not respond to metabolic acidosis with an appropriate ventilatory response because of insufficient respiratory reserve. Such imposition of respiratory acidosis on metabolic acidosis can lead to severe acidemia and a poor outcome. When metabolic acidosis and metabolic alkalosis coexist in the same patient, the pH may be normal or near normal. When the pH is normal, an elevated anion gap denotes the presence of a metabolic acidosis. A discrepancy in the AG (prevailing minus normal AG) and the HCO_3^- (normal minus prevailing HCO_3^-) indicates the presence of a mixed high-gap acidosis—metabolic alkalosis. A diabetic patient with ketoacidosis may have renal dysfunction resulting in simultaneous metabolic acidosis. Patients who have ingested an overdose of drug combinations, such as sedatives and salicylates may have mixed disturbances as a result of the acid-base response to the individual drugs (metabolic acidosis mixed with respiratory acidosis or respiratory alkalosis, respectively). Even more complex are triple acid-base disturbances. For example, patients with metabolic acidosis due to alcoholic ketoacidosis may develop metabolic alkalosis due to vomiting and superimposed respiratory alkalosis due to the hyperventilation of hepatic dysfunction or alcohol withdrawal.

CASE STUDIES

CASE STUDY 1

Theme: Diagnosis of Acid-base Imbalance

A 35-year-old type I insulin-dependent diabetic had the flu for the previous week. He presented with hypotension, dry mucous membranes, and poor skin turgor. The patient was tachypneic and his breath had a fruity odor. He had the following laboratory findings:

- Serum albumin = 6.0 g/dL
- Serum calcium = 9.0 mg/dL
- Serum phosphorus = 5 mg/dL
- Serum blood urea nitrogen (BUN) = 60 mg/dL
- Serum creatinine = 2 mg/dL
- Serum glucose = 800 mg/dL
- Serum sodium = 132 mEq/L
- Serum potassium = 6.0 mEq/L
- Serum chloride = 92 mEq/L
- Serum bicarbonate = 17 mEq/L.

Urinalysis: Dipstick urine for glucose and ketones is strongly positive; the dipstick protein is 1 + (SSA 1+).

Explain the biochemical basis of the results of all the laboratory investigations.

CASE DISCUSSION

1. **Dehydration:** The patient is volume depleted. His blood pressure is low owing to a mixed hypotonic loss of fluid in his urine (more water than salt) from osmotic diuresis induced by glucosuria. Poor skin turgor and dry mucous membranes also indicate the loss of salt and water from the interstitial space within the extracellular fluid compartment.
2. **Prerenal azotemia:** The serum albumin is elevated owing to hemoconcentration of albumin secondary to a reduction in plasma volume. The serum BUN and creatinine are disproportionately elevated and the BUN/creatinine ratio is 30/1 (normal, 10/1); urea is filtered and reabsorbed in the proximal tubule, the latter being dependent on the glomerular filtration rate (GFR). The lower the GFR, the greater is the amount of urea reabsorption. Creatinine is filtered by the kidney and neither reabsorbed nor secreted. Therefore, when hypovolemia is present and the GFR is reduced, the serum BUN increases as more urea is reabsorbed in the proximal tubules and the creatinine increases only slightly from the reduction in clearance of the analyte from plasma. This condition is called prerenal azotemia.
3. **Metabolic acidosis:** The patient has an increased anion gap metabolic acidosis secondary to an increase in keto acids. This situation is the result of poor glucose control when the patient was sick with the flu. A lack of insulin results in the release of glucagon and other counterregulatory hormones (cortisol, catecholamines). Glucagon increases glycogenolysis and gluconeogenesis, hence there is a resultant increase in blood glucose. It also stimulates hormone-sensitive lipase in the adipose tissue, causing the release of free fatty acids and glycerol (which is converted to glycerol-3-phosphate in the liver and is used as a substrate for gluconeogenesis). Fatty acids undergo (β-oxidation) in the mitochondria, leading to an increase in acetyl-CoA, which is converted in the liver to ketone bodies [acetone (fruity odor of breath)], acetoacetate, and (β-hydroxybutyric acid). ketoacids are responsible for the patient's increased AG metabolic acidosis. The AG in this patient is 23 mEq/L [132 – (92 + 17) = 23].
4. **Hyperkalemia:** Hyperkalemia is due to the metabolic acidosis and the buffering of excess hydrogen ions by cells in exchange for potassium in order to maintain electroneutrality. This transcellular shift of potassium underscores the importance of how pH alters serum potassium and obscures the patient's true total body potassium status. Once the patient is treated with insulin, the potassium will drop dramatically, often into hypokalemic range, as it enters muscle and adipose along with the glucose. Hypokalemia is common in this setting owing to the loss of potassium along with sodium and water in the urine secondary to osmotic diuresis.
5. **Hyponatremia:** The serum sodium is always lower in the presence of hyperglycemia, since glucose establishes an osmotic gradient favoring the movement of water out of the intracellular fluid (ICF) compartment into the ECF, where it dilutes the sodium. The correction for sodium for the dilutional effect of glucose is as follows: Corrected serum sodium = measured serum sodium + (serum glucose/100 × 1.6), which in this case is 145 mEq/L [132 + (800/100) × 1.6)]. The reason the patient's serum sodium is at the upper limit of the normal range for sodium when the dilutional effect of glucose is eliminated is that osmotic diuresis produces a hypotonic loss of fluid, which over time produces hypernatremia (the measured rather than the corrected serum sodium is utilized when calculating the AG in the presence of metabolic acidosis).
6. **Proteinuria:** The patient has proteinuria which may indicate the presence of diabetic glomerulosclerosis. Captopril, an angiotensin-converting enzyme inhibitor, is useful in this situation, since it blocks the vasoconstrictor effect of angiotensin II on the efferent arteriole, hence reducing the pressure on the glomerular capillaries. Diabetic nephropathy may be associated with the nephrotic syndrome owing to the increased permeability of the glomerular capillaries to protein from nonenzymatic glycosylation of their basement membranes.

CASE STUDY 2

Theme: Causes, Compensation, and Clinical Implications of Metabolic Acidosis (Lactic Acidosis)

A 60-year-old man was brought to hospital in a very serious condition. The patient complained of constant vomiting from the previous 2 days containing large amount of dark brown fluid plus several episodes of melena. Past history of alcoholism, cirrhosis, portal hypertension, and a previous episode of bleeding varices were there. Sclerotherapy for the varices had been performed several months earlier at another hospital.

Physical examination: The patient had jaundice and was in distress, sweaty, clammy, and tachypneic. Blood pressure (BP): 98/50 mm Hg, pulse: 120 beats/min. Heart sounds—systolic murmur. Peripheries were cold. Abdomen was soft and nontender. Signs of chronic liver disease were present (spider nevi, gynecomastia, and testicular atrophy).

Laboratory investigations: Na^+ 131 mmol/L, Cl^- 85 mmol/L, K^+ 4.2 mmol/L, "total CO_2" 5.1, glucose 52 mg/dL, urea 38.6 mg/dL, creatinine 1.24 mg/dL, lactate 20.3 mmol/L, Hb 6.2 g%, and WBC 18 × 10^3/mm^3.

Arterial blood gases:

- pH—7.10
- pCO_2—13.8 mm Hg
- pO_2—103 mm Hg
- HCO_3^-—4.1 mmol/L.

What is the probable diagnosis?

CASE DETAILS

The patient is severely ill with circulatory failure and gastrointestinal (GI) bleeding on a background of known cirrhosis with portal hypertension.

The very low pH indicates a severe acidosis. The combination of a low pCO_2 and low bicarbonate indicates either a metabolic acidosis or a compensatory respiratory alkalosis (or both). As this patient has a severe acidosis, so the most probable diagnosis is metabolic acidosis. The anion gap is 41 indicating the presence of a high anion gap disorder. The lactate level of 20.3 mmol/L is extremely high and this confirms the diagnosis of a severe lactic acidosis. Hemoglobin is very low consistent with the history of bleeding and hypovolemia. Urea and creatinine are elevated (renal failure) but at these levels, there would not be retention of anions sufficient to result in a renal acidosis. Hence, lactic acidosis can be suspected. The respiratory efforts may be due to the distress or as a consequence of a metabolic acidosis (i.e., compensatory).

Clinical Diagnosis

Cirrhosis and portal hypertension with bleeding varices and sepsis, resulting in shock, lactic acidosis, anemia, and renal failure.

Patients with chronic liver disease do not develop lactic acidosis unless additional factors are present, which depress hepatic lactate metabolism or increase peripheral lactate production. The typical situation is a patient with cirrhosis who develops sepsis or hypovolemic shock (especially due to gastrointestinal bleeding). The combination of cirrhosis and lactic acidosis predicts a very high mortality.

BASIC CONCEPT

Lactic acidosis

The underlying etiology of metabolic acidosis is classically categorized into those that cause an elevated anion gap (AG) and those that do not. Lactic acidosis, identified by a state of acidosis and an elevated plasma lactate concentration, is one type of high anion gap metabolic acidosis and may result from numerous conditions. Patients with critical illness can be considered to have normal lactate concentrations of <2 mmol/L. Hyperlactatemia is defined as a mild-to-moderate persistent increase in blood lactate concentration (2–5 mmol/L) without metabolic acidosis, whereas lactic acidosis is characterized by persistently increased blood lactate levels (usually >4–5 mmol/L) in association with metabolic acidosis.

Etiology and Pathogenesis

Lactate, a product of anaerobic glucose metabolism, is generated from pyruvate with lactate dehydrogenase as a catalyst. Pyruvate is in a state of equilibrium with lactate that, under certain conditions, can shift toward the overproduction of lactate. Lactic acidosis results from an increase in blood lactate levels when lactate production exceeds consumption and body buffer systems become overburdened. This occurs when tissue oxygenation is inadequate to meet metabolic requirements as a result of either hypoperfusion or hypoxia. Lactate is cleared from blood, primarily by the liver, with the kidneys (10–20%) and skeletal muscles to a lesser degree.

Types of Lactic Acidosis

1. **Type A**—secondary to poor tissue perfusion: The most frequent cause of lactic acidosis is poor tissue perfusion, which is induced by various shock states causing tissue hypoxia. In ischemic tissues of the skeletal muscle (and less significantly intestine, erythrocytes,

and brain), production of lactate is accelerated with a concomitant fall in lactate consumption by the liver, kidney, and myocardium. Examples are:
- Circulatory insufficiency (shock, cardiac failure)
- Severe anemia, mitochondrial enzyme defects, and
- Inhibitors (carbon monoxide, cyanide).

2. **Type B**—an increase in plasma L-lactate may be secondary to aerobic disorders:
   - Malignancies
   - Nucleoside analog reverse transcriptase inhibitors in HIV
   - Diabetes mellitus
   - Renal or hepatic failure
   - Thiamine deficiency
   - Severe infections (cholera, malaria), seizures
   - Drugs/toxins (biguanides, ethanol, methanol, propylene glycol, isoniazid, and fructose). Propylene glycol may be used as a vehicle for IV medications including lorazepam and toxicity has been reported in several settings
   - Unrecognized bowel ischemia
   - Infarction in a patient with severe atherosclerosis
   - Cardiac decompensation receiving vasopressors is a common cause of lactic acidosis
   - Pyroglutamic acidemia has been reported in critically ill patients receiving acetaminophen, which is associated with depletion of glutathione.

Lactic acid exists in two forms—the L-lactate and D-lactate:
1. L-lactate is the most commonly measured level, as it is the only form produced in human metabolism. Its excess represents increased anaerobic metabolism due to tissue hypoperfusion.
2. D-lactate is a byproduct of bacterial metabolism and may accumulate in patients with short gut syndrome or in those with a history of gastric bypass or small-bowel resection.

Incidence

The overall incidence of lactic acidosis in critically ill patients is unknown; however, increasing acid-base evaluations of critically ill patients indicate its persistence, which increases associated morbidity and mortality.

Mortality/Morbidity

Patients exhibiting a disorder of lactate metabolism are typically significantly ill and are at risk for developing multiple organ failure. The mortality rate of patients, with a serum lactate level greater than 2 mmol/L, persisting after 24 hours, with an associated acidemia approaches nearly 70%.

Clinical Manifestations

History

No single historical feature itself is indicative of the presence of lactic acidosis, as symptoms are dependent on the underlying etiology. Nevertheless, a careful history is vital to determine the underlying pathology. The onset of acidosis may be rapid (i.e., within minutes to hours) or progressive (i.e., over a period of several days).

Physical Findings

The physical examination also depends on the underlying cause of lactic acidosis. Signs of cardiovascular compromise frequently include cyanosis, cool extremities, tachycardia, hypotension, dry mucous membranes, dyspnea, confusion, lethargy, stupor, or coma. Hyperventilation is common as a compensatory mechanism causing respiratory alkalosis.

Laboratory Investigations

Biochemical markers of impaired tissue perfusion may be useful because they are indicative of end-organ failure, whereas hemodynamic patterns can vary in different patient groups.

- AG: Calculation from serum electrolytes [AG = sodium – (CO_2 + chloride)].
- Arterial blood gas (ABG) analysis: The base deficit, derived from blood gas analysis, gives an approximation of tissue acidosis; however, the presence of an acidemia is required for the diagnosis.
- Serum lactate level:
  - The normal serum lactate level is approximately 1 mmol/L with a range up to 2 mmol/L. Values above 4–5 mmol/L in the setting of acidemia are indicative of lactic acidosis.
  - In hypoperfused states, persistent lactate elevation is associated with excessive mortality. If circulatory failure develops, serial lactate values are helpful in following the course of the hypoperfusion state and the response to therapeutic interventions.
  - Other tests: Additional laboratory tests may be selected on the basis of the suspected underlying etiology of lactic acidosis.

Treatment

1. The underlying condition that disrupts lactate metabolism must first be corrected; tissue perfusion must be restored when inadequate.
2. Vasoconstrictors should be avoided, if possible, since they may worsen tissue perfusion.
3. **Alkali therapy:** It is generally advocated for acute, severe acidemia (pH <7.15) to improve cardiac function and lactate utilization. However, $NaHCO_3$ therapy may paradoxically depress cardiac performance and exacerbate acidosis by enhancing lactate production (HCO_3^- stimulates phosphofructokinase). A reasonable approach is to infuse sufficient $NaHCO_3$ to raise the arterial pH to no more than 7.2 over 30–40 minutes. When the underlying cause of the lactic acidosis can be remedied, blood lactate will be converted to HCO_3^- and may result in an **overshoot alkalosis.**

Prognosis

Lactate levels have been well-described to correlate with the presence of tissue hypoperfusion in shock. The duration and degree of increased serum lactic acid appear to predict morbidity and mortality. Elevated levels have been shown to be correlated with increased mortality.

CLINICAL NOTE

While the use of alkali in moderate lactic acidosis is controversial, it is generally agreed that attempts to return the pH or (HCO_3^-) to normal by administration of exogenous $NaHCO_3$ are deleterious. A reasonable approach is to infuse sufficient $NaHCO_3$ to raise the arterial pH to no more than 7.2 over 30–40 minutes.

CLINICAL PEARLS

1. Lactic acidosis is characterized by an excess of serum lactate due to lactate production that exceeds systemic consumption.
2. Numerous etiologies may be responsible for its presence, most commonly circulatory failure and hypoxia.
3. Elevated levels have been shown to be correlated with increased mortality.
4. Identification and discontinuation of any offending agents and treatment of known pathology should occur promptly.
5. Although treatment with buffering agents remains controversial, their use should be considered in certain instances with the assistance of critical care consultation.

CASE STUDY 3

Theme: Causes, Compensation, and Clinical Implications of Metabolic Alkalosis

A 28-year-old man was admitted to the hospital with a week long history of severe vomiting. He confessed to self-medication for his chronic heart burns and indigestion. He was clinically severely dehydrated and had shallow respiration.

Initial biochemical results were:

Arterial blood gases:

H^+	pCO_2	pO_2
28 nmol/L ↓	7.2 kPa	1.5 kPa

Serum electrolytes composition in mEq/L:

Na^+ K^+	Cl^-	HCO_3^-
146 2.8	83	41

Blood urea—41 mg/dL

Serum creatinine—1.8 mg/dL

Comment on acid-base status.

What could be the possible cause for all these biochemical findings?

CASE DETAILS

The low (H^+) concentration and high HCO_3^- concentration denote that the patient has metabolic alkalosis. This would have been caused by severe vomiting. The ingestion of alkali would not have lead to this degree of alkalosis, although it would have aggravated the situation. The severe vomiting has caused dehydration that has resulted in prerenal uremia. The hypokalemia is due to two reasons: Firstly due to loss in vomiting and secondly due to internalization of K^+ from extracellular fluid (ECF) to intracellular fluid (ICF) as a result of metabolic alkalosis. Shallow respiration is due to compensatory hypoventilation which has lead to the increase in pCO_2.

Metabolic alkalosis

Metabolic alkalosis is primary increase in HCO_3^- with or without compensatory increase in pCO_2; pH may be high or nearly normal. Common causes include prolonged vomiting, hypovolemia, diuretic use, and hypokalemia.

Renal impairment of HCO_3^- excretion must be present to sustain alkalosis.

Pathophysiology

The organ systems involved are mainly the kidneys and gastrointestinal (GI) tract. The pathogenesis of metabolic alkalosis involves two processes: The onset of metabolic alkalosis and the maintenance of metabolic alkalosis, events that usually overlap. Abnormalities that generate HCO_3^- within the body are called "initiation factors" of metabolic alkalosis, whereas abnormalities that promote renal conservation of HCO_3^- are called "maintenance factors". Metabolic alkalosis may remain even after the initiation factors have disappeared.

- **Onset of metabolic alkalosis:** Metabolic alkalosis may be generated by one of the following mechanisms:
  - **Loss of hydrogen ions:** Whenever a hydrogen ion is excreted, a bicarbonate ion is gained into the extracellular space. Hydrogen ions may be lost through the kidneys or the GI tract. Vomiting or nasogastric (NG) suction generates metabolic alkalosis by the loss of gastric secretions, which are rich in hydrochloric acid (HCl). Renal losses of hydrogen ions occur in the presence of excess aldosterone, which stimulates the electrogenic epithelial sodium channel (ENaC) in the collecting duct. As this channel reabsorbs sodium ions, the tubular lumen becomes more negative, leading to the secretion of hydrogen ions and potassium ions into the lumen.
  - **Shift of hydrogen ions into the intracellular space:** This mainly develops with hypokalemia. As the extracellular potassium concentration decreases, potassium ions move out of the cells. To maintain neutrality, hydrogen ions move into the intracellular space.
  - **Alkali administration:** Administration of sodium bicarbonate in amounts that exceed the capacity of the kidneys to excrete this excess bicarbonate may cause metabolic alkalosis. This capacity is reduced when a reduction in filtered bicarbonate occurs, as observed in renal failure, or when enhanced tubular reabsorption of bicarbonate occurs, as observed in volume depletion.
  - **Contraction alkalosis:** Loss of bicarbonate-poor, chloride-rich extracellular fluid, as observed with thiazide diuretic or loop diuretic therapy or chloride diarrhea, leads to contraction of extracellular fluid volume. Because the original bicarbonate mass is now dissolved in a smaller volume of fluid, an increase in bicarbonate concentration occurs. This increase in bicarbonate causes, at most, a 2–4 mEq/L rise in bicarbonate concentration.
- **Maintenance of metabolic alkalosis:** The following factors are believed to maintain the alkalosis:
  - **Decrease in renal perfusion:** Decreased perfusion to the kidneys, caused by either volume depletion or a reduction in effective circulating blood volume (e.g., edematous states, such as heart failure or cirrhosis), stimulates the renin-angiotensin-aldosterone system. This increases renal sodium ion reabsorption throughout the nephron. This results in enhanced hydrogen ion secretion. Whenever a hydrogen ion is secreted into the tubular lumen, a bicarbonate ion is gained into the systemic circulation via the basolateral Cl^-/HCO_3^- exchanger.
  - **Chloride depletion:** Chloride depletion may occur through the GI tract by loss of gastric secretions which are rich in chloride ions, or through the kidneys with loop diuretics or thiazides.
  - **Hypokalemia:** Many of the causes of metabolic alkalosis are also associated with hypokalemia which maintains metabolic alkalosis by different mechanisms. These include the following:
    - Shift of hydrogen ions intracellularly.
    - Stimulation of the apical H^+/K^+-ATPase in the collecting duct.
    - Stimulation *of renal ammonia genesis*: Ammonium ions (NH_4^+) are produced in the proximal tubule from the metabolism of glutamine. During this process, first glutamate and then alpha-ketoglutarate is produced, the metabolism of which generates bicarbonate that is returned to the systemic circulation.
    - Impaired *chloride ion reabsorption in the distal nephron*: This results in an increase in luminal electronegativity, with subsequent enhancement of hydrogen ion secretion.
    - Reduction in glomerular filtration rate (GFR): In the presence of volume depletion, this impairs renal excretion of the excess bicarbonate.

Frequency

Metabolic alkalosis is the most common acid-base disturbance observed in hospitalized patients, accounting for approximately 50% of all acid-base disorders.

Causes

The most common causes of metabolic alkalosis are the use of diuretics and the external loss of gastric secretions. Causes of metabolic alkalosis can be divided into chloride-responsive alkalosis (urine chloride <20 mEq/L), chloride-resistant alkalosis (urine chloride >20 mEq/L), and other causes including alkali-loading alkalosis.

- **Chloride-responsive alkalosis** (urine chloride <20 mEq/L):
  - Loss of gastric secretions—vomiting, NG suction

- Loss of colonic secretions
- Thiazides and loop diuretics (after discontinuation)
- Posthypercapnia
- Cystic fibrosis (due to loss of chloride in the sweat)
- Ingestion of large doses of nonabsorbable antacids.

During respiratory acidosis, the kidneys reabsorb bicarbonate and secrete chloride to compensate for the acidosis; urine chloride becomes high and can lead to chloride depletion. In the posthypercapnia state, the kidneys cannot excrete the excess bicarbonate because of the low luminal chloride.

- **Chloride-resistant alkalosis** (urine chloride >20 mEq/L):
  - With hypertension:
    - Primary hyperaldosteronism
    - 11-beta-hydroxysteroid dehydrogenase type 2 deficiency
    - Current use of diuretics in hypertension
    - Cushing syndrome
    - Exogenous mineralocorticoids or glucocorticoids
    - Liddle syndrome (unregulated reabsorption of Na^+)
    - Renovascular hypertension
    - Renin- or deoxycorticosterone-secreting tumors
  - Without hypertension:
    - Bartter syndrome (salt depletion and stimulation of the renin-angiotensin-aldosterone system)
    - Gitelman syndrome (salt depletion and stimulation of the renin-angiotensin-aldosterone system)
    - Severe potassium depletion
    - Current use of thiazides and loop diuretics
    - Hypomagnesemia (through hypokalemia)
- Other causes (alkali-loading alkalosis):
  - Exogenous alkali administration: Sodium bicarbonate therapy in the presence of renal failure
  - Milk-alkali syndrome (hypercalcemia increases renal bicarbonate reabsorption)
  - Hypercalcemia (enhanced bicarbonate reabsorption in the proximal tubule)
    - Intravenous penicillin (through hypokalemia)
  - Refeeding alkalosis (enhanced metabolism of ketoacids to bicarbonate)
  - Massive blood transfusion (citrate in the transfused blood is converted to bicarbonate)
  - End-stage renal disease (hemodialysis using high bicarbonate dialysate)
  - Recovery from lactic or ketoacidosis (when the patient recovers, the beta-hydroxybutyrate and lactate are metabolized to bicarbonate and the original bicarbonate deficit is recovered. The administered bicarbonate now becomes a surplus).
  - Hypoproteinemic alkalosis: Metabolic alkalosis has been reported in patients with hypoproteinemia. The mechanism of alkalosis is not clear, but it may be related to loss of negative charges of albumin. A decrease in plasma albumin of 1 g/dL is associated with an increase in plasma bicarbonate of 3.4 mEq/L.

Compensation

Respiratory mechanism: Excess of bicarbonate causes an increase in the ratio of bicarbonate to carbonic acid, pH is also increased. The respiratory center is inhibited by alkalosis causing shallow, irregular breathing. This reduced ventilation results in CO_2 retention and increase in H_2CO_3 level. The ratio is restored back to normal as the levels of both in blood are increased. However, decreased ventilation raises pCO_2, which tends to stimulate the respiratory center.

Renal mechanism: The following changes are brought about:

- Decreased excretion of H^+ ions
- Increased excretion of K^+ ions in the distal tubules
- Increased bicarbonate excretion
- Decreased ammonia formation

Biochemical characteristics:

a. Uncompensated phase:
  - Disproportionate increase in (HCO_3^-)↑
  - Increase in (H_2CO_3)↑, pCO_2↑
  - Increase in total CO_2 content
  - Increase in pH↑.

b. Fully compensated phase:
  - CO2 content is high
  - Increase in (HCO_3^-)↑ and (H_2CO_3)↑ is proportionate
  - Ratio and pH remain normal.

Symptoms and Signs

Symptoms and signs of mild alkalemia are usually related to the underlying disorder. More severe alkalemia increases protein binding of ionized Ca^{++}, leading to hypocalcemia and subsequent headache, lethargy, and neuromuscular excitability, sometimes with delirium, tetany, and seizures. Concomitant hypokalemia may cause weakness. Physical examination is helpful to establish the cause of metabolic alkalosis. Important aspects of the physical examination include the evaluation of hypertension and volume status assessment.

Complications

- Severe alkalosis causes diffuse arteriolar constriction with reduction in tissue perfusion. By decreasing cerebral blood flow, alkalosis may lead to tetany, seizures, and decreased mental status.
- Metabolic alkalosis also decreases coronary blood flow and predisposes persons to refractory arrhythmias.
- Metabolic alkalosis causes hypoventilation which may cause hypoxemia, especially in patients with poor respiratory reserve and it may impair weaning from mechanical ventilation.
- Alkalosis decreases the serum concentration of ionized calcium by increasing calcium ion binding to albumin. In addition, metabolic alkalosis is almost always associated with hypokalemia, which can cause neuromuscular weakness and arrhythmias and by increasing ammonia production; it can precipitate hepatic encephalopathy in susceptible individuals.

Mortality/Morbidity

Severe metabolic alkalosis (i.e., blood pH >7.55) is a serious medical problem. Mortality rates have been reported as 45% in patients with an arterial blood pH of 7.55 and 80% when the pH was greater than 7.65.

Laboratory Investigations

Diagnosis is made by obtaining serum electrolytes and an arterial blood gas analysis. The arterial blood pH and bicarbonate are elevated. The arterial pCO_2 is increased due to compensatory hypoventilation. Serum potassium and chloride are decreased. There may be an increased anion gap.

- **Urinary chlorides:** If the etiology of metabolic alkalosis is not clear from the clinical history and physical examination, including drug use and the presence of hypertension, then a urine chloride ion concentration can be obtained.
- **Urinary K^+:** Urinary K^+ <30 mEq/day signifies hypokalemia. Urinary K^+ >30 mEq/day without hypertension suggests diuretic abuse or Bartter- or Gitelman syndrome. Urinary K^+ >30 mEq/day with hypertension requires evaluation for hyperaldosteronism, mineralocorticoid excess, and renovascular disease.
- **Measurement of urine sodium ion concentration:** It is used in many conditions to determine volume status, especially in patients with oliguria.
- **Plasma renin activity and aldosterone level:** Plasma renin activity and aldosterone level may help to find the etiology of metabolic alkalosis.
- **Primary hyperaldosteronism:** Measure aldosterone levels in a 24-hour urine collection after salt loading to diagnose primary hyperaldosteronism.
- **Cushing syndrome:** Evaluate plasma cortisol at midnight during sleep, 24-hour urine-free cortisol, or dexamethasone suppression test in Cushing syndrome.

Imaging Studies

- Perform adrenal imaging studies (e.g., CT scan, MRI) to find the etiology of primary hyperaldosteronism and Cushing syndrome.
- Renal Doppler ultrasound, MRI, and renal angiography are helpful in diagnosing renovascular hypertension (i.e., significant renal artery stenosis).

Other Tests

- **Gene analysis:** It is helpful to diagnose inherited causes of hypokalemic alkalosis. Examples are Liddle syndrome, glucocorticoid-remediable hypertension, Bartter syndrome, and Gitelman syndrome.

Treatment

Mild alkalosis is generally well-tolerated. Severe or symptomatic alkalosis (pH >7.60) requires urgent treatment.

a. **Chloride-responsive metabolic alkalosis:** Therapy for chloride-responsive metabolic alkalosis is aimed at correction of extracellular volume deficit. Depending on the degree of hypovolemia, adequate amounts of 0.9% NaCl and KCl should be administered. Discontinuation of diuretics and administration of H2-blockers in patients whose alkalosis is due to nasogastric suction can be useful. If impaired pulmonary or cardiovascular status prohibits adequate volume repletion, acetazolamide can be used. One must be alert to the possible development of hypokalemia, since potassium depletion can be induced by forced natriuresis via bicarbonaturia. Administration of acid can be used as emergency therapy. Patients with marked renal failure may require dialysis.

b. **Chloride-resistant metabolic alkalosis:** Therapy for chloride-resistant metabolic alkalosis includes surgical removal of a mineralocorticoid-producing tumor and blockage of aldosterone effect with an ACE inhibitor or with spironolactone. Metabolic alkalosis in primary aldosteronism can be treated only with potassium repletion. If renal artery stenosis or Cushing syndrome is present, correction of the underlying cause will reverse the alkalosis.

Prognosis

Mortality rates have been reported as 45% in patients with an arterial blood pH of 7.55 and 80% when the pH was greater than 7.65.

CLINICAL NOTE

Alkalosis decreases the serum concentration of ionized calcium by increasing calcium ion binding to albumin. In addition, metabolic alkalosis is almost always associated with hypokalemia, which can cause neuromuscular weakness and arrhythmias.

CLINICAL PEARLS

1. Metabolic alkalosis is primary increase in HCO_3^- with or without compensatory increase in pCO_2; pH may be high or nearly normal.
2. Causes of metabolic alkalosis can be divided into chloride-responsive alkalosis (urine chloride <20 mEq/L), chloride-resistant alkalosis (urine chloride >20 mEq/L), and other causes including alkali-loading alkalosis.
3. Hypocalcemia, hypoventilation, and hypokalemia are diagnostic of metabolic alkalosis. The arterial blood pH and bicarbonate are elevated. The arterial pCO_2 is increased. There may be an increased anion gap.
4. Mild alkalosis is generally well-tolerated. Severe or symptomatic alkalosis (pH >7.60) requires urgent treatment.
5. Severe metabolic alkalosis (i.e. blood pH >7.55) is a serious medical problem. Mortality rates have been reported as 45% in patients with an arterial blood pH of 7.55 and 80% when the pH was greater than 7.65.

CASE STUDY 4

Theme: Anion Gap and Causes, Compensation, and Clinical Implications of Metabolic Acidosis

A 5-year-old girl displayed increased appetite, increased urinary frequency, and thirst. Her physician suspected new-onset diabetes mellitus.

The diagnosis was confirmed from the laboratory investigations:

Fasting blood sugar—246 mg/dL
pH—7.33
Serum bicarbonate—12.0 mmol/L
Arterial pCO_2—21 mm Hg
Urine—glucose ++++
Ketones— + (Present)

What is the acid-base status of the patient?

CASE DETAILS

The child is in a state of compensated metabolic acidosis. The cause of acidosis is diabetic ketoacidosis, as is evident from the hyperglycemia, low pH, and positive urine for glucose and ketone bodies. Low pCO_2 is a result of respiratory compensation.

Metabolic Acidosis

Metabolic acidosis is a primary decrease in serum HCO_3^- concentration and in its pure form, manifests as acidemia (pH <7.40). Rarely, metabolic acidosis can be part of a mixed or complex acid-base disturbance in which 2 or more separate metabolic or respiratory derangements occur together. In these instances, pH may not be reduced or the HCO_3^- concentration may not be low.

Etiology and Pathophysiology

Metabolic acidosis is acid accumulation from increased acid production or acid ingestion, decreased acid excretion, or GI or renal HCO_3^- loss. Acidemia (arterial pH <7.35) results when acid load overwhelms respiratory compensation. Causes are classified by their effect on the anion gap.

Anion Gap in Metabolic Acidosis

Plasma, like any other body fluid compartment, is neutral; total anions match total cations. The major plasma cation is Na^+, and major plasma anions are Cl^- and HCO_3^-. Extracellular anions present in lower concentrations include phosphate, sulfate, and some organic anions, while other cations present include K^+, Mg^{2+}, and Ca^{2+}. The AG is the difference between the concentration of the major measured cation Na^+ and the major measured anions Cl^- and HCO_3^-. Normal values for those ions are 140, 108, and 24 mEq/L, respectively and the gap is usually between 6 mEq/L and 12 mEq/L. The AG represents the difference between unmeasured anions and unmeasured cations as shown in the following:

$$AG = (Na^+) - [(Cl^-) + (HCO_3^-)] = \text{Unmeasured anions} - \text{Unmeasured cations}$$

This equation indicates that an increase in the AG can result from either a decrease in unmeasured cations (e.g., hypokalemia, hypocalcemia, and hypomagnesemia) or an increase in unmeasured anions (e.g., hyperphosphatemia, high albumin levels).

$$HA + NaHCO_3 \rightarrow NaA + H_2CO_3 \rightarrow CO_2 + H_2O$$

This reaction indicates that the addition of an acid (HA, where H^+ is combined with an unmeasured anion A^-) results in the consumption of HCO_3^- with an addition of anions that will account for the increase in the AG.

Metabolic acidosis is classified on the basis of AG into normal (also called non-AG or hyperchloremic metabolic acidosis) and high-AG metabolic acidosis.

Causes of Metabolic Acidosis

A. High anion gap acidosis: The most common causes of a high anion gap metabolic acidosis are:

- **Ketoacidosis:** It is a common complication of type 1 diabetes mellitus, but it also occurs with chronic alcoholism, undernutrition, and to a lesser degree, fasting. In these conditions, the body converts glucose to free fatty acid (FFA) metabolism; FFAs are converted by the liver into ketoacids, acetoacetic acid, and β-hydroxybutyrate (all unmeasured anions). Ketoacidosis is also a rare manifestation of congenital isovaleric acid and methylmalonic acidemia.
- **Lactic acidosis:** It is the most common cause of metabolic acidosis in hospitalized patients. Lactate accumulation results from a combination of excess formation and decreased utilization of lactate. Excess lactate production occurs during states of anaerobic metabolism. The most serious form occurs during the various types of shock. Decreased utilization generally occurs with hepatocellular dysfunction from decreased liver perfusion or as a part of generalized shock.
- **Renal failure:** It causes anion gap acidosis by decreased acid excretion and decreased HCO_3^- reabsorption. Accumulation of sulfates, phosphates, urate, and hippurate accounts for the high anion gap.
- **Toxins or Toxic ingestions:** It may have acidic metabolites or trigger lactic acidosis. Rhabdomyolysis is a rare cause of metabolic acidosis and thought to be due to release of protons and anions directly from muscle **(Table 19.1)**.

B. Normal anion gap acidosis: The most common causes of normal anion gap acidosis are:

- GI or renal HCO_3^- loss
- Impaired renal acid excretion
- Ingestion and parenteral infusion of drugs.

Normal anion gap metabolic acidosis is also called **hyperchloremic acidosis,** because instead of reabsorbing HCO_3^- with Na^+, the kidney reabsorbs Cl^-.

Many GI secretions are rich in HCO_3^- (e.g., biliary, pancreatic, and intestinal fluids); loss from diarrhea, tube drainage, or fistulas can cause acidosis. In ureterosigmoidostomy (insertion

TABLE 19.1: Causes of metabolic acidosis (summary).

Examples	
A. High anion gap	
1. Ketoacidosis	• Diabetes • Chronic alcoholism • Undernutrition • Fasting.
2. Lactic acidosis (from physiologic processes)	• Shock • Primary hypoxia due to lung disorders • Seizures
3. Lactic acidosis (from exogenous toxins)	• Carbon monoxide • Cyanide • Iron • Isoniazid.
4. Renal failure	• —
5. Toxins metabolized to acids	• Alcohol • Methanol (formate) • Ethylene glycol (oxalate) • Paraldehyde (acetate, chloroacetate) • Salicylates.
6. Rhabdomyolysis (rare)	• —
B. Normal anion gap (hyperchloremic acidosis)	
1. GI HCO_3^- loss	• Colostomy • Diarrhea • Enteric fistulas • Ileostomy.
2. Urologic procedures	• Ureterosigmoidostomy
3. Renal HCO_3^- loss	• Tubulointerstitial renal disease • Renal tubular acidosis • Hyperparathyroidism.
4. Ingestions	• Acetazolamide • $CaCl_2$ • Magnesium sulfate ($MgSO_4$)
5. Parenteral infusion	• Ammonium chloride (NH_4Cl) • Rapid NaCl infusion
6. Other	• Hypoaldosteronism • Hyperkalemia

of ureters into the sigmoid colon after obstruction or cystectomy), the colon secretes and loses HCO_3^- in exchange for urinary Cl^- and absorbs urinary ammonium, which dissociates into ammonia (NH_3^+) and hydrogen ion (H^+).
The renal tubular acidosis either impairs H^+ secretion or HCO_3^- absorption.

Impaired acid excretion and a normal anion gap also occur in early renal failure, tubulointerstitial renal disease, and when carbonic anhydrase inhibitors (e.g., acetazolamide) are given **(Table 19.1)**.

Compensation

If primary deficit of bicarbonate occurs, the ratio of bicarbonate: carbonic acid is decreased (normal 20:1). There are two compensatory mechanisms to restore the ratio back to normal:

a. **Primary compensatory mechanism:** As a compensatory mechanism, metabolic acidosis leads to alveolar hyperventilation due to stimulation of respiratory center causing deep and rapid (Kussmaul) breathing. This increased ventilation results in CO_2 loss and a fall in $PaCO_2$. The ratio of bicarbonate: carbonic acid is restored back to normal with the reduction in carbonic acid content.
   However, increased ventilation will result in reduction in $PaCO_2$, which in turn depresses the respiratory center. Normally, $PaCO_2$ falls by 1–1.3 mm Hg for every 1 mEq/L fall in serum HCO_3^- concentration, a compensatory response that can occur fairly quickly. If the change in $PaCO_2$ is not within this range, then a mixed acid-base disturbance is present. For example, if the decrease in $PaCO_2$ is <the expected change, then a primary respiratory acidosis also is present.
   During the early stage of alkali deficit, the person is in a stage of compensated acidosis, but as the condition progresses and if the primary cause is not treated, the alkali deficit becomes more pronounced, the primary compensatory mechanism fails, and the condition becomes one of the uncompensated acidosis with the increase in H^+ ion concentration in blood.
b. **Secondary compensated mechanism (renal mechanism):** Renal mechanisms attempt to correct the disturbance as follows:
   - By conserving cations.
   - By increasing:
     - NH_3 formation
     - H^+ excretion compared to K^+ excretion in distal tubules
     - Bicarbonate reabsorption.

Mortality/Morbidity

The causes of metabolic acidosis are varied and the morbidity and mortality of this disorder are primarily related to the underlying condition.

Clinical Manifestations

Symptoms and signs are primarily those of the cause. Mild acidemia is itself asymptomatic. More severe acidemia (pH < 7.10) may cause nausea, vomiting, and malaise. Symptoms may appear at higher pH if acidosis develops rapidly. The most characteristic sign is hyperpnea (long, deep breaths at a normal rate), reflecting a compensatory increase in alveolar ventilation.

Severe, acute acidemia predisposes to cardiac dysfunction with hypotension and shock, ventricular arrhythmias, and coma. Chronic acidemia causes bone demineralization disorders (rickets, osteomalacia, and osteopenia).

Laboratory Diagnosis

The investigations are carried out either to confirm the diagnosis or to determine the cause of acidosis. The investigations of importance are:

1. **Blood gas analysis:** pH may be markedly low or slightly subnormal with compensatory reduction in pCO_2.
2. **Serum electrolytes:** Metabolic acidosis is indicated by a decreased serum HCO_3^- concentration observed when serum electrolytes are measured; however, a decreased serum (HCO_3^-) level can be observed as a compensatory response to respiratory alkalosis also. A (HCO_3^-) level <15 mEq/L, however, almost always is due, at least in part, to metabolic acidosis. The only definitive way to diagnose metabolic acidosis is by simultaneous measurement of serum electrolytes and ABGs, which shows both pH and $PaCO_2$ to be low; calculated HCO_3^- also is low.
3. **High anion gap:** The cause of an elevated anion gap may be clinically obvious (e.g., hypovolemic shock), but if not, blood testing should include glucose, BUN, creatinine, lactate, and tests for possible toxins.
4. **Normal anion gap:** If the anion gap is normal and no cause is obvious (e.g., marked diarrhea), urinary electrolytes are measured and the urinary anion gap is calculated as (Na^+) + (K^+) – (Cl^-). A normal urinary anion gap (including in patients with GI losses) is 30–50 mEq/L; an elevation suggests renal HCO_3^- loss (for evaluation of renal tubular acidosis).
5. **Osmolar gap:** The osmolar gap can also help to determine the nature of the anion in high-AG acidosis because some osmotically active toxins also cause a high-AG acidosis. Methanol, ethylene glycol, and acetone are classic poisons that increase the osmolar gap and AG; measuring the osmolar gap can help narrow the differential diagnosis of high-AG acidosis.

$$\text{Osmolar gap} = \text{Measured plasma osmolality} - \text{Calculated plasma osmolality}$$

Plasma osmolality P_{osm} can be calculated using the following equation:

$$P_{osm} = (2 \times Na^{+}) + (\text{glucose in mg/dL})/18 + (\text{BUN in mg/dL})/2.8$$

Plasma osmolality (P_{osm}) can also be measured in the laboratory and because other solutes normally contribute minimally to serum osmolality, the difference between the measured and the calculated value (osmolar gap) is no more than 10–15 mOsm/kg.

Treatment

- Primary cause treated
- $NaHCO_3$ rarely indicated.

Treatment of acidemia with $NaHCO_3$ is clearly indicated only in certain circumstances and is probably deleterious in others. When metabolic acidosis results from loss of HCO_3^- or accumulation of inorganic acids (i.e., normal anion gap acidosis), HCO_3^- therapy is generally safe and appropriate. However, when acidosis results from organic acid accumulation (i.e., high anion gap acidosis), HCO_3^- therapy is controversial; it does not clearly improve mortality in these conditions and there are several possible risks. With treatment of the underlying condition, lactate and ketoacids are metabolized back to HCO_3^-; exogenous HCO_3^- loading may, therefore, cause an "overshoot" metabolic alkalosis. In any condition, HCO_3^- may also cause Na^+ and volume overload, hypokalemia, and by inhibiting respiratory drive, hypercapnia. Furthermore, because HCO_3^- does not diffuse across cell membranes, intracellular acidosis is not corrected and may paradoxically worsen because some of the added HCO_3^- is converted to CO_2, which does cross into the cell and is hydrolyzed to H^+ and HCO_3^-.

Despite these and other controversies, most experts still recommend HCO_3^- IV for severe metabolic acidosis (pH <7.00), with a target pH of 7.20.

- K^+ depletion, common in the treatment of metabolic acidosis, should be identified through frequent serum K^+ monitoring and treated as needed with oral or parenteral KCl.
- **Hemodialysis:** It is required for renal failure and sometimes for ethylene glycol, methanol, and salicylate poisoning.

CLINICAL NOTE

In high-AG acidosis secondary to accumulation of organic acids, lactate, and ketones, these anions are eventually metabolized to HCO_3^-. When the underlying disorder is treated, the serum pH corrects; thus, caution should be exercised in these patients when providing alkali to raise the pH much higher than 7.20 because an overshoot alkalosis may occur.

CLINICAL PEARLS

1. Metabolic acidosis is primary reduction in HCO_3^-, typically with compensatory reduction in pCO2; pH may be markedly low or slightly subnormal.
2. Metabolic acidosis is categorized as high or normal anion gap based on the presence or absence of unmeasured anions in serum.
3. Causes include accumulation of ketones and lactic acid, renal failure, and drug or toxin ingestion (high anion gap) and GI or renal HCO_3^- loss (normal anion gap).
4. Symptoms and signs in severe cases include nausea and vomiting, lethargy, and hyperpnea.
5. Diagnosis is clinical and with ABG and serum electrolyte measurement. The cause is treated; IV $NaHCO_3$ may be indicated when pH is very low.

CASE STUDY 5

Theme: High Anion Gap Metabolic Acidosis

A 19-year-old boy was brought to the emergency department with loss of consciousness. Apparently, the patient was a homeless found on the street.

Vital signs at the first visit were—blood pressure 90/60 mm Hg, respiratory rate 12 breaths/min, pulse rate 71 beats/min, and axillary temperature was 36.8°C.

On physical examination: The pupils were bilaterally dilated, fixed, and nonreactive. The lungs were symmetrically clear and S1 and S2 were heard without murmur or gallop. Bowel sounds were present and abdomen was soft without distention.

On fundoscopy: He had bilateral papilledema with disk hyperemia.

BLOOD BIOCHEMISTRY

Arterial blood gases:
- pH 7.33, pCO_2 28 mm Hg, pO_2 117 mm Hg, and HCO_3^- 14 mmol/L.

Rest of the laboratory data:
- BUN—43 mg/dL
- Creatinine—0.9 mg/dL
- Na—132 mmol/L
- K—3.7 mmol/L
- Chloride—103 mmol/L
- Calcium—9.3 mg/dL
- Blood sugar—156 mg/dL

Computed tomography (CT) scanning of the brain without contrast revealed generalized brain edema with bilateral infarction in basal ganglia and hemorrhagic transformation in the left lentiform nucleus. The blood level of methanol was 0.4 mg/dL.
What is your diagnosis?

CASE DETAILS

The patient is suffering from metabolic acidosis as is evident from the low pH and low bicarbonate levels. Low pCO_2 and high pO_2 signifies that the patient is in a state of respiratory compensation. The anion gap is 15. So, it is high anion gap acidosis. Blood urea nitrogen (BUN) and creatinine are near normal. High blood methanol levels, bilateral papilledema with disk hyperemia, and CT scan findings clearly indicate that the cause of metabolic acidosis is methanol poisoning.

Methanol Poisoning

Methanol (methyl alcohol) is an uncommon but life-threatening poison. Despite knowledge of its toxicity, methanol is rarely substituted for ethyl alcohol by unscrupulous winemakers. Toxicity usually occurs from intentional overdose or accidental ingestion and results in metabolic acidosis, neurologic sequelae, and even death. Methanol toxicity remains a common problem in many parts of the developing world, especially among members of lower socioeconomic classes.

Pathophysiology

Methanol has a relatively low toxicity. Upon ingestion, methanol is quickly absorbed in the gastrointestinal tract and metabolized in the liver. In the first step of degradation, methanol is transformed to formaldehyde via the enzyme alcohol dehydrogenase (ADH) **(Fig. 19.6)**. This reaction is slower than the next step, the transformation of formaldehyde to formic acid via the enzyme aldehyde dehydrogenase. This may explain the reason for the latency of symptoms between ingestion and effect. The half-life of formaldehyde is estimated to be 1–2 minutes.

Formic acid is further oxidized to carbon dioxide and water in the presence of tetrahydrofolate. The metabolism of formic acid is very slow; thus, it often accumulates in the body, which results in metabolic acidosis.

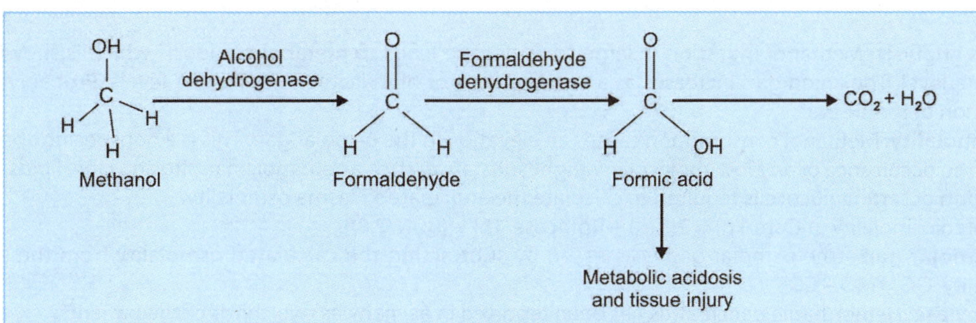

Fig. 19.6: Metabolism of methanol.

The eye damage caused by methanol has been well-described; however, the mechanism behind this phenomenon is not well-understood. The major damage occurs to the optic nerve. Little to no change is seen in the retina.

Methanol also affects the basal ganglia. With severe intoxication, common problems are hemorrhagic and nonhemorrhagic damage of the putamen.

Methanol blood levels peak at 30–90 minutes following ingestion and are often not correlated with time to symptom appearance. The minimal lethal dose in adults is believed to be 1 mg/kg of body weight.

Mortality/Morbidity

- Prognosis is correlated with the degree of metabolic acidosis (and the quantity of methanol ingested); more severe acidosis confers a poorer prognosis.
- Direct correlation exists between the formic acid concentration and the morbidity and mortality.

Clinical Manifestations

The clinical manifestations of methanol poisoning vary significantly from patient to patient. Initial symptoms result from toxicity of methanol itself and late signs are due to its metabolic product, formic acid. Initial symptoms generally appear 12–24 hours after ingestion.

- **Neurological manifestations:**
  - Initial symptoms from methanol poisoning are akin to those of ethanol intoxication, often with disinhibited behavior and ataxia.
  - After a latent period, headache, nausea, vomiting, or epigastric pain may appear.
  - In later stages, drowsiness may rapidly proceed to a depressed level of consciousness (obtundation) and coma.
  - Seizures may appear, usually as a result of metabolic complications or brain damage.
- **Vision loss:**
  - Blindness
  - Formic acid accumulates within the optic nerve, causing typical visual symptoms of blurring and flashes of light.
  - Formic acid-induced impairment of mitochondrial function in the optic nerve is believed to be the cause of vision loss. Hyperemia, edema, optic nerve atrophy, and optic nerve demyelination result from the damage caused by formic acid.
  - Immediate therapeutic intervention can help revert the symptoms; however, complete loss of vision is the usual outcome.
- **Metabolic acidosis:** Metabolic acidosis is manifested as tachycardia, tachypnea, hypertension, and altered mental status.
- **Respiratory complications**: Pulmonary edema and acute respiratory distress may occur necessitating intubation.
- **Cardiovascular complications**: Depressed cardiac contractility, circulatory collapse, heart failure, and cardiac arrhythmias may occur after consumption of a substantial amount of methanol.

Causes of Methanol poisoning

- Accidental overconsumption can be observed in children. Methanol is commonly found in perfumes, paint solvents, antifreeze, photocopying fluid, and windshield washing fluid, all of which are readily available.
- Chronic alcoholics commonly consume methanol as an alternative to ethanol. Excessive consumption can then lead to toxicity.
- In several areas of the developing world, methanol is usually a part of "bootlegged alcohol", which is manufactured in rural areas. People of lower socioeconomic classes often consume it due to its lower cost.
- Inhalation of methanol fumes is a risk in the industrial setting. It is used in the shellac processing and production of formaldehyde. Additionally, it is used as an extractant in chemical processes and as a denaturant in ethanol.
- Suicidal attempts using methanol are not frequent.

Laboratory Studies

- **Blood gas analysis**: Methanol ingestion in large toxic dosage leads to metabolic acidosis which is shown by a low serum bicarbonate level. The anion gap increases as a consequence of high lactate and ketone levels. Probably this is due to the accumulation of formic acid.
- **Serum osmolality**: Methanol consumption causes an elevation in the osmolar gap. This is a nonspecific observation as it may represent the occurrence of any low-molecular-weight substance, such as ethanol, mannitol, glycine, lipids, or proteins.
  - Estimation of serum glucose is required to calculate the anticipated plasma osmolality.
  - Calculated osmolality (mOsm/kg) = $2(Na^+) + [(glucose/18) + (BUN/2.8)]$.
  - **The osmolar gap**—the osmolar gap is assessed by subtracting the calculated osmolality from the measured plasma osmolality. OG = MO – CO
- **Serum amylase**: Hemorrhagic pancreatitis has been reported in as many as two-thirds of the patients.
- **Serum methanol level:** The confirmation of the diagnosis of methanol toxicity requires a discrete increase in the serum methanol level estimated by gas chromatography. The highest concentrations are attained 60–90 minutes after ingestion, but they do not correlate with the level of toxicity and thus are good predictors of prognosis.

Imaging Studies

- **CT scanning:**
  - CT scanning may show the typical changes of bilateral putaminal necrosis with hemorrhage of variable degrees. Additionally, cerebral white matter is also involved. However, the lesions are not well-localized when compared with MRI findings.
  - Furthermore, often the earlier CT scan is normal and lesions become evident after several days of intoxication.

- **Magnetic resonance imaging:**
  - Typical findings are bilateral putaminal necrosis with or without hemorrhage, probably resulting from the direct toxic effects of metabolites of methanol. This observation is certainly not characteristic of methanol toxicity as it can be observed with certain other diseases,, such as Wilson disease, Leigh disease, and stroke.

Treatment

Objectives

The three primary goals of therapy include treatment of metabolic acidosis, inhibition of the methanol metabolism, and enhanced elimination of the unmetabolized compound and existing toxic metabolites.

Gastric decontamination is unlikely to be beneficial because methanol is rapidly and completely absorbed from the gut. Ipecac-induced emesis is contraindicated due to the risk of rapid loss of consciousness. It is doubtful that activated charcoal has the ability to absorb significant amounts of methanol; however, it may be useful if a coingestant is suspected. Gastric lavage would need to be performed soon after ingestion to be beneficial. Stabilization of the critical patient must be performed before other therapies can be instituted. Correcting acid-base status should be a priority because serious metabolic acidosis is common and a pH <7 is associated with poor prognosis. Sodium bicarbonate should be administered to correct serum pH. Fluid and electrolyte replacement, airway management, and the treatment of serious cardiovascular and neurological signs,, such as hypotension and seizures should also be a primary concern.

The elimination of methanol may be enhanced by administering folic acid, a cofactor in the conversion of formic acid to carbon dioxide and by performing hemodialysis.

Prognosis

Outcomes are excellent when asymptomatic methanol-poisoned patients are treated promptly.

CLINICAL NOTE

Vision loss in methanol poisoning is thought to be caused by interruption of mitochondrial function in the optic nerve, resulting in hyperemia, edema, and optic nerve atrophy.

CLINICAL PEARLS

1. Methanol is relatively nontoxic; however, it is metabolized to highly toxic compound formic acid that is responsible for the acidosis and blindness characteristic of methanol poisoning.
2. Formic acid also inhibits cellular respiration leading to lactic acidosis.
3. Severe metabolic acidosis in conjunction with visual effects is the hallmark of methanol poisoning.
4. Signs and symptoms may be shallow respiration, cyanosis, tachypnea, coma, seizures, electrolyte disturbances, and various hemodynamic changes including profound hypotension and cardiac arrest. There may be mild-to-profound loss of memory, confusion, and agitation, which may progress to stupor and coma as the severity of the acidosis increases. In severe cases, death is possible.
5. The three primary goals of therapy include treatment of metabolic acidosis, inhibition of the methanol metabolism, and enhanced elimination of the unmetabolized compound and existing toxic metabolites.

CASE STUDY 6

Theme: Causes, Compensation, and Clinical Implications of Respiratory Acidosis

A 56-year-old man who smoked heavily for many years, developed worsening cough with purulent sputum and was admitted to the hospital because of difficulty in breathing. He was drowsy and cyanosed.

His arterial blood gas analysis was as follows:

pH—7.2

pCO_2—70 mm Hg

HCO_3^-—26 mmol/L

pO_2—50 mm Hg

What is the likely diagnosis?

CASE DETAILS

Difficulty in breathing, cough, and purulent sputum signifies the underlying lung pathology. Low pH and high pCO_2 indicate respiratory acidosis as a result of hypoventilation. The low pO_2 is due to associated hypoxia. Slightly high HCO_3^- may be due to compensation as a result of increased reabsorption from the kidney. The patient is, thus, in a state of compensated respiratory acidosis.

The treatment is based on treating the primary cause; O_2 and mechanical ventilation are often needed.

RESPIRATORY ACIDOSIS

Pathophysiology

Respiratory acidosis is CO_2 accumulation (hypercapnia) from a decrease in respiratory rate, respiratory volume (hypoventilation), or both. It can be due to severe pulmonary disease, respiratory muscle fatigue, or abnormalities in ventilatory control and is recognized by an increase in $PaCO_2$ and decrease in pH. Respiratory acidosis may be acute or chronic. Distinction is based on the degree of metabolic compensation. In acute respiratory acidosis, there is an immediate compensatory elevation (due to cellular buffering mechanisms) in HCO_3^-, which increases 1 mmol/L for every 10 mm Hg increase in $PaCO_2$. In chronic respiratory acidosis (>24 hours), renal adaptation increases the (HCO_3^-) by 4 mmol/L for every 10 mm Hg increase in $PaCO_2$. The serum HCO_3^- usually does not increase above 38 mmol/L. Respiratory acidosis does not have a great effect on electrolyte levels. Some small effects occur in calcium and potassium levels. Acidosis decreases binding of calcium to albumin and tends to increase serum ionized calcium levels. In addition, acidemia causes an extracellular shift of potassium, but respiratory acidosis rarely causes clinically significant hyperkalemia.

Causes

Respiratory acidosis is also called **"primary (H_2CO_3) excess"**. The underlying abnormality is increase in H_2CO_3 content in the blood which follows decreased elimination of CO_2 in the pulmonary alveoli (high pCO_2). This may result from:

- Breathing air containing abnormally high percentage of CO_2.
- Conditions in which the elimination of CO_2 is reduced, hypoxia typically accompanies hypoventilation. Some of the common causes are as follows:

A. Central: Depression of the respiratory center by a variety of drugs, injuries, or diseases can produce respiratory acidosis. Acutely, this may occur with general anesthetics, sedatives, and head trauma. Chronically with sedatives, alcohol, intracranial tumors, and the syndromes of sleep-disordered breathing include the primary alveolar and obesity—hypoventilation syndromes.

B. **Airway obstruction:** Restrictive disorders involving both the chest wall and the lungs which can cause respiratory acidosis because the high metabolic cost of respiration causes ventilatory muscle fatigue.
   Acute hypercapnia follows sudden occlusion of the upper airway or generalized bronchospasm as in severe asthma, anaphylaxis, inhalational burn, or toxin injury.
   Chronic hypercapnia and respiratory acidosis occur in end-stage obstructive lung disease.

C. **Parenchymatous damage:** This is due to loss of ventilatory functions and due to an increase in intrathoracic pressure or loss of elasticity.
   1. Emphysema
   2. Pneumoconiosis
   3. Bronchitis
   4. Adult respiratory distress syndrome
   5. Barotraumas
   6. Pleurisy

D. **Neuromuscular:** Abnormalities or disease in the motor neurons, neuromuscular junction, and skeletal muscle can cause hypoventilation via respiratory muscle fatigue.
   1. Poliomyelitis
   2. Kyphoscoliosis
   3. Myasthenia
   4. Muscular dystrophies

E. Miscellaneous:
   1. Certain congenital heart diseases.
   2. Mechanical ventilation, when not properly adjusted and supervised, may result in respiratory acidosis, particularly if CO_2 production suddenly rises (because of fever, agitation, sepsis, or overfeeding) or alveolar ventilation falls because of worsening pulmonary function.
   3. Rebreathing from a closed space

Mechanism of Respiratory Acidosis

When the elimination of CO_2 is reduced, CO_2 accumulates in blood, resulting in excess H_2CO_3 formation. As a result, the ratio of bicarbonate to carbonic acid is reduced, pH is lowered, and the respiratory acidosis sets in.

Compensation

In respiratory acidosis, the respiratory mechanism becomes secondary and the renal mechanism becomes primary.

a. **Respiratory mechanism:** The respiratory center is stimulated by the high pCO_2; the rate of ventilation increases. But this mechanism is less effective since the defect may be at the level of respiratory center or at the level of lungs and hyperventilation might not be possible to that extent to normalize the disturbed ratio.
b. **Renal mechanism:** It is of prime importance. More HCO_3^- are reabsorbed from tubules in response to raised pCO_2 in blood and the ratio of HCO_3^-: H_2CO_3 is restored back to normal.

Clinical Manifestations

The clinical features vary according to the severity and duration of the respiratory acidosis, the underlying disease, and whether there is accompanying hypoxemia.

- A rapid increase in $PaCO_2$ may cause anxiety, dyspnea, confusion, psychosis, and hallucinations and may progress to coma.
- Lesser degrees of dysfunction in chronic hypercapnia include sleep disturbances, loss of memory, daytime somnolence, personality changes, impairment of coordination, and motor disturbances, such as tremor, myoclonic jerks, and asterixis.
- Headaches and other signs that mimic raised intracranial pressure, such as papilledema, abnormal reflexes, and focal muscle weakness, are due to vasoconstriction secondary to loss of the vasodilator effects of CO_2.

Mortality/Morbidity

The morbidity and mortality of respiratory acidosis depends on the underlying cause of the respiratory acidosis, associated conditions, the patient's compensatory mechanisms, and effectiveness of medical care.

Laboratory studies

- **Arterial blood gas determination:** Acidemia is documented by the presence of a decreased pH (<7.35) shown on arterial blood gas analysis. The presence of an increased $PaCO_2$ (>45 mm Hg) indicates a respiratory etiology of the acidemia.
- **Serum chemistries:** The most common finding in chronic respiratory acidosis is the presence of a compensatory increase in serum bicarbonate concentration.
- **Hypothyroidism:** Some patients have hypothyroidism as a cause for their obesity (and resulting hypoventilation due to associated obstructive sleep apnea) leading to chronic respiratory acidosis. A thyrotropin and free T4 level should be obtained.
- **Complete blood cell count:** Many patients with chronic hypercapnia and respiratory acidosis also are hypoxemic. These patients may have secondary polycythemia.
- **Drug screens:** Drug and toxicology screens should be performed in patients presenting with unexplained hypercapnia and respiratory acidosis. Screening for specific drugs including opiates, barbiturates, and benzodiazepines should be performed.

Imaging studies

- **Chest radiography:** Chest radiography should be performed to help rule out pulmonary disease as a cause of hypercapnia and respiratory acidosis.
- **CT scanning of the chest:** A CT scan of the chest may be obtained if the results of chest radiography are inconclusive or if a pulmonary disorder remains high on the differential diagnosis.
- **CT scanning of the brain:** Imaging of the brain is performed if a central cause of hypoventilation and respiratory acidosis is suspected. Specific etiologies that may be diagnosed using brain CT scanning include stroke, central nervous system (CNS) tumor, and CNS trauma.
- **MRI of the brain:** If a central cause of hypoventilation and respiratory acidosis is suspected and initial findings after brain CT scanning are negative or inconclusive, consider MRI of the brain. The MRI may disclose abnormalities not observed on CT scans, particularly in the brainstem.

Other tests

- Pulmonary function testing
- **Electromyography and nerve conduction velocity:** Electromyography (EMG) and nerve conduction velocity (NCV) are useful in diagnosing neuromuscular disorders which can cause ventilatory muscle weakness.

Treatment

The management of respiratory acidosis depends on its severity and rate of onset. Acute respiratory acidosis can be life-threatening and measures to reverse the underlying cause should be undertaken simultaneously with restoration of adequate alveolar ventilation. This may necessitate tracheal intubation and assisted mechanical ventilation. Oxygen administration should be titrated carefully in patients with severe obstructive pulmonary disease and chronic CO_2 retention who are breathing spontaneously. When oxygen is used injudiciously, these patients may experience progression of the respiratory acidosis. Aggressive and rapid correction of hypercapnia should be avoided, because the falling $PaCO_2$ may provoke the cardiac arrhythmias, reduced cerebral perfusion, and seizures. The $PaCO_2$ should be lowered gradually in chronic respiratory acidosis, aiming to restore the $PaCO_2$ to baseline levels and to provide sufficient Cl^- and K^+ to enhance the renal excretion of HCO_3^-.

Chronic respiratory acidosis is frequently difficult to correct, but measures aimed at improving lung function can help some patients and forestall further deterioration in most.

Prevention

- Smoking cessation is an important aspect in the long-term treatment, especially in COPD patients.
- Weight loss is very helpful especially in patients with obesity-hypoventilation syndrome. It improves daytime symptoms and the pCO_2. In patients with obstructive sleep apnea, weight loss decreases the number of apneas and hypopneas.

Complications

- Patients with chronic respiratory acidosis, by definition, have a component of alveolar hypoventilation. The patients have increased $PaCO_2$ and bicarbonate levels. They also have obligatory decreases in PaO_2. Complications are often related to the chronic hypoxemia.
- Chronic hypoxemia can result in increased erythropoiesis leading to polycythemia.
- Chronic hypoxia is a well-known cause of pulmonary vasoconstriction. This physiologic response can in the long-term, lead to pulmonary hypertension, right ventricular failure, and cor pulmonale.
- The hypopneas and apneas during sleep lead to impaired sleep quality and cerebral vasodilation, causing morning headaches, daytime fatigue, and somnolence.
- High levels of $PaCO_2$ can lead to confusion, often referred to as carbon dioxide narcosis. As a late complication of cerebral vasodilation, patients may have papilledema.

Prognosis

The prognosis for patients with respiratory acidosis varies and depends on the severity of the underlying pathophysiological process.

CLINICAL NOTE

Aggressive and rapid correction of hypercapnia should be avoided because the falling $PaCO_2$ may provoke the cardiac arrhythmias, reduced cerebral perfusion, and seizures.

CLINICAL PEARLS

1. Respiratory acidosis is primary increase in pCO_2 with or without compensatory increase in HCO_3^-; pH is usually low but may be near normal.
2. Cause is a decrease in respiratory rate, volume (hypoventilation), or both from CNS, pulmonary, or iatrogenic conditions.
3. Respiratory acidosis can be acute or chronic; the chronic form is asymptomatic, but the acute, or worsening form causes headache, confusion, and drowsiness.
4. Signs include tremor, myoclonic jerks, and asterixis. Diagnosis is clinical and with ABG and serum electrolyte measurements.
5. The cause is treated; O_2 and mechanical ventilation are often required.

SUMMARY OF THE CAUSES OF RESPIRATORY ACIDOSIS

A. Central:
- Drugs—sedatives, alcohol, and general anesthetic agents
- Infections
- Injuries—head trauma
- Diseases—intracranial tumor
- Syndromes of sleep-disordered breathing including the primary alveolar and obesity-hypoventilation syndromes.

B. Airway obstruction:
- Severe asthma
- Anaphylaxis

- Inhalational burn
- Toxic injury
- Laryngeal obstruction
- End-stage obstructive lung disease

C. Parenchymatous damage/inflammation:
- Emphysema
- Bronchitis
- Pneumoconiosis
- Adult respiratory distress syndrome
- Pleurisy
- Barotrauma

D. Neuromuscular:
- Poliomyelitis
- Kyphoscoliosis
- Myasthenia gravis
- Muscular dystrophies

E. Miscellaneous:
- Certain congenital heart diseases
- Mechanical ventilation
- Rebreathing from a closed space

Chapter 20

Molecular Biology

LEARNING OBJECTIVES

To understand:
- Types and effects of mutations
- Mechanism of action and clinical applications of topoisomerases
- DNA damage and repair mechanisms
- Clinical implications of unrepaired DNA damage

CASE STUDIES

CASE STUDY 1

Theme: Types and Effects of Mutations

An 8-year-old boy was brought to his pediatrician by his mother because she was concerned that he was having language-speech problems, was hyperactive, and was told by teachers that he might be having mental retardation. The mother reported a strong family history of mental retardation in males of the family.

The boy on examination was found to have a large jaw, prominent ears, and enlarged testes (macroorchidism). The patient underwent a series of blood tests and was scheduled to see a genetic counselor, who expressed that the etiology of the genetic defect was likely transmitted from his mother. The genetic counselor stated that his mother likely had a silent mutation.

What is the most likely diagnosis?
Which chromosome is likely to be affected?
What are mutations?
What is the biochemical basis for the different types of mutations?

CASE DETAILS

The child is most probably suffering from fragile X syndrome.

Fragile X syndrome, also termed as **Martin–Bell syndrome or marker X syndrome**, is the most common cause of inherited mental retardation and is the second most common cause of genetically associated mental deficiencies after trisomy 21.

It affects males primarily. The clinical presentation can vary, but usually the affected male has moderate-to-severe mental retardation, hyperactivity, typical facies , such as large jaw and large ears. Pigmented skin lesions (café au lait) can also be seen. Because females have two copies of the X chromosome, they are "resistant" to mutations on one gene. Fragile X affects the long arm of the X chromosome, with multiple copies of triplicate repeats, usually CGG, leading to methylation of the deoxyribonucleic acid (DNA). The fragile X mental retardation (FMR) gene product is affected and, through a little-understood mechanism, leads to mental retardation.

BASIC CONCEPT

Mutations

Replication often produces changes in the chemical makeup of DNA. Many of these changes are easily repaired; however, those alterations in the DNA base sequence that do not get repaired are referred to as mutations.

Types of Mutations

There are various types of mutations including-point mutations, deletions, and insertions **(Table 20.1)**.

TABLE 20.1: Examples of mutational events.

SILENT MUTATION					
Codon	*Amino acid*	*Codon*	*Amino acid*	*Codon*	*Amino acid*
GCC	Alanine	GCC	Alanine	GCU	Alanine
GCU	Alanine				
GCA	Alanine				
GCG	Alanine				

MISSENSE MUTATION							
β-chain of normal hemoglobin	*GGU*	*CAC*	*CUG*	*ACU*	*CCU*	*GAG*	*GAG*
	Gly	His	Leu	Thr	Pro	Glu	Glu
A missense mutation found in	GGU	CAC	CUG	ACU	CCU	GUG	GAG
β-chain of sickle cell hemoglobin	Gly	His	Leu	Thr	Pro	Val	Glu

NONSENSE MUTATION							
Normal	GGC	CUG	ACA	GGG	CAA	AAA	CUG
	Gly	Leu	Thr	Gly	Gln	Lys	Leu
A nonsense mutation found in	GGC	CUG	ACA	GGG	UAA	AAA	CTG
Duchenne muscular dystrophy	Gly	Leu	Thr	Gly	STOP		

Point mutations

Point mutations arise when one base pair is substituted for another, and they are the most common types of mutations. Point mutations may be transition type (when purine is changed to purine or when a pyrimidine is changed by another pyrimidine) or they may be transversion type (when a given purine is replaced by a pyrimidine and vice versa).

Point mutations can be further subdivided into three categories: silent, missense, and nonsense **(Table 20.1)**.

- **Silent mutations** do not affect the translated mRNA or final protein product—thus the name silent. The genetic code is degenerate, which means that most amino acids are encoded by several different codons or triplets of DNA/RNA bases. Therefore, it is possible to switch a single base but not alter the resulting protein product.
- **Missense mutation:** The sickle cell trait is a result of a missense mutation. This type of point mutation actually does alter the protein product. In the case of sickle cell hemoglobin, an adenine is replaced by a thymine, causing a hydrophilic glutamic acid to be replaced with a hydrophobic valine in the resulting protein.
- **Nonsense mutation:** In a nonsense mutation, the mutation brings about a premature stop in the gene of interest because the altered codon now represents a stop codon. These are commonly seen in muscular dystrophies and some cystic fibrosis cases. Aminoglycosides are currently being used to treat premature stop codons as they affect the translational accuracy of transfer ribonucleic acids (tRNAs), thereby allowing recognition of incorrect codons including the stop codon. Ultimately, the translation machinery reads through the premature stop codon because of altered amino acid insertion by the tRNAs and produces full-length protein instead of a truncated protein or degraded mRNA.

Deletion

Another type of mutation is a deletion in which one or more DNA bases have been removed.

Insertion

An insertion is a mutation where one or more DNA bases have been added.

Frameshift mutations:

These two types of mutations can cause a shift in the open reading frame, called frameshift mutations, of a gene, if the insertion or deletion is a multiple of one or two bases. Typically, a frameshift mutation will result in disease either as result of altering the protein product, leaving it nonfunctional, or generation of a premature stop codon, which confers a truncated form of the altered protein. Both cases present major problems because the altered protein will not likely be able to carry out the normal duties required of it. Since codons are read as multiples of three, an insertion or deletion of three or a multiple of three may/may not be as deleterious to the gene as multiples of one or two. In this situation, the resulting protein could include extra amino acids in the case of insertions or lose amino acids in the case of deletions. It is possible that this could hinder the protein from normally functioning.

Frameshift mutation

Frameshift resulting in altered protein:

CCC	*GCA*	*UAU*	*CAU*	*UUU*	*ACC*
Pro	Ala	Tyr ↓	His	Phe	Thr
		Deletion of UA			
CCC	GCA	UCA	UUU	UAC	
Pro	Ala	Ser	Phe	Tyr	

Frameshift causing premature stop:

CCC	*GCA*	*UAU*	*CAU*	*UUU*	*ACC*
Pro	Ala	Tyr ↓	His	Phe	Thr
		Deletion of UC			
	CCC	GCA	UAA		
	Pro	Ala	STOP		

Many forms of fragile X syndrome are examples of insertions in multiples of three where the outcome is detrimental not because of altered amino acid sequence but rather a loss of protein expression.

Deletions and insertions typically occur in highly repetitive sequences, and this is exactly what is seen in fragile X.

FRAGILE X SYNDROME

Fragile X syndrome is the most common form of inherited mental retardation.

Incidence

It affects approximately 1 in 4,000 males and 1 in 8,000 females. Mutations of the X chromosome, including fragile X, may account for the higher number of male patients in mentally handicapped facilities.

Basic Defect

The fragile X mental retardation 1 (*FMR1*) gene is highly conserved.

Normal individuals have 7 to 60 (CGG) repeats in the 5′-untranslated region, and the repeats are often broken up by AGG. Many fragile X individuals have an increase in the number of CGG repeats, which may expand to over 230 repeats. This is termed as the ***full mutation***. Repeats ranging from 60 to 230 are called a **premutation**. The premutation carrier has normal fragile X mental retardation protein (FMRP) levels, but the gene is unstable in its passage to offspring. The FMRP is a regulatory protein that binds messenger RNA (mRNA) in neurons and dendrites. In patients with a full mutation in the *FMR1* gene, FMRP is not manufactured and brain development is impaired primarily because of abnormal synapse connections. The FMRP is present in other tissues; however, its role is less understood.

The fragile X phenotype is mainly caused by the loss of FMRP resulting from CGG trinucleotide repeat expansion of the *FMR1* gene. However, some point mutations and deletions in the *FMR1* gene show the same phenotype as the repeat expansion. The alteration arising from the trinucleotide repeat expansion within the promoter region of *FMR1* leads to enhanced local methylation and ultimately transcriptional silencing. DNA methylation causes protrusions in the DNA helix where the methylated cytosines interfere with transcription factor binding. This is a common property used for gene regulation.

However, in the case of fragile X, the methylation signals to halt all expression of FMRP. Loss of FMRP gives the phenotypical characteristics commonly seen in fragile X patients.

Some people have chromosomes that, when studied in a laboratory, have a tendency to "break" or "tear". The damage to these aberrant chromosomes typically occurs in particular regions, called fragile sites.

Most of the time, these fragile sites are not associated with medical problems, but a pronounced gap in one such region, at the end of the long arm of the X chromosome, is associated with fragile X syndrome **(Fig. 20.1)**. For unexplained reasons, fragile X syndrome does not behave in the typical manner of an X-linked trait. Nearly 20% of fragile X males are silent carriers, who are unaffected by the syndrome, but can pass the fragile X chromosome to their female offspring. About one-third of female fragile X carriers, who would be expected to be asymptomatic, exhibit some symptoms of the disorder.

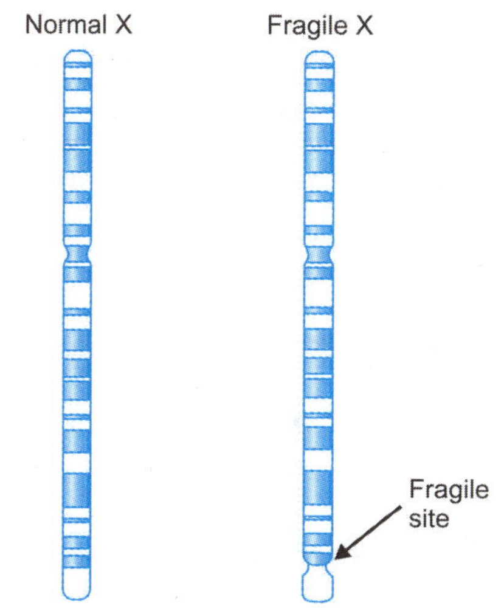

Fig. 20.1: Fragile sites on fragile X chromosome.

Mortality/Morbidity

Aside from the morbidity associated with mental retardation and cognitive, behavioral, and neuropsychological problems, the morbidity and mortality associated with fragile X syndrome are unremarkable. Life span is generally unaffected by the disorder.

Symptoms of Fragile X Syndrome

In addition to moderate-to-severe mental retardation, other characteristics of individuals with fragile X syndrome may include large ears, large testes (macroorchidism), **large jaw (prognathism), speech delays, prominent forehead, double-jointedness, autistic symptoms, and occasional self-mutilation.**

The face is typically long and narrow, and a high-arched palate, large ears, otitis media, strabismus, and dental problems are present.

Other common characteristics include hyperextensible joints, hypotonia, and heart problems including mitral valve prolapse. In males, abnormally large testes are a distinctive feature.

In young children, delayed motor development, hyperactivity, behavioral problems, toe walking, and occasional seizures can occur. Autism is suggested by poor eye contact, hand flapping, hand biting, and self-stimulating behaviors.

Poor sensory skills and mathematical ability are sometimes found in conjunction with good reading skills. Speech and language problems can include echolia, perseveration, poor language content, and cluttering (dropping of letters or syllables when speaking).

Affected girls tend to be shy and socially withdrawn, and to have particular difficulty with mathematics.

Diagnosis

Imaging studies

- Radiography of the spine is recommended in patients with fragile X syndrome to evaluate for scoliosis.
- Echocardiography is recommended to exclude mitral valve prolapse.

Other Tests

- **Cytogenetics:**
  - Cytogenetic testing for fragile X syndrome is not as sensitive as molecular testing, with a false-negative result rate of approximately 20%. Thus, DNA testing for fragile X syndrome is recommended.
  - Karyotyping may reveal other chromosomal anomalies, and both a standard karyotype and DNA testing are suggested when a possible diagnosis of fragile X syndrome is considered.
- **Molecular genetics:** The criterion standard diagnostic test involves molecular genetic techniques. The exact number of CGG triplet repeats can be determined. Southern blot and polymerase chain reaction (PCR) are the 2 methods of genetic analysis that are currently available.
  - Southern blot analysis provides a more accurate estimation of the number of CGG triplet repeats, if a full mutation is present (with a large CGG expansion). It can also be used to evaluate the degree of methylation at the CGG repeat site.
  - PCR is faster, requires a minimal sample, and is less expensive than Southern blot analysis. Additionally, PCR more accurately estimates the number of CGG triplet repeats, if a premutation is present (with small-to-moderate increases in CGG repeats). Recent success with fluorescent methylation-specific PCR and GeneScan analysis may further expand diagnostic options.
- A comprehensive developmental evaluation by a speech and language therapist, physical therapist, and occupational therapist is recommended to assess weaknesses and to identify areas in which improvement is needed most. As the patient matures, repeat evaluation may be necessary.
- Ophthalmology examinations are required.
- Routine auditory examinations are advised; otolaryngology referral for chronic otitis media and evaluation for pressure equalization (PE) tube placement are recommended.

Treatment

Standard treatment includes special education, speech, occupational, and sensory integration training; and behavior modification programs. Surgical correction of heart defects is sometimes necessary. Genetic counseling will benefit families of affected persons. Other treatment is symptomatic and supportive.

Folic acid has been found to improve hyperactivity and attention deficits in some preadolescent males with fragile X syndrome.

Complications

- Scoliosis
- Mitral valve prolapse (most frequently encountered cardiac defect).

Prognosis

Life expectancy is normal.

CLINICAL NOTE

The fragile X phenotype is mainly caused by the loss of FMRP resulting from CGG trinucleotide repeat expansion of the *FMR1* gene.

CLINICAL PEARLS

1. Fragile X syndrome, also termed Martin–Bell syndrome or marker X syndrome, is the most common cause of inherited mental retardation and is the second most common cause of genetically associated mental deficiencies after trisomy 21.
2. Mutations of the X chromosome, including fragile X, may account for the higher number of male patients in mentally handicapped facilities.
3. The fragile X phenotype is mainly caused by the loss of FMRP resulting from CGG trinucleotide repeat expansion of the *FMR1* gene.
4. Symptoms of fragile X syndrome may include mental retardation, large ears, large testes (macroorchidism), large jaw (prognathism), speech delays, prominent forehead, double-jointedness, autistic symptoms, and occasional self-mutilation.
5. The exact number of CGG triplet repeats can be determined by Southern blot and polymerase chain reaction (PCR). Treatment is symptomatic.

CASE STUDY 2

Theme: Effects of Mutations (Codon Deletion)

A 3-year-old boy was brought to the clinic for a chronic productive cough not responding to antibiotics given in the recent past. There was no history of fever, but his medical history was significant for abdominal distention, failure to pass stool, and emesis as an infant. History revealed that the child frequently passed bulky and foul-smelling stools. No diarrhea was present. He had several relatives with chronic lung and "stomach" problems, and some had even died at a young age.

The examination revealed an ill-appearing, slender child in moderate distress. The lung examination revealed poor air movement in the base of lungs, bilateral and coarse rhonchi throughout both lung fields. Chest X-ray showed signs consistent with bronchopneumonia. A quantitative pilocarpine iontophoresis sweat test was performed and the serum chloride was 70 mEq/L (>60 mEq/L is a positive test); the test was repeated a few days later with similar results.

What is the probable diagnosis?
What is the mechanism of the disease?

CASE DETAILS

The child has a history of chronic pulmonary and gastrointestinal problems and has a positive chloride sweat test. A family history of similar symptoms is also present. The most probable diagnosis is cystic fibrosis, which is an autosomal recessive disorder resulting in defective chloride ion channels of exocrine glands and epithelial tissues of the pancreas, sweat glands, and mucous glands in the respiratory, digestive, and reproductive tracts.

BASIC CONCEPT

Cystic Fibrosis

Cystic fibrosis (CF) is a monogenic disorder that presents as a multisystem disease. This disease is characterized by chronic bacterial infection of the airways that ultimately lead to bronchiectasis and bronchiolectasis, exocrine pancreatic insufficiency and intestinal dysfunction, abnormal sweat gland function, and urogenital dysfunction.

Incidence

It affects about one in 3,200 whites; 1 in 25 is a carrier. It is the most common cause of severe chronic lung disease in young adults and the most common fatal hereditary disorder of whites in the United States.

Pathogenesis

Cystic fibrosis (CF) is an autosomal recessive disease resulting from mutations in the gene that encodes the CF transmembrane conductance regulator (CFTR) protein located on chromosome 7. **The mutations in the CFTR gene fall into four major classes: Classes I–III mutations are considered "severe", as indexed by pancreatic insufficiency and high sweat NaCl values and Class IV mutations can be "mild", i.e., associated with pancreatic sufficiency and intermediate/normal sweat NaCl values.** Class I mutations that encode for premature stop codons are important to identify, as they may in the future be treated with agents that promote "read-through" of the stop codon with production of functional CFTR.

The most common mutation in the CF gene (~70% of CF chromosomes) is a 3-bp deletion (a Class III mutation) that results in an absence of phenylalanine at amino acid position 508 (F508) of the CF gene protein product, known as CFTR. The large number (>1,400) of relatively uncommon (<2% each) mutations identified in the CF gene makes it difficult to use DNA diagnostic technologies for identifying heterozygotes in populations at large.

CFTR Protein

The CFTR protein is a single polypeptide chain, containing 1,480 amino acids, that appears to function both as a cyclic AMP-regulated Cl^- channel and, as its name implies, a regulator of other ion channels. The fully processed form of CFTR is found in the plasma membrane in normal epithelia. Biochemical studies indicate that the F508 mutation leads to improper processing and intracellular degradation of the CFTR protein. Thus, absence of CFTR in the plasma membrane is central to the molecular pathophysiology of the ΔF508 mutation and other Classes I–II mutations. However, Classes III–IV mutations produce CFTR proteins that are fully processed, but are nonfunctional or only partially functional in the plasma membrane.

The abnormalities in the membrane chloride channel [the cystic fibrosis transmembrane conductance regulator (CFTR) protein] result in altered chloride transport and water flux across the apical surface of epithelial cells. Almost all exocrine glands produce abnormal mucus that obstructs glands and ducts. Obstruction results in glandular dilation and damage to tissue. In the respiratory tract, inadequate hydration of the tracheobronchial epithelium impairs mucociliary function. Over 1,400 mutations in the gene that encode CFTR have been described, and at least 230 mutations are known to be associated with clinical abnormalities. **The mutation referred to as ΔF508 accounts for about 70% of cases of cystic fibrosis.**

Organ-specific Pathophysiology

Lung

The diagnostic hallmark of CF airway epithelia is the raised transepithelial electric potential difference (PD). CF airway epithelia exhibit abnormalities in both active Na^+ absorption and active Cl^- secretion. The central hypothesis of CF airways pathophysiology is that the faulty regulation of Na^+ absorption and inability to secrete Cl^- via CFTR reduce the volume of liquid on airway surfaces; i.e., they are "dehydrated". Both the thickening of mucus and the depletion of the periciliary liquid lead to adhesion of mucus to the airway surface. Mucus adhesion leads to a failure to clear mucus from the airways both by ciliary and airflow-dependent (cough) mechanisms. Mucus clearance is the primary innate airways defense mechanism against infection by inhaled bacteria. Normal airways vary the rates of active Na^+ absorption and Cl^- secretion to adjust the volume of liquid (water), i.e., "hydration", on airway surfaces for efficient mucus clearance.

The infection that characterizes CF airways involves the mucus layer rather than epithelial or airway wall invasion. The predisposition of CF airways to chronic infection by *Staphylococcus aureus* and *Pseudomonas aeruginosa* is consistent with failure to clear mucus.

Gastrointestinal Tract

The gastrointestinal effects of CF are diverse.

- In the exocrine pancreas, the absence of the CFTR, Cl^- channel in the apical membrane of pancreatic ductal epithelia limits the function of an apical membrane Cl^--HCO_3^- exchanger to secrete bicarbonate and Na^+ (by a passive process) into the duct. The failure to secrete Na^+ HCO^- and water leads to retention of enzymes in the pancreas and ultimately destruction of virtually all pancreatic tissue.

- The CF intestinal epithelium, because of the lack of Cl^- and water secretion, fails to flush secreted mucins and other macromolecules from intestinal crypts. The diminished CFTR-mediated secretion of liquid may be exacerbated by excessive absorption of liquid, reflecting abnormalities of CFTR-mediated regulation of Na^+ absorption (both mediated by Na^+ channels and possibly other Na^+ transporters, e.g., Na^+-H^+ exchangers). Both dysfunctions lead to desiccated intraluminal contents and obstruction of both the small and large intestine.
- In the hepatobiliary system, defective hepatic ductal salt (Cl^-) and water secretion causes thickened biliary secretions, focal biliary cirrhosis, and bile duct proliferation in approximately 25–30% of patients with CF. The inability of the CF gallbladder epithelium to secrete salt and water can lead to both chronic cholecystitis and cholelithiasis.

Sweat Gland

Cystic fibrosis patients secrete nearly normal volumes of sweat in the sweat acinus. However, CF patients are not able to absorb NaCl from sweat, as it moves through the sweat duct due to the inability to absorb Cl^- across the ductal epithelial cells. This dysfunction in the sweat gland is typically measured by collecting sweat after iontophoresing a cholinergic agonist into the forearm.

Note: The epithelia affected by CF exhibit different functions in their native state, i.e., some are volume-absorbing (airways and distal intestinal epithelia), and some are salt- but not volume-absorbing (sweat duct), whereas others are volume-secretory (proximal intestine and pancreas). Given this diversity of native activities, it is not surprising that CF produces organ-specific effects on electrolyte and water transport. However, the unifying concept is that all affected tissues express abnormal ion transport function.

Clinical Manifestations

Most patients with CF present with signs and symptoms of the disease in childhood. Approximately 20% of patients present within the first 24 hours of life with gastrointestinal obstruction, termed *meconium ileus*. Other common presentations within the first year or two of life include respiratory tract symptoms, most prominently cough and/or recurrent pulmonary infiltrates, and failure to thrive. A significant proportion of patients (~5%), however, are diagnosed after age of 18.

Cystic fibrosis should be suspected in a young adult with a history of chronic lung disease (especially bronchiectasis), pancreatitis, or infertility. Cough, sputum production, decreased exercise tolerance, and recurrent hemoptysis are typical complaints. Patients also often complain of facial (sinus) pain or pressure and purulent nasal discharge. Steatorrhea, diarrhea, and abdominal pain are also common.

Complications of Cystic Fibrosis

Because of the wide range of alterations seen in the CFTR protein structure and function, cystic fibrosis in adults may present with a variety of pulmonary and nonpulmonary manifestations. Pulmonary manifestations in adults include acute and chronic bronchitis, bronchiectasis, pneumonia, atelectasis, and peribronchial and parenchymal scarring. Pneumothorax and hemoptysis are common. Hypoxemia, hypercapnia, and cor pulmonale occur in advanced cases. Biliary cirrhosis and gallstones may occur. Nearly all men with cystic fibrosis have congenital bilateral absence of the vas deferens with azoospermia. Patients with cystic fibrosis have an increased risk of malignancies of the gastrointestinal tract, osteopenia, and arthropathies.

Laboratory Findings

Arterial blood gas studies often reveal hypoxemia and, in advanced disease, a chronic, compensated respiratory acidosis. Pulmonary function studies show a mixed obstructive and restrictive pattern.

Imaging

Hyperinflation is seen early in the disease process. Peribronchial cuffing, mucus plugging, bronchiectasis (ring shadows and cysts), increased interstitial markings, small rounded peripheral opacities, and focal atelectasis may be seen separately or in various combinations. Pneumothorax can also be seen. Thin-section CT scanning may confirm the presence of bronchiectasis.

Diagnosis

The quantitative pilocarpine iontophoresis sweat test reveals elevated sodium and chloride levels (>60 mEq/L) in the sweat of patients with cystic fibrosis. Two tests on different days are required for accurate diagnosis. A normal sweat chloride test does not exclude the diagnosis. Genotyping or other alternative diagnostic studies (, such as measurement of nasal membrane potential difference, semen analysis, or assessment of pancreatic function) should be pursued, if the test is repeatedly negative but there is a high clinical suspicion of cystic fibrosis. Standard genotyping is a limited diagnostic tool because it screens for only a fraction of the known cystic fibrosis mutations, although complete genetic testing is available.

Treatment

The major objectives of therapy for CF are to promote clearance of secretions and control infection in the lung, provide adequate nutrition, and prevent intestinal obstruction. Ultimately, therapies that restore the processing of misfolded mutant CFTR or gene therapy may be the treatments of choice.

Lung Diseases

- Clearance of lower airway secretions should be promoted.
- Sputum viscosity in cystic fibrosis is increased by the large quantities of extracellular DNA that result from chronic airway inflammation and autolysis of neutrophils. Inhaled recombinant human deoxyribonuclease (rhDNase) cleaves extracellular DNA in sputum.
- Inhalation of hypertonic saline has been associated with small improvements in pulmonary function and fewer pulmonary exacerbations.
- Antibiotics are used to treat active airway infections based on results of culture and susceptibility testing of sputum.
- Inhaled bronchodilators should be considered in patients who demonstrate an increase of at least 12% in FEV1 after an inhaled bronchodilator.
- Vaccination against pneumococcal infection and annual influenza vaccination are advised. Screening of family members and genetic counseling are suggested.
- Lung transplantation is currently the only definitive treatment for advanced cystic fibrosis. Double-lung or heart-lung transplantation is required.
- Investigational therapies for cystic fibrosis include anti-inflammatory agents (e.g., ibuprofen, pentoxifylline, and antiproteases), protein modification agents (e.g., milrinone, phenylbutyrate), ion transport agents (e.g., amiloride), and gene therapy.

Gastrointestinal Diseases

- Maintenance of adequate nutrition is critical for the health of the CF patient.
- Most (>90%) CF patients require pancreatic enzyme replacement.
- Replacement of fat-soluble vitamins, particularly vitamins E and K, is usually required.
- Hyperglycemia most often becomes manifest in the adult and typically requires insulin treatment.
- Cholestatic liver disease occurs in about 8% of CF patients. End-stage liver disease occurs in about 5% of CF patients and can be treated by transplantation.
- Persistent symptoms may indicate a diagnosis of gastrointestinal malignancy, which is increased in incidence in patients with CF.

Prognosis

The longevity of patients with cystic fibrosis is increasing, and the median survival age is over 30 years. Death occurs from pulmonary complications (e.g., pneumonia, pneumothorax, or hemoptysis) or as a result of terminal chronic respiratory failure and cor pulmonale.

CLINICAL NOTE

The quantitative pilocarpine iontophoresis sweat test reveals elevated sodium and chloride levels (>60 mEq/L) in the sweat of patients with cystic fibrosis.

CLINICAL PEARLS

1. Cystic fibrosis (CF) is a monogenic disorder that presents as a multisystem disease.
2. CF is an autosomal recessive disease resulting from mutations in the gene that encode the CF transmembrane conductance regulator (CFTR) protein located on chromosome 7.
3. This disease is characterized by chronic bacterial infection of the airways that ultimately lead to bronchiectasis and bronchiolectasis, exocrine pancreatic insufficiency and intestinal dysfunction, abnormal sweat gland function, and urogenital dysfunction.
4. Arterial blood gas analysis, pulmonary function tests, sweat chloride test, and DNA analysis are the tools for the diagnosis of cystic fibrosis.
5. The objective of the treatment is to promote clearance of secretions and control infection in the lung, provide adequate nutrition, and prevent intestinal obstruction.

CASE STUDY 3

Theme: Mechanism of Action and Clinical Applications of Topoisomerases

A 40-year-old female presented to the emergency with complaints of fever, lower abdominal pain, some nausea, and vomiting increasing over the previous 2 days. She denied diarrhea or sick contacts. There was no previous history of such like episode.

On examination, she had a temperature of 38.9°C (102°F) and appeared ill. She had moderate bilateral lower abdominal tenderness and minimal guarding without rebound or distention. Bowel sounds were present and were normal. Pelvic examination revealed a foul-smelling discharge through cervix with severe cervical motion tenderness and bilateral adnexal tenderness. Cervical cultures were obtained. A diagnosis of PID (pelvic inflammatory disease) was made and the patient was begun on a quinolone antibiotic. **What is the mechanism of action of the quinolone?**

CASE DETAILS

Pelvic inflammatory disease (PID) is usually an acute infection affecting the fallopian tubes and possibly the uterus and ovaries. It is generally sexually transmitted, caused by organisms , such as *Chlamydia* or *Neisseria gonorrhoeae* (gonorrhea). The treatment is with antibiotics.

QUINOLONE ANTIBIOTICS

The **quinolones are broad-spectrum synthetic antibiotic** drugs that contain the **4-quinolone ring**. Antibacterial agents, such as all antimicrobial drugs, are directed against unique targets not present in mammalian cells. The goal is to limit toxicity to the host and maximize chemotherapeutic activity affecting invading microbes only.

The quinolones, including nalidixic acid and its fluorinated derivatives (ciprofloxacin, levofloxacin, and moxifloxacin), are synthetic compounds that inhibit the activity of the A subunit of the bacterial enzyme DNA gyrase as well as topoisomerase IV. DNA gyrase and topoisomerases are responsible for negative supercoiling of DNA—an essential conformation for DNA replication in the intact cell. Inhibition of the activity of DNA gyrase and topoisomerase IV is lethal to bacterial cells. The antibiotic *novobiocin* also interferes with the activity of DNA gyrase, but it interferes with the β subunit. The quinolone antibiotics target bacterial DNA gyrase in many gram-negative bacteria, such as *Escherichia coli*, *Klebsiella pneumoniae*, *Pseudomonas aeruginosa*, and the like.

BASIC CONCEPT

The normal biological functioning of DNA-like ribonucleic acid (RNA) transcription and DNA replication occurs only if it is in the proper topological state.

Supercoiling

In duplex DNA, the two strands are wound about each other once every 10 bp, that is, once every turn of the helix. Double-stranded circular DNA can form either negative supercoils when the strands are underwound or positive supercoils when they are overwound. Negative supercoiling introduces a torsional stress that promotes unwinding or separation of the right-handed B-DNA double helix, while positive supercoiling overwinds such a helix **(Fig. 20.2)**.

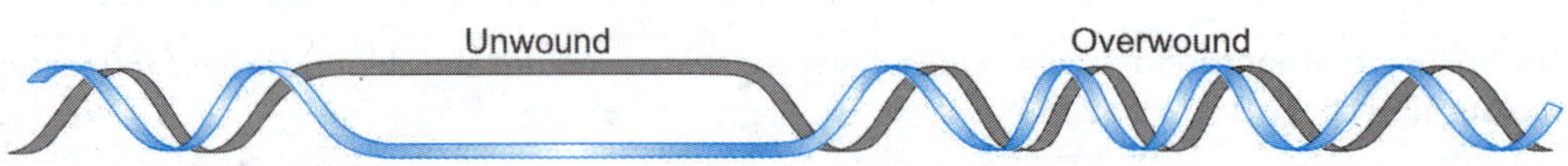

Fig. 20.2: Negative and positive supercoils.

A right-handed coil is assigned a negative number (negative supercoiling) and a left-handed coil is assigned a positive number (positive supercoiling). Most naturally occurring DNA molecules are negatively supercoiled **(Fig. 20.3)**. What is the basis for this prevalence? As already stated, negative supercoiling arises from the unwinding or underwinding of the DNA. In essence, negative supercoiling prepares DNA for processes requiring separation of the DNA strands, , such as replication or transcription. Positive supercoiling condenses DNA as effectively, but it makes strand separation more difficult.

The supercoiling is controlled by a remarkable group of enzymes known as topoisomerases. Supercoiling markedly alters the overall form of DNA.

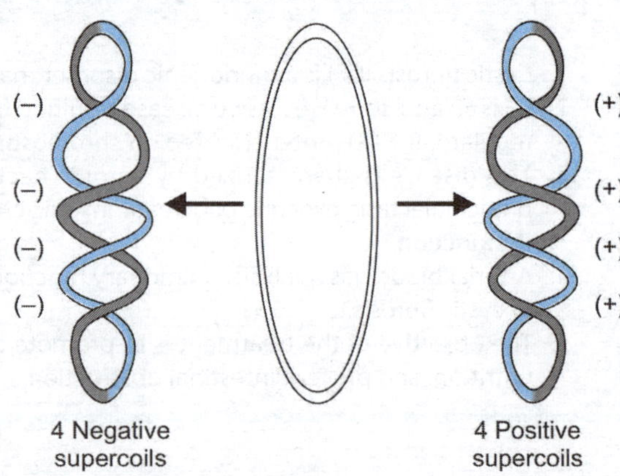

Fig. 20.3: Negative and positive supercoils.

Topoisomerases

There are two classes of topoisomerases. These enzymes act by catalyzing a three-step process: (1) the *cleavage* of one or both strands of DNA, (2) the *passage* of a segment of DNA through this break, and (3) the *resealing* of the DNA break.

a. **Type I topoisomerases** relax DNA from negative supercoils by creating transient single-strand breaks in DNA without any expense of ATP. The Type I enzymes have been further subdivided into Type IA and Type IB subfamilies based on their reaction mechanism. Type I topoisomerases, which form covalent linkages to the 5′ end of the DNA break, are members of the Type IA subfamily and Type I enzymes, which form covalent linkages to the 3' end of DNA break, are members of the Type IB subfamily. With the backbone of one strand cleaved, the DNA can now rotate around the remaining strand, driven by the release of the energy stored because of the supercoiling. The rotation of the DNA unwinds supercoils. The enzyme controls the rotation, so that the unwinding is not rapid.

b. **Type II topoisomerases** change DNA topology by making transient double-strand breaks in DNA and require ATP consumption **(Fig. 20.4)**.
c. A topoisomerase III has been described, which makes transient single-strand DNA breaks and is therefore a Type I enzyme.
d. A topoisomerase IV has been described, which makes transient double-strand DNA breaks and is therefore a member of the Type II enzyme family.

All Type II topoisomerases require ATP while Type I topoisomerases do not.

The DNA is covalently linked to the enzyme only during a short period of time during the catalytic cycle. In the cell, this is a transient linkage and readily reversible. The complex of DNA and a covalently bound topoisomerase molecule has been referred to as a "cleavable complex".

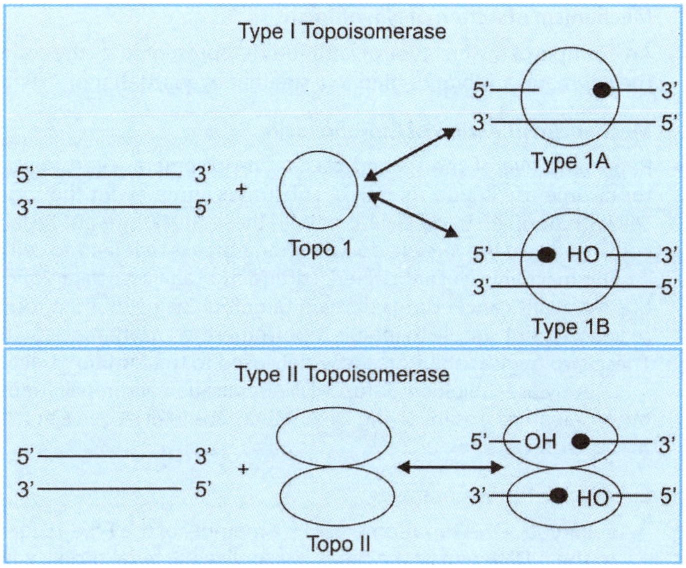

Fig. 20.4: Action of two types of topoisomerases—Type I and Type II.

Prokaryotic Topoisomerases

1. ***Escherichia coli* DNA topoisomerase I:** The enzyme is a monomer of 97 kDa (kilo-Daltons) and is coded for by the *topA* gene. It has a preference for binding at single-strand regions of DNA. This explains why the enzyme readily relaxes negatively, but not positively supercoiled DNA, as single-stranded areas tend to be present in negatively supercoiled (underwound) DNA but not in positively supercoiled DNA.
2. ***E. coli* DNA topoisomerase III:** The gene coding for topo III is referred to as *topB*. Topo III is a Type I enzyme and is therefore only capable of making transient DNA single-strand breaks.
3. ***E. coli* DNA gyrase and DNA topoisomerase IV:** The Type II topoisomerases are represented in *E. coli* by DNA gyrase and topoisomerase IV (topo IV). Unlike the Type I topoisomerases, the Type II enzymes all require ATP for catalysis.

DNA gyrase was discovered prior to topo IV. As a Type II enzyme, it requires ATP. DNA gyrase is a heterotetramer composed of two A and two B subunits to yield an A2B2 holoenzyme. The A subunit is the product of the *gyrA* gene and has a molecular weight of 97 kDa. The B subunit is the product of the *gyrB* gene and has a molecular weight of 90 kDa. Gyrase is unique among topoisomerases because it is able to supercoil DNA. This supercoiling reaction is unique to prokaryotes. No active supercoiling activity has yet been described in higher organisms.

Like gyrase, topoisomerase IV is a heterodimer and consists of two C encoded subunits and two E encoded subunits giving a molecular structure for the enzyme of C2E2. The enzyme is a potent decatenate and plays a critical role in decatenating DNA after replication to allow proper partitioning of daughter chromosomes.

During DNA replication, Type II topoisomerase, or topo II, plays an important role in the fork progression by continuous removal of the excessive positive supercoils that stem from the unwinding of the DNA strands. Topo II has the ability to cut both strands of a double-stranded DNA molecule, pass another portion of the duplex through the cut, and reseal the cut in a process that uses ATP. Hydrolysis of ATP by topo IIs inherent ATPase activity powers the conformational changes that are critical for the enzyme's operation. Based on the DNA substrate, topo II can change a positive supercoil into a negative supercoil or increase the number of negative supercoils by two.

During transcription, positive supercoils accumulate in front of the transcription machinery, which can be removed by gyrase, and negative supercoils accumulate behind. It may be that a major function of *E. coli* topo I is to relax underwound DNA, which accumulates behind an active RNA polymerase.

Drugs Targeting The Prokaryotic Type Ii Topoisomerases

DNA gyrase and topoisomerase IV are the molecular targets of two distinct groups of antibiotics—the coumarins (novobiocin) and the quinolones (ciprofloxacin). These two classes of drugs work by different mechanisms and are analogous to the mechanism of action of the two broad classes of anticancer drugs that target the eukaryotic enzymes. In general, topoisomerase-targeting drugs, as antibiotics or anticancer drugs, either inhibit the catalytic activity of the enzyme or impair the ability of the enzyme to religate DNA after cleavage. Although drugs of the latter type necessarily inhibit catalysis as well, it is thought that the inhibition of DNA religation after cleavage leaves a cell with drug-stabilized DNA breaks, which are eventually converted into chromosomal breaks, which result in cell death.

Mechanism of Action of Novobiocin

An example of the first type of antibiotic is represented by the coumarins. These drugs inhibit the ATPase activity of gyrase. Because the coumarin antibiotics bind to a site that overlaps that of ATP on the B subunit, they are competitive inhibitors.

Mechanism of Action of Ciprofloxacin

Representative of the second class of topoisomerase-targeting drugs is the quinolone. Theses drugs interact with gyrase or topoisomerase IV and their DNA substrates and prevent the topoisomerase from religating DNA after cleavage. This leaves the cell with double-strand DNA breaks. If these breaks are not repaired, they interact with other intracellular proteins and become converted into irreversible double-strand breaks that lead to cell death.

This mechanism of antibacterial drug action against prokaryotic Type II topoisomerases is reminiscent of the mechanism of action of several anticancer drugs that are targeted against human topoisomerase II. In both instances, the drug's primary mechanism of action is not simply to inhibit topoisomerase enzymatic activity, but rather to convert the enzyme to a DNA-damaging agent. These two gyrase inhibitors are widely used to treat urinary tract and other infections.

DNA gyrase inhibition disrupts DNA replication and repair, transcription, bacterial chromosome separation during division, and other cell processes involving DNA. Mutations in *gyrA* gene that encodes the A subunit of the polypeptide can confer resistance to these drugs.

Eukaryotic Topoisomerases

1. Eukaryotic DNA topoisomerase I is a member of the Type 1B family because when it cleaves DNA, it becomes covalently attached to the 3′ DNA end of the break site, unlike bacterial topo I, which becomes attached to the 5′ DNA terminus. The gene for the human enzyme is located on chromosome 20. Eukaryotic topo I does not share homology with *E. coli* topo I and carries out its topoisomerization reactions in a different manner. Eukaryotic topo I is located in areas of active RNA transcription and may function ahead of the transcription apparatus to relieve superhelical stress generated during mRNA synthesis. A role for the enzyme in the synthesis of rRNA has also been suggested as topo I has been shown to interact with RNA polymerase I. In addition, the enzyme has been observed to associate with mitotic chromosomes and may play a structural role in chromosome organization.
2. **Eukaryotic DNA Topoisomerase III:** For many years, it was thought that eukaryotic topo I was the only Type I topoisomerase in higher organisms. This is incorrect as a new Type I enzyme, more similar to the *E. coli* Type I topoisomerases than to eukaryotic topo I, has been readily documented to exist in a number of higher organisms. The function of topo III in higher organisms may be important for normal embryological development and during meiosis.
3. **Eukaryotic DNA Topoisomerase II:** Eukaryotic cells lack DNA gyrase but have a similar type of topoisomerase that can remove positive supercoils from eukaryotic DNA to prevent its tangling during replication.

Eukaryotic topoisomerase II (topo II) is a homodimer of identical subunits. Although eukaryotic topo II has an ATP requirement, the enzyme has never been shown to supercoil DNA. The activity of this enzyme is necessary to untangle intertwined chromosomes after DNA synthesis to allow for proper chromosomal segregation into daughter cells. The ATP requirement probably provides the energy necessary for the enzyme to control the topology of DNA. Knotted and catenated DNA structures, which would normally be present at equilibrium, could provide a hindrance to chromosomal segregation; it appears that topo II may use the energy of ATP to unknot and decatenate DNA to an untangled state, which would then allow for efficient separation of chromosomes. The enzyme may carry out this role as a component of the nuclear matrix. Topo II is one of the major proteins isolated from the nuclear scaffold where it may also help to anchor chromosomal loops. Thus, the enzyme may play a structural as well as a catalytic role in the cell.

Quinolones inhibit eukaryotic topoisomerase at much higher concentrations (100–1,000 µg/mL).

Chemotherapy

Topo I-targeted Chemotherapy

Camptothecin: Mechanism of action

One of the more exciting developments in clinical oncology has been the identification of the topoisomerases as the molecular targets of a variety of anticancer drugs. Presently, there have been described a wide variety of drugs, which interact with eukaryotic Topo I, many of which have anticancer properties. The drugs targeting Topo I that are now currently in clinical use are derivatives of Camptothecin, Topo I is the sole molecular target of the camptothecins. By preventing efficient religation after cleavage, the Camptothecin drugs prolong the half life of the normal cleaved DNA intermediate. This act alone probably does not result in cell death, but when the drug stabilized single strand break encounters a replication fork, the single DNA strand break is converted into a double DNA strand break, which kills the cell. The drugs therefore work by a novel mechanism. They convert the Topo I molecule into a DNA-damaging agent.

Topo II-targeted Chemotherapy

Anticancer drugs targeting topo II are some of the most widely used chemotherapeutic agents. These drugs include doxorubicin, etoposide, mitoxantrone, and others. In a broad sense, the drugs targeting Topo II can be classified as either topoisomerase "poisons" or topoisomerase catalytic inhibitors. As previously discussed, a transient double-strand DNA break is characteristic of the topo II enzymatic reaction.

The Topo II poisons increase the steady state levels of this transient intermediate. They do this either by increasing the rate of DNA cleavage (ellipticine and genistein) or by inhibiting the rate of DNA religation (etoposide, amsacrine, and teniposide). In either case, these drugs convert the enzyme into a DNA-damaging agent.

On the other hand, the Topo II catalytic inhibitors act like other types of anti-cancer drugs and inhibit the activity of the enzyme. Drugs interfering with the catalytic activity of the enzyme deprive the cell of the enzyme's ability to decatenate chromosomal DNA strands prior to mitosis. Cell growth is therefore altered.

Thus to summarize, the topoisomerases are important enzymes of biological system. They are important for DNA replication, RNA transcription, DNA recombination, DNA repair, and DNA organization. The bacterial topoisomerases are the targets for antibiotics while the eukaryotic topoisomerases are the targets for anticancer drugs.

CLINICAL NOTE

DNA gyrase inhibition disrupts DNA replication and repair, transcription, bacterial chromosome separation during division, and other cell processes involving DNA.

CLINICAL PEARLS

1. The quinolones, including nalidixic acid and its fluorinated derivatives (ciprofloxacin, levofloxacin, and moxifloxacin), are synthetic compounds that inhibit the activity of the A subunit of the bacterial enzyme DNA gyrase as well as topoisomerase IV.
2. DNA gyrase and topoisomerases are responsible for negative supercoiling of DNA—an essential conformation for DNA replication in the intact cell. Inhibition of the activity of DNA gyrase and topoisomerase IV is lethal to bacterial cells.
3. Camptothecin drugs work by a novel mechanism, they convert the Topo I molecule into a DNA-damaging agent.
4. The drugs targeting Topo II act as either topoisomerase "poisons" or topoisomerase catalytic inhibitors.
5. The bacterial topoisomerases are the targets for antibiotics, while the eukaryotic topoisomerases are the targets for anticancer drugs.

CASE STUDY 4

Theme: DNA Damage and Repair System

A 12-year-old boy presented at a dermatology clinic with a skin tumor on his right cheek. He had always avoided exposure to sunlight because it made his skin blister. His skin had scattered areas of hyperpigmentation and other areas where it looked mildly atrophied. Because of the presence of a skin tumor at such a young age, the history of avoidance of sunlight and other milder skin lesions, the dermatologist made a tentative diagnosis of xeroderma pigmentosum.

What is the defect in this disease?
What is the biochemical basis for all these presenting symptoms?

CASE DETAILS

Xeroderma pigmentosum (XP) is a group of rare autosomal-recessive inherited disorders characterized by extreme skin sensitivity to ultraviolet (UV) light, abnormal skin pigmentation, and high frequency of skin cancers, especially on sun-exposed skin.

Xeroderma Pigmentosum

Pathophysiology

Xeroderma pigmentosum is due to defective nucleotide excision repair (NER) leading to deficient repair of DNA damaged by UV radiation. Seven xeroderma pigmentosum repair genes, *XPA* through *XPG*, have been identified. A xeroderma pigmentosum variant has also been described. The defect in this condition is not in NER, but is instead in postreplication repair (see the details of repair system below). In the xeroderma pigmentosum variant, a mutation occurs in DNA polymerase.

The UV radiation induces cross-linking (dimerization) between thymine nucleotides. After exposure to UV light, normal cells identify and excise the UV-induced thymine dimers and insert undamaged nucleotides after DNA synthesis and ligation. This repair process, known as unscheduled DNA synthesis, is deficient in xeroderma pigmentosum.

Xeroderma pigmentosum is a multisystem disorder; sun-exposed skin and eyes (i.e., eyelids and conjunctivae) are the most affected tissues. Cutaneous photosensitivity and early development of skin cancer are caused by defective DNA repair. Unrestored damage to DNA causes mutations. In case mutations impinge on significant genes, such as tumor suppressor genes (for instance p53 or proto-oncogenes), then this form of disorder could cause cancer. Patients display high risk of getting cancer like basal cell carcinoma. Multiple basaliomas and other forms of malignancies affecting the skin are very common at a very juvenile age. In extreme situations, it becomes indispensable to keep away from sunlight totally. The two prevalent reasons behind fatalities for XP sufferers are metastatic malignant melanoma and squamous cell carcinoma.

Central nervous system (CNS) involvement is due to premature neuronal death. Necrosis in tissues that are not exposed to UV light suggests that these cells in patients with xeroderma pigmentosum are unable to repair DNA damage from other mutagens (e.g., reactive oxygen species and other free radicals). Neurodegeneration probably results from accumulating mutations due to cells' inability to repair DNA damage. Increased oxidative damage in neurons is due to abnormal function of free radical scavengers, such as superoxide dismutase. The presence of neurological abnormalities correlates with the degree of NER repair defect; patients with the greatest impairment of DNA repair are more prone to develop neurodegeneration.

Frequency

The worldwide frequency of xeroderma pigmentosum is estimated at 1 case in 250,000 population.

Clinical Manifestations

Xeroderma pigmentosum is a clinical diagnosis that is based on a history of sun hypersensitivity and skin neoplasms. Dermatologic symptoms precede neurologic manifestations, and diagnosis is typically straightforward. Some of the prevalent symptoms of XP involve:

- Abnormally intense sunburn subsequent to a small sun exposure
- Appearance of several freckles in a juvenile age
- Uneven dark patches over the surface of the skin or splotchy pigmentation
- Skin appearing thin
- Undue skin drying
- Rough-textured growths or solar keratoses and cancers affecting the skin
- Eyes are excruciatingly sensitive on exposure to the sun
- Blister formations or freckles appearing on the least extent of exposure to the sun
- Untimely, early aging appearing on the skin, lips, eyes, mouth, and tongue areas
- Spider-like appearance of the blood vessels (telangiectasia)
- Raw skin surface that oozes
- Less hair growth on the chest area and the legs
- Skin cancer is detected in approximately 50% of patients by age 14 years.

An examination of the eye would reveal:

- Cloudiness of the cornea
- Keratitis
- Lid tumors
- Blepharitis

Laboratory Investigations

The below stated tests could aid in diagnosing the condition in an infant prior to birth:

- Amniocentesis
- Chorionic villus sampling
- Amniotic cell culture

The following testing methods could aid in diagnosing the disorder subsequent to the child being born:

- Skin fibroblasts culture
- Skin biopsy

  Removal of a small section of tissue sample to be analyzed microscopically.

Treatment

- The vital aspect of management of this condition is to reduce sun exposure. Infants having this condition need complete safeguard from the sun's rays. Even the light percolating via the windows and through fluorescent bulbs is detrimental for them. The person concerned should always make it a point to wear protective clothes when heading outdoors. High sun protection SPF of thirty or above must be used and quite dark UV-protective sun glasses must be worn.

- The amounts of keratoses could be lowered by the use of isotretinoin (though it has some major side effects). Treatment of existent keratoses involves the use of cryotherapy or fluorouracil.
- Cryotherapy is the use of intense cold for obliterating anomalous or malignant tissues.
- Fluorouracil or 5-FU alike several cancer-combatant drugs can be used, fluorouracil could be utilized as a topical cream for treatment of solar keratoses and some forms of basal cell carcinomas affecting the skin.

Prognosis

Lesser than 40% of people having this disease have a survival of twenty plus years of age, while those with the milder version of the disease could have survival lasting past middle age.

Complications

- Skin disfigurement
- Skin cancer

Prevention

Experts suggest gene therapy for individuals those who desire to bear children, but are having a family history of xeroderma pigmentosum.

CLINICAL NOTE

Dermatologic symptoms precede neurological manifestations in xeroderma pigmentosum.

CLINICAL PEARLS

1. Xeroderma pigmentosum is due to defective nucleotide excision repair (NER) leading to deficient repair of DNA damaged by UV radiation.
2. It is a multisystem disorder; sun-exposed skin and eyes (i.e., eyelids and conjunctivae) are the most affected tissues. Cutaneous photosensitivity and early development of skin cancer are caused by defective DNA repair.
3. Xeroderma pigmentosum is a clinical diagnosis that is based on a history of sun hypersensitivity and skin neoplasms.
4. Fibroblast culture and skin biopsy can be undertaken to confirm the diagnosis.
5. The vital aspect of management of this condition is to reduce sun exposure. Isotretinoin, 5-fluorouracil, and cryotherapy can also be undertaken depending upon the status of the patient.

OVERVIEW OF DNA DAMAGE AND REPAIR

DNA in the living cell is subject to many chemical alterations. If the genetic information encoded in the DNA is to remain uncorrupted, any chemical changes must be corrected. A failure to repair DNA produces a mutation.

AGENTS THAT DAMAGE DNA

- Certain wavelengths of radiation:
  - Ionizing radiation, such as gamma rays and X-rays
  - Ultraviolet rays, especially the UV-C rays (~260 nm) that are absorbed strongly by DNA, but also the longer-wavelength UV-B that penetrates the ozone shield
- Highly-reactive oxygen radicals produced during normal cellular respiration as well as by other biochemical pathways
- Chemicals in the environment:
  - Many hydrocarbons, including some found in cigarette smoke
  - Some plant and microbial products, e.g., the aflatoxin produced in moldy peanuts
- Chemicals used in chemotherapy, especially chemotherapy of cancers.

Types of DNA Damage

DNA in cells suffers a wide range of damage:
- Purine bases are lost by spontaneous fission of the base-sugar link
- Cytosines, and occasionally adenines, spontaneously deaminate to produce uracil and hypoxanthine, respectively

- Many chemicals, for example alkylating agents, form adducts with DNA bases
- Reactive oxygen species in the cell attack purine and pyrimidine rings
- Errors in DNA replication result in incorporation of a mismatched base
- Ionizing radiation causes single- or double-strand breaks
- Errors in replication or recombination leave strand breaks in DNA
- Crosslinks covalent linkages can be formed between bases on the same DNA strand ("intrastrand") or on the opposite strand ("interstrand"). Ultraviolet light causes adjacent thymines to form a stable chemical dimer.

All these lesions must be repaired, if the cell is to survive. The importance of effective DNA repair systems is highlighted by the severe diseases affecting people with deficient repair systems.

THE MAJOR PATHWAYS OF DNA REPAIR

To cope with all these forms of damage, cells must be capable of several different types of DNA repair. DNA repair seldom involves simply undoing the change that caused the damage. Almost always a stretch of DNA containing the damaged nucleotide(s) is excised and the gap is filled by re-synthesis.

All proteins, from bacterial to human, involved in DNA repair can be grouped into the following major functional categories: (1) damage reversal, (2) base excision repair (BER), (3) nucleotide excision repair (NER), (4) mismatch repair (MMR), and (5) strand break repairs **(Fig. 20.5)**.

DAMAGE REVERSAL

The direct reversal of DNA damage is by far the simplest repair mechanism described until now. It consists of a single-polypeptide chain, with enzymatic properties, binding to the damage and restoring the DNA genome to its normal state in a single-reaction step. The major polypeptides involved in this pathway are:

i. DNA photolyase, which is the enzyme responsible for removing cyclobutane pyrimidine dimers from DNA in a light-dependent process denominated photo reactivation.
ii. O6-methylguanine-DNA methyltransferase I and II (MGMT), also called DNA-alkyltransferases, remove the modified bases, such as O6-alkylguanine and O4-alkylthymine.

The photolyase protein is not found in all living cells. However, the DNA-alkyltransferases are widespread in nature.

Some of the drugs used in cancer chemotherapy also damage DNA by alkylating. Some of the methyl groups can be removed MGMT enzyme; however, the enzyme can only do it once, so the removal of each methyl group requires another molecule of enzyme.

EXCISION OF DNA DAMAGE

There are three major pathways of DNA excision repair: (i) BER, (ii) NER, and (iii) MMR. In these reactions, a nucleotide segment containing base damage, double-helix distortion or mispaired bases is replaced by the normal nucleotide sequence in a new DNA polymerase synthesis process. All of these pathways have been characterized in both bacterial and eukaryotic organisms.

Base Excision Repair

Base excision repair (BER) is initiated by DNA glycosylases, which catalyze the hydrolysis of the N-glycosidic bonds, linking particular types of chemically altered bases to the deoxyribose-phosphate backbone. Thus, DNA damage is excised as free bases, generating sites of base loss called apurinic or apyrimidinic (AP) sites. Another means of AP site generation is the depurination or depyrimidination of DNA, due to spontaneous hydrolysis of N-glycosidic bonds **(Fig. 20.6)**. The AP sites are substrates for AP endonucleases. These enzymes produce incisions in duplex DNA as a result of the hydrolysis of a phosphodiester bond immediately 5′ or 3′ to each AP site. The ribose-phosphate backbone is then removed from the DNA through the action of a specific exonuclease called deoxyribophosphodiesterase or dRpase. Finally, the DNA polymerase and a ligase catalyze the incorporation of a specific deoxyribonucleotide into the repaired site, enabling correct base pairing **(Fig. 20.6)**.

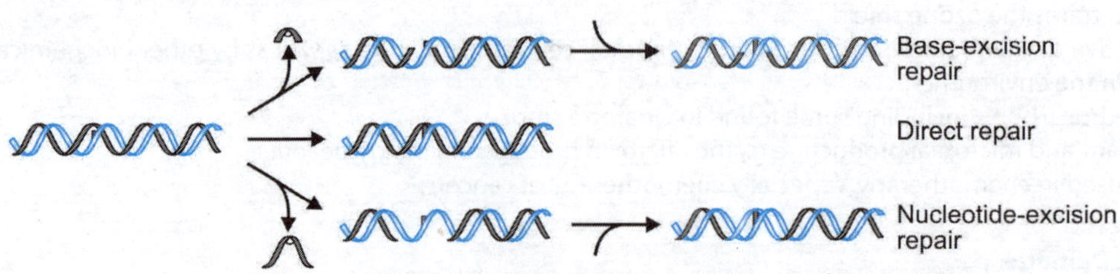

Fig. 20.5: DNA repair mechanisms.

Base excision repair is a multiple enzymatic DNA repair mechanism in which each enzyme works separately; this scenario has been maintained during evolution. The BER is essential to protect DNA from various types of lesions, , such as uracil, hydroxymethyluracil, methyl cytosine, hypoxanthine, G-T mispairs, 3-methyladenine, 7-methylguanine, 3-methylguanine, and pyrimidine dimers. Each of these is recognized by a specific DNA glycosylase.

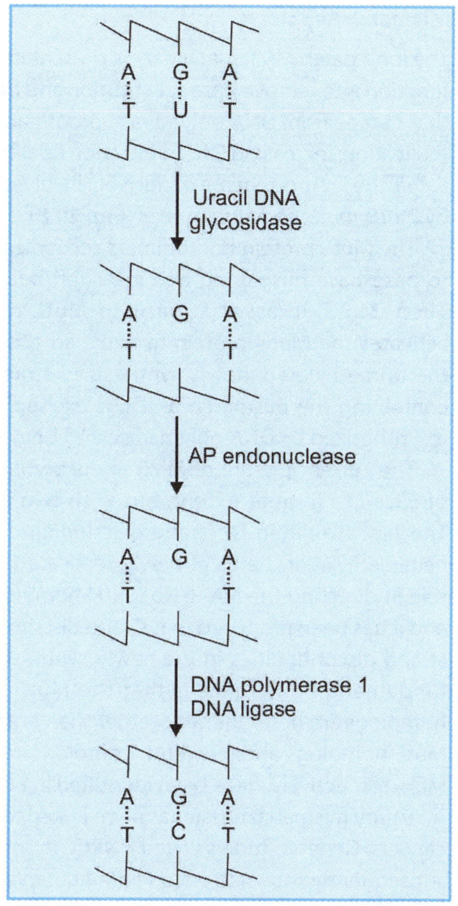

Fig. 20.6: Mechanism of basic excision repair system.

Nucleotide Excision Repair

Several types of agents generate bulky base adducts in DNA, leading to a significant distortion of the DNA helix. The most widely studied of these DNA damaging agents is UV radiation, responsible for thymine dimers, which produce a bend of ~30° in the DNA. Some chemical agents form DNA cross-links, which are particularly hazardous. These cross-links produce conformational distortions in DNA; they are substrates for DNA endonucleases that make an incision in DNA, several nucleotides to each side of the damage, generating a potential oligonucleotide fragment. Subsequent helicase reactions promote the excision of this fragment. The resulting gap is filled by DNA polymerase synthesis and covalently sealed by DNA ligase. These sequential enzymatic reactions, initiated by a specific endonuclease that recognizes the DNA distortion, are called NER. This pathway was originally described in the repair of DNA in cells exposed to UV radiation, which produces lesions , such as pyrimidine dimers and 6-4 photoproducts that are enzymatically excised from DNA as intact nucleotides rather than as free bases. NER is a much more complex biochemical process than BER, especially in eukaryotic cells. Several gene products are required in a multiple step process, during which the ordered assembly of DNA proteins provides an enzymatic complex that discriminates damaged from undamaged DNA.

In *Escherichia coli*, there are three specific proteins, called UvrA, B, and C, involved in lesion recognition and endonuclease incision. An assembly of two UvrA and one UvrB protein binds to DNA nonspecifically; this assembly translocates unidirectionally in the genome, driven by the energy of ATP hydrolysis. This mechanism allows constant monitoring for base damage in living cells. It has been suggested that when a damaged site is found, UvrA proteins dissociate and a stable UvrB-DNA complex is formed. Then the UvrC protein associates with high affinity to the UvrB-DNA site and induces a conformational change that enables bound UvrB protein to nick the DNA at the fourth nucleotide, 3′ to the site of damage. This reaction requires the binding of ATP by UvrB protein; however, no ATP hydrolysis occurs at this time. Following the 3′ incision, UvrC protein catalyzes nicking of the DNA at the seventh nucleotide, 5′ to the damage. Thus, a stretch of 12 nucleotides is held in the DNA by only hydrogen bonds. This fragment is released by UvrD helicase action, generating a gap that is finally submitted to repair synthesis **(Fig. 20.7)**.

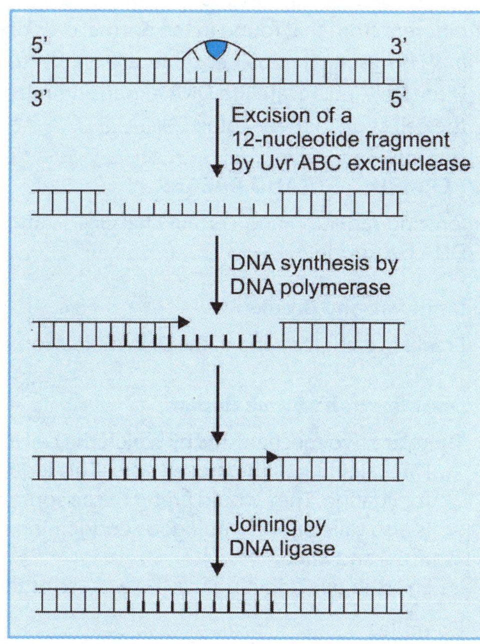

Fig. 20.7: Mechanism of nucleotide excision repair.

Transcription-coupled NER

Nucleotide-excision repair proceeds most rapidly:

- In cells whose genes are being actively transcribed
- On the DNA strand that is serving as the template for transcription.
- This enhancement of NER involves XPB, XPD, and several other gene products. The genes for two of them are designated *CSA* and *CSB* (mutations in them cause an inherited disorder called Cockayne's syndrome).

The CSB product associates in the nucleus with RNA polymerase II, providing a molecular link between transcription and repair.

If RNA polymerase II, tracking along the template (antisense) strand, encounters a damaged base, it can recruit other proteins, e.g., the CSA and CSB proteins, to make a quick fix before it moves on to complete transcription of the gene.

Mismatch Repair

The long patch MMR machinery is present in several organisms. Its function is to remove base substitution and frame shift mismatches that escape from DNA polymerase proofreading activity after DNA replication, increasing DNA replication fidelity 100- to 1,000-fold. In *E. coli*, the factors that are exclusively involved in MMR are encoded by *mutS, mutL, and mutH* genes **(Fig. 20.8)**.

The MutS protein homodimers recognize and bind specifically to base-base mispairing and insertion/deletion loop-outs (IDL). Then, MutS, in association with MutL protein homodimers, activates the MutH protein to make an excision-initiating nick in the unmethylated, newly synthesized strand. The nicked strand containing the mismatch or IDL is excised by exonucleases and resynthesized by DNA polymerase and DNA ligase.

The current picture of MMR in eukaryotic cells resembles that of *E. coli* to a great extent, but with two important differences. The first is related to strand discrimination. In eukaryotes, the hemimethylation status of newly replicated DNA does not play a role in directing the MMR. No MutH homolog has been identified and it has been proposed that strand discrimination is mediated by strand discontinuities in the newly synthesized DNA. The second fundamental difference is that the MutS and MutL functional homologs are heterodimeric rather than homodimeric. At least six MutS homologs and five MutL homologs, referred to as MSH and MLH, respectively, have been identified in eukaryotes.

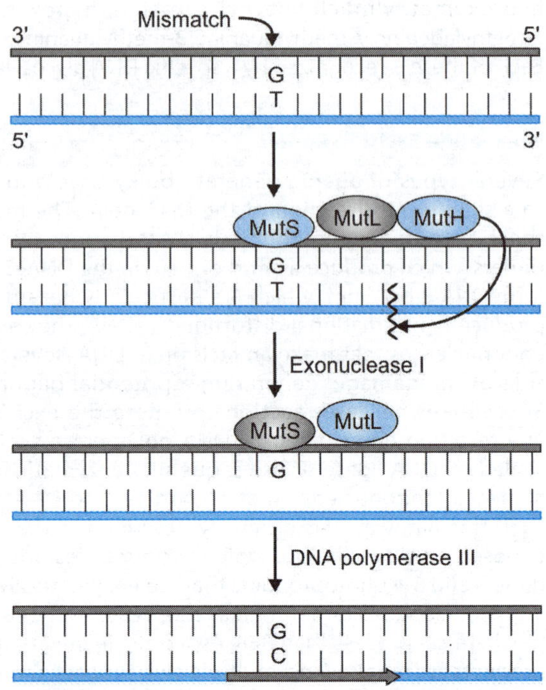

Fig. 20.8: Mechanism of mismatch repair system.

Faulty mismatch repair has been linked to hereditary nonpolyposis colon cancer (HNPCC), one of the most common inherited cancers. Genetic studies linked HNPCC in some families to a region of chromosome 2. The gene located, designated *hMSH2*, was subsequently shown to encode the human analog of the *E. coli* MutS protein that is involved in mismatch repair above. Mutations of *hMSH2* account for 50–60% of HNPCC cases. Another gene, *hMLH1*, is associated with most of the other cases. *hMLH1* is the human analog of the bacterial mismatch repair gene MutL. How does faulty mismatch repair result in colon cancer? The human genes were localized because microsatellite instability was detected. That is, the cancer cells had a microsatellite of a length different from that found in the normal cells of the individual. It appears that the affected cells, which harbor a mutated *hMSH2* or *hMLH1* mismatch repair enzyme, are unable to remove small loops of unpaired DNA, and the microsatellite thus increases in size. Ultimately, microsatellite DNA expansion must affect either the expression or the function of a protein critical in surveillance of the cell cycle in these colon cells.

REPAIRING STRAND BREAKS

Ionizing radiation and certain chemicals can produce both single-strand breaks (SSBs) and double-strand breaks (DSBs) in the DNA backbone.

Single-strand Breaks

Breaks in a single strand of the DNA molecule are repaired using the same enzyme systems that are used in base excision repair (BER).

Double-strand Break Repair

There are two mechanisms by which the cell attempts to repair a complete break in a DNA molecule:

1. Direct joining of the broken ends: This requires proteins that recognize and bind to the exposed ends and bring them together for ligating. They would prefer to see some complementary nucleotides but can proceed without them, so this type of joining is also called nonhomologous end-joining (NHEJ). A protein called Ku is essential for NHEJ. Ku is a heterodimer of the subunits Ku70 and Ku80.

   Errors in direct joining may be a cause of the various translocations that are associated with cancers.

Examples:
- Burkitt's lymphoma
- The Philadelphia chromosome in chronic myelogenous leukemia (CML)
- B-cell leukemia.

Generation of Antibody Diversity

Some of the same enzymes used to repair DSBs by direct joining are also used to break and reassemble the gene segments used to make antibody variable regions; that is, to accomplish V(D)J joining of different antibody classes; that is, to accomplish class switching.

2. **Homologous recombination:** Here, the broken ends are repaired using the information on the intact—
   - Sister chromatid, or on the
   - Homologous chromosome (in G1; that is, before each chromosome has been duplicated). This requires searching around in the nucleus for the homolog—a task sufficiently uncertain and G1 cells usually prefer to mend their DSBs by NHEJ or on the same chromosome, if there are duplicate copies of the gene on the chromosome oriented in opposite directions (head-to-head or back-to-back).

   Two of the proteins used in homologous recombination are encoded by the genes *BRCA1* and *BRCA2*. Inherited mutations in these genes predispose women to breast and ovarian cancers.

Meiosis also involves DSBs

Recombination between homologous chromosomes in meiosis I also involves the formation of DSBs and their repair. So, it is not surprising that this process uses the same enzymes. Meiosis I with the alignment of homologous sequences provides a mechanism for repairing damaged DNA; that is, mutations.

DISEASES ASSOCIATED WITH DEFECTIVE DNA REPAIR SYSTEM

Some of the examples include:

- Ataxia telangiectasia
- Bloom syndrome
- Cockayne's syndrome
- Progeria (Hutchinson–Gilford progeria syndrome)
- Rothmund–Thomson syndrome
- Trichothiodystrophy
- Werner syndrome
- Xeroderma pigmentosum
- Hereditary nonpolyposis colon cancer

Chapter 21

Organ Function Tests

LEARNING OBJECTIVES

To understand significance of organ function tests in the diagnosis and management of:

- ❖ Acute renal failure
- ❖ Chronic renal failure
- ❖ Diabetic nephropathy
- ❖ Nephrotic syndrome
- ❖ Acute myocardial infarction, and
- ❖ Liver diseases.

CASE STUDIES

CASE STUDY 1

Theme: Diagnosis and Management of Acute Renal Failure

A 50-year-old patient was seen in the emergency room for treatment of serious bilobar pneumonia. He was considered a high-risk patient due to his poorly controlled diabetes and therefore the team wanted to admit him for a few days of intravenous antibiotics rather than treat him as an outpatient. On admission, his blood urea nitrogen (BUN) was 53, probably reflecting dehydration from 4 days of illness, but his serum creatinine was 2.8, representing underlying kidney disease, which was probably a result of his long-standing diabetes.

On day 1 of admission, despite receiving 2 L of fluid in the emergency room, his BUN increased to 59 and his creatinine to 3.0. While these changes could represent a laboratory error, it was of concern that his creatinine and BUN were increasing, despite the fluid challenge. Over the day, his urine output which was initially brisk fell to 500 mL over a 24-hour period. On day 2, he developed shortness of breath and lower-extremity edema. The fluids were discontinued and laboratories revealed that his creatinine had risen to 6.3 and his BUN had increased to 90. He failed to respond to diuretics and a renal consult was called. The patient was immediately taken for hemodialysis.

What is the probable diagnosis?

CASE DETAILS

The patient is suffering from **"acute renal failure"**. A brief history, the rising BUN, and creatinine despite the fluid challenge: Oliguria, edema, and the failed response to diuretics all signify the underlying renal functional impairment. Retention of nitrogenous waste products, oliguria (urine output <400 mL/day contributing to extracellular fluid overload), and electrolyte and acid-base abnormalities are frequent clinical features of acute renal failure. Acute renal failure (ARF) is usually asymptomatic and diagnosed when biochemical monitoring of hospitalized patients reveals a new increase in blood urea and serum creatinine concentrations. ARF is often considered to be reversible, although a return to baseline serum creatinine concentrations postinjury might not be sufficiently sensitive to detect clinically significant irreversible damage that may ultimately contribute to chronic kidney disease.

ACUTE RENAL FAILURE

Basic Concept

ARF or acute kidney injury (AKI) is characterized by a rapid decline in glomerular filtration rate (GFR) over hours to days.

Classification of Acute Renal Failure

AKI may be classified into three general categories as follows:

1. Prerenal—as an adaptive response to severe volume depletion and hypotension, with structurally intact nephrons (~55%).
2. Intrinsic—in response to cytotoxic, ischemic, or inflammatory insults to the kidney, with structural and functional damage (~40%).
3. Postrenal—from obstruction to the passage of urine (~5%).

Etiology and Pathophysiology

Prerenal ARF (Prerenal Azotemia)

Prerenal azotemia is the most common cause of acute renal failure. It is owing to renal hypoperfusion. If the hypoperfusion is immediately reversed with restoration of renal blood flow, renal parenchymal damage does not occur. More severe or prolonged hypoperfusion may lead to ischemic injury, often termed as acute tubular necrosis or ATN. Thus, prerenal ARF and ischemic ATN fall along a spectrum of manifestations of renal hypoperfusion. Prerenal ARF can complicate any disease that induces hypovolemia (volume depletion), low cardiac output, systemic vasodilatation, or selective intrarenal vasoconstriction.

Causes of decreased renal perfusion:

1. **Causes of volume depletion (hypovolemia) include:**
   a. Increased extracellular fluid losses: Hemorrhage
   b. Gastrointestinal fluid loss: Vomiting, diarrhea
   c. Renal fluid loss: Diuretics, osmotic diuresis, and nephrogenic diabetes insipidus
   d. Extravascular sequestration: Burns, pancreatitis, and severe hypoalbuminemia (hypoproteinemia)
   e. Decreased intake: Dehydration, altered mental status.
2. **Altered renal hemodynamics resulting in hypoperfusion:**
   a. Low cardiac output state: Diseases of the myocardium, valves, and pericardium (including tamponade); pulmonary hypertension or massive pulmonary embolism leading to right and left heart failure
   b. Systemic vasodilation: Sepsis, antihypertensive, and anaphylaxis
   c. Renal vasoconstriction: Hypercalcemia, catecholamines
   d. Impairment of renal autoregulatory responses: Cyclo-oxygenase inhibitors (e.g., nonsteroidal anti-inflammatory drugs), angiotensin-converting enzyme inhibitors, or angiotensin II receptor blockers
   e. Hepatorenal syndrome.

Hepatorenal syndrome (HRS) is a unique form of prerenal ARF that frequently complicates advanced cirrhosis as well as acute liver failure. In HRS, the kidneys are structurally normal but fail due to splanchnic vasodilation and arteriovenous shunting, resulting in profound renal vasoconstriction. Correction of the underlying liver disease (e.g., by liver transplantation) results in resolution of the acute renal failure.

In states of mild hypoperfusion, glomerular perfusion and the filtration fraction are preserved through several compensatory mechanisms. With more severe hypoperfusion, these compensatory responses are overwhelmed and GFR falls, leading to prerenal ARF.

Intrinsic ARF

Intrinsic causes of ARF can be conceptually divided based on the predominant compartment of the kidney that is affected:

a. **Renovascular obstruction** (bilateral, or unilateral in the setting of one kidney):
   - Renal artery obstruction—atherosclerotic plaque, thrombosis, embolism, and dissection aneurysm
   - Renal vein obstruction—thrombosis or compression.

b. **Diseases of the glomeruli or vasculature:**
   - Glomerulonephritis or vasculitis
   - Others—thrombotic microangiopathy, malignant hypertension, and collagen vascular diseases.

c. **ATN:**
   - Ischemia—causes are the same as for prerenal ARF, but generally the insult is more severe and/or more prolonged
   - Infection, with or without sepsis syndrome
   - Nephrotoxins—antibiotics (e.g., aminoglycoside), chemotherapy (e.g., cisplatin), antifungal (e.g., amphotericin B), ethylene glycol, rhabdomyolysis, and hemolysis.

d. **Interstitial nephritis:**
   - Allergic—antibiotics (β-lactams, sulfonamides, quinolones, and rifampin), nonsteroidal anti-inflammatory drugs, diuretics, and other drugs

- Infection—pyelonephritis (if bilateral)
- Infiltration—lymphoma, leukemia, and sarcoidosis.

Prerenal ARF and ischemic ATN are both due to renal hypoperfusion. In its most extreme form, ischemia leads to bilateral renal cortical necrosis and irreversible renal failure. ATN differs from prerenal ARF in that the renal tubular epithelial cells are injured in the latter. Recovery typically takes 1–2 weeks after normalization of renal perfusion, as it requires repair and regeneration of renal cells.

A physiologic hallmark of ATN is a failure to maximally dilute or concentrate urine (isosthenuria). This defect is not responsive to pharmacologic doses of vasopressin. The injured kidney fails to generate and maintain a high medullary solute gradient, because the accumulation of solute in the medulla depends on normal distal nephron function. Failure to excrete concentrated urine even in the presence of oliguria is a helpful diagnostic clue in distinguishing prerenal from intrinsic renal disease; in prerenal azotemia, urine osmolality is typically >500 mOsm/kg, whereas in intrinsic renal disease, urine osmolality is less than 300 mOsm/kg.

Postrenal ARF (Obstruction)

Causes:

a. **Ureteric (bilateral, or unilateral in the case of one kidney)**—calculi, blood clots, cancer, and external compression (e.g., retroperitoneal fibrosis)
b. **Bladder neck**—neurogenic bladder, prostatic hypertrophy, calculi, blood clots, and cancer
c. **Urethra**—stricture or congenital valves.

If the site of obstruction is unilateral, then a rise in the serum creatinine level may not be apparent due to contralateral renal function. Although the serum creatinine level may remain low with unilateral obstruction, a significant loss of GFR occurs and patients with partial obstruction may develop progressive loss of GFR, if the obstruction is not relieved. Patients who develop anuria typically have obstruction at the level of the bladder or downstream to it.

Risk Factors

People with the following conditions are at a higher risk for developing AKI:

- Hypertension
- Congestive cardiac failure
- Diabetes
- Multiple myeloma
- Chronic infection
- Myeloproliferative disorder

Diagnosis

Distinguishing AKI from chronic renal failure is important. If review of laboratory records demonstrates that the rise in blood urea nitrogen and creatinine is recent, this suggests that the process is acute. A history of chronic symptoms—fatigue, weight loss, anorexia, nocturia, and pruritus—suggests chronic renal failure. Once a diagnosis of ARF has been established, the etiology of ARF needs to be determined.

History

History should include:

- History of nephrotoxic drug ingestion
- Blood loss or transfusions
- History of trauma or unaccustomed exertion
- Exposure to toxic substances, such as ethyl alcohol or ethylene glycol, mercury vapors, lead, cadmium, or other heavy metals
- Urine output history can be useful. Oliguria generally favors AKI. Abrupt anuria suggests acute urinary obstruction, acute and severe glomerulonephritis, or embolic renal artery occlusion. A gradually diminishing urine output may indicate a urethral stricture or bladder outlet obstruction due to prostate enlargement.

Clinical Manifestations

- Symptoms of prerenal ARF include thirst and orthostatic dizziness.
- Physical signs of orthostatic hypotension, tachycardia, reduced jugular venous pressure, decreased skin turgor, and dry mucous membranes suggest prerenal ARF.
- Fever, arthralgia, and a pruritic erythematous rash following exposure to a new drug suggest allergic interstitial nephritis, although systemic features of hypersensitivity are frequently absent.
- Flank pain may be a prominent symptom following occlusion of a renal artery or vein and with other parenchymal diseases distending the renal capsule (e.g., severe glomerulonephritis or pyelonephritis).
- ARF in association with oliguria, edema, and hypertension, with an "active" urine sediment (nephritic syndrome), suggests acute glomerulonephritis or vasculitis.

- Malignant hypertension may result in ARF, often in association with hypertensive injury to other organs (e.g., papilledema, neurologic dysfunction, and left ventricular hypertrophy) and may mimic glomerulonephritis in its other clinical manifestations.
- Postrenal ARF may present with suprapubic and flank pain due to distention of the bladder and of the renal collecting system and capsule, respectively. Colicky flank pain radiating to the groin suggests acute ureteric obstruction. Prostatic disease is likely if there is a history of nocturia, frequency, hesitancy and enlargement of the prostate on rectal examination.

Laboratory Investigations

Several laboratory tests are useful for assessing the etiology of AKI and the findings can aid in proper management. These tests include serum biochemistries, urine analysis with microscopy, and urine electrolytes.

- **Blood urea nitrogen (BUN) and serum creatinine:**
  - Although increased levels of BUN and creatinine are the hallmarks of renal failure, the rate of rise is dependent on the degree of renal insult as well as protein intake with respect to BUN.
  - The **ratio of BUN to creatinine** is an important finding because the ratio can exceed 20:1 in conditions in which enhanced reabsorption of urea is favored (e.g., in volume contraction); this suggests prerenal AKI.
  - BUN may be elevated in patients with GI or mucosal bleeding, steroid treatment, or protein loading.
  - As a general rule, if serum creatinine increases to >1.5 mg/dL/day, rhabdomyolysis must be ruled out.
- **Blood biochemistry and serological tests:**
  - The presence of myoglobin or free hemoglobin, increased serum uric acid level, and other related findings may help further define the etiology of AKI.
  - Serum electrolytes can be measured to know the extent of electrolyte imbalance since hyponatremia, hyperkalemia, hyperphosphatemia, hypocalcemia, hypermagnesemia, and metabolic acidosis are frequently present in patients of ARF.
  - Serologic tests for antinuclear antibody (ANA), hepatitis, antistreptolysin O (ASO), and complement levels may help include and exclude glomerular disease.
- **Urine analysis:**
  - Findings of granular, muddy-brown casts are suggestive of tubular necrosis.
  - Reddish brown or cola-colored urine suggests the presence of myoglobin or hemoglobin.
  - Significant proteinuria may be there, which would suggest glomerular or interstitial disease.
  - The presence of RBCs in the urine is always pathologic.
  - The presence of WBCs or WBC casts suggests pyelonephritis or acute interstitial nephritis.
  - The presence of eosinophils suggests interstitial nephritis but can also be seen in urinary tract infections, glomerulonephritis, and atheroembolic disease.
  - The presence of uric acid crystals may represent ATN associated with uric acid nephropathy.
  - Calcium oxalate crystals are usually present in cases of ethylene glycol poisoning.
- **Urine electrolytes:** Urine electrolyte findings also can serve as valuable indicators of functioning renal tubules.
- **Imaging studies:**
  In some cases, renal imaging is useful, especially if renal failure is secondary to obstruction.
  - Ultrasonography—renal ultrasonography is useful for evaluating existing renal disease and obstruction of the urinary collecting system.
  - Ultrasonographic scans or other imaging studies showing small kidneys suggest chronic renal failure.
  - CT or MRI scan can be of diagnostic significance.
- **Doppler ultrasonography:**
  - Doppler scans are useful for detecting the presence and nature of renal blood flow and in the diagnosis of thromboembolic or renovascular disease.
- **Nuclear scans:**
  - Radionuclide imaging with technetium-99m mercaptoacetyltriglycine can be used to assess renal blood flow and tubular functions.
- **Aortorenal angiography**—it can be helpful in establishing the diagnosis of renal vascular diseases including renal artery stenosis, renal atheroembolic disease, and atherosclerosis with aortorenal occlusion.
  Renal biopsy: Biopsy is reserved for patients in whom prerenal and postrenal ARF have been excluded and the cause of intrinsic ARF is unclear.

Complications

ARF is frequently complicated by intravascular volume overload, hyponatremia, hyperkalemia, hyperphosphatemia, hypocalcemia, hypermagnesemia, and metabolic acidosis. In addition, patients are unable to excrete nitrogenous waste products and are prone to develop the uremic syndrome. The speed of development and the severity of these complications reflect the degree of renal impairment and catabolic state of the patient.

- Expansion of extracellular fluid volume is an inevitable consequence of diminished salt and water excretion in oliguric or anuric individuals. The continued volume expansion may precipitate life-threatening pulmonary edema. Excessive administration of free water, either through ingestion and nasogastric administration or as hypotonic saline or isotonic dextrose solutions, can induce hypoosmolality and hyponatremia, which, if severe, lead to neurologic abnormalities, including seizures.

- Hyperkalemia is a frequent complication of ARF. Coexistent metabolic acidosis may exacerbate hyperkalemia by promoting potassium efflux from cells. Mild hyperkalemia (<6.0 mmol/L) is usually asymptomatic. Higher levels may trigger electrocardiographic abnormalities and/or arrhythmias.
- ARF is typically complicated by metabolic acidosis, often with an increased anion gap. Acidosis can be particularly severe when endogenous production of hydrogen ions is increased by other mechanisms (e.g., diabetic or fasting ketoacidosis; lactic acidosis complicating generalized tissue hypoperfusion, liver disease, or sepsis; and metabolism of ethylene glycol or methanol).
- Hyperphosphatemia is an almost invariable complication of ARF. Metastatic deposition of calcium phosphate can lead to hypocalcemia, particularly with elevation of serum calcium (mg/dL) and phosphate (mg/dL) concentrations. Other factors that contribute to hypocalcemia include tissue resistance to the actions of parathyroid hormone and reduced levels of 1,25-dihydroxyvitamin D.
- Anemia develops rapidly in ARF and is usually multifactorial in origin. Contributing factors include impaired erythropoiesis, hemolysis, bleeding, hemodilution, and reduced red cell survival time.
- Prolongation of the bleeding time is also common. Common contributors to the bleeding diathesis include mild thrombocytopenia, platelet dysfunction, and/or clotting factor abnormalities (e.g., factor VIII dysfunction).
- Infection is a common and serious complication of ARF.
- Cardiopulmonary complications of ARF include arrhythmias, pericarditis.
- Protracted periods of severe ARF are invariably associated with the development of the uremic syndrome.
- A vigorous diuresis can occur during the recovery phase of ARF, which may be inappropriate on occasion and leads to intravascular volume depletion.
- Hypernatremia can also complicate recovery if water losses via hypotonic urine are not replaced or if losses are inappropriately replaced by relatively hypertonic saline solutions.

Treatment

- Aggressive treatment should begin at the earliest indication of renal dysfunction. A large proportion of the renal mass is damaged before any biochemical evidence of renal dysfunction is appreciated because the relationship between the GFR and the serum creatinine level is exponential, not linear. The rise of serum creatinine may not be evident before 50% of the GFR is lost.
- Recognizing the presence of AKI and promptly initiating therapy aimed at minimizing the damage to the remaining functional renal mass are important considerations. This may also aid in reversing the renal damage that has already occurred. Reversing renal damage can be accomplished only by identifying the underlying cause and directing the appropriate therapy.
- Maintenance of volume homeostasis and correction of biochemical abnormalities remain the primary goals of treatment.
- All nephrotoxic agents (e.g., radiocontrast agents, antibiotics with nephrotoxic potential, heavy metal preparations, cancer chemotherapeutic agents, and NSAIDs) are either avoided or used with extreme caution. Similarly, all medications cleared by renal excretion should be avoided or their doses should be adjusted appropriately.
- Correcting acidosis with bicarbonate administration is important. It cannot be overstated that the current treatment of AKI is mainly supportive in nature and no therapeutic modalities to date have shown efficacy in treating the condition.
- Hyperkalemia which can be life-threatening should be treated by decreasing the intake of potassium, delaying the absorption of potassium, exchanging potassium across the gut lumen using potassium-binding resins, controlling intracellular shifts, and instituting dialysis.
- Correcting hematologic abnormalities (e.g., anemia, platelet dysfunction) warrant appropriate measures, including transfusions and administration of desmopressin or estrogens.

Diet

- Dietary modulation is an important facet of the treatment of AKI. Diet and fluid restriction become crucial in the management of oliguric renal failure, wherein the kidneys do not adequately excrete either toxins or fluids.
- Calculation of the nitrogen balance can be challenging especially in the presence of volume contraction, hypercatabolic states, gastrointestinal bleeding, and diarrheal disease.

Medication

Diuretics, vasodilators, calcium channel blockers, and N-acetylcysteine can be given depending upon the state of the patient.

Dialysis

During ARF, dialysis is often used to support renal function until renal repair/recovery occurs. Absolute indications for dialysis include symptoms or signs of the uremic syndrome and management of refractory hypervolemia, hyperkalemia, or acidosis.

Mortality/Morbidity of Acute Renal Failure

The mortality rate estimates for ARF vary from 25 to 90%. The in-hospital mortality rate is 40–50%; in intensive care settings, the rate is 70–80%. Increments of 0.3 mg/dL in serum creatinine have important prognostic significance.

On long-term follow-up, (1–10 years), approximately 12.5% of ARF survivors are dialysis-dependent and 19–31% of them have chronic kidney disease.

CLINICAL NOTE

A large proportion of the renal mass is damaged before any biochemical evidence of renal dysfunction is appreciated because the relationship between the GFR and the serum creatinine level is exponential, not linear.

CLINICAL PEARLS

1. ARF or AKI is characterized by a rapid decline in GFR over hours to days.
2. AKI may be classified into three general categories: Prerenal—as an adaptive response to severe volume depletion and hypotension, with structurally intact nephrons, intrinsic—in response to cytotoxic, ischemic, or inflammatory insults to the kidney, with structural and functional damage, and postrenal—from obstruction to the passage of urine.
3. The laboratory tests for the diagnosis include serum biochemistries, urine analysis with microscopy, and urine electrolytes.
4. ARF is frequently complicated by intravascular volume overload, hyponatremia, hyperkalemia, hyperphosphatemia, hypocalcemia, hypermagnesemia, and metabolic acidosis.
5. Recognizing the presence of AKI and promptly initiating therapy aimed at minimizing the damage to the remaining functional renal mass are important considerations.

CASE STUDY 2

Theme: Diagnosis and Management of Chronic Renal Failure

A 53-year-old male was admitted to the hospital with loss of appetite, nausea, vomiting, difficulty in breathing, and fatigability. History revealed that he was hospitalized for the second time. He was diagnosed of hypertension and kidney failure 5 years back. He was admitted due to body weakness and severe anemia. He was a chronic smoker and he consumed 8 sticks/day. He was also an occasional drinker.

On examination: His initial vital signs were as follows: Body temperature—36.8°C, respiratory rate—22 breaths/min, pulse rate—64 beats/min, and BP—170/100 mm Hg. Marked pallor was there, chest and lungs—with bilateral basal rales.

Abdomen—soft, flat, and tender. No other abnormality was detected.

The patient was admitted and he was advised to have laboratory examination.

Blood biochemistry revealed:
- Serum creatinine—2.5 mg%
- Blood urea—67 mg%
- Serum calcium—6.5 mg%
- Serum potassium—4.78 mmol/L
- Serum Na—137 mmol/L.

Urine examination revealed:
- Color—light yellow
- pH—5.0
- Specific gravity—1.020
- Appearance—turbid
- Volume—600 mL/24 h
- Albumin—3+
- Sugar—negative
- Pus cells—1–3/HPF
- Red blood cells—1–2/HPF
- Epithelial cells—rare.

What is the probable diagnosis? Comment on the laboratory findings.

CASE DETAILS

The characteristic symptoms and laboratory findings in this patient (high blood urea and creatinine level, hypocalcemia, anemia, proteinuria, and electrolyte imbalance) are suggestive of renal functional impairment.

The patient is most probably suffering from chronic renal disease. The past history of hypertension and hospitalization with kidney failure exclude the possibility of acute renal failure.

BASIC CONCEPT

Chronic Kidney Disease

Chronic kidney disease is long-standing, progressive deterioration of renal function. Symptoms develop slowly and include anorexia, nausea, vomiting, stomatitis, nocturia, lassitude, fatigue, pruritus, decreased mental acuity, muscle twitches and cramps, water retention, undernutrition, GI ulceration and bleeding, peripheral neuropathies, and seizures. Diagnosis is based on laboratory testing of renal function, sometimes followed by renal biopsy. Treatment is primarily directed at the underlying condition but includes fluid and electrolyte management, erythropoietin for anemia, and often dialysis or transplantation.

Etiology

Major causes of chronic renal failure are as follows:

a. **Glomerulopathies:**
   - Primary glomerular diseases:
     - Focal and segmental glomerulosclerosis
     - Membranoproliferative glomerulonephritis
     - IgA nephropathy
     - Membranous nephropathy.
   - Secondary glomerular diseases:
     - Diabetic nephropathy
     - Amyloidosis
     - Postinfectious glomerulonephritis
     - HIV-associated nephropathy
     - Collagen-vascular diseases
     - Sickle cell nephropathy
     - HIV-associated membranoproliferative glomerulonephritis.

b. **Tubulointerstitial nephritis:**
   - Drug hypersensitivity
   - Heavy metals
   - Analgesic nephropathy
   - Reflux/chronic pyelonephritis
   - Idiopathic.

c. **Hereditary diseases:**
   - Polycystic kidney disease:
     - Medullary cystic disease
     - Alport's syndrome.

d. **Obstructive nephropathies:**
   - Prostatic disease
   - Nephrolithiasis
   - Retroperitoneal fibrosis/tumor
   - Congenital

e. **Vascular diseases:**
   - Hypertensive nephrosclerosis
   - Renal artery stenosis

The most common cause is diabetic nephropathy, followed by hypertensive nephroangiosclerosis and various primary and secondary glomerulopathies. Metabolic syndrome, in which hypertension and type 2 diabetes are present, is a large and growing cause of renal damage.

Incidence

Chronic kidney disease affects up to 20 million Americans, or one in nine adults. Most are unaware of the condition because they remain asymptomatic until the disease has significantly progressed.

Pathophysiology

Chronic kidney disease can be classified as—decreased renal reserve, renal insufficiency, or renal failure (end-stage renal disease). Initially, as kidney starts losing function, there are only a few alterations as the residual tissue enhances its performance (renal functional adaptation), a loss of approximately 75% of renal tissue produces a fall in GFR to only 50% of normal.

Decreased renal function affects the ability of the kidney to maintain fluid and electrolyte balance. **The concentrating ability decreases early, which is followed by a decrease in the ability to excrete phosphate, acid, and K.** With advanced renal failure (GFR ≤ 10 mL/min/1.73 m^2), the ability to dilute urine is lost; thus, urine osmolality is usually fixed close to that of plasma (300–320 mOsm/kg) and variations in water intake do not readily affect the urinary volume. As the GFR falls, the plasma levels of urea and creatinine start rising, as they are much dependent on glomerular filtration. Initially, there are minimum alterations, but as the GFR falls below 10 mL/min/1.73 m^2 (standard = 100 mL/min/1.73 m^2), their levels start rising rapidly and are associated with systemic manifestations (uremia). The clinical signs in uremia are not due to elevated levels of urea and creatinine. However, these levels mark the elevation of other toxic substances that cause the symptoms.

Although GFR decreases, yet by increased fractional loss of sodium and normal physiological response to thirst, the Na and water homeostasis is well-maintained. Therefore, unless dietary intake of sodium or water is varied, the plasma levels of sodium are characteristically within the normal range and hypervolemia is rare. Na and water overload can cause heart failure, especially in patients with decreased cardiac reserve. As K secretion is regulated chiefly through distal nephron secretion, its plasma level is maintained within the normal limits by renal functional adaptation until renal failure has progressed.

Variations in the levels of calcium, phosphate, and parathyroid hormone (PTH) are observed. Similarly, impairment in the metabolism of vitamin D and renal osteodystrophy can also occur. Hypocalcemia and hyperphosphatemia are frequently seen, while hypocalcemia is the outcome of decreased renal activation of vitamin D and hyperphosphatemia occurs due to reduced excretion of phosphates.

Secondary hyperparathyroidism frequently develops in renal failure even before the onset of variations in Ca or phosphate levels.

Renal osteodystrophy (aberrant bone mineralization) may result secondary to vitamin D deficiency, hyperparathyroidism, high phosphate, or low serum calcium levels. The bone turnover may be high, as in hyperparathyroidism, or low, such as in adynamic bone disease due to increased parathyroid suppression, or osteomalacia. Osteopenia or osteomalacia may develop secondary to calcitriol deficiency.

Metabolic acidosis (low plasma HCO_3^- content in the range of 15–20 mmol/L) and anemia are characteristic of renal failure. The anemia of CKD is usually caused by reduced erythropoietin production secondary to a reduced functional renal mass. It is normochromic-normocytic, with an hematocrit (Hct) of 20–30% (35–50% in patients with polycystic kidney disease). Anemia due to deficiencies of iron, folate, and vitamin B_{12} can also be observed.

Chronic kidney disease leads to a progressive functional decline. It is rarely reversible and the decline occurs despite the elimination of the triggering event. Hypertrophy of the remaining nephrons with hyperfiltration happens in response to a reduction in renal mass.

In these nephrons, the glomerular filtration rate is at supranormal levels for a short time. These alterations put a load on the remaining nephrons causing progressive glomerular sclerosis and interstitial fibrosis. Thus, implying that hyperfiltration may even worsen renal function.

Symptoms and Signs

Patients with slightly decreased renal reserve generally have no symptoms. Even with mild-to-moderate renal insufficiency symptoms may be absent despite the raised BUN and creatinine levels. **Nocturia** is frequently observed, chiefly resulting from a failure to concentrate the urine. **Malaise, fatigue, loss of appetite, and reduced mental acuity are the common earliest symptoms of uremia.**

With the setting of more severe renal insufficiency (e.g., creatinine clearance <10 mL/min for patients without diabetes and <15 mL/min for those with diabetes), **neuromuscular symptoms may develop, such as coarse muscular twitches, muscle cramps, peripheral neuropathies (sensory and motor), hyperreflexia, and seizures.** The seizures develop secondary to hypertensive or metabolic encephalopathy.

Loss of appetite, nausea, vomiting, loss of weight, stomatitis, and an unpleasant taste in the mouth are almost always present. The skin may become yellow-brown in color due to the crystallization of urea from sweat on the skin (uremic frost). Pruritus is frequently present and causes much discomfort. Generalized tissue wasting due to **undernutrition** is a prominent feature of chronic uremia.

In advanced CKD, pericarditis, gastrointestinal ulceration, and hemorrhages are very common. Hypertension is present in majority (>80%) of patients with advanced CKD. It is usually related to hypervolemia and occasionally occurs as a result of activation of the renin-angiotensin-aldosterone system. Cardiomyopathy (hypertensive, ischemic) and renal retention of Na and water can lead to dependent edema and heart failure.

Diagnosis

- Electrolytes
- BUN, creatinine

- Phosphate, Ca
- CBC
- Urinalysis (including urinary sediment examination)
- Ultrasonography, and
- Renal biopsy

The suspicion of CKD arises when serum creatinine starts rising. The first step is to identify whether the renal failure is acute, chronic, or acute superimposed on chronic. The etiology of renal failure is also determined. The duration of renal failure helps to investigate the cause; at times, the cause can be easily defined than the period and identifying the cause helps to determine the length of time.

Laboratory investigations include **urinalysis with an examination of the urinary sediment, serum electrolytes, blood urea nitrogen, creatinine, phosphate, Ca, and CBC.** Specific serologic tests are sometimes required to determine the cause. Differentiation of acute from chronic renal failure can be carried out by a history of an elevated creatinine level or abnormal urinalysis. The findings of urinalysis are based on the nature of the underlying defect, but broad (>3 WBC diameters wide) or especially waxy casts often are predominantly found in the advanced renal failure of any etiology.

An ultrasound examination of the kidneys generally helps in evaluating for obstructive uropathy and in differentiating acute from chronic renal failure depending on kidney size. Exempting certain conditions, patients with chronic renal failure often have small shrunken kidneys (usually <10 cm in length) with thinned, hyperechoic cortex. Making a specific diagnosis becomes increasingly challenging as renal function touches values nearly those of end-stage renal disease.

The confirmation of the diagnostic is done by **renal biopsy**, but when ultrasonography indicates small, fibrotic kidneys, renal biopsy is not recommended.

Classification

Staging of chronic kidney disease is a process of assessing the severity of CKD. Chronic kidney disease has been classified into five stages:

- Stage 1: Normal GFR (>90 mL/min/1.73 m^2) plus either continuous albuminuria or known the structural or hereditary renal disease
- Stage 2: GFR 60–89 mL/min/1.73 m^2
- Stage 3: GFR 30–59 mL/min/1.73 m^2
- Stage 4: GFR 15–29 mL/min/1.73 m^2
- Stage 5: GFR <15 mL/min/1.73 m^2

Treatment

- Management of primary defect
- Restriction of dietary protein, phosphate, and potassium
- Supplementation with vitamin D
- Treatment of anemia, acidosis, and heart failure
- Adjustment of all doses of drugs as required
- Dialysis in patients with severely decreased GFR, uremic symptoms, hyperkalemia, or heart failure.

The primary defect and contributory factors need to be managed. Specifically, regulating blood glucose concentration in patients with diabetic nephropathy and controlling hypertension in all patients considerably slows the deterioration of GFR. BP should be maintained at about 110–130/<80 mm Hg. ACE inhibitors and angiotensin II receptor blockers are recommended to decrease the rate of decline in GFR in patients with most causes of chronic kidney disease, particularly those with proteinuria.

Physical activity should be restricted, although fatigue and malaise usually limit a patient's capacity for exercise. Pruritus due to hyperphosphatemia may respond to phosphate binders. If not response occurs, ultraviolet phototherapy can help.

Nutrition: Extreme protein restriction in renal disease is contentious. However, moderate restriction (0.8 g/kg/day) is justified and convenient for most patients to tolerate. Many uremic symptoms are grossly reduced when protein catabolism and urea production are reduced. Adequate carbohydrate and fat are recommended to meet energy requirements and prevent ketosis.

As dietary restrictions may decrease optimum vitamin intake, therefore, patients should be prescribed at least water-soluble vitamins. Vitamin D, as 1,25-dihydroxyvitamin D, should be supplemented as identified by PTH concentrations.

Dietary modification may benefit hypertriglyceridemia. In patients with hypercholesterolemia, statins are effective. Correction of hypercholesterolemia can decrease the progression of the underlying renal disease and lessen coronary risk.

Fluid and electrolytes: Water intake is reduced only when serum Na concentration is <135 mmol/L.

Na restriction of 2 g/day helps patients, especially those with edema, heart failure, or hypertension.

K intake: Hyperkalemia is less common until end-stage renal failure, when intake may need to be decreased to ≤50 mmol/day.

Phosphate restriction to <1 g/day is generally sufficient to maintain phosphate level in the required range during the early phase of stages 3 and 4 chronic kidney disease. However, in the later stages, phosphate binders, such as Ca salts are often required.

Mild **acidosis** (pH 7.30–7.35) needs no treatment. However, most patients with chronic metabolic acidosis with a pH <7.3 have a plasma HCO_3^- content <15 mmol/L and symptoms of anorexia, lassitude, dyspnea, heightened protein catabolism and renal osteodystrophy. $NaHCO_3$ 1–2 g per orally twice/day is recommended and the dose is increased slowly until HCO_3^- level is about 20 mEq/L or until evidence of Na overloading prevents further therapy.

Anemia and coagulation disorders: Anemia is treated to maintain the Hb between 11 and 12 g/dL. Anemia gradually responds to recombinant human erythropoietin. Due to increased iron utilization with stimulated erythropoiesis, iron stores should be replaced, generally with parenteral iron. Iron levels, iron-binding capacity, and ferritin levels should be followed carefully. Blood transfusion is not recommended unless anemia is severe (Hb <8 g/dL) or causes symptoms. The bleeding tendency in CKD infrequently needs treatment.

Heart failure: Symptomatic heart failure is managed with Na restriction and diuretics. Sometimes, dialysis can be required to control heart failure.

Dialysis: Dialysis is started when GFR reaches ≤10 mL/min in a patient without diabetes or ≤15 mL/min in a patient with diabetes. Patients with uremic symptoms, such as anorexia, vomiting, weight loss, pericarditis, pleuritis, or fluid overload who have no other conditions that explain these symptoms should be started on dialysis even if GFR has not reached these levels. Other indications for dialysis in chronic kidney disease include hyperkalemia that causes ECG changes or that is persistent (K >6 mmol/L) despite dietary restriction, heart failure, poorly controlled with drugs, and metabolic acidosis that is difficult to control.

Transplantation: If a living kidney donor is available, better long-term outcomes occur when a patient receives the transplanted kidney early, even before beginning dialysis.

Prognosis

The most common cause of death is cardiac dysfunction (45%). Other causes include infection (14%), cerebrovascular disease (6%), and malignancy (4%). Diabetes, age, a low serum albumin, lower socioeconomic status, and inadequate dialysis are all significant predictors of mortality.

For those who require dialysis to sustain life but elect not to undergo dialysis, death ensues within days to weeks.

CLINICAL NOTE

Sometimes determining the duration of renal failure helps determine the cause; sometimes, it is easier to determine the cause than the duration and determining the cause helps determine the duration.

CLINICAL PEARLS

1. Chronic kidney disease is long-standing, progressive deterioration of renal function.
2. Symptoms develop slowly and include anorexia, nausea, vomiting, stomatitis, nocturia, lassitude, fatigue, pruritus, decreased mental acuity, muscle twitches and cramps, water retention, undernutrition, GI ulceration and bleeding, peripheral neuropathies, and seizures.
3. Diagnosis is based on laboratory testing of renal function, sometimes followed by renal biopsy.
4. Treatment is primarily directed at the underlying condition but includes fluid and electrolyte management, erythropoietin for anemia, and often dialysis or transplantation.
5. Dialysis is initiated when GFR reaches ≤10 mL/min in a patient without diabetes or ≤15 mL/min in a patient with diabetes.

RENAL CLEARANCE

Renal clearance is a measurement to analyze the functions of the kidney. By definition, clearance is **the volume of plasma from which a substance is completely removed by the excretion through kidney in a given amount of time** (usually a minute). For example, the clearance for urea is 75 mL/min. This means that the kidney removes all of the urea in 75 mL of plasma in 1 minute.

Every minute approximately 625 mL of plasma flows to the kidney. This is the renal plasma flow. Some of the fluid leaves the kidney in the plasma while some leaves the kidney as urine. There are only two ways for a substance to end up in the urine: Either it is **filtered** at the glomerulus and then not **reabsorbed** from the tubules, or the substance is not filtered but is **secreted** by the **peritubular capillaries** into the tubules **(Fig. 21.1)**. In either instance, the substance ends up in the collecting duct and is excreted into the urine.

Of the 625 mL/min of plasma that goes to the glomerulus, 125 mL/min is filtered into Bowman's capsule forming the filtrate (the rate of filtration is known as the glomerular filtration rate—GFR). The remaining 500 mL/min enters into the **peritubular capillaries.** Of the 125 mL/min filtered, almost all of the water in this fluid is reabsorbed back into the blood. The composition of the filtrate in Bowman's capsule is **identical** to the composition of the plasma, except that the filtrate has no or very little amount of proteins.

Any substance which is freely filtered by the glomerulus and is neither reabsorbed nor secreted, ends up in the urine. Thus, all the plasma that gets filtered is **cleared** of **that substance** (that is, all the **substance** in the filtrate gets excreted) while the **substance** that is not filtered (and thus remains in the plasma) is not excreted. Since clearance is defined as the volume of plasma "cleared" of a substance in 1 minute, the clearance for **that substance** would be 125 mL/min. This means that out of the 625 mL of plasma that come to the kidney in 1 minute, 125 mL (the fraction that is filtered) has all of the **substance** removed from it in that minute, the other 500 mL (the fraction that is not filtered) keeps it as there is no way for the **substance** to get into the urine as it is not secreted.

The GFR is typically recorded in units of *volume per time*, e.g., milliliters per minute (mL/min).

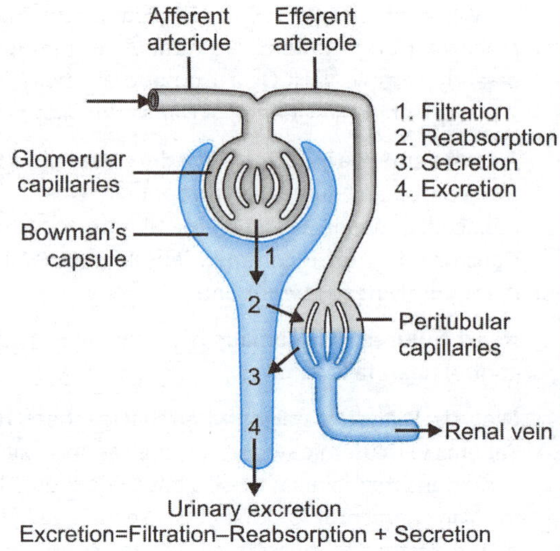

Fig. 21.1: Basic renal process of filtration, reabsorption, secretion, and excretion.

$$GFR = \frac{\text{Urine concentration} \times \text{Urine flow}}{\text{Plasma concentration}}$$

The compound **inulin is cleared in the same as mentioned above.** All of the plasma that is filtered is cleared of inulin so that if one has to measure the clearance of inulin, it would be equal to the amount of plasma filtered in a minute, the **glomerular filtration rate**. Therefore, the clearance of inulin is equal to the **glomerular filtration rate,** the volume of plasma filtered in 1 minute. Inulin is not a normal metabolite of the body; it is, in fact, administered to determine the functional status of the kidney.

The clearance of any other substance is not similar to clearance of inulin. For example, glucose, like inulin, is freely filtered. Thus, glucose is present in Bowman's capsule. However, glucose does not appear in urine because glucose is completely reabsorbed as it passes through the tubules. Inulin is not reabsorbed. This means all of the glucose that comes to the kidney is saved and leaves the kidney in the plasma and that no glucose is excreted into the urine. The clearance of glucose is, therefore, 0 mL/min as no plasma has its glucose removed as it passes through the kidney. This would be true for any substance that is completely reabsorbed. Hence, if the clearance of tryptophan (an amino acid) is 0 mL/min, it can be inferred that tryptophan must be completely reabsorbed (as long as it is freely filtered).

Taking the example of another substance, para-aminohippuric acid (PAH), it is freely filtered, not reabsorbed, and is completely secreted by the kidney. Thus, all of the PAH entering the kidney ends up in the urine, both the PAH that is filtered and that is not filtered. This means that all the plasma entering the kidneys would be cleared of PAH. Since the **renal plasma flow** is about 625 mL/min in a "normal" kidney, the clearance of PAH must be 625 mL/min. Therefore, the PAH clearance is equal to the **renal plasma flow**. PAH clearance is used to determine whether the kidneys have an adequate plasma flow.

Now, if the clearance of a substance is 625 mL/min, this would suggest that the kidney completely secretes this substance (that is, the kidney "treats" this substance the same as PAH which is known to be completely secreted). Using similar logic, a clearance value of 125 would suggest that the kidney neither reabsorbs nor secretes the substance and a clearance value of 0 suggests that the kidney completely reabsorbs the substance (assuming that the substance is freely filterable in the glomerulus).

The urea clearance has been measured to be 75 mL/min. What does the kidney "do" with urea (does it reabsorb, secrete, or neither)? Well if urea is completely reabsorbed, its clearance should be like that of glucose (0 mL/min) and if urea is not reabsorbed at all (and not secreted), its clearance should be 125 mL/min. Since the value of urea clearance is 75 mL/min, which means urea is partially reabsorbed. Note that the common belief concerning kidney function is that it removes urea from the blood yet the nephron partially reabsorbs urea. Thus, urea clearance is not a true predictor of glomerular filtration rate as is inulin clearance.

In clinical practice, however, **creatinine clearance** or estimates of creatinine clearance based on the serum creatinine level are used to measure GFR. Creatinine is produced naturally by the body (creatinine is a breakdown product of creatine phosphate, which is found in muscle). It is freely filtered by the glomerulus, but also actively secreted by the peritubular capillaries in very small amounts such that creatinine clearance overestimates actual GFR by 10–20%. This margin of error is acceptable, considering the ease with which creatinine clearance is measured. Unlike precise GFR measurements involving constant infusions of inulin, creatinine is already at a steady-state concentration in the blood, and so measuring creatinine clearance is much less cumbersome.

CASE STUDY 3

Theme: Diagnosis and Management of Diabetic Nephropathy

A 35-year-old African male was seen in the nephrology clinic on the advice and referral of his primary care physician. A recent fasting lipoprotein analysis revealed a low-density lipoprotein (LDL) cholesterol level of 145 mg/dL, a high-density lipoprotein (HDL) cholesterol level of 36 mg/dL, a triglyceride level of 420 mg/dL, and a total cholesterol level of 280 mg/dL.

At the time of presentation to the clinic, his blood pressure was high (190/100 mm Hg), although there was no evidence of coronary heart disease (CHD) or peripheral vascular disease.

A fasting serum glucose level drawn in the clinic revealed a level of 212 mg/dL and a glycosylated hemoglobin level of 10.5%. A urine dipstick test with Micral-Test II strips (specific for detecting microalbuminuria) showed an albumin excretion of 135 mg/L. To confirm this finding, a 24-hour urine collection was performed that revealed an albumin excretion of 90 µg/min (130 g/day). Serum blood urea nitrogen (BUN) and creatinine level were checked and revealed a value of 28 mg/dL and 1.9 mg/dL, respectively. Baseline serum creatinine was found to be 0.9 mg/dL.

His past medical history was relatively benign except for a 13-year history of type 1 insulin-dependent diabetes mellitus. He never had any previous hospitalizations. His medications included isophane insulin suspension (NPH) [Novolin (R) N] 22 units every morning before breakfast along with the use of a regular insulin sliding scale, depending on the results of his home blood glucose monitoring.

What is the probable diagnosis?

The patient is suffering from diabetic nephropathy.

Diabetic nephropathy (*nephropatia diabetica*), also known as Kimmelstiel–Wilson syndrome and intercapillary glomerulonephritis, is a progressive kidney disease, caused by angiopathy of capillaries in the kidney glomeruli and it is characterized by nephrotic syndrome and diffuse glomerulosclerosis. It is due to long-standing diabetes mellitus and is a prime cause for dialysis in many Western countries.

BASIC CONCEPT

Diabetic Nephropathy

The chronic complications of diabetes mellitus (DM) affect many organ systems and are responsible for the majority of morbidity and mortality associated with the disease. Chronic complications can be divided into vascular and nonvascular complications. The vascular complications of DM are further subdivided into microvascular (retinopathy, neuropathy, and nephropathy) and macrovascular complications [coronary artery disease (CAD), peripheral arterial disease (PAD), and cerebrovascular disease)]. Nonvascular complications include problems, such as gastrointestinal, infections, and skin changes.

Incidence

Diabetic nephropathy is the principal cause of end-stage renal disease (ESRD) in the Western world. According to reports, in the past 2 decades, there has been a continual increase in the incidence of ESRD among patients with diabetes. However, because of the incidence of type 2 diabetes mellitus being fivefold higher than type 1, greater than 500/0 of patients in ESRD programs have this form of diabetes. Diabetic nephropathy with proteinuria rarely develops before 10 years duration of diabetes.

Etiology

Like other microvascular complications, the pathogenesis of diabetic nephropathy is related to chronic hyperglycemia. The mechanisms by which chronic hyperglycemia leads to ESRD, though incompletely defined, involve the effects of soluble factors (growth factors, angiotensin II, endothelin, and AGEs), hemodynamic alterations in the renal microcirculation (glomerular hyperfiltration or hyperperfusion, increased glomerular capillary pressure), and structural changes in the glomerulus (increased extracellular matrix, basement membrane thickening, mesangial expansion, and fibrosis). Some of these effects may be mediated through angiotensin II receptors.

The earliest detectable change in the course of diabetic nephropathy is a thickening in the glomerulus. At this stage, the kidney may start allowing more albumin than normal in the urine (albuminuria) and this can be detected by sensitive medical tests for albumin. This stage is called "microalbuminuria". After 5–10 years of type 1 DM, ~40% of individuals begin to show microalbuminuria. Microalbuminuria is defined as 30–300 mg/day of albumin in a 24-hour collection of urine. As diabetic nephropathy progresses, increasing numbers of glomeruli are destroyed by nodular glomerulosclerosis. Although the appearance of microalbuminuria in type 1 DM is an important risk factor for progression to overt proteinuria (in >300 mg/day), only ~50% of individuals will progress to macroalbuminuria over the next 10 years. In some individuals with type 1 diabetes and microalbuminuria of short duration, the microalbuminuria regresses. Once macroalbuminuria is present, there is a steady decline in GFR and ~50% of individuals reach ESRD in 7–10 years. Once macroalbuminuria develops, blood pressure rises slightly and the pathologic changes are likely to be irreversible. At this stage, a kidney biopsy clearly shows diabetic nephropathy.

Clinical Manifestations

Kidney failure provoked by glomerulosclerosis leads to fluid filtration deficits and other disorders of kidney function. There is an increase in blood pressure and fluid retention in the body causing edema. Other complications may be arteriosclerosis of the renal artery and proteinuria.

Throughout its early course, diabetic nephropathy has no symptoms. They develop in late stages and may be a result of excretion of high amounts of protein in the urine or due to renal failure:

- Edema—swelling, usually around the eyes in the mornings; later, general body swelling may result, such as swelling of the legs
- Foamy appearance or excessive frothing of the urine (caused by the proteinuria)
- Unintentional weight gain (from fluid accumulation)
- Anorexia
- Nausea and vomiting
- Malaise
- Fatigue
- Headache
- Frequent hiccups
- Generalized itching.

Laboratory Diagnosis

The first laboratory abnormality is a positive microalbuminuria test. Most often, the diagnosis is suspected when a routine urinalysis of a person with diabetes shows too much protein in the urine (proteinuria). The urinalysis may also show glucose in the urine, especially if blood glucose is poorly controlled. Serum creatinine and BUN may increase as kidney damage progresses. Dyslipidemia is a common associated finding. A renal biopsy confirms the diagnosis.

The nephropathy that develops in type 2 DM differs from that of type 1 DM in the following respects: (1) microalbuminuria or macroalbuminuria may be present when type 2 DM is diagnosed, reflecting its long asymptomatic period; (2) hypertension more commonly accompanies microalbuminuria or macroalbuminuria in type 2 DM; and (3) microalbuminuria may be less predictive of diabetic nephropathy and progression to macroalbuminuria in type 2 DM.

Treatment

The optimal therapy for diabetic nephropathy is prevention by control of glycemia. As a part of comprehensive diabetes care, microalbuminuria detection and measurement of the serum creatinine to estimate GFR should be done at an early stage, when effective therapies can be instituted.

Interventions effective in slowing progression from microalbuminuria to macroalbuminuria include: (1) normalization of glycemia, (2) strict blood pressure control, and (3) administration of angiotensin-converting enzyme (ACE) inhibitors or angiotensin II receptor blockers (ARBs) dyslipidemia should also be treated. Modest restriction of protein and fat intake is recommended. Once macroalbuminuria ensues, the likelihood of ESRD is very high. Survival after the onset of ESRD is shorter in the diabetic population compared to nondiabetics with similar clinical features. Dialysis may be necessary once end-stage renal disease develops. At this stage, kidney transplantation must be considered. Another option for type 1 diabetes patients is a combined kidney-pancreas transplant.

CLINICAL NOTE

Microalbuminuria detection and measurement of the serum creatinine to estimate GFR should be done at an early stage, when effective therapies can be instituted to prevent the onset and progression of diabetic nephropathy.

CLINICAL PEARLS

1. Diabetic nephropathy (*nephropatia diabetica*), also known as Kimmelstiel–Wilson syndrome and intercapillary glomerulonephritis, is a progressive kidney disease, caused by angiopathy of capillaries in the kidney glomeruli and it is characterized by nephrotic syndrome and diffuse glomerulosclerosis.
2. There is an increase in blood pressure and fluid retention in the body causing edema.
3. The first laboratory abnormality is a positive microalbuminuria test.
4. The optimal therapy for diabetic nephropathy is prevention by control of glycemia.
5. Once macroalbuminuria ensues, the likelihood of ESRD is very high.

SCREENING FOR DIABETIC NEPHROPATHY (FIG. 21.2)

All patients of type 1 diabetes mellitus of 5 years duration and all diagnosed cases of type 2 diabetes are required to be screened for the early detection of type 2 diabetes mellitus.

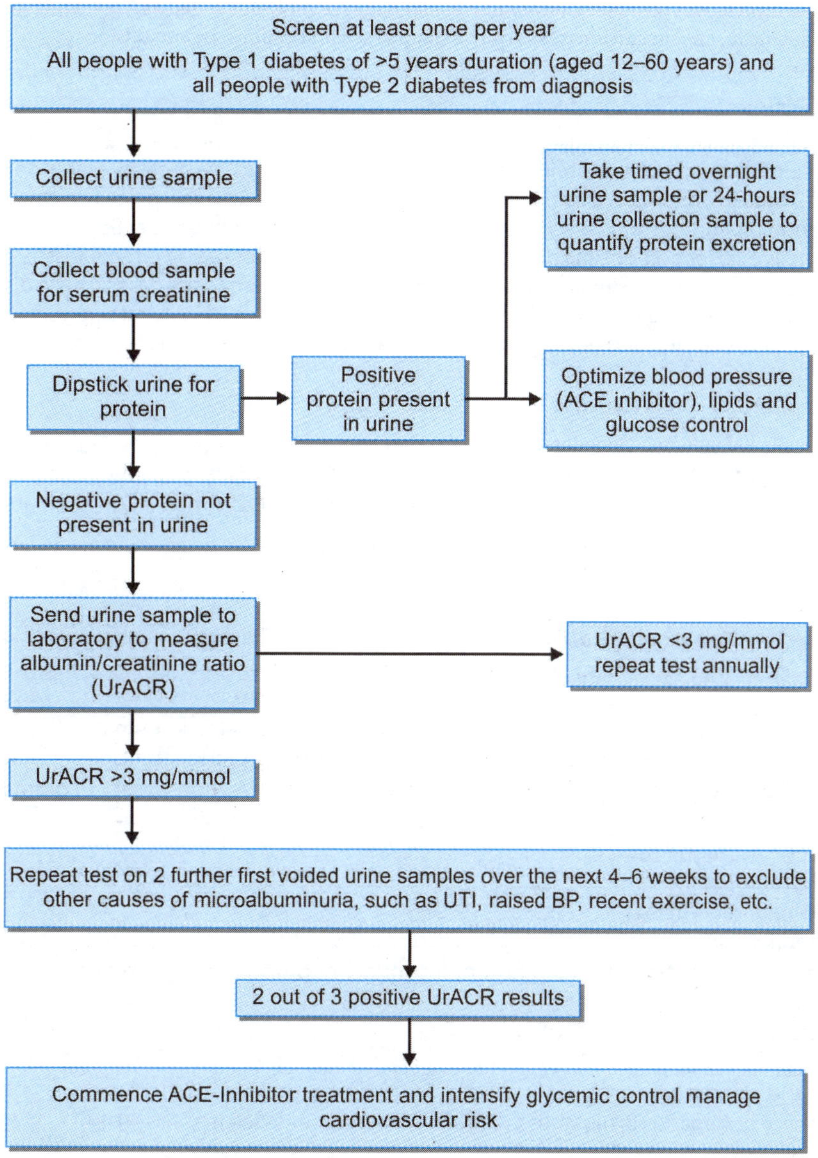

Fig. 21.2: Screening for diabetic nephropathy.

CASE STUDY 4

Theme: Diagnosis and Management of Nephrotic Syndrome

A 53-year-old hypertensive man reported to the physician for consultation. He claimed of dry, painful eyes and xerostomia that started a few weeks ago. He was afebrile, with blood pressure of 140/92 mm Hg, pulse of 80 bpm, with no respiratory distress. He had no organomegalies but facial and lower limbs edema was identified. He had hyperglycemia (FBS-256 mg/dL), glycosuria (reducing sugars +++), severe proteinuria (14 g/24 h), hypoalbuminemia (2 g/dL), hypercholesterolemia (243 mg/dL), and acute renal failure (creatinine 2 mg/dL; urea 102 mg/dL). Serum immunoglobulins were within normal limit. Tests for hepatitis B virus surface antigen, hepatitis C, and HIV antibody were negative. Culture for bacteria and fungi revealed no microbiological growth. Serum/urinary immunoelectrophoresis disclosed no monoclonal proteins. Abdominal ultrasonography and chest X-rays were normal. **What is the probable diagnosis?**

CASE DETAILS

Proteinuria, hypoalbuminemia, hypercholesterolemia, acute renal failure, and edema signify the presence of nephrotic syndrome. Since there is hyperglycemia and glycosuria, so the patient has diabetes mellitus which was probably not diagnosed earlier. The cause of nephrotic syndrome seems to be secondary to hypertension or diabetes mellitus. The other secondary causes have been eliminated from the specific tests. The confirmation of the diagnosis can be done by renal biopsy.

NEPHROTIC SYNDROME

Nephrotic syndrome (NS), also known as nephrosis, is defined by the presence of nephrotic-range proteinuria, edema, hyperlipidemia, and hypoalbuminemia. Nephrotic-range proteinuria in adults is characterized by protein excretion of 3.5 g or more per day. Nephrotic-range proteinuria in children is protein excretion of >40 $mg/m^2/h$. A urine protein/creatinine value of >2–3 mg/mg indicates nephrotic-range proteinuria and correlates with results from 24-hour urine collection.

Nephrotic syndrome is a collection of clinical findings that are the result of massive renal losses of protein. Thus, nephrotic syndrome is not a disease itself, but the manifestation of many different glomerular diseases. These diseases might be acute and transient, such as postinfectious glomerulonephritis, or chronic and progressive, such as focal segmental glomerulosclerosis (FSGS). Still other diseases might be relapsing and remitting, such as minimal-change nephrotic syndrome (MCNS).

Incidence

Nephrotic syndrome may affect adults and children of both sexes and of any race but it is 15 times more common in children than adults. The incidence is 2–3/100,000 children per year and the vast majority of affected children have steroid-sensitive minimal change disease. Diabetic nephropathy with nephrotic syndrome is the most common, at an estimated rate of at least 50 cases per million populations.

Classification

1. **Classification based on the pathological cause:** Nephrotic syndrome can be primary; being a disease specific to the kidneys, or it can be secondary, being a renal manifestation of a systemic general illness. In all cases, injury to glomeruli is an essential feature.
   a. **Primary nephrotic syndrome:** Primary nephrotic syndrome (PNS), also known as idiopathic nephrotic syndrome (INS), is associated with glomerular diseases intrinsic to the kidney. The subcategories of INS are based on histological descriptions, but clinical-pathological correlations have been made. A wide variety of glomerular lesions can be seen in INS.
      - Minimal-change nephropathy
      - Focal glomerulosclerosis
      - Membranous nephropathy
      - Hereditary nephropathies

   b. **Secondary nephrotic syndrome:** By definition, secondary nephrotic syndrome refers to an etiology extrinsic to the kidney.
      - Diabetes mellitus
      - Lupus erythematosus
      - Amyloidosis and paraproteinemias
      - Viral infections [e.g., hepatitis B, hepatitis C, and human immunodeficiency virus (HIV)]
      - Pre-eclampsia
      - Vasculitis
      - Henoch-Schönlein purpura (HSP)
      - Drug exposure (heroin, mercury, and others)
      - Medication can cause nephrotic syndrome. This includes the very infrequent occurrence of minimal-change nephropathy with NSAID use and the occurrence of membranous nephropathy with the administration of gold and penicillamine, which are older drugs used for rheumatic diseases; there have also been reports of focal glomerulosclerosis in association with bisphosphonates.

      The above causes of nephrotic syndrome are largely those for adults.

   c. Congenital and hereditary focal glomerulosclerosis may result from mutations of genes that code for podocyte proteins, including nephrin or podocin.
2. **Classification from a therapeutic perspective:**
   Nephrotic syndrome may be classified as:
   - Steroid sensitive
   - Steroid resistant
   - Steroid dependent.

Pathophysiology

Glomerular permeability: In a healthy individual, <0.1% of plasma albumin may traverse the glomerular filtration barrier.

The glomerular capillaries are lined by a fenestrated endothelium that lies on the glomerular basement membrane which in turn is covered by glomerular epithelium, or podocytes, which envelop the capillaries with cellular extensions called foot processes. In between the foot processes are the filtration slits. These three structures—the fenestrated endothelium, glomerular basement membrane, and glomerular epithelium—are the glomerular filtration barrier.

Proteinuria: The glomerular structural changes that may cause proteinuria are: (1) damage to the endothelial surface, (2) damage to the glomerular basement membrane, and/or (3) damage of the podocytes. One or more of these mechanisms may be seen in any one type of nephrotic syndrome.

Albuminuria alone may occur, or, with greater injury, leakage of all plasma proteins (i.e., proteinuria) may take place.

Proteinuria that is >85% albumin is selective proteinuria. Albumin has a net negative charge and it is proposed that loss of glomerular membrane negative charges could be important in causing albuminuria. Nonselective proteinuria, being a glomerular leakage of all plasma proteins would not involve changes in glomerular net charge but rather a generalized defect in permeability. This construct does not permit clear-cut separation of causes of proteinuria, except in minimal-change nephropathy, in which proteinuria is selective.

Pathogenesis of edema: An increase in glomerular permeability leads to albuminuria and eventually to hypoalbuminemia. In turn, hypoalbuminemia lowers the plasma colloid osmotic pressure causing greater transcapillary filtration of water throughout the body and thus the development of edema.

Capillary hydrostatic pressure and the gradient of plasma to interstitial fluid oncotic pressure determine the movement of fluid from the vascular compartment to the interstitium. The oncotic pressure is mainly determined by the protein content. The flux of water across the capillary wall can be expressed by the following formula:

$$Q_w = K(P_c - P_i) - (p_p - p_i)$$

In this formula, Q_w is net flux of water, K is the capillary filtration coefficient, P_c is capillary hydrostatic pressure, and P_i is the interstitial fluid hydrostatic pressure, while p_p is the plasma oncotic pressure and p_i is the interstitial fluid oncotic pressure. With a high enough capillary hydrostatic pressure or a low enough intravascular oncotic pressure, the amount of fluid filtered exceeds the maximal lymphatic flow and edema occurs.

The reduction in intravascular volume decreases renal perfusion pressure, activating the renin-angiotensin-aldosterone system, which stimulates tubular reabsorption of sodium. The reduced intravascular volume also stimulates the release of antidiuretic hormone, which enhances the reabsorption of water in the collecting duct. Because of the decreased plasma oncotic pressure, fluid shifts into the interstitial space, exacerbating the edema.

Metabolic Consequences of Proteinuria

Hyperlipidemia: In the nephrotic syndrome, levels of serum lipids are usually elevated. This can occur via: (1) hypoproteinemia that stimulates protein including lipoprotein, synthesis by the liver, and (2) diminution of lipid catabolism caused by reduced plasma levels of lipoprotein lipase. Apolipoprotein (apo)-B containing lipoproteins are elevated, including very-low-density lipoprotein (VLDL), intermediate-density lipoprotein (IDL), LDL and lipoprotein(a), with resultant increase in total cholesterol and LDL-cholesterol. High-density lipoprotein (HDL)-cholesterol is normal or low. Elevations in triglycerides occur with severe hypoalbuminemia.

Hypercoagulable state: The loss of antithrombin III and plasminogen occur via urine, along with the simultaneous increase in clotting factors, especially factors I, VII, VIII, and X, increasing the risk for venous thrombosis and pulmonary embolism.

Hypovitaminosis D: Vitamin D-binding protein may be lost in the urine, leading to hypovitaminosis D, with malabsorption of calcium and development of bone disease.

Immunodeficiency: Urinary immunoglobulin losses may lower the patient's resistance to infections and increase the risk of sepsis and peritonitis.

Clinical Manifestations

- Edema is the predominant feature of nephrotic syndrome and initially develops around the eyes and legs. With time, the edema becomes generalized and may be associated with an increase in weight, the development of ascites, or pleural effusions.
- Hematuria may be present in a minority of patients.
- Foamy urine may be a presenting feature.
- A thrombotic complication, such as deep vein thrombosis of the calf veins or even a pulmonary embolus, may be the first clue indicating nephrotic syndrome.
- Additional historical features that appear can be related to the cause of nephrotic syndrome and as a result of whether or not renal function impairment exists.

- Thus, the recent start of a nonsteroidal anti-inflammatory drug (NSAID) or a 10-year history of diabetes may be very relevant. In the case of long-standing diabetes, there may be diabetic retinopathy, which correlates closely with diabetic nephropathy. If the kidney function is reduced, there may be hypertension and/or anemia.

Laboratory Findings

Urinalysis: Proteinuria occurs as a result of an alteration of the negative charge in the glomerular basement membrane. The screening test for proteinuria is the urinary dipstick analysis; however, this test indicates albumin only. The addition of sulfosalicylic acid to the urine sediment allows abnormal paraproteins to be detected.

Urine dipstick testing can detect as little as 15 mg/dL of protein, but the results must be interpreted along with the urine specific gravity.

Microscopically, the urinary sediment has relatively few cellular elements or casts. However, if marked hyperlipidemia is present, patients can have oval fat bodies in the urine. These represent lipid deposits in sloughed renal tubular epithelial cells. They appear as "grape clusters" under light microscopy and "Maltese crosses" under polarized light.

Blood Chemistries

Serum total and differential protein: A decreased serum albumin (<3 g/dL) and total serum protein <6 g/dL may be observed.

Lipid profile: Hyperlipidemia occurs in over 50% of those with early nephrotic syndrome. The degree of hyperlipidemia increases with the degree of protein loss.

ESR and serum fibrinogen levels: Patients can also have an elevated erythrocyte sedimentation rate as a result of alterations in some plasma components, such as increased levels of fibrinogen.

Renal function tests: Blood urea nitrogen (BUN) and serum creatinine rise in the setting of renal failure.

Miscellaneous tests: Other less common tests may be necessary depending on the patient's clinical presentation, including complement levels, serum, and urine protein electrophoresis, ANA, and serologic tests for hepatitis. Patients may become deficient in vitamin D, zinc, and copper from loss of binding proteins in the urine; they are prone to infection, in part from urinary losses of immunoglobulins.

Renal biopsy: Specimens are examined by light microscopy, with immunofluorescent stains and by electron microscopy. Renal biopsy is often performed in adults with new-onset idiopathic nephrotic syndrome if a primary renal disease that may require drug therapy (e.g., corticosteroids, cytotoxic agents) is suspected. Significantly elevated creatinine levels may indicate irreversible renal disease mitigating the usefulness of renal biopsy. Disease due to amyloid or diabetes mellitus often does not need to be biopsied, since nephrotic-range proteinuria in these diseases represents irreversible damage, although bone marrow transplant with high-dose chemotherapy can be considered in some patients with amyloid. The role of biopsy for other systemic renal diseases is debated. However, it can be useful for prognosis and treatment. An occasional unexpected diagnosis is made, such as membranous nephropathy due to lupus erythematosus without serologic evidence of that illness.

Management of Nephrotic Syndrome

Protein loss: The daily total dietary protein intake should replace the daily urinary protein losses so as to avoid negative nitrogen balance. Protein malnutrition often occurs with urinary protein losses greater than 10 g/day protein. A restriction of proteins to 0.6 g/kg/day in patients with a GFR <25 mL/min is recommended prior to starting dialysis.

Edema: Dietary salt restriction is essential for managing edema; most patients also require diuretic therapy. Commonly used diuretics include thiazide and loop diuretics. Both are highly protein bound. With hypoalbuminemia, diuretic delivery to the kidney is reduced and patients often require large doses. The combination of loop and thiazide diuretics can potentiate the diuretic effect. This may be needed for patients with refractory fluid retention associated with pleural effusions and ascites.

Hyperlipidemia: Hypercholesterolemia and hypertriglyceridemia occur as outlined above. Dietary management in patients with nephrotic syndrome is of little value; however, dietary modification and exercise should be advocated. Aggressive pharmacologic treatment should be pursued.

Hypercoagulable state: Patients with serum albumin <2 g/dL can become hypercoagulable. Nephrotic patients have urinary losses of antithrombin III, protein C, protein S and increased platelet activation. Patients are prone to renal vein thrombosis and other venous thromboemboli, particularly with membranous glomerulopathy. Anticoagulation therapy is warranted for at least 3–6 months in patients with evidence of thrombosis. Patients with renal vein thrombosis and recurrent thromboemboli require indefinite anticoagulation.

Specific Treatment

Specific treatment of nephrotic syndrome depends on the disease's cause. Thus, glucocorticosteroids, such as prednisone, are used for minimal-change nephropathy. Prednisone and cyclophosphamide are useful in some forms of lupus nephritis. Secondary amyloidosis with nephrotic syndrome may respond to anti-inflammatory treatment of the primary disease.

Diet

- For patients with nephrotic syndrome, their diet should provide adequate energy (caloric) intake and adequate protein (1–2 g/kg/day). Supplemental dietary protein is of no proven value.
- A diet with no added salt will help to limit fluid overload.
- Management of hyperlipidemia could be of some importance if the nephrotic state is prolonged.
- Fluid restriction *per se* is not required.

Prognosis

The prognosis varies depending on the cause of the nephrotic syndrome, the person's age, and the type and degree of kidney damage. Symptoms may disappear completely if the nephrotic syndrome is caused by a treatable disorder, such as an infection, cancer, or drugs. This situation occurs in about half the cases in children but less often in adults. If the underlying disorder responds to corticosteroids, sometimes progression of the disease is halted and less often the condition partially, or rarely, completely reverses. When the syndrome is caused by HIV infection, it usually progresses relentlessly, often resulting in complete kidney failure in 3 or 4 months. Children born with the nephrotic syndrome rarely live beyond their first birthday, although a few have survived by means of dialysis treatments or a kidney transplant.

When the cause is systemic lupus erythematosus or diabetes mellitus, drug treatment often stabilizes or decreases the amount of protein in the urine. However, some people do not respond to drug treatment and develop progressive kidney failure within a few years.

In cases of nephrotic syndrome resulting from conditions, such as an infection, allergy, or intravenous heroin use, the prognosis varies, depending on how early and effectively the underlying condition is treated.

CLINICAL NOTE

Nephrotic syndrome is not a disease itself, but the manifestation of many different glomerular diseases. These diseases might be acute and transient, such as postinfectious glomerulonephritis, or chronic and progressive, such as FSGS. Still other diseases might be relapsing and remitting, such as MCNS.

CLINICAL PEARLS

1. NS, also known as nephrosis, is defined by the presence of nephrotic-range proteinuria, edema, hyperlipidemia, and hypoalbuminemia.
2. Nephrotic syndrome can be primary; being a disease specific to the kidneys, or it can be secondary, being a renal manifestation of a systemic general illness. In all cases, injury to glomeruli is an essential feature.
3. Edema is the predominant feature of nephrotic syndrome and initially develops around the eyes and legs. With time, the edema becomes generalized and may be associated with an increase in weight, the development of ascites, or pleural effusions. Hematuria may be present in a minority of patients.
4. Treatment is based on treating the protein loss, edema, hyperlipidemia, hypercoagulable state, associated nutritional deficiencies, and protection from infections.
5. The prognosis varies depending on the cause of the nephrotic syndrome, the person's age, and the type and degree of kidney damage.

CASE STUDY 5

Theme: Renal and Liver Function Tests in Preeclampsia

A 26-year-old woman in her 31st week of pregnancy presented with a 2.8 kg weight gain in 1 week, dependent pitting edema in her feet, a blood pressure of 150/100 mm Hg on three separate readings, and a urine dipstick test demonstrating 2+ proteinuria [sulfosalicylic acid (SSA) method 2+]. No casts or RBCs were noted in the urine sediment examination.

Important laboratory test results are as follows:

BUN = 18 mg/dL
Serum creatinine = 1.2 mg/dL
Serum uric acid = 6.8 mg/dL
Serum aspartate aminotransferase (AST) = 100 U/L
Serum alanine transaminase (ALT) = 150 U/L

Serum alkaline phosphatase (AP) = 150 U/L
Serum gamma-glutamyl transferase (GGT) = 37 U/L
Serum total bilirubin = Normal

Are the serum BUN, creatinine, and uric acid levels really "normal" in this patient?
What is the significance of the elevated liver function tests?

CASE DISCUSSION

The patient has a classic presentation of **pre-eclampsia** (weight gain, pitting edema, and hypertension), which most commonly occurs in the third trimester. In pregnancy, the plasma volume is increased greater than the increase in red blood cell (RBC) mass. This is responsible for a slight drop in the Hb concentration; an increase in the creatinine clearance; and increased clearance of urea, creatinine, and uric acid. Hence, in pregnancy, serum BUN >10 mg/dL, serum creatinine >1.0 mg/dL, and uric acid >5 mg/dL are abnormal even though the values are all in the "normal" range for an adult. The renal disease associated with pre-eclampsia is associated with a reduction in the creatinine clearance and an increase in serum BUN, creatinine, and uric acid, since they are not filtered and cleared from the plasma as in a normal pregnancy.

The elevated serum AP is normal for pregnancy and is of placental origin. In this case, it should not be construed as indicating cholestatic liver disease, since the GGT is normal. Elevation of the transaminases may occur in pre-eclampsia owing to mild periportal (zone I) necrosis of hepatocytes. Diffuse liver cell disease or cholestasis must be present for the total bilirubin to be elevated. With the treatment of pre-eclampsia, the enzyme levels revert back to normal.

A positive dipstick for protein is always confirmed by an SSA precipitation test. The dipstick for protein detects albumin but not globulins, while the SSA detects both albumin and globulins. Hence, the equal results in both tests (2+) indicate that albumin is mainly being lost in the urine. Proteinuria in pre-eclampsia may sometimes be in the nephrotic range (>3.5 g/24 h), in which case there would be fatty casts in the urine and more advanced pitting edema owing to hypoalbuminemia and the loss in plasma oncotic pressure.

CASE STUDY 6

Theme: Diagnosis and Management of Acute Myocardial Infarction

A 51-year-old male presented to the emergency room with chest pain. He stated that he had chest discomfort or pressure intermittently over the last year especially with increased activity. He described the chest pain as a pressure behind his breastbone that spreads to the left side of his neck. Unlike previous episodes, he was lying down, watching television. The chest pain lasted approximately 15 minutes and then subsided on its own. He also noticed that he was nauseated and had sweating during the pain episode. He had no medical problems that he was aware of and had not been to a physician for several years.

On examination, he was in no acute distress with normal vital signs. His lungs were clear to auscultation bilaterally and his heart had a regular rate and rhythm with no murmurs. An electrocardiogram (ECG) revealed ST-segment elevation and peaked T waves in leads II, III, and aVF. Serum troponin I and T levels are elevated.

What is the most likely diagnosis?

CASE DISCUSSION

The patient is most probably suffering from acute myocardial infarction as is evident from clinical manifestations, ECG changes, and the laboratory report.

ACUTE MYOCARDIAL INFARCTION

Myocardial infarction (MI) is the rapid development of myocardial necrosis caused by a critical imbalance between oxygen supply and demand of the myocardium. This usually results from plaque rupture with thrombus formation in a coronary vessel, resulting in an acute reduction of blood supply to a portion of the myocardium. More rarely, infarction may result from prolonged vasospasm, inadequate myocardial blood flow (e.g., hypotension), or excessive metabolic demand. Very rarely, myocardial infarction may be caused by embolic occlusion, vasculitis, aortic root or coronary artery dissection, or aortitis.

Pathophysiology

The most common cause of MI is narrowing of the epicardial blood vessels due to atheromatous plaques. Approximately 90% of myocardial infarctions result from an acute thrombus that obstructs an atherosclerotic coronary artery. Plaque rupture is considered to be the major trigger of coronary thrombosis. Following plaque rupture, platelet activation, and aggregation, coagulation pathway activation and endothelial vasoconstriction occur and lead to coronary thrombosis and occlusion. This can result in partial or complete occlusion of the vessel and subsequent myocardial ischemia. Total occlusion of the vessel for >4–6 hours results in irreversible myocardial necrosis, but reperfusion within this period can salvage the myocardium and reduce morbidity and mortality.

Nonatherosclerotic causes of MI include coronary vasospasm as seen in variant (Prinzmetal) angina and in patients using cocaine and amphetamines; coronary emboli from sources, such as an infected heart valve; occlusion of the coronaries due to vasculitis; or other causes leading to mismatch of oxygen supply and demand, such as acute anemia from GI bleeding.

Acute myocardial infarction is classified as ST (STEMI) or non-ST-segment elevation (NSTEMI), based on the presenting ECG. ST elevation connotes an acute coronary occlusion and thus warrants immediate reperfusion therapy. Patients without ST elevation are more likely to be older, have multivessel disease, and more vascular disease in general; thus, this population is at higher risk for adverse outcomes following hospital discharge.

The location and extent of infarction depend on the anatomic distribution of the occluded vessel, the presence of additional stenotic lesions, and the adequacy of collateral circulation. Thrombosis in the anterior descending branch of the left coronary artery results in infarction of the anterior LV and interventricular septum. Occlusion of the left circumflex artery produces anterolateral or posterolateral infarction. Right coronary thrombosis leads to infarction of the posteroinferior portion of the LV and generally involves the RV myocardium if the obstruction is proximal. The arteries supplying the AV node and the sinus node more commonly arise from the right coronary artery; thus, AV block at the nodal level and sinus node dysfunction occur more frequently during inferior or right-sided infarctions.

Causes of Acute MI

a. **Atherosclerosis with occlusive or partially occlusive thrombus formation:** The risk factors for atherosclerosis are as follows:
- Nonmodifiable risk factors for atherosclerosis:
  - Age
  - Sex
  - Family history of premature coronary heart disease.
- Modifiable risk factors for atherosclerosis:
  - Smoking or other tobacco use
  - Diabetes mellitus
  - Hypertension
  - Dyslipidemia
  - Obesity
- Other risk factors for atherosclerosis:
  - Elevated homocysteine levels
  - Male pattern baldness
  - Sedentary lifestyle and/or lack of exercise
  - Psychosocial stress
  - Presence of peripheral vascular disease
  - Poor oral hygiene.

b. **Nonatherosclerotic causes:**
- Vasculitis
- Coronary emboli
- Congenital coronary anomalies
- Coronary trauma
- Coronary spasm
- Drug use (cocaine)
- Factors that increase oxygen requirement, such as heavy exertion, fever, or hyperthyroidism
- Factors that decrease oxygen delivery, such as hypoxemia of severe anemia.

Incidence

MI continues to be a significant problem in industrialized countries and is becoming an increasingly significant problem in developing countries.

MI is a leading cause of morbidity and mortality in the United States. Approximately 1.3 million cases of nonfatal MI are reported each year, for an annual incidence rate of approximately 600 cases per 100,000 people. The proportion of patients diagnosed with NSTEMI compared with STEMI has progressively increased.

Sex

- A male predominance in incidence exists up to age 70 years.
- Premenopausal women appear to be somewhat protected from atherosclerosis, effects of estrogen may be the reason.

Age

Incidence of MI increases with advancing age. MI most commonly occurs in persons older than 45 years. However, some persons younger than 45 years can also be at risk, especially drug addicts, people with type 1 diabetes, persons with dyslipidemia, and those with a positive family history of premature coronary artery disease. A positive family history encompasses any family member, such as a first-degree male relative of age 40–45 years or younger or any first-degree female relative of age 50–55 years or younger who experienced a myocardial infarction in the past.

Clinical Manifestations

- **Chest pain** is felt across the anterior precordium and is typically expressed as crushing, compressing, or gripping pain.
- The pain usually radiates to left arm (some patients may even experience pain in both the arms), jaw, neck, back, and epigastrium.
- Chest pain may be accompanied by dyspnea, or dyspnea may be the only chief complaint especially in old-elderly persons or in diabetics. Dyspnea signifies poor ventricular compliance in the phase of acute ischemia.
- The patients can present with nausea, vomiting, and upper abdominal pain, especially in the inferior or posterior wall infarcts.
- Anxiety, diaphoresis, and lightheadedness with or without syncope may be present.
- Some patients present with cough and wheezing,
- Elderly patients present with extreme fatigue, weakness, syncope, altered mental state, and dementia of recent origin, with no recollection of current symptoms.
- In almost half of the patients with MI, the classic symptoms are absent (silent MI). Therefore, the diagnosis of MI can be skipped. The suspicion of MI should be kept in mind while evaluating elderly patients, female patients with diabetes, and patients with a history of heart failure.

Physical Examination

The physical examination can often be unremarkable.

- Patients with ongoing symptoms usually lie quietly in bed and appear pale and diaphoretic.
- Hypertension may precipitate MI, or it may reflect elevated catecholamine levels due to anxiety, pain, or exogenous sympathomimetics.
- Hypotension may indicate ventricular dysfunction due to ischemia. Hypotension in the setting of MI usually indicates a large infarct secondary to either decreased global cardiac contractility or a right ventricular infarct.
- Acute valvular dysfunction may be present. Valvular dysfunction usually results from infarction that involves the papillary muscle. Mitral regurgitation due to papillary muscle ischemia or necrosis may be present.
- Rales may represent congestive heart failure.
- Neck vein distention may represent pump failure. With right ventricular failure, cannon jugular venous a waves may be noted.
- Third heart sound (S3) may be present.
- A fourth heart sound is a common finding in patients with poor ventricular compliance that is due to pre-existing heart disease or hypertension.
- Dysrhythmias may present as an irregular heartbeat or pulse.
- Low-grade fever is not uncommon. Edema is usually not present. Cyanosis and cold temperature indicate low output. The peripheral pulses should be noted, since later shock or emboli may alter the examination.

Diagnosis

Electrocardiography: The ECG is the most important tool in the initial evaluation. It is confirmatory of the diagnosis in approximately 80% of cases.

- An ECG should be obtained as soon as possible after presentation to the emergency department (ED).
- Results that indicate high probability of MI are ST-segment elevation greater than 1 mm in 2 anatomically contiguous leads or the presence of new Q-waves.
- Results that indicate intermediate probability of MI are ST-segment depression, T-wave inversion, and other nonspecific ST-T-wave abnormalities.
- Results that indicate low probability of MI are normal findings on ECG; however, normal or nonspecific findings on ECG do not exclude the possibility of MI.

Laboratory Studies

A number of laboratory tests are available. None is completely sensitive and specific for myocardial infarction particularly in the hours following onset of symptoms. Timing is important, as are correlation with patient symptoms, electrocardiograms, and angiographic studies.

The following tests are available as markers for acute myocardial infarction:

1. **Creatine kinase—total:** The total creatine kinase (CK) is a simple and inexpensive test that is readily available using many laboratory instruments. However, an elevation in total CK is not specific for myocardial injury, because most CK is located in skeletal muscle and elevations are possible from a variety of noncardiac conditions.
2. **Creatine kinase—MB fraction:** Creatine kinase has three isoenzymes—MM, MB, and BB. The MM fraction is present in both cardiac and skeletal muscle, but the MB fraction is much more specific for cardiac muscle: About 15–40% of CK in cardiac muscle is MB, while <2% in skeletal muscle is MB. The BB fraction (found in brain, bowel, and bladder) is not routinely measured.

   Thus, CK-MB is a very good marker for acute myocardial injury, because of its excellent specificity and it rises in serum within 2–8 hours of onset of acute myocardial infarction. Serial measurements every 2–4 hours for a period of 9–12 hours after the patient is first seen will provide a pattern to determine whether the CK-MB is rising, indicative of myocardial injury. The CK-MB is also useful for diagnosis of reinfections or extensive of an MI because it begins to fall after a day, dissipating in 1–3 days, so subsequent elevations are indicative of another event. A "cardiac index" can provide a useful indicator for early MI. This is calculated as a ratio of total CK to CK-MB and is a sensitive indicator of myocardial injury when the CK-MB is elevated. Occasionally, very small infarcts can be missed by CK-MB; therefore, a troponin level should be measured for patients suspected of having had MI who have negative serial CK-MBs.
3. **Troponins:** Troponins have the greatest sensitivity and specificity in detecting MI. The test result is both diagnostic as well as prognostic of outcome. Troponin I and T are structural components of cardiac muscle. They are released into the bloodstream with myocardial injury. They are highly specific for myocardial injury—more so than CK-MB—and help to exclude elevations of CK with skeletal muscle trauma. Troponins will begin to increase following MI within 3–12 hours, about the same time frame as CK-MB. However, the rate of rise for early infarction may not be as dramatic as for CK-MB.

   Troponins will remain elevated longer than CK—up to 5–9 days for troponin I and up to 2 weeks for troponin T. This makes troponins a superior marker for diagnosing myocardial infarction in the recent past—better than lactate dehydrogenase (LDH). However, this continued elevation has the disadvantage of making it more difficult to diagnose reinfarction or extension of infarction in a patient who has already suffered from an initial MI. Troponin T lacks some specificity because elevations can appear with skeletal myopathies and with renal failure.
4. **Myoglobin:** Myoglobin is a low-molecular-weight heme protein found in skeletal and cardiac muscle which binds oxygen. It is a very sensitive indicator of muscle injury. The rise in myoglobin can help to determine the size of an infarction. A negative myoglobin can help to rule out myocardial infarction. It is elevated even before CK-MB. The marker has high sensitivity but poor specificity and can be elevated with any form of injury to skeletal muscle. When performed in conjunction with other studies, it may be useful for the early detection of MI.
5. **Lactate dehydrogenase:** LDH begins to rise in 12–24 hours following MI and peaks in 2–3 days, gradually dissipating in 5–14 days. Measurement of LDH isoenzymes is necessary for greater specificity for cardiac injury. There are 5 isoenzymes (1 through 5). Ordinarily, isoenzyme 2 is greater than 1, but with myocardial injury, this pattern is "flipped" and 1 is higher than 2. LDH-5 from liver may be increased with centrilobular necrosis from passive congestion with congestive heart failure following ischemic myocardial injury.
6. **Complete blood cell count:** Complete blood cell (CBC) count is indicated if anemia is suspected as a precipitant. Transfusion with packed red blood cells may be indicated. Leukocytosis may be observed within several hours after an AMI. It peaks in 2–4 days and returns to levels within the reference range within 1 week.
7. **Chemistry profile:**
   - Potassium and magnesium levels should be monitored and corrected.
   - Creatinine levels must be considered before using an angiotensin-converting enzyme (ACE) inhibitor.
8. **Lipid profile:** This may be helpful if obtained upon presentation because levels can change after 12–24 hours of an acute illness.
9. **C-reactive protein (CRP) levels:** Consider measuring CRP levels and other markers of inflammation upon presentation if an acute coronary syndrome is suspected.
10. Erythrocyte sedimentation rate (ESR) rises above reference range values within 3 days and may remain elevated for weeks.
11. Plasma homocysteine levels may be elevated in some of the patients.

Imaging Studies

- Chest radiography:
  - Chest radiography may provide clues to an alternative or complicating diagnosis (e.g., aortic dissection, pneumothorax). Other imaging studies, such as a contrast chest CT scan or transesophageal echocardiography should be used to differentiate MI from aortic dissection in patients in whom the diagnosis is in doubt. Chest radiography also reveals complications of MI, such as pulmonary edema secondary to heart failure.
- Echocardiography:
  - Echocardiography can identify complications of MI (e.g., valvular insufficiency, ventricular dysfunction, and pericardial effusion).
- Technetium-99m sestamibi scan:
  - Technetium-99m is a radioisotope that is taken up by the myocardium in proportion to the blood flow and is only minimally redistributed after initial uptake. This allows for time delay between injection of the isotope and imaging.

- It has potential use in identifying infarct in patients with atypical presentations or in patients with ECGs that are not interpretable.
- Normal scan findings are associated with an extremely low risk of subsequent cardiac events.

- **Thallium scanning:** Thallium accumulates in the viable myocardium.
- Perfusion imaging has been used in risk stratification after MI and for measurement of infarct size to evaluate reperfusion therapies. Novel "hot spot" imaging radiopharmaceuticals that visualize infarction or ischemia are currently undergoing evaluation and hold promise for the future.
- Recent advances include dual-source 64-slice CT scanning that can do a full scan in 10 seconds and produce high-resolution images that allow fine details of the patient's coronary arteries to be seen. This technology allows for noninvasive and early diagnosis of coronary artery disease and thus earlier treatment before the coronary arteries become more or completely occluded. It allows direct visualization of not only the lumen of the coronary arteries but also plaque within the artery.
- Whereas the use of CT coronary angiography (CTCA) as the primary noninvasive testing for coronary artery disease seems very attractive and is becoming more popular, the evidence for its diagnostic accuracy and clinical utility is still being evaluated in several prospective studies.
- MRI can identify wall thinning, scar, delayed enhancement (infarction), and wall motion abnormalities (ischemia). Currently, this is not a primary diagnostic modality for MI, but coronary artery assessment may be enhanced by magnetic resonance angiography (MRA) in the future.
- Coronary artery calcium scoring is an emerging technique for identifying patients at low risk for coronary artery disease. The test appears to add some predictive value in patients at low risk for coronary artery disease. However, in high-risk patients or those who have established coronary artery disease, the test does not appear to be helpful at this time.

Treatment

Specific prehospital care includes the following:

- Intravenous access, supplemental oxygen, and pulse oximetry
- Immediate administration of aspirin *en route*
- Nitroglycerin for active chest pain, given sublingually or by spray
- Telemetry and prehospital ECG, if available.

Initial therapy for acute myocardial infarction is directed toward restoration of perfusion as soon as possible to salvage as much of the jeopardized myocardium as possible. This may be accomplished through medical or mechanical means, such as percutaneous coronary intervention (PCI) or coronary artery bypass grafting.

A. **Medical therapy:** The main goals of ED medical therapy are rapid intravenous thrombolysis and/or rapid referral for PCI, optimizing oxygenation, decreasing cardiac workload, and controlling pain.

1. **Antithrombotic agents:** These agents prevent the formation of thrombus associated with myocardial infarction and inhibit platelet function by blocking cyclo-oxygenase and subsequent aggregation. Antiplatelet therapy has been shown to reduce mortality rates by reducing the risk of fatal myocardial infarctions, fatal strokes, and vascular death.
   - **Aspirin:** Low-dose aspirin has shown substantial benefit for primary prevention of myocardial infarction and stroke, but its use must be weighed against the risk for hemorrhagic stroke and gastrointestinal bleeding. Clopidogrel (Plavix) is used in case of aspirin allergy.
   - **Heparin:** Heparin augments activity of antithrombin III and prevents conversion of fibrinogen to fibrin. It does not actively lyse preformed clot, but is able to inhibit further thrombogenesis after thrombolysis. Heparin should be administered to patients undergoing PCI. Benefit as adjunctive therapy for streptokinase is not clear.
   - **Low-molecular-weight heparins (LMWH):** Produced by partial chemical or enzymatic depolymerization of unfractionated heparin (UFH). Binds to antithrombin III, enhancing its therapeutic effect. The heparin-antithrombin III complex binds to and inactivates activated factor X (Xa) and factor II (thrombin). It does not actively lyse but is able to inhibit further thrombogenesis. It prevents reaccumulation of clot after spontaneous fibrinolysis and is commonly used because of convenient dosing and reliable therapeutic levels, but there have been no definitive trials of LMWH in patients with STEMI to provide a firm basis for recommendations. Low-molecular-weight heparin should not be used as an alternative to unfractionated heparin as ancillary therapy to fibrinolytics in patients aged older than 75 years or in patients with significant renal dysfunction (serum creatinine level >2.5 mg/dL in men or >2 mg/dL in women).
2. **Vasodilators:** These agents oppose coronary artery spasm which augments coronary blood flow and reduces cardiac work by decreasing preload and afterload.
   - Nitrates are useful for preload reduction and symptomatic relief but have no apparent impact on mortality rate in MI. Systolic BP <90 mm Hg, HR <60 beats/min or >100 beats/min and RV infarction are a contraindications to nitrate use. Intravenous nitroglycerin is indicated for relief of ongoing ischemic discomfort, control of hypertension, or management of pulmonary congestion. Nitrates should not be administered to patients who have taken any phosphodiesterase inhibitor for erectile dysfunction within the last 24 hours (extend time frame to 48 hours for tadalafil). Nitrates cause relaxation of vascular smooth muscle by stimulating intracellular cyclic guanosine monophosphate production. Result is decrease in blood pressure.

3. **Beta-adrenergic blockers:** These agents inhibit chronotropic, inotropic, and vasodilatory responses to beta-adrenergic stimulation and reduce blood pressure which decreases myocardial oxygen demand. Greatest benefit is achieved when given within 8 hours of symptom onset. Metoprolol is the standard and is a selective beta-1-adrenergic receptor blocker that decreases automaticity of contractions. Beta-blockers reduce the rates of reinfarction and recurrent ischemia and may also reduce mortality.
4. **Thrombolytic agents:** Thrombolytic agents by preventing thrombus formation help in reversing the hemodynamic alterations. Additionally, they clear away undissolved pathologic intraluminal thrombus or embolus. Ideally, they should be given within 12 hours of the onset of symptoms and then they can revive the patency of the obstructed arteries, reverse the myocardial changes, and decrease the rate of morbidity and mortality associated with acute MI. Thrombolytic therapy needs to be started within 30 minutes of admission (door-drug time). Best results are observed when administered within 1–3 hours of the onset of symptoms in patients with: (i) ST-segment elevation >1 mm in 2 or more anatomically adjacent ECG leads, (ii) new or presumed new left bundle branch block, or (iii) anterior ST depression where posterior infarction is suspected. With ST-segment elevation, the diagnosis is almost confirmed; therefore, initiation of reperfusion therapy should not be delayed for the results of cardiac markers.
   Alteplase (tPA—tissue plasminogen activator): With a short half-life of 5 minutes, it acts by activating plasminogen to plasmin. During the first 24–48 hours, adjuvant therapy with IV heparin is required to maintain the patency of the blood vessels.
   Tenecteplase: It is formed by the modification of alteplase and can be administered as a single bolus over 5-second infusion instead of 90 minutes with alteplase. It is known to cause less in intracranial bleeding; however, the risk of intracranial bleeding and stroke is almost the same as alteplase.
   Anistreplase: It acts by activating the conversion of plasminogen to plasmin, which degrades fibrin, fibrinogen, and other procoagulant proteins into soluble fragments. These effects cause thrombolysis; it is, therefore, a nonfibrin-specific agent. It is known for a higher rate of allergic reactions and hemorrhagic complications. Nevertheless, it is easier to administer that tPA has a reasonable cost and does not require adjunct therapy with heparin.
   Streptokinase: It is also a nonfibrin-specific agent and acts by converting plasminogen to plasmin, which degrades fibrin clots as well as fibrinogen and other plasma proteins. It has a half-life of 23 minutes and the fibrinolytic effects are observed with intravenous infusion of streptokinase. The need for adjunct therapy with heparin is contentious.
   Reteplase: It is a recombinant plasminogen activator which forms plasmin after promoting cleavage of endogenous plasminogen.
5. **Platelet aggregation inhibitors:** These agents act by preventing platelet aggregation.
   Clopidogrel: It is an inhibitor of ADP-induced aggregation of platelets and acts by selectively inhibiting binding of adenosine diphosphate (ADP) to platelet receptor and then inhibiting ADP-mediated activation of glycoprotein GPIIb/IIIa complex resulting in inhibition of aggregation of platelets.
   Eptifibatide: It is an inhibitor of the platelet glycoprotein (GP) IIb/IIIa receptor and reversibly inhibits binding of von Willebrand factor, fibrinogen, and other adhesion ligands to the GP IIb/IIIa receptor, thereby causing inhibition of platelet aggregation.
   Tirofiban: It is also an inhibitor of the platelet GP IIb/IIIa receptor and reversibly prevents von Willebrand factor, fibrinogen, and other adhesion ligands from binding to the GP IIb/IIIa receptor, thereby inhibiting platelet aggregation.
   Abciximab: It is a recombinant human-murine monoclonal antibody, which binds to the receptor with high affinity and decreases platelet aggregation by almost 80% for as long as 48 hours after infusion. It prevents acute cardiac ischemic complications in unstable angina, which are nonresponsive to conventional therapy.
6. **Analgesics:** These agents reduce pain, promote pulmonary toilet, and because of their sedating properties, help to reduce the chest discomfort resulting from myocardial infarction.
   Morphine sulfate: It is a drug of choice for pain relief and its reliable and anticipated effects, safety profile, and convenience of reversibility with naloxone. Various IV doses are used that are commonly titrated until expected effects are obtained.
7. **ACE inhibitors:** These agents prevent the conversion of angiotensin I to angiotensin II, which is a potent vasoconstrictor and causes lowered aldosterone secretion.
   An ACE inhibitor (Captopril) is given orally in the following conditions: (i) within the first 24 hours of STEMI, (ii) patients with anterior infarction, (iii) pulmonary congestion, or (iv) left ventricular ejection fraction (LVEF) <40% in the absence of hypotension.
8. **An angiotensin receptor blocker (valsartan or candesartan)** is administered to patients with STEMI who cannot tolerate ACE inhibitors and patients with either clinical or radiological signs of heart failure or LVEF <40%.
9. **Calcium channel blockers:** Their role is controversial based on the recent reports of adverse effects caused by calcium channel blockers. Diltiazem and verapamil need to be avoided in patients with pulmonary edema or severe left ventricular (LV) dysfunction.

B. **Surgical care:**

- Percutaneous coronary intervention
- Coronary artery graft bypass surgery.

Complications

- A number of arrhythmias occur after myocardial infarction, ranging from benign to fatal. Arrhythmias are common in the setting of myocardial infarction and are a major cause of morbidity and mortality.
- Conduction abnormalities may result from ischemia.
- Recurrent ischemia may be due to incomplete reperfusion. Postinfarct angina occurs in 20–30% of patients. This is an indication to proceed to cardiac catheterization followed by mechanical revascularization as needed.
- Congestive heart failure can occur.
- Cardiogenic shock.

Prevention

- Patients should avoid risk factors when possible and act upon treatable risk factors.
- Seeking medical attention with the first symptoms or signs of angina may initiate the cascade of interventions that will ultimately prevent or limit damage to the myocardium. All patients should be educated as to these symptoms and signs.
- Daily low-dose aspirin may be helpful, but the decision to prescribe aspirin as a preventative measure for MI must be made considering his or her overall condition and risk-benefit ratio.

Prognosis

- Acute myocardial infarction is associated with a 30% mortality rate; half of the deaths occur prior to arrival at the hospital.
- An additional 5–10% of survivors die within the first year after their myocardial infarction.
- Approximately half of all patients with a myocardial infarction are rehospitalized within 1 year of their index event.
- Overall, prognosis is highly variable and depends largely on the extent of the infarct, the residual LV function, and whether the patient underwent revascularization.

CLINICAL NOTE

While heart attacks can occur at any time, more heart attacks occur between 4:00 AM and 10:00 AM because of the higher blood levels of adrenaline released from the adrenal glands during the morning hours. Increased adrenaline may contribute to rupture of cholesterol plaques.

CLINICAL PEARLS

1. MI is the irreversible necrosis of heart muscle secondary to prolonged ischemia resulting from an imbalance of oxygen supply and demand.
2. This usually results from plaque rupture with thrombus formation in a coronary vessel, resulting in an acute reduction of blood supply to a portion of the myocardium.
3. The appearance of cardiac enzymes in the circulation generally indicates myocardial necrosis.
4. The ECG is the most important tool in the initial evaluation. It is confirmatory of the diagnosis in approximately 80% of cases.

Initial therapy for acute myocardial infarction is directed toward restoration of perfusion as soon as possible to salvage as much of the jeopardized myocardium as possible. This may be accomplished through medical or mechanical means, such as percutaneous coronary intervention or coronary artery bypass grafting.

CASE STUDY 7

Theme: Diagnostic Significance of Liver Function Tests

A 32-year-old white female was referred to a hepatologist for a liver biopsy. Past history was remarkable for a needlestick injury (the patient was a registered critical care nurse), from a patient believed to be infected with non-A, non-B hepatitis. 6 weeks subsequent to the needlestick, she had become ill with a mild flu-like syndrome.

She was not icteric and no laboratory tests were obtained.

The attending physician examined the patient and ordered for liver function tests. On physical examination, the patient was found to be well-developed, well-nourished, and in no acute distress. Lymph nodes were negative, chest was clear to auscultation, and there was no hepatosplenomegaly. No spider angioma or palmar erythema was present and there was no edema of the extremities. The patient was very active and did not complain of fatigue or malaise. There was no evidence or history of decompensated liver disease or cirrhosis.

Liver function tests were abnormal, with an AST of 48 U/L and an ALT of 60 U/L. In light of these elevated LFTs, a complete hepatitis profile was obtained. The patient was found to be hepatitis C virus (HCV) antibody positive. She subsequently tested positive for HCV by polymerase chain reaction (PCR). The patient was referred to a hepatologist who procured a percutaneous liver biopsy to establish baseline liver condition. Interferon alpha (IFN) therapy was initiated after careful consideration of side effects versus possible benefits. The patient began a drug regimen of 3 million international units (MIU) administered subcutaneously three times a week. After 4 weeks of therapy, LFTs were normalized and HCV was not detectable in the serum after 16 weeks of drug therapy.

What are the different causes, clinical manifestations, and the laboratory methods to diagnose different types of hepatitis? What are the other liver function tests, which can be carried out to detect different hepatic disorders?

CASE DETAILS

The patient is suffering from hepatitis C, acquired by needleprick injury.

VIRAL HEPATITIS

Basic Concept

Hepatitis can be caused by many drugs and toxic agents as well as by numerous viruses, the clinical manifestations of which may be quite similar. Viruses causing hepatitis are: (1) hepatitis A virus (HAV), (2) hepatitis B virus (HBV), (3) HCV, (4) hepatitis D virus (HDV) (delta agent), and (5) hepatitis E virus (HEV) (an enterically transmitted hepatitis seen in epidemic form in Asia, North Africa, and Mexico). Hepatitis G virus (HGV) rarely, if ever, causes frank hepatitis. A DNA virus designated the TT virus (TTV) has been identified in up to 7.5% of blood donors and found to be transmitted readily by blood transfusions, but an association between this virus and liver disease has not been established. A related virus known as SEN-V has been found in 2% of US blood donors is transmitted by transfusion and may account for some cases of transfusion-associated non-ABCDE hepatitis.

Clinical Manifestations

The clinical picture of viral hepatitis is extremely variable, ranging from asymptomatic infection without jaundice to a fulminating disease and death in a few days.

Symptoms: The onset may be abrupt or insidious, with general malaise, myalgia, arthralgia, easy fatigability, upper respiratory symptoms, and anorexia. A distaste for smoking, paralleling anorexia may occur early. Nausea and vomiting are frequent and diarrhea or constipation may occur. Serum sickness may be seen early in acute hepatitis B. Fever is generally present but is low-grade, except in occasional cases of hepatitis A. Defervescence and a fall in pulse rate often coincide with the onset of jaundice.

Abdominal pain is usually mild and constant in the right upper quadrant or epigastrium, often aggravated by jarring or exertion and rarely may be severe enough to simulate cholecystitis.

Jaundice occurs after 5–10 days but may appear at the same time as the initial symptoms. In many patients, jaundice never develops. With the onset of jaundice, prodromal symptoms often worsen, followed by progressive clinical improvement. Stools may be acholic during this phase.

The acute illness usually subsides over 2–3 weeks with complete clinical and laboratory recovery by 9 weeks in hepatitis A and by 16 weeks in hepatitis B. In 5–10% of cases, the course may be more protracted, but <1% will have a fulminant course. In some cases of acute hepatitis A, clinical, biochemical, and serologic recovery may be followed by one or two relapses, but recovery is the rule.

Signs

Hepatomegaly is present in about half of cases; however, it is rarely marked. The liver is usually tender. Splenomegaly is observed in about 15% of patients and soft, large lymph nodes—especially in the cervical or epitrochlear area may be observed. Systemic toxicity is usually seen in hepatitis A. Mild neurocognitive alterations have been reported in patients with chronic hepatitis C.

Laboratory Diagnosis

- White blood cell count is normal to low, especially before the onset of clinical jaundice. Large atypical lymphocytes may infrequently be seen. Rarely, aplastic anemia may follow an episode of acute hepatitis not resulting from any of the known hepatitis viruses.
- Mild proteinuria is frequent and bilirubinuria often precedes the onset of jaundice.
- Extremely elevated AST or ALT levels are found early, followed by elevations of bilirubin and alkaline phosphatase; in a few patients, the raised levels of bilirubin and alkaline phosphatase may persist even after aminotransferase levels have normalized.
- Cholestasis is sometimes marked in acute hepatitis A.
- Marked prolongation of the prothrombin time in severe hepatitis may increase mortality.

Treatment

Bed rest is recommended only if symptoms are severe. If nausea and vomiting are severe or if oral intake is markedly reduced, intravenous 10% glucose is recommended. Encephalopathy or severe coagulopathy signifies impending acute hepatic failure and hospitalization at a liver transplant center is compulsory.

Dietary management consists of balanced palatable meals as accepted, without overfeeding; breakfast is generally best tolerated. Extreme physical exertion, alcohol, and hepatotoxic agents are prohibited. Small doses of oxazepam are safe, as hepatic metabolism is inhibited; morphine sulfate is avoided.

Corticosteroids are of no use in patients with viral hepatitis including those with the fulminant disease. Treatment of acute hepatitis C patients with peginterferon or interferon alfa for 6–24 weeks considerably reduces the risk of chronic hepatitis. In general, patients infected with HCV genotype 1 require a 24-week course of treatment, whereas those infected with genotypes 2, 3, or 4 require 8–12 weeks of therapy. As 20% of patients with acute hepatitis C, especially those who are symptomatic, clear the virus without such treatment, reserving it for patients in whom serum HCV RNA levels fail to clear after 3–4 months may be advisable. Ribavirin may be supplemented if HCV RNA fails to clear after 3 months of peginterferon or interferon alfa. Antiviral therapy is generally not needed in patients with acute hepatitis B.

Prognosis

In most patients, clinical recovery is complete in 3–6 months. Laboratory evidence of liver dysfunction may persist for a longer period, but most patients recover completely. The overall mortality rate is <1%, but the rate is reportedly higher in older people.

Liver Function Tests

Several biochemical tests are useful in the evaluation and management of patients with hepatic dysfunction. These tests can be used to: (1) detect the presence of liver disease (diagnosis), (2) distinguish among different types of liver disorders (differential diagnosis), (3) gauge the extent of known liver damage (prognostic), and (4) follow the response to treatment (therapeutic monitoring).

The liver carries out thousands of biochemical functions, most of which cannot be easily measured by blood tests. Laboratory tests measure only a limited number of these functions. Liver tests rarely suggest a specific diagnosis; rather, they suggest a general category of liver disease, such as hepatocellular or cholestatic, which then further directs the evaluation. To increase both the sensitivity and the specificity of laboratory tests in the detection of liver disease, it is best to use them as a battery. The tests usually employed in clinical practice include the bilirubin, aminotransferases, alkaline phosphatase, albumin, and prothrombin time tests.

Based on the functions of liver, the classification of the liver function tests is as follows:

1. **Tests based on detoxification and excretory functions:**
   a. **Serum bilirubin:** Bilirubin, a breakdown product of the porphyrin ring of heme-containing proteins, is found in the blood in two fractions—conjugated and unconjugated. The unconjugated fraction, also termed the indirect bilirubin, is insoluble in water and is bound to albumin in the blood. The conjugated (direct) bilirubin fraction is water soluble and can, therefore, be excreted by the kidney. When measured by the original van den Bergh method, the normal total serum bilirubin concentration is <17 mol/L (1 mg/dL). Up to 30% or 5.1 mol/L (0.3 mg/dL) of the total is direct-reacting (or conjugated) bilirubin.
      - **Unconjugated hyperbilirubinemia:** Elevation of the unconjugated fraction of bilirubin is rarely due to liver disease. An isolated elevation of unconjugated bilirubin is seen primarily in hemolytic disorders and in a number of genetic conditions, such as Crigler–Najjar and Gilbert's syndromes.
      - **Conjugated hyperbilirubinemia:** Conjugated hyperbilirubinemia almost always implies liver or biliary tract disease. The rate-limiting step in bilirubin metabolism is not conjugation of bilirubin, but rather the transport of conjugated bilirubin into the bile canaliculi. Thus, elevation of the conjugated fraction may be seen in any type of liver disease.
      - **Mixed hyperbilirubinemia:** In most liver diseases, both conjugated and unconjugated fractions of the bilirubin tend to be elevated.

      Except in the presence of a purely unconjugated hyperbilirubinemia, fractionation of the bilirubin is rarely helpful in determining the cause of jaundice.

   b. **Urine bilirubin:** Unconjugated bilirubin always binds to albumin in the serum and is not filtered by the kidney. Therefore, any bilirubin found in the urine is conjugated bilirubin; the presence of bilirubinuria implies the presence of liver disease. In patients recovering from jaundice, the urine bilirubin clears prior to the serum bilirubin.

   c. **Blood ammonia:** Ammonia is produced in the body during normal protein metabolism and by intestinal bacteria, primarily those in the colon. The liver plays a role in the detoxification of ammonia by converting it to urea which is excreted by the kidneys. Striated muscle also plays a role in detoxification of ammonia which is combined with glutamic acid to form glutamine.

Indications for estimating blood ammonia levels:

- Patients with advanced liver disease typically have significant muscle wasting which likely contributes to hyperammonemia in these patients.

- Blood ammonia is estimated for detecting encephalopathy or for monitoring hepatic synthetic function.
- It can be occasionally useful for identifying occult liver disease in patients with mental status changes.
- The ammonia can be elevated in patients with severe portal hypertension and portal blood shunting around the liver even in the presence of normal or near-normal hepatic function.
- Elevated arterial ammonia levels have been shown to correlate with outcome in fulminant hepatic failure.

2. **Serum enzymes in liver diseases:** The liver contains thousands of enzymes, some of which are also present in the serum in very low concentrations. These enzymes have no known function in the serum (nonfunctional enzymes). The elevation of a given enzyme activity in the serum is thought to primarily reflect its increased rate of entrance into serum from damaged liver cells.

   Classification of serum enzymes: Serum enzyme tests can be grouped into three categories: (1) enzymes whose elevation in serum reflects damage to hepatocytes, (2) enzymes whose elevation in serum reflects cholestasis, (3) tests that measure biosynthetic function of the liver.

1. **Enzymes that reflect damage to hepatocytes:** The aminotransferases (transaminases) are sensitive indicators of liver cell injury and are most helpful in recognizing acute hepatocellular diseases, such as hepatitis. They include the AST and the ALT. AST is found in the liver, cardiac muscle, skeletal muscle, kidneys, brain, pancreas, lungs, leukocytes, and erythrocytes in decreasing order of concentration. ALT is found primarily in the liver. The aminotransferases are normally present in the serum in low concentrations. These enzymes are released into the blood in greater amounts when there is damage to the liver cell membrane resulting in increased permeability. Liver cell necrosis is not required for the release of the aminotransferases and there is a poor correlation between the degree of liver cell damage and the level of the aminotransferases. Thus, the absolute elevation of the aminotransferases is of no prognostic significance in acute hepatocellular disorders.

   Diagnostic significance: Any type of liver cell injury can cause modest elevations in the serum aminotransferases.
   - Levels of up to 300 U/L are nonspecific and may be found in any type of liver disorder.
   - Striking elevations—i.e., aminotransferases >1,000 U/L—occur almost exclusively in disorders associated with extensive hepatocellular injury such as: (1) viral hepatitis, (2) ischemic liver injury (prolonged hypotension or acute heart failure), or (3) toxin- or drug-induced liver injury.
   - In most acute hepatocellular disorders, the ALT is higher than or equal to the AST.
   - An AST: ALT ratio >2:1 is suggestive while a ratio >3:1 is highly suggestive of alcoholic liver disease.
   - The AST in alcoholic liver disease is rarely >300 U/L and the ALT is often normal. A low level of ALT in the serum is due to an alcohol-induced deficiency of pyridoxal phosphate.
   - In obstructive jaundice, the aminotransferases are usually not greatly elevated. One notable exception occurs during the acute phase of biliary obstruction caused by the passage of a gallstone into the common bile duct. In this setting, the aminotransferases can briefly be in the 1,000–2,000 U/L range. However, aminotransferase levels decrease quickly and the liver function tests rapidly evolve into one typical of cholestasis.

2. **Enzymes that reflect cholestasis:** The activities of three enzymes—alkaline phosphatase, 5′-nucleotidase, and γ-glutamyl transpeptidase (GGT)—are usually elevated in cholestasis. Alkaline phosphatase and 5′-nucleotidase are found in or near the bile canalicular membrane of hepatocytes, while GGT is located in the endoplasmic reticulum and in bile duct epithelial cells.
   - **GGT:** Reflecting its more diffuse localization in the liver, GGT elevation in serum is less specific for cholestasis than are elevations of alkaline phosphatase or 5′-nucleotidase. GGT estimation is done to identify patients with occult alcohol use.
   - **Alkaline phosphatase:** The normal serum alkaline phosphatase consists of many distinct isoenzymes found in the liver, bone, placenta, and, less commonly, small intestine.

   Physiological variations:
   - Patients over age 60 years can have a mildly elevated alkaline phosphatase (1–1.5 times normal).
   - Individuals with blood types O and B can have an elevation of the serum alkaline phosphatase after eating a fatty meal due to the influx of intestinal alkaline phosphatase into the blood.
   - It is also nonpathologically elevated in children and adolescents undergoing rapid bone growth, because of bone alkaline phosphatase.
   - It is also high late in normal pregnancy due to the influx of placental alkaline phosphatase.
   - Pathological variations:
   - Elevation of liver-derived alkaline phosphatase is not totally specific for cholestasis and less than threefold elevation can be seen in almost any type of liver disease.
   - Alkaline phosphatase elevations greater than four times normal occur primarily in patients with cholestatic liver disorders, infiltrative liver diseases, such as cancer and amyloidosis, and bone conditions characterized by rapid bone turnover (e.g., Paget's disease).
   - In bone diseases, the elevation is due to increased amounts of the bone isoenzymes.
   - In liver diseases, the elevation is almost always due to increased amounts of the liver isoenzyme.
   - In the absence of jaundice or elevated aminotransferases, an elevated alkaline phosphatase of liver origin often, but not always suggests early cholestasis and, less often, hepatic infiltration by tumor or granulomata.
   - Other conditions that cause isolated elevations of the alkaline phosphatase include Hodgkin's disease, diabetes, hyperthyroidism, congestive heart failure, amyloidosis, and inflammatory bowel disease.

- **Intrahepatic cholestasis:** Values are increased in drug-induced hepatitis, primary biliary cirrhosis, rejection of transplanted livers, and, rarely, alcohol-induced steatonecrosis.
- **Extrahepatic cholestasis:** Very high values are found in obstructive jaundice due to cancer, common duct stone, sclerosing cholangitis, or bile duct stricture.
- The level of serum alkaline phosphatase elevation is not helpful in distinguishing between intrahepatic and extrahepatic cholestasis.
- Values are also greatly elevated in hepatobiliary disorders seen in patients with acquired immunodeficiency syndrome (AIDS) (e.g., AIDS cholangiopathy due to cytomegalovirus or cryptosporidial infection and tuberculosis with hepatic involvement).

Fractionation of alkaline phosphatase isoenzymes: This is required, if an elevated serum alkaline phosphatase is the only abnormal finding in an apparently healthy person, or if the degree of elevation is higher than expected in the clinical setting. The identification of the source of elevated isoenzymes can be determined by fractionation, which can be done by the following methods:

- **Electrophoresis:** Fractionation of the alkaline phosphatase can be done by electrophoresis.
- **Heat stability:** Other than electrophoresis, the second approach is based on the observation that alkaline phosphatase from individual tissues differs in susceptibility to inactivation by heat. The finding of an elevated serum alkaline phosphatase level in a patient with a heat-stable fraction strongly suggests that the placenta or a tumor is the source of the elevated enzyme in serum. Susceptibility to inactivation by heat increases, respectively, for the intestinal, liver, and bone alkaline phosphatases, bone being by far the most sensitive.
- **Estimation of liver-specific enzymes:** The third, best substantiated, and most available approach involves the measurement of serum 5′-nucleotidase or GGT. These enzymes are rarely elevated in conditions other than liver disease.

3. **Tests that measure biosynthetic function of the liver:**
   - **Serum albumin:** Serum albumin is synthesized exclusively by hepatocytes. Hypoalbuminemia is more common in chronic liver disorders, such as cirrhosis and usually reflects severe liver damage and decreased albumin synthesis. Serum albumin has a long half-life: 18–20 days, with ~4% degraded per day; because of this slow turnover, the serum albumin is not a good indicator of acute or mild hepatic dysfunction; only minimal changes in the serum albumin are seen in acute liver conditions, such as viral hepatitis, drug-related hepatoxicity, and obstructive jaundice. In hepatitis, albumin levels <3 g/dL should raise the possibility of chronic liver disease. However, hypoalbuminemia is not specific for liver disease and may occur in protein malnutrition of any cause, as well as protein-losing enteropathies, nephrotic syndrome, and chronic infections that are associated with prolonged increase in levels of serum interleukin 1 and/or tumor necrosis factor, cytokines that inhibit albumin synthesis.
   - **Serum globulins:** Serum globulins are a group of proteins produced by B lymphocytes and the globulins produced primarily in hepatocytes. Globulins are increased in chronic liver disease, such as chronic hepatitis and cirrhosis. In cirrhosis, the increased serum gamma-globulin concentration is due to the increased synthesis of antibodies, some of which are directed against intestinal bacteria. This occurs because the cirrhotic liver fails to clear bacterial antigens that normally reach the liver through the hepatic circulation.
   - Increases in the concentration of specific isotypes of globulins are often helpful in the recognition of certain chronic liver diseases. Diffuse polyclonal increases in IgG levels are common in autoimmune hepatitis. Increases in the IgM levels are common in primary biliary cirrhosis, while increases in the IgA levels occur in alcoholic liver disease.
   - **Coagulation factors:** With the exception of factor VIII, the blood clotting factors are made exclusively in hepatocytes. Their serum half-lives are much shorter than albumin, ranging from 6 hours for factor VII to 5 days for fibrinogen. Because of their rapid turnover, measurement of the clotting factors is the single best acute measure of hepatic synthetic function and helpful in both the diagnosis and assessing the prognosis of acute parenchymal liver disease. Useful for this purpose is the serum prothrombin time, which collectively measures factors II, V, VII, and X. Biosynthesis of factors II, VII, IX, and X depends on vitamin K. The prothrombin time may be elevated in hepatitis and cirrhosis as well as in disorders that lead to vitamin K deficiency, such as obstructive jaundice or fat malabsorption of any kind. Marked prolongation of the prothrombin time, >5 s above control and not corrected by parenteral vitamin K administration, is a poor prognostic sign in acute viral hepatitis and other acute and chronic liver diseases.
4. **Other diagnostic tests:**
   - **Percutaneous liver biopsy:** Percutaneous biopsy of the liver is of proven value in the following situations: (1) hepatocellular disease of uncertain cause, (2) prolonged hepatitis with the possibility of chronic active hepatitis, (3) unexplained hepatomegaly, (4) unexplained splenomegaly, (5) hepatic filling defects by radiologic imaging, (6) fever of unknown origin, and (7) staging of malignant lymphoma. Liver biopsy is most accurate in disorders causing diffuse changes throughout the liver.
   - **Ultrasonography:** Ultrasonography is the first diagnostic test to use in patients whose liver tests suggest cholestasis, to look for the presence of a dilated intrahepatic or extrahepatic biliary tree, or to identify gallstones. In addition, it shows space-occupying lesions within the liver.

Significance of Liver Function Tests in Hepatobiliary Disorders:

1. **Hemolysis/Gilbert's syndrome:** In hemolytic disorders, bilirubin rises up to 5 mg/dL. Since bilirubin is unconjugated so it does not appear in urine. Aminotransferases are slightly high but alkaline phosphatase is normal. Synthetic functions of liver are intact so there is no change in the concentration of serum albumin and prothrombin time is also normal.
2. **Acute hepatocellular necrosis (viral and drug hepatitis, hepatotoxins, and acute heart failure):** Mixed type of hyperbilirubinemia, both unconjugated and conjugated fractions are present in serum. Bilirubinuria is also there. Aminotransferases are elevated (ALT >AST). Alkaline phosphatase is high. Serum albumin is normal. Prothrombin time is prolonged.
3. **Chronic hepatocellular disorders:** Both fractions may be elevated, bilirubinuria is present, aminotransferases are elevated, but usually <300 IU, alkaline phosphatase is elevated normal to <3 times. Serum albumin is decreased and prothrombin time is prolonged which cannot be corrected by vitamin K.
4. **Alcoholic hepatitis cirrhosis:** Both fractions may be elevated, bilirubinuria is there. Aminotransferases are raised (AST >ALT 2:1). Alkaline phosphatase is high, serum albumin is decreased, and prothrombin time is prolonged which cannot be corrected by vitamin K.
5. **Intra- and extrahepatic cholestasis (obstructive jaundice):** Both fractions are present, bilirubinuria is also there. Aminotransferases are moderately elevated; alkaline phosphatase is elevated 4 times the normal. Serum albumin may be normal or slightly decreased. Prothrombin time is prolonged but it can be corrected by vitamin K administration.
6. **Infiltrative diseases (tumor, granulomata); partial bile duct obstruction:** Bilirubin is usually normal, aminotransferases are normal or slightly elevated, alkaline phosphatases are 4 times the normal, serum albumin is normal, and prothrombin time is also normal.

CLINICAL NOTE

The serum albumin is not a good indicator of acute or mild hepatic dysfunction; only minimal changes in the serum albumin are seen in acute liver conditions, such as viral hepatitis. In hepatitis, albumin levels <3 g/dL should raise the possibility of chronic liver disease.

CLINICAL PEARLS

1. Viruses causing hepatitis are: (1) HAV, (2) HBV, (3) HCV, (4) HDV (delta agent), and (5) HEV and HGV rarely, if ever, causes frank hepatitis.
2. The clinical picture of viral hepatitis is extremely variable, ranging from asymptomatic infection without jaundice to a fulminating disease and death in a few days.
3. In most patients, clinical recovery is complete in 3–6 months. Laboratory evidence of liver dysfunction may persist for a longer period, but most patients recover completely.
4. Liver tests rarely suggest a specific diagnosis; rather, they suggest a general category of liver disease, such as hepatocellular or cholestatic which then further directs the evaluation.
5. The liver function tests usually employed in clinical practice include the bilirubin, aminotransferases, alkaline phosphatase, albumin, and prothrombin time tests.

CASE STUDY 8

Theme: Interpretation of Impaired Liver Function Tests

A 25-year-old man with a long history of intravenous drug abuse and chronic hepatitis B presented with jaundice. Physical examination revealed a malnourished man with ascites, dependent pitting edema, spider angiomata, female secondary sex characteristics, and bilateral gynecomastia. Rectal examination reveals yellow-brown stool and a negative stool guaiac. External hemorrhoids were present. The patient had poor concentration, but no asterixis was present.

He had the following biochemical profile:

Total protein 8.2 g/dL, serum albumin 2.6 g/dL, and serum globulins 5.6 g/dL
Serum calcium 6.8 mg/dL, serum phosphorus 2.5 mg/dL
Serum BUN 6 mg/dL, serum creatinine 0.9 mg/dL
Serum sodium 131 mEq/L, serum potassium 3.0 mEq/L, and serum chloride 91 mEq/L
Serum bicarbonate 20 mEq/L
Serum total bilirubin 6.0 mg/dL
Serum AST 200 U/L

Serum ALT 350 U/L, serum alkaline phosphatase 180 U/L
Serum LDH 300 U/L

Urinalysis: Positive for bilirubin.

CBC: Macrocytic anemia with hypersegmented neutrophils, mild neutropenia, and mild thrombocytopenia.

Coagulation: Prothrombin time (PT) was prolonged and did not correct with intramuscular vitamin K administration.

What is the clinical significance of his abnormal liver function tests, hypoalbuminemia, and prolonged prothrombin time that does not correct with intramuscular vitamin K?
What is your interpretation of the electrolyte abnormalities in this patient?
What is the clinical significance of hypocalcemia in this patient?
Why does he have a low serum BUN?
What is the most likely cause of the macrocytic anemia?

CASE DISCUSSION

The patient is most probably suffering from chronic end-stage liver disease secondary, most likely, to chronic hepatitis B.

1. **Transaminases:** The transaminases are moderately elevated and ALT is higher than AST. In acute hepatitis, the transaminases would be higher owing to the presence of more liver tissue; however, in chronic hepatitis, the loss of hepatocytes and replacement by fibrosis result in less of an increase.
2. **Hypoalbuminemia and a prolonged PT** are markers of increased severity of liver disease, since both depend on the ability of the liver to synthesize proteins (albumin and coagulation factors). Inability to correct the PT with vitamin K documents that the liver is unable to synthesize the precursor vitamin K-dependent factors II, VII, IX, and X for (γ-carboxylation by vitamin K into functional coagulation factors). So, the synthetic functions of liver are impaired.
3. **Electrolyte imbalance:** The electrolytes reveal hyponatremia, hypokalemia, and a mild increased AG metabolic acidosis. Since the patient has ascites and dependent pitting edema, the total body Na must be increased; therefore, in order for there to be hyponatremia, there must be a hypotonic gain of fluid [serum Na TBNa/(TBW)]. This finding is expected owing to reduced venous return to the right heart (fluid is in the interstitial space) with a subsequent drop in the cardiac output. This decreases the effective arterial blood volume which initiates the release of ADH, aldosterone (activation of the renin-angiotensin-aldosterone system), and increased renal reabsorption of a hypotonic fluid containing a little more water than salt (in the same proportions as depicted in the serum sodium relationship above). Hence, when the hypotonic fluid reabsorbed by the kidneys encounters the reduced oncotic pressure (hypoalbuminemia) in the capillary and venular system, it is driven into the interstitial space by Starling's forces without restoring the cardiac output. In addition, some of the fluid contributes to the formation of ascitic fluid. The increased AG metabolic acidosis may be secondary to ketoacidosis from starvation and lactic acidosis from liver disease.
4. **Hypocalcemia:** The total serum calcium represents the calcium that is bound to albumin (40%), other anions (13%), and free (ionized calcium; 47%). A low ionized calcium may result in tetany. Therefore, in the presence of hypoalbuminemia, the most common cause of hypocalcemia, the total calcium is decreased while the ionized calcium is normal, so tetany is not present. Hypocalcemia is partly due to hypoalbuminemia and to hypovitaminosis D secondary to his liver disease. The liver is responsible for the first hydroxylation step in vitamin D metabolism after its reabsorption from the small bowel. Hypocalcemia is a stimulus for secondary hyperparathyroidism, which is likely to be present in this patient as well.
5. **Prerenal azotemia:** Because of the decrease in cardiac output, the reduction in the glomerular filtration rate would be expected to increase the reabsorption of urea in the proximal tubule, leading to prerenal azotemia. However, owing to location of the urea cycle in the liver, the presence of liver disease seriously hampers the normal function of disposing of ammonia in the urea cycle. Hence, in chronic liver disease, the serum BUN is low while the ammonia level is increased.
6. **Macrocytic anemia:** The macrocytic anemia with hypersegmented neutrophils in this patient is more likely secondary to folate rather than to B_{12} deficiency owing to the 3- to 4-month supply of folate in the liver versus the 6- to 9-year supply of B_{12}. This is easily verified by measurement of serum folate, RBC folate, and B_{12}. The elevated serum LDH is most likely secondary to destruction of the macrocytic RBCs (which contain increased LDH1 isoenzyme) in the bone marrow by macrophages (ineffective erythropoiesis).

Chapter 22

Water and Electrolyte Balance and Imbalance

LEARNING OBJECTIVES

To understand:
- Normal water and electrolyte balance
- Regulatory mechanisms, and
- Conditions causing water and electrolyte imbalance

CASE STUDIES

CASE STUDY 1

Theme: Normal water and electrolyte balance and the implication of dehydration

A man was trapped in a collapsed building after an earthquake. He had sustained no injuries or blood loss. He had no access to food or water until he was rescued after 72 hours.

What would have happened to his body fluid compartments?

CASE DETAILS

After 2 days or so, the kidneys would have adapted to the decreased input and conserved sodium, potassium and water. However, the patient continued to lose water insensibly, and as a result, the intracellular fluid (ICF) and the extracellular fluid (ECF) would have contracted in equal proportion.

After 3 to 4 days, usually the contraction becomes critical when the ECF is insufficient to maintain the circulation, and if the correction is not done, it leads to death of the individual. Since the patient has been rescued after 72 hours, hence in the present situation the person is having pure water deletion.

BASIC CONCEPT

Distribution of body water: Water and Na balance are closely interdependent. Total body water (TBW) is about 60% of body weight (ranging from about 50% in obese people to 70% in lean people). The body water can be visualized to be distributed in two "compartments." Almost 2/3 of TBW is in the intracellular compartment (intracellular fluid, or ICF); the other 1/3 of TBW is in the extracellular compartment (extracellular fluid, or ECF). Normally, about 25% of the ECF is in the intravascular compartment; the other 75% of the ECF is in the interstitial fluid.

Distribution of electrolytes in the body: Nonelectrolytes,, such as glucose, urea, etc., do not dissociate in solution. while substances like NaCl and KCl in solution dissociate into Na^+, K^+, and Cl^- respectively, they are called as electrolytes. Fluids in any body compartment will contain equal number of positively and negatively charged ions.

Electrolyte composition of ECF: Both plasma in vitro fertilization (IVF) and tissue fluid (ITF) may be considered as one single compartment for all practical purposes as both resemble each other and both grossly differ from ICF. Electrolyte composition of tissue fluid is same as plasma except that Cl^- largely replaces proteins as anions. Predominant cation is Na^+, with an average concentration of 140 mEq/L and the chief anion is chloride. The concentration of chloride in plasma is 103 mEq/L, while in tissue fluid, it is 116 mEq/L.

Electrolyte composition of ICF: The major intracellular cation is K, with an average concentration of 140 mEq/L. The extracellular K concentration is 3.5 to 5 mEq/L. Magnesium is the other major intracellular cation. These cations are balanced by the chief anions phosphates and proteins. The intracellular Na concentration is 12 mEq/L. About 2/3 of K within the cells is protein bound, while the remaining 1/3 is free which is exchanged with ECF. The chloride, bicarbonate, and sodium are present only in small concentrations. Total electrolyte concentration is higher than ECF.

Osmotic forces: The concentration of combined solutes in water is osmolarity (amount of solute per liter of solution), which, in body fluids, is similar to osmolality (amount of solute per kg of solution). Plasma osmolality can be measured in the laboratory or estimated according to the formula given as follows:

$$\text{Plasma osmolality (mOsm/kg)} = 2\,(\text{plasma Na}) + \frac{(\text{Glucose})}{18} + \frac{(\text{BUN})}{2.8}$$

Where serum Na is expressed in mEq/L and glucose and BUN are expressed in mg/dL. Osmolality of body fluids is normally between 275 and 290 mOsm/kg. Na is the major determinant of serum osmolality. Apparent changes in osmolality may result from errors in the measurement of Na with electrodes that are not ion selective. An osmolar gap is present when measured osmolality exceeds estimated osmolality by ≥10 mOsm/kg. It is caused by unmeasured osmotically active substances present in the plasma. The most common substances are alcohols (ethanol, methanol, isopropanol, and ethylene glycol), mannitol, and glycine.

Water crosses cell membranes freely from areas of low solute concentration to areas of high solute concentration. Thus, osmolality tends to equalize across the various body fluid compartments, resulting primarily from movement of water, not solutes. Solutes, such as urea that freely diffuse across cell membranes have little or no effect on water shifts (little or no osmotic activity), whereas solutes that are restricted primarily to one fluid compartment,, such as Na and K, have the greatest osmotic activity. Tonicity, or effective osmolality, reflects osmotic activity and determines the force drawing water across fluid compartments (the osmotic force). Osmotic force can be opposed by other forces. For example, plasma proteins have a small osmotic effect that tends to draw water into the plasma; this osmotic effect is normally counteracted by vascular hydrostatic forces that drive water out of the plasma.

Normal Water Balance

Body water is constantly exchanged with external environment

1. **Water intake:** The average daily fluid intake is about 2.5 L. It includes water ingested, water taken in cooked food, and the metabolic water formed from oxidation of food stuffs.
2. **Output of water:** Water is lost from the body constantly from various routes:
    - Via kidney as urine
    - Via skin as "insensible perspiration". Sweat losses can be significant during environmental heat exposure or excessive exercise.
    - Via lungs in the expired air
    - Through feces (GI losses are usually negligible, except when marked vomiting, diarrhea, or both occur).

Normally in health, the intake of water is more than the loss via skin, lungs, and feces, and the surplus is excreted by the kidneys. Thus in health, the urinary volume largely depends on intake of water. If the intake of water is less or excessive amounts are lost via extrarenal sites, the excretion of urine is diminished until only sufficient is excreted to eliminate the "waste products" of metabolism. Urinary volume may be reduced to 500 to 600 mL in 24 hours and this is called minimum excretory volume. The exact quantity depends on the:

- Concentrating power of the kidney
- The quantity of the solute load.

Renal concentrating capacity is lost in:

- The elderly
- Patients with diabetes insipidus, certain renal disorders, hypercalcemia, severe salt restriction, chronic over hydration, or hyperkalemia
- People who ingest ethanol, phenytoin, lithium, demeclocycline, or amphotericin B
- People with osmotic diuresis (e.g., due to high-protein diets or hyperglycemia).

Obligatory water losses are mostly insensible losses from the lungs, skin, and feces and the minimum excretory volume of the kidney to eliminate the waste products. All this averages about 1,600 mL approximately. With fever, another 50 to 75 mL/day may be lost for each degree centigrade of temperature elevation above normal. These losses continue till the person is surviving. The amount needed to replace losses from the urine and other sources is about 1 to 1.5 L/day in healthy adults. However, on a short-term basis, an average young adult with normal kidney function may ingest as little as 500 mL of water each day to excrete the nitrogenous and other wastes generated by cellular metabolism. More is needed in people with any loss of renal concentrating capacity.

In normal health, the electrolyte balance is maintained by gastrointestinal tract and the kidneys. This process of regulation is called "Internal recirculation of salts".

- **Gastrointestinal (GI) tract:** About 8 L of fluid of different electrolytes enter GI tract every day and are absorbed almost completely. The fluid loss is 100 to150 mL, Na^+ loss is 10 to 30 mEq/L, and K^+ loss is 10 mEq/L.
- **Kidneys:** A volume of 180 L of fluid is filtered everyday and 99.4% is reabsorbed. The fluid loss is 1 L and approximately 100 mEq of sodium is lost. Na^+ is exchanged with H^+ and NH^+ in proximal and distal tubules, respectively.

Regulatory Mechanisms

Water intake is regulated by thirst. Thirst is triggered by receptors in the anterolateral hypothalamus that respond to increased serum osmolality (as little as 2%) or decreased body fluid volume. Rarely hypothalamic dysfunction decreases the capacity for thirst. A deficient intake of water with continuing "obligatory losses" leads to concentration of body fluids with respect to solutes and a rise in osmotic pressure. This tends to draw water from ICF; the dehydration of the cells seems to be the main stimulus for thirst mechanisms.

Water and electrolyte excretion by the kidneys is regulated primarily by:

1. **Antidiuretic hormone (ADH) (vasopressin):** Antidiuretic hormone (ADH) is released by the posterior pituitary and results in increased water reabsorption in the distal nephron. Antidiuretic hormone (ADH) release is stimulated by any of the following:
    - Increased serum osmolality
    - Decreased blood volume
    - Decreased BP
    - Stress

    Antidiuretic hormone (ADH) release may be impaired by certain substances (e.g., ethanol, phenytoin, and central diabetes insipidus). Water intake decreases serum osmolality. Low serum osmolality inhibits ADH secretion, allowing the kidneys to produce dilute urine. The action of ADH is mediated through cAMP.
2. **Aldosterone:** Aldosterone increases the rate of tubular absorption of Na^+. It has the most important effect on mineral metabolism. It stimulates the water absorption from the tubules by stimulating the hypothalamus to release ADH and by creating an osmotic gradient across the tubular membrane. When the electrolytes are absorbed, water is also absorbed passively through the membrane. Aldosterone increases the reabsorption of chlorides also but at the same time it promotes the excretion of K^+. This may result from the elimination of K^+ in exchange of the reabsorbed Na^+.
3. **Kinins:** Kinins produced in the kidney increases salt and water excretion (natriuretic and diuretic effects). Action of Kinins is just opposite to ADH and aldosterone.
4. **Atrial natriuretic peptide (ANP):** Atrial natriuretic peptide (ANP) causes natriuresis by decreasing Na reabsorption of the renal collecting duct. Besides this, it causes increase in GFR, diuresis, decrease in renin and angiotensin secretion, and decrease in blood pressure.

Overview of Sodium Balance

Sodium is actively pumped out of cells by the Na^+, K^+-ATPase pump. As a result, 85–90% of all Na^+ is extracellular, and the ECF volume is a reflection of total body Na^+ content. Normal volume regulatory mechanisms ensure that Na^+ loss balances Na^+ gain. If this does not occur, conditions of Na^+ excess or deficit ensue and are manifest as edematous or hypovolemic states, respectively. It is important to distinguish between disorders of osmoregulation and disorders of volume regulation since water and Na^+ balance are regulated independently. Changes in Na^+ concentration generally reflect disturbed water homeostasis, whereas alterations in Na^+ content are manifested as ECF volume contraction or expansion and imply abnormal Na^+ balance.

Sodium Intake

Individuals eating a typical Western diet consume approximately 150 mmol of NaCl daily. This normally exceeds basal requirements. As sodium is the principal extracellular cation, therefore, dietary intake of Na^+ results in ECF volume expansion, which in turn promotes enhanced renal Na^+ excretion to maintain steady state Na^+ balance.

Sodium Excretion

The regulation of Na^+ excretion is multifactorial and is the major determinant of Na^+ balance. A Na^+ deficit or excess is manifested as a decreased or increased effective circulating volume, respectively. Changes in effective circulating volume tend to lead to parallel changes in glomerular filtration rate (GFR). However, tubule Na^+ reabsorption, and not GFR, is the major regulatory mechanism controlling Na^+ excretion. Almost two-thirds of filtered Na^+ is reabsorbed in the proximal convoluted tubule; this process is electroneutral and is osmotic. Further reabsorption (25–30%) occurs in the TALH via the apical Na^+-K^+-$2Cl^-$ cotransporter; this is an active process and is also electroneutral. Distal convoluted tubule reabsorption of Na^+ (5%) is mediated by the thiazide-sensitive Na^+-Cl^- cotransporter. Final Na^+ reabsorption occurs in the cortical and medullary collecting ducts; the amount excreted being reasonably equivalent to the amount ingested per day.

The abnormalities of water and electrolyte balance lead to dehydration and water intoxication.

CASE DISCUSSION

In the present situation, the person has been deprived of water so he is having dehydration (pure water dehydration). Since, there is a loss of water without simultaneous loss of sodium, it results in contraction of both ECF and ICF, and such a condition is known as "hypertonic contraction."

DEHYDRATION

Dehydration is a disturbance of water balance in which the output exceeds the intake, causing reduction of water below the normal level. Dehydration may be the result of:
- Pure water depletion
- Pure salt depletion
- Mixed type in which both occur

Dehydration can be categorized according to osmolarity and severity. Serum sodium is a good surrogate marker of osmolarity assuming the patient has normal serum glucose. Dehydration may be isonatremic (130–150 mEq/L), hyponatremic (<130 mEq/L), or hypernatremic (>150 mEq/L). Isonatremic dehydration is the most common (80%). Hypernatremic and hyponatremic dehydration each comprises 5–10% of cases. Variations in serum sodium reflect the composition of the fluids lost and have different pathophysiological effects.
- **Isonatremic (isotonic) dehydration:** Mixed water and salt depletion occurs when the lost fluid is similar in sodium concentration to the blood. Sodium and water losses are of the same relative magnitude in both the intravascular and extravascular fluid compartments.
- **Hyponatremic (hypotonic) dehydration:** Pure salt depletion occurs when the lost fluid contains more sodium than the blood (loss of hypertonic fluid). Relatively more sodium than water is lost. Because the serum sodium is low, intravascular water shifts to the extravascular space, exaggerating intravascular volume depletion for a given amount of total body water loss.
- **Hypernatremic (hypertonic) dehydration:** Pure water depletion occurs when the lost fluid contains less sodium than the blood (loss of hypotonic fluid). Relatively less sodium than water is lost. Because the serum sodium is high, extravascular water shifts to the intravascular space, minimizing intravascular volume depletion for a given amount of total body water loss.

Pure Water Depletion

Pure water depletion is also called primary dehydration. Pure water depletion occurs when water intake is stopped or water intake is inadequate, and there is no parallel loss of salt in the secretions from the body.

Causes

- When a person is too weak or too ill to satisfy his water needs
- In mental patients who refuse to drink
- In cases of coma and dysphagia
- In individuals lost in deserts or at places where water is not available (present case)
- Diabetes insipidus

Pathophysiology

Water depletion occurs almost always due to lack of intake, rather than because of losses from the body. Body water stores are depleted due to the ongoing "obligatory losses" and later on supplemented by the continued excretion of 'minimal volume" of required for excretion of "metabolic loads." Only source of water is the metabolic water obtained from the food stuffs. With the continuation of obligatory water losses, the ECF becomes hypertonic, and water flows from ICF to ECF. Thus, the ECF volume remains constant at the expense of ICF, which is grossly reduced in volume causing intracellular dehydration. Clinical manifestations of dehydration are most closely related to intravascular volume depletion. As dehydration progresses, hypovolemic shock ultimately ensues, resulting in end organ failure and death.

Diagnosis

History: The following should be considered in patients with dehydration:
- Intake of fluids, including the volume, and frequency
- Urine output, including the frequency of voiding, presence of concentrated or dilute urine, hematuria
- Stool output, frequency of stools, stool consistency, presence of blood or mucus in stools.

Clinical Manifestations

The signs and symptoms of dehydration range from minor to severe.
- Increased thirst: It is the earliest symptom due to intracellular dehydration
- Dry mouth, swollen tongue and pinched facies
- Dizziness
- Palpitations
- Confusion

- Sluggishness
- fainting
- Inability to sweat
- Neurological manifestations in severe dehydration
- **Decreased urine output:** Hyperosmolality stimulates the release of ADH, which causes reabsorption of water from renal tubules, causing a decreased output of urine.
- Death occurs when the water losses amount to approximately 15% of body weight (about 22% of total body water), which happens on the 7th to 10th day of complete water deprivation.

Physical Examination

A complete physical examination may assist in determining the underlying cause of the patient's dehydration and in defining the severity of dehydration. In general, physical signs of dehydration have poor precision and accuracy. The determination of dehydration severity should be based on the overall constellation of symptoms. Literature reviews have suggested that delayed capillary refill, delayed skin turgor, and abnormal respiratory pattern are the most reliable clinical signs of dehydration.

The estimation of water losses should be done based on the clinical features which is as follows:
Early (Mild) dehydration: The most important feature is thirst. There is approximately water loss of 2% of body weight.

Moderately severe (72–96 hours without water): Thirst, dry mouth, and pinched facies are the most important features. Weakness, oliguria, and neurological symptoms can be there. Water deficit is 6% of body weight.

Very severe: All the clinical symptoms mentioned above, along with diminution of mental and physical capabilities, hallucination and delirium. Water deficit is 7–14% of body weight.

Laboratory Investigations

No definitive laboratory test for dehydration is available. Laboratory data are generally not required if the etiology is apparent and mild-to-moderate dehydration is present. With severe dehydration, the following laboratory studies are suggested:

- Serum sodium is high, in pure water dehydration ECF remains hypertonic, plasma volume is normal, there is no increase in blood viscosity and there is no hemoconcentration.
- Plasma and urinary osmolality—both will be high
- Blood lactate may be high.
- Glucose may be dangerously low because of poor intake or extremely elevated in diabetic ketoacidosis (DKA).
- Blood urea nitrogen (BUN) and creatinine levels may be elevated because of renal hypoperfusion.
- Urine specific gravity may be elevated in patients with dehydration, but should not be relied on because it is not an accurate diagnostic test for dehydration.
- Urinalysis may show reduced volume. Urinary sodium and chlorides are elevated, ketone bodies may be present.

Treatment

Fluid replacement: Water through mouth or 5% glucose by I/V, S/C, or intraperitoneal routes depending on the case (For more details see hypernatremia).

Pure Salt Depletion

Pure salt depletion occurs when fluid of high Na^+ or Cl^- content is lost from the body and is replaced by salt-deficient fluids (see details of hyponatremia).

Mixed Water and Salt Depletion

In clinical practice, depletion of both water and sodium is more common than depletion of either alone. The clinical picture is a mixture of the two. The ECF is initially hypotonic; in the continuation of water loss, it becomes hypertonic later. The patient appears dehydrated and complains of thirst.

There may be hemoconcentration, blood urea is raised, and urinary output and urinary sodium are low. It is treated by a mixture of saline and 5% glucose in the proportion of 1:1or 1:2.

MORTALITY/MORBIDITY

Mortality and morbidity generally depend on the severity of dehydration and the promptness of oral or intravenous rehydration. If treatment is rapidly and appropriately obtained, morbidity and mortality are low.

CLINICAL NOTE

Water depletion occurs almost always due to lack of intake, rather than because of losses from the body.

CLINICAL PEARLS

1. Dehydration is a disturbance of water balance in which the output exceeds the intake, causing reduction of water below the normal level.
2. Dehydration may be the result of—pure water depletion, pure salt depletion, or mixed type in which both occur.
3. Dehydration may be isonatremic (130–150 mEq/L), hyponatremic (<130 mEq/L), or hypernatremic (>150 mEq/L). Isonatremic dehydration is the most common (80%).
4. The signs and symptoms of dehydration range from minor to severe. Increased thirst—is the earliest symptom due to intracellular dehydration. Dry mouth, swollen tongue, pinched facies, dizziness, palpitations, confusion sluggishness, and fainting may be there.

Laboratory data are generally not required if the etiology is apparent and mild-to-moderate dehydration is present. Treatment is symptomatic and fluid or saline replacement depending upon the cause.

CASE STUDY 2

Theme: Causes and consequences of hyponatremia

A 64-year-old woman was admitted with anorexia, weight loss, and anemia. Carcinoma of the colon was diagnosed. She was normotensive and did not have edema.

The following biochemical results were obtained shortly after admission:

Na^+	K^+	Cl^-	HCO_3^-	Urea	Creatinine
[			mmol/L		]
	[μmol/L				
123	3.8	88	21	6.2	115

Serum osmolality was measured as 247 mOsm/kg.
Urinary osmolality was 176 mOsm/kg.

What is the probable diagnosis of this patient?
What is the significance of urinary osmolality in this patient?

CASE DETAILS

These urea and electrolytes are typical of dilutional hyponatremia. Her normal blood pressure and serum urea and creatinine concentrations exclude significant sodium depletion. The absence of edema excludes a significance increase in her total body sodium. These results are characteristic of the so-called "syndrome of inappropriate antidiuresis" and are due to secretion of arginine vasopressin (AVP) in response to nonosmotic stimuli.

BASIC CONCEPT

Hyponatremia

Hyponatremia: Hyponatremia is a decrease in serum Na concentration <136 mEq/L caused by an excess of water relative to solute. Common causes include diuretic use, diarrhea, heart failure, and renal disease. Clinical manifestations are primarily neurologic (due to an osmotic shift of water into brain cells causing edema), especially in acute hyponatremia, and include headache, confusion, and stupor; seizures and coma may occur. Diagnosis is by measuring serum Na. Serum and urine electrolytes and osmolality help determine the cause. Treatment involves restricting water intake and promoting its loss, replacing any Na deficit, and treating the cause.

Pathophysiology

Serum sodium concentration is regulated by stimulation of thirst, secretion of antidiuretic hormone (ADH), feedback mechanisms of the renin–angiotensin–aldosterone system, and variations in renal handling of filtered sodium. Increases in serum osmolarity above the normal range (280–300 mOsm/kg) stimulate hypothalamic osmoreceptors, which, in turn, cause an increase in thirst and in circulating levels of ADH. Antidiuretic hormone (ADH) increases free water reabsorption from the urine, yielding urine of low volume and relatively high osmolarity and, as a result, returning serum osmolarity to normal. Antidiuretic hormone (ADH) is also secreted in response to hypovolemia, pain, fear, nausea, and hypoxia.

Aldosterone, synthesized by the adrenal cortex, is regulated primarily by serum potassium but also is released in response to hypovolemia through the renin–angiotensin–aldosterone axis. Aldosterone causes absorption of sodium at the distal renal tubule. Sodium retention obligates free water retention, helping to correct the hypovolemic state. The healthy kidney regulates sodium balance independently of ADH or aldosterone by varying the degree of sodium absorption at the distal tubule. Hypovolemic states,, such as hemorrhage or dehydration, prompt increases in sodium absorption in the proximal tubule. Increases in vascular volume suppress tubular sodium reabsorption, resulting in natriuresis and helping to restore normal vascular volume. Generally, disorders of sodium balance can be traced to a disturbance in thirst or water acquisition, ADH, aldosterone, or renal sodium transport.

Hyponatremia is physiologically significant when it indicates a state of extracellular hyposmolarity and a tendency for free water to shift from the vascular space to the intracellular space. Although cellular edema is well tolerated by most tissues, it is not well tolerated within the rigid confines of the bony calvarium. Therefore, clinical manifestations of hyponatremia are related primarily to cerebral edema. The rate of development of hyponatremia plays a critical role in its pathophysiology and subsequent treatment. When serum sodium concentration falls slowly, over a period of several days or weeks, the brain is capable of compensating by extrusion of solutes and fluid to the extracellular space. Compensatory extrusion of solutes reduces the flow of free water into the intracellular space, and symptoms are much milder for a given degree of hyponatremia.

When serum sodium concentration falls rapidly, over a period of 24–48 hours, this compensatory mechanism is overwhelmed and severe cerebral edema may ensue, resulting in brainstem herniation and death.

Etiology

Hyponatremia reflects an excess of total body water (TBW) relative to total body Na content.

1. **Hypovolemic hyponatremia:** Total body water (TBW) decreases; total body sodium (Na^+) decreases to a greater extent. The extracellular fluid (ECF) volume is decreased.

   Hypovolemic hyponatremia develops as sodium and free water are lost and replaced by inappropriately hypotonic fluids,, such as tap water, half-normal saline, or dextrose in water. Sodium can be lost through renal or nonrenal routes. Nonrenal routes include GI losses, excessive sweating, third spacing of fluids (e.g., ascites, peritonitis, pancreatitis, burns), and cerebral salt-wasting syndrome.

   a. **Renal causes:**
      - Acute or chronic renal insufficiency, in which the patient may be unable to excrete adequate amounts of free water.
      - Salt-wasting nephropathy—salt-losing nephropathy encompasses a loosely defined group of intrinsic renal disorders with primarily renal tubular dysfunction. This group includes interstitial nephritis, medullary cystic disease, partial urinary tract obstruction, and, occasionally, polycystic kidney disease.
      - Diuretics may also produce hypovolemic hyponatremia. Thiazide diuretics, in particular, decrease the kidneys' diluting capacity and increase Na excretion. Once volume depletion occurs, the nonosmotic release of ADH causes water retention and worsens hyponatremia. Concomitant hypokalemia shifts Na intracellularly and enhances ADH release, thereby worsening hyponatremia.

   b. **Extrarenal causes:**
      - Excess fluid losses (e.g., vomiting, diarrhea, excessive sweating, GI fistulas or drainage tubes, pancreatitis, and burns) that have been replaced primarily by hypotonic fluids.
      - Cerebral salt-wasting syndrome seen in patients with traumatic brain injury, aneurysmal subarachnoid hemorrhage, and intracranial surgery. Cerebral salt-wasting must be distinguished from syndrome of inappropriate antidiuretic hormone (SIADH) because both conditions can cause hyponatremia in neurosurgical patients, and yet the pathophysiology and treatment are different.
      - Prolonged exercise in a hot environment, especially in patients who hydrate aggressively with hypoosmolar fluids during exertion.

      Renal causes of hypovolemic hyponatremia can usually be differentiated from extrarenal causes by the history. Patients with ongoing renal fluid losses can also be distinguished from patients with extrarenal fluid losses because the urine Na concentration is inappropriately high (>20 mEq/L). In extrarenal causes of hypovolemia, because the normal renal response to volume loss is Na conservation, urine Na concentration is typically <10 mEq/L.

2. **Euvolemic hyponatremia:** Total body water (TBW) increases while total sodium remains normal. The ECF volume is increased minimally to moderately but without the presence of edema.

   This occurs in patients who take in excess fluids.

   - Primary polydipsia can cause hyponatremia only when water intake overwhelms the kidneys' ability to excrete water. Because normal kidneys can excrete up to 25 L urine/day, hyponatremia due solely to polydipsia results only from the ingestion of

large amounts of water or from defects in renal capacity to excrete free water. Patients affected include those with psychosis or more modest degrees of polydipsia plus renal insufficiency.
- Administration of hypotonic intravenous or irrigation fluids in the immediate postoperative period.
- Infants who may have been given inappropriate amounts of free water.
- SIADH.
- Euvolemic hyponatremia may also result from excessive water intake in the presence of Addison's disease or hypothyroidism.

3. **Hypervolemic hyponatremia:** Total body sodium increases, but TBW increases to a greater extent. The ECF is increased markedly, with the presence of edema.
   - This may result from renal causes, such as acute or chronic renal failure, when dysfunctional kidneys are unable to excrete the ingested sodium load. It also may occur in response to states of decreased effective intravascular volume.
   - History of hepatic cirrhosis, congestive heart failure, or nephrotic syndrome, in which patients are subject to insidious increases in total body sodium and free water stores. In each of these disorders, a decrease in effective circulating volume results in the release of ADH and angiotensin II. The following factors contribute to hyponatremia:
   - The antidiuretic effect of ADH on the kidneys
   - Direct impairment of renal water excretion by angiotensin II
   - Decreased glomerular filtration rate (GFR)
   - Stimulation of thirst by angiotensin II.

   Urine Na excretion is usually <10 mEq/L, and urine osmolality is high relative to serum osmolality.
4. **Redistributive hyponatremia:** Water shifts from the intracellular to the extracellular compartment, with a resultant dilution of sodium. The TBW and total body sodium are unchanged. This condition occurs with hyperglycemia or administration of mannitol.
5. **Pseudohyponatremia:** The aqueous phase is diluted by excessive proteins or lipids. The TBW and total body sodium are unchanged. This condition is seen with hypertriglyceridemia and multiple myeloma. Pseudohyponatremia may be due to interference with Na measurement by elevated lipids.

Incidence

Hyponatremia is the most common electrolyte disorder, with a marked increase among hospitalized patients. Hyponatremia has also been observed in approximately 30% of patients treated in the intensive care unit (ICU).

MORTALITY/MORBIDITY

Pathophysiological differences between patients with acute and chronic hyponatremia engender important differences in their morbidity and mortality.
- Patients with acute hyponatremia (developing over 48 hours or less) are subjected to more severe degrees of cerebral edema for a given serum sodium level. The primary cause of morbidity and death is brainstem herniation and mechanical compression of vital midbrain structures. Rapid identification and correction of serum sodium level is necessary in patients with severe acute hyponatremia to avert brainstem herniation and death.
- Patients with chronic hyponatremia (developing over more than 48 hours) experience milder degrees of cerebral edema for a given serum sodium level. Brainstem herniation has not been observed in patients with chronic hyponatremia. The principal causes of morbidity and death are status epilepticus (when chronic hyponatremia reaches levels of 110 mEq/L or less) and cerebral pontine myelinolysis (an unusual demyelination syndrome that occurs in association with chronic hyponatremia).
- The distinction between acute hyponatremia and chronic hyponatremia has critical implications in terms of morbidity and mortality and in terms of proper corrective therapy.

Age

Hyponatremia is the most common in the extremes of age; these groups are less able to experience and express thirst and less able to regulate fluid intake autonomously.

CLINICAL MANIFESTATIONS

- Symptoms mainly involve central nervous system (CNS) dysfunction.
- However, when hyponatremia is accompanied by disturbances in total body Na content, signs of ECF volume depletion or overload also occur.
- In general, older chronically-ill patients with hyponatremia develop more symptoms than younger otherwise healthy patients.
- Symptoms are also more severe with faster-onset hyponatremia.
- Symptoms generally occur when the effective plasma osmolality falls to <240 mOsm/kg.
- Symptoms can be subtle and consist mainly of changes in mental status, including altered personality, lethargy, and confusion.
- As the serum Na falls to <115 mEq/L, stupor, neuromuscular hyperexcitability, hyperreflexia, seizures, coma, and death can result.

- Severe cerebral edema may occur in premenopausal women with acute hyponatremia, perhaps because estrogen and progesterone inhibit brain Na^+ and K^+-ATPase and decrease solute extrusion from brain cells. Sequelae include hypothalamic and posterior pituitary infarction and occasionally brainstem herniation.

Diagnosis

Hyponatremia is occasionally suspected in patients who have neurologic abnormalities and are at risk. However, because findings are nonspecific, hyponatremia is often recognized only after serum electrolyte measurement.

Laboratory tests should include:

- Serum and urine osmolality and electrolytes. Hypoosmolality in euvolemic patients causes excretion of a large volume of dilute urine (e.g., osmolality <100 mOsm/kg and specific gravity <1.003).
- Euvolemic patients should also have thyroid and adrenal function tested.
- Serum Na concentration and serum osmolality that are low and urine osmolality that is inappropriately high (120–150 mmol/L) with respect to the low serum osmolality suggest volume overload, volume contraction, or SIADH.
- Falsely low levels of sodium—Serum Na may be low when severe hyperglycemia increases osmolality and water moves out of cells into the ECF. Serum Na concentration falls about 1.6 mEq/L for every 100 mg/dL (5.55 mmol/L) rise in the serum glucose concentration above normal. This condition is often called translocational hyponatremia because it is caused by translocation of Na across cell membranes. Pseudohyponatremia with normal serum osmolality may occur in hyperlipidemia or extreme hyperproteinemia, because the lipid or protein occupies space in the volume of serum taken for analysis; the concentration of Na in serum itself is not affected. Newer methods of measuring serum electrolytes with ion-selective electrodes circumvent this problem.
- Volume overload and volume contraction are differentiated. When neither volume overload or volume contraction appears likely, SIADH is considered. Patients with SIADH are usually euvolemic or slightly hypervolemic.
- Blood urea nitrogen (BUN) and creatinine values are normal, and serum uric acid is generally low.
- Urine Na concentration is usually >30 mmol/L, and fractional excretion of Na is >1%.
- In patients with hypovolemia and normal renal function, Na reabsorption results in a urine Na of <20 mmol/L. Urine Na >20 mmol/L in hypovolemic patients suggests mineralocorticoid deficiency or salt-losing nephropathy.
- Hyperkalemia suggests adrenal insufficiency.

TREATMENT

- When hypovolemic, 0.9% saline
- When hypervolemic, fluid restriction and sometimes a diuretic
- When euvolemic, treatment of cause
- Rarely, cautious correction with hypertonic (3%) saline

Rapid correction of hyponatremia, even mild hyponatremia, risks neurologic complications. Except possibly in the first few hours of treatment of severe hyponatremia, Na should be corrected no faster than 0.5 mEq/L/h. Even with severe hyponatremia, increase in serum Na concentration should not exceed 10 mEq/L over the first 24 hours. Any identified cause of hyponatremia is treated concurrently.

Osmotic demyelination syndrome: Osmotic demyelination syndrome (previously called central pontine myelinolysis) may follow too-rapid correction of hyponatremia. Demyelination may affect the pons and other areas of the brain. Lesions are more common in patients with alcoholism, under nutrition, or other chronic debilitating illness. Flaccid paralysis, dysarthria, and dysphagia can evolve over a few days or weeks. The lesion may extend dorsally to involve sensory tracts and leave patients with a locked-in syndrome (an awake and sentient state in which patients, because of generalized motor paralysis, cannot communicate, except possibly by coded eye movements). Damage often is permanent. When Na is replaced too rapidly (e.g., >14 mEq/L/8 hours) and neurologic symptoms start to develop, it is critical to prevent further serum Na increases by stopping hypertonic fluids. In such cases, inducing hyponatremia with hypotonic fluid may mitigate the development of permanent neurologic damage.

Complications

- Complications related to hyponatremia include rhabdomyolysis, seizures, permanent neurologic sequelae related to ongoing seizures or cerebral edema, respiratory arrest, and death.
- Complications related to therapy of hyponatremia include fluid overload and the osmotic demyelination syndrome.

Prognosis

Prognosis is dependent on the underlying condition and the severity of disease.

CLINICAL NOTE

Rapid correction of hyponatremia, even mild hyponatremia, risks neurologic complications.

CLINICAL PEARLS

1. Hyponatremia is a decrease in serum Na concentration <136 mEq/L caused by an excess of water relative to solute.
2. Serum sodium concentration is regulated by stimulation of thirst, secretion of ADH, feedback mechanisms of the renin–angiotensin–aldosterone system, and variations in renal handling of filtered sodium.
3. Symptoms can be subtle and consist mainly of changes in mental status, including altered personality, lethargy, and confusion. As the serum Na falls to <115 mEq/L, stupor, neuromuscular hyperexcitability, hyperreflexia, seizures, coma, and death can result.
4. Mild, asymptomatic hyponatremia (i.e., serum Na >120 mEq/L) requires restraint because small adjustments are generally sufficient.
5. Complications related to therapy of hyponatremia include fluid overload and the osmotic demyelination syndrome.

CASE STUDY 3

Theme: Causes and consequences of hypernatremia

A 76-year-old man with depression and very severe incapacitating disease was admitted as an acute emergency. He was clinically dehydrated. His skin was lax and his lips and tongue were dry and shriveled looking. His pulse was 104 beats/min, and his blood pressure was 95/65 mm Hg. The following biochemical results were obtained on admission:

Na^+	K^+	Cl^-	HCO_3^-	Urea	Creatinine
[—			mmol/L	—]	[μmol/L
162	3.6	132	18	23	155

Comment on these biochemical findings. What is the probable diagnosis of this patient?

CASE DETAILS

The biochemical results strongly suggest prerenal uremia, as there is marked increase in serum urea and a modest increase in serum creatinine. He has a very severe hypernatremia and these two observations indicate that the patient is primarily suffering from water depletion. The serum potassium is normal as is his anion gap. These results would, therefore, indicate the presence of profound uncomplicated water depletion.

In a case, such as this, it is essential to exclude nonketotic, diabetic precoma. His blood glucose and ketones are required to be estimated. It is rapidly established from the clinical history that the patient did not have access to water for many days. A diagnosis of pure water depletion can be established on the basis of history, clinical findings, and biochemical features.

BASIC CONCEPT

Hypernatremia

Hypernatremia is the serum Na concentration >145 mEq/L. It implies a deficit of total body water relative to total body Na, caused by water intake being less than water losses. A major symptom is thirst; other clinical manifestations are primarily neurologic (due to an osmotic shift of water out of brain cells), including confusion, neuromuscular excitability, seizures, and coma. Diagnosis requires measurement of serum Na and sometimes other tests. Treatment is usually controlled water replacement. When the response is poor, testing (e.g., monitored water deprivation or administration of vasopressin) is directed at detecting causes other than decreased water intake.

Pathophysiology

Net water loss accounts for most cases of hypernatremia. Hypertonic sodium gain usually results from clinical interventions or accidental sodium loading. As a result of increased extracellular sodium concentration, plasma tonicity increases. This increase in tonicity induces the movement of water across cell membranes, causing cellular dehydration.

The following three mechanisms may lead to hypernatremia, alone or in concert:
1. Pure water depletion (e.g., diabetes insipidus)
2. Water depletion exceeding sodium depletion (e.g., diarrhea)
3. Sodium excess (e.g., salt poisoning)

Sustained hypernatremia can occur only when thirst or access to water is impaired. Therefore, the groups at highest risk are infants and intubated patients.

Because of certain physiologic characteristics, infants are predisposed to dehydration. They have a large surface area in relation to their height or weights compared with adults and have relatively large evaporative water losses. In infants, hypernatremia usually results from diarrhea and sometimes from improperly prepared infant formula or inadequate mother–infant interaction during breastfeeding.

Hypernatremia causes decreased cellular volume as a result of water efflux from the cells to maintain equal osmolality inside and outside the cell. Brain cells are especially vulnerable to complications resulting from cell contraction. Severe hypernatremic dehydration induces brain shrinkage, which can tear cerebral blood vessels, leading to cerebral hemorrhage, seizures, paralysis, and encephalopathy.

In patients with prolonged hypernatremia, rapid rehydration with hypotonic fluids may cause cerebral edema, which can lead to coma, convulsions, and death.

Incidence

In developing nations, the reported incidence is 1.5–20%. Hypernatremia is primarily a hospital-acquired condition occurring in children of all ages who have restricted access to fluids, mostly due to significant underlying medical problems, such as a chronic disease, neurologic impairment, a critical illness, or prematurity. Hospital-acquired hypernatremia accounts for 60% of hypernatremia cases in children. Gastroenteritis contributes to the hypernatremia in only 20% of cases. The group most affected is intubated, critically-ill patients.

Mortality/Morbidity

In children with acute hypernatremia, mortality rates are as high as 20%. Neurologic complications related to hypernatremia occur in 15% of patients. In cases of chronic hypernatremia in children, the mortality rate is 10%.

Clinical Manifestations

The major symptom of hypernatremia is thirst. The absence of thirst in conscious patients with hypernatremia suggests an impaired thirst mechanism. Patients with difficulty communicating may be unable to express thirst or obtain access to water.

The major signs of hypernatremia result from central nervous system (CNS) dysfunction due to brain cell shrinkage. Confusion, neuromuscular excitability, hyperreflexia, seizures, or coma may result; cerebrovascular damage with subcortical or subarachnoid hemorrhage and venous thrombosis are common in patients who died from severe hypernatremia.

In chronic hypernatremia, osmotically active substances occur in CNS cells (idiogenic osmoles) and increase intracellular osmolality. Therefore, the degree of brain cell dehydration and resultant CNS symptoms are less severe in chronic than in acute hypernatremia.

When hypernatremia occurs with abnormal total body Na, the typical symptoms of volume depletion or overload are present. A large volume of hypotonic urine is characteristically excreted in patients with renal concentrating defects. When losses are extrarenal, the route of water loss is often evident (e.g., vomiting, diarrhea, and excessive sweating), and the urinary Na concentration is low.

Physical Examination

- Skin turgor is a physical finding in patients with hypernatremia. Extracellular and plasma volumes tend to be maintained in hypernatremic dehydration until dehydration is severe (i.e., when the patient loses >10% of body weight).
- When dehydration is severe, skin turgor is reduced, and the skin develops a characteristic doughy appearance.

Causes of Hypernatremia

Hypernatremia reflects a deficit of total body water (TBW) relative to total body Na content. Because total body Na content is reflected by extracellular fluid (ECF) volume status, hypernatremia must be considered along with status of the ECF volume: hypovolemia, euvolemia, and hypervolemia. Note that the ECF volume is not the same as effective plasma volume. For example, decreased effective plasma volume may occur with decreased ECF volume, but it may also occur with an increased ECF volume (e.g., in heart failure, hypoalbuminemia, and capillary leak syndrome).

Hypernatremia usually implies either an impaired thirst mechanism or limited access to water. The severity of the underlying disorder that results in an inability to drink in response to thirst and the effects of brain:

Description	*Category*	*Examples*
Hypovolemic hypernatremia		
Decreased TBW and Na with a relatively greater decrease in TBW	GI losses	Diarrhea
	Skin losses	Vomiting Burns
	Renal losses	Excessive sweating Intrinsic renal disease Loop diuretics Osmotic diuresis (glucose, urea, mannitol)
Euvolemic hypernatremia		
Decreased TBW with near-normal total body Na	Extrarenal losses from respiratory tract	
	Extrarenal losses from skin	Tachypnea Fever
	Renal losses	Central diabetes insipidus
	Other	Nephrogenic diabetes insipidus Inability to access water Primary hypodipsia Reset osmostat
Hypervolemic hypernatremia	Hypertonic fluid administration	Hypertonic saline
Increased Na with normal or increased TBW		
		$NaHCO_3$ TPN
	Mineralocorticoid excess	Adrenal tumors secreting deoxycorticosterone
		Congenital adrenal hyperplasia (caused by 11-hydroxylase defect)

TBW = total body water.

Hyperosmolality is thought to be responsible for a high mortality rate in hospitalized adults with hypernatremia. There are several common causes of hypernatremia.

Principal Causes of Hypernatremia (Fig. 22.1)

a. **Hypovolemic hypernatremia:** Hypernatremia associated with hypovolemia occurs with Na loss accompanied by a relatively greater loss of water from the body. Common extrarenal causes include most of those that cause hyponatremia and volume depletion; either hypernatremia or hyponatremia can occur with severe volume loss, depending on the relative amounts of Na and water lost and the amount of water ingested before presentation.

   Renal causes of hypernatremia and volume depletion include therapy with diuretics. Loop diuretics inhibit Na reabsorption in the concentrating portion of the nephron and can increase water clearance. Osmotic diuresis can also impair renal concentrating capacity because of a hypertonic substance present in the tubular lumen of the distal nephron. Glycerol, mannitol, and occasionally urea can cause osmotic diuresis resulting in hypernatremia. The most common cause of hypernatremia due to osmotic diuresis is hyperglycemia in patients with diabetes. Because glucose does not penetrate cells in the absence of insulin, hyperglycemia further dehydrates the intracellular fluid (ICF) compartment. The degree of hyperosmolality in hyperglycemia may be obscured by the lowering of serum Na resulting from movement of water out of cells into the ECF (translational hyponatremia). Patients with renal disease can also be predisposed to hypernatremia when their kidneys are unable to maximally concentrate urine.

b. **Euvolemic hypernatremia:** Hypernatremia with euvolemia is a decrease in TBW with near-normal total body Na (pure water deficit). Extrarenal causes of water loss,, such as excessive sweating, result in some Na loss, but because sweat is hypotonic, hypernatremia can result before significant hypovolemia. A deficit of almost purely water also occurs in central and nephrogenic diabetes insipidus.

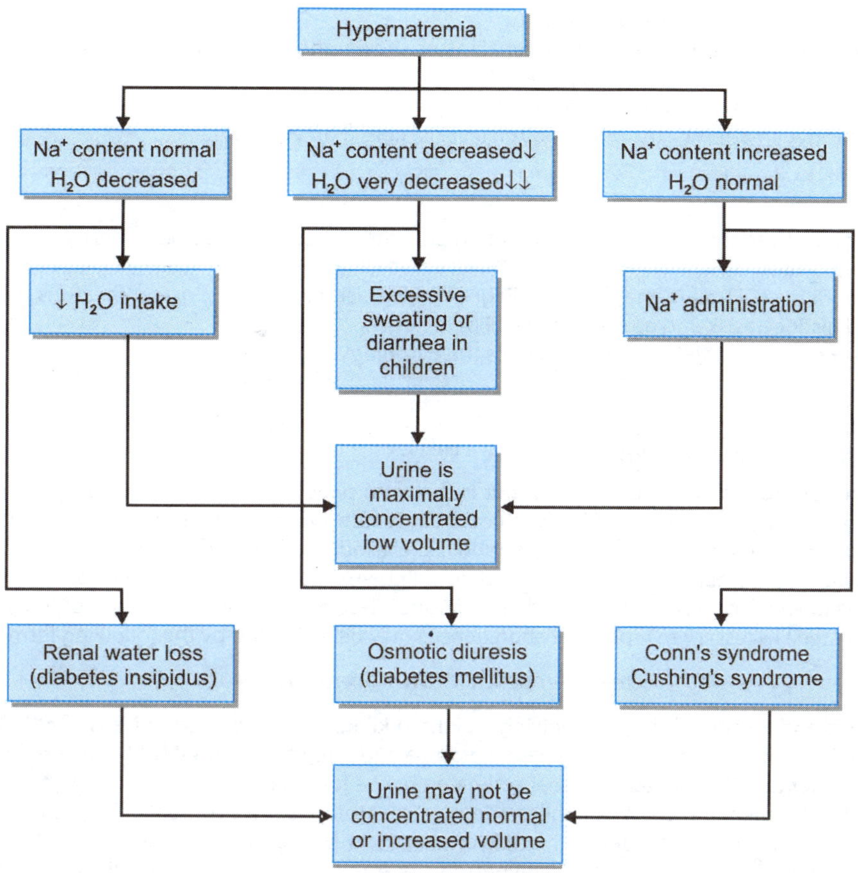

Fig. 22.1: Causes of hypernatremia.

Essential hypernatremia (primary hypodipsia) occasionally occurs in children with brain damage and in chronically-ill elderly adults. It is characterized by an impaired thirst mechanism (e.g., caused by lesions of the brain's thirst center). Altered osmotic trigger for antidiuretic hormone (ADH) release is another possible cause of euvolemic hypernatremia; some lesions cause both an impaired thirst mechanism and an altered osmotic trigger. The nonosmotic release of ADH appears intact, and these patients are generally euvolemic.

c. **Hypervolemic hypernatremia:** Hypernatremia in rare cases is associated with volume overload. In this case, hypernatremia results from a grossly elevated Na intake associated with limited access to water. One example is the excessive administration of hypertonic $NaHCO_3$ during treatment of lactic acidosis. Hypernatremia can also be caused by the administration of hypertonic saline or incorrectly formulated hyperalimentation.
d. **Hypernatremia in the elderly:** Hypernatremia is common in the elderly, particularly postoperative patients and those receiving tube feedings or parenteral nutrition. Other contributing factors may include the following:
   - Dependence on others to obtain water
   - Impaired thirst mechanism
   - Impaired renal concentrating capacity (due to diuretics, impaired ADH release, or nephron loss accompanying aging or other renal disease)
   - Impaired angiotensin II production (which may contribute directly to the impaired thirst mechanism).

Laboratory Studies

The following studies are indicated in patients with suspected hypernatremia:

- Serum Na

The diagnosis is clinical and by measuring serum Na. In patients who do not respond to simple rehydration or in whom hypernatremia recurs despite adequate access to water, further diagnostic testing is warranted. Determination of the underlying disorder requires assessment of urine volume and osmolality, particularly after water deprivation.

In those with increased urine output, a water deprivation test is occasionally used to differentiate among several polyuric states,, such as central and nephrogenic diabetes insipidus.

- Blood urea nitrogen (BUN), and creatinine levels are also measured to check the kidney status.

- Urine tests of sodium concentration and osmolality
  - In cases of hypovolemic hypernatremia, extrarenal losses show urine sodium levels of less than 20 mEq/L, and in cases of renal losses, urine sodium values are more than 20 mEq/L.
  - In euvolemic hypernatremia, urine sodium data vary.
  - In hypervolemic hypernatremia, the urine sodium level is more than 20 mEq/L.

Imaging studies

- Imaging studies of the head should be considered in alert patients with severe hypernatremia to rule out a hypothalamic lesion affecting the thirst center.
- Computed tomography (CT) scans may help in diagnosing intracranial tumors, granulomatous diseases (e.g., sarcoidosis, tuberculosis, and histiocytosis), and other intracranial pathologies.
- Magnetic resonance imaging (MRI) further delineates the pathology.

TREATMENT

Replacement of Intravascular Volume and of Free Water

Replacement of intravascular volume and of free water is the main goal of treatment. Oral hydration is effective in conscious patients without significant gastrointestinal (GI) dysfunction. In severe hypernatremia or in patients unable to drink because of continued vomiting or mental status changes, IV hydration is preferred. Hypernatremia that lasts <24 hours should be corrected within 24 hours. However, hypernatremia that is chronic or of unknown duration should be corrected over 48 hours, and the serum osmolality should be lowered at a rate of no faster than 2 mOsm/L/h to avoid cerebral edema caused by excess brain solute. The amount of water (in liters) necessary to replace existing deficits may be estimated by the following formula:

$$\text{Free water deficit} = \text{TBW} \times [(\text{serum Na}/140) - 1]$$

Where TBW is in liters and is estimated by multiplying weight in kilograms by 0.6; serum Na is in mEq/L. This formula assumes constant total body Na content. In patients with hypernatremia and depletion of total body Na content (i.e., who have volume depletion), the free water deficit is greater than that estimated by the formula.

1. In patients with hypernatremia and ECF volume overload (excess total body Na content), the free water deficit can be replaced with 5% D/W, which can be supplemented with a loop diuretic. However, too-rapid infusion of 5% D/W may produce glycosuria, thereby increasing salt-free water excretion and hypertonicity, especially in patients with diabetes mellitus. Other electrolytes, including serum K, should be monitored and should be replaced as needed.
2. In patients with hypernatremia and euvolemia, free water can be replaced using either 5% D/W or 0.45% saline. Treatment of patients with central diabetes insipidus and nephrogenic diabetes insipidus is specifically done.
3. In patients with hypernatremia and hypovolemia, particularly in patients with diabetes with nonketotic hyperglycemic coma, 0.45% saline can be given as an alternative to a combination of 0.9% normal saline and 5% D/W to replenish Na and free water. Alternatively, ECF volume and free water can be replaced separately, using the formula given previously to estimate the free water deficit. When severe acidosis (pH <7.10) is present, $NaHCO_3$ solution can be added to 5% D/W or 0.45% saline, as long as the final solution remains hypotonic.

Diet

In diabetes insipidus, a sodium-restricted and protein-restricted diet should be prescribed.

Medication

The medications described below are used in patients with diabetes insipidus who have hypernatremia.

Vasopressin and Vasopressin Analogs

Desmopressin is a synthetic ADH with actions mimicking vasopressin. These agents are used to treat diabetes insipidus, which deprives the kidney of its capacity to produce concentrated urine. This effect results in large volumes of dilute urine (polyuria) and excessive thirst (polydipsia). Serum sodium concentrations may be elevated, but hypernatremia is most likely to be severe when fluid is restricted.

Desmopressin Acetate

Structural analog of vasopressin (ADH), the endogenous posterior pituitary hormone, that maintains serum osmolality in a physiologically acceptable range, works in neurohypophysial (e.g., central) diabetes insipidus and exerts similar antidiuretic effects. Vasopressin increases resorption of water at level of renal collecting duct, reducing urinary flow and increasing urine osmolality.

Diuretics

These drugs promote the excretion of water and electrolytes by the kidneys. They are used in patients with nephrogenic diabetes insipidus.

Prevention

- Parents and caregivers should avoid making oral rehydration solutions at home or adding salt to any commercial infant formula.
- Treat the underlying cause.

Complications

- Seizures can occur because of hypernatremia *per se*, which is rare. They usually occur during the treatment of hypernatremia because of a rapid decline in serum sodium levels. Therefore, slowly correcting hypernatremia is important.
- Other complications include the following:
  - Mental retardation
  - Intracranial hemorrhage
  - Intracerebral calcification
  - Cerebral infarction
  - Cerebral edema, especially during treatment
  - Hypocalcemia
  - Hyperglycemia

Prognosis

- Patients usually recover from hypernatremia.
- Patients with recurrent hypernatremic dehydration develop neurologic sequelae, especially infants with diabetes insipidus.

CLINICAL NOTE

Hypernatremia causes decreased cellular volume as a result of water efflux from the cells to maintain equal osmolality inside and outside the cell.

CLINICAL PEARLS

1. Hypernatremia is a serum Na concentration of >145 mEq/L. It implies a deficit of total body water relative to total body Na, caused by water intake being less than water losses.
2. A major symptom is thirst; other clinical manifestations are primarily neurologic (due to an osmotic shift of water out of brain cells), including confusion, neuromuscular excitability, seizures, and coma.
3. Diagnosis requires measurement of serum Na and sometimes other tests.
4. Treatment is usually controlled water replacement.
5. When the response is poor, testing (e.g., monitored water deprivation or administration of vasopressin) is directed at detecting causes other than decreased water intake.

CASE STUDY 4

Theme: Causes and consequences of hyperkalemia

A 55-year-old man was trapped for 7 hours in a railway accident. He sustained severe multiple injuries including crush injuries to both thighs, fractures of the pelvis and scalp lacerations. On arrival at accident and emergency center, he was still conscious and breathing spontaneously.

His pulse rate was 130 beats/minute and his blood pressure (BP) was 60/40 mm Hg. The laboratory report was as follows:

Serum Na^+	142 mmol/L
Serum K^+	8.1 mmol/L
Serum Cl^-	108 mmol/L
Blood urea	38 mg/dL
Serum creatinine	1.2 mg/dL

What is the probable diagnosis?
What are the priorities in managing this patient?

CASE DISCUSSION

As in all cases of acute trauma, the priorities are A, B, and C; ensure a patent airway, ensure that the patient is breathing and ensure that the patient's circulation is intact. These are the principles of resuscitation. From a biochemical point of view, the patient has dangerously high serum potassium. This is due to release of potassium from damaged tissues. This will require immediate treatment with calcium given I/V as calcium gluconate or calcium chloride to counteract the dangers of hyperkalemia and the steps are needed to lower potassium levels. This will involve the use of insulin and glucose infusion in the first instance and it is likely that such a patient may require to be dialyzed. The other feature to note is low serum bicarbonate and high serum anion gap. From the history and these results, one can make a diagnosis of lactic acidosis due to tissue hypoxia. The treatment of lactic acidosis will depend on establishing a satisfactory circulation and tissue oxygenation.

BASIC CONCEPT

Potassium Metabolism and Its Significance in the Body

Potassium is the principal intracellular cation of the body and is a significant determinant of intracellular osmolality. Only 2% of total body K is extracellular; the rest of the K is present within the cell. The considerable amount of K is contained within muscle cells; therefore, the total body K is practically proportional to lean body mass. An average 60-kg adult has about 3,000 mEq of K.

The cell membrane polarization that influences the conduction of nerve impulses and muscle (including myocardial) contraction is strongly affected by the ratio between ICF and ECF potassium concentrations. Therefore, even small changes in serum K levels can have profound clinical manifestations.

In the absence of factors that promote movement of K in or out of cells, the serum K concentration corresponds closely with total body K content. In the presence of stable intracellular and extracellular levels, a decrease in serum K concentration of about 1 mEq/L signifies an overall K deficit of about 200 to 400 mEq. Patients with K <3 mEq/L characteristically have a significant K deficit.

a. K shifts: Factors that promote movement of K in or out of cells include the following:
- Plasma insulin levels
- β-adrenergic activity
- Plasma pH.

1. **Plasma insulin levels**—K shifts into cells in the presence of high concentrations of insulin, thereby lowering serum K concentration. Low insulin concentrations, as in diabetic ketoacidosis, cause movement of K to out of cells, thus raising serum K; however, there may even be total body K deficiency.
2. **β-Adrenergic agonists**, especially selective β_2-agonists, promote K movement into cells, whereas β-blockade and α-agonists promote movement of K out of cells.
3. **Plasma pH**—Acute metabolic acidosis causes movement of K out of cells, whereas acute metabolic alkalosis causes movement of K into cells. However, changes in serum HCO_3 concentration may be more important than changes in pH; acidosis caused by the accumulation of mineral acids (normal anion gap, hyperchloremic acidosis) is more likely to raise serum K. In contrast, metabolic acidosis due to the collection of organic acids (high anion gap acidosis) is not associated with hyperkalemia. Therefore, the hyperkalemia observed in diabetic ketoacidosis results in more from insulin deficiency rather than from acidosis. Acute respiratory acidosis and alkalosis affect serum K concentration less than metabolic acidosis and alkalosis. However, serum K concentration needs to be interpreted in the context of the plasma pH (and HCO_3 concentration) **(Fig. 22.2)**.

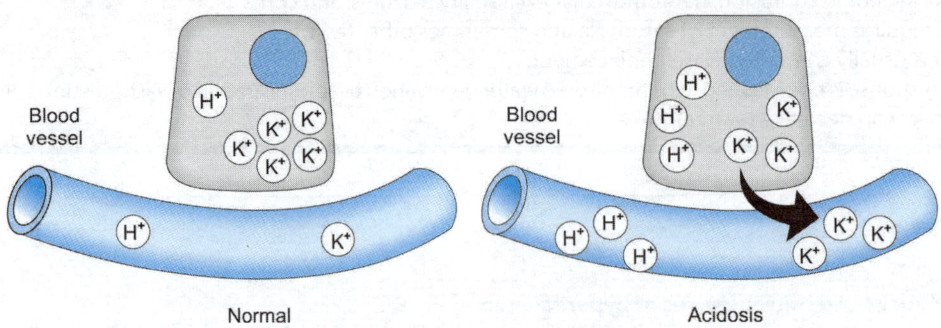

Fig. 22.2: Acidosis-induced hyperkalemia.

b. K metabolism—Dietary intake of K varies typically between 40 and 150 mEq/day. In the stable state, fecal losses are usually close to 10% of intake. Urinary excretion contributes to the maintenance of K balance.

When K intake is >150 mEq/day, about 50% of the excess K is found in the urine over the next several hours. Most of the remainder is transferred into the intracellular compartment, thus minimizing the increase in serum K levels. When higher K intake continues, **aldosterone secretion is stimulated,** and thus, renal K excretion is increased. Also, K absorption from gut seems to be under some regulation and may fall by 50% in chronic K excess.

When K intake falls, intracellular K again serves to minimize wide variations in serum K concentration. **Renal K conservation develops** relatively slowly in response to decreases in dietary K and is far less efficient than the kidneys' ability to conserve Na.

Thus, K loss is a frequent clinical problem. Urinary K excretion of 10 mEq/day highlights a near-maximal renal K conservation and implies significant K loss.

Acute acidosis affects K excretion, whereas chronic acidosis and acute alkalosis can promote K excretion. Increased delivery of Na to the distal nephrons, as occurs with high Na intake or loop diuretic therapy, promotes K excretion.

c. **False K concentrations**:

1. **Pseudohypokalemia** or falsely low serum K levels occasionally occur in patients with chronic myelocytic leukemia with a WBC count $>10^5/\mu L$. If the sample remains at room temperature before being processed, serum K shows low levels because of the uptake of serum K by abnormal leukocytes in the sample. It is prevented by prompt separation of plasma or serum in blood samples.
2. **Pseudohyperkalemia,** or falsely elevated serum K, is more common, typically occurring due to hemolysis and release of intracellular K. Pseudohyperkalemia can also result from platelet count >400,000/μL due to the release of K from platelets during clotting. In cases of pseudohyperkalemia, the plasma K (unclotted blood), as opposed to serum K, is normal.

HYPERKALEMIA

Hyperkalemia is the serum K concentration of >5.5 mEq/L resulting from excess total body K stores or abnormal movement of K out of cells. There are usually several simultaneous contributing factors, including increased K intake, drugs that impair renal K excretion, and acute or chronic kidney disease. It can also occur in metabolic acidosis as in diabetic ketoacidosis. Clinical manifestations are generally neuromuscular, resulting in muscle weakness and cardiac toxicity that, when severe, can degenerate to ventricular fibrillation or asystole. Diagnosis is by measuring serum K. Treatment may involve decreasing K intake, adjusting drugs, giving a cation exchange resin and, in emergencies, Ca gluconate, insulin, and dialysis.

Etiology

Potassium is a major ion of the body. Nearly 98% of potassium is intracellular, with the concentration gradient maintained by the sodium-and potassium-activated adenosine triphosphatase (Na^+/K^+ –ATPase) pump. Minute-to-minute levels of potassium are controlled by intracellular to extracellular exchange, mostly by this sodium-potassium pump that is controlled by insulin and β2 receptors. A balance of GI intake and renal potassium excretion achieves long-term potassium balance.

Hyperkalemia is defined as a potassium level greater than 5.5 mEq/L. Ranges are as follows:

- 5.5–6.0 mEq/L—mild
- 6.1–7.0 mEq/L—moderate
- 7.0 mEq/L and greater—severe.

Causes

- Pseudohyperkalemia
  - Hemolysis (in laboratory tube) most common
  - Thrombocytosis
  - Leukocytosis
  - Venipuncture technique (i.e., ischemic blood draw from prolonged tourniquet application)
- Redistribution
  - Acidosis
  - Insulin deficiency
  - Beta-blocker drugs
  - Acute digoxin intoxication or overdose
  - Succinylcholine
  - Arginine hydrochloride
  - Hyperkalemic familial periodic paralysis
- Excessive endogenous potassium load
  - Hemolysis
  - Rhabdomyolysis
  - Internal hemorrhage
- Excessive exogenous potassium load
  - Parenteral administration
  - Excess in diet
  - Potassium supplements
  - Salt substitutes
- Diminished potassium excretion
  - Decreased glomerular filtration rate (e.g., acute or end-stage chronic renal failure)
  - Decreased mineral corticoid activity
  - Defect in tubular secretion (e.g., renal tubular acidosis II and IV)
  - Drugs (e.g., NSAIDs, cyclosporine, and potassium-sparing diuretics)
- Laboratory error

Incidence

Hyperkalemia is diagnosed in up to 8% of hospitalized patients.

Mortality/Morbidity

- The primary cause of morbidity and death is potassium's effect on cardiac function.
- The mortality rate can be as high as 67% if severe hyperkalemia is not treated rapidly.

Diagnosis

Hyperkalemia can be difficult to diagnose clinically because complaints may be vague.

A. The history is most valuable in identifying conditions that may predispose to hyperkalemia.
  - Hyperkalemia frequently is discovered as an incidental laboratory finding.
  - Hyperkalemia is suggested in any patient with a predisposition toward elevated potassium level. Potential potassium level elevation is observed in the following:
    - Acute or chronic renal failure, especially in patients who are on dialysis
    - Trauma, including crush injuries (rhabdomyolysis), or burns
    - Ingestion of foods high in potassium (e.g., bananas, oranges, high-protein diets, tomatoes, and salt substitutes). This alone is not likely to cause clinically significant hyperkalemia in most people; it is often a contributing factor to an acute potassium elevation.
    - Medications—potassium supplements, potassium-sparing diuretics, nonsteroidal anti-inflammatory drugs (NSAIDs), beta-blockers, digoxin, succinylcholine, and digitalis glycosides.
    - Medication combinations (i.e., spironolactone and ACE inhibitors)
    - Redistribution—metabolic acidosis [diabetic ketoacidosis (DKA)], catabolic states.

B. Clinical manifestations
  - Patients may be asymptomatic or report the following:
    - Generalized fatigue
    - Weakness
    - Paresthesias
    - Paralysis
    - Palpitations
    - Cardiac and neurologic symptoms predominate
    - Cardiac examination may reveal extrasystoles, pauses, or bradycardia
    - Neurologic examination may reveal diminished deep tendon reflexes or decreased motor strength
    - In rare cases, muscular paralysis and hypoventilation may be observed
    - Signs of renal failure,, such as edema, skin changes, and dialysis sites may be there
    - Signs of trauma that could put the patient at risk for rhabdomyolysis can be there
    - Evaluation of vital signs is essential to determine hemodynamic stability and presence of cardiac arrhythmias related to the hyperkalemia.

C. Laboratory investigations
  - Serum K measurement
  - Electrocardiogram (ECG)
  - Assessment of the cause

1. **Serum potassium:** Hyperkalemia (serum K >5.5 mEq/L) may be found on routine serum electrolyte measurement. It should be suspected in patients with typical changes on an ECG or patients at high risk,, such as those with renal failure, advanced heart failure treated with ACE inhibitors and K-sparing diuretics, or urinary obstruction.
2. **Electrocardiogram (ECG):** Electrocardiogram (ECG) should be done on patients with hyperkalemia.
   - Electrocardiogram (ECG) changes are frequently visible when serum K is >5.5 mEq/L. Slowing of conduction characterized by an increased P–R interval and shortening of the QT interval as well as tall, symmetric, peaked T waves are visible initially **(Figs. 22.3A and B)**.
   - K >6.5 mEq/L produces further slowing of conduction with widening of the QRS interval, disappearance of the P wave, and nodal and escape ventricular arrhythmias.
   - Finally, the QRS complex degenerates into a sine wave pattern, and ventricular fibrillation or asystole ensues.
3. **Diagnosis of the cause:** Pseudohyperkalemia should be considered in patients without risk factors or ECG abnormalities. Hemolysis may be reported by the laboratory. When pseudohyperkalemia is suspected, K concentration should be repeated, taking measures to avoid hemolysis of the sample. Diagnosis of the cause of hyperkalemia requires a detailed history, including a review of drugs, a physical examination with emphasis on volume status, and measurement of the following:
   - Blood urea nitrogen (BUN) and creatinine level—for evaluation of renal status

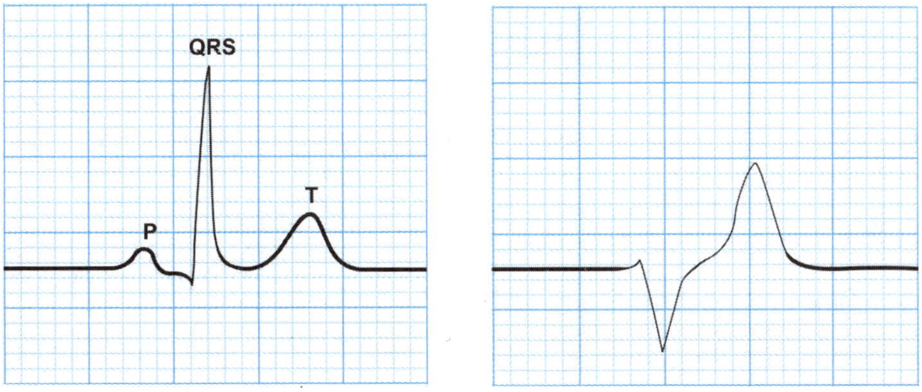

Figs. 22.3A and B: (A) Normal ECG; and (B) ECG (hyperkalemia) widened QRS complex and peaked T waves.

- Calcium level—if patient has renal failure (because hypocalcemia can exacerbate cardiac rhythm disturbances)
- Glucose level—in patients with diabetes mellitus
- Digoxin level—if patient is on a digitalis medication
- Arterial or venous blood gas—if acidosis is suspected urinalysis—if signs of renal insufficiency without an already known cause are present (to look for evidence of glomerulonephritis)
- In cases in which renal failure is present, additional tests, including renal ultrasonography to exclude obstruction, are needed
- Cortisol and aldosterone levels—to check for mineralocorticoid deficiency when other causes are eliminated.

TREATMENT

Direct treatment is aimed at stabilizing the myocardium, shifting potassium from the extracellular environment to the intracellular compartment, and promoting the renal excretion and GI loss of potassium.

1. **Electrolyte supplements:** These agents are used to treat hyperkalemia and to reduce the risk of ventricular fibrillation caused by hyperkalemia. They act quickly and can be lifesaving, and thus, they are the first-line treatment for severe hyperkalemia when the ECG shows significant abnormalities (e.g., widening of QRS interval, loss of P wave, and cardiac arrhythmias). Calcium usually is not indicated when the ECG shows only peaked T waves.
2. **Calcium chloride or calcium gluconate:** Calcium increases threshold potential, thus restoring normal gradient between threshold potential and resting membrane potential, which is elevated abnormally in hyperkalemia. Doses should be titrated with constant monitoring of ECG changes during administration; dose is repeated if ECG changes do not normalize within 3 to 5 minutes.
3. **Antidotes:** Insulin is administered with glucose to facilitate the uptake of glucose into the cell, bringing potassium with it. Glucose and insulin temporarily shift K^+ into cells.
4. **Alkalinizing agents:** These agents increase the pH, which results in a temporary potassium shift from the extracellular to the intracellular environment. Sodium bicarbonate is used for this purpose. Bicarbonate ion neutralizes hydrogen ions and raises urinary and blood pH.
5. **Beta-2-adrenergic agonists:** These agents promote cellular reuptake of potassium, possibly via the cyclic GAMP receptor cascade.
6. **Diuretics:** These agents cause the loss of potassium through the kidney.
7. **Binding resins:** These agents promote exchange of potassium for sodium in GI system.

Prevention

- Avoid foods high in potassium
- Avoid medications that predispose to hyperkalemia.

Complications

- Life-threatening cardiac arrhythmias may ensue
- Hypokalemia may result from the treatment of hyperkalemia.

Prognosis

- Full resolution is expected with correction of the underlying etiology
- Reduction of plasma potassium should begin within the first hour of initiation of treatment.

CLINICAL NOTE

The treatment of hyperkalemia is aimed at stabilizing the myocardium, shifting potassium from the extracellular environment to the intracellular compartment, and promoting the renal excretion and GI loss of potassium.

CLINICAL PEARLS

1. Hyperkalemia is the serum K concentration of >5.5 mEq/L resulting from excess total body K stores or abnormal movement of K out of cells.
2. There are usually several simultaneous contributing factors, including increased K intake, drugs that impair renal K excretion, and acute or chronic kidney disease.
3. Clinical manifestations are generally neuromuscular, resulting in muscle weakness and cardiac toxicity that, when severe, can degenerate to ventricular fibrillation or asystole.
4. Diagnosis is by measuring serum K.
5. Treatment may involve decreasing K intake, adjusting drugs, giving a cation exchange resin and, in emergencies, Ca gluconate, insulin, and dialysis.

CASE STUDY 5

Theme: Causes and consequences of hypokalemia

A 62-year-old female who was having an acute exacerbation of Crohn's disease presented to the clinic. She complained of severe and frequent diarrhea over the previous 4 days. She experienced dizziness when she stood up.

Her physical examination revealed dry mucous membranes. In the supine position, her blood pressure (BP) was 110/65 mm Hg, while in the upright position her BP was 90/45 mm Hg and her pulse rate was140 beats/minute.

Her laboratory report was as follows:
Serum Na^+—132 mEq/L
Serum K^+—2.9 mEq/L
Serum Cl^-—92 mEq/L
pCO_2—31 mm Hg
BUN—25 mg/dL
Serum creatinine—1.0 mg/dL

What is the problem with this patient?
What is the cause of alteration in biochemical parameters?

CASE DISCUSSION

The patient has extracellular volume depletion (ECVD) due to prolonged diarrhea. The diagnosis is supported by her physical assessment and postural hypotension and her BUN/Cr is >20:1.The diarrhea has resulted in a loss of fluid and sodium chloride. Some potassium was lost directly in the stools, but the main cause of her hypokalemia is her ECVD which has induced a metabolic alkalosis (contraction alkalosis.) The alkalosis contributed to her hypokalemia by two mechanisms. Some potassium has moved to the intracellular compartment but much of it has been lost in the urine where potassium wasting occurs secondary to chloride deficit. Administration of normal saline with potassium chloride will correct her fluid and electrolyte problems (and alkalosis.)

BASIC CONCEPT

Hypokalemia

Hypokalemia is the serum potassium (K) concentration of <3.5 mEq/L caused by a deficit in total body K stores or abnormal movement of K into cells. The most common causes are excess losses from the kidneys or GI tract. Clinical features include muscle weakness and polyuria; cardiac hyperexcitability may occur with severe hypokalemia. Diagnosis is by serum measurement. Treatment is the administration of K and addressing the cause.

Incidence

As many as 20% of hospitalized patients are hypokalemic; however, hypokalemia is clinically significant in only about 4% to 5% of these patients. Severe hypokalemia is relatively uncommon. Up to 14% of outpatients who undergo laboratory testing are found to be mildly hypokalemic. Approximately 80% of patients who are receiving diuretics become hypokalemic. Incidence is equal in males and females.

Causes

Hypokalemia can be caused by decreased intake of K but is usually caused by excessive losses of K in the urine or from the GI tract.

- Renal losses—various disorders can increase renal K excretion. Excess mineralocorticoid effect can directly increase K secretion by the distal nephrons. The renal losses of K occur in any of the following:
  - Renal tubular acidosis
  - Adrenal steroid excess that is due to Cushing's syndrome, primary hyperaldosteronism, rare renin-secreting tumors, glucocorticoid-remediable aldosteronism (a rare inherited disorder involving abnormal aldosterone metabolism), and congenital adrenal hyperplasia.
  - Ingestion of substances, such as glycyrrhizin (present in natural licorice and used in the manufacture of chewing tobacco), which inhibits the enzyme 11β-hydroxysteroid dehydrogenase (11β-HSDH), preventing the conversion of cortisol, which has some mineralocorticoid activity, to cortisone, which does not, resulting in high circulating concentrations of cortisol and renal K wasting.
  - Bartter and Gitelman's syndromes are uncommon genetic disorders characterized by renal K and Na wasting, excessive production of renin and aldosterone, and normotension. Bartter syndrome is caused by mutations in a loop diuretic–sensitive ion transport mechanism in the loop of Henle. Gitelman's syndrome is caused by loss of function mutations in a thiazide-sensitive ion transport mechanism in the distal nephron.
  - Liddle syndrome is a rare autosomal dominant disorder characterized by severe hypertension and hypokalemia. Liddle syndrome is caused by unrestrained Na reabsorption in the distal nephron due to one of several mutations found in genes encoding for epithelial Na channel subunits. Inappropriately high reabsorption of Na results in both hypertension and renal K wasting.
  - Renal K wasting can also be caused by numerous congenital and acquired renal tubular diseases,, such as the renal tubular acidosis and Fanconi syndrome, an unusual syndrome resulting in renal wasting of K, glucose, phosphate, uric acid, and amino acids.
  - Hypomagnesemia is a common correlate of hypokalemia. Much of this is attributable to common underlying causes (i.e., diuretics and diarrhea), but hypomagnesemia itself may also result in increased renal K losses.
  - Leukemia (mechanism uncertain)
- GI losses—abnormal GI K losses occur in all of the following:
  - Vomiting
  - Diarrhea
  - Enemas or laxative use
  - Ileal loop
  - Protracted gastric suction (which removes volume and HCl, causing the kidneys to excrete HCO_3 and to electrically balance lost HCO_3, K)
  - Rarely, villous adenoma of the colon, which causes massive K secretion
  - GI K losses may be compounded by concomitant renal K losses due to metabolic alkalosis and stimulation of aldosterone due to volume depletion.
- Medication effects
  - Diuretics (most common cause): Diuretics are by far the most commonly used drugs that cause hypokalemia. K-wasting diuretics that block Na reabsorption proximal to the distal nephron include:
    - i. Thiazides
    - ii. Loop diuretics
    - iii. Osmotic diuretics
  - Beta-adrenergic agonists—there is stimulation of the sympathetic nervous system, particularly with β_2-agonists (e.g., albuterol and terbutaline), which may increase cellular K uptake
  - Steroids
  - Theophylline
  - Aminoglycosides
  - By inducing diarrhea, laxatives, especially when abused, can cause hypokalemia. Surreptitious diuretic or laxative abuse or both is a frequent cause of persistent hypokalemia, particularly among patients preoccupied with weight loss and among healthcare practitioners with access to prescription drugs.
- Transcellular shift—the transcellular shift of K into cells may also cause hypokalemia. This shift can occur in any of the following:
  - Insulin administration
  - α-adrenergic antagonists
  - Glycogenesis during TPN or enteral hyperalimentation (stimulating insulin release)
  - Thyrotoxicosis (occasionally) due to excessive β-sympathetic stimulation (hypokalemic thyrotoxic periodic paralysis)

    - Familial periodic paralysis is a rare autosomal dominant disorder characterized by transient episodes of profound hypokalemia thought to be due to sudden abnormal shifts of K into cells. Episodes frequently involve varying degrees of paralysis. They are typically precipitated by a large carbohydrate meal or strenuous exercise.
    - Metabolic alkalosis
- Malnutrition or decreased dietary intake, parenteral nutrition and clay ingestion.
- Pseudohypokalemia

Clinical Features

The clinical manifestations of K^+ depletion vary greatly between individual patients, and their severity depends on the degree of hypokalemia. Symptoms seldom occur unless the plasma K^+ concentration is <3 mmol/L.

- Fatigue, myalgia, and muscular weakness of the lower extremities are common complaints and are due to a lower (more negative) resting membrane potential.
- More severe hypokalemia may lead to progressive weakness, hypoventilation (due to respiratory muscle involvement), and eventually complete paralysis.
- Impaired muscle metabolism and the blunted hyperemic response to exercise associated with profound K^+ depletion increase the risk of rhabdomyolysis.
- Smooth-muscle function may also be affected and manifest as paralytic ileus.
- Hypokalemia may also predispose to digitalis toxicity.
- Hypokalemia is often associated with acid-base disturbances related to the underlying disorder. In addition, K^+ depletion results in intracellular acidification and an increase in net acid excretion or new HCO_3^- production. This is a consequence of enhanced proximal HCO_3 reabsorption, increased renal ammonia genesis, and increased distal H^+ secretion. This contributes to the generation of metabolic alkalosis frequently present in hypokalemic patients.
- Glucose intolerance may also occur with hypokalemia and has been attributed to either impaired insulin secretion or peripheral insulin resistance.

Laboratory Investigations

- **Serum K measurement:** Hypokalemia (serum K <3.5 mEq/L) may be found on routine serum electrolyte measurement. It should be suspected in patients with typical changes on an ECG or who have muscular symptoms and risk factors and confirmed by blood testing.
- **Electrocardiogram (ECG):** Electrocardiogram should be done on patients with hypokalemia. The electrocardiographic changes of hypokalemia are due to delayed ventricular depolarization and do not correlate well with the plasma K^+ concentration. Cardiac effects of hypokalemia are usually minimal until serum K concentrations are <3 mEq/L. Hypokalemia produces sagging of the ST segment, depression of the T wave, and elevation of the U wave **(Fig. 22.4)**. With marked hypokalemia, the T wave becomes progressively smaller and the U wave becomes increasingly larger. Sometimes, a flat or positive T wave merges with a positive U wave, which may be confused with QT prolongation. Hypokalemia may produce premature ventricular and atrial contractions, ventricular and atrial tachyarrhythmias, and 2nd- or 3rd-degree atrioventricular block. Such arrhythmias become more severe with increasingly severe hypokalemia; eventually, ventricular fibrillation may occur. Patients with significant preexisting heart disease and patients receiving digoxin are at risk of cardiac conduction abnormalities even from mild hypokalemia.

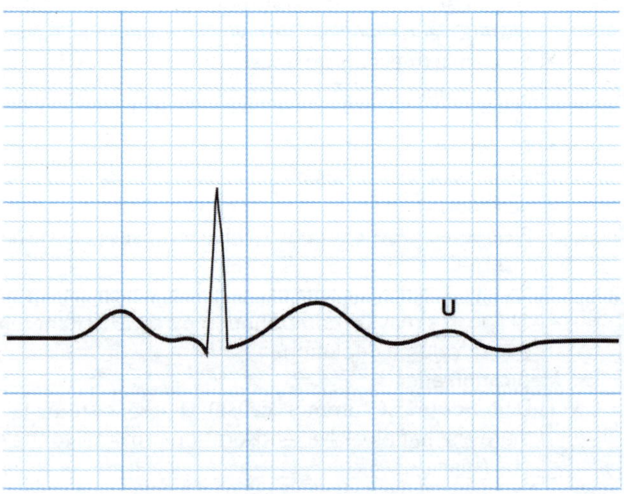

Fig. 22.4: Electrocardiogram (ECG) changes in hypokalemia (Flattened T wave and prominent U wave).

- **Diagnosis of cause:** The cause is usually apparent by history (particularly the medication history); when it is not, further investigation is warranted. After acidosis and other causes of intracellular K shift (increased β-adrenergic effect, hyperinsulinemia) have been eliminated, 24-hour urinary K and serum Mg concentrations are measured. In hypokalemia, K secretion is normally <15 mEq/L. Extrarenal (GI) K loss or decreased K ingestion is suspected in chronic unexplained hypokalemia when renal K secretion is <15 mEq/L. Secretion of >15 mEq/L suggests a renal cause for K loss. Unexplained hypokalemia with increased renal K secretion and hypertension suggests an aldosterone-secreting tumor or Liddle syndrome. Unexplained hypokalemia with increased renal K loss and normal BP suggests Bartter or Gitelman's syndrome, but hypomagnesemia, surreptitious vomiting, and diuretic abuse are more common and should also be considered.

TREATMENT

The therapeutic goals are to correct the K deficit and to minimize ongoing losses. With the exception of periodic paralysis, hypokalemia resulting from transcellular shifts rarely requires intravenous K^+ supplementation, which can lead to rebound hyperkalemia. It is generally safer to correct hypokalemia via the oral route. The degree of K^+ depletion does not correlate well with the plasma K^+ concentration. A decrement of 1 mmol/L in the plasma K^+ concentration (from 4.0 to 3.0 mmol/L) may represent a total body K deficit of 200 to 400 mmol, and patients with plasma levels under 3.0 mmol/L often require in excess of 600 mmol of K^+ to correct the K deficit. Furthermore, factors promoting K^+ shift out of cells (e.g., insulin deficiency in diabetic ketoacidosis) may result in underestimation of the K deficit. Therefore, the plasma K^+ concentration should be monitored frequently when assessing the response to treatment. Potassium chloride is usually the preparation of choice and will promote more rapid correction of hypokalemia and metabolic alkalosis. Potassium bicarbonate and citrate (metabolized to HCO^-) tend to alkalinize the patient and would be more appropriate for hypokalemia associated with chronic diarrhea or RTA.

Patients with severe hypokalemia or those unable to take anything by mouth require intravenous replacement therapy with KCl. The maximum concentration of administered K^+ should be no more than 40 mmol/L via a peripheral vein or 60 mmol/L via a central vein. The rate of infusion should not exceed 20 mmol/h unless paralysis or malignant ventricular arrhythmias are present. Ideally, KCl should be mixed in normal saline since dextrose solutions may initially exacerbate hypokalemia due to insulin-mediated movement of K^+ into cells. Rapid intravenous administration of K^+ should be used judiciously and requires close observation of the clinical manifestations of hypokalemia (electrocardiogram and neuromuscular examination).

Prevention

Routine K replacement is not necessary in most patients receiving diuretics. However, serum K should be monitored during diuretic use when risk of hyperkalemia or of its complications is high. Risk is high in:

- Patients with decreased left ventricular function
- Patients taking digoxin
- Patients with diabetes (in whom insulin concentrations can fluctuate)
- Patients with asthma who are taking β2-agonists.

When hypokalemia develops, K supplementation, usually with oral KCL, is indicated.

The pseudohypokalemia can be avoided by storing the blood sample on ice or rapidly separating the plasma (or serum) from the cells.

CLINICAL NOTE

Diuretics are by far the most commonly used drugs that cause hypokalemia. .

CLINICAL PEARLS

1. Hypokalemia is the serum K concentration of <3.5 mEq/L caused by a deficit in total body K stores or abnormal movement of K into cells.
2. Hypokalemia can be caused by decreased intake of K, but is usually caused by excessive losses of K in the urine or from the GI tract.
3. Fatigue, myalgia, and muscular weakness of the lower extremities are common complaints and are due to a lower (more negative) resting membrane potential.
4. Hypokalemia produces sagging of the ST segment, depression of the T wave, and elevation of the U wave. With marked hypokalemia, the T wave becomes progressively smaller and the U wave becomes increasingly larger.
5. Rapid intravenous administration of K^+ should be used judiciously and requires close observation of the clinical manifestations of hypokalemia (electrocardiogram and neuromuscular examination).

Chapter 23

Biochemistry of Cancer

LEARNING OBJECTIVES

To understand:
- Types and mechanism of action of tumor suppressor genes
- Mechanism of activation of proto-oncogenes
- Mechanism of action of anticancer drugs

CASE STUDIES

CASE STUDY 1

Theme: Tumor Suppressor Genes and Oncogenes

A 36-year-old female presented to the clinic with concerns over a recently detected right breast lump. A mammogram performed, revealed a right breast mass measuring 2 cm with numerous microcalcifications suggestive of breast cancer. On further questioning, she revealed that her sister was also diagnosed with breast cancer at the age of 39, her mother who passed away at age 40 years was also suffering with ovarian cancer, and a maternal aunt also had both breast and colon cancer.

Patient underwent an examination, which revealed a fixed and nontender breast mass on right side measuring 2 cm with mild right axillary lymphadenopathy. No skin involvement was noted. The biopsy revealed intraductal carcinoma.

What cancer gene might be associated with this clinical scenario?
What is the likely mechanism of the cancer gene in this case?

CASE DETAILS

The patient had breast cancer at the young age of 35 years. She had two first-degree relatives with breast and/or ovarian cancer prior to menopause that means she had genetic predisposition for breast cancer.

Cancer arises through a series of somatic alterations in deoxyribonucleic acid (DNA) that result in unrestrained cellular proliferation. Most of these alterations involve actual sequence changes in DNA (i.e., mutations). They may arise as a consequence of random replication errors, exposure to carcinogens (e.g., radiation), or faulty DNA repair processes. While most cancers arise sporadically, familial clustering of cancers occurs in certain families that carry a germline mutation in a cancer gene. Human breast cancer is a clonal disease; a single transformed cell—the product of a series of somatic (acquired) or germline mutations—is eventually able to express full malignant potential.

Breast cancer is a malignant proliferation of epithelial cells lining the ducts or lobules of the breast. Not more than 10% of human breast cancers can be linked directly to germline mutations. Several genes have been implicated in familial cases.

BASIC CONCEPT

Classes of cancer genes: There are two major classes of cancer genes. The first class comprises genes that directly affect cell growth either positively (oncogenes) or negatively (tumor suppressor genes). These genes exert their effects on tumor growth through their ability to control cell division (cell birth) or cell death (apoptosis). Oncogenes are tightly regulated in normal cells. In cancer cells, oncogenes acquire mutations that relieve this control and lead to increased activity of the gene product. In contrast, the normal function of tumor suppressor genes is to restrain cell growth, and this function is lost in cancer. Because of the diploid nature of mammalian cells, both alleles must be inactivated to completely lose the function of a tumor suppressor gene, leading to a recessive mechanism at the cellular level.

The second class of cancer genes, the caretakers, does not directly affect cell growth but rather affects the ability of the cell to maintain the integrity of its genome. Cells with deficiency in these genes have an increased rate of mutations in all the genes, including oncogenes and tumor suppressor genes.

CANCER GENES

Some of the cancer-causing genes are as follows:

a. **Tumor suppressor genes:**
   1. ***BRCA1*:** Tumor suppressor gene, *BRCA1*, has been identified at the chromosomal locus 17q21; this gene encodes a zinc finger protein, and the product therefore may function as a transcription factor. The gene appears to be involved in gene repair. Women who inherit a mutated allele of this gene from either parent have at least a 60–80% lifetime chance of developing breast cancer and about a 33% chance of developing ovarian cancer. Men who carry a mutant allele of the gene have an increased incidence of prostate cancer and breast cancer.
   2. ***BRCA2:*** This gene has been localized to chromosome 13q12; it is also associated with an increased incidence of breast cancer in men and women.
   3. ***P53* gene:** The *p53* mutation is present in nearly 40% of human breast cancers as an acquired defect. The *p53* tumor suppressor gene acts as the "Guardian of the Genome". It encodes a protein of molecular weight 53 kDa. This protein is nuclear in location and is subjected to phosphorylation and dephosphorylation. The *p53* has following four major effects:
      i. It acts as a transcriptional activator regulating certain genes involved in the cell cycle.
      ii. It acts as G1 checkpoint control for the DNA damage. If excess damage to the DNA has occurred, it causes inhibition of the cell cycle, allowing time for repair. If the cell cycle proceeds without repair, DNA damage would be replicated, introducing permanent mutations in to the genome. If the *p53* is inactivated or mutated as happens in certain tumors, DNA damage accumulates and the DNA becomes unstable.
      iii. *p53* also participates in apoptosis. The purpose of this function is that it hastens the death of the potentially dangerous cells, e.g., those damaged by ultraviolet (UV) light, which have the potential to become cancer cells.
      iv. Besides all this *p53* also combines with certain viral proteins.

   Mutations in the *p53* gene are the most common genetic alterations in human cancer and are frequent in breast, colon, and lung cancers.
   4. ***PTEN*:** Acquired mutations in *PTEN* occur in about 10% of the cases. The gene appears to be located on chromosome 10 and appears to be an important "tumor suppressor" and when mutated, it allows the cells to grow out of the control and become malignant. This gene is also called "*MMAC1*"; mutations in this gene also play an important role in the aggressiveness of the tumor.

b. **Oncogenes in human cancer:** Other genetic mechanisms of cancer include oncogenes, which are abnormal genes that cause cancer usually by mutations. Proto-oncogenes are normal genes that are present in normal cells and involved in normal growth and development, but if mutations occur, they may become oncogenes.

Oncogenes found in human cancers were initially discovered through their presence in the genome of retroviruses capable of causing cancers in chickens, mice, and rats. The cellular homologs of these viral genes are often targets of mutation or aberrant regulation in human cancer. Whereas many oncogenes were discovered because of their presence in retroviruses, other oncogenes, particularly those involved in translocations characteristic of particular leukemias and lymphomas, were isolated through genomic approaches. In the normal cellular environment, proto-oncogenes have crucial roles in cell proliferation and differentiation **(Fig. 23.1)**. The normal growth and differentiation of cells are controlled by growth factors that bind to receptors on the surface of the cell. The signals generated by the membrane receptors are transmitted inside the cells through signaling cascades involving kinases, G proteins, and other regulatory proteins **(Fig. 23.2)**. Ultimately, these signals affect the activity of transcription factors in the nucleus, which regulate the expression of genes crucial in cell proliferation, cell differentiation, and cell death. Proto-oncogene products have been found to function at critical steps in these pathways and inappropriate activation of these pathways can lead to tumorigenesis.

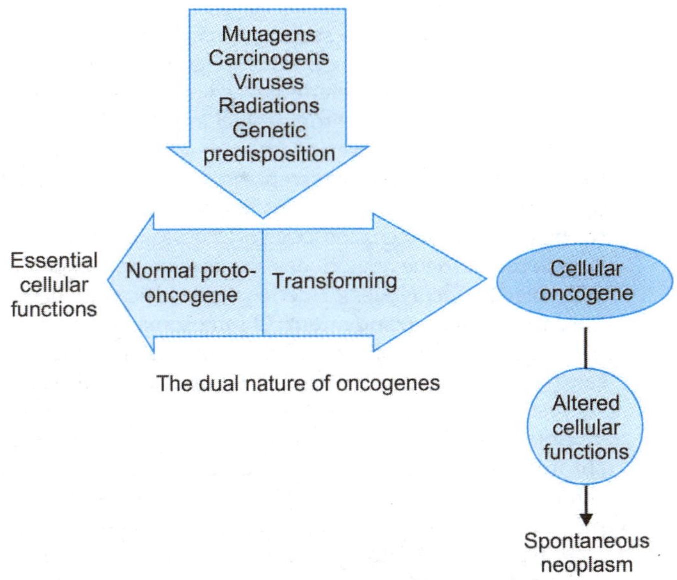

Fig. 23.1: Effects of proto-oncogenes and oncogenes.

Mechanisms of Oncogene Activation

Mechanisms that upregulate (or activate) cellular oncogenes (proto-oncogenes) fall into three broad categories: point mutation, gene amplification, and chromosomal rearrangement.

1. **Point mutation:** Point mutation is a common mechanism of oncogene activation. For example, mutations in one of the RAS genes (*HRAS*, *KRAS*, or *NRAS*) are present in up to 85% of pancreatic cancers and 50% of colon cancers, but are relatively uncommon in other cancer types. Most of the activated *RAS* genes contain point mutations in codons 12, 13, or 61 (which convey resistance to GAP, a protein that interacts with *RAS* and inactivates it through substitution of the GTP cofactor with GDP) **(Fig. 23.2)**.

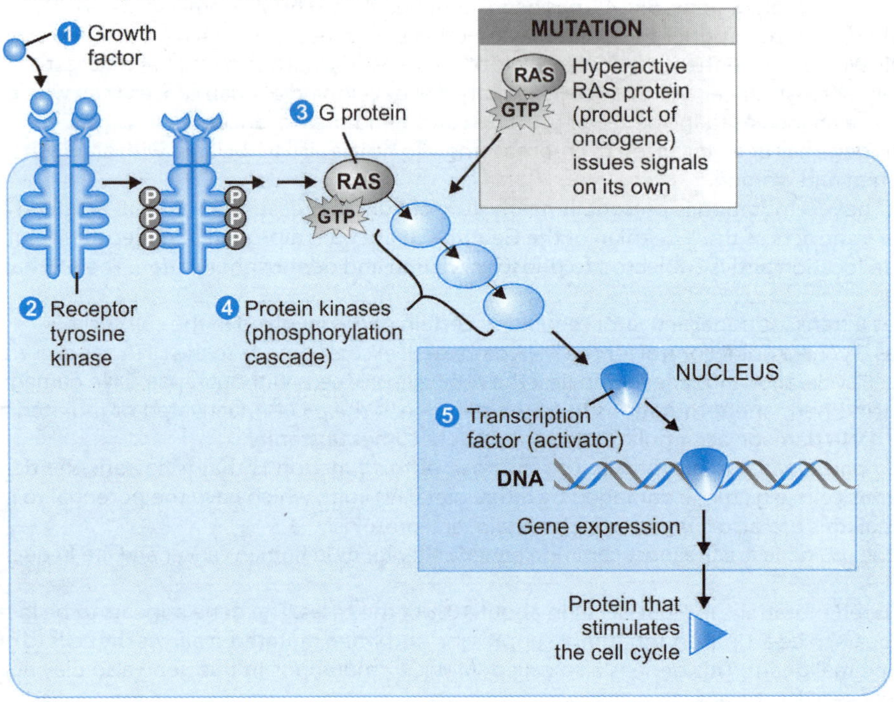

Fig. 23.2: Effects of activates RAS protein.

2. **Gene amplification:** The second mechanism for activation of oncogenes is DNA sequence amplification, leading to overexpression of the gene product **(Fig. 23.3)**. This increase in DNA copy number may cause cytologically recognizable chromosome alterations referred to as homogeneous staining regions (HSRs), if integrated within chromosomes, or double minutes (dmins), if extrachromosomal in nature. The recognition of DNA amplification is accomplished through various cytogenetic techniques, such as comparative genomic hybridization (CGH) and fluorescence in situ hybridization (FISH), which allow the visualization of chromosomal aberrations using fluorescent dyes. With these techniques, the entire genome can be surveyed for gains and losses of DNA sequences, thus pinpointing chromosomal regions likely to contain genes important in the development or progression of cancer. Noncytogenetic and molecular techniques for identifying amplifications have more recently become available.
3. **Chromosomal rearrangement:** Chromosomal alterations provide important clues to the genetic changes in cancer. The chromosomal alterations in human solid tumors, such as carcinomas are heterogeneous and complex and likely reflect selection for the loss of tumor suppressor genes on the involved chromosome. In contrast, the chromosome alterations in myeloid and lymphoid tumors are often simple translocations, i.e., reciprocal transfers of chromosome arms from one chromosome to another. The breakpoints of recurring chromosome abnormalities usually occur at the site of cellular oncogenes. Translocations are particularly common in lymphoid tumors, probably because these cell types normally rearrange their DNA to generate antigen receptors. Indeed, antigen receptor genes are commonly involved in the translocations, implying that an imperfect regulation of receptor gene rearrangement may be involved in the pathogenesis.

An example is Burkitt's lymphoma, a B cell tumor characterized by a reciprocal translocation between chromosomes 8 and 14. Molecular analysis of Burkitt's lymphomas demonstrated that the breakpoints occurred within or near the MYC locus on chromosome 8 and within the

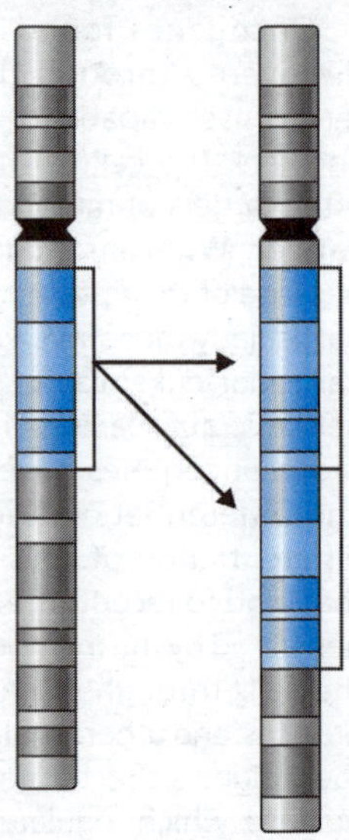

Fig. 23.3: Gene amplification.

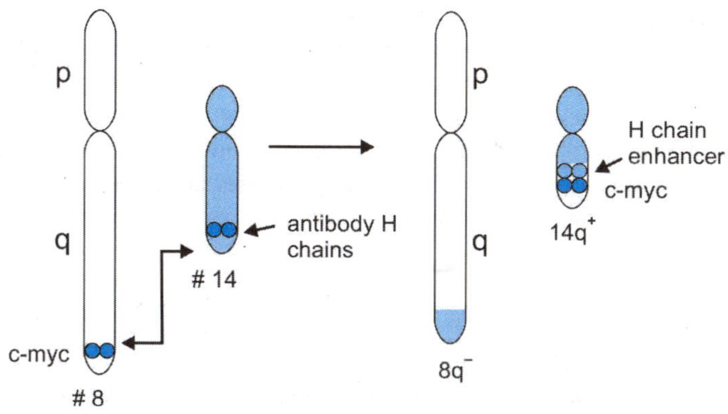

Fig. 23.4: Chromosomal translocation in Burkitt's lymphoma.

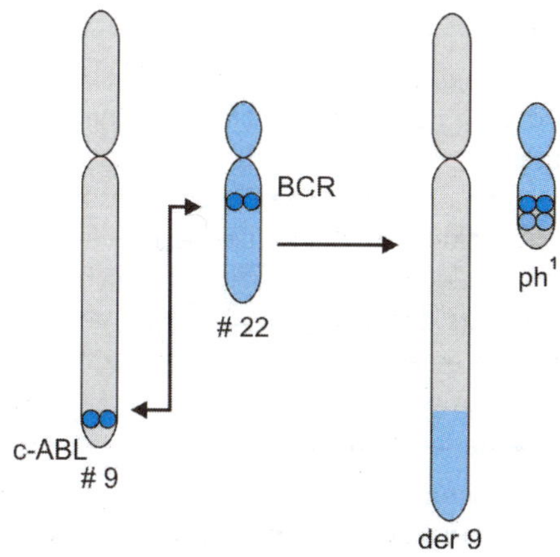

Fig. 23.5: Philadelphia chromosome in CML.

immunoglobulin heavy chain locus on chromosome 14, resulting in the transcriptional activation of MYC **(Fig. 23.4)**. Enhancer activation by translocation, although not universal, appears to play an important role in malignant progression. In addition to transcription factors and signal transduction molecules, translocation may result in the overexpression of cell cycle regulatory proteins, such as cyclins and of proteins that regulate cell death, such as BCL-2.

The first reproducible chromosome abnormality detected in human malignancy was the Philadelphia chromosome detected in Chronic myeloid leukemia. This cytogenetic abnormality is generated by reciprocal translocation involving the *ABL* oncogene, a tyrosine kinase on chromosome 9, being placed in proximity to the *BCR* (breakpoint cluster region) on chromosome 22 **(Fig. 23.5)**. The consequence of expression of the *BCR-ABL* gene product is the activation of signal transduction pathways leading to cell growth independent of normal external signals. Imatinib, a drug that specifically blocks the activity of *BCR-ABL*, has shown remarkable efficacy with little toxicity in patients with CML. Thus, by a variety of mechanisms, the proto-oncogenes are activated to oncogenes (see the summary of processes involved in the activation of proto-oncogenes to oncogenes in **Figure 23.6**).

Summary of Mechanisms of Oncogene Activation

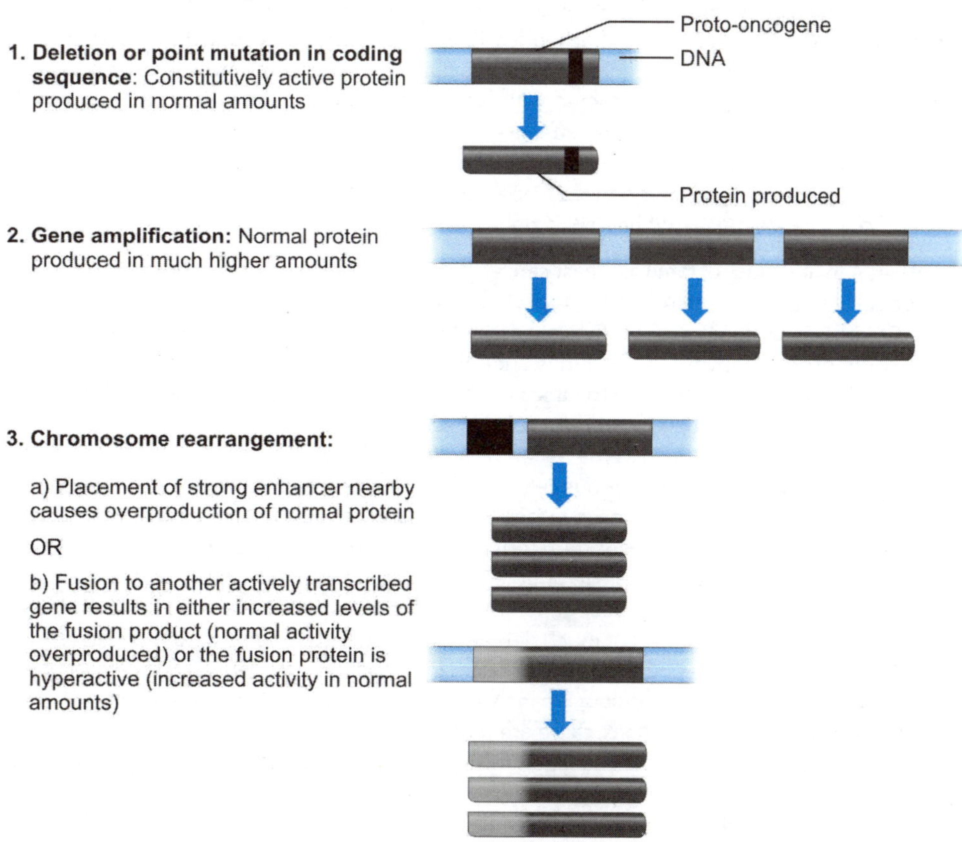

Fig. 23.6: Summary of mechanism of oncogene activation.

Mechanisms of Tumor Suppressor Inactivation

The two major types of somatic lesions observed in tumor suppressor genes during tumor development are point mutations and large deletions. Point mutations in the coding region of tumor suppressor genes will frequently lead to truncated protein products or otherwise nonfunctional proteins. Similarly, deletions lead to the loss of a functional product and sometimes encompass the entire gene or even the entire chromosome arm, leading to loss of heterozygosity (LOH) in the tumor DNA compared to the corresponding normal tissue DNA. LOH in tumor DNA is considered a hallmark for the presence of a tumor suppressor gene at a particular locus, and LOH studies have been useful in the positional cloning of many tumor suppressor genes. Gene silencing, which occurs in conjunction with hypermethylation of the promoter, is another mechanism of tumor suppressor gene inactivation. Silencing is an epigenetic change rather than a sequence alteration.

Familial Cancer Syndromes

A small fraction of cancers occurs in patients with a genetic predisposition. In these families, the affected individuals have a predisposing loss-of-function mutation in one allele of a tumor suppressor gene or caretaker gene. The tumors in these patients show a loss of the remaining normal allele as a result of somatic events (point mutations or deletions) in agreement with the Knudson hypothesis, i.e., both normal alleles must be inactivated (two hits) for the development of the tumor. In familial cases, one defective allele is inherited and the other is normal. Tumor develops after the loss of normal allele, while in sporadic cases, both normal alleles are lost for the development of tumor. Thus, most cells of an individual with an inherited loss-of-function mutation in a tumor suppressor gene are functionally normal, and only the rare cells that develop a mutation in the remaining normal allele will exhibit uncontrolled growth. The current paradigm states that the genes mutated in familial syndromes can also be targets for somatic mutations in sporadic (noninherited) tumors.

Roughly, 100 syndromes of familial cancer have been reported, although many are rare. The majority are inherited as autosomal dominant. Breast cancer is also considered as familial, although it is multifactorial in origin.

Genetic Testing for Familial Cancers

The discovery of cancer susceptibility genes raises the possibility of DNA testing to predict the risk of cancer in individuals of affected families. Once a mutation is discovered in a family, subsequent testing of asymptomatic family members can be crucial in patient management. A negative gene test in these individuals can prevent years of anxiety in the knowledge that their cancer risk is no higher than that of the general population. On the other hand, a positive test may lead to alteration of clinical management,, such as increased frequency of cancer screening and, when feasible and appropriate, prophylactic surgery. Potential negative consequences of a positive test result include psychological distress (anxiety and depression) and discrimination (insurance and employment). Testing should therefore not be conducted without counseling before and after disclosure of the test result. In addition, the decision to test should depend on whether effective interventions exist for the particular type of cancer to be tested. Despite these caveats, genetic cancer testing for some cancer syndromes already appears to have greater benefits than risks, and many companies now offer testing for various genes associated with the predisposition to breast cancer (*BRCA1* and *BRCA2*), melanoma (*p16INK4*), and colon cancer (*APC* and the *HNPCC* genes).

***BRCA1* and breast cancer:** A major cause of familial breast cancer results from mutation in the breast cancer susceptibility gene, *BRCA1*. *BRCA1* gene product is a nuclear protein. *BRCA1* functioned as a cell cycle regulator in response to DNA damage.

Cells defective in *BRCA1* possesses numerous cytological and biological features that have been correlated with perturbation in the maintenance of chromosome stability. This includes aneuploidy, centrosome amplification, spontaneous chromosome breakage, aberrant recombination events, sensitivity to ionizing radiation, and impaired cell cycle checkpoints.

In addition, a variety of experiments have demonstrated roles for *BRCA1*, in enforcing the G2/M cell cycle transition, homologous recombination between sister chromatids, as well as the restart of stalled replication in S phase.

The *BRCA1* tumor suppressor interacts with numerous cellular proteins in large complexes. This includes a variety of proteins implicated in various DNA repair and cell cycle processes. In fact, *BRCA1* has been reported to interact with as many as 50 proteins! Moreover, *BRCA1* has been shown to function in various transcriptional mechanisms, suggesting that the function of this important protein may go well beyond its well-documented role in double-strand break repair. How the inactivation of *BRCA1*, a gene that appears to operate in DNA repair pathways that appear generic to various cell types and predisposes women to inherited forms of breast cancer, remains a mystery and the subject of much debate. Given that *BRCA1* appears to have key roles in transcriptional regulation, it has been suggested that *BRCA1* could influence mammary tissue through pathways that impinge on the biology of estrogen and estrogen-related metabolites. In addition, it has been suggested that breast tissue differs from other tissues in the types of DNA repair processes that are used. Perhaps, there are redundant DNA repair pathways in nonmammary tissue. In any event, the complex behavior of *BRCA1* promises to challenge future researchers as they search for the underlying mechanisms that initiate familial breast cancer.

CLINICAL NOTE

The recognition of DNA amplification is accomplished through various cytogenetic techniques, such as comparative genomic hybridization (CGH) and fluorescence in situ hybridization (FISH), which allow the visualization of chromosomal aberrations using fluorescent dyes.

CLINICAL PEARLS

1. Cancer arises through a series of somatic alterations in DNA that result in unrestrained cellular proliferation.
2. While most cancers arise sporadically, familial clustering of cancers occurs in certain families that carry a germline mutation in a cancer gene.
3. There are two major classes of cancer genes. The first class comprises genes that directly affect cell growth either positively (*oncogenes*) or negatively (*tumor suppressor genes*). The other class is *caretaker genes*.
4. Proto-oncogenes are activated to oncogenes by point mutation, gene amplification, or by chromosomal rearrangements.
5. Tumor suppressor genes are inactivated by point mutations, gene deletions, or gene silencing by hypermethylation of DNA.

CASE STUDY 2

Theme: Mechanism of Action of Anticancer Drugs

A 32-year-old female, diagnosed with choriocarcinoma of the ovary and getting methotrexate as a treatment, presented with complaints of oral mucosal ulcers. The patient recalled being advised not to take folate-containing vitamins during therapy. An uncomplicated surgical exploration was performed with removal of the affected ovary. The patient had been taking methotrexate from the previous 2 weeks but she never had any of the above symptoms before.

On examination, patient was afebrile, pale, and appeared ill. Several mucosal ulcers were seen in her mouth. The patient also had some upper abdominal tenderness. Her platelet count was decreased at 60,000/mm^3 (normal 150,000–450,000/mm^3).

What is the most likely cause of her symptoms?
What is the biochemical explanation of her symptoms?

CASE DETAILS

Chemotherapeutic agents are used to treat various types of cancers. Although some are specific for cancer cells, most chemotherapeutic agents are toxic for both normal and cancer cells. Methotrexate acts as a folate antagonist, affecting deoxyribonucleic acid (DNA) synthesis. Because cancer cells divide faster than normal cells, a higher proportion of these neoplastic cells will die. Nevertheless, normal cells that also are rapidly dividing,, such as the gastrointestinal mucosa, the oral mucosa, and the bone marrow cells, may be affected. The patient was advised to avoid folate during therapy, since folate would be an "antidote", and would allow the cancer cells to escape cell kill. Hence, the likely cause of her symptoms is side effects of methotrexate (antimetabolite chemotherapy) affecting rapidly dividing cells, such as oral mucosa.

BASIC CONCEPT

Cancer Treatment

The goal of cancer treatment is first to eradicate the cancer. If this primary goal cannot be accomplished, the goal of cancer treatment shifts to palliation, the amelioration of symptoms, and preservation of quality of life while striving to extend life. When cure of cancer is possible, cancer treatments may be undertaken despite the certainty of severe and perhaps life-threatening toxicities. Every cancer treatment has the potential to cause harm, and treatment may be given that produces toxicity with no benefit.

Cancer treatments are divided into four main types: surgery, radiation therapy (including photodynamic therapy), chemotherapy (including hormonal therapy and molecularly targeted therapy), and biological therapy (including immunotherapy and gene therapy). The modalities are often used in combination, and agents in one category can act by several mechanisms. Surgery and radiation therapy are considered local treatments, though their effects can influence the behavior of tumor at remote sites. Chemotherapy and biological therapy are usually systemic treatments. In many ways, cancer mimics an organ attempting to regulate its own growth. However, cancers have not set an appropriate limit on how much growth should be permitted.

Cancer drug treatments are of four broad types: chemotherapeutic agents, targeted agents, hormonal treatments, or biological agents. They can induce cancer cell death, resulting in tumor shrinkage with corresponding improvement in patient survival, or increase the time until the disease progresses.

Commonly Used Cancer Chemotherapy Agents

1. Direct DNA-interacting agents:
    - Cyclophosphamide
    - Mechlorethamine
    - Chlorambucil
    - Melphalan
    - Carmustine
    - Lomustine (CCNU)
    - Ifosfamide
    - Procarbazine
    - Dacarbazine (DTIC)
    - Temozolomide
    - Cisplatin
2. Antitumor antibiotics:
    - Bleomycin
    - Actinomycin D
    - Mitomycin C
    - Etoposide
    - Doxorubicin and daunorubicin
    - Idarubicin
    - Epirubicin
3. Indirect DNA-interacting agents:
   Antimetabolites:
    - Deoxycoformycin
    - 6-Mercaptopurine
    - 6-Thioguanine
    - Azathioprine
    - 2-Chlorodeoxyadenosine
    - Hydroxyurea
    - Methotrexate
    - 5-fluorouracil
    - Cytosine arabinoside
    - Azacytidine
    - Asparaginase
4. Antimitotic agents:
    - Vincristine
    - Vinblastine
    - Paclitaxel
5. Molecularly targeted agents
    - Tretinoin
    - Bexarotene

Methotrexate

Methotrexate is an antimetabolite. A broad definition of antimetabolites would include compounds with structural similarity to precursors of purines or pyrimidines, or compounds that interfere with purine or pyrimidine synthesis. Antimetabolites can cause DNA damage indirectly, through misincorporation into DNA, abnormal timing or progression through DNA synthesis, or altered function of pyrimidine and purine biosynthetic enzymes. They tend to convey greatest toxicity to cells in S-phase, and the degree of toxicity increases with duration of exposure. Common toxic manifestations include stomatitis, diarrhea, and myelosuppression.

Mechanism of action: Methotrexate inhibits dihydrofolate reductase, which regenerates reduced folates from the oxidized folates produced when thymidine monophosphate is formed from deoxyuridine monophosphate. Without reduced folates, cells die a "thymine-less" death.

Overview of role of folic acid in DNA synthesis: Folate is an essential vitamin, found in green leafy vegetables. It is essential for many biochemical processes in the body, including DNA synthesis and red blood cell synthesis; tetrahydrofolate (THF) derived from the vitamin folic acid is the major source of 1-carbon units, used in the biosynthesis of many important biological molecules. This cofactor is a carrier of activated 1-carbon units at various oxidation levels (methyl, methylene, formyl, formimino, and methenyl). These compounds can be interconverted as required by the cellular process **(Fig. 23.7)**.

1. **Role of folic acid in the synthesis of pyrimidine nucleotides:** All cells, especially rapidly growing cells, must synthesize thymidylate (dTMP) for DNA synthesis. The difference between (T) and (U) is one methyl group at the carbon-5 position.

Thymidylate is synthesized by the methylation of uridylate (dUMP) in a reaction catalyzed by the enzyme thymidylate synthase. This reaction requires a methyl donor and a source of reducing equivalents, which are both provided by N5,N10-methylene-THF **(Fig. 23.8)**. For this reaction, to continue, the regeneration of THF from dihydrofolate (DHF) must occur.

$$\text{Dihydrofolate} + \text{NADPH} + \text{H}^+ \xrightarrow[\textit{Dihydrofolate reductase}]{} \text{THF} + \text{NADPH}^+$$

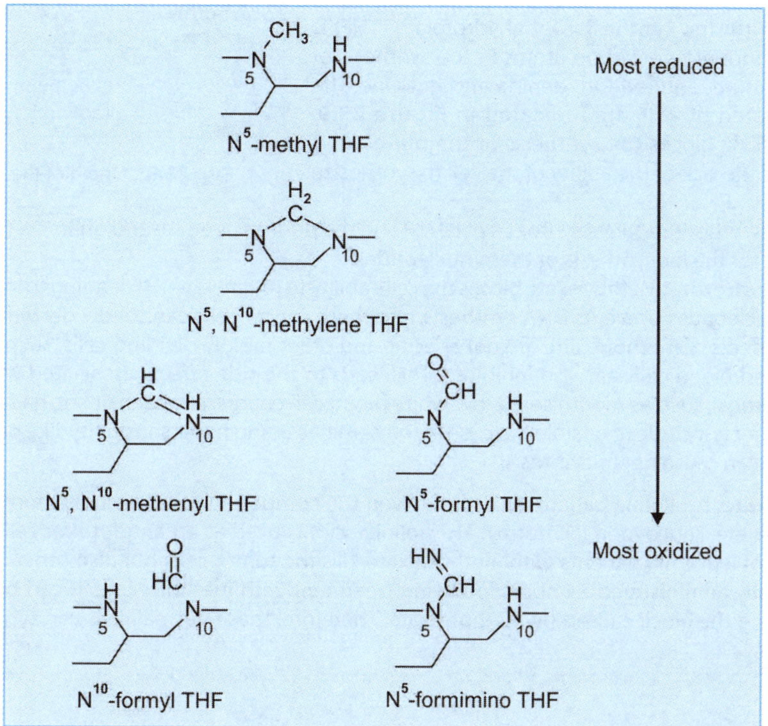

Fig. 23.7: Structures of the various 1-carbon carriers of tetrahydrofolate (THF).

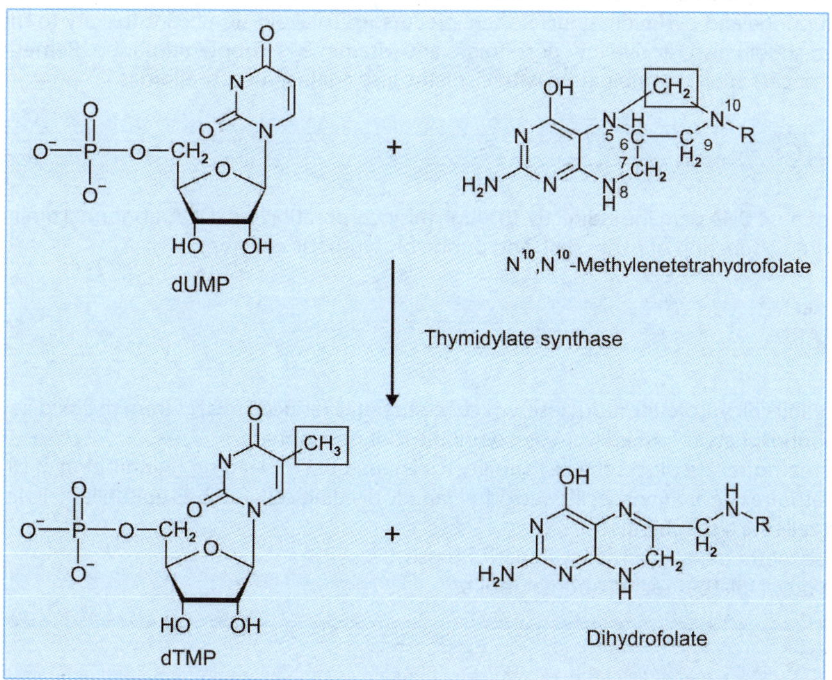

Fig. 23.8: Thymidylate synthesized by the methylation of uridylate (dUMP) in a reaction catalyzed by the enzyme thymidylate synthase.

The enzyme dihydrofolate reductase (DHFR) catalyzes this reaction, which is a target of the anticancer drugs aminopterin and methotrexate.

These drugs are analogs of DHF and act as competitive inhibitors of DHFR. Inhibition of this enzyme prevents the regeneration of THF and blocks dTMP synthesis because of the lack of the methyl donor required for the reaction of thymidylate synthase.

2. **Role of folic acid in purine synthesis:** Tetrahydrofolate (THF) is also required as a donor of two carbon atoms in the synthesis of the purine ring structure required for adenine and guanine. The carbon atoms donated by THF are indicated in **Figure 23.9**. Therefore, a lack of THF blocks the synthesis of the purine ring structure because of the lack of the ability of the cell to synthesize N10-formyl-THF.

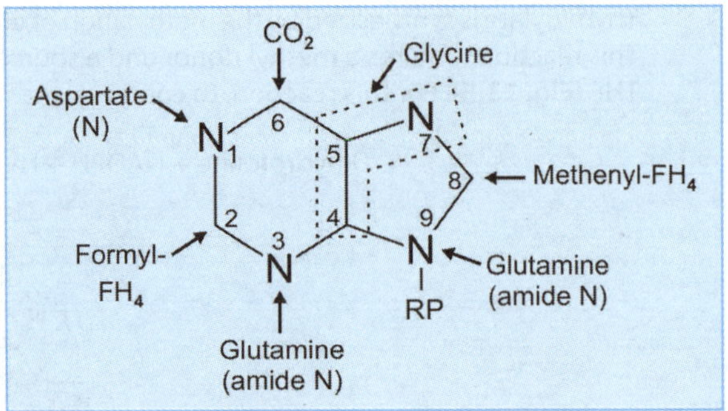

Fig. 23.9: Origin of the atoms of the purine base.

In summary, DNA synthesis requires synthesis of dTMP and the purines adenine and guanine. THF, derived from the vitamin folic acid, is required for the biosynthesis of these nucleotides.

Adverse effects of methotrexate: Methotrexate blocks the cell's ability to regenerate THF, leading to inhibition of these biosynthetic pathways. The lack of nucleotides prevents DNA synthesis, and these cancer cells cannot divide without DNA synthesis.

Unfortunately, the effects of methotrexate are nonspecific and other rapidly dividing cells, such as epithelial cells in the oral cavity, intestine, skin, and blood cells are also inhibited. This leads to the side effects associated with methotrexate (and other cancer chemotherapy drugs), such as mouth sores, low white blood cell counts, stomach upset, hair loss, skin rashes, and itching. Less frequent adverse effects include reversible increase in transaminases and hypersensitivity-like pulmonary syndrome. Chronic low-dose methotrexate can cause hepatic fibrosis.

Antidote of methotrexate: Leukemia patients are often given the compound leucovorin (N5-formyl THF) following treatment with the drug methotrexate. Leucovorin (N5-formyl THF, folinic acid) is used as an antidote for cells that have decreased levels of folic acid. Treatment of leukemia patients with methotrexate kills the tumor cells but also other normal rapidly dividing cells. N5-formyl THF is normally administered 24 hours following treatment with methotrexate; it can be converted to THF by these normal cells by bypassing the block caused by methotrexate. Therefore, these normal cells can synthesize deoxythymidine and carry out DNA synthesis.

Alternative Drug

Pemetrexed is a novel folate-directed antimetabolite. It is "multitargeted" in that it inhibits the activity of several enzymes, including thymidylate synthetase, dihydrofolate reductase, and glycinamide ribonucleotide formyltransferase, thereby affecting the synthesis of both purine and pyrimidine nucleic acid precursors. To avoid significant toxicity to the normal tissues, patients receiving pemetrexed should also receive low-dose folate and vitamin B12 supplementation. Pemetrexed has notable activity against certain lung cancers and, in combination with cisplatin, also against mesotheliomas.

CLINICAL NOTE

Antimetabolites can cause DNA damage indirectly, through misincorporation into DNA, abnormal timing or progression through DNA synthesis, or altered function of pyrimidine and purine biosynthetic enzymes.

CLINICAL PEARLS

1. Methotrexate inhibits dihydrofolate reductase, which regenerates reduced folates from the oxidized folates produced when thymidine monophosphate is formed from deoxyuridine monophosphate.
2. Treatment with methotrexate blocks the cell's ability to regenerate THF, leading to inhibition of DNA synthesis.
3. The effects of methotrexate are nonspecific and other rapidly dividing cells, such as epithelial cells in the oral cavity, intestine, skin, and blood cells are also inhibited.
4. Chronic low-dose methotrexate can cause hepatic fibrosis.
5. Pemetrexed is a novel folate-directed antimetabolite.

CASE STUDY 3

Theme: Tumor Markers

CASE DETAILS

A 78-year-old male was brought to emergency with difficulty in passing urine and weight loss. The attending urologist suspected carcinoma prostate.
Which molecular marker would help in the confirmation of diagnosis?

CASE DISCUSSION

Prostatic acid phosphatase (PAP) is a nonspecific enzyme synthesized in prostate epithelial cells and its level proportionally increases with prostate cancer progression. PAP had been the biochemical diagnostic marker for prostate cancer until the introduction of prostate-specific antigen (PSA), which improved the detection of early-stage prostate cancer and largely displaced PAP.

BASIC CONCEPT

Tumor/Oncogenic Markers

Tumor markers are hormones, enzymes, peptides, or proteins abnormally synthesized and released by the cancer cells, or are produced by the host cells in response to cancerous growth.

Tumor markers may be present in the body fluids, blood, cell membranes, or in the cytoplasm of the cell.

Clinical Significance of Tumor Markers

They are used for:
- Screening of cancer in asymptomatic individuals
- Clinical staging of the cancerous condition
- Monitoring during cancer treatment
- Early detection of recurrence of the cancerous process.

Classification of Tumor Markers

The clinically important tumor markers are as follows:

1. **Tumor-associated antigens:** These are also called **oncofetal proteins/antigens**. The tumor-associated antigens are produced in large amount in fetal life, but after birth, these antigens disappear and are present in very minute amount in adults. In malignant cells, the synthesis of oncofetal antigens is reactivated and their concentration in blood and cancer cells is increased.

   Examples of oncofetal antigens:
   a. **Carcinoembryonic antigen (CEA):** Gastrointestinal cancer, ovarian, breast, cervical, and lung cancers, best marker of colorectal carcinoma.
   b. **Alpha-fetoprotein (AFP):** Germ cell tumor and hepatocellular carcinoma
   c. **Tissue polypeptide antigen:** Colonic cancer, breast, and prostatic cancer.

   Other less important antigens are:
   - Pancreatic oncofetal antigen
   - Colon-specific antigen
   - Beta-oncofetal antigen

2. **Carbohydrate antigens:**
   These antigens are more specific in determining the site of tumor. They are organ and tissue specific.
   Examples of important carbohydrate antigens are:
   a. **CA 125:** Mainly ovarian cancer, but may also be elevated in endometrial cancer, fallopian tube cancer, lung cancer, breast cancer, and gastrointestinal cancer.
   b. **CA 15-3:** Breast cancer
   c. **CA 19-9:** Mainly pancreatic cancer, but also colorectal cancer and other types of gastrointestinal cancers.
   d. **CA 27-29:** Breast cancer

3. **Pregnancy-associated antigens:**
   a. **Human chorionic gonadotropin-β-subunits (β-hCG):** It is a placental hormone, synthesized by the syncytiotrophoblastic cells of placental villi. In the nonpregnant state, it is present only in very minute concentration in the serum, but it is markedly elevated in pregnancy. The peak level is attained at 12 weeks of pregnancy, then it declines slowly to reach 1/5th of peak at the end of 20 weeks and continues at a very low level for a few days even after parturition.

      Measurement of hCG in serum and urine is undertaken to diagnose pregnancy.

      Chemically, it has two subunits—**α- and β-subunits.**

      The β-subunit is typically measured, because of its increased specificity and because some tumor cells secrete only β-subunit.

      Its high level is an ideal marker of gestational trophoblastic and germ cell tumors of testes and ovaries.

      Its high level is also observed in seminoma, embryonal carcinoma, teratocarcinoma, and choriocarcinoma.
   b. **Placental-like alkaline phosphatase (Regan isoenzyme, PLAP):** The Regan isoenzyme is a placental-type alkaline phosphatase that is expressed in a number of human tumors, particularly in gonadal and urological cancers.
   c. **Other antigens:**
      - Human placental lactogen (HPL)
      - Sex hormone-binding protein (SHBG)
      - Steroid-binding β-globulin (SBBG)
      - α2–pregnancy-associated globulin (α2-PAG)
4. **Mammary-associated antigens:**
   - MCA (mucin-like carcinoma-associated antigen): Breast cancer
   - Mammaglobin: Breast cancer
   - MSA (mammary serum antigen): Breast cancer
   - MAP (mitogen activated protein kinase): Breast cancer
5. **Hormones used as tumor markers:**
   - ACTH: Lung cancer, medullary carcinoma of thyroid, and pancreatic carcinoma
   - Calcitonin: Medullary carcinoma of thyroid
   - Catecholamines: Pheochromocytoma
   - Gastrin: Gastrinoma
   - Insulin: Insulinoma
   - Glucagon: Glucagonoma
   - Serotonin: Carcinoid syndrome.
6. **Enzymes and isoenzymes used as tumor markers:**
   a. **Lactate dehydrogenase (LDH):**
      - Total LDH: Lymphoma, leukemia, germ cell tumor, breast, and lung cancer
      - LDH-1: Germ cell tumors, ovarian carcinoma, osteosarcoma
      - Lactate dehydrogenase: Leukemia
      - LDH-5: Hepatoma, breast cancer, colorectal cancer, and other benign liver diseases.
   b. **Alkaline phosphatase (ALP):**
      - Liver isoenzyme: Metastatic liver cancer
      - Bone isoenzyme: Metastatic bone disease and benign bone disease
      - Regan isoenzyme: Lung cancer, ovarian cancer, breast cancer, colonic cancer, and uterine cancer
      - Nagao isoenzyme: Metastatic carcinoma of pleural surfaces, adenocarcinoma of pancreas, and bile duct.
   c. **Acid phosphatase:**
      - Prostatic acid phosphatase: Prostate cancer
   d. **Creatine kinase:**
      - Creatine phospho kinase: Adenocarcinoma and prostatic carcinoma
   e. **α1-antitrypsin:** Germ cell tumor of testes and ovaries.
   f. **Neuron-specific enolase:** Neuroblastoma and lung cancer
7. **Miscellaneous tumor markers:**
   - Prostate-specific antigen: Carcinoma prostate
   - Monoclonal immunoglobulins
   - Polyamines

A summary of important tumor markers with their clinical significance is presented in the **Table 23.1**.

TABLE 23.1: Summary of tumor markers.

Sl. No.	Tumor marker	Significance
1.	**Carcinoembryonic antigen (CEA)**	Gastrointestinal cancer, ovarian, breast, cervical and lung cancers. Best marker of colorectal carcinoma
2.	**Alpha-fetoprotein (AFP)**	Germ cell tumor and hepatocellular carcinoma
3.	**Tissue polypeptide antigen**	Colonic cancer, breast, and prostatic cancer
4.	**CA 125**	Mainly ovarian cancer, but may also be elevated in endometrial cancer, fallopian tube cancer, lung cancer, breast cancer, and gastrointestinal cancer
5.	**CA 15-3**	Breast cancer
6.	**CA 19-9**	Mainly pancreatic cancer, but also colorectal cancer and other types of gastrointestinal cancers
7.	**β-hCG**	Gestational trophoblastic and germ cell tumors of testes and ovaries
8.	**MAP (mitogen-activated protein kinase)**	Breast cancer
9.	**ACTH**	Lung cancer, medullary carcinoma of thyroid, and pancreatic carcinoma
10.	**Calcitonin**	Medullary carcinoma of thyroid
11.	**Catecholamines**	Pheochromocytoma
12.	**Gastrin**	Gastrinoma
13.	**Insulin**	Insulinoma
14.	**Glucagon**	Glucagonoma
15.	**Serotonin**	Carcinoid syndrome
16.	**Total LDH**	Lymphoma, leukemia, germ cell tumor, breast, and lung cancer
17.	**Alkaline phosphatase (ALP)**	Metastatic liver cancer, bone disease, lung, and gonadal cancers
18.	**Acid phosphatase**	Prostate cancer
19.	**Prostate-specific antigen**	Prostate cancer

CLINICAL NOTE

Tumor markers are used for screening, clinical staging, monitoring during treatment, and early detection of recurrence of cancerous process.

CLINICAL PEARLS

1. Tumor markers are hormones, enzymes, peptides, or proteins abnormally synthesized and released by the cancer cells, or are produced by the host cells in response to cancerous growth.
2. Tumor markers may be present in the body fluids, blood, cell membranes, or in the cytoplasm of the cell.
3. Tumor-associated antigens (oncofetal antigens), carbohydrate antigens, pregnancy-associated antigens, mammary associated antigens, certain hormones, and enzymes act as clinically important tumor markers.

Chapter 24

Biochemical Techniques

LEARNING OBJECTIVES

To understand the principle, types, procedure, and applications of:

- Electrophoresis
- Chromatography
- Western blotting
- Southern blotting
- Polymerase chain reaction
- Enzyme-linked immunosorbent assay (ELISA)
- Colorimetry
- Newborn screening

CASE STUDIES

CASE STUDY 1

Theme: Principle, types, mechanism, and applications of electrophoresis

A 28-year-old female presents to her obstetrician at 12-weeks' gestation for her second prenatal visit. This is her second pregnancy, and she is concerned about her baby and the risk of inheriting a "blood" disease, such as her first child. The patient reports a personal history of mild anemia, but nothing as severe as her younger brother who required frequent transfusions and died at age of 13 years. The patient was told by her physician that she did not need to take iron supplementation for her anemia. Patient denies having any anemic symptoms. Her physical examination is consistent with a 12-week pregnancy and ultrasound confirmed an intrauterine pregnancy at 12-weeks' gestation.

The patient's hemoglobin level (Hb: 9 g/dL) shows a hypochromic, microcytic anemia and hemoglobin electrophoresis demonstrated increased hemoglobin A2 level (4.0%) and increased fetal hemoglobin level (HbF), a pattern consistent with β-thalassemia minor.

What is the diagnostic significance of Hb electrophoresis in this case?
What is the basic principle and applications of electrophoresis?

CASE DETAILS

Hemoglobin electrophoresis is used as a screening test to identify variant and abnormal hemoglobins, including hemoglobin A1 (HbA1), hemoglobin A2 (HbA2), hemoglobin F (HbF; fetal hemoglobin), hemoglobin C (HbC), and hemoglobin S (HbS).

The reference ranges are as follows:
HbA1: 95%–98%
HbA2: 1.5%–3.5%
HbF: <2% (age-dependent)
HbC: Absent
HbS: Absent

The patient in the given case is suffering from β-thalassemia minor. β-thalassemias are usually caused by point mutations rather than deletions. These mutations result in premature chain termination of RNA and ultimately result in reduced or absent β-globin chain synthesis. The molecular defects leading to β-thalassemia are numerous and heterogeneous. Defects that result in absent globin chain expression are termed β°, whereas those causing reduced synthesis are termed β^+. The reduced β-globin chain synthesis in β-thalassemia results in a relative increase in the percentages of hemoglobins A2 and F compared to hemoglobin A, as the β-like goblins (δ and γ) substitute for the missing β chains.

Hemoglobin electrophoresis (using quantitative techniques) in β^+ may show an elevation of hemoglobin A2 to 4–8% and occasional elevations of hemoglobin F to 1–5%.

β-thalassemia major produces severe anemia, and without transfusion, the hematocrit may fall to less than 10%. Little or no hemoglobin A is present. Variable amounts of hemoglobin A2 are seen, and the major hemoglobin present is hemoglobin F.

BASIC CONCEPT

ELECTROPHORESIS

Electrophoresis is the movement of charged particles through an electrolyte when subjected to an electric field.

- Cations move toward cathode.
- Anions move toward anode.
- By this technique, solutes are separated by their different rates of travel through an electric field.
- Commonly used in biological analysis, particularly in the separations of proteins, peptides and nucleic acids.

Factors affecting electrophoresis

The rate of migration of a solute in an electric field depends on the following factors:

1. Net charge on the particle
2. Mass and shape of the particles
3. pH of the medium
4. Strength of electric field
5. Properties of supporting medium
6. Temperature

Electrophoretic Mobility

Electrophoretic mobility is defined as the rate of migration (cm/second) per unit field strength (volts/cm)

$\mu = Q/6\,\pi r \eta$

where μ—electrophoretic mobility

Q—net charge on the ion

r—ionic radius of the solute

η—viscosity of the medium

The electrophoretic mobility is directly proportional to net charge and inversely proportional to molecular size and viscosity of the electrophoresis medium.

Effect of pH

The pH of solution affects the mobility of the ion by determining the amount and nature of charge.

- Proteins, nucleic acids, nucleotides, and amino acids bear charged polar groups making them suitable groups for electrophoresis.
- Carbohydrates carrying no charged groups are first bound to charged groups, such as borate or sulfite ions and then electrophoresis is carried out.
- Lipids are not electrophoresed because electrophoretic current requires polar solvents in which most lipids are insoluble.

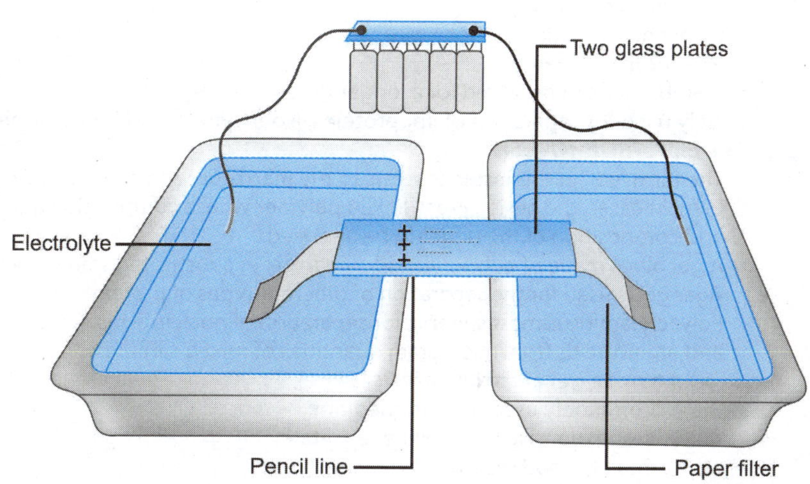

Fig. 24.1: Apparatus for electrophoresis.

Electrophoresis Apparatus

Electrophoresis apparatus **(Fig. 24.1)** consists of:

1. Buffer tank to hold the buffer

2. Buffer
3. Electrodes made of platinum or carbon
4. Power supply
5. Support media
   - The electrophoresis support on which separation takes place may contact the buffer directly or by means of wicks.
   - The entire apparatus is covered to minimize separation.
   - Choice of buffer depends on the nature of substance to be separated and the electricity is supplied at a constant current and voltage.

Support media for electrophoresis

1. Filter paper
2. Cellulose acetate membrane
3. Agar or Agarose gel
4. Starch gel
5. Polyacrylamide gel

Types of Electrophoresis

1. Horizontal
2. Vertical

   Vertical electrophoresis is mainly used for polyacrylamide gel electrophoresis.

Based on the nature of the support medium used, the different types of electrophoresis are as follows:

A. **PAPER ELECTROPHORESIS**
   - The support medium is a filter paper.
   - Frequently used in isolating proteins, amino acids, and oligopeptides.

   Procedure

   a. A long strip of filter paper is moistened with a suitable buffer solution of the desired pH and the sample is applied transversely across the central part of the strip.
   b. Ends are fixed to dip in buffer solutions in two troughs fitted with electrodes.
   c. Electric field of about 20 volts/cm is established.
   d. The charged particles of sample migrate along the strip toward respective electrodes of opposite polarity, according to net charges, sizes, and interactions with the solid matrix.
   e. Homogeneous group of particles migrate as a separate band.
   f. The electrophoresis is carried out for 16–18 hours.
   g. Separated proteins are fixed to a solid support using a fixative, such as acetone or methanol.
   h. Proteins are stained to make them visible.
   i. The separated proteins appear as distinct bands.

   Drawback: Long time interval and blurring of margins.

B. **CELLULOSE ACETATE MEMBRANE ELECTROPHORESIS**
   - Preferred solid support media
   - Less time consuming
   - Excellent separation
   - No blurring of margins
   - Membranes can be stored for a longer time.

   Widely used for separation of lipoproteins, isoenzymes, and hemoglobin.

C. **GEL ELECTROPHORESIS**
   - The term "gel" in this instance refers to the matrix used to contain, and then separate the target molecules.
   - In most cases, the gel is a cross-linked polymer whose composition and porosity are chosen based on the specific weight and composition of the target to be analyzed.
   - A gel block made of polyacrylamide, agarose, or substituted starch gel is used in this method as the solid support.
   - Agar gel is used for the separation of different types of protein mixtures as well as nucleic acids.
   - Polyacrylamide is most suitable for separation of nucleic acids. It is also frequently used in separating proteins, peptides, and amino acids from microgram quantities of mixed samples

   i. **Agarose gel electrophoresis**
      - Commonly used support medium.
      - Less expensive than cellulose acetate
      - Equally good separation
      - Agar is a complex acidic polysaccharide containing monomers of sulfated galactose.
      - Agarose is a sulfate free fraction of Agar.
      - Gel is prepared in buffer and spread over a microscopic slide.

- ◊ A small sample of serum or biological fluid is applied by cutting into the gel with a sharp edge.
- ◊ The electrophoretic rum takes about 90 minutes.

ii. **Polyacrylamide Gel Electrophoresis: PAGE**

- ◊ Most popular type
- ◊ Polyacrylamide is a polymer formed when acrylamide is heated with a variety of catalysts with/without cross-linking agents.
- ◊ It is thermostable, transparent, strong, and relatively chemically inert.
- ◊ Gels are uncharged and are prepared in a variety of pore sizes.
- ◊ Proteins are separated on the basis of charge to mass ratio and molecular size, a phenomenon called molecular sieving.

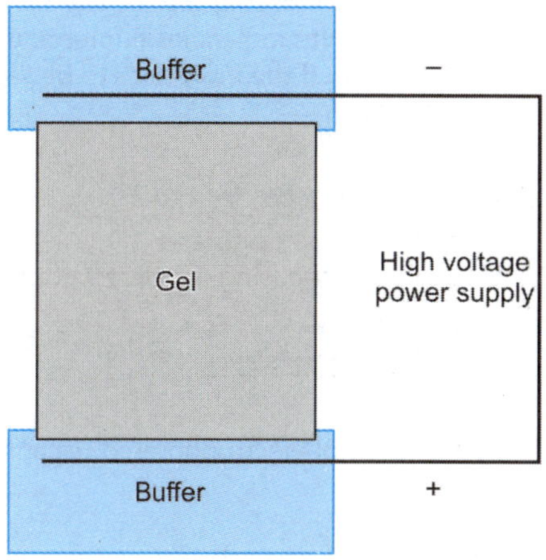

Fig. 24.2: Apparatus for polyacrylamide gel electrophoresis.

Classification of PAGE

PAGE can be classified according to the separation conditions into:

- **Native-PAGE:**
  - Separation is based upon charge, size, and shape of macromolecules.
  - Useful for separation and/or purification of mixture of proteins.
  - This was the original mode of electrophoresis.
- **Denatured-PAGE or SDS-PAGE**
  - Separation is based upon the molecular weight of proteins.
  - The most common method for determining MW of proteins.
  - Very useful for checking purity of protein samples.

Procedure

- The gel of different pore sizes is cast into a column inside a vertical tube, often with large pore gel at the top and small pore gel at the bottom **(Fig. 24.2)**.
- Microgram quantity of the sample is placed over the top of the gel column and covered by a buffer solution having such a pH so as to change sample components into anions.
- The foot of the gel column is made to dip in the same buffer in the bottom reservoir.
- Cathode and anode are kept above and below the column to impose an electric field through the column **(Fig. 24.2)**.
- Macromolecular anions move toward the anode down the gel column.
- There is no external solvent space; all the migratory particles have to pass through the gel pores.
- Rate of migration depends on the charge to mass ratio.
- Different sample components get separated into discrete migratory bands along the gel column on the basis of electrophoretic mobility and gel filtration effect.
- PAGE may yield 20 or more fractions and may be used to study individual proteins and nucleic acids in serum especially genetic variants and isoenzymes.

SDS-PAGE

- SDS-PAGE, sodium dodecyl sulfate polyacrylamide gel electrophoresis, is a technique widely used in biochemistry, forensics, genetics, and molecular biology to separate proteins according to their electrophoretic mobility.
- SDS coats protein molecules giving all proteins a constant charge to mass ratio.
- Due to masking of charges of proteins by the large negative charge on SDS binding with them, the proteins migrate along the gel in order of increasing sizes or molecular weights.
- Molecular weight of a given protein can be determined by comparing the relative electrophoretic mobility of sample with that of standard protein of known molecular weight, when both the sample and the standard proteins are electrophoresed side by side in the same gel slab.
- In oligomeric proteins, SDS-PAGE usually gives the molecular weight of separated monomer chains of the proteins because SDS cleaves the noncovalent bonds interlinking the monomer chains in the intact molecule.

Slab PAGE

- The polyacrylamide gel is cast as a thin rectangular slab inside a plastic frame and this slab is placed vertically on a buffer solution taken in a reservoir **(Figs. 24.3A and B)**.

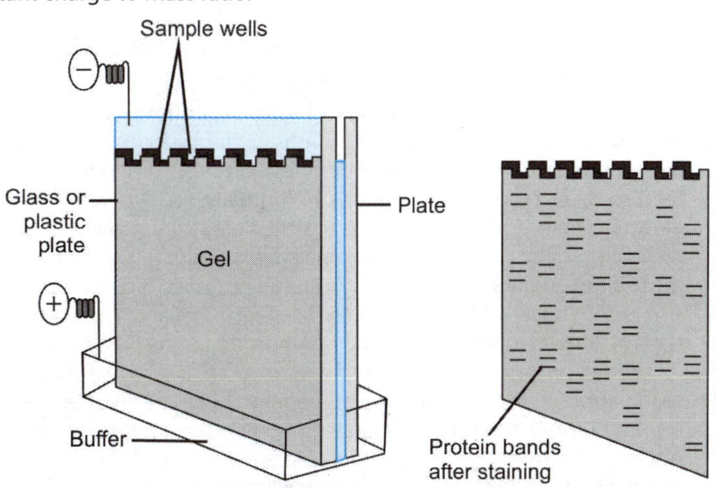

Figs. 24.3A and B: Slab electrophoresis. (A) The gel is poured vertically between two glass plates; (B) Protein bands are separated on the basis of relative molecular weight and visualized with stains.

- Several samples dissolved in dense sucrose solution or glycerol are placed in separate wells cut into the upper edge of the slab and are covered by the same buffer solution. Cathode and anode are above and below to produce electric field effect. Different components migrate simultaneously down parallel lanes in the slab and get separated in to bands **(Figs. 24.3A and B)**.

Visualization
- After the electrophoresis is complete, the molecules in the gel can be stained to make them visible.
- Ethidium bromide, silver, or Coomassie blue dye may be used for this process.
- Other methods may also be used to visualize the separation of the mixture's components on the gel.
- If the analyte molecules fluoresce under ultraviolet light, a photograph can be taken of the gel under ultraviolet lighting conditions. If the molecules to be separated contain radioactivity added for visibility, an autoradiogram can be recorded of the gel.

Other Capillary Electrophoresis
- Immunoelectrophoresis
- Isoelectric focusing (isoelectrophoresis)

CLINICAL NOTE

Lipids are not electrophoresed because electrophoretic current requires polar solvents in which most lipids are insoluble.

CLINICAL PEARLS

1. Electrophoresis is the movement of charged particles through an electrolyte when subjected to an electric field.
2. The rate of migration of a solute in an electric field depends on the net charge on the particle, mass and shape of the particles, pH of the medium, strength of electric field, properties of supporting medium, and temperature.
3. Horizontal and vertical are the main types of electrophoresis. Vertical electrophoresis is mainly used for polyacrylamide gel electrophoresis.
4. Based on nature of support medium, the types of electrophoresis are: paper, cellulose acetate membrane, and gel electrophoresis.
5. Proteins, nucleic acids, nucleotides, and amino acids bear charged polar groups making them suitable groups for electrophoresis. Carbohydrates carrying no charged groups are first bound to charged groups, such as borate or sulfite ions and then electrophoresis is carried out.

CASE STUDY 2

Theme: Principle, types, mechanisms, and applications of Chromatography

Mr XX is a retired 70-year-old man with a 5-year history of type 2 diabetes. Referred by his family physician to the diabetes specialty clinic, he presents with recent weight gain, suboptimal diabetes control, and foot pain. He has been trying to lose weight and increase his exercise for the past 6 months without success. He had been started on glyburide (Diabeta), 2.5 mg every morning, but had stopped taking it because of dizziness, often accompanied by sweating and a feeling of mild agitation, in the late afternoon. He also takes atorvastatin (Lipitor), 10 mg daily, for hypercholesterolemia (elevated LDL cholesterol, low HDL cholesterol, and elevated triglycerides). He has tolerated this medication and adheres to the daily schedule. During the past 6 months, he has also taken chromium picolinate, gymnema sylvestre, and a "pancreas elixir" in an attempt to improve his diabetes control. He stopped these supplements when he did not see any positive results.

He does not test his blood glucose levels at home and expresses doubt that this procedure would help him improve his diabetes control. "What would knowing the numbers do for me?" he asks. "The doctor already knows the sugars are high."

His diet history reveals excessive carbohydrate intake in the form of bread and pasta. The medical documents that Mr XX brings to this appointment indicate that his hemoglobin A1c (A1C) has never been <8%. His blood pressure has been measured at 150/70 mm Hg, 148/92 mm Hg, and 166/88 mm Hg on separate occasions during the past year at the local senior center screening clinic. Although he was told that his blood pressure was "up a little," he was not aware of the need to keep his blood pressure ≤130/80 mm Hg for both cardiovascular and renal health.

Laboratory Results

Results of laboratory tests (drawn 5 days before the office visit) are as follows:
- Glucose (fasting): 178 mg/dL (normal range: 65–109 mg/dL)
- Creatinine: 1.0 mg/dL (normal range: 0.5–1.4 mg/dL)
- Blood urea nitrogen: 18 mg/dL (normal range: 7–30 mg/dL)
- Sodium: 141 mg/dL (normal range: 135–146 mg/dL)
- Potassium: 4.3 mg/dL (normal range: 3.5–5.3 mg/dL)
- Lipid panel
- Total cholesterol: 162 mg/dL (normal: <200 mg/dL)
- HDL cholesterol: 43 mg/dL (normal: ≥40 mg/dL)
- LDL cholesterol (calculated): 84 mg/dL (normal: <100 mg/dL)
- Triglycerides: 177 mg/dL (normal: <150 mg/dL)
- Cholesterol-to-HDL ratio: 3.8 (normal: <5.0)
- HbA1C: 8.1% (normal: 4–6%)
- Urine microalbumin: 45 mg (normal: <30 mg)
- **What is the most probable diagnosis?**
- **What is the significance of HbAlc?**
- **What are different methods of estimation of HbAlc?**

CASE DETAILS

Based on his medical history, records, physical examination, and laboratory results, he can be assessed as follows:
- Uncontrolled type 2 diabetes (A1C >7%)
- Hyperlipidemia (controlled with atorvastatin)
- Hypertension (by previous chart data and examination)
- Elevated urine microalbumin level
- Self-care management/lifestyle deficits
- Limited exercise
- High carbohydrate intake
- Poor understanding of diabetes

Mr XX is suffering from uncontrolled diabetes mellitus and associated comorbidities, such as dyslipidemia and hypertension.

Significance of HbAlc estimation

Hemoglobin becomes glycated by ketoamine reactions between glucose and other sugars and the free amino groups on the alpha and beta chains. Only glycation of the N-terminal valine of the beta chain imparts sufficient negative charge to the hemoglobin molecule to allow separation by charge-dependent techniques. These charges separated hemoglobin are collectively referred to as hemoglobin A1 (HbA1).

The major form of HbA1 is hemoglobin A1c (HbA1c) where glucose is the carbohydrate. HbA1c comprises 4–6% of total hemoglobin A1. The remaining HbA1 species contain fructose-1, 6 bisphosphate (HbA1a1); glucose-6-phosphate (HbA1a2); and unknown carbohydrate moiety (HbA1b). The hemoglobin A1c fraction is abnormally elevated in diabetic persons with chronic hyperglycemia.

Since glycohemoglobins circulate within red blood cells whose lifespan lasts up to 120 days, they generally reflect the state of glycemia over the preceding 8–12 weeks, thereby providing an improved method of assessing diabetic control. Measurements should be made in patients with either type of diabetes mellitus at 3- to 4-month intervals so that adjustments in therapy can be made. In patients monitoring their own blood glucose levels, HbA1c values provide a valuable check on the accuracy of monitoring.

Methods for measuring HbA1c include electrophoresis, cation-exchange chromatography, boronate affinity chromatography, and immunoassays. Office-based immunoassays using capillary blood give a result in about 9 minutes and this allows for immediate feedback to the patients regarding their glycemic control.

The major method of estimation of HbAlc is cation exchange chromatography.

BASIC CONCEPT

Chromatography

The word chromatography is derived from two Greek words—*Chroma* means—color and *graphein* to write. Chromatography is the collective term for a family of laboratory techniques for the separation of mixtures.

Chromatography, literally "color writing," was used—and named—in the first decade of the 20th century, primarily for the separation of plant pigments, such as chlorophyll.

Chromatography is a misnomer since it is no longer limited to the separation of the colored substances.

Principle

Chromatography is based on the principle of the partition of the solute between two phases/solvents. It usually consists of a **mobile phase** and a **stationary phase.** The mobile phase usually refers to the mixture of the substances to be separated dissolved in a liquid or a gas. The stationary phase is a porous solid matrix through which the sample contained in the mobile phase percolates. The interaction between the mobile and the stationary phases results in the separation of the compounds from the mixture. These interactions include the physico-chemical principles, such as the adsorption, ion-exchange, molecular sieving, and affinity.

Classification

There are two ways to classify the methodology of chromatography:

A. Based on nature of stationary phase or mobile phase

It is of two types:

1. Planar—it may be paper or thin layer
2. Column—it may be gas or liquid.

B. Based on nature of interactions between the sample components and the stationary phase, whereby the components are retarded to different degrees in their migration with the mobile phase and are consequently separated from each other. Following are the different types of chromatographic procedures:

1. Partition chromatography
2. Adsorption chromatography
3. Ion-exchange chromatography
4. Gel filtration chromatography
5. Affinity chromatography
6. High-performance liquid chromatography

A. Classification based on nature of stationary phase or mobile phase

1. Planar chromatography:

- Planar chromatography is a separation technique in which the stationary phase is present as or on a plane.
- The plane can be a paper, serving as such or impregnated by a substance as the stationary bed (paper chromatography) or a layer of solid particles spread on a support, such as a glass plate (thin-layer chromatography).
- Different compounds in the sample mixture travel different distances according to how strongly they interact with the stationary phase as compared to the mobile phase.
- The specific retardation factor (R_f) of each chemical can be used to aid in the identification of an unknown substance.

2. Column Chromatography

- Column chromatography is a separation technique in which the stationary bed is within a tube.
- The particles of the solid stationary phase or the support coated with a liquid stationary phase may fill the whole inside volume of the tube (packed column) or be concentrated on or along the inside tube wall leaving an open, unrestricted path for the mobile phase in the middle part of the tube (open tubular column).
- Differences in rates of movement through the medium are calculated to different retention times of the sample.

B. Classification based on nature of interactions between the sample components and the stationary phase

1. Partition Chromatography

This is more commonly used for the separation of mixture of amino acids and peptides. The molecules of a mixture get partitioned between the stationary and the mobile phase depending on the relative affinity of each one of the phases.

a. Paper chromatography

Paper chromatography is an analytical technique for separating and identifying mixtures that are or can be colored, especially pigments. This method has been largely replaced by thin layer chromatography; however, it is still a powerful technique. It is a liquid–liquid partition chromatography. The **stationary phase** is water held on a solid support of filter paper (cellulose). The **mobile phase** is a mixture of immiscible solvents which are mixtures of water, a non-polar solvent, and an acid or base, e.g., butanol, acetic acid water, or phenol-water-ammonia.

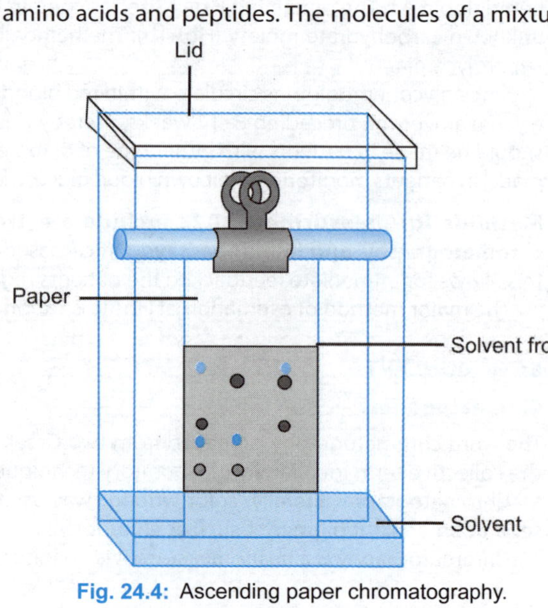

Fig. 24.4: Ascending paper chromatography.

Technique (Fig. 24.4)

- A small concentrated spot of solution that contains the sample of the solute is applied to a strip of chromatography paper about 2 cm away from the base of the plate.
- This sample is absorbed onto the paper and may form interactions with it.

- Any substance that reacts or bonds with the paper cannot be measured using this technique.
- The paper is then dipped into a suitable solvent, such as ethanol or water, taking care that the spot is above the surface of the solvent, and placed in a sealed container.
- The solvent moves up the paper by capillary action, which occurs as a result of the attraction of the solvent molecules to the paper **(Fig. 24.4)**.
- As the solvent rises through the paper, it meets and dissolves the sample mixture, which will then travel up the paper with the solvent solute sample.
- Different compounds in the sample mixture travel at different rates due to differences in solubility in the solvent, and due to differences in their attraction to the fibers in the paper.
- Paper chromatography takes anywhere from several minutes to several hours.
- In some cases, paper chromatography does not separate pigments completely; this occurs when two substances appear to have the same values in a particular solvent.
- In these cases, two-way chromatography is used to separate the multiple-pigment spots.

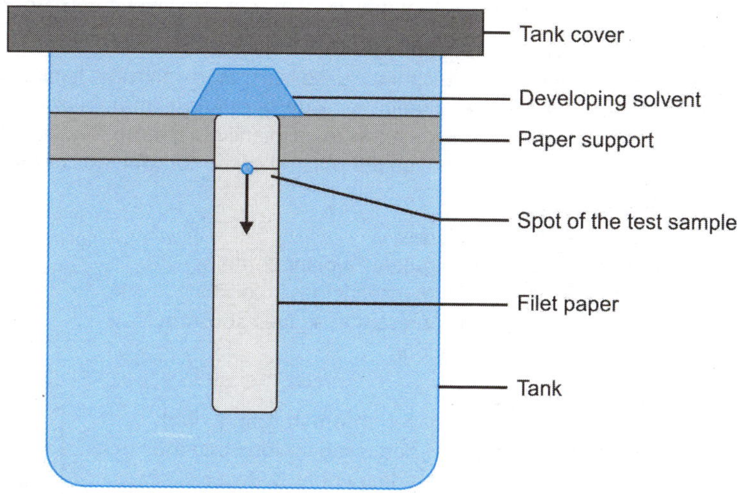

Fig. 24.5: Descending paper chromatography. The developing solvent is placed in a trough at the top which is usually made up of an inert material. The paper is then suspended in the solvent. Substances that cannot be separated by ascending method, can be separated by the above descending method.

Ascending Chromatography

In this method, the solvent is in pool at the bottom of the vessel in which the paper is supported. It rises up the paper by capillary action against the force of gravity (Fig. 24.4).

Descending Chromatography

In this method, the solvent is kept in a trough at the top of the chamber and is allowed to flow down the paper. The liquid moves down by capillary action as well as by the gravitational force. In this case, the flow is more rapid as compared to the ascending method. Because of this rapid speed, the chromatography is completed in a comparatively shorter time **(Fig. 24.5)**.

Analysis

After development, the spots corresponding to different compounds may be located by their color, ultraviolet light, ninhydrin, or by treatment with iodine vapors. The paper remaining after the experiment is known as the chromatogram.

Composition of Filter Paper

The original work in paper chromatography was carried on Whatman No. 1 filter paper. These days paper for chromatography is made from cotton cellulose.

R_f value

The components which have been separated differ in their retention factor, i.e., ratio of distance traveled from the spot or origin by the solute component to that of the distance traveled from the spot or origin by the solvent. Retention factor can never be greater than one.

R_f = distance traveled by the sample/distance traveled by the solvent.

The final chromatogram can be compared with other known mixture chromatograms to identify sample mixes using the R_f value in an experiment. The retention values found can be compared to known values, and from that conclusions can be drawn.

R_f values are usually expressed as a fraction of two decimal places.

If R_f value of a solution is zero, the solute remains in the stationary phase and thus, it is immobile. If R_f value = 1, then the solute has no affinity for the stationary phase and travels with the solvent front.

a. Two-dimensional chromatography

Sometimes, it is difficult to separate a complex mixture of substances by a single run with one solvent system. In such a case, a second run is carried out by a different solvent system, in a direction perpendicular to the first run. This is referred to as two-dimensional chromatography which enhances the separation of a mixture in to individual components **(Fig. 24.6)**.

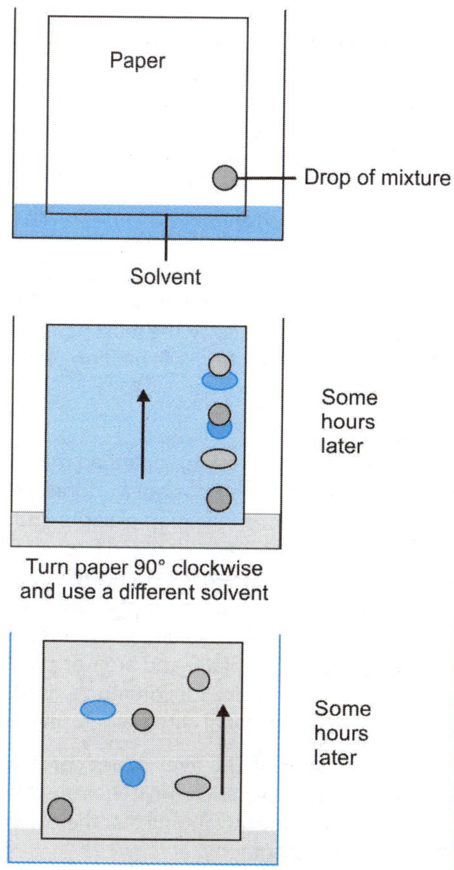

Fig. 24.6: Two-dimensional paper chromatography.

Importance

1. Paper chromatography is a very easy, simple, rapid, and highly efficient method of separation.
2. It can be applied even in microgram quantities of the sample.
3. It can also be used for the separation of a wide variety of materials, such as amino acids, oligopeptides, sugars, oligosaccharides, glycosides, purines and pyrimidines, steroids, vitamins, and some alkaloids like penicillin, tetracycline, and streptomycin.
4. It is not preferred for separating proteins because they are not soluble in many of the solvent systems and are also denatured by them. Paper chromatography is inferior to thin layer chromatography in resolving power.

b. Thin layer chromatography (TLC)

TLC is a chromatographic technique used to separate mixtures. It involves a *stationary phase* consisting of a thin layer of adsorbent material, usually silica gel, aluminum oxide, or cellulose immobilized onto a flat, inert carrier sheet. A *liquid phase* consisting of the solution to be separated is then dissolved in an appropriate solvent and is drawn up the plate via capillary action, separating the experimental solution based on the polarity of the components of the compound in question.

Importance of TLC

Its wide range of uses includes:

- Determination of the pigments a plant contains
- Detection of pesticides or insecticides in food
- Identifying compounds present in a given substance
- Monitoring organic reaction

Technique

The process is similar to paper chromatography with the advantage of faster runs, better separations, and the choice between different stationary phases. Because of its simplicity and speed, TLC is often used for monitoring chemical reactions and for the qualitative analysis of reaction products.

A small spot of solution containing the sample is applied to a plate, about 1 cm from the base. The plate is then dipped into a suitable solvent, such as hexane or ethyl acetate, and placed in a sealed container. The solvent moves up the plate by capillary action and meets the sample mixture, which is dissolved and is carried up the plate by the solvent. Different compounds in the sample mixture travel at different rates due to the differences in their attraction to the stationary phase, and because of differences in solubility in the solvent **(Fig. 24.7)**.

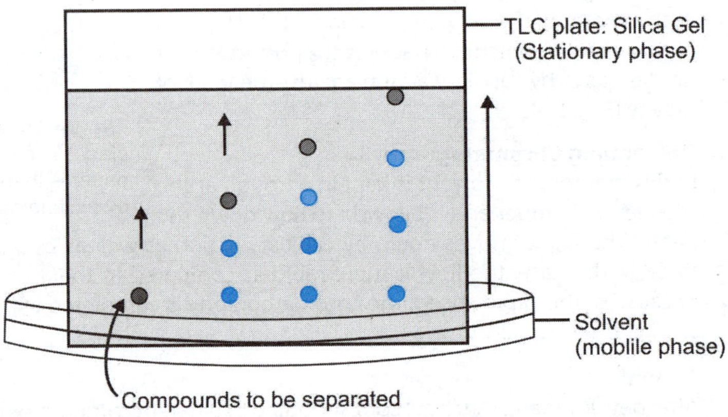

Fig. 24.7: Mechanism of thin layer chromatography.

Separation of compounds is based on the competition of the solute and the mobile phase for binding places on the stationary phase. For instance, if normal phase silica gel is used as the stationary phase, it can be considered polar. Given two compounds which differ in polarity, the most polar compound has a stronger interaction with the silica and is therefore more capable to dispel the mobile phase from the binding places. Consequently, the less polar compound moves higher up the plate (resulting in a higher Rf value).

Analysis

As the chemicals being separated may be colorless, several methods exist to visualize the spots:

- Often a small amount of a fluorescent compound, usually manganese-activated zinc silicate, is added to the adsorbent that allows the visualization of spots under a blacklight (UV_{254}).
- Iodine vapors are a general unspecific color reagent.
- Ninhydrin is used for amino acids and proteins.
- Sulfuric acid is used for phospholipids.

Once visible, the R_f value, or retention factor, of each spot can be determined. These values depend on the solvent used, and the type of TLC plate, and are not physical constants. The Rf value for compounds (amino acids, peptides, sugars, fatty acids, phospholipids, etc.) for commonly used solvent systems has been calculated and available for comparison. TLC can also be used for two-dimensional chromatography using the same plate with two solvent systems, as in the case of paper chromatography.

Advantages of TLC over paper chromatography

1. In case of paper chromatography, it takes 14–16 hours, for the separation of the components, but in TLC, It takes only 3–4 hours.
2. TLC has the advantage that the corrosive reagents, such as sulfuric acid can also be used which pose a limitation for the paper chromatography.
3. It is easier to separate and visualize the components by this method.

4. It has the capacity to analyze multiple samples in a single run.
5. It is relatively a low cost.

2. **Adsorption chromatography**
   - In this technique, the separation is based on differences in adsorption at the surface of the solid stationary medium.
   - The adsorbents, such as silica gel, charcoal powder, and calcium hydroxyapatite are packed into a column in a glass tube.
   - This serves as the stationary phase. The sample mixture in a solvent is loaded on this column.
   - The individual components get differentially adsorbed on to the adsorbent **(Fig. 24.8)**.
   - The elution is carried out by a buffer system (mobile phase).
   - The most weakly held fraction moves fastest, followed by others, according to the order of tightness in adsorption.
   - The individual compounds come out of the column at different rates which may be separately collected and identified.

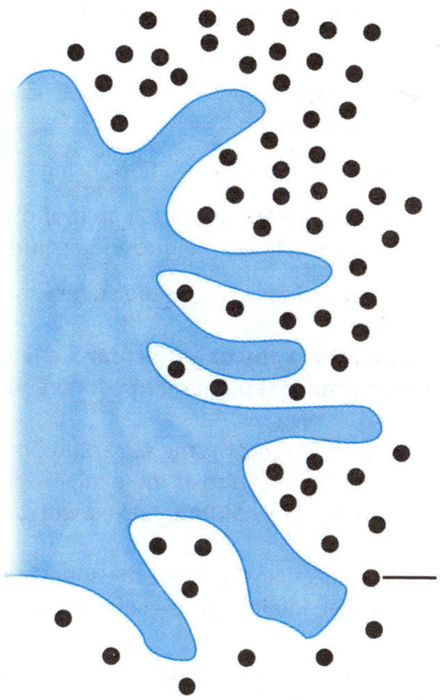

Fig. 24.8: Adsorption chromatography.

3. **Ion-exchange chromatography**
   - Ion-exchange chromatography (or *ion chromatography*) is a process that allows the separation of ions and polar molecules based on the charge properties of the molecules **(Fig. 24.9)**.
   - It can be used for almost any kind of charged molecule including large proteins, small nucleotides, and amino acids.
   - The solution to be injected is usually called a *sample*, and the individually separated components are called *analytes*. It is often used in protein purification, water analysis, and quality control.
   - Ion-exchange chromatography retains analyte molecules based on coulombic (ionic) interactions.
   - The stationary phase surface displays ionic functional groups that interact with analyte ions of opposite charge. This type of chromatography is further subdivided into cation exchange chromatography and anion exchange chromatography. The ionic compound consisting of the cationic species and the anionic species can be retained by the stationary phase.

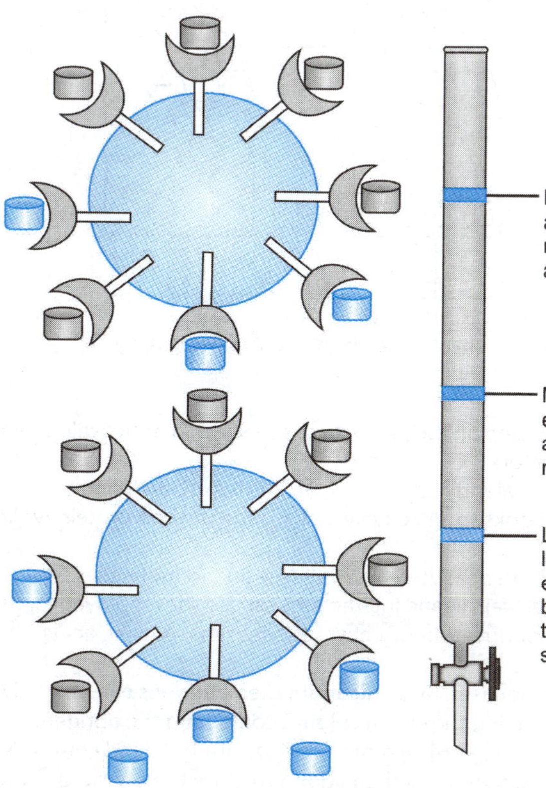

Fig. 24.9: Ion-exchange chromatography.

Cation exchange chromatography retains positively charged cations because the stationary phase displays a negatively charged functional group.

Cation exchange resins: Polystyrene sulfonate resins, CM-sephadex gel, CM—cellulose, these bear acidic groups and immobilize cations from adjacent solutions.

Anion exchange chromatography retains anions using positively charged functional group.

Anion exchangers: DEAE cellulose, trimethyl aminopolystyrene, DEAE-sephadex. All these bear basic groups ionize into fixed positions and immobilize anions from neighboring solutions.

The ionic groups in cation exchange resins are sulfonic and carboxyl groups, while the anion exchange resins have a quaternary nitrogen.

4. **Gel filtration chromatography or Molecular Sieve chromatography:**
   - This is extremely useful in separating ribosomes, viruses, nucleic acids, and proteins depending on their particle sizes and shapes.
   - In gel filtration chromatography, the separation of the particles is based on their size, shape, and molecular weight.
   - This technique is also referred to as molecular exclusion chromatography.
   - The apparatus consists of a column packed with sponge-like gel beads (usually cross-linked polysaccharides) containing pores.
   - The gels serve as molecular sieves for the separation of smaller and bigger molecules.
   - The solution mixture containing molecules of different sizes (say protein) is applied to the column and eluted with a buffer **(Fig. 24.10)**.
   - The larger molecules cannot pass through the pores of a gel and therefore move faster.
   - On the other hand, the smaller molecules enter the gel beads and are left behind which come out slowly.
   - By selecting the gel beads of different porosity, the molecules can be separated.
   - The commercially available gels include (G-10, G-25, G-100), Biogel (P-10, P-30, P-100), and Sepharose (6B, 4B, 2B).
   - The gel filtration chromatography can be used for an approximate determination of molecular weights.
   - This is done by using a calibrated column with substances of known molecular weights.

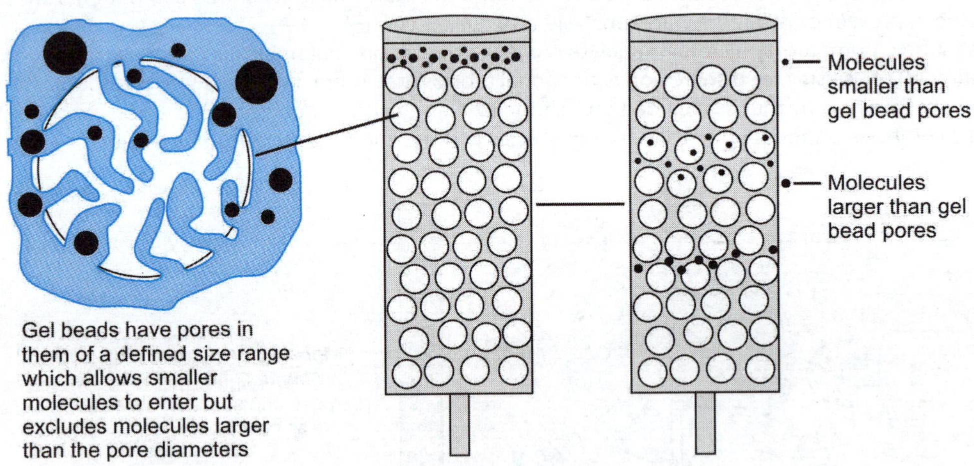

Fig. 24.10: Mechanism of molecular sieve chromatography.

5. **Affinity Chromatography**
   - The principle of affinity chromatography is based on the property of specific and noncovalent binding of proteins to other molecules, referred to as substrates or cofactors.
   - The technique involves the use of ligands covalently attached to an inert and porous matrix in a column.
   - The immobilized ligands act as molecular hooks to selectively pick up the desired protein while the remaining proteins pass through the column.
   - The desired protein captured by the ligand can be eluted by using free ligand molecules.
   - Alternatively, some reagents that can break protein ligand interactions can also be employed for the separation **(Fig. 24.11)**.
   - Affinity chromatography is useful for the purification of enzymes, vitamins, nucleic acids, drugs, hormone receptors, antibodies, etc.
   - For example, NAD is used to purify dehydrogenases. By using antibodies, antigens can be easily separated.
   - Conversely, antibodies can be purified by passing through a column containing the antigen.
   - It is also widely used for the estimation of glycated Hb. Normal Hb does not bind and comes out first, while glycated Hb binds with the boronic acid used as a ligand. Sorbitol is then added to elute the glycated Hb which can be quantitated then.

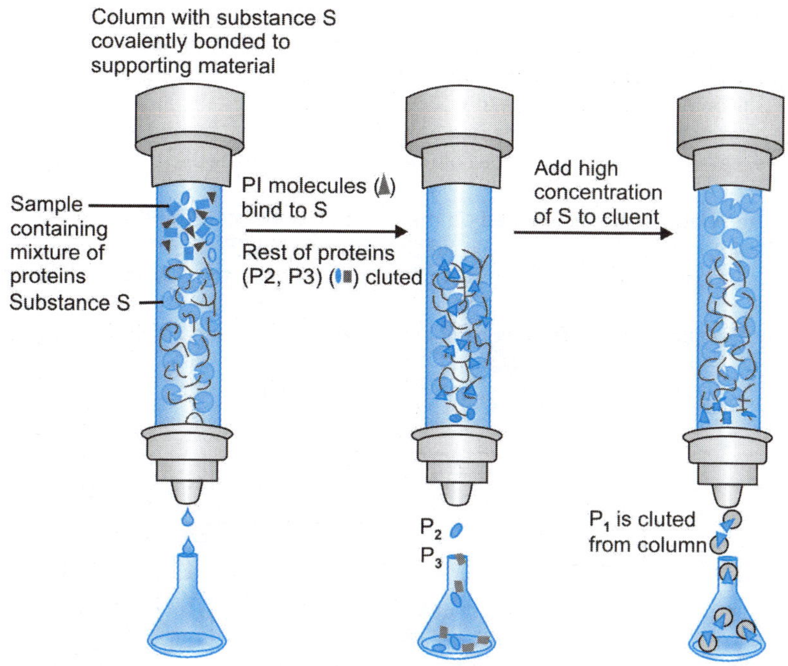

Fig. 24.11: Mechanism of affinity chromatography.

6. **High-performance liquid chromatography**
   - In general, chromatographic techniques are slow and time-consuming.
   - The separation can be greatly improved by applying high pressure in the range of 5,000–10,000 pounds per square inch; hence, this technique is also referred to as high pressure liquid chromatography.
   - HPLC requires the use of non-compressible resin materials and strong metal columns.
   - The eluents of the columns are detected by methods, such as UV absorption and fluorescence.
   - It can be applied in the form of partition, adsorption, ion exchange, or molecular sieve chromatography.
   - The stationary phase consists of an immobilized thin layer of a liquid on the micro glass or plastic beads, tightly packed in to a narrow column **(Fig. 24.12)**.
   - The mobile phase consists of a buffered solvent system which is passed under high pressure through the column for eluting the solutes of the sample.

Due to rapidity in action, it is used for assaying amino acids, peptides, proteins, carbohydrates, lipids, nucleic acids and related compounds, vitamins, hormones, metabolites, and drugs, such as anti-arrhythmic, antibiotics, antiepileptics, analgesics, bronchial smooth muscle relaxants, and anti-depressants.

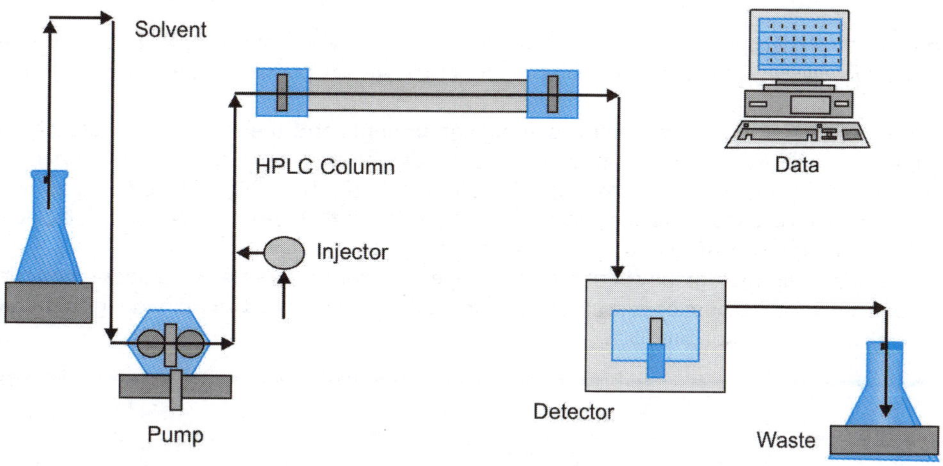

Fig. 24.12: Apparatus for high-performance liquid chromatography.

7. Gas liquid chromatography

- This is the method of choice for the separation of volatile substances or volatile derivatives of certain in volatile substances.
- In GLC, the stationary phase is an inert solid material (diatomaceous earth or powdered firebrick), impregnated with a nonvolatile liquid (silicon or polyethylene glycol).
- This is packed in a narrow column and maintained at high temperature (around 200°C).
- A mixture of volatile material is injected into the column along with the mobile phase, which is an inert gas (argon, helium, or nitrogen).
- The separation of the volatile material is based on the partition of the components between the mobile phase(gas) and stationary phase(liquid), hence, the name gas liquid chromatography **(Fig. 24.13)**.
- The separated compounds can be identified and quantitated by a detector. Gas liquid chromatography is sensitive, rapid, and reliable.

It is frequently used for the quantitative estimations of biological materials, such as lipids, drugs, and vitamins.

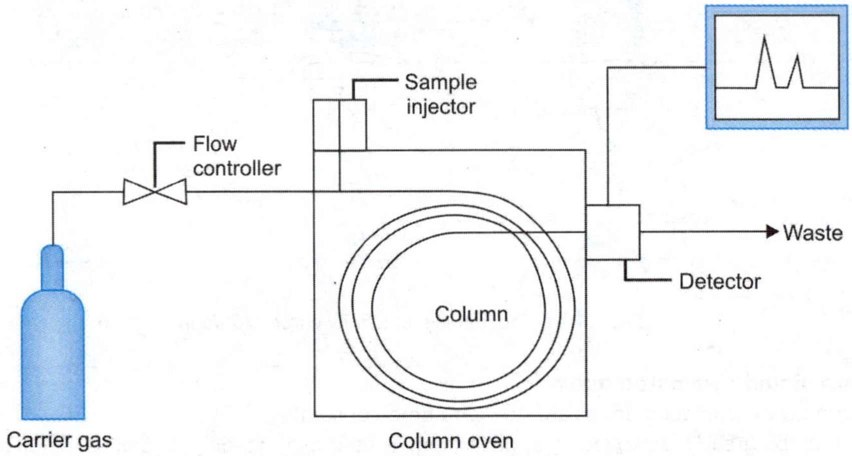

Fig. 24.13: Apparatus for gas liquid chromatography.

CLINICAL NOTE

Paper chromatography is not preferred for separating proteins because they are not soluble in many of the solvent systems and are also denatured by them. It is inferior to thin layer chromatography in resolving power.

CLINICAL PEARLS

1. Chromatography is the collective term for a family of laboratory techniques for the separation of mixtures.
2. Based on nature of stationary phase or mobile phase, it is of two types: (i) planar—paper or thin layer and (ii) column—gas or liquid.
3. Based on nature of interactions between the sample components and the stationary phase, the different types of chromatographic procedures are: partition chromatography, adsorption chromatography, ion-exchange chromatography, gel filtration chromatography, affinity chromatography, and high-performance liquid chromatography.
4. Paper chromatography is used for separating and identifying mixtures that are or can be colored, especially pigments. This method has been largely replaced by thin layer chromatography.
5. TLC is similar to paper chromatography with the advantage of faster runs, better separations, and the choice between different stationary phases. Because of its simplicity and speed, TLC is often used for monitoring chemical reactions and for the qualitative analysis of reaction products.

CASE STUDY 3

Theme: Principle, procedure, and applications of Western Blotting technique

A 25-year-old female is sexually active with a new partner and would like to have an HIV test. The current standard for HIV testing is to start with an enzyme-linked immunosorbent assay (ELISA). HIV antigens are coated on a plate, and the patient's serum is added. If the patient has HIV antibodies, binding of these antibodies to the antigens on the plate will be detected. If the ELISA test is positive, a confirmatory test is done. In this confirmatory test, the patient's serum is added to HIV antigens, which are on a nitrocellulose membrane. This confirmatory test is a:

A. Northern blot
B. Southern blot
C. Western blot
D. Gel electrophoresis
E. Polymerase chain reaction

CASE DETAILS

The correct response is C. Western blot

Demonstration of antibodies is the simplest and most widely employed technique for the diagnosis of HIV infection. However, it takes 2–8 weeks to months for the antibodies to appear in circulation and during that period the person may be highly infectious.

ELISA: ELISA is the most frequently used method for screening of blood samples for HIV antibody. The sensitivity and specificity of the presently available commercial systems approach 100%, but false positive and false negative reactions occur.

Western blotting: Western blots are regarded as the gold standard and seropositivity is diagnosed when antibodies against both the env and the gag proteins are detected. The sensitivity of the test systems is currently being improved by the use of recombinant antigens.

Western Blotting

The term "blotting" refers to the transfer of biological samples from a gel to a membrane and their subsequent detection on the surface of the membrane. Western blotting (also called immunoblotting, because an antibody is used to specifically detect its antigen) is now a routine technique for protein analysis. The specificity of the antibody–antigen interaction forms the basis of identification of a target protein amidst a complex protein mixture.

Overview of Western Blotting

- **Gel electrophoresis:** The first step in a western blotting procedure is to separate the macromolecules in a sample using gel electrophoresis **(Fig. 24.14)**.
- **Protein transfer:** Subsequently, the separated molecules are transferred or blotted onto a second matrix, generally a nitrocellulose or polyvinylidene difluoride (PVDF) membrane **(Fig. 24.14)**.
- **Blocking nonspecific sites:** Next, the membrane is blocked to prevent any nonspecific binding of antibodies to the surface of the membrane.
- **Hybridization:** The transferred protein is then probed with a combination of antibodies: one antibody specific to the protein of interest (primary antibody) and another antibody specific to the host species of the primary antibody (secondary antibody). Often the secondary antibody is complexed with an enzyme, which when combined with an appropriate substrate, will produce a detectable signal.
- **Visualization:** Chromogenic substrates produce a precipitate on the membrane resulting in colorimetric changes visible to the eye.
- **Detection:** The most sensitive detection methods use a chemiluminescent substrate that produces light as a byproduct of the reaction with the enzyme conjugated to the antibody. The light output can be captured using film. Digital imaging instruments based on charge-coupled device (CCD) cameras are becoming popular alternatives to film for capturing chemiluminescent signal. Alternatively, fluorescently-tagged antibodies can be used, which require detection using an instrument capable of capturing the fluorescent signal.

Procedural details (Fig. 24.15):

a. Electrophoretic separation of proteins

- Proteins are commonly separated using polyacrylamide gel electrophoresis (PAGE) to characterize individual proteins in a complex sample or to examine multiple proteins within a single sample.
- PAGE is a powerful analytical tool providing information on the mass, charge, purity, or presence of a protein.
- Nondenaturing PAGE, or native PAGE, separates proteins according to their mass to charge ratios. In contrast, sodium dodecyl sulfate-PAGE, or SDS-PAGE, separates proteins according to mass due to the negative charge imparted on proteins bound to the ionic SDS detergent.

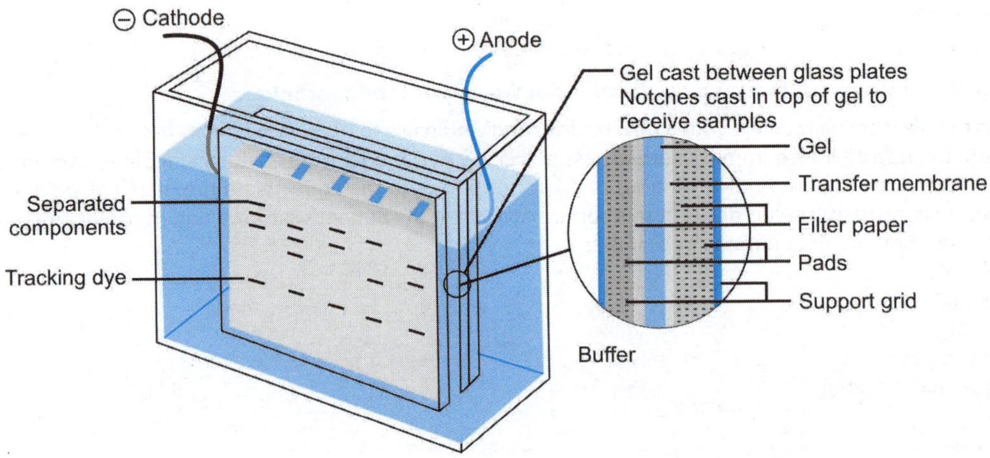

Fig. 24.14: Western blot apparatus showing the assembly of a typical western blot apparatus with the position of the gel, transfer membrane, and direction of protein in relation to the electrode position.

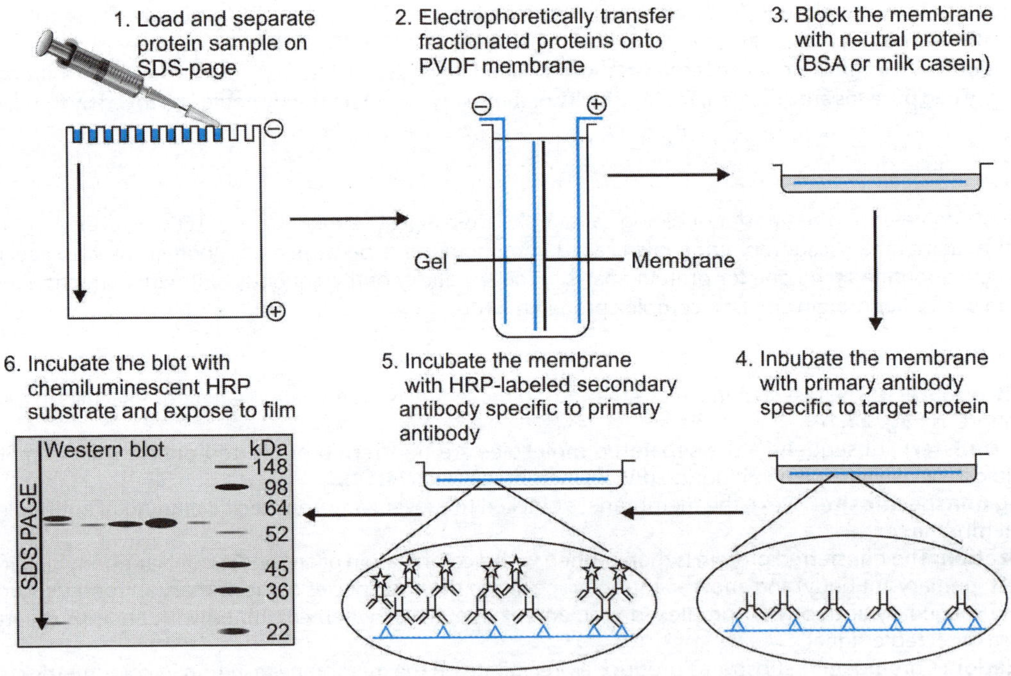

Fig. 24.15: Steps involved in western blotting technique.

b. Transferring proteins to a membrane

- Following electrophoresis, the protein must be transferred from the gel to a membrane.
- The types of methods include: diffusion transfer, capillary transfer, vacuum blotting transfer, and electroelution.
- Electroelution or electrophoretic transfer is the most commonly used method because of its speed and transfer efficiency. This method uses the electrophoretic mobility of proteins to transfer them from the gel to the membrane.
- Electrophoretic transfer of proteins involves placing a protein-containing polyacrylamide gel in direct contact with a piece of nitrocellulose or other suitable, protein-binding support and "sandwiching" this between two electrodes submerged in a conducting solution.
- The process involves the use of porous pads and filter paper to facilitate the transfer. When an electric field is applied, the proteins move out of the polyacrylamide gel and onto the surface of the membrane, where the proteins become tightly attached. The result is a membrane with a copy of the protein pattern that was originally in the polyacrylamide gel.
- Transfer efficiency varies among proteins, based upon the ability of a protein to migrate out of the gel and its ability to bind to the membrane under a particular set of conditions.

- The efficiency of transfer depends on factors, such as the composition of the gel, complete contact of the gel with the membrane, the position of the electrodes, the transfer time, size and composition of proteins, field strength, and the presence of detergents and alcohol in the buffer.
- After transfer and before proceeding with the western blot, total protein on the membrane is often stained with a dye, such as Ponceau S or amido black 10B, to check the transfer efficiency.
- Because dyes may interfere with antibody binding and detection, a protein stain that is easily removable is ideal.

c. Blocking nonspecific sites

- The membrane supports used in western blotting have a high affinity for proteins. Therefore, after the transfer of the proteins from the gel, it is important to block the remaining surface of the membrane to prevent nonspecific binding of the detection antibodies during subsequent steps.
- A variety of blocking buffers ranging from milk or normal serum to highly purified proteins have been used to block free sites on a membrane.
- No single blocking agent is ideal for every experiment since each antibody–antigen pair has unique characteristics.

d. Primary and secondary antibodies

- Western blotting is typically performed by probing the blocked membrane with a primary antibody that recognizes a specific protein or epitope on a group of proteins.
- The choice of a primary antibody for a western blot depends on the antigen to be detected and availability of the antibodies against that antigen.
- In general, the primary antibody that recognizes the target protein in a western blot is not directly detectable. Therefore, tagged secondary antibodies are used as the means of ultimately detecting the target antigen (indirect detection).
- A wide variety of labeled secondary antibodies can be used for western blot detection. The choice of secondary antibody depends on either the species of animal in which the primary antibody was raised (the host species) or any tag linked to the primary antibody [e.g., biotin, histidine (His), hemagglutinin (HA), etc.] For example, if the primary antibody is an unmodified mouse monoclonal antibody, then the secondary antibody must be an anti-mouse IgG secondary (or non-IgG) antibody obtained from a non-mouse host **(Fig. 24.16)**.
- Antibodies for western blotting are typically used as dilute solutions, ranging from a 1/100–1/500,000 dilution from a 1 mg/mL stock solution.

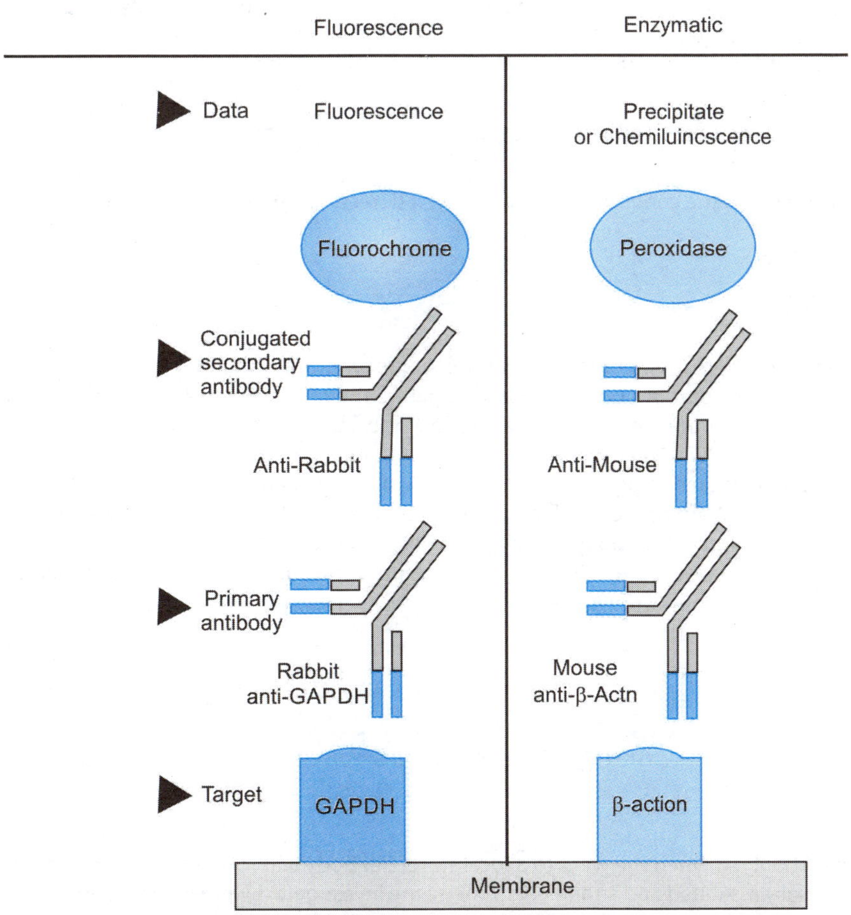

Fig. 24.16: Primary and secondary antibodies in western blotting (GAPDH—glyceraldehyde-3-P dehydrogenase), and fluorescent versus enzymatic labels.

e. Detection methods

- Many different tags can be conjugated to a secondary or primary antibody.
- Radioisotopes were used extensively in the past, but they are expensive, have a short shelf-life, and require special handling and disposal.
- Alternative labels are enzymes and fluorophores.
- Enzymatic labels are most commonly used for western blotting and, can be extremely sensitive when optimized with an appropriate substrate. Horseradish peroxidase (HRP), and to a lesser extent, alkaline phosphatase (AP) are the two enzymes used most extensively as labels for protein detection.
- An array of chromogenic, fluorogenic, and chemiluminescent substrates are available for use with either enzyme.
- Enzyme-conjugated antibodies offer the most flexibility in detection and documentation methods for western blotting because of the variety of substrates available.
- Chemiluminescent blotting substrates differ from other substrates in that the signal is a transient product of the enzyme–substrate reaction and persists only as long as the reaction is occurring. If either the substrate is used up or the enzyme loses activity, then the reaction will cease, and signal will be lost. However, in well-optimized assays using proper antibody dilutions and sufficient substrate, the reaction can produce stable output of light for 1 to 24 hours depending on the substrate, allowing consistent and sensitive detection that may be documented with X-ray film or digital imaging equipment.
- The use of fluorophore-conjugated antibodies requires fewer steps because there is no substrate development step in the assay. This method requires special equipment in order to detect and document the fluorescent signal due to the need for an excitation light source. Recent advances in digital imaging and the development of newer generation fluorophores, such as infrared, near-infrared, and quantum dots have increased the sensitivity and popularity of using fluorescent probes for western blotting and other immunoassays.

Applications of Western Blotting

- To determine the size and amount of protein in a given sample.
- Disease diagnosis: detects antibody against virus or bacteria in serum.
- Western blotting technique is the confirmatory test for HIV. It detects anti-HIV antibody in patient's serum.
- Useful to detect defective proteins, e.g., Prions disease.
- Definitive test for Creutzfeldt-Jakob disease, Lyme disease, Hepatitis B, and Herpes.

CLINICAL NOTE

Western blotting technique is the confirmatory test for HIV. It detects anti-HIV antibody in patient's serum.

CLINICAL PEARLS

1. Western blotting (also called immunoblotting) is a technique for protein analysis.
2. The first step in a western blotting procedure is to separate the macromolecules in a sample using gel electrophoresis. Subsequently, the separated molecules are transferred or blotted onto a second matrix, generally a nitrocellulose or polyvinylidene difluoride (PVDF) membrane.
3. Next, the membrane is blocked to prevent any nonspecific binding of antibodies to the surface of the membrane.
4. The transferred protein is then probed with a combination of antibodies: one antibody specific to the protein of interest (primary antibody) and another antibody specific to the host species of the primary antibody (secondary antibody).
5. Chromogenic substrates produce a precipitate on the membrane resulting in colorimetric changes visible to the eye.

CASE STUDY 4

Theme: Southern Blotting—principle, steps, and applications

CASE DETAILS

A 16-year-old girl was abducted when she went to a local store. Her body was found the next morning and the autopsy revealed that she had been sexually assaulted and strangled. Crime scene investigators were able to collect a semen sample from vaginal fluid as well as tissue samples from underneath the victim's fingernails. DNA samples were obtained from three suspects besides the victim. A variable number of tandem repeats (VNTR) analysis were performed on the DNA samples from the evidence collected, the victim, and the suspect and the results were compared.

Which of the following techniques is the most appropriately applied for this analysis?

A. Thin layer chromatography
B. Polyacrylamide gel electrophoresis
C. Northern blot
D. Southern blot
E. Western blot

CASE DETAILS

The correct option is D. Southern blot.

Variable numbers of tandemly repeated (VNTR) units are types of "insertions" that result in an RFLP (restriction fragment length polymorphism).

Every individual has different numbers of VNTRs. The VNTRs can be inherited, in which case they are useful in establishing genetic association with a disease in family or kindred; or they can be unique to an individual and thus serve as a molecular fingerprint of that person.

Treatment of genomic DNA from different individuals with a single restriction enzyme does not always give the same set of fragments because some restriction sites are polymorphic, being present in some individuals but absent in others, usually because a point change in the nucleotide sequence changes the restriction site into a sequence not recognized by the restriction enzyme **(Fig. 24.17)**.

VNTR analysis is performed by Southern blotting (Southern hybridization).

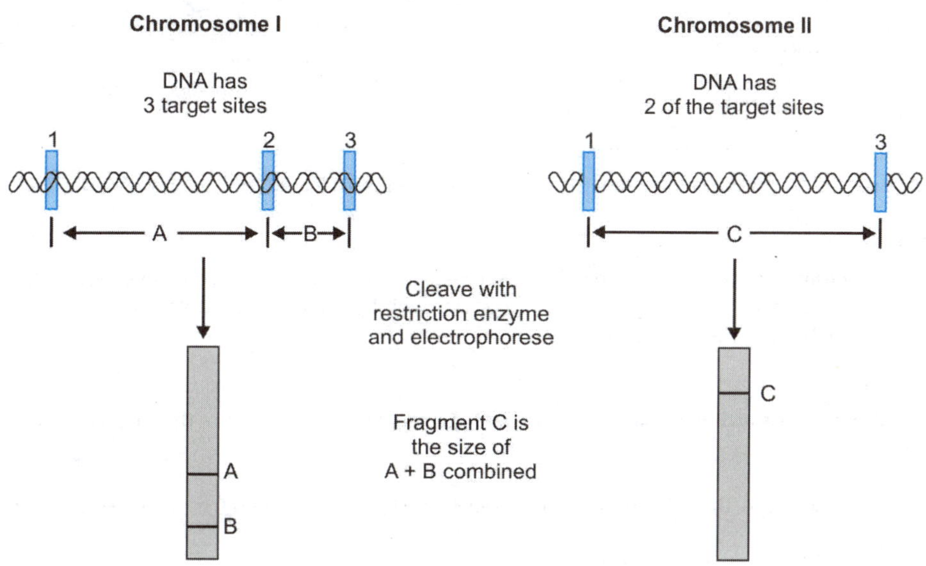

Fig. 24.17: Restriction fragment length polymorphism (RFLP).

Southern Blotting

Principle

Southern blotting is named for the person who developed the technique [Edward M. Southern (1975)]. It is a hybridization technique for identification of specific DNA (carrying the gene of interest) from a mixture of other similar molecules. **Northern** and **Western** blot transfer procedures are based on the detection of specific RNA and proteins, respectively.

This technique involves transfer of DNA molecules from an electrophoresis gel to a nitrocellulose or nylon membrane, in such a way that the DNA banding pattern present in the gel is reproduced on the membrane. During transfer or as a result of subsequent treatment, the DNA becomes immobilized on the membrane and can be used as a substrate for hybridization analysis with labeled DNA or RNA probes that specifically target individual restriction fragments in the blotted DNA. Southern blotting is thus a method for "detection of a specific restriction fragment against a background of many other restriction fragments."

Steps of Southern Blotting

The steps involved **(Fig. 24.18)** in southern blotting are:

Step I: Restriction digestion

1. DNA is extracted from the cell.
2. It is partially digested by a restriction endonuclease (RE) that cuts the DNA at a specific site generating fragments (obtaining complete fragmentation of DNA at the intended restriction enzyme sites is a critical step in Southern blot analysis).
3. The fragments of DNA obtained by restriction digestion are amplified by PCR.

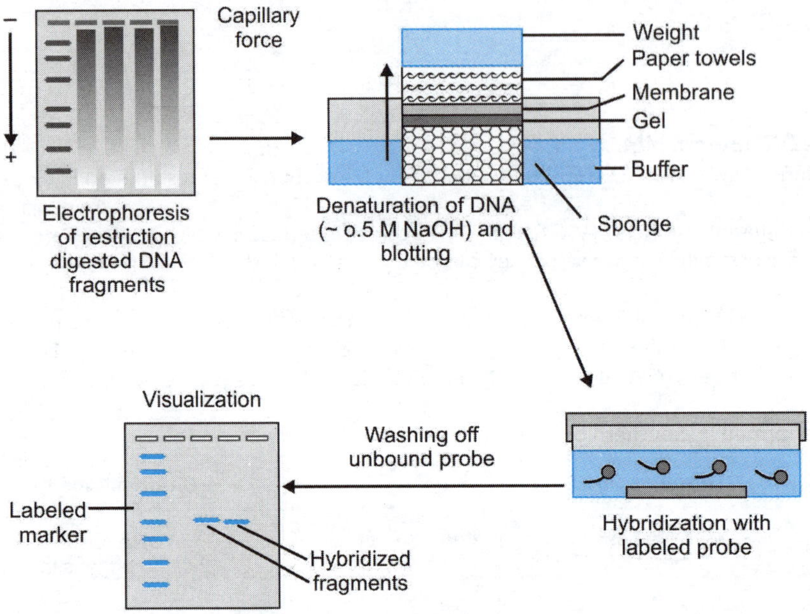

Fig. 24.18: Steps of Southern blotting.

Step II: Gel electrophoresis

4. The resulting DNA fragments are separated by electrophoresis. Fragmented DNA is typically electrophoresed on an agarose gel to separate the fragments according to their molecular weights. Acrylamide gels can alternatively be used for good resolution of smaller DNA fragments (<800 bp).

Step III: Denaturation

5. The gel after electrophoresis is then soaked in alkali (NaOH) or acid (HCl) to denature the double-stranded DNA fragments.

Step IV: Blotting

6. Without altering their positions, the separated bands of ssDNA are transferred to a nitrocellulose filter by the process of blotting.

Step V: Baking and blocking

7. After the DNA of interest is bound on the membrane, it is baked on autoclave to fix in the membrane. The membrane is then treated with casein or bovine serum albumin (BSA) which saturates all the binding site of membrane

Step VI: Hybridization with labeled probes

8. The DNA bound to membrane is then treated with labeled probe. The probe binds with complementary DNA on the membrane since all other nonspecific binding sites on the membrane are blocked by BSA or casein. The probe can be labeled with radioactivity, fluorescent dye, or an enzyme that can generate a chemiluminescent signal when incubated with the appropriate substrate.

Step VII: Visualization by Autoradiogram

9. The membrane bound DNA labeled with probe can be visualized under autoradiogram which give pattern of bands.
10. In the detection step, the bound, labeled probe is detected using the method required for the particular label used. For example, radiolabeled probes may be detected using X-ray film or a phosphor imaging instrument, and enzymatically labeled probes are typically detected by incubating with a chemiluminescent substrate and exposing the blot to X-ray film.

Applications of Southern blot

- Southern blotting has many applications in molecular biology, including the identification of one or more restriction fragments that contain a gene or other DNA sequence of interest and in the detection of RFLPs used in construction of genomic maps.

- DNA finger printing is an example of southern blotting.
- Used for paternity testing, criminal identification, and victim identification.
- To identify mutation or gene rearrangement in the sequence of DNA.
- Used in diagnosis of diseases caused by genetic defects.
- Used to identify infectious agents.

In the current situation **(Fig. 24.19)**, the identity of the criminal (suspect 2) has been confirmed by this method, the electrophoretic pattern of sample DNA is similar to suspect 2.

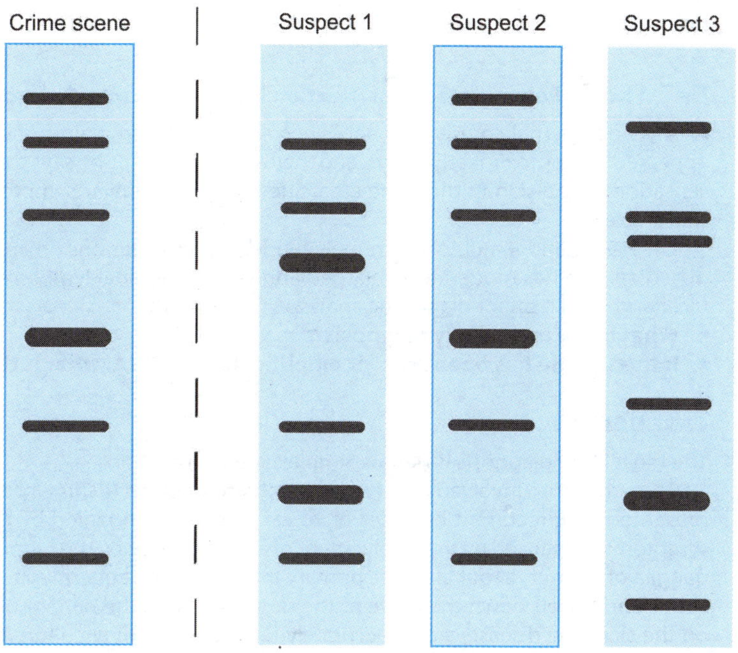

Fig. 24.19: Electrophoretic pattern of sample DNA and three suspects.

As regard other options

A. Thin layer chromatography

Thin-layer chromatography (TLC) is a chromatography technique used to separate nonvolatile mixtures. It can also be used to monitor the progress of a reaction, identify compounds present in a given mixture, and determine the purity of a substance.

B. Polyacrylamide gel electrophoresis

Polyacrylamide gel electrophoresis (PAGE) is a technique widely used to separate biological macromolecules, usually proteins or nucleic acids, according to their electrophoretic mobility.

C. Northern blot

The northern blot is a technique used in molecular biology to study gene expression by detection of RNA (or isolated mRNA) in a sample. Northern blotting involves the use of electrophoresis to separate RNA samples by size and detection with a hybridization probe complementary to part of or the entire target sequence. They can be DNA, RNA, or oligonucleotides with a minimum of 25 complementary bases to the target sequence.

D. Western blot

The western blot (also called the immunoblot) is a widely used analytical technique used to detect specific proteins in a sample of tissue homogenate or extract. It uses gel electrophoresis to separate native proteins by 3D structure or denatured proteins by the length of the polypeptide. The proteins are then transferred to a membrane (typically nitrocellulose), where they are hybridized with antibodies specific to the target protein.

CLINICAL NOTE

The VNTRs can be inherited, in which case they are useful in establishing genetic association with a disease in family or kindred; or they can be unique to an individual and thus serve as a molecular fingerprint of that person.

CLINICAL PEARLS

1. The DNA fragments are separated on the basis of size and charge during electrophoresis.
2. Separated DNA fragments are transferred on nylon membrane.
3. The desired DNA is detected using specific DNA probe that is complementary to the target DNA.
4. A hybridization probe is a short (100–500 bp), single-stranded DNA. The probes are labeled with a marker so that they can be detected after hybridization.
5. The membrane-bound DNA labeled with probe can be visualized under autoradiogram which give pattern of bands.

CASE STUDY 5

Theme: Polymerase Chain Reaction (PCR)—Principle, Procedure, Types, and applications

A 24-year-old female presents to her gynecologist with complaints of very painful vulvar ulcers. The patient states the symptoms appeared for approximately 3 days, and they are worsening. She says that prior to the ulcerations, there was a burning and tingling sensation of the skin in the same area. She has noted similar symptoms like this before and has been told these are sexually transmitted.

On examination, multiple extremely tender, vesicular lesions on an erythematous base on both labia majora of the vulva are observed. She has moderately enlarged and tender inguinal lymph nodes bilaterally. The physician uses a swab to sample the ulcer and send it off for diagnostic analysis.

- **What is the most likely diagnosis?**
- **If the sample has been sent for amplification of DNA, what is the procedure involved?**

CASE DETAILS

The most likely diagnosis is Herpes Simplex virus-2 infection.

The procedure involved is **polymerase chain reaction (PCR)** which is a very sensitive diagnostic technique. The patient has presented with recurrent episodes of vulvar ulcers accompanied by burning and tingling sensation in the same region. These symptoms are caused by the involvement of afferent nerve by the herpes simplex virus. The herpes virus lies dormant in the dorsal ganglia of the nerve root after the primary infection. Subsequently, in times of stress or for unknown reasons, the virus becomes active and travels down the nerve to the skin. Therefore, the patient often has neurological symptoms well before the outbreak on the skin. The disease can be accurately diagnosed by viral culture, alternatively, and even in a better way, polymerase chain reaction can be used for the confirmation of the diagnosis.

Polymerase Chain Reaction

Polymerase chain reaction (PCR) is a molecular technique to copy or amplify small segments of DNA or RNA. It is an efficient and cost-effective technique that combines the principles of complementary nucleic acid hybridization with those of nucleic acid replication that are applied repeatedly through numerous cycles. It results in the exponential production of the specific target DNA/RNA sequences by a factor of 10^7 within a relatively short period.

Components of Polymerase Chain Reactions (PCRs)

- DNA template (the sample DNA that contains the target sequence to amplify)
- Deoxyribonucleoside triphosphates (dNTPs)
- PCR buffer
- Primers (forward and reverse)
- Taq polymerase

Steps of procedure

The PCR is carried out in a single test tube containing all the necessary components. The extracted sample (which contains target DNA template) is added to the tube containing primers, free nucleotides (dNTPs), and Taq polymerase. The PCR mixture is placed in a PCR machine, that increases and decreases the temperature of the PCR mixture in automatic, programed steps and the copies of the target sequence are generated exponentially.

The PCR amplification occurs by repeated cycles of three temperature-dependent steps called denaturation, annealing, and elongation **(Fig. 24.20)**.

1. **Denaturation (strand separation)**: Native DNA exists as a double helix; therefore, the first step, denaturation, of the process separates the two DNA chains by heating the reaction mixture to 90°C to 95°C (194°F to 203°F).
2. **Annealing (primer binding)**: In the second step, annealing, the reaction mixture is cooled to 45°C to 60°C (113°F to 140°F) so that the oligonucleotide primers can bind or anneal to the separated strands of the target DNA.
3. **Extension (synthesis of new DNA)**: In the final step of the process, elongation, the DNA polymerase adds nucleotides to the 3′ ends of the primers to complete a copy of the target DNA template.

These three steps are repeated 20–30 times in an automated thermocycler that can heat and cool the reaction mixture in tube within very short time. This results in exponential accumulation of specific DNA fragments. Therefore, PCR is a method able to amplify any DNA sequence virtually without limit and allows the separation of the nucleic acid of interest from its context.

The doubling of number of DNA strands corresponding to target sequences can be estimated by amplification number associated with each cycle using the formula.

Amplification = 2n, where n = no. of PCR cycles **(Fig. 24.21)**.

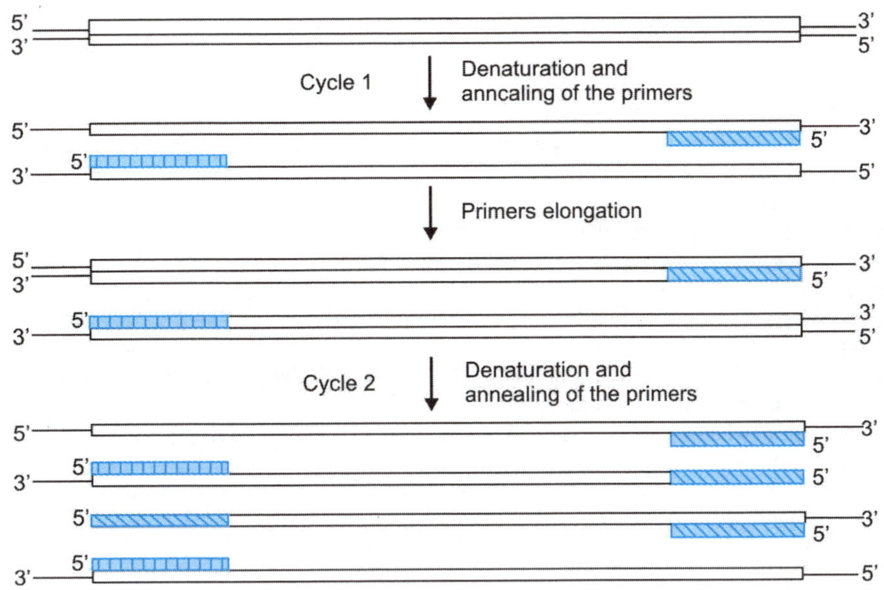

Fig. 24.20: Steps of polymerase chain reaction.

PCR Cycles	*Target Copies*
1	2
2	4
3	8
4	16
5	32
6	64
7	128
8	256
9	512
10	1024
15	32,768
20	1,048,576
25	33,554,432
30	1,073,741,842

Fig. 24.21: Each new DNA strand can act as a new template in the next cycle, yielding approximately one million copies of a target DNA after 20 cycles.

PCR can amplify desired DNA sequences of any origin hundred or millions time in a matter of hour, which is very short in comparison to recombinant DNA technology.

PCR is especially valuable because the reaction is highly specific, easily automated, and very sensitive. It is widely used in the fields like—clinical medicine for medical diagnosis, diagnosis of genetic diseases, forensic science; DNA finger printing, evolutional biology.

Factors affecting PCR

i. Primer

- A short segment of nucleotides (15–30 bases long) which is complementary to a section of the DNA or RNA, which is to be amplified in the PCR.
- Two short DNA sequences designed to bind to the start (forward primer) and end (reverse primer) of the target sequence are used in PCR.

- Primers are designed in such a way that at 3′ end they do not have more than two bases complementary to each other as this results in primer–dimer formation.
- The G+C contents are in the range of 40–60%.
- The melting temperature (Tm) of both forward and reverse primer is usually the same.
- Low concentration of primer results in poor yield while high concentration may result in nonspecific amplification. Hence, optimal concentration of primer is needed, i.e., 0.1–1 μ.

ii. Amount of Template DNA

- Optimal amount of template DNA usually is in nanogram.
- Higher concentrations inhibit or result in nonspecific amplification.

iii. Taq DNA polymerase:

- A heat-stable DNA polymerase obtained from the thermophilic bacterium, *Thermus aquaticus*, is used to synthesize the new strands in most PCR reactions.
- Since this Taq DNA polymerase works best at around 72°C (161.6°F), the temperature of the PCR mixture is raised to that temperature for elongation to proceed efficiently.
- Taq DNA polymerase has both 5′-3′ polymerase and 5′-3′ exonuclease activities. But it lacks 3′-5′ exonuclease activity (proofreading activity).

Detection of PCR products

Labeled probe that is specific for the target gene sequence is used to detect PCR amplified gene product (also known as amplicon). Based on the nature of the reporter molecule used, probe generates radioactive, colorimetric, fluorometric, or chemiluminescent signals. Probe-based detection of amplicons serves two purposes:

1. It allows visualization of the PCR product.
2. It provides specificity by ensuring that the amplicon is the target sequence of interest and not the result of nonspecific amplification.

Apart from DNA-based hybridization method, sometimes simple gel electrophoresis method is sufficient to confirm the presence of specific amplicons.

Types of PCR

1. PCR techniques based on thermocycling techniques

Thermocycling techniques use temperature cycling to drive repeated cycles of DNA synthesis.

a. **Multiplex PCR:** Multiplex PCR is a type of PCR technique which allows an amplification of many target sequences concurrently in the same reaction mixture.

b. **Nested PCR:** Nested PCR is used to increase the specificity of a DNA amplification reducing unspecific products. This technique utilizes two sets of primers. The first set allows a first polymerase chain reaction. The product of this reaction serves as a source of target DNA to a second PCR using the second set of primers.

c. **Hot-start PCR:** This type of polymerase chain reaction serves to reduce nonspecific amplification during the initial set-up stages. Hot-start PCR technique keeps the DNA polymerase in an inactive state at temperatures lower than an annealing temperature.
This modification prevents the amplification during reaction setup when primers bind to DNA sequences with low homology.

d. **Touchdown PCR:** Touchdown PCR is another technique to reduce non-specific amplification. It is achieved by raising the annealing temperature above the melting temperature of the used primers in the initial cycles and lowering in the later cycles. The higher temperatures during the initial cycles help primers to bind to DNA templates with greater specificity while the lower temperatures allow more efficient amplification from the produced amplicons.

e. **Ligase Chain Reaction (LCR):** This type of PCR technique uses four primers for DNA amplification (two primers for each strand of the DNA target). Ligase Chain Reaction primers are much longer than usual PCR primers and designed to cover the entire sequence to be amplified. The main advantage of Ligase Chain Reaction is that a single point mutation near the junction in the original template DNA can prevent the reaction and an absence of product can be an indicator of mutations.

f. **Quantitative PCR (qPCR):** The amount of product that is synthesized during a set number of cycles of a polymerase chain reaction depends on the number of DNA molecules that are present in the starting mixture. This enables PCR to be used to quantify the number of DNA molecules present in an extract.
In quantitative PCR, the amount of product synthesized during a test PCR is compared with the amounts synthesized during PCRs with known quantities of starting DNA.

g. **Real-time PCR:** It is a modification of the standard PCR technique in which synthesis of the product is measured over time. More frequently, this method is used to measure RNA amounts, for example, to determine the expression of a particular gene in cancerous cells. This method allows monitoring the development of cancer.

h. **Reverse transcription PCR:** To carry out polymerase chain reaction where RNA is the starting material, this method uses reverse transcriptase, a process called RT-PCR (reverse transcriptase polymerase chain reaction). The first step in this method is to convert the RNA molecules into single-stranded complementary DNA (cDNA). After this step, the experiment proceeds as in the standard technique.

i. **TaqMan PCR:** TaqMan PCR is one of the real-time PCR techniques. It uses an oligonucleotide probe which is complementary to an internal sequence within the amplified strands. It has a fluorescent group at one end and a quencher at another end. As long as both fluorophore and quencher stay within the oligonucleotide probe, no fluorescence is emitted. During DNA amplification, the oligonucleotide probe, and the primers will bind to newly synthesized strands. The polymerase will destroy the probe due to the intrinsic 5′→3′ exonuclease activity and release the fluorophore. The intensity of the fluorescence is proportional to the amount of generated product.

j. **Assembly PCR:** Assembly PCR or Polymerase Cycling Assembly was developed to produce novel long nucleic acid sequences. The main difference from traditional polymerase chain reaction is the length and quantity of primers. To synthesize artificial oligonucleotide, assembly PCR is performed on long, up to 50 nucleotides, primers. These primers have short overlapping segments and alternate between sense and antisense directions covering the entire target sequence.

During successive cycles, the primers hybridize by complementary segments and then polymerase increases the length of fragments producing the final long nucleic acid sequence.

2. **PCR technique based on isothermal amplification of DNA**

Isothermal techniques do not rely on thermocycling. They are easier to operate and require less energy than standard PCR methods. These types of PCR utilize DNA polymerases with strand-displacement activity.

a. **Loop-mediated isothermal amplification (LAMP)**

PCR reaction mixture for loop-mediated isothermal amplification has strand displacement-type DNA synthetase instead of Taq polymerase. The mixture is held at a constant temperature (about 65°C) to promote the reaction.

b. **Rolling Circle Amplification (RCA)**

With Rolling Circle Amplification, first two ends of the DNA of interest are joined together using a DNA ligase to form a circular single-stranded DNA template. The primer is attached to this template during an annealed step. The amplification is carried out to complete the circle. The synthesized strand is displaced due to the property of the polymerase with strand-displacement activity. The main advantage is that the synthesis can occur at room temperature.

c. **Helicase-Dependent DNA Amplification (HDA)**

Helicase-dependent DNA Amplification relies on a DNA helicase to separate the double-stranded DNA. The major advantage is that the helicase can operate at room temperature.

Applications of PCR:

1. Forensic science: DNA finger printing, paternity testing, and criminal identification.
2. Diagnosis: Identification and characterization of infectious agents
   - Direct detection of microorganisms in patient specimens
   - Identification of microorganisms grown in culture
   - Detection of antimicrobial resistance
   - Investigation of strain relatedness of pathogen of interest
3. Detection of mutation (investigations of genetic diseases)
4. Evolution study: Evolutionary biology
5. Fossil study: Paleontology
6. Gene cloning and expression
7. Gene sequencing
8. Vaccine production by recombinant DNA technology
9. Drug discovery
10. Human genome project

Diagnostic Significance of PCR

PCR is becoming the leading method for detection of the continuously increasing number of human pathogens. Examples include herpes simplex virus (HSV), human papillomavirus, human immunodeficiency virus (HIV), human T lymphotropic virus type I and type II, cytomegalovirus (CMV), Epstein-Barr virus, human herpesvirus-6 (HHV-6), hepatitis B virus, B16 parvovirus, JC and BK viruses, rubella virus, mycobacteria, *Toxoplasmosis gondii*, *Trypanosoma cruzi*, and malaria.

Advantages of PCR over other diagnostic procedures

1. Sensitivity and specificity: PCR can be applied as a detection method for virtually any pathogen for which even limited nucleotide sequence information is known and for which even a very small amount of a specimen of infected tissue is available.
2. Discriminative: In most cases, PCR assays are more discriminative than conventional serology. For example, it is difficult to distinguish HSV-I from HSV-II or HIV-1 from HIV-2 by serology, yet such distinctions can be readily made on the basis of PCR amplification of type-specific genetic sequences.
3. PCR yields rapid results, typically in 1 to 2 days in a clinical setting. The results are specific, faster, and accurate.
4. It is applicable to a wide variety of clinical, pathologic, or forensic specimens, as well as to formalin-fixed tissue, inactivated bacterial cultures, and archeological specimens.

CLINICAL NOTE

PCR is widely used in the fields, such as clinical medicine for medical diagnosis, diagnosis of genetic diseases, forensic science; DNA finger printing, evolutional biology.

CLINICAL PEARLS

1. It is an efficient and cost-effective technique that combines the principles of complementary nucleic acid hybridization with those of nucleic acid replication that are applied repeatedly through numerous cycles.
2. The PCR amplification occurs by repeated cycles of three temperature-dependent steps called denaturation, annealing, and elongation.
3. Labeled probe that is specific for the target gene sequence is used to detect PCR amplified gene product (also known as amplicon).
4. PCR can be applied as a detection method for virtually any pathogen for which even limited nucleotide sequence information is known and for which even a very small amount of a specimen of infected tissue is available.
5. PCR yields rapid results, typically in 1 to 2 days in a clinical setting. The results are specific, faster, and accurate.

CASE STUDY 6

Theme: ELISA—Enzyme-linked Immunosorbent Assay

A 24-year-old female became ill and exhibited lymphadenopathy, exanthema, and fever. A provisional diagnosis of a possible viral infection was made. Laboratory test revealed a positive ELISA against HIV-1 and a dubious immunoblot. This became fully positive 2 weeks later. Follow-up counseling revealed several unprotected sexual contacts.

- **What is the diagnostic significance of ELISA in HIV infection?**
- **What is the principle, procedure, and significance of ELISA?**

CASE DETAILS

The patient is suffering from HIV infection. Based on molecular and antigenic differences, two types of HIV have been recognized. The original isolates of HIV and the related strains present all over the world belong to HIV type 1. The HIV strains, first isolated from West Africa, which react with HIV type I antiserum very weakly or not at all have been termed as HIV type 2. It has 40% genetic similarity and is more closely related to Simian immunodeficiency virus than to HIV-1. It can cause AIDS but is less pathogenic and is less common.

HIV is transmitted when the virus enters the body, usually by injecting infected cells or semen. There are several possible ways in which the virus can enter.

1. **Sexual contact:** In 75% cases, transmission is by sexual contact.
2. **Parenteral:** In 15 % cases, it is by blood transfusion or blood product transfusion.
3. **From mother to child:** Women can transmit HIV to their babies during pregnancy or birth, when infected maternal cells enter the baby's circulation.

Laboratory procedures for the diagnosis of HIV infection include tests for immunodeficiency as well.

ELISA is the most frequently used method for screening of blood samples for HIV antibody. The sensitivity and specificity of the presently available commercial systems approach 100% but false positive and false negative reactions occur as specific tests for HIV.

ELISA

Enzyme-linked immunosorbent assay (ELISA) is a very sensitive immunochemical technique which is used to assess the presence and quantification of a specific protein (antigen or antibody) in the given sample. It is also called solid-phase enzyme immunoassay as it employs an enzyme-linked antigen or antibody as a marker for the detection of specific protein. An enzyme conjugated with an antibody reacts with a colorless substrate to generate a colored reaction product. A number of enzymes have been employed for ELISA, including alkaline phosphatase, horseradish peroxidase, and B-galactosidase.

Principle

ELISA is based on the immunochemical principles of Ag–Ab reaction. The specific interactions between specific antigens and antibodies are used here to detect/quantitate the specific components of a biological fluid, using the enzyme labeled antibodies. The substrate of the enzyme is added, coupled with a color reagent; which is colorless in the beginning, but during the course of the reaction becomes colored. The intensity of the color formed predicts the concentration of the Ag/Ab present in the given sample. Along with the enzyme-labeling of antigens or antibodies, the technique involves following three principles in combination which make it one of the most specific and sensitive than other immunoassays to detect the biological molecule:

a. **An immune reaction,** i.e., antigen–antibody reaction.
b. **Enzymatic chemical reaction,** i.e., enzyme catalyzes the formation of colored (chromogenic) product from colorless substrate.
c. **Signal detection and quantification,** i.e., detection and measurement of color intensity of the colored products generated by the enzyme and added substrate.

Types of ELISA

There are three types of ELISA on the basis of binding structure between the antibody and the antigen:

- Sandwich ELISA
- Indirect ELISA
- Competitive ELISA

Steps of ELISA

A. Sandwich ELISA (antigen detection): A specific antibody is fixed to the well of a micro titer plate **(Fig. 24.22)**. Nonspecific binding sites are blocked using bovine serum albumin. The patient's serum is added in the well and incubated for 30 minutes at 37-degree Celsius. During this time, if the serum contains the antigen, it is fixed on the antibody. Excess antigens and other unwanted proteins are washed out. Then antibodies tagged with horse radish peroxidase (HRP) enzyme are added. If the antigen is already fixed, the Ab-HRP conjugate will be fixed in the well. Then a color reagent, containing hydrogen peroxide (H_2O_2) and diamino benzidine (DAB), are added. The reaction is as follows:

i. $H_2O_2 \longrightarrow H_2O +$ Nascent oxygen (o)
The reaction is catalyzed by Horse radish peroxidase enzyme.

ii. Diamino benzidine (colorless) ⟶ Oxidized DAB (brown color)

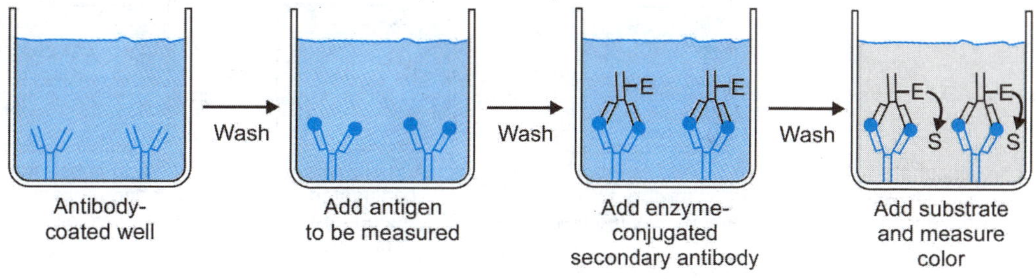

Fig. 24.22: Sandwich ELISA.

The reaction takes place in the presence of Nascent oxygen (o).

Thus, in the above reaction, antigen is sandwiched between Ab (solid phase) and the enzyme-labeled antibody. Development of brown color indicates that the antigen is originally present in the patient's serum. Color developed is proportional to the antigen in the serum. Therefore, intensity of the color is measured from which the concentration of the antigen can be calculated. Other chromogens that can be used in ELISA are NBT (nitro blue tetrazolium-blue color) and NPP (nitro phenyl phosphate-yellow color).

Advantages

- High specificity because the antigen/analyte is specifically captured and detected.
- Suitable for complex (or crude/impure) samples as the antigen does not require purification prior to measurement.
- Flexible and sensitive

B. Indirect ELISA (Antibody detection)

This is useful to detect small quantities of antibodies in the blood, e.g., to detect HIV antibodies in the patient's serum, this test can be undertaken by the following method: Antigen from HIV is coated in the well of a multiwell microtiter plate. Patient's serum is added and incubated. If it contains the antibodies, it is fixed. The wells are washed. This is done to remove excess unbound antibodies. Then a second antibody (antibody against human immunoglobulin) conjugated with HRP is added. Then color reagent containing hydrogen peroxide and diamino benzidine is poured over. Development of brown color indicates the presence of antibodies in the patient's serum. The color developed is proportional to the antibody concentration. Thus, from the intensity of color, the concentration of Ab can be determined **(Fig. 24.23)**.

ELISA is less specific for HIV so the confirmation by other methods is necessary for the final diagnosis of AIDS.

Advantages

- A wide variety of labeled secondary antibodies are available commercially.
- Versatile because many primary antibodies can be made in one species and the same labeled secondary antibody can be used for detection.
- Maximum immunoreactivity of the primary antibody is retained because it is not labeled.
- Sensitivity is increased because each primary antibody contains several epitopes that can be bound by the labeled secondary antibody, allowing for signal amplification.

Disadvantages

- Cros-sreactivity might occur with the secondary antibody, resulting in nonspecific signal.
- An extra incubation step is required in the procedure.

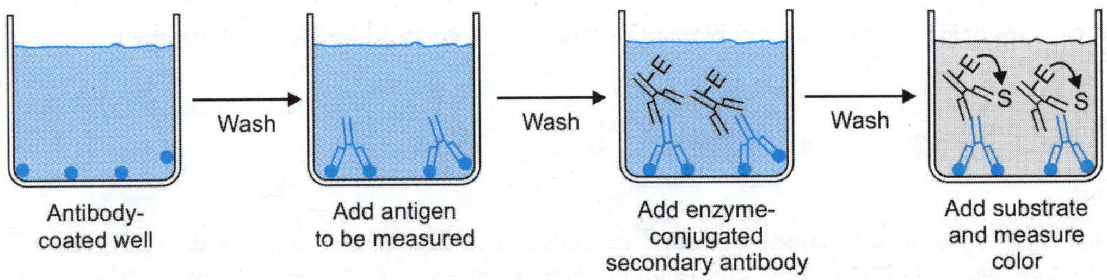

Fig. 24.23: Indirect ELISA.

C. Competitive ELISA

There is a competitive reaction between the sample antigen and antigen bound to the wells of microtiter plate with the primary antibody **(Fig. 24.24)**.

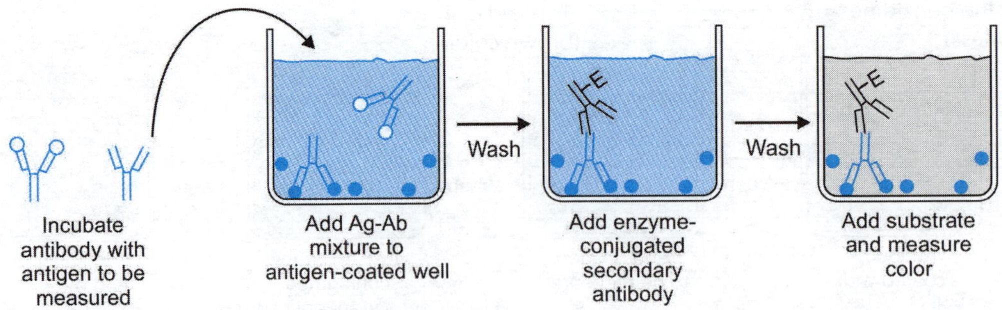

Fig. 24.24: Competitive ELISA.

First, the primary antibody is incubated with the sample. This results in the formation of Ag–Ab complexes which are then added to the wells that have been coated with the same antigens. After an incubation, unbound antibodies are washed off. More the antigen in the sample, more primary antibody will bind to the sample antigen. Therefore, there will be a smaller amount of primary antibody available to bind to the antigen coated on well. Secondary antibody conjugated to an enzyme is added, followed by a substrate to elicit a chromogenic signal. The intensity of color is inversely proportional to the amount of antigen present in the sample.

Advantage

It is highly sensitive even when the specific detecting antibody is present in relatively small amounts.

Applications of ELISA

The ELISA techniques are widely used for:

1. **Quantitative estimation of:**
   - Hormones
   - Amino acids
   - Growth factors
   - Tumor markers, and
   - Other analytes which are present in very small concentration in biological fluids.
2. **Qualitative detection of:**
   - Bacterial or viral antigens
   - Antibodies against microbes
   - Any antigen, or antibody present in small concentration in the biological fluid/tissues.

Advantages of ELISA

- The test can be undertaken to detect antigens or antibodies present in very small quantities in tissues or blood.
- It is highly economical and a sensitive method.
- An enzyme is used as a label, so it is nonisotopic immune assay.
- It is more sensitive than radioimmuno assay and there is no risk of radiation hazards.

CLINICAL NOTE

ELISA is the most frequently used method for screening of blood samples for HIV antibody. The sensitivity and specificity of the presently available commercial systems approach 100%, but false positive and false negative reactions occur as specific tests for HIV.

CLINICAL PEARLS

1. Enzyme-linked immunosorbent assay (ELISA) is a very sensitive immunochemical technique which is used to assess the presence and quantification of a specific protein (antigen or antibody) in the given sample.
2. There are three types of ELISA—sandwich, indirect, and competitive ELISA based on the binding structure between the antibody and the antigen.
3. ELISA can be used for the quantitative estimation of hormones, amino acids, growth factors, tumor markers, and other analytes which are present in very small concentration in biological fluids.
4. It is also used for the qualitative detection of bacterial or viral antigens, antibodies against microbes and any antigen, or antibody present in small concentration in the biological fluid/tissues.
5. It is highly economical, sensitive, nonisotopic immunoassay and there is no risk of radiation hazards.

CASE STUDY 7

Theme: Principle, procedure, and significance of Colorimetry

A 48-year-old woman with a long history of obesity, diabetes, dyslipidemia, and reactive airway disease presented to the hospital emergency department with a 5-day history of weakness, fever, productive cough, nausea, and vomiting. Patient report and chart review confirmed that 2 years before this presentation, her diabetes had been managed with diet alone.

On examination,

- Temperature—99.1°F
- Blood pressure—98/64 mm Hg
- Pulse rate—136 beats/minute
- Respiratory rate—36 breaths/minute
- The patient was drowsy but cogent with strong smell of ketones in the breath.
- Her lung sounds were clear without wheezes or rhonchi.
- Her heart sounds were normal.
- The abdominal examination revealed mild epigastric tenderness to deep palpation but no rebound tenderness or guarding.

Laboratory Investigations

Urine Examination
Urine sugar ++++
Ketone bodies- +++
Blood chemistry
Random blood sugar—400 mg/dL
Arterial blood gas analysis

- pH—7.12
- pCO_2—12 mm Hg
- pO_2—95 mm Hg
- HCO_3^-—11.2 meq/L
- Serum sodium—139 mEq/L
- S. potassium of 5.0 mEq/L
- S. chloride—112 mEq/L

Her chest X-ray revealed no infiltrate.

What might be the likely diagnosis?
Which of these biomolecule/s can be estimated by colorimetric method?
What is the principle, procedure, and significance of colorimetric technique?

CASE DETAILS

The patient is suffering from diabetic ketoacidosis.

DKA is defined as a plasma glucose level >250 mg/dL, plasma bicarbonate <15 mEq/L, pH < 7.35, ketonemia, and an elevation in the anion gap. This patient clearly meets the criteria for DKA based on her blood glucose of 400 mg/dL, HCO_3^- of 11.2, pH of 7.12, anion gap of 15.8, and obvious ketonemia.

Blood glucose can be estimated by the colorimetric method.

Colorimetry

Introduction

A colorimeter is a device used in colorimetry. The word generally refers to the device that measures the absorbance of particular wavelengths of light by a specific solution. This device is most commonly used to determine the concentration of a known solute in a given solution by the application of the Beer-Lambert law.

Principle of colorimetry

Colored solutions have the property of absorbing light of definite wavelengths. The amount of light absorbed or transmitted by a colored solution is in accordance with the Beer-Lambert law.

Beer's law: The intensity of the color is directly proportional to the concentration of the colored particles in the solution.

Lambert's law: The amount of light absorbed by a colored solution depends on the length of the column or the depth of the depth of the liquid through which the light passes.

Equations

When a monochromatic light with an original intensity ("Io") passes through a solution that can absorb radiant energy, (Is) will be less than the (Io).

Some of the radiant energy is reflected back by the cell containing the solution or absorbed by the cell wall or the solvent. The amount of radiation absorbed may be measured in a number of ways:

i. **By measuring transmittance**
ii. **By measuring absorbance**

i. **The transmittance (T) is defined as**
   T = Is/Io
   The ratio is expressed as percentage, thus
   %T = Is/ Io X 100
   As the concentration of the compound increases, less light is transmitted.
   %T varies inversely and logarithmically with the concentration.
ii. **Absorbance measurement is convenient than transmittance.**
   Absorbance (A) or optical density is directly proportional to the concentration.

The relationship between absorbance and transmittance can be expressed as:

$A = -\log Is/Io = -\log T = \log 1/T$

To convert T to % T,

$A = \log 1/T \times 100/100 = \log (100)/\%T = \log 100 - \log\%T = 2 - \log \%T$

Thus,

$A = 2 - \log \%T$

In other words, absorbance (optical density) and transmittance (T) are reciprocally related.

So, if all the light passes through a solution *without* any absorption, then absorbance is zero, and percent transmittance is 100%. If all the light is absorbed, then percent transmittance is zero, and absorption is infinite **(Fig. 24.25)**.

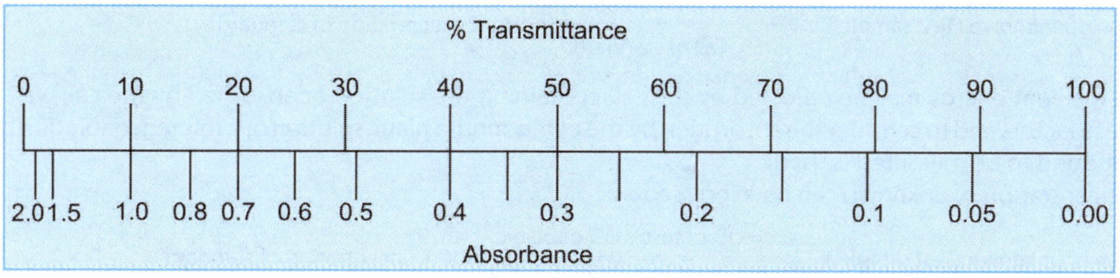

Fig. 24.25: Transmittance and absorbance are reciprocally related.

Lambert-Beer's law

The mathematical expression at a given wavelength can be represented as follows:

$OD = A = \Sigma cl$

Since,

$OD = -\log Is/Io$

(Absorption has no units, since, it is a ratio)

Thus:

$-\log Is/Io = cl$

or $Is/Io = e\ \Sigma cl$

where $= \Sigma$ is a constant. It is the molar extinction coefficient (molar absorptivity).

C = concentration of the colored substance

l = the path length of the sample, that is, the path length of the cuvette in which the sample is contained.

e = base of the natural logarithm.

Since Is/Io is known as transmittance (T)

Thus,

$T = e\ \Sigma cl$

Taking logarithm:

$-\log 10T = \Sigma cl$

As per equation:

$-\log T = A$

Hence,

$A = OD = \Sigma cl$

Since the thickness of the layer of solution is constant in the instrument, optical density is proportional to the concentration. When optical density is plotted against concentration "c," a straight line passing through the origin should be obtained, because the absorbance is directly proportional to the concentration **(Fig. 24.26)**.

The concentration of an unknown solution can be readily determined by measurement of its absorbance and interpolation of its concentration from the graph of the standards.

When %T is plotted versus concentration, a curvilinear relationship is obtained.

The linear relationship between concentration and absorbance is both simple and straightforward, which is why it is preferred to express the Beer-Lambert law using absorbance as a measure of the absorption rather than %T.

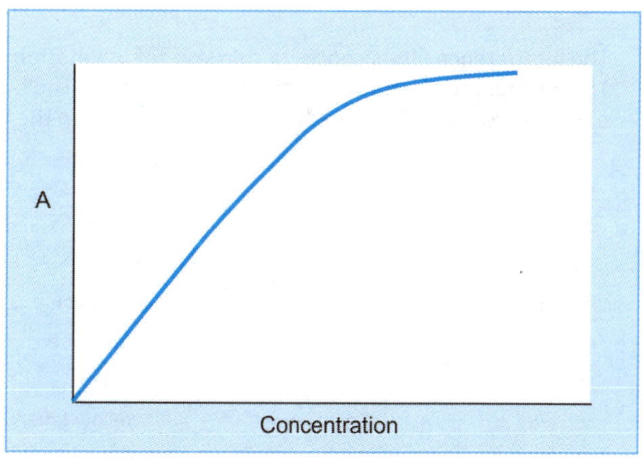

Fig. 24.26: Relationship of absorbance and concentration of a solute in a solution.

Calculation of unknown concentration in the test sample

Since there is a linear relationship between absorbance and concentration, it is possible to calculate the unknown concentration of a substance in the test sample by simple proportional equation:

$$\frac{\text{Absorbance of unknown}}{\text{Absorbance of standard}} = \frac{\text{Concentration of unknown}}{\text{Concentration of standard}}$$

$$\text{Concentration of unknown} = \frac{\text{Absorption of unknown}}{\text{Absorption of standard}} \times \text{Concentration of standard}$$

Thus,

$$\text{Concentration of unknown (Test sample T)} = \frac{\text{OD of test}}{\text{OD of standard}} \times \text{Concentration of standard}$$

Some of the incident energy may be reflected by the cell containing the solution or absorbed by the cell wall or the solvent. To eliminate these factors and to consider the absorption by the compound, a blank solution or a reference solution having everything, but the compound to be measured is used.
Thus, the concentration of unknown can be expressed as:

$$\text{Concentration of unknown (Test sample T)} = \frac{\text{OD of test} - \text{OD of blank}}{\text{OD of standard} - \text{OD of blank}} \times \text{Concentration of standard}$$

Deviations from Beer's law are observed when a very large concentration of an unknown substance is measured or when the incident light is not monochromatic light.

Components of a photo colorimeter

1. **Light source**
   The light source is usually a tungsten lamp for wavelength in the visible range (320–700 nm) and a deuterium or hydrogen lamp for ultraviolet light (below 350 nm). Hydrogen lamp is usually preferred to UV range.
2. **Monochromators**
   This is for the selection of sufficiently narrow wave band. The monochromator consists of an entrance slit to exclude unwanted, followed by absorption or interference filters, prisms, or diffraction grating for wavelength selection **(Fig. 24.27)**.

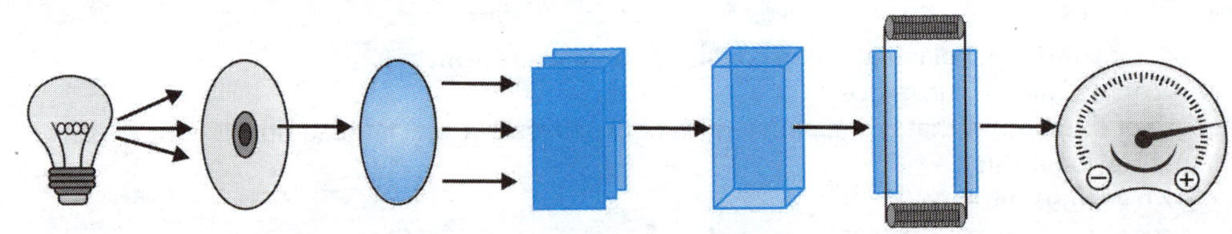

Fig. 24.27: Components of a colorimeter.

The interference filters consist of thin layer of magnesium fluoride crystals with a semitransparent coating of silver on each side. The interference filters have a bandpass of 5–8 nm. The bandpass is defined as the width of the spectrum that will be isolated by a monochromator. The choice of filter depends upon the final color of the solution formed.

Wavelength (nm)	*Filter used/color absorbed*	*Color of solution*
350–430	Violet	Yellow blue
430–475	Blue	Yellow
475–495	Green blue	Orange
495–505	Blue green	Red
505–555	Green	Purple
555–575	Yellow green	Violet
575–600	Yellow	Blue
600–650	Orange	Green blue
650–700	Red	Blue green

3. **Lens**
   Instruments using filters as wavelength selectors require lenses to focus correctly the light from the source through the filter and cuvette to the detector. In the ultraviolet range, quartz or fused silica is essential because the glass does not transmit light efficiently at wavelength shorter than 340 nm.
   An exit slit at the end of monochromator allows only a narrow fraction of the spectrum of reach the sample cuvette.
4. **Sample cuvette**
   For accurate and precise reading, cuvette must be transparent, clean, and devoid of any scratches. The optical path of the cuvette is always 1 cm. Glass cuvettes are used for reading in the visible light range while quartz or fused silica cuvettes are used for UV range.
5. **Photosensitive detectors**
   These detectors contain a light sensitive surface that releases electrons in number proportional to the intensity of light on it, converting light energy into electrical energy. Different detectors used are:
   a. Barrier layer cells
   b. Photosensitive tubes
   c. Photomultiplier tubes
   d. Photoconductive cells
6. **Read-out devices**: The detector response can be measured by any of the following read-out devices:
   a. Galvanometer
   b. Ammeter
   c. Recorder
   d. Digital read out
      The signal may be transmitted to computer or print-out device. Most modern instruments are of direct reading type where the amplified detector signal operates a galvanometer.

Spectrophotomerty

In contrast to colorimeter, spectrophotometer is an instrument that is capable of splitting the incident radiation into spectrum producing a radiation of defined wavelength, and subsequently measuring the intensity of that radiation. In place of colored filters, a diffraction grating or glass prism or quartz prism is fitted, which disperses the white light in to a continuous spectrum **(Fig. 24.28)**. Total wavelength at which measurements can be made includes the visible spectrum (400–750 nm) and extends to each side in to the near ultraviolet (360–400 nm) and near infrared (750–1,000 nm). It is thus possible to eliminate substances which are more or less colorless in the visible region, but which absorb light and are therefore colored, in the ultraviolet or infrared region.

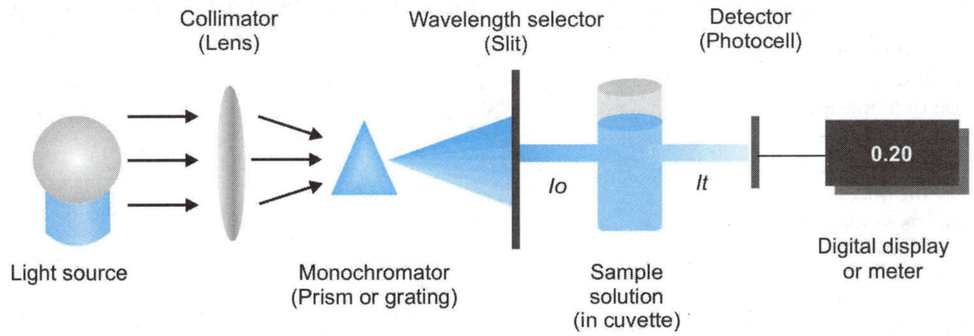

Fig. 24.28: Components of a spectrophotometer. First a collimator (lens) transmits a straight beam of light (photons) that passes through a monochromator (prism) to split it into several component wavelengths (spectrum). Then a wavelength selector (slit) transmits only the desired wavelength.

CLINICAL NOTE

If all the light passes through a solution *without* any absorption, then absorbance is zero, and percent transmittance is 100%. If all the light is absorbed, then percent transmittance is zero, and absorption is infinite.

CLINICAL PEARLS

1. Colorimetry is most commonly used to determine the concentration of a known solute in a given solution by the application of the Beer-Lambert law.
2. **Beer's law:** The intensity of the color is directly proportional to the concentration of the colored particles in the solution.
3. **Lambert's law:** The amount of light absorbed by a colored solution depends on the length of the column or the depth of the liquid through which the light passes.
4. The bandpass is defined as the width of the spectrum that will be isolated by a monochromator.
5. In contrast to colorimeter, spectrophotometer is an instrument that is capable of splitting the incident radiation in to spectrum producing a radiation of defined wavelength, and subsequently measuring the intensity of that radiation.

CASE STUDY 8

Theme: Newborn screening tests

A newborn male infant on screening was diagnosed as having phenylketonuria (PKU), and immediately placed on a diet low in phenylalanine (Phe); careful compliance with the diet and frequent monitoring of the patient's plasma phenylalanine level resulted in the level being maintained at the lower limit of the normal range.

a. **What is the goal of newborn screening?**
b. **What are the steps involved in newborn screening?**

Newborn Screening

Newborn screening is essential for the early detection of several congenital disorders. The main aim is to (i) Identify and manage the affected newborns and (ii) impede the morbidity, mortality, and disabilities associated with an inherited metabolic disorder.

At its establishment, newborn screening has been driven by the selection of genetic diseases whose clinical manifestations developed postnatally, such as phenylketonuria, galactosemia, and hypothyroidism. The latest advances in laboratory techniques including, tandem mass spectrometry (MS/MS), which is more specific, sensitive, reliable, and comprehensive than traditional assays, has increased the number of congenital conditions that can be diagnosed through neonatal screening programs. With a single dried filter paper blood spot, MS/MS can identify more than 30 inherited metabolic disorders in around 2 to 3 minutes.

This comprehensive system includes:
- Examination and testing
- Confirmation of diagnosis
- Management of symptoms
- Treatment of the specific defect
- Evaluation of prognosis
- Education of the family, and
- Follow-up

Disease criteria

According to the WHO Wilson–Jungner criteria, a disease which has the following properties should be screened:
- Should be a significant health problem.
- The natural history of the disease should be sufficiently known.
- It should be identifiable in the early phases.
- There should be a reasonable test or examination system.
- The test should be acceptable to the population.
- Intervals for reiterating the test should be determined.
- There should be a rational treatment for patients.
- Amenities for diagnosis and treatment should be available.
- There should be an approved policy concerning whom to treat as patients; and
- The expenses of case finding should be economically balanced against the benefits.

Metabolic disorders detected by newborn screening

a. **Amino acid disorders**
Phenylketonuria (PKU) is one of the most frequently screened metabolic disorders. It can quickly and accurately be identified by mass spectroscopy (MS/MS). Early diagnosis of phenylketonuria immediately after birth can prevent the irrevocable mental retardation. This necessitates extensive newborn screening in all populations across the world. A special low-phenylalanine diet for the entire lifetime is recommended to the infants diagnosed with PKU.

b. **Fatty acid oxidation disorders**
Medium chain acyl-CoA dehydrogenase (MCAD) deficiency is the most common disorder of fatty acid oxidation. Infants with MCAD deficiency appear to develop normally, but secondary to acute vomiting or fasting, present with rapidly severe hypoglycemia. MCAD deficiency can reliably be detected by MS/MS analysis and is currently included in most expanded newborn screening programs worldwide. Newborn screening has been effective in substantially reducing the risk of disability or death resulting from MCAD.

c. **Organic acidemias**
Methylmalonic acidemia (MMA): MMA is one of the most common organic acidurias worldwide. It is a disorder of the metabolic pathway of propionate characterized by the accumulation of methylmalonic acid in body fluids. There is an inability to convert L-methyl malonyl-CoA to succinyl-CoA. This autosomal recessive disorder results either from a deficiency of methylmalonyl-CoA mutase or its cofactor deoxyadenosyl cobalamin. Clinically, the patients present with acute or chronic neurological symptoms, progressive mental retardation, osteoporosis, and progressive renal failure, due to the accumulation of toxic compounds proximal to the metabolic block. The disease is associated with pernicious anemia and metabolic ketoacidosis, which are hallmarks of MMA. The treatment includes restriction of sources of methylmalonate, protein restriction, and supplementation with L-carnitine and vitamin B12.

d. **Cystic Fibrosis:** The results of neonatal screening for cystic fibrosis report that there are distinct advantages associated with presumptive diagnosis, but also that there are some inherent problems related to genetic testing for complex autosomal recessive diseases that are common and are caused by a rather large number of mutations (>1,500) of a single gene. The definitive diagnostic test for CF is the measurement of concentrations of chloride in sweat, a test that is not practical during the first week of life. Neonates with CF usually have elevations in whole blood trypsinogen. This test allows the screening of neonates at risk for CF. Unfortunately, trypsinogen as a screening test has a high false-positive rate, an unfavorable feature that generates extreme anxiety among newborn parents and families and is costly because of the time and expense for medical follow-up. DNA analysis for mutations that cause CF reduces the size of the suspect group and identifies neonates with a higher likelihood of disease. This two-tiered strategy identifies a manageable number of infants on whom to perform sweat tests.

e. **Hemoglobinopathies**
Any condition that results in the production of abnormal hemoglobin is included under the broad category of hemoglobinopathies. Worldwide, it is estimated that 7% of the population may carry a hemoglobinopathy with clinical significance. The most well-known condition in this group is sickle cell disease.
Sickle cell disease, easily detected using liquid chromatography or isoelectric focusing, can be treated more effectively if it is diagnosed before clinical signs appear.

f. **Urea cycle disorders**
Disorders of the distal urea cycle, such as citrullinemia, argininosuccinic aciduria, and argininemia are included in newborn screening programs in many jurisdictions that using tandem mass spectrometry to identify key amino acids.

g. **Hearing loss**
Undiagnosed hearing loss in a child can have serious effects on many developmental areas, including language, social interactions, emotions, cognitive ability, academic performance, and vocational skills, any combination of which can have negative impacts on the quality of life. The serious impacts of a late diagnosis, combined with the high incidence (estimated at 1–3 per 1000 live births, and as high as 4% for neonatal intensive care unit patients) have been the driving forces behind screening programs designed to identify infants with hearing loss as early as possible. Early identification allows these patients and their families to access needed resources to help them develop normally.
Newborn hearing testing is done at the bedside using transiently evoked otoacoustic emissions, automated auditory brainstem responses, or a combination of both techniques.

h. **Congenital heart defects (CHD)**
In some cases, critical congenital heart defects (CCHD) are not identified by prenatal ultrasound or postnatal physical examination. Pulse oximetry has been recently added as a bedside screening test for critical CHD at 24–48 hours after birth. However, not all heart problems can be detected by this method, which relies only on blood oxygen levels.

i. **Severe combined immunodeficiency**
Severe combined immunodeficiency (SCID) caused by T-cell deficiency is a disorder that was recently added to newborn screening programs in some regions of the United States. Identification of infants with SCID is done by detecting T-cell receptor excision circles (TRECs) using real-time polymerase chain reaction (qPCR). TRECs are decreased in infants affected with SCID. SCID has not been added to newborn screening in a wide scale for several reasons. It requires technology that is not currently used in most newborn screening labs, as PCR is not used for any other assays included in screening programs. Follow-up and

treatment of affected infants also require skilled immunologists, which may not be available in all regions. Treatment for SCID is a stem-cell transplant, which cannot be done in all centers.

j. **Endocrinopathies**
The most commonly included disorders of the endocrine system are congenital hypothyroidism (CH) and congenital adrenal hyperplasia (CAH). Testing for both disorders can be done using blood samples collected on the standard newborn screening card. Screening for CH is done by measuring thyroxin (T4), thyrotropin (TSH), or a combination of both analytes. Elevated 17α-hydroxyprogesterone (17α-OHP) is the primary marker used when screening for CAH, most commonly done using enzyme-linked immunosorbent assays, with many programs using a second-tier tandem mass spectrometry test to reduce the number of false positive results.

k. **Other conditions**
Duchenne muscular dystrophy (DMD) is an X-linked disorder caused by defective production of dystrophin. Many jurisdictions around the world have screened for or attempted to screen for DMD using elevated levels of creatine kinase measured in dried blood spots. Because universal newborn screening for DMD has not been undertaken, affected individuals often have a significant delay in diagnosis.

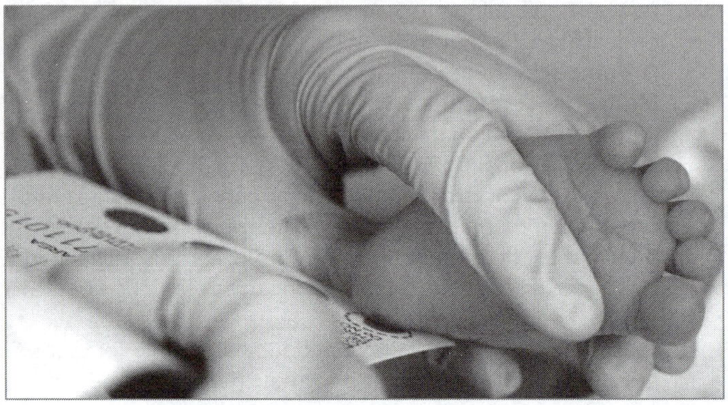
Fig. 24.29: Sample collection for newborn screening.

Sample Collection

Newborn screening tests are most commonly done from whole blood samples. Within the first few days of life (between 24 hours to 7 days after birth), a few drops of blood are taken from an infant's heel and placed on a special card **(Fig. 24.29)**. The card is sent to a laboratory for testing. In most regions, the newborn screening card (which contains demographic information as well as attached filter paper for blood collection) is supplied by the organization carrying out the testing, to remove variations from this source.

Laboratory Testing

Because newborn screening programs test for a number of different conditions, a number of different laboratorial methodologies are used, including the bedside testing. For example:

a. **Evoked otoacoustic emissions and automated auditory brainstem responses** for hearing loss.
b. **Pulse oximetry** for congenital heart defects.
c. **Bacterial inhibition assays:** The first disorder detected by modern newborn screening programs was phenylketonuria. Robert Guthrie developed a simple method using a bacterial inhibition assay that could detect high levels of phenylalanine in blood shortly after a baby was born. Guthrie also pioneered the collection of blood on filter paper which could be easily transported, recognizing the need for a simple system if the screening was going to be done on a large scale. Newborn screening around the world is still done using a similar filter paper.
d. **Mass spectrometry:** the technology allowed rapid determination of a number of acylcarnitines and amino acids from a single dried blood spot. This increased the number of conditions that could be detected by newborn screening.
e. **Enzyme assays** are used to screen for galactosemia and biotinidase deficiency.
f. **Immunoassays** measure thyroid hormones for the diagnosis of congenital hypothyroidism and 17α-hydroxyprogesterone for the diagnosis of congenital adrenal hyperplasia.
g. **Molecular techniques** are used for the diagnosis of cystic fibrosis and severe combined immunodeficiency.
Tandem mass spectrometry (MS/MS) is a technically advanced method in which many compounds are initially fragmented and separated by molecular weight. Each compound is then fragmented again. Identification of compounds is based upon characteristic fragments. The process requires roughly 2 minute per sample and can detect 20 or more inborn errors of metabolism.

The effects of prematurity, neonatal illness, and intensive neonatal management on metabolites in blood complicate the interpretation of results. The MS/MS permits a diagnosis to be made before clinical illness develops and has revolutionized the purpose and ability of newborn screening. MS/MS is not directed toward diseases defined as treatable, but it is directed toward all of the diseases, each of which is rare, that the technique can identify. Electrospray MS/MS permits the detection of rare inborn errors of metabolism and has been introduced as a newborn screening tool all around the world.

Around 40 disorders can be detected through the aforementioned analytes. The severity of metabolic disorders can range from mild to severe. In an attempt to standardize newborn screening programs, the American College of Medical Genetics recommends that every baby born in the United States be screened for a core panel of 29 disorders **(Table 24.1)**.

TABLE 24.1: Standardize newborn screening programs, the American College of Medical Genetics.

Sl. No	*Disease*
1.	Isovaleric acidemia
2.	Glutaric aciduria type 1
3.	3-Hydroxy-3-methylglutaricaciduria
4.	Multiple coenzyme A (CoA) carboxylase deficiency
5.	Methylmalonic acidemia (mutase deficiency)
6.	3-Methylcrotonyl-CoA carboxylase deficiency
7.	Methylmalonic acidemia [cobalamin (Cbl) A, B]
8.	Propionic acidemia
9.	β-Ketothiolase deficiency
10.	Medium-chain acyl-CoA dehydrogenase deficiency
11.	Very-long-chain acyl-CoA dehydrogenase deficiency
12.	Long-chain L-3-hydroxy acyl-CoA dehydrogenase deficiency
13.	Trifunctional protein deficiency
14.	Carnitine uptake deficiency
15.	Phenylketonuria
16.	Maple syrup urine disease
17.	Homocystinuria (because of cystathionine β-synthase deficiency)
18.	Citrullinemia
19.	Argininosuccinic acidemia
20.	Tyrosinemia type 1
21.	Sickle cell anemia (Hb SS disease)
22.	Hemoglobin (Hb) S/β-thalassemia
23.	Hb S/C disease
24.	Congenital hypothyroidism
25.	Biotinidase deficiency
26.	Congenital adrenal hyperplasia (21-hydroxylase deficiency)
27.	Classical galactosemia
28.	Hearing loss
29.	Cystic fibrosis

An additional 25 conditions were recommended as secondary targets because they may be identified while screening for the core panel disorders.

Advantages of using MS/MS for newborn screening

The benefits of using MS/MS include the following:

a. The assay can be performed on minimal amounts of blood or other body fluids.
b. The analytic procedure uses two mass spectrometers simultaneously. The first one is used to segregate the components of the mixture, therefore, eliminating or diminishing prior chromatographic separation.
c. The time needed for the analysis of each sample is thus reduced to approximately 2 to 3 minutes; and
d. The procedure can be automated, allowing an analysis of roughly 600 samples per 24 hours, with a very reasonable cost per sample.

Reporting of results

The results of the blood tests are sent to the pediatrician. The goal is to report the results within a short period. If any of the tests show positive results, further testing is done to make a diagnosis. The confirmatory test varies depending on the positive results on the initial screen. Confirmatory testing can include analyte specific assays to confirm any elevations detected, functional studies to determine enzyme activity, and genetic testing to identify disease-causing mutations.

In some cases, a positive newborn screen can also trigger testing on other family members, such as siblings who did not undergo newborn screening for the same condition or the baby's mother, as some maternal conditions can be identified through results on the baby's newborn screen. Depending on the likelihood of the diagnosis and the risk of delay, the specialist initiates treatment and provides information to the family. Follow-up testing is typically coordinated between geneticists and the infant's pediatrician or primary care physician.

Status of newborn screening

Many countries screen all newborns for PKU and hypothyroidism, while in some of the more developed countries, the routine screening panels include 20 or more conditions. In Australia, all disorders detectable by MS/MS analysis are screened; in the United States, nearly all of the 4.3 million newborns are screened for more than 30 metabolic conditions; in the Netherlands, 17 disorders are screened; in Denmark, the panel includes 13 metabolic disorders; in Germany, 12 disorders; and the United Kingdom (UK) screens only for PKU and MCAD deficiency.

Controversies of newborn screening

The expansion of the screening test menu raises several issues:

- The cost of implementation can be significant because multiple MS/MS systems are required.
- Staffing the laboratory with qualified technical personnel to run the MS/MS system and qualified clinical scientists to interpret the profiles can be a challenge.
- A number of false-positive results will also be obtained with these newborn screening programs.
- Many of these findings are the result of parenteral nutrition, biologic variation, or treatment, and are not the result of an inborn error of metabolism.
- Consequently, qualified staff will be needed to ensure that patients with abnormal results are contacted and receive follow-up testing and counseling, if needed.

Ethical issues

- **Diseases with no treatment:** Many of the new diseases being tested for are rare and have no known treatment, while some of the diseases need not be treated until later in life. This raises more issues, such as: if there is no available treatment for the disease should we test for it at all? Moreover, if we do, what do we tell the families of those with children bearing one of the untreatable diseases?
- **Parent–child bonding:** Ten percent of parents whose children were diagnosed with a false-positive still worried that their child was fragile and/or sickly even though they were not, potentially preventing the parent–child bond forming as it would have otherwise. As a result, some parents may begin to opt out of having their newborns screened.

CLINICAL NOTE

With a single dried filter paper blood spot, MS/MS can identify more than 30 inherited metabolic disorders in around 2 to 3 minutes.

CLINICAL PEARLS

1. The main aim of newborn screening is to (i) identify and manage the affected newborns and (ii) prevent the morbidity, mortality, and disabilities associated with an inherited metabolic disorder.
2. Within the first few days of life (between 24 hours to 7 days after birth), a few drops of blood are taken from an infant's heel and placed on a special card.
3. If any of the tests show positive results, further testing is done to make a diagnosis. The confirmatory test varies depending on the positive results on the initial screen.
4. Many countries screen all newborns for PKU and hypothyroidism, while in some of the more developed countries, the routine screening panels include 20 or more conditions.
5. Depending on the likelihood of the diagnosis and the risk of delay, the specialist initiates treatment and provides information to the family. Follow-up testing is typically coordinated between geneticists and the infant's pediatrician or primary care physician.

Chapter 25

Case Studies for Self-assessment

CASE STUDIES

CASE STUDY 1

An infant girl was hospitalized because of respiratory difficulty, myopathy, brain damage, and poor growth. When she was fed with a high-carbohydrate diet, the urine contained large quantities of short-chain fatty acids. A liver biopsy revealed that almost no acetyl-CoA carboxylase activity was present, whereas propionyl-CoA carboxylase activity was within the normal range.

What metabolic processes would be defective in this child? What is the cause of respiratory difficulty in this patient?

CASE STUDY 2

A 35-year-old male came into the physician's office because his hands and feet were "swelling", and his face had coarse features with oily skin. On examination, he was above the 95th percentile for height at his age. He was noted to have some coarse facial features including large nose, large tongue, and frontal bossing of his forehead. His hands were enlarged with soft tissue swelling, and his heel pad was thickened. He was noticed to have a slightly enlarged liver and spleen. The remainder of the examination was otherwise normal.

What is the most likely diagnosis?
What is the biochemical mechanism of this disorder?

CASE STUDY 3

A 20-year-old healthy male college student went to celebrate his birthday with some friends at a bar. His friends convinced him to have his first beer since he just turned 20. After consuming the beer, he began to experience intense, worsening abdominal pain that was nonspecific in location and described as cramping. Nausea and vomiting then ensued and he was taken to the emergency room (ER). Upon arrival to the ER, he was found to be very anxious with hallucinations. He was noted to be hypertensive, tachycardic, and diaphoretic. Peripheral neuropathy was also noticed on examination. Initial laboratory test revealed a normal complete blood count (CBC). Serum and urine aminolevulinic acid (ALA) and porphobilinogen (PBG) were both found to be elevated.

What is the likely diagnosis?
What is the underlying biochemical problem?

CASE STUDY 4

A 66-year-old man had a postoperative cardiac arrest.

Past history of hypertension treated with an angiotensin-converting enzyme (ACE) inhibitor was there. There was no past history of ischemic heart disease. Following reversal and extubation, myocardial ischemia was noticed on electrocardiogram (ECG). He was transferred to intensive care unit (ICU) for overnight monitoring. On arrival in ICU, blood pressure (BP) was 90/50 mm Hg, pulse 80 beats/min, and respiratory rate was 16 breaths/min. During handover to intensive care unit (ICU) staff, he developed ventricular fibrillation, which reverted to sinus rhythm with a single 200-J countershock. Soon after, blood gases were obtained from a radial arterial puncture:

Arterial blood gases:
pH—7.27
PCO_2—55.4 mm Hg

PO_2—144 mm Hg
HCO_3—24.3 mmol/L

Biochemistry results (all in mmol/L): Na^+—138, K^+—4.7, Cl^-—103, urea—6.4, and creatinine—0.07.
What is the probable diagnosis?

CASE STUDY 5

An adolescent presents with abdominal discomfort, abdominal fullness, excess gas, and weight loss. Blood glucose, cholesterol, and alkaline phosphatase levels are normal. There is no jaundice or elevation. The stool test is positive for reducing substances.

What is the probable diagnosis?
What is the biochemical basis for these symptoms?
What is the nature of reducing substance present in stool?

CASE STUDY 6

A 55-year-old man was admitted to the emergency department in coma. Apparently, he had become increasingly depressed after death of his daughter 2 months ago. Previously, before her death, he had been moderate drinker, but consumption of alcohol had increased markedly over last a few weeks. He had also been eating poorly, his other married daughter had dropped around to see him on Sunday morning and found him unconscious in the living room couch with two empty bottles of whisky. Two more bottles were also found on the living room table.

On examination, he could not be roused, his breathing was deep and noisy, alcohol could be smelt in his breath, and his temperature was 35.6°C.

Laboratory findings were:

- Blood alcohol—500 mg/dL
- Blood glucose—50 mg/dL
- Blood lactate—8 mmol/L
- pH—7.21

What is the biochemical basis for all the laboratory findings in this patient?

CASE STUDY 7

A 4-year-old child with a previous fracture in right foot had a serum alkaline phosphatase (AP) of 850 U/L, a serum phosphate of 4.5 mg/dL, and a serum gamma-glutamyl transferase (GGT) of 33 U/L. After the clotted blood was spun down in the test tube, the serum was visibly hemolyzed owing to difficulty in obtaining the specimen. The physical examination of the child is unremarkable.

Why is the normal range of AP higher in children than in adults?
What is the significance of a hemolyzed serum sample and the elevated serum AP? What is the most likely cause of the elevated AP?

CASE STUDY 8

A 23-year-old medical student complained of excessive fatigue and a poor appetite over the past a few months. He had some vague right upper quadrant pain on deep palpation; however, the liver was not enlarged on physical examination.

A biochemical profile revealed a serum ALT of 125 U/L and a normal serum aspartate aminotransferase (AST; SGOT), total bilirubin, AP, and GGT.

What is the significance of an isolated elevation in transaminase in this medical student?
What tests, if any, are required to further evaluate this patient?

CASE STUDY 9

A 3-year-old female was brought for consultation by her mother who was troubled by her daughter's continuous fatigue, dizziness, and loss of weight. The patient was 5 feet 5 inches tall and weighed 103 pounds.

Laboratory results revealed leukopenia, blood glucose = 50 mg%, and elevated ketones.

Further questioning revealed that the young women had been virtually fasting for 4 months hoping to obtain a "skinny face" as a prelude to a career in modeling.

What is the problem with the patient?
What is the cause of hypoglycemia?

CASE STUDY 10

A 48-year-old menopausal woman reports to her physician with symptoms of fatigue. She has been previously healthy except for osteopenia, for which she is taking Fosamax, 70 mg once a week, and also estrogen replacement therapy. She reports no back pain, no polydipsia, polyuria, no slurred speech, and no lethargy.

Examination revealed mild pallor. The rest of the examination was normal, including the absence of percussion tenderness over the thoracic and lumbar spine. A complete blood count (CBC) revealed hemoglobin of 10.9 g/dL. The white blood cell count was normal, and the platelet count was 110,000. Serum chemistry revealed a serum calcium level of 12.5 mg/dL. Creatinine was slightly elevated at 1.2 mg/dL.

Further evaluation revealed a monoclonal IgG kappa protein in the serum, measuring 2.5 g/dL. A 24-hour urine protein electrophoresis showed a monoclonal kappa free light chain measuring 500 mg per 24 hours. A skeletal survey revealed equivocal skull lesions and osteopenia of the thoracic and lumbar spine and pelvis. A bone marrow examination revealed 30% plasma cells.

What is the probable diagnosis?

CASE STUDY 11

A 16-year-old man hospitalized in a coma after an automobile accident was started on intravenous hyperalimentation. Although a complete vitamin mixture was present in the solution, fat was omitted in the diet because of solubility problems. After 3 months, the patient developed skin lesions and hematuria. Plasma lipid analysis revealed normal cholesterol level but a very low level of arachidonic acid. Analysis of a 24-hour urine collection indicated a low excretion of prostaglandin metabolites. A corn and soybean emulsion was added to the intravenous solution, and the symptoms and chemical abnormalities gradually resolved during the next month.

What is the cause of this problem?

Why did the treatment correct the low level of plasma arachidonic acid and low urinary output of prostaglandin metabolites?

CASE STUDY 12

A 2-year-old girl was brought by her mother to the outpatient department (OPD) of the local hospital. The mother had four children, the youngest of whom was 3 months of age and still being breastfed. The father had broken his leg in an accident during the previous year and had not been able to work since. Family income was thus low, and they were not able to buy milk and meat on a regular basis. Their main food was a starchy gruel, high in carbohydrate and low in protein. The mother stated that the daughter had been eating poorly from the past month, had intermittent diarrhea for some time, and had recently developed a cough and a fever, and had become very irritable and apathetic.

On examination, the girl was found to be both underweight for her height and small for her age. She was pale, very weak, and drowsy. Her temperature was 40.5°C. Her skin was flaky and her hair was brittle and dry. The abdomen was distended and the liver was moderately enlarged. Generalized edema was evident. Rales were heard over the lower lobe of the left lung.

What is the likely diagnosis for this patient?

CASE STUDY 13

A young black man reported to the physician with complaints of bloating and diarrhea. His eyes were sunken and the physician noted other signs of dehydration also. The patient's temperature was normal. He explained that the episode occurred previously also following a birthday party in which he participated in an ice cream eating contest. The patient reported prior episodes of similar nature following ingestion of a significant amount of the dairy products. This clinical picture is due to which disease?

What is the defect in this?

CASE STUDY 14

A 67-year-old man had an intermittent history of constipation and diarrhea and a weight loss of 18 pounds over the last 4 months. He stated that he had a dragging sensation in his right upper abdomen. The past history included the transfusion of 5 units of blood, 10 years ago after his spleen, was ruptured in a car accident. Positive physical findings include a slightly enlarged, nontender liver and an anal fissure. The laboratory findings are listed below:

Serum alkaline phosphatase = 125 U/L
Serum GGT = 100 U/L
Serum LDH = 250 U/L
Serum AST, ALT, and total bilirubin are normal
Serum iron = 40 µg/dL

Serum ferritin = 280 ng/mL
CBC: Mild normocytic anemia; corrected reticulocyte count is 2%.

What is the likely diagnosis?
What is the significance of the liver function test abnormalities?

CASE STUDY 15

A 35-year-old woman presented to her obstetrician/gynecologist with complaints of irregular periods, hirsutism, and mood swings from the previous 6–8 months. She also reported weight gain and easy bruising even after a minor trauma.

On examination, she was having truncal obesity, a round "moon" face, ecchymoses, and abdominal striae. The pulse was 78 beats/min and blood pressure was 170/100 mm Hg. The patient was given a dexamethasone suppression test, which revealed an elevated level of cortisol.

What is the most likely diagnosis?

CASE STUDY 16

A 23-year-old male was seen in the emergency department after suffering a concussion and head trauma from a motor vehicle accident. The patient was stabilized in the emergency department and transferred to the intensive care unit (ICU) for observation. The patient had computed tomography (CT) scan of the head that revealed a small amount of cerebral edema, but was otherwise normal. During the 2nd day in the ICU, the nurse informed that the patient had a large amount of urine output in the last 24 hours. The nursing records reported his urine output over the previous 24 hours to be 6,000 cc. He had not been given any diuretic medications. A urine osmolality was ordered and was found to be low. His physician remarked that the kidneys were not concentrating urine normally.

What is the most likely diagnosis for the increasing dilute urine output?
Which biochemical mediator is responsible for this disorder?

CASE STUDY 17

A 72-year-old male with diabetes mellitus was evaluated in the emergency room because of lethargy, disorientation, and long and deep breaths (Kussmaul respiration). Initial chemistries on venous blood demonstrated high-glucose level at 380 mg/dL, pH of 7.3, bicarbonate—15 mM, and PCO_2—30 mm Hg.

What is the diagnosis for this patient?
How will you treat such a patient?
What is the biochemical basis for all these symptoms?

CASE STUDY 18

A 47-year-old female is brought to the emergency department with complaints of malaise, nausea and vomiting, and fatigue. The patient reveals a long history of alcohol abuse for the last 10 years requiring drinks daily especially in the morning as an "eye opener". She has been to rehab on several occasions for alcoholism but has not been able to stop drinking. She is currently homeless and jobless. She denies cough, fever, chills, upper respiratory symptoms, sick contacts, recent travel, hematemesis, or abdominal pain. She reports feeling hungry and has not eaten very well in a long time. On physical examination, she appears malnourished but in no distress. Her physical examination is normal. Her blood count reveals a normal white blood cell count but does show an anemia with large red blood cells. Her amylase, lipase, and liver function tests were normal.

What is the most likely cause of her anemia?
What is the molecular basis for the large erythrocytes?

CASE STUDY 19

A 10-year-old boy received a sulfonamide antibiotic as prophylaxis for recurrent urinary tract infections. Although he was previously healthy and well-nourished, he became progressively ill and presented with pallor and irritability. A blood count revealed that he was severely anemic with jaundice due to hemolysis of the red blood cells.

What is the problem with the boy?
What is the cause of anemia and jaundice in this boy?
What is the simplest way for the diagnosis of this problem?

CASE STUDY 20

A 24-year-old male suffering from malaria was put on primaquine. He developed malaise, fatigue, and yellow discoloration of sclera and skin.

On examination, there was pallor ++, icterus ++, pulse was 100 beats/min, and temperature was 102°F. Liver and spleen were palpable.

The investigation report was as follows: hemoglobin (Hb)—5 g%, total leukocyte count (TLC)—13,000 cmm esp. polymorphs, serum bilirubin was 6 mg% (direct—4.2 mg% and indirect—1.8 mg%), urine had hemoglobin and urobilinogen. The color of the urine was brownish black.

What is the probable diagnosis?
What is the relationship of primaquine intake and the present manifestations?

CASE STUDY 21

A 22-year-old soldier collapsed from dehydration during maneuvers in the desert and was sent to a military hospital. Prior to enlisting, a physician observed a high level of glucose in his urine during an examination. At first, he was not allowed to enlist because he was suspected of being a diabetic. Further tests, however, determined that his insulin level was normal. A glucose tolerance test exhibited a normal pattern. Laboratory tests following his dehydration episode repeated the previous findings, but further testing of the urine reveals that only D-glucose is elevated. Other sugars were not elevated.

What is the cause of patient's elevated urinary glucose and his dehydration episode?

CASE STUDY 22

A 7-year-old boy was hospitalized with fever, vomiting, and diarrhea that were thought to be due to viral gastroenteritis. His blood chemistry revealed pH—7.2 and bicarbonate—13.9 mM, and an elevated glycerol content in the plasma (2.5 mM, normal 0.02–0.28 mM). Urinary glycerol was 90 mM (normal <0.2 mM). The episode reoccurred over the next a few years, and on occasions, he became unconscious. His brother was similarly affected.

What is the nature of this genetic disorder?

CASE STUDY 23

A 25-year-old woman presented with a 4-month history of increased sweating and palpitations with weight loss of 6 kg. On examination, she was a nervous, agitated woman with an obvious, diffuse, nontender, smooth enlargement of thyroid, over which a bruit could be heard. She had a fine tremor of her fingers and a resting pulse rate of 150 beats/min. She had no evidence of exophthalmos. A maternal aunt had suffered from "thyroid disease".

On investigation, she had a raised serum T3 of 4.8 nmol/L (NR 0.8–2.4) and a T4 of 48 nmol/L (NR 9–23). Measurement of her thyroid-stimulating hormone showed that this was low normal, 0.4 mU/L (NR 0.4–5 mU/L). The biochemical findings pointed to primary thyroid disease rather than pituitary overactivity. Circulating antibodies to thyroid peroxidase (titer 1/3,000; 200 IU/mL) were detected by agglutination.

What is the most likely diagnosis?

CASE STUDY 24

A female, 60 years of age, suffering from pernicious anemia reported to the consultant for a routine visit. She complained of constipation and fatigue. For pernicious anemia, she was receiving 1 (one) mg cyanocobalamin intramuscularly every 3 months from the previous 10 years. On further questioning, she reported that she had started forgetting the things and all that was taking longer to recall about the routine assignments.

The patient was found with a puffy swollen face, dry and cold skin, and sparse hair.

The heart rate was 55 beats/min.

A series of blood tests revealed the following: High levels of microsomal autoantibodies against the thyroid gland and autoantibodies against her parietal cells. Thyroid-stimulating hormone (TSH) concentration in the plasma was high, whereas the T4 was low.

What is the probable diagnosis?
What is the connection between pernicious anemia and the other condition?

CASE STUDY 25

A 35-year-old male presented to the clinic with complaints of a sore throat. He reported numerous upper respiratory infections over the past 3 months. Patient stated that he required antibiotics for some of the infections. The patient's sore throat had been present for 4 days and was progressively worsening. He was no longer able to eat solid foods because of the pain. Nobody else in contact with him had been ill. Patient gave a history of intravenous (IV) drug use in the past, but no other significant medical history was given. On examination, patient was found to have a temperature of 37.8°C (100.0°F) and was in minimal distress from the sore throat. His pharynx was erythematous and had numerous white plaques coating the throat. There was also prominent cervical lymph node enlargement. His chest was clear to auscultation and heart had regular rate and rhythm. A CD4 T lymphocyte cell count was performed and was less than 200 cells/mm^3 (normal >500 cells/mm^3). The responsible organism is composed of ribonucleic acid (RNA) genome.

What is the most likely diagnosis?
What is the biochemical mechanism that the pathogen uses to affect the patient's cells?
What enzyme is required for this pathogen to affect the host genome?

CASE STUDY 26

A 26-year-old male presented with complaints of heat intolerance, heavy sweating, tremulousness, and feeling of "jittery inside". Physical examination revealed reddened conjunctiva and warm and moist palms, but the thyroid gland was not visibly enlarged.

Which of the following tests would be most helpful to obtain an accurate diagnosis?

A. Electrocardiogram
B. Free thyroxine level
C. Serum cortisol levels
D. Serum electrolytes
E. Serum glucose level

CASE STUDY 27

An 18-year-old man had numbness and tingling around his mouth and in his finger tips. The problem was intermittent usually occurring during times of great stress. Aside from this problem, he had been in good health. His physical examination was normal, as were his laboratory values, especially his total calcium concentration was 2.4 mM, with ionized calcium of 1.2 mM (normal: 2.1–2.6 mM and 1.14 and 1.30 mM, respectively). After breathing rapidly for about 3 minutes at 30 breaths per minute, he stated that it provoked the episode. At this time, he had increased irritability of his seventh cranial nerve (Chovstek's sign) and carpal spasm on oxygen deprivation of his hand (Trousseau's sign), both indicating clinical hypocalcemia. His plasma calcium concentration during an episode remained at 2.4 mM but his ionized calcium level fell to 0.9 mM.

What is the cause for all these symptoms?
How this patient can be treated?

CASE STUDY 28

A 65-year-old man presented to his family doctor with complaints of frequent episodes of dizziness and of numbness in his legs. During a routine history and physical examination, the doctor finds that the patient leads a sedentary lifestyle, is obese (body mass index of 32), and has hypertension (blood pressure of 200/120 mm Hg). The patient is asked to return to the clinic a week later in the fasting state, during which time a blood specimen is obtained, and a glucose tolerance test is performed. Humoral analysis reveals fasting hyperglycemia, hyperinsulinemia, dyslipidemia, and glucose intolerance.

What is the probable diagnosis?

CASE STUDY 29

An 8-year-old boy was brought to the emergency room by his parents after 2 days of worsening nausea/vomiting and abdominal pain. The abdominal pain was located in the epigastric region and radiated to his back. He had several episodes of similar pain in the past but none of them was as severe. There was no history of fever/chills and change in bowel habits. On further questioning, the father reported having high triglyceride levels and several members of the mother's family had early heart disease. In the emergency room, the patient was afebrile, but was in moderate distress. Several small yellow–white papules were noted on his back and buttocks.

Both the liver and spleen appeared to be enlarged and he had epigastric tenderness. Laboratory tests revealed elevated amylase, and lipase levels laboratory tests performed after hospitalization revealed elevated triglyceride levels and reduced lipoprotein lipase activity.

What is etiology of the boy's abdominal pain?
What is the likely underlying biochemical disorder?
What is the role of lipoprotein lipase?

CASE STUDY 30

A 54-year-old man presented to the emergency department with a 1 week history of chest pain and shortness of breath. He complained that his face and extremities had a blue color. History revealed that he was a known patient of chronic unstable angina for which he was taking nitroglycerin and isosorbide dinitrate. Blood obtained for analysis was chocolate-colored.

What is the most likely diagnosis?

CASE STUDY 31

A 6-year-old child was rushed to emergency as he had accidentally consumed wood alcohol (methanol). He was complaining of severe headache, nausea, and abdominal pain.

The child was in a state of confusion and was slightly drowsy, but he was responsive to the surroundings.

There was slight distension of the abdomen, but it was not tender to touch. There was no other apparent finding except for some difficulty in breathing.

The attending duty doctor admitted the child for observation.

The child was given ethanol as a part of treatment.

What is the possible toxicity with methanol?
Why was ethanol given as a part of treatment?
What is the acid–base status of the patient?

CASE STUDY 32

A 3-day-old case of myocardial infarction comes to the outpatient department (OPD). His enzyme profile is done. Which of the following enzymes would be raised and why?
AST (Aspartate amino transferase)
CPK (Creatine phospho kinase)
LDH (Lactate dehydrogenase)

When would the above enzymes peak?
What are the other nonenzymatic cardiac markers?

CASE STUDY 33

A 6-year-old boy developed marked edema over a period of a few days and his parents had noted that his urine had become frothy. His general practitioner detected proteinuria on doing urine test and arranged admission to the hospital where the results of chemical investigations were as follows:

Laboratory test	*Patient's result*	*Reference range*
Serum		
Creatinine	58	55–120 μmol/L
Urea	3.4	2.5–6.4 mmol/L
Sodium	136	135–145 mmol/L
Potassium	4.0	3.5–5.1 mmol/L
Total protein	34	60–80 g/L
Albumin	14	35–50 g/L
Cholesterol	**11**	3.2–5.2 mmol/L
Triglycerides	**15**	0.5–2.27 mmol/L
Urine		
24 hours urine protein	**12**	0.03–0.10 g

What is the probable diagnosis?

CASE STUDY 34

A 40-year-old woman, 5 feet 1 inch tall and weighing 188 pounds, came for consultation to a physician. She was too worried for her weight. Her waist measured 41 inches and hip measured 39 inches. Physical examination and laboratory data were all within the normal range. Her only child was 14 years old, her sister and both of the parents were overweight. The patient recalled that she had been obese throughout her childhood and adolescence. Over the past 5 years, she had been on seven different diets for periods of 2 weeks to 3 months, losing from 5–25 pounds. On discontinuation of each diet, she regained weight returning to 185–190 pounds.

How will you describe this patient?
What are the health risks associated with obesity?

CASE STUDY 35

A 4-year-old girl presented to the clinic with megaloblastic anemia and failure to thrive. Enzyme measurements of white blood cells revealed a deficiency of enzyme orotate phosphoribosyltransferase and abnormally high activity of enzyme aspartate transcarbamoylase.

What is the probable diagnosis?
Which biochemical pathway is affected?

CASE STUDY 36

A 20-year-old college student was brought to the emergency room with extreme pain. He was feeling well previously but had severe pain in the middle of his back. His medical history revealed a seizure disorder that had been present for past 10 years for which he used to take phenobarbital.

An X-ray of the spine revealed a compression fracture of the first lumber vertebra. In addition, there was diffuse loss of calcification in all bones visible on the film. A CAT scan of the spine showed density of the bone to be only 55% of the normal for his age and sex. Laboratory value showed a serum calcium concentration of 8.6 mg/dL (normal: 8.5–10.6) and a serum phosphate of 5.6 mg/dL (normal: 3.5–5). The serum PTH was normal, but the serum 25-hydroxyvitamin D level was 4 ng/mL (normal: 8–55).

What was the defect and what was the cause of low 25-hydroxyvitamin D level?

CASE STUDY 37

A 40-year-old lawyer was found by his physician to have a blood pressure of 165/110 mm Hg. The patient's main complaint was of excessive sweating. Glucose was detected on examination of his urine.

Suggest two possible diagnoses.
What biochemical investigations should now be requested?

CASE STUDY 38

A 55-year-old man presented to the medical OPD with painful blisters on the back of his hands. He was a football player and stated that the blisters appeared a few days back only after a week long session in the playground. He was not on any new medication and he did not even try any new soap or cosmetics. There was no previous history of such episodes of blistering. He admitted that almost every day he was taking a small amount of beer. The patient's urine was reddish orange. A 24-hour urine collection showed elevated uroporphyrins.

What is the most likely diagnosis?

CASE STUDY 39

A blood sample was collected from a 65-year-old woman to check her serum potassium concentration as she had been on thiazide diuretics for some time. General practitioner (GP) left the specimen in his car and dropped it off at the laboratory on the way to the surgery next morning. Immediately on analyzing the sample, the biochemist was on the phone to the GP as the pattern of the results obtained was; as serum urea—58 mg/dL, sodium—130 mmol/L, and potassium—6.7 mmol/L.

What could be the possible urgency and why?

CASE STUDY 40

A 65-year-old woman with rheumatoid arthritis presented with a history of increased pain and stiffness in her hands and generalized fatigue. She had increased the dose of nonsteroidal anti-inflammatory drugs (NSAIDs) over the last few months without relief of pain. Physical examination revealed swelling and tenderness of the second and third metatarsophalangeal joints in hands, pale palmar creases, and pale conjunctiva. Her stool guaiac was positive. She had the following pertinent laboratory data:

Serum total protein = 8.5 g/dL
Serum albumin = 3.0 g/dL
Serum globulins = 5.5 g/dL
Serum iron = 40 μg
Serum ferritin = 50 ng/mL
CBC: Hb = 7.0 g/dL rouleaux are present as are a mild normocytic anemia and an absolute monocytosis.

Why the total protein is increased and serum albumin decreased?
What is the cause of anemia in this patient?
What is the significance of an absolute monocytosis?

CASE STUDY 41

A 19-year-old woman came to the emergency department after taking an overdose of Midol (ingredients: 454 mg aspirin, 14.9 mg cinnamedrine hydrochloride, and 32.4 mg caffeine) in a suicide attempt. She reported that she had ingested 25–30 Midol tablets about 2 hours before coming to the emergency department. She complained of severe nausea, shortness of breath, vertigo, and tinnitus.

On examination, the patient was in moderate distress due to nausea and shortness of breath. The physical examination was normal, as were the electrocardiogram and chest radiograph. Laboratory results included a hemoglobin level of 14 g/dL (140 g/L); serum sodium—145 mEq/L (145 mmol/L); potassium—3.6 mEq/L (3.6 mmol/L); chloride—109 mEq/L (109 mmol/L), and carbon dioxide content—17 mEq/L (17 mmol/L). An arterial blood gas determination, obtained while the patient was breathing 2 L of oxygen/minute, showed a pH of 7.47, PO_2 of 123 mm Hg, PCO_2 of 19, and serum bicarbonate level of 14 mEq/L (14 mmol/L). Salicylate level at the time of admission was 38.2 mg/dL (2.75 mmol/L).

What is the biochemical basis for the clinical symptoms and abnormal laboratory results in this condition?

CASE STUDY 42

A 6-year-old boy was brought to his pediatrician with profound mental retardation. Upon questioning, the mother revealed that several members of both the mother's and father's family had mental retardation. She also had noticed that he appeared very active and restless frequently getting into trouble in school. On examination, the boy appeared restless and his speech was significantly delayed and incomprehensible. The boy had coarse facial features but otherwise has a normal examination. Laboratory tests revealed an elevated level of heparan sulfate.

What is the most likely diagnosis?
What is the inheritance pattern of this disorder?

CASE STUDY 43

A 16-year-old girl reported to the dermatologist with a minor scalp injury. History revealed that all this occurred after a visit to her hair stylist. Her hair dresser used rollers and applied some lotion to create permanent waves for her hair. Immediately after that she started having burning sensation and itching in the scalp.
On local examination, the scalp was found to be red, tender, and a little ulcerated.
It was a minor allergic reaction to the styling lotion.
A local ointment and antibiotic supplementation was given and the girl was sent back home.

What is the basis for permanent hair waving?
Is the permanent wave truly permanent?
What is the nature of the solution used for permanent hair waving?

CASE STUDY 44

A 59-year-old smoker had an onset of mental alterations including loss of memory from the past few days. His physical examination revealed scattered rhonchi that cleared with coughing. The skin turgor was normal, and the mucous membranes were moist. His biochemical profile revealed the following:

Serum BUN = 6 mg/dL
Serum uric acid = 3.0 mg/dL
Serum sodium = 110 mEq/L
Serum potassium = 4.0 mEq/L
Serum chloride = 79 mEq/L
Serum bicarbonate = 20 mEq/L
Random urine sodium = 80 mEq/L
Chest X-ray: Centrally located mass in the left hilar area
CT scan of the brain: No focal lesions

What is the cause of hyponatremia in this patient?
What is the cause of mental alterations in this patient?
What would be a nonpharmacological treatment for the hyponatremia?

CASE STUDY 45

A patient stung by a bee is rushed to the hospital with a variety of symptoms including increasing difficulty to breathing due to vaso- and bronchoconstriction. The treatment with antihistamines to block the effects of histamine and other acute phase reactants released by mast cells was immediately started.

The attempt was also undertaken to block the slow reactive substances of anaphylaxis (SRS-A), which is the most potent constrictor of muscle enveloping the bronchial passages.

What is SRS-A composed of?

CASE STUDY 46

A Jewish couple of eastern European descent presented to the clinic for prenatal counseling after their only child died early in childhood. The family could not remember the name of the disorder but said it was common in their ancestry. Their first child was normal at birth, a slightly larger than normal head circumference, an abnormal "eye finding", and a severe progressive neurological disease with decreased motor skills and eventually death. The autopsy was consistent with Tay-Sachs disease.

What type of inheritance is this disorder?
What is the biochemical cause of the disorder?

CASE STUDY 47

A 7-year-old child was brought to the pediatrician by his parents after they noticed that he felt very fatigued. They also noted that his abdomen seemed to be enlarged. Further history revealed that he had been taking vitamins and iron supplements over the last few months. Examination revealed an enlarged spleen. Laboratory tests revealed a microcytic anemia and elevated iron levels in tissues.

What is the probable diagnosis?

CASE STUDY 48

A 23-year-old Mediterranean female presented to her obstetrician at 16 weeks of gestation for her first prenatal visit. That was her first pregnancy, and she was concerned about her baby and the risk of inheriting a "blood" disease, such as others in her family. The patient reported a personal history of mild anemia, but nothing as severe as her brother who required frequent transfusions and died at age of 12 years. The patient was told by her physician that she should not take iron supplementation for her anemia. Patient denied having any anemic symptoms. Her physical examination was consistent with a 16-week pregnancy and ultrasound confirmed an intrauterine pregnancy at 16-week gestation. The patient's hemoglobin level revealed a hypochromic, microcytic (small-sized red cell) anemia (hemoglobin—9 g/dL) and hemoglobin electrophoresis demonstrated increased hemoglobin A2 level (4.0%) and increased fetal hemoglobin level.

What is the cause of anemia in this patient?
What is the nature of the inherited disease in the family?
What is the risk to the growing baby?

CASE STUDY 49

A boy aged 5 was brought to the hospital with a complaint of swelling in the abdomen and history of reeling sensation often. On examination, the liver was found to be enlarged. Blood biochemistry revealed—high serum uric acid, serum cholesterol, and free fatty acid levels, but low sugar levels. There was no rise in blood sugar level even after intravenous administration of glucagon. A liver biopsy showed increase in the glycogen content.

What is the probable diagnosis?
What is the biochemical defect in this?

CASE STUDY 50

A newborn with tachypnea is found to have a blood pH of 7.1. Serum bicarbonate is measured as 12 mM, but the blood gas machine that would determine the partial pressure of oxygen (PO_2) and carbon dioxide (PCO_2) is broken. Given the following values, the pKa of 6.1 for carbonic acid (reflecting the HCO_3^-/CO_2 equilibrium in blood) and the fact that the blood CO_2 concentration is equal to the PCO_2 in mm Hg (normal value = 40 mm Hg) multiplied by 0.03, diagnose the problem and suggest the treatment plan for the baby.

CASE STUDY 51

A 20-year-old female after delivery of a baby bleeds profusely due to atonic uterus. She becomes breathless, starts shivering, and is very anxious.

On examination:
Pulse: Feeble, 120 beats/min
Pallor: +++
Blood pressure: Systolic—70 mm Hg
Diastolic: Not recordable
Skin: Cold clammy
Urine output: 300 mL/day

Investigations
Blood:
Hb: 4 g%
TLC: 12,000/mm^3
Urea: 100 mg%
Creatinine: 3 mg%
Na: 162 mEq/L
K: 5.5 mEq/L
Calcium: 6 mg%
Phosphorus: 6 mg%

Urine:
Volume: 300 mL/day
Specific gravity: 1.002
Color: Yellow
Proteins: Traces

What is the probable diagnosis?

CASE STUDY 52

A mother seeks help for her child with the complaint that the urine becomes dark on standing and diapers used are stained black. Urine examination shows the following:

Benedict's test: Positive
Glucose oxidase test: Negative
Ferric chloride test: Positive

What is the probable diagnosis?
What is the defect in this disease?
What is the basis for the laboratory results?

CASE STUDY 53

A patient of long-standing diabetes mellitus on treatment presents with recurrent fractures and generalized weakness.

On examination:
Pallor: ++
Puffiness around the eyes: +
Blood pressure: 160/100 mm Hg

Laboratory investigations
Urine:
Specific gravity: 1.010
Proteins: ++
Sugar: Nil

Blood:
Fasting sugar: 110 mg%
Urea: 100 mg%
Creatinine: 6 mg%
Uric acid: 8.8 mg%
Calcium: 6 mg%
Hb: 6 g%

What is your diagnosis?

CASE STUDY 54

A patient comes to the OPD with complaints of increased thirst, increased frequency and volume of urine. He had a tendency to drink lots of chilled water.

His 24-hour urine analysis shows the following findings:
- Volume: 5 L/day
- Pale color and odorless
- Specific gravity: 1.002
- Urinary chlorides: 6 g/day

Serum electrolytes reveal as follows:
- Serum Na: 160 mEq/L
- Serum potassium: 5.5 mEq/L
- Serum osmolality: 330 mOsm/kg water

What is the probable diagnosis?
What is the possible defect in this disease?
Comment on the osmolality of urine; will it same as serum or different?

CASE STUDY 55

Based on the following clinical laboratory data, give the most probable diagnosis:
Serum total proteins: 4.5 g%
Serum albumin: 2.3 g%
Serum total cholesterol: 323 mg%
Urinary proteins: +++
Urinary sugar: ++++
What is the biochemical basis for high serum total cholesterol in this patient?
What type of diet will you recommend to this patient?

CASE STUDY 56

Following are the laboratory findings of a patient brought to the hospital in a state of coma:
Random blood sugar: 370 mg%
Blood pH: 7.2
Serum bicarbonates: 16 mmol/L
Urine test: Reducing sugars, ++; Ketones, +; proteins traces.

What is the probable diagnosis?
What is the biochemical basis for all these findings?

CASE STUDY 57

An adult male of 50 years presents with recurrent attacks of painful arthritis of great toe associated with lethargy, low-grade fever, and involvement of other joints. Attacks are of variable period and separated by symptom-free intervals.

Physical examination:
Pulse: 90 beats/min
Temperature: 100°F
First metatarsophalangeal joint: Hot, red, and swollen

Laboratory investigations:
Hb: 13 g%
TLC: 14,000/m^3
Serum uric acid: 11 mg%
24 hours urine: 1.3 g of uric acid
Microscopic examination of synovial fluid aspirated from joint space under polarized light reveals birefringent crystals.

What is the likely diagnosis?

CASE STUDY 58

An Rh-negative mother delivers a baby who develops jaundice immediately after birth.

General examination reveals:

Heart rate	80 beats/min
Icterus	+
Irritability	+
Liver	Palpable

Laboratory investigations:
Serum
Bilirubin

Total	10 mg%
Indirect	7 mg%
Direct	3 mg%
Alkaline phosphatase	50 U/L
Urine	
Urobilinogen	+++
Feces	
Stercobilinogen	+++

What is your likely diagnosis?

CASE STUDY 59

A middle-aged woman complains of loss of weight, anxiety, palpitations, tremors, and sweating in hands. Her thyroid function tests show the following:
T_4: 11.5 µg/dL
T_3: 150 µg/dL
Thyroid-stimulating hormone (TSH): 0.05 mU/L

Comment on the result.
What would be the BMR in this patient?

CASE STUDY 60

A 26-week-old baby was brought to pediatric clinic because of increasing lethargy and cyanosis. The infant had been in good health at birth, and the mother attempted breastfeeding. Since the mother's milk flow had ceased, the family physician had recommended formula feeding. The child was unwell since then. The blood sample was collected and a positive test for methemoglobin was obtained.

A diagnosis of methemoglobinemia was made. The baby was treated for 2 days. At the time of discharge, child was alert and there was no cyanosis. The child was discharged with instructions to the mother concerning formula prepared with distilled water.

What is the cause for methemoglobinemia?
What type of treatment was given to the baby?

CASE STUDY 61

A 2-year-old boy was brought by his mother to the hospital. The child had been eating poorly for the past 1 month and had intermittent diarrhea for sometime and had become irritable and apathetic.

On examination:

The patient was found to be both underweight for height and small for his age. He was pale and weak. His skin was flaky. His hair was dry and brittle.

Abdomen was distended and liver was moderately enlarged. Generalized edema was present. The laboratory investigations revealed:

Hb: 6 g%
Serum total proteins: 4.4 g%
Serum albumin: 2 g%

What is the probable diagnosis?

CASE STUDY 62

A 40-year-old fat female presents with intolerance to fatty foods, pain in the right side of abdomen, yellowness of eyes, and passage of clay-colored stools.

Laboratory investigations revealed:

Serum
Total bilirubin: 20 mg%
Direct bilirubin: 16 mg%
ALP (Alkaline phosphatase): 800 U(KA)
SGPT (Serum glutamate pyruvate transaminase): 90 IU/L

Urine
Color: Deep yellow
Bilirubin: ++
Urobilinogen: Absent

Stools
Clay colored
Stercobilinogen: Absent

What is the likely diagnosis?
Which other enzymes are likely to increase?

CASE STUDY 63

A fair chubby boy was brought to the hospital with the complaint that he has mental retardation. Blood chemistry revealed that phenylalanine was abnormally high. Phenylpyruvate was present in appreciable amounts in urine.

What is the probable diagnosis?
Which other metabolites can be found in urine?
What would be the other clinical manifestations and laboratory findings in this patient?
What would be the dietary advice to the patient?

CASE STUDY 64

Based on the following clinical laboratory data, give the most probable diagnosis:

Serum bilirubin: 8 mg%
Direct bilirubin: 0.2 mg%
Serum alkaline phosphatase: 6 U(KA)
SGOT: 30 IU/L
SGPT: 26 IU/L
Urine bilirubin: Negative
Urine bile salts: Negative

CASE STUDY 65

A 45-year-old male presents with vague illness, generalized weakness, and lack of energy. He further complains of breathlessness on exertion, anorexia, nausea and vomiting, pruritis, and bone pains.

The general examination reveals:
Pallor: ++
Skin pigmentation: +
Respiratory rate: 22 breaths/min
Blood pressure: 180/120 mm Hg

Biochemical findings are as:
Hb: 7 g%
TLC: 13,000/mm^3
Blood urea: 110 mg%
Serum creatinine: 6 mg%
Serum uric acid: 7 mg%
Serum calcium: 7 mg%
Serum inorganic phosphorus: 6 mg%
Serum total proteins: 5 g%

Urine examination:
Urine output: 3,000 mL/24 hours
Proteins: ++
RBC: +

What is your likely diagnosis?
Plan the diet for this patient.
What will be the status of lipid profile in this patient?
Suggest the investigations for the confirmation of the diagnosis.

CASE STUDY 66

A 32-year-old man underwent surgery for a fractured hip. Due to immobilization, pulmonary embolism occurred and shortness of breath developed rapidly (respiratory rate increased). Blood chemistry revealed the following results:
PCO_2: 25 mm Hg
PO_2: 30 mm Hg
pH: 7.5
HCO_3^-: 23.0 mmol/L
Cl^-: 95 mmol/L
K^+: 4.1 mmol/L
Na^+: 143 mmol/L

What is the acid–base status of the patient?
What is the first line of defense, in case required?

CASE STUDY 67

A 5-year-old boy was brought to the hospital by the mother with complaints of slow growth and pain in the bones.

On examination:
Pallor: ++
Frontal bossing: +
Bowing of the legs: +
Swelling of costochondral junctions: +
Laboratory investigations revealed:
Serum ALP: 180 U(KA)
Serum calcium: 7 mg%
Serum inorganic phosphorus: 2 mg%

What is the diagnosis?
What is the treatment for this disease?

CASE STUDY 68

A 50-year-old woman had 8-day history of loss of appetite, nausea, and flu-like symptoms. She had noticed that her urine had been dark in color over the past 2 days. On examination, she had tenderness in the right upper quadrant. Laboratory investigations showed:

Serum total bilirubin: 4.5 mg%
Direct bilirubin: 2.5 mg%
Indirect bilirubin: 2.0 mg%
Serum AST: 40 IU/L
Serum ALT: 115 IU/L
Serum ALP: 20 U(KA)

What is the probable diagnosis?
What will be the observation regarding bile pigments and salt in the urine?

CASE STUDY 69

A 6-year-old girl was brought to the hospital with vision problems. She was found to have downward dislocation of the left lens. Her mother indicated that the child was born normally, but she lagged in development. She was unable to crawl until she was 1 year old and did not walk until she was 2 years old. Speech was also delayed. She had long thin bones.

X-ray of the lower femur showed signs of osteoporosis. An older brother had similar symptoms, but had been diagnosed as having Marfan's syndrome. A similar cyanide–nitroprusside test of the patient's urine was positive, suggesting homocystinuria, not Marfan's syndrome. This was confirmed by amino acid analysis of the plasma, which revealed presence of homocysteine.

What is the probable diagnosis?

CASE STUDY 70

A 32-year-old man presented with severe pain, swelling, and loss of vision in his left eye after excessive exposure to sunlight. He reported multiple, recurrent, and discrete blisters developing on sun-exposed areas that healed with scarring and passing red-colored urine for more than 25 years. Multiple hypopigmented scars of variable size were present on his face, the upper part of his chest, his forearms, and the dorsa of his hands and feet. In addition, hypertrichosis of his face and extremities, resorption of the distal phalanges in his hands, destruction of the ear lobules and cartilaginous part of his nose, and hepatosplenomegaly were present. Ocular examination revealed proptosis, tense eyelid, nonreactive pupil, cataract, and a lack of light perception in his left eye. Excessive concentrations of porphyrins were measured in the urine, erythrocytes, and feces. The patient was advised to avoid sunlight, prescribed ascorbic acid and beta carotene, and advised to have all skin infections treated promptly. 10 days later, he returned because of intense pain in his left eye. The eye was enucleated.

What is the probable diagnosis?

CASE STUDY 71

A 71-year-old man had a 3-week history of weakness, polyuria, intense thirst, difficulty in speaking and understanding commands, staggering walk, confusion, and a weight loss of 10 kg. For 1 month, he took 200,000 units of vitamin D each day because he had severe osteoarthritis. His plasma calcium was 3.38 mmol/L (13.5 mg/dL).

What is the most probable diagnosis?

CASE STUDY 72

A 29-year-old laborer developed chest pain while operating a pneumatic hammer on a construction project. The pain was of moderate intensity, but he felt well enough to continue to work. As the day continued, he experienced sharp pain on respiration and a tight feeling across the chest wall. He was rushed to the emergency room of a local hospital and was admitted after a brief examination. Electrocardiographic and chest X-ray examination were negative. However, the blood analysis revealed an elevated plasma LDH level of 400 IU/L. The high plasma LDH persisted during the next 4 days, no other laboratory or physical abnormalities appeared and the chest pain gradually improved with bed rest.

What is the reason for rise in LDH level?
What is the probable diagnosis?

Chapter 26

Explanations of Case Studies

1. Acetyl-CoA carboxylase deficiency drastically alters the ability of the patient to synthesize fatty acids. Acetyl-CoA carboxylase-mediated formation of malonyl-CoA is the first step of fatty acid synthesis. Palmitate is the major end product of *de novo* fatty acid synthesis. All processes dependent upon *de novo* synthesis of fatty acid are affected.

   In the present case, the respiratory difficulty is due to reduced surfactant synthesis. Dipalmitoylphosphatidylcholine (surfactant) is deficient as a result of palmitic acid deficiency. Palmitic acid can be present in the diet also; but if enough feeding is not there, the lungs depend mainly on *de novo* fatty acid synthesis. Developmental delay and the neurological problems are all due to impaired fatty acid synthesis.
2. The patient is suffering from acromegaly.
3. The patient is suffering from acute intermittent porphyria.
   Alcohol ingestion induces increased activity of ALA synthase significantly in the liver and moderately in peripheral tissues. This effect is mediated by alleviating the negative regulation of ALA synthase by free heme. Mitochondrial concentrations of free heme are diminished by increased heme utilization and/or reduced activity of downstream pathway enzymes. In the liver, the demand for heme is exacerbated by requirement for heme incorporation into alcohol-eliminating cytochromes P450. Upon increased activity of ALAS, a genetic defect in either ALAD or PBGD would cause the rapid accumulation of ALA or both ALA and PBG, resulting in ALAD deficiency porphyria (very rare) or acute intermittent porphyria, respectively. During an attack, excess ALA and PBG produced in the liver are secreted into systemic circulation and are later excreted in the urine. In circulation, these neurotoxic compounds have the greatest effect on the autonomic and peripheral nervous systems resulting in the peripheral neuropathy and neurovisceral symptoms, that is, abdominal pain, nausea and vomiting, tachycardia, and hypertension.
4. Acid–base diagnosis
   i. **pH:** Low, acidosis is present.
   ii. **PCO_2:** High, hypoventilation (the residual depressant effect of the anesthetic agents is considered the most likely cause).
   iii. **Bicarbonate:** Near normal
   iv. **PO_2—high:** This is because the patient is breathing a high inspired oxygen concentration. If the patient was breathing room air ($FiO_2 = 0.21$), then a depression of alveolar PO_2 must occur if the PCO_2 is elevated (as predicted from the alveolar gas equation). Most ill patients in hospital are breathing supplemental oxygen, so, it is common for the PO_2 to be elevated on blood gas results.
   v. An acidemia with the pattern of elevated PCO_2 and normal HCO_3 is consistent with an acute respiratory acidosis.
   vi. **Anion gap:** The anion gap is about 11, which is normal so no evidence of a high-anion gap acidosis.

   Diagnosis: Acute respiratory acidosis.
   Cause: Resuscitation from postoperative ventricular fibrillation.
5. Milk intolerance may be due to milk protein allergies during infancy, but it is commonly caused by lactase deficiency in older individuals. Intestinal lactase hydrolyzes the milk sugar lactose into galactose and glucose, both reducing sugars that can be detected as reducing substances in stool. The symptoms of lactose intolerance and other conditions involving intestinal malabsorption include diarrhea, abdominal cramps, and flatulence due to water retention and bacterial action in the gut.
6. The patient has hypoglycemia and acidosis due to alcohol intoxication as evident from history and blood levels. Oxidation of ethanol by alcohol dehydrogenase leads to formation of acetaldehyde, which is oxidized by aldehyde dehydrogenase, producing acetate. The increased (NADH)/(NAD^+) ratio causes increased (lactate)/(pyruvate), resulting in hyperlactic acidemia, which decreases excretion of uric acid, aggravating gout. Alcohol impairs gluconeogenesis in the liver, resulting in a fall in the amount of glucose produced from glycogen and decreased oxidation of fatty acids. This contributes to hypoglycemia and an increase in fat accumulation in liver cells. In healthy individuals, these changes are reversible, but with repeated exposure to ethanol, more severe changes in the liver occur, including alcohol-induced hepatitis, perivenular sclerosis, and cirrhosis, with the latter observed in an estimated 15% of alcoholics. Lactate accumulation produces lactic acidosis (metabolic acidosis).
7. The normal range for serum AP is three to five times higher in children than in adults owing to increased osteoblastic activity in active bone growth.

A hemolyzed serum sample does not significantly alter the alkaline phosphatase activity; however, it would falsely increase the serum potassium, serum lactate dehydrogenase, and serum aspartate transaminase (AST/SGOT) because these enzymes are located within red blood cells.

Since the serum GGT is normal, the serum AP is not of liver origin. Serum AP and GGT are indices of cholestasis (blockage to bile flow) in liver disease; hence, both should be elevated, if the AP is of liver origin. The elevated AP over normal for age is due to healing of the bone fracture.

8. The transaminases, ALT and AST, are indices of liver cell necrosis that are released into the circulation with diffuse liver cell injury. With the exception of alcoholic hepatitis, ALT is invariably higher than AST and is also more specific for liver cell injury than AST, which is also present in high concentration in muscle and RBCs. Hence, the patient must have a resolving hepatitis, in which the AST would be expected to return to normal before the ALT. This possibility can be documented with hepatitis serologic testing, i.e., anti-HAV IgM and IgG, HBsAg, anti-HBc IgM, and anti-HCV antibodies. It is likely that the patient has resolving hepatitis A, unless there is a history of needle puncture or intimate contact with a person having active disease.
9. The patient shows many signs of anorexia nervosa, which is an eating disorder. The etiology of AN is unknown but appears to involve a combination of psychological, biological, and cultural risk factors. The condition is characterized by aversion to food that leads to a state of fasting and emaciation. Patients often have a distorted image of their own body weight or shape and are unconcerned by the serious health consequences of their low weight. As weight loss progresses, the fear of gaining weight grows; dieting becomes stricter; and psychological, behavioral, and medical aberrations increase.

   After several months of near starvation, the blood glucose in these patients is maintained by gluconeogenesis, primarily from amino acids mobilized from tissue proteins. The patients develop potential vitamin deficiencies liver glycogen is exhausted in the first day of fasting. Gluconeogenesis depletes the supply of oxaloacetate, which is essential for the entry of acetyl-CoA into the citric acid cycle. Consequently, the liver produces large quantities of ketone bodies, which are released into the blood. After several weeks of starvation, ketone bodies become the major fuel of the brain. The impaired conversion of amino acids into glucose is responsible for producing hypoglycemia in these patients. A person's survival time is mainly determined by the size of the triacylglycerol depot.

   The diagnosis of AN is based on the presence of characteristic behavioral, psychological, and physical attributes. Psychotherapy, medication, or hospitalization is required to treat these patients.
10. The patient is suffering from multiple myeloma.
11. It is a case of essential fatty acid deficiency.

   Basic concept: Three polyunsaturated fatty acids—linoleic acid, linolenic acid, and arachidonic acid—are called "essential fatty acids". They cannot be synthesized in the body and must be provided in the diet. Linoleic acid is most important as, arachidonic acid, can be synthesized from linoleic acid. The introduction of additional double bonds in unsaturated fatty acid is limited to the area between –COOH group and the existing double bond, and it is not possible to introduce a double bond between the $-CH_3$ group at the opposite end of the molecule and the first unsaturated linkage. The essential fatty acids form structural elements of tissues, gonads, and mitochondrial membrane. Arachidonic acid is a precursor of prostanoids (prostaglandins, prostacyclins, and thromboxane) and leukotrienes. Essential fatty acids lower serum cholesterol levels and prevent fatty liver formation. They are required for general body growth and vision. Normal dietary allowance of PUFA (polyunsaturated fatty acids) is 2–3% of total calories.

   Case details: The history is suggestive of essential fatty acid deficiency.

   Clinical features: This deficiency is manifested in the human beings by eczema like dermatitis, fatty liver, growth retardation, acanthosis, hypercholesterolemia, and hemolytic anemia.

   Since the patient was on intravenous fluid therapy and the fats were omitted in the diet, so this leads to essential fatty acid deficiency. Since arachidonic acid was low in the body, hence, the prostaglandins were less synthesized and less of their metabolites were excreted in urine. Arachidonic acid can be synthesized in the body, if the other fatty acids are supplied in the diet. The corn oil and soybean oil are rich in linoleic acid, so supplementation with these oils will help in correcting the arachidonic acid deficiency and thereby improve the synthesis and the metabolism of prostaglandins also.
12. The child is suffering from kwashiorkor (PEM: protein–energy malnutrition).
13. The person is suffering from lactose intolerance. The symptoms of abdominal distension, bloating diarrhea, and dehydration following consumption of dairy products clearly indicate that the person has lactase deficiency and is unable to metabolize lactose, which is the predominant sugar present in milk or dairy products. Many of the symptoms of lactase deficiency are related to the interaction of colonic bacteria and nonabsorbed lactose. The diagnosis can be confirmed by hydrogen breath test or by stool acidity test. The treatment is by supplementation with lactose-free, lactose-reduced milk or soy milk. Calcium and vitamin D supplementations are also recommended.
14. Case discussion
   - **Diagnosis:** The history of alternating constipation and diarrhea, a positive stool guaiac, hepatomegaly, and weight loss, suggests colon cancer with metastatic disease to the liver, which would produce the LFT findings noted in this case.
   - **The liver function tests (LFTs):** These are characteristic of focal disease because of the absence of transaminase elevation (transaminases are markers of cell necrosis in diffuse injury) and the normal total bilirubin levels. Therefore, it is unlikely that the patient has liver disease resulting from his previous transfusions (since, hepatitis C is the most common cause of post-transfusion hepatitis).
   - **Lactate dehydrogenase (LDH):** An increase in serum LDH is frequently associated with an underlying malignancy, since, it is a nonspecific enzyme marker of malignancy.

- **The iron deficiency anemia:** It might be due to blood loss.
- **The elevated serum alkaline phosphatase:** It is of liver, owing to the increase in serum GGT. Unlike the transaminases, which are released with cell injury, both AP and GGT are synthesized when there is compression of the bile ducts by an extrinsic mass.
- **A positive stool guaiac:** It should always be evaluated even if it appears that an anal fissure or hemorrhoids are the most likely source of the bleeding. Since the patient is over 50 years of age, colon cancer must be ruled out as the cause of a positive stool guaiac.
- **The rectosigmoid adenocarcinoma:** It could be there and might be responsible for the constipation and diarrhea.
- **Imaging studies:** It can confirm the presence of metastasis to the liver.

15. Cushing's syndrome
16. The patient is suffering from diabetes insipidus.
17. **Hint:** The man is acidotic as defined by pH lower than normal 7.4. His hyperventilation with Kussmaul respiration can be interpreted as compensation by lungs to blow off CO_2, lower PCO_2, increase $(HCO_3^-)/(CO_2)$ ratio, and raise pH. The man has compensated his metabolic acidosis (caused by accumulation of ketone bodies) by increasing his respiratory rate and volume.
18. Folic acid deficiency
19. The child is suffering from glucose-6-phosphate dehydrogenase deficiency.
20. The patient is suffering from glucose-6-phosphate dehydrogenase deficiency.
21. The patient probably has deficiency of glucose transporter required for reabsorption of glucose from the renal tubules. Since there is no reabsorption of glucose, it is excessively excreted in urine. Glycosuria is responsible for polyuria and polydipsia and this results in dehydration. The symptoms are same as diabetes mellitus but there is no hyperglycemia and the other tests are also normal.
22. The present case is of glycerol kinase deficiency. Glycerol kinase enzyme is the enzyme for conversion of glycerol to glycerol-3-phosphate. The glycerol kinase gene is located on the X chromosome, locus Xp21, between that for the dystrophin gene in Duchenne's muscular dystrophy and that involved in congenital adrenal hyperplasia. Persons with these genetic diseases are frequently deficient in glycerol kinase and similarly persons with deficiency of glycerol kinase defect show symptoms of either muscular dystrophy or congenital adrenal hyperplasia as seen in this case by vomiting and diarrhea that reflect adrenal dysfunction.
23. The patient is suffering from autoimmune thyrotoxicosis (Graves' disease).
24. The patient is suffering from Hashimoto"s thyroiditis, an autoimmune disorder. Pernicious anemia is also as a result of autoimmune process.
25. This patient acquired HIV infection by sharing needles with an infected individual. The HIV genome is composed of single-stranded RNA. Reverse transcription of the viral RNA is required to infect the host cells. HIV causes immunosuppression because it has a propensity for attaching to helper T cells (CD4 cells), the cells that support cell-mediated immunity. Initially, an HIV infection may cause systemic flu-like symptoms, lymphadenopathy, and fatigue. During this phase, the patient experiences a viremia. The next phase is largely asymptomatic as the virus slowly causes attrition of the CD4 helper T cells. When the levels of these important cells drop to low levels, the patient will not be able to fend off organisms. Treatment for HIV infection includes agents that attack the unique aspects of the virus such as nucleoside analog reverse transcriptase inhibitors and protease inhibitors.
26. The patient is suffering from hyperthyroidism. Free thyroxin can be estimated to confirm the diagnosis.
27. Symptoms of perioral and fingertip paresthesias are typical of hypocalcemia. When seen intermittently such as this, such symptoms are almost caused by hyperventilation. More than 50% of the circulating calcium is bound to plasma proteins via anionic sites that are highly dependent on the pH of blood. Small increase in pH creates more anionic sites for the binding of calcium. Since, it can occur in just a few seconds, PTH is unable to compensate for the hypocalcemia and the symptoms may occur. Hyperventilation can acutely reduce the carbon dioxide of the blood and raise the pH, dropping the ionized calcium by up to 30% without altering the total plasma calcium concentration. In this patient, the hyperventilation is related with anxiety, and the therapy should be directed at lowering the patient's anxiety. Counseling may be necessary for this. Meanwhile, the patient must treat his symptoms by preventing the diminished CO_2 that accompanies the hyperventilation. He can do this simply by breathing into paper bag, thereby increasing the CO_2 of the inspired air.
28. The patient is suffering from metabolic syndrome (syndrome X).
29. The child is suffering from acute pancreatitis. The underlying defect is deficiency of lipoprotein lipase enzyme.

    Lipoprotein lipase (LPL) is an enzyme found on the capillary endothelial surface of adipose tissue, heart, and skeletal muscle and is required, along with apoC-II, for the hydrolysis of triglycerides. ApoC-II, found on the surface of chylomicrons and VLDL, serves as an activator of LPL. A deficiency in LPL results in elevated levels of triglycerides (VLDL and chylomicrons). The cholesterol level may be normal or slightly elevated. LPL deficiency is inherited in an autosomal recessive pattern. Patients with LPL deficiency often present with recurrent episodes of pancreatitis in their childhood and may have other clinical signs of hypertriglyceridemia such as xanthomas, hepatosplenomegaly, and lipemia retinalis. Reduced serum LPL activity, after an injection of intravenous heparin, confirms the diagnosis of either LPL or apoC-II deficiency. The initial therapeutic intervention consists primarily of dietary modification (reduction of fat intake).
30. The patient is suffering from methemoglobinemia. Oxidation of the ferrous component of heme to ferric state forms methemoglobin. This may be caused due to the action of certain drugs such as nitrates. The methemoglobinemia is characterized by chocolate cyanosis (a brownish-brown coloration of the skin and membranes) and chocolate-colored blood due to the presence of dark-colored methemoglobin. Symptoms are related to tissue hypoxia and include anxiety, headache, and dyspnea and in severe cases, coma and death can also occur.

31. Methanol toxicity
32. Acute myocardial infarction (LDH)
33. Nephrotic syndrome
34. The patient has an apple (android) pattern of fat distribution. Her waist to hip ratio is 41/39 = 1.05. Apple shape is defined as a waist to hip ratio of more than 0.8 in women, and more than 1.0 in men. She has, therefore, apple pattern of fat distribution, which is common in males. Compared with other women of same body weight who have gynecoid fat pattern, the presence of increased visceral or intra-abdominal adipose tissue places her at greater risk for diabetes, hypertension, dyslipidemia, and coronary heart disease.

    For this patient BMI = Weight (kg)/height (m^2)
    $= 85.5/(1.55)^2$
    $= 35.6\ kg/m^2$

    The result indicates that the patient is classified as obese.

    Individuals, with marked obesity and a history dating to early childhood, have an adipose depot made up of too many adipocytes, each fully loaded with triacylglycerols. Most successful programs employ a multidisciplinary approach to weight loss, with hypocaloric diets, behavior modification to change eating behavior, aerobic exercise, and social support. Emphasis must be on maintenance of weight loss.
35. The baby is suffering from orotic aciduria.
36. It is a case of osteomalacia due to phenobarbital-induced vitamin D deficiency.

    Phenobarbital and diphenylhydantoin are known to cause increased activity of hepatic cytochrome P450 enzymes. This causes vitamin D to be more rapidly metabolized to polar, inactive metabolites. Severe osteomalacia is associated with weak bones. In particular, weight-bearing bones, such as vertebral bodies may fracture without a history of significant trauma. Treatment with 10,000 U of vitamin D daily will allow the bones to remineralize to normal density.
37. The patient is having hypertension, but it is important to consider other secondary causes especially in a relatively young patient. Acromegaly and pheochromocytoma may present with the combination of hypertension, excessive sweating, and glycosuria. The saliva sample of acromegaly is readily recognized; however, the signs of pheochromocytoma apart from the episodic sweating are not readily recognized.

    Metabolites of catecholamine are measured in urine. If diagnosed, the other family members are also screened since it is familial in nature.
38. The patient is suffering from porphyria cutanea tarda. The biochemical defect in this disease is deficiency of uroporphyrinogen decarboxylase enzyme. The clinical presentation of this disease is influenced by alcoholism, hepatic iron overload, exposure to sunlight, and the presence of hepatitis B or C or HIV infections. Clinical onset is during the fourth or fifth decade of life. Porphyrin accumulation leads to cutaneous manifestations and urine becomes red to brown. The disease becomes worst on exposure to sunlight.
39. The delay in processing the sample (removing serum from the clot) has made the potassium and sodium concentrations unreliable as these ions moved out of and into the erythrocytes along their concentration gradients. The pattern of the results obtained suggested that the patient might be sodium depleted with prerenal uremia and hyperkalemia. This pattern, if correct, is typical of Addison's disease, which is an endocrine emergency. Thus, another sample is required to know the exact status of the patient.
40. **Case discussion:** The total proteins are the sum of the serum albumin and the globulins. In general, an elevated total protein is due to an increase in globulins. The increase in globulins is primarily secondary to an increase in γ globulins, particularly IgG. IgG is not only the most abundant γ globulin, but also the one most often increased in chronic inflammation owing to increased synthesis by many different clones of plasma cells. Since the patient has rheumatoid arthritis, a chronic disease, she most likely has an increase in IgG causing the increase in total protein. Hypoalbuminemia is present in the patient owing to reduced synthesis of albumin by the hepatocytes as a way to conserve amino acids for synthesis of acute-phase reactants.

    The patient has a chronic disease and a positive stool guaiac, both anemia of chronic disease (ACD) and iron deficiency may be present. The serum iron is decreased in both of these anemias, so it cannot differentiate the two when both are present. ACD is characterized by iron blockade in macrophages (serum ferritin is increased), whereas iron deficiency is associated with absent iron stores (low serum ferritin). In inflammation, interleukin-1 (IL-1) released from macrophages stimulates the synthesis and release of acute-phase reactants from the liver, one of which is ferritin. Hence, in inflammation, the serum ferritin may be increased even though the ferritin stores in the bone marrow are depleted. A bone marrow examination would be required to document whether the iron stores are adequate.

    Since the NSAIDs are likely responsible for the positive stool guaiac (they produce gastric erosions), they should be discontinued and the patient followed to see whether the stool guaiac becomes negative. If not, further workup of the GI tract would be indicated to document the source of the bleeding.

    Absolute monocytosis is expected in patients with chronic disease. Just as neutrophils are the key inflammatory cells in acute inflammation, monocytes and macrophages share the same notoriety in chronic inflammation. They contain growth factors and have phagocytic properties that are important in the healing process.
41. The patient is suffering from salicylate toxicity.
42. The boy is suffering from Sanfilippo syndrome. Accumulation of glycosaminoglycans results in mucopolysaccharidoses. Common causes of this disorder include Hunter syndrome, Hurler syndrome, and Sanfilippo syndrome. Sanfilippo syndrome is inherited in an autosomal recessive pattern and clinically evident by profound mental retardation, lack of normal developmental milestones,

and significant language delay. Sanfilippo syndrome results in an excess of heparan sulfate and can be caused by a variety of enzyme deficiencies.

43. A hair is an array of many α-keratin filaments. When hair is exposed to moist heat, it can be stretched. At molecular level, the α-keratins of hair are stretched out until they arrive at the fully extended β conformation. On cooling, they spontaneously revert to the α-helical conformation. The characteristic "stretchability" of α-keratins, as well as numerous disulfide cross-linkages, are the basis of permanent waving. The hair to be waved or curled is first bent around a form of appropriate shape. A solution of a reducing agent, thiol or sulfhydryl group (–SH), is then applied with heat. The reducing agent then cleaves the cross-linkages by reducing each disulfide bond to form two Cys residues. The moist heat breaks hydrogen bonds and causes the α-helical structure of the polypeptide chains to uncoil. After a time, the reducing solution is removed, and an oxidizing agent is added to establish new bond between pairs of Cys residues of adjacent polypeptide chains, but not the same pairs as before the treatment. After the hair is washed and cooled, the polypeptide chains revert to there α-helical conformation. The hair fibers now curl in the desired fashion because the new disulfide cross-linkages exert same torsion or twist on the bundle of α-helical coils in the hair fibers. A permanent wave is not truly permanent because the hair grows; in the new hair replacing the old, the α-keratin has the natural, nonwavy pattern of disulfide bonds **(Fig. 26.1)**.

44. With a history of smoking and a centrally located mass in the lungs, the patient most likely has the inappropriate ADH syndrome (SIADH) secondary to secretion of ADH by a small-cell carcinoma of the lung.

The patient has severe hyponatremia in the presence of normal skin turgor, hence the total body Na (TBNa) must be normal. Therefore, the hyponatremia must be secondary to a gain of pure water (dilutional hyponatremia). The increase in reabsorption of free water in the kidneys by ADH produces a dilutional hyponatremia favoring the movement of water into the ICF compartment by osmosis. Cerebral edema would explain the patient's mental alterations. Eventually, the plasma volume increases, which increases the cardiac output and the effective arterial blood volume (EABV). Unfortunately, ADH cannot be suppressed. However, there is no stimulus for activation of the renin-angiotensin-aldosterone system, and the proximal tubules of the kidneys are unable to reabsorb salt owing to the increase in peritubular capillary hydrostatic pressure. Hence, the random urine sodium is increased. Since ADH is present (it should be suppressed when the EABV is increased), the free water is being reabsorbed rather than eliminated, so urine concentration rather than dilution is occurring in the patient. This explains why the urine osmolality is often higher than the plasma osmolality in SIADH.

A nonpharmacological method of managing SIADH is water restriction without restriction of salt intake, since, the TBNa is normal in these patients.

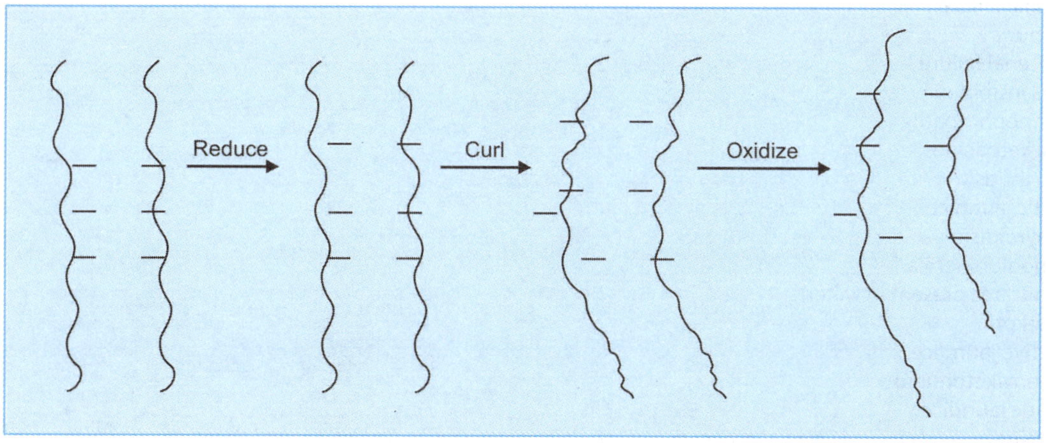

Fig. 26.1: The application in a sequence of reducing agent, moist heat and oxidizing agent allow the hair fibers to curl in a desired fashion.

45. **Basic concept:** Leukotrienes C4, D4, and E4 together compose the slow reacting substance of anaphylaxis (SRS-A), which is thought to be the cause of asphyxiation in individuals not treated rapidly enough following an anaphylactic shock. These leukotrienes are responsible for intense bronchoconstriction, vasodilatation, and increased vascular permeability seen in anaphylactic or allergic reactions. SRS-A is up to 1,000 times more effective than histamines in causing bronchial muscle constriction. Leukotrienes are synthesized from arachidonic acid by lipoxygenase pathway.

Case details: In the present case, the clinical signs are suggestive of allergic symptoms/anaphylaxis due to the release of histamine, SRS-A, and other mediators of inflammation. Acute treatment involves epinephrine injected subcutaneously initially and then intravenously antihistamines, such as diphenhydramine are administered intravenously or intramuscularly. Anti-inflammatory steroids are usually given intravenously to end bronchoconstriction. The steroids block phospholipase A2 action, preventing the synthesis of leukotrienes from arachidonic acid. Lipoxygenase pathway is not inhibited by aspirin or other anti-inflammatory drugs. In fact, prolonged use of aspirin for certain conditions like arthritis, etc., depresses cyclooxygenase system and enhances lipoxygenase system. As a result, synthesis of prostaglandins is reduced while the synthesis of leukotrienes is increased, which may lead to aspirin-induced bronchial asthma.

Selective lipoxygenase inhibitors are currently used for various ailments. Zileuton, a selective 5-lipoxygenase inhibitor, is currently under trial to be used for ulcerative colitis.

46. The child is suffering from Tay-Sachs disease. Tay-Sachs disease is a genetic disease that is the result of a deficiency of hexosaminidase A enzyme that is involved in the degradation of gangliosides in the lysosomes. The disease is prevalent in Jewish children of Eastern European descent and leads to a buildup of ganglioside GM2 in nerve cells of the brain and causes neuronal dysfunction.
47. The child is suffering from thalassemia major.
48. The lady is suffering from thalassemia minor and her brother was suffering most probably from thalassemia major.
49. The child is suffering from von Gierke's disease (type I glycogen storage disease).
50. The blood pH is 7.1 (acidosis), serum bicarbonate—12 mmol/L (low).
    It is metabolic acidosis. Both the findings can be there in compensated respiratory acidosis also. To rule out the possibility, PCO_2 level is required to be calculated from the given values.
    Calculation of PCO_2
    The equilibrium between an acid and conjugated base is defined by Henderson–Hasselbalch equation:

$$pH = pKa + \log (base)/(acid) \text{ or } pH = 6.1 + \log (HCO_3^-)/(CO_2)$$

$$pH - 6.1 = \log (HCO_3^-)/(CO_2)$$

$$7.1 - 6.1 = 1 = \log (10) = \log (HCO_3^-)/(CO_2)$$

In the case of carbonic acid, the CO_2 is effective acid and HCO^- is conjugated base due to complete dissociation in water.

$$CO_2 = 0.03 \times PCO_2 = PCO_2 \times 0.03$$

(Normal PCO_2 is 40 mm Hg multiplied by 0.03) comes out to be 1.2 mM

Since, the (HCO_3^-) is 12 mM?

So, log (10) = log (10) = 1

i.e., the actual value of PCO_2 is also 40 mm Hg.

Since PCO_2 is within the normal range, so this rules out the possibility of compensated respiratory acidosis, in which it should have been higher. The baby has tachypnea. It might be the compensatory hyperventilation to restore the ratio of bicarbonate: carbonic acid back to normal. Keeping in view all the laboratory results, i.e., low pH, low bicarbonate, relatively low PCO_2, low ratio of bicarbonate to carbonic acid, the diagnosis is uncompensated metabolic acidosis. The baby can be treated by treating the primary cause for acidosis and by supplementation with sodium bicarbonate.

51. Acute renal failure
52. Alkaptonuria
53. Chronic renal failure
54. Diabetes insipidus
55. Diabetic nephropathy
56. Diabetic ketoacidosis
57. Gouty arthritis
58. Hemolytic jaundice
59. Hyperthyroidism
60. Methemoglobinemia
    (Cause nitrates present in water)
61. Kwashiorkor
62. Obstructive jaundice
63. PKU (Phenylketonuria)
64. Prehepatic jaundice
65. Renal failure
66. Respiratory alkalosis
67. Rickets
68. Viral hepatitis
69. Homocysteinemia
70. Congenital erythropoietic porphyria
71. Vitamin D intoxication
72. Muscular injury

Chapter 27

Multiple Choice Questions for Self-Assessment

1. **A 25-year-old female with acute appendicitis undergoing a halothane inhaled anesthetic with acute onset of hyperthermia, tachypnea, respiratory acidosis, hyperkalemia, and family history of similar events. The provisional diagnosis is malignant hyperthermia (MH). Which of the following processes gets affected by halothane?**
   A. Inhibition of NADH-Q oxidoreductase (Complex I)
   B. Inhibition of Q-cytochrome *c* oxidoreductase (Complex III)
   C. Inhibition of succinate Q reductase (Complex II)
   D. Inhibition of ADP/ATP transporter
   E. Uncoupling of oxidative phosphorylation

2. **A 7-year-old girl is brought to the emergency department by her parents with complaints of severe polyuria and polydipsia. Laboratory examination reveals ketones in her urine. Which of the following is the most likely source of ketones?**
   A. Fatty acid breakdown
   B. Protein breakdown
   C. Glycogenolysis
   D. Gluconeogenesis
   E. Glycolysis

3. **The major metabolic product produced under normal circumstances by erythrocytes and by muscle cells during intense exercise is recycled through liver in the Cori cycle. The metabolite is:**
   A. Oxaloacetate
   B. Alanine
   C. Glycerol
   D. Lactate
   E. Pyruvate

4. **A 45-year-old obese man complains of having to get up frequently to urinate at night-time. He has also noticed that he is constantly thirsty and hungry. The patient is diagnosed with type 2 diabetes mellitus. If this is a problem at the level of glucose transporters, which tissue would be most affected?**
   A. Liver
   B. Red blood cells
   C. Muscle and adipose tissue
   D. Brain tissue
   E. β cells of pancreas

5. **A 30-year-old woman is enduring her second trimester of pregnancy. The greater affinity fetal hemoglobin acquires oxygen released from the lesser affinity maternal hemoglobin due to the effect of an allosteric modifier, which is:**
   A. Fr-2,6 bisphosphate
   B. 2,3-Bisphosphoglycerate
   C. Citrate
   D. Acetyl-CoA
   E. Fr-1,6 bisphosphoglycerate

6. **A 14-year-old high-school girl who is extremely conscious about her appearance has gone a full-day fasting to fit into a dress she intentionally brought a size smaller than her actual size for a dance party. Which of the following organs/tissues contributes to the glucose that is being synthesized through gluconeogenesis during periods of prolonged fasting?**
   A. Spleen
   B. Red blood cells
   C. Skeletal muscle
   D. Liver
   E. Brain

7. **A 35-year-old woman presents with crushing substernal chest pain and shortness of breath. A coronary artery is occluded due to an atherosclerotic plaque, and she is diagnosed with having myocardial infarction. Her serum cholesterol level is 700 mg/dL. The family history is positive for high cholesterol level and she seems to be having familial hypercholesterolemia. What is the possible biochemical defect in this genetic disorder?**
   A. High activity of HMG CoA reductase
   B. Low activity of 7-α hydroxylase
   C. Abnormal LDL receptors
   D. More conversion of VLDL to LDL
   E. Less concentration of HDL

8. **A 23-year-old female presents with low red blood cell count, corneal opacities, and kidney insufficiency. She is diagnosed with lecithin: cholesterol acyltransferase (LCAT) deficiency. In which of the following reactions, LCAT is involved?**
   A. Transfer of cholesterol esters from HDL to VLDL
   B. Hydrolysis of HDL
   C. Uptake of cholesterol from liver cells
   D. Converting cholesterol to cholesteryl esters
   E. Promoting uptake of HDL in to liver cells

9. **A 16-year-old extremely slender girl presents with a body weight that is 35% below expected. She still feels herself to be obese and severely restricts her food intake. She is diagnosed with anorexia nervosa. In this patient, due to improper dietary intake, the breakdown of fatty acids is required to provide energy. Which of the following substance is formed in the first step of the beta oxidation of fatty acids?**
   A. ATP
   B. CoA
   C. Fatty acyl-CoA
   D. Carnitine
   E. Malonyl CoA

10. **A 20-year-old woman has a myocardial infarct and is given an aspirin to chew. Taking aspirin has been shown to be cardioprotective in myocardial infarction. Aspirin is a nonsteroidal anti-inflammatory drug that inhibits cyclo-oxygenase enzyme (COX). Cyclo-oxygenase is required for the production of which of these?**
    A. Thromboxane from arachidonic acid
    B. Leukotrienes from arachidonic acid
    C. Arachidonic acid from linoleic acid
    D. Release of arachidonic acid from membrane phospholipids
    E. Hydroperoxyeicosatetraenoic acid (HPETEs) from arachidonic acid

11. **A 23-year-old woman is seen for a lump in her breast that she palpated on self-breast examination. History reveals that her mother and her aunt both had breast and ovarian cancer. Given this presentation, you suspect that the patient may have a mutation in which of the following genes involved in DNA repair?**
    A. *BRCA-1*
    B. ras
    C. bcl-2
    D. p53
    E. Rb

12. **A 65-year-old man presents to the physician complaining of unwellness and easy fatigue. The routine set of tests demonstrates a white blood cell count of 95,000/mL (normal 3,000–10,000/mL). Molecular studies suggest that he has chronic myelogenous leukemia. A chromosomal translocation is responsible for this disease. Which of the following translocations is associated with this disorder?**
    A. t (8;14)
    B. t (14;18)
    C. t (11;14)
    D. t (9;22)
    E. t (15;17)

13. **A 54-year-old postmenopausal woman presented to internist for care of hot flashes that had returned 2 years after menopause. The symptoms occurred mostly after meals, when she drank wine, or when she went for running. There was history of hypertension and frequent diarrheas also. The 24-hour urine levels of 5-HIAA (5-hydroxyindoleacetic acid), a breakdown product of serotonin was found to be highly elevated. What is the probable diagnosis for this patient?**
    A. Pheochromocytoma
    B. Carcinoid tumor
    C. Hartnup disease
    D. Hyperpituitarism
    E. Medullary carcinoma of thyroid gland

14. **A 50-year-old male is seen in the emergency with severe headache. His blood pressure is 210/130 mm Hg. An evidence of retinal hemorrhage and epistaxis is also there. He has been given an infusion of nitroprusside. Which of the following processes is directly affected by the active metabolite of this drug?**
    A. Phospholipase A2
    B. Phospholipase C
    C. Guanylate cyclase
    D. Phosphodiesterase
    E. Adenylate cyclase

15. **A child with tall stature, loose joints, and detached retinas is found to have a mutation in collagen. Which of the following amino acids is the recurring amino acid most likely to be altered in mutations that distort collagen molecules?**
    A. Glycine
    B. Tyrosine
    C. Tryptophan
    D. Tyrosine
    E. Alanine

16. The drug Fluorouracil is recommended for the treatment of cancers. It undergoes a series of changes and then binds to thymidylate synthase enzyme resulting in its inhibition and blockage of cell division. This mode of inhibition is most probably due to:

A. Allosteric inhibition
B. Competitive inhibition
C. Noncompetitive inhibition
D. Suicidal inhibition
E. Uncompetitive inhibition

17. A 64-year-old female presents with severe back pain for the past three weeks. Imaging reveals a compression fracture of one of the vertebrae and diffuse osteoporosis, which is a common condition resulting from calcium depletion in bones. As a treatment, she should be prescribed:

A. Oxytocin
B. Parathyroid hormone
C. Estradiol
D. Calcitonin
E. Prolactin

18. An underweight 4-year-old boy was brought to the emergency department in a semi-conscious state. His blood glucose, urea, and glutamine were abnormally low, acetoacetate was elevated but lactate was normal. He was admitted to ICU where his blood glucose was increased by injection glucagon. Which metabolic pathway is most likely deficient in this child?

A. Hepatic gluconeogenesis
B. Skeletal muscle glycogenolysis
C. Adipose tissue lipolysis
D. Skeletal muscle proteolysis
E. Hepatic glycogenolysis

19. A pregnant woman is able to transfer oxygen to her fetus because fetal hemoglobin has a greater affinity for oxygen than does adult hemoglobin. Why is the affinity of fetal hemoglobin for oxygen higher?

A. The tense form of hemoglobin is more prevalent in the circulation of the fetus
B. There is less 2, 3-BPG in the fetal circulation as compared to maternal circulation
C. Fetal hemoglobin binds 2, 3-BPG with fewer ionic bonds than the adult form
D. The Bohr effect is enhanced in the fetus
E. The oxygen-binding curve of fetal hemoglobin is shifted to the right

20. A 16-month-old girl was found to have ingested approximately 30 mL of an acetonitrile-based cosmetic nail remover when she vomited 15 minutes post ingestion. The poison control center was contacted, but no treatment was recommended because it was confused with an acetone-based nail polish remover. The child was put to bed at her normal time, which was 2 hours post ingestion. Respiratory distress developed sometimes after the child was put to bed, and she was found dead the next morning.

Inhibition of which of the following enzymes was the most likely cause of this child's death?

A. Cytochrome c reductase
B. Cytochrome oxidase
C. Coenzyme Q reductase
D. NADH dehydrogenase
E. Succinate dehydrogenase

21. A 48-year-old man with bronchiectasis presents to the hospital emergency room with 3 days of increasing cough, sputum, and dyspnea. About 1 month ago, his arterial blood gas analysis showed pH 7.38, PaO_2 55 mm Hg, $PaCO_2$ 65 mm Hg, and HCO_3- 32 mEq/L. His current vital signs are BP 117/65 mm Hg, pulse 123 beats/min, and temperature 100°F. His current ABG (blood gas analysis) in the emergency room is pH 7.28, $PaCO_2$ 70 mm Hg, PaO_2 50 mm Hg, and HCO_3- 23 mEq/L. Which of the following best characterizes the current acid–base status?

A. Compensated metabolic acidosis
B. Compensated metabolic alkalosis
C. Uncompensated metabolic acidosis
D. Uncompensated respiratory acidosis
E. Uncompensated respiratory alkalosis

22. A 50-year-old chronic alcoholic is brought to the emergency room in a semiconscious state. Blood pressure is 100/50 mm Hg, heart rate 120 beats/min, respiratory rate 35 breaths/min, and his temperature is 104°F (40°C).

Blood chemistry reveals: sodium 150 mEq/L (135–145), potassium 2.5 mEq/L (3.5–5.0), chloride 107 mEq/L (95–105), bicarbonate 10 mEq/L (24–26), pH 7.2 (7.35–7.45), PCO_2 25 mm Hg (35–45), alcohol 40 mmol/L (0), osmolality 370 mOsm/L (280–295), glucose 50 mg/dL (60–110), BUN 40 mg/dL (5–22). What is the acid–base status?

A. Metabolic acidosis
B. Metabolic alkalosis
C. Respiratory acidosis
D. Respiratory alkalosis
E. Metabolic acidosis with respiratory compensation

23. A 24-year female reported to the emergency department with difficulty in breathing. History revealed that she had ingested some unknown drug. The blood chemistry revealed the following: PH-7.1; PCO_2-55 mm Hg; PO_2-42 mm Hg, and HCO_3— 17 mEq/L. Which of the following is the most appropriate acid–base imbalance in the above said condition?

A. Metabolic acidosis with respiratory acidosis
B. Respiratory acidosis
C. Respiratory alkalosis
D. Metabolic alkalosis
E. None of the above

24. A 23-year-old male, golden gloves boxing contender presents with a metabolic disorder. He describes his training regimen that involves consuming a dozen raw eggs a day for a protein. Raw eggs contain a protein called Avidin, with an extremely high affinity for a cofactor, required by propionyl-CoA carboxylase, Acetyl-CoA carboxylase, and pyruvate carboxylase. The patient is deficient in which of the following cofactors?

A. Cobalamin
B. Biotin
C. Folic acid
D. Pyridoxal phosphate
E. TPP

25. Oral contraceptives are known to lower blood levels of vitamin B6. Which of the following conversion process might be directly affected?

A. Phenylalanine to tyrosine
B. Pyruvate to oxaloacetate
C. Dopamine to norepinephrine
D. Histidine to histamine
E. Pyruvate to lactate

26. A 20-year-old female, a known alcoholic, has been brought to the emergency department with respiratory distress. Bilateral crepitations are felt in the lungs, neck veins are engorged, and X-ray chest shows dilated heart. She has been diagnosed with "Cardiac Beri-Beri." Which of the following reactions might have been affected?

A. Pyruvate to malic acid
B. Pyruvate to acetyl-CoA
C. Pyruvate to oxaloacetate
D. Pyruvate to lactate
E. Pyruvate to alanine

27. A 60-year-old chronic smoker and alcoholic man presents with epigastric discomfort and recurrent diarrhea. Clinical examination reveals memory disorientation, stomatitis, glossitis, esophagitis, and exfoliative dermatitis. Treatment with nicotinamide 500 mg daily has been initiated. Which of the following conversions might not have been affected?

A. Succinate to fumarate
B. Malate to oxaloacetate
C. Pyruvate to acetyl-CoA
D. Pyruvate to lactate
E. Dihydrofolate to tetrahydrofolate

28. A 10-year-old male presents with muscle cramping and dark urine after rigorous exercise. He is found to have a deficiency of lactate dehydrogenase. This enzyme catalyzes interconversion of lactate and pyruvate based upon the availability/absence of oxygen. Which of the following coenzymes is needed for this action?

A. NAD^+
B. FAD
C. TPP
D. Adenosylcobalamin
E. Pyridoxal-P

29. A 30-year-old pregnant female presents to her obstetrician for a prenatal visit. She has been conscious of her weight gain and has not been taking a multivitamin. Her red blood cells are found to have decreased transketolase function. Transketolase requires:

A. TPP
B. Pyridoxine
C. Folate
D. B_{12}
E. FAD

30. A 27-year-old female with epilepsy has been taking phenytoin to control her seizures. She is pregnant and considering the risk of potential bleeding episodes in the infant, her physician is considering changing her medicine. What biochemical activity might be deficient in the baby if her medication is continued as such?

A. Hydroxylation of proline
B. Gamma carboxylation of glutamic acid residues
C. Glucuronidation of bilirubin
D. Oxidation of lysine
E. Oxidation of glutathione

31. A 75-year-old female is seen in the emergency room with fractured arm. Physical examination reveals multiple bruises, perifollicular hemorrhages, and bleeding gums. Her diet consisted mainly of plain buns, pasta, rolls, and coffee. Laboratory result indicates microcytic hypochromic anemia. Which of the following enzymes should be less active than the normal in this patient?

A. Glutathione peroxidase
B. Prolyl hydroxylase
C. Gamma glutamyl transferase
D. ALA synthase
E. Glutathione reductase

32. Failure of downregulation of extrahepatic receptors for oxidized LDL is mainly responsible for the formation of foam cells and for triggering the process of atherosclerosis. This process can be prevented by timely supplementation of antioxidants. Which of the following should be considered the best choice to be considered as an antioxidant?

A. Vitamin B_6
B. Vitamin K
C. Vitamin D
D. Vitamin E
E. Folic acid

33. In the fed state after a very heavy meal, there is active lipogenesis in the adipose tissue. Glycolysis must go on at the same pace to provide which of the following intermediate from glycolysis required for fat storage?

A. Acetyl-CoA
B. Pyruvate
C. Glucose-6-P
D. Glycerol
E. Dihydroxyacetone phosphate

34. A 56-year-old man with a history of genetic disease underwent hip replacement surgery for arthritis. During surgery, black stains were observed in the cartilage. These stains are usually observed in patients suffering from ochronosis, a condition initially characterized by darkening of urine upon standing (alkaptonuria). There is deficiency of homogentisic acid oxidase in this condition. Which of the following vitamins acts as a coenzyme for the above said enzyme?

A. Vitamin B_{12}
B. Folic acid
C. Ascorbic acid
D. Niacin
E. Riboflavin

35. A 45-year-old man presents with multiple gunshot wounds to the abdomen. He undergoes emergent surgery during which a part of his intestine is resected. After surgery he is placed on total parenteral nutrition (TPN), an intravenous form of nutrition. TPN supplies essential fatty acids also in the diet. Which of the following is an essential fatty acid?

A. Palmitic acid
B. Linoleic acid
C. Elaidic acid
D. Oleic acid
E. Erucic acid

36. A 43-year-old man with a long history of poorly controlled hypertension presents to the emergency with a severe headache. His blood pressure is found to be dramatically elevated at 220/150 mm Hg. Which of the following products derived from amino acids might bring down his highly elevated blood pressure?

A. Melanin
B. Nitric oxide
C. GABA
D. Dopamine
E. Serotonin

37. A 40-year-old obese woman presents with acute pain in the right upper quadrant of her abdomen as well as vomiting. She is diagnosed with gallstones and is placed on ursodeoxycholate, a bile salt used to inhibit the formation of cholesterol gallstones by facilitating dissolution of cholesterol.

Which of the following is also a bile salt?

A. HMG CoA
B. Mevalonate
C. Lanosterol
D. Squalene
E. Glycocholate

38. A young infant, who was nourished with a synthetic formula, had a sugar in the blood and urine. This compound gave a positive reducing sugar test but was negative when measured with glucose oxidase (specific test for detection or estimation of glucose). Treatment of blood and urine with acid (which cleaves glycosidic bonds) did not increase the amount of reducing sugar measured. Which of the following compounds is most likely to be present in this infant's blood and urine?

A. Glucose
B. Fructose
C. Maltose
D. Sorbitol
E. Lactose

39. A 3-year-old Caucasian female presents with chronic diarrhea and a failure to thrive. Stools were oily. History reveals that she was breastfed and had no problems until she was weaned. Which of the enzymes would be expected to be deficient following stimulation with secretin?

A. Cholesteryl esterase
B. Gastric lipase
C. Hormone sensitive lipase
D. Lipoprotein lipase
E. Pancreatic lipase

40. A known alcoholic was found lying semiconscious by his landlady at the bottom of a stairwell with a broken arm; he was then taken to the emergency room. Initial laboratory studies showed relatively large anion gap of 34 (normal = 9 to 15). His blood alcohol was elevated at 245 mg/dL (intoxication level = 150 to 300 mg/dL), and his blood glucose was 38 mg/dL (low normal). The patient/s large anion gap and hypoglycemia can best be explained by which of the following?

A. Decreased secretion of glucagon
B. Increased secretion of insulin
C. Increased urination resulting from the diuretic effect of alcohol
D. Inhibition of dehydrogenase enzymes by NADH
E. Inhibition of glycogenolysis by ethanol

41. A 30-month-old female child whose growth rate has been in the lower 10th percentile over the last year presents with chronic, nonproductive cough, and diarrhea with foul-smelling stools. She is diagnosed as having cystic fibrosis. For which of the following vitamins is this child most likely to be at risk of deficiency?

A. Ascorbic acid (vitamin C)
B. Biotin
C. Folic acid
D. Retinol (vitamin A)
E. Riboflavin (vitamin B_2)

42. Leukemia patients are often given the compound Leucovorin (N5-formyl THF) following treatment with the drug methotrexate. Why is Leucovorin useful as part of this treatment protocol?

A. It facilitates the uptake of methotrexate by cells
B. It can be converted to THF by bypassing DHFR
C. It acts as an activator of thymidylate synthase
D. It prevents the uptake of methotrexate by normal cells
E. It stimulates cells of the immune system

43. A 3-year-old boy is brought to the emergency room with abdominal pain, mental status changes, and fatigue. On taking history, the physician finds the child belongs to a very poor family and lives in an old house and has the habit of licking the paint chips that have crumbled in the window sills. The physician suspects lead poisoning. Lead typically interferes with which of the following enzymes?

A. Cytochrome oxidase
B. Protoporphyrinogen oxidase
C. ALA synthase
D. Coproporphyrinogen oxidase
E. ALA dehydratase

44. A 10-year-old boy comes to the ER after eating wild mushrooms. The poison associated with these mushrooms most likely DIRECTLY inhibits the synthesis of the following:

A. hnRNA
B. tRNA
C. DNA
D. mRNA
E. rRNA

45. A couple of African-American descent gives birth to a boy after an otherwise uneventful pregnancy. The child is exceptionally fair skinned and has almost white hair. Further examination reveals red pupils. A postnatal screen is likely to confirm the deficiency of which of the following enzymes?

A. Glutathione reductase
B. Glutathione peroxidase
C. Tyrosinase
D. Methionine synthase
E. Cystathionine beta synthase

46. During a medical rotation, a medical student volunteered for a respiratory physiology examination that determines basal metabolic rate and the respiratory quotient. She followed the protocol for a resting individual in the postabsorptive state. Which of the following amino acids would be found in the highest concentration in the serum?

A. Alanine and glutamine
B. Arginine and ornithine
C. Glutamate and aspartate
D. Branched chain amino acids
E. Hydrophobic amino acids

47. A 56-year-old diabetic with end-stage renal disease receives a kidney transplant from his son. His nephrologist is concerned for the possibility of transplant rejection and puts the patient on mycophenolic acid that inhibits which of the following enzymes in the synthesis of nucleotides?

A. PRPP synthetase
B. IMP dehydrogenase
C. Adenylosuccinate synthetase
D. Ribonucleotide reductase
E. Adenylosuccinase

48. A 73-year-old woman is transferred to intensive care unit after she is found to be in septic shock. It is believed that she originally had a urinary tract infection and that the bacteria seeded her blood stream. The critical care fellow is concerned she may not have an adequate stress response in this situation. He orders a cosyntropin test, which evaluates the body's ability to produce which of the following hormones?

A. Oxytocin
B. Vasopressin
C. Cortisol
D. Corticotropin releasing hormone
E. Adrenocorticotropic hormone (ACTH)

49. A 75-year-old woman with osteoporosis complains of back pain. A magnetic resonance imaging (MRI) scan of her back confirms a compressing fracture of the L3 vertebra. The attending physician begins treating the patient with morphine for pain control. Morphine is an analgesic that works similarly to which of the following endogenously produced substances?

A. ACTH
B. POMC
C. MSH
D. Endorphin
E. Lipotropin

50. A 23-year-old young woman, who recently began taking birth control pills, presents to the emergency room with cramping abdominal pain, anxiety, hallucinations, and paranoid behavior. A surgical evaluation, including ultrasound and computed tomography (CT) scan, has failed to demonstrate any abdominal process. Examination reveals vesicles and bullae on the skin of arms and face. Urine analysis reveals the presence of porphyrins (ALA, PBG, Uro, and Coproporphyrins). What is the possible diagnosis for this patient?

A. Variegate porphyria
B. Acute intermittent porphyria
C. Congenital erythropoietic porphyria
D. Hereditary coproporphyria
E. Porphyria cutanea tarda

KEY TO ANSWERS

1. **E.** Uncoupling of oxidative phosphorylation
2. **A.** Fatty acid breakdown
3. **D.** Lactate
4. **C.** Muscle and adipose tissue
5. **B.** 2,3 Bisphosphoglycerate
6. **C.** Skeletal muscle
7. **C.** Abnormal LDL receptors
8. **D.** Converting cholesterol to cholesteryl esters
9. **C.** Fatty acyl-CoA
10. **A.** Thromboxane from arachidonic acid
11. **A.** BRCA-1
12. **D.** t (9;22)
13. **B.** Carcinoid tumor
14. **C.** Guanylate cyclase
15. **A.** Glycine
16. **D.** Suicidal inhibition
17. **D.** Calcitonin
18. **A.** Hepatic gluconeogenesis
19. **B.** There is less 2, 3-BPG in the fetal circulation as compared to maternal circulation
20. **B.** Cytochrome oxidase
21. **D.** Uncompensated respiratory acidosis
22. **E.** Metabolic acidosis with respiratory compensation
23. **A.** Metabolic acidosis with respiratory acidosis
24. **B.** Biotin
25. **D.** Histidine to histamine
26. **B.** Pyruvate to acetyl-CoA
27. **A.** Succinate to fumarate
28. **A.** NAD^+
29. **A.** TPP
30. **B.** Gamma carboxylation of glutamic acid residues
31. **B.** Prolyl-hydroxylase
32. **D.** Vitamin E
33. **E.** Dihydroxyacetone phosphate
34. **C.** Ascorbic acid
35. **B.** Linoleic acid
36. **B.** Nitric oxide
37. **E.** Glycocholate
38. **B.** Fructose
39. **E.** Pancreatic lipase
40. **D.** Inhibition of dehydrogenase enzymes by NADH
41. **D.** Retinol (vitamin A)
42. **B.** It can be converted to THF by bypassing DHFR
43. **E.** ALA dehydratase
44. **A.** hnRNA
45. **C.** Tyrosinase
46. **A.** Alanine and glutamine
47. **B.** IMP dehydrogenase
48. **C.** Cortisol
49. **D.** Endorphin
50. **A.** Variegate porphyria

Chapter 28

Quick Revisions

SUMMARY CHART 1

Acid–base Imbalance

Primary disorder	*Defect*	*Causes*	*Effect on pH and ratio of bicarbonate: carbonic acid*	*Compensatory responses*
Metabolic acidosis Primary HCO_3^- deficiency	Gain in H^+ or HCO_3^- loss	**(A) High anion gap (acid gain)** 1. **Ketoacidosis** • Diabetes • Chronic alcoholism • Under nutrition • Fasting 2. **Lactic acidosis** • Shock • Primary hypoxia due to lung disorders • Seizures 3. **Renal failure** 4. **Toxins metabolized to acids** • Alcohol • Methanol (formate) • Ethylene glycol (oxalate) • Salicylates **(B) Normal anion gap acidosis (bicarbonate loss—hyperchloremic acidosis)** 1. **GI HCO_3—loss** • Colostomy • Diarrhea • Enteric fistulas • Ileostomy 2. **Urologic procedures** 3. **Renal HCO_3—loss** • Renal tubular acidosis 4. **Ingestions** • Acetazolamide	pH—decreased Ratio—decreased	**Respiratory mechanism** Respiratory alkalosis (hyperventilation) $PaCO_2$ decreased (transient compensation) **Renal mechanisms** 1. Increased excretion of H+ ions 2. Decreased excretion of K^+ ions in the distal tubules 3. Decreased bicarbonate excretion 4. Increased ammonia formation 5. Increased acid phosphate excretion

Primary disorder	*Defect*	*Causes*	*Effect on pH and ratio of bicarbonate: carbonic acid*	*Compensatory responses*
Metabolic alkalosis HCO_3^- increased	Gain in HCO_3^- or loss of H^+	**Chloride-responsive alkalosis** • Loss of gastric secretions – vomiting, NG suction • Loss of colonic secretions • Thiazides and loop diuretics (after discontinuation) • Cystic fibrosis (due to loss of chloride in the sweat) • Ingestion of large doses of nonabsorbable antacids **Chloride-resistant alkalosis** • Primary hyperaldosteronism • Cushing syndrome • Exogenous mineralocorticoids or glucocorticoids • Reno vascular hypertension • Renin- or deoxycorticosterone-secreting tumors • Current use of thiazides and loop diuretics • Milk alkali syndrome	pH—increased Ratio—increased	**Respiratory mechanism** Respiratory acidosis (hypoventilation) $PaCO_2$ increased **Renal mechanisms** 1. Decreased excretion of H^+ ions 2. Increased excretion of K^+ ions in the distal tubules 3. Increased bicarbonate excretion 4. Decreased ammonia formation 5. Decreased acid phosphate excretion
Respiratory acidosis $PaCO_2$ increased	CO_2 retention	**(A) Central** • Drugs—sedatives, alcohol, general anesthetic agents • Infections • Injuries—head trauma • Diseases— intracranial tumor • Syndromes of sleep-disordered breathing, including the primary alveolar and obesity-hypoventilation syndromes **(B) Airway obstruction** • Severe asthma • Anaphylaxis • Inhalational burn • Toxic injury • Laryngeal obstruction • End-stage obstructive lung disease **(C) Parenchymatous damage/ inflammation** • Emphysema • Bronchitis • Adult respiratory distress syndrome • Pleurisy • Barotrauma	pH—decreased Ratio—decreased	Metabolic alkalosis HCO_3^- increased **Renal mechanisms** 1. Increased excretion of H^+ ions 2. Decreased bicarbonate excretion 3. Increased ammonia formation 4. Increased acid phosphate excretion
		(D) Neuromuscular • Poliomyelitis • Kyphoscoliosis • Myasthenia gravis • Muscular dystrophies **(E) Miscellaneous** • Certain congenital heart diseases • Mechanical ventilation • Rebreathing from a closed space		

Primary disorder	*Defect*	*Causes*	*Effect on pH and ratio of bicarbonate: carbonic acid*	*Compensatory responses*
Respiratory alkalosis $PaCO_2$ decreased	CO_2 washout	**(A) Central nervous system** • Pain • Hyperventilation syndrome • Anxiety • Psychosis • Fever • Cerebrovascular accident • Meningitis • Encephalitis • Tumor • Trauma • **Hypoxia** – High altitude – Severe anemia • **Drugs** – Salicylates – Catecholamines – Nicotine • **Endocrine** – Pregnancy – Hyperthyroidism • **Pulmonary** – Pneumothorax/hemothorax – Pneumonia – Pulmonary edema – Pulmonary embolism – Aspiration – Interstitial lung disease – Asthma – Emphysema – Chronic bronchitis • **Miscellaneous** – Sepsis – Hepatic failure – Mechanical ventilation – Heat exhaustion – Recovery phase of metabolic acidosis – Congestive heart failure	pH—increased Ratio—increased	Metabolic acidosis HCO_3^- decreased **Renal mechanisms** 1. Decreased excretion of H^+ ions 2. Increased bicarbonate excretion 3. Decreased ammonia formation 4. Decreased phosphate excretion

SUMMARY CHART 2

Disorders of Amino Acid Metabolism—Quick Revision

Disease	*Biochemical defect and pathogenesis*	*Laboratory findings*	*Clinical manifestations*	*Treatment*
Alkaptonuria	Deficiency of **homogentisic acid oxidase** Homogentisic acid accumulates in the body and slowly and progressively gets deposited causing discoloration of connective tissue (including bone, cartilage, and skin). This condition is called **ochronosis** The polymerized homogentisic acid products are excreted in large amounts in urine imparting black color to urine.	Diagnosis can be confirmed by demonstrating the presence of homogentisic acid in the urine. This may be done by paper chromatography or thin-layer chromatography.	The earliest signs are **thickening of the ear cartilage and blue-black coloration of the skin** Bones and cartilage of the lower back, knees, shoulders, and hips are most affected. Deposits around the trachea, larynx, and bronchi may cause **shortness of breath and difficulty in breathing. Deposits around the heart and blood vessels can calcify and lead to atherosclerotic plaques** **Urine exposed to air can become dark**; this is useful for diagnosing young children using diapers **Sclera becomes pigmented, but this does not affect the vision**	**Reducing intake of the amino acid phenylalanine and tyrosine to the minimum** **Vitamin C** can slow down the conversion of homogentisic acid to the polymeric deposits in cartilage and bone
Albinism	A defect of melanin production that results in little or no color (pigment) in the skin, hair, and eyes There are three main categories of albinism in humans: **Oculocutaneous albinism**—pigment is lacking in the eyes, skin, and hair **Ocular albinism**—only the eyes lack pigment. The skin and hair color are normal **Patchy albinism**—patches of depigmentation are observed on skin and hair	The diagnosis of the condition is based on the appearance of skin, hair, and eyes **Genetic testing** offers the most accurate way to diagnose albinism and its type	Absence of coloring from the hair, skin, or iris of the eye. Long-term sun exposure greatly increases the risk of skin damage and skin cancers, including an aggressive form of skin cancer called melanoma	Symptomatic treatment Sun screen lotions and sun glasses are very helpful Genetic counseling is recommended if the disease runs in families
Phenylketonuria (PKU)	Deficiency of the enzyme phenylalanine hydroxylase or of its cofactor tetrahydrobiopterin causes accumulation of phenylalanine in body fluids and the central nervous system (CNS)	In classic PKU, levels may range from 6 to 80 mg/dL, but are usually greater than 30 mg/dL **Identification and measurement of phenylketones in the urine** Identification of phenylketones in the urine by **ferric chloride** may offer a simple test for diagnosis of infants with developmental and neurologic abnormalities	**Classical PKU** The infants are normal at birth, **mental retardation** may develop gradually, **vomiting**, sometimes severe enough to be misdiagnosed as pyloric stenosis, may be an early symptom. Older untreated children become hyperactive with **purposeless movements** On physical examination these infants are **fairer in their complexion** than unaffected siblings About 25% of children have **seizures,** and more than 50% have **electroencephalographic abnormalities** **Microcephaly, prominent maxilla with widely spaced teeth, enamel hypoplasia, and growth retardation** are other common findings in untreated children	**The goal of PKU treatment is to maintain the blood level of phenylalanine between 2 and 10 mg/dL**. Some phenylalanine is needed for normal growth. This requires a diet that has **some phenylalanine but in much lower amounts than normal**. Because phenylalanine is not synthesized by the body, "over treatment" may lead to phenylalanine deficiency manifested by lethargy, failure to thrive, anorexia, anemia, rashes, diarrhea, and even death; moreover, **tyrosine becomes an essential amino acid in this disorder and its adequate intake must be ensured** **Oral administration of the cofactor (BH4)** to patients with milder forms of hyperphenylalaninemia from phenylalanine hydroxylase deficiency may produce significant reductions

Disease	*Biochemical defect and pathogenesis*	*Laboratory findings*	*Clinical manifestations*	*Treatment*
Hartnup disease	It is caused by **impaired neutral (i.e., monoamino monocarboxylic) amino acid transport** in the apical brush border membrane of the small intestine and the proximal tubules of the kidney. Excessive amounts of amino acids, such as tryptophan, are excreted in the urine. The body is thus left with inadequate amounts of amino acids	**Urine analysis** - Neutral amino acids, Tryptophan, Indole derivatives and Tryptophan degradation products are present in urine	Patients present with **pellagra like skin eruptions, cerebellar ataxia, nystagmus, tremor, failure to thrive, photosensitivity, and gross aminoaciduria**. Symptoms may be triggered by sunlight, fever, drugs, emotional or physical stress	A **high-protein diet** can overcome the deficient transport of neutral amino acids in most patients. **Avoiding excessive exposure to sunlight**, wearing protective clothing, and using physical and chemical sunscreens are mandatory, daily **supplementation with nicotinic acid or nicotinamide** reduces both number and severity of attacks
Maple syrup urine disease	MSUD is caused by a deficiency of the branched-chain alpha-keto acid dehydrogenase complex (BCKDH), leading to a buildup of the branched-chain amino acids (leucine, isoleucine, and valine) and their toxic by-products in the blood and urine	Blood and urine in this disease have elevated levels of branched amino acids and their keto derivatives. The keto derivatives cause acidosis	**Poor feeding, vomiting, dehydration, lethargy, hypotonia, seizures, ketoacidosis, opisthotonos, pancreatitis, coma, and neurological decline** The disease is characterized in an infant by the presence of **sweet-smelling urine**, with an odor similar to that of maple syrup Infants with this disease seem healthy at birth but if left untreated suffer **severe brain damage**, and eventually **die**	A diet with minimal levels of the amino acids leucine, isoleucine, and valine must be maintained in order to prevent neurological damage. As these three amino acids are required for proper metabolic functions, specialized protein preparations containing substitutes and adjusted levels of the amino acids have been synthesized and tested, allowing MSUD patients to meet normal nutritional requirements without causing harm
Cystinuria	The amino acid transporter for cystine and other amino acids , such as arginine, ornithine, and lysine is defective both in the intestine and in PCT of nephron. This leads to retention of cystine and other amino acids in urine. Cystine gets precipitated in acidic pH	**1) Sodium cyanide nitroprusside test**—in the presence of cystine a purple-red color is observed **2)** Flat X-ray of the kidney, ureters, and bladder (KUB) is undertaken to visualize the stones 3) **Microscopic examination of urine** reveals flat hexagonal crystals of cystine	**Recurrent nephrolithiasis** Possible complications include obstruction of the urinary tract, which can predispose to infection of the urine, fever may be apparent, and white blood cells are noted in the urine Unrelieved obstruction leads to renal dysfunction, renal failure and the need for dialysis are quite rare	Medical therapy is directed toward **dissolution of existing calculi** and **prevention of new stone formation. Increasing urine volume by generous oral fluid** intake is beneficial. Cystine solubility can be improved by urinary **alkalinization** and where necessary by the administration of **thiol chelators, particularly D-penicillamine or mercaptopropionyl glycine**
Carcinoid syndrome	**Carcinoid syndrome** refers to the array of symptoms that occur secondary to Carcinoid tumors Many of the symptoms of carcinoid syndrome are produced by serotonin or its metabolites	**24-hour urine levels of 5-HIAA** (5-hydroxyindoleacetic acid), a breakdown product of serotonin Patients with carcinoid syndrome usually excrete >25 mg of 5-HIAA per day For localization of both primary lesions and metastasis, the initial imaging method is **octreoscan**	Flushing, pellagra like rash, **secretory diarrhea, and abdominal cramps** are also characteristic features of the syndrome When the diarrhea is intensive, it may lead to electrolyte disturbance and dehydration Other associated symptoms are **nausea and vomiting** About 50% of patients have **cardiac abnormalities**, caused by serotonin-induced fibrosis of the tricuspid and pulmonary valves	Symptomatic treatment, **octreotide** (a somatostatin analogue that neutralizes serotonin and decreases urinary 5-HIAA), **methysergide maleate** (antiserotonin agent but not used because of serious side effect of retroperitoneal fibrosis), **cyproheptadine** (an antihistamine drug). **Surgical resection of tumor and chemotherapy** (5-FU and doxorubicin) are the alternative treatments

Disease	*Biochemical defect and pathogenesis*	*Laboratory findings*	*Clinical manifestations*	*Treatment*
Homocystinuria (homocysteinemia)	Three major forms of homocysteinemia and homocystinuria have been identified: 1) Homocystinuria due to cystathionine beta synthetase deficiency, (classical homocystinuria), 2) The other forms can be caused by defective methionine synthase or reduced availability of two essential cofactors, 5-methyltetrahydrofolate and methylcobalamine (methyl-vitamin B_{12})	Elevations of both methionine and homocysteine in body fluids are the diagnostic laboratory findings. Total plasma homocysteine is extremely elevated (usually >100) Cystine is low or absent in plasma The diagnosis may be established by assay of the enzyme in liver biopsy specimens, cultured fibroblasts	**Failure to thrive and developmental delay** **Subluxation of the ocular lens (ectopia lentis)** occurs This causes severe **myopia and iridodonesis** (quivering of the iris), astigmatism, glaucoma, cataracts, retinal detachment, and optic atrophy may develop later in life **Progressive mental retardation** is common, skeletal abnormalities resemble those of **Marfan syndrome** Patients usually have **fair complexions, blue eyes, and a peculiar malar flush** **Generalized osteoporosis, especially of the spine,** is the main radiographic finding **Thromboembolic episodes** involving both large and small vessels, especially those of the brain, are common and may occur at any age	Supplementation with pyridoxine, **folic acid, B12 or trimethyl glycine (betaine)** reduces the concentration of homocysteine considerably in the blood stream Those who do not respond require a **low methionine diet**
Cystinosis	Abnormal lysosomal cystine transporter (**cystinosin**), due to a mutation in the gene CTNS, located on chromosome 17 The abnormal transport of cystine from lysosomes results in a massive intralysosomal cysteine accumulation in tissues. Via an as yet unknown mechanism, lysosomal cysteine amplifies and alters apoptosis in such a way that cells die inappropriately, leading to loss of renal epithelial cells. This results in renal Fanconi syndrome and similar loss in other tissues can account for the short stature, retinopathy, and other features of the disease	Definitive diagnosis and treatment monitoring are most often performed through measurement of white blood cell cystine level using tandem mass spectrometry	Symptoms are first seen at about 3 to 18 months of age with profound polyuria (excessive urination), followed by poor growth, photophobia, and ultimately kidney failure by age 6 years in the nephropathic form. The other forms are intermediate cystinosis (juvenile) and non-nephropathic or ocular cystinosis (adult) forms	The drug **cysteamine** slows the progression of cystinosis by removing the cystine from cells, but for the drug treatment to be effective, it must be taken every 6 hours Without specific treatment, these children progress to end-stage renal failure by an average age of 9 years Cystinosis is a common cause of the Fanconi syndrome, a renal tubular disease

SUMMARY CHART 3

Disorders of Carbohydrate Metabolism

Sl.No.	*Disease*	*Biochemical defect and pathogenesis*	*Inheritance and classification*	*Clinical manifestations*	*Laboratory investigations*	*Treatment*
1.	**Lactose intolerance**	**Deficiency of lactase** Uncleaved lactose present in ingested dairy products passes intact into the colon producing osmotic effects and undergoes fermentation to produce a variety of abdominal manifestations	Three major types of lactose intolerance: 1. **Primary lactose intolerance** begins after age 2 2. **Secondary lactose intolerance**—mucosal damage resulting from certain gastrointestinal diseases, or from medications 3. **Congenital lactase deficiency**—present at birth, autosomal recessive inheritance	Abdominal pain, bloating, gas, diarrhea and nausea	**1 Hydrogen breath test**—Normally, very little hydrogen is detectable in the breath, but undigested lactose produces high levels of hydrogen 2. **Stool acidity test**—Undigested lactose creates lactic acid and other fatty acids that can be detected in a stool sample Glucose may also be present in the stool as a result of undigested lactose	**Lactose-free, lactose-reduced milk**, soy milk, **lactase enzyme** drops or tablets and **calcium** supplementation
2.	**Pyruvate kinase deficiency (PKD)** An erythrocyte enzymopathy involving glycolysis	A discrepancy between erythrocyte energy requirements and ATP-generating capacity produces irreversible membrane injury, resulting in cellular distortion, rigidity, and dehydration This leads to **premature erythrocyte destruction** by the spleen and liver with the resultant anemia	Autosomal recessive	Severe anemia, jaundice, kernicterus, chronic leg ulcers, growth failure and failure to thrive	Hb, serum bilirubin and confirmation by enzyme assays	Mild-to-moderate only supportive treatment Severe case—blood transfusion or bone marrow transplantation can be done Splenectomy is indicated only in severe anemia
3.	**PDH complex deficiency** Pyruvate dehydrogenase complex (PDC) converts pyruvate to acetyl-coenzyme A (CoA)	A deficiency in this enzymatic complex limits the production of citrate Because citrate is the first substrate in the citric acid cycle, the cycle cannot proceed Malfunction of this cycle deprives the body of energy An abnormal lactate buildup results in nonspecific symptoms	X-linked	Severe lethargy, poor feeding, tachypnea), especially during times of illness, stress, or high carbohydrate intake Progressive neurological symptoms, such as developmental delay, intermittent ataxia, poor muscle tone, abnormal eye movements, or seizures are present in early infancy	High serum lactate and pyruvate levels, high urinary and serum alanine levels MRI for detection of neurological damage	**Symptomatic treatment**—Low carbohydrate diet, thiamine supplementation, ketogenic diet, and oral citrate to correct acidosis

Sl.No.	Disease	Biochemical defect and pathogenesis	Inheritance and classification	Clinical manifestations	Laboratory investigations	Treatment
4	**Glucose-6-phosphatase dehydrogenase (G6PD) deficiency**	Glucose 6-phosphate dehydrogenase (G6PD) is an enzyme critical in the redox metabolism of all aerobic cells. In red cells, it is the only source of reduced nicotinamide adenine dinucleotide phosphate (NADPH), which, directly and via reduced glutathione (GSH), defends these cells against oxidative stress With the help of the enzyme glutathione peroxidase, reduced glutathione converts harmful hydrogen peroxide to water. Deficiency leads to hemolytic anemia	X-linked disorder	The vast majority of people remain asymptomatic throughout life other develop hemolytic anemia in response to oxidative challenges Acute hemolytic anemia develops in response to ingestion of fava beans, drugs and infections Typically, a hemolytic attack starts with malaise, weakness, and abdominal or lumbar pain After an interval of several hours to 2–3 days, the patient develops jaundice and often dark urine, due to hemoglobinuria The onset can be extremely abrupt, especially with favism in children	Hb low—The anemia is moderate to extremely severe, usually normocytic and normochromic associated with hemoglobinuria, LDH is high and so is the unconjugated bilirubin The confirmation is done by measuring the actual enzyme activity	Identification and discontinuation of the precipitating agent Oxygen and bed rest for symptomatic relief Prevention of drug-induced hemolysis is possible in most cases by choosing alternative drugs
5.	**Hereditary galactosemia**	Galactose-1-phosphate uridyl transferase (GALT) deficiency is the most common enzyme deficiency that causes Galactosemia The other enzyme deficiencies which can produce galactosemia are: galactokinase and uridine diphosphate (UDP) galactose-4-epimerase enzyme deficiencies	Autosomal recessive	The cardinal features of classic galactosemia are **hepatomegaly, cataracts, and mental retardation** Poor growth, liver dysfunction and jaundice are also present	1) **Urine test for reducing sugar** is positive. The confirmation is done by thin layer chromatography 2) A **galactose tolerance test** is abnormal in these patients. There is much higher than normal rise in blood galactose after the administration of galactose, and the elevation persists for a much longer time than normal 3) **Serum bilirubin and transaminases may** be high 4) Confirmation is by enzyme estimation in erythrocytes.	Galactose free diet is recommended to prevent the accumulation of galactose

Sl.No.	Disease	Biochemical defect and pathogenesis	Inheritance and classification	Clinical manifestations	Laboratory investigations	Treatment
6.	**Hereditary fructose intolerance**	Hereditary fructose intolerance is caused by mutation in the gene encoding aldolase B enzyme The rate of phosphorylation by fructokinase is very high and in the presence of aldolase B deficiency ATP depletion takes place which is manifested in the form of hyperuricemia, lactic acidemia and liver dysfunction	An autosomal recessive trait	These patients are healthy and asymptomatic until fructose or sucrose (table sugar) is ingested (usually from fruit, sweetened cereal, or sucrose-containing formula). Clinical features include recurrent abdominal pain, vomiting and hypoglycemia Long-term exposure leads to liver and kidney failure	Urine test is positive for reducing sugar, aminoaciduria, proteinuria and phosphaturia may also be associated Liver and kidney function tests may be abnormal The confirmation is done by enzyme estimation	Total avoidance of fructose containing foods
7.	**Essential pentosuria**	Deficiency of xylitol dehydrogenase enzyme This enzyme converts L-xylulose to xylitol Failure to convert leads to accumulation of L-xylulose in blood and is also excreted excessively in urine	Autosomal recessive	Asymptomatic, just a chance finding	Urine test is positive for reducing sugar. Confirmation by Bial's test and loading test by D-glucuronic acid	No treatment is needed

SUMMARY CHART 4

Glycogen Storage Diseases

Type	*Name*	*Enzyme deficiency*	*Clinical and biochemical features*
0	-	Glycogen synthase	Hypoglycemia, ketosis, and early death
I	**Von Gierke's disease**	Glucose 6-phosphatase	High glycogen content (normal structure) in liver and renal tubule cells, hepatomegaly, growth retardation, hypoglycemia, lactic acidosis, ketosis, hyperuricemia, and hyperlipidemia
II	**Pompe's disease**	Lysosomal α1à4 and α 1à6 Glucosidase (acid maltase)	Juvenile onset variant- accumulation of glycogen in lysosomes, muscle hypotonia, early death from heart failure by age 2; adult onset variant-muscle dystrophy
III	**Limit dextrinosis, Forbe's or Cori's disease**	Debranching enzyme	Accumulation of abnormal glycogen (characteristic branched polysaccharide), fasting hypoglycemia, and hepatomegaly
IV	**Amylopectinosis, Andersen's disease**	Branching enzyme	Accumulation of abnormal glycogen (polysaccharide with few branch points), hepatosplenomegaly, and early death from heart or liver failure
V	**Myophosphorylase deficiency, McArdle's syndrome**	Muscle phosphorylase	Muscle glycogen abnormally high (2.5%–4%), reduced exercise tolerance, post exercise blood lactate extremely low
VI	**Hers' disease**	Liver phosphorylase	Accumulation of glycogen (normal structure) in liver, hepatomegaly, mild hypoglycemia and good prognosis in treated cases
VII	**Tarui's disease**	Muscle and erythrocyte phospho fructokinase 1	Abnormally high muscle glycogen content (2.5%–4%), reduced exercise tolerance, very low post exercise blood lactate level and hemolytic anemia
VIII	-	Liver phosphorylase kinase	Accumulation of glycogen in liver (normal structure), hepatomegaly and mild hypoglycemia
IX	-	Liver and muscle phosphorylase kinase	Accumulation of glycogen in liver and muscle (normal structure), hepatomegaly, mild hypoglycemia and good prognosis
X	-	cAMP-dependent protein kinase A	Accumulation of normal glycogen in liver and hepatomegaly

SUMMARY CHART 5

Major metabolic pathways—Regulatory mechanisms
Carbohydrate Metabolism

Enzyme	Pathway	Effect of substrate concentration	Allosteric modification/feedback Inhibition	Induction/repression	Clinical significance
Hexokinase	Glycolysis		Feedback inhibition by glucose-6-P	-	Deficiency causes hemolytic anemia
Glucokinase	Glycolysis	Stimulated by high carbohydrate diet Activity decreases during fasting	-	Induced by insulin Repressed by glucagon	Activity low in diabetes mellitus
Phosphofructokinase-1	Glycolysis	Stimulated by high carbohydrate diet Activity decreases during fasting	**Activators**-5'AMP, fructose 6-phosphate, fructose 2,6-bisphosphate **Inhibitors**—Citrate, ATP	**Induced by** insulin **Repressed by** glucagon	Activity low in diabetes mellitus
Pyruvate kinase	Glycolysis	Stimulated by high carbohydrate diet Activity decreases during fasting	**Activators**—Fructose 1,6-bisphosphate, insulin **Inhibitors**—ATP, alanine, acetyl CoA glucagon	**Induced by** Insulin **Repressed by** glucagon	Deficiency causes hemolytic anemia
Pyruvate dehydrogenase	Pyruvate to acetyl CoA	Stimulated by high carbohydrate diet Activity decreases during fasting	**Activators**—CoA, NAD^+, insulin, ADP, pyruvate **Inhibitors**—Acetyl CoA, NADH, ATP (fatty acids, ketone bodies)		Deficiency causes lactic acidosis
Pyruvate carboxylase	Gluconeogenesis	Inhibited by high carbohydrate diet Stimulated during fasting	**Activator**—Acetyl CoA **Inhibitor**—ADP	**Induced by** glucocorticoids, glucagon, epinephrine **Repressed by** insulin	Activity increases in diabetes mellitus
Fructose 1,6 bisphosphatase	Gluconeogenesis	Inhibited by high carbohydrate diet Stimulated during fasting	**Activator**—Citrate **Inhibitor**—AMP, Fr 2,6 bisphosphate	**Induced by** glucocorticoids, glucagon, and epinephrine **Repressed by** insulin	Activity increases in diabetes mellitus

Enzyme	Pathway	Effect of substrate concentration	Allosteric modification/feedback Inhibition	Induction/repression	Clinical significance
Glucose-6-P dehydrogenase	HMP pathway	Stimulated by high carbohydrate diet Activity decreased during fasting	**Activator**—$NADP^+$	**Induced by** insulin	Deficiency causes hemolytic anemia
Glycogen Synthase	Glycogenesis	Stimulated by high carbohydrate diet Activity decreased during fasting	**Activator**—Glucose and glucose-6-P and insulin (by causing dephosphorylation) **Inhibitor**—Glucagon (by cAMP-mediated phosphorylation)		Deficiency cause Type-0 glycogen Storage disease
Glycogen phosphorylase	Glycogenolysis	Stimulated during fasting Inhibited in the fed state	**Activator**—Ca^{++}, low glucose concentration, glucagon (by cAMP-mediated phosphorylation) **Inhibitor**—**Insulin** (by causing dephosphorylation)		**Muscle phosphorylase deficiency** causes—Type V glycogen storage disease (McArdle's syndrome) **Liver phosphorylase** deficiency causes Type VI glycogen storage disease (Her's disease)

SUMMARY CHART 6

Disorders of lipoprotein metabolism

(A) Hyperlipoproteinemia

a. **Primary hyperlipoproteinemia**

Type	*Classification*	*Biochemical defect*	*Inheritance*	*Plasma lipids and lipoproteins*	*Clinical features*
I.	**Familial lipoprotein lipase deficiency (Hyperchylomicronemia)**	Deficiency of lipoprotein lipase. A variant of this disease can be produced by deficiency of apo CII.	Autosomal recessive	TG↑, cholesterol may also be increased, chylomicrons ++, VLDL↑, HDL and LDL ↓ Refrigeration test confirms the presence of chylomicrons in serum	Present in early childhood, eruptive xanthomas, recurrent abdominal pain, no premature cardiovascular disease
II.	**Familial hypercholesterolemia (FHC)**	Defective LDL receptor (impaired degradation of LDL)	Autosomal dominant	LDL ↑, total cholesterol ↑, VLDL and TG are also raised	Xanthomas, corneal arcus, and increased risk of premature cardiovascular disease
III.	**Familial dysbeta lipoproteinemia, also called broad beta band disease, "remnant removal disease"**	Increase concentration of apo-E, increased synthesis of apo B, conversion of normal VLDL to IDL and its degradation without conversion to LDL. Defect in remnant removal	Autosomal dominant	LDL↑, VLDL↑, actual rise in IDL which appears as **broad beta band** on electrophoresis. TG↑, cholesterol may also be increased	Tuberous and palmar xanthomas, increased risk of premature cardiovascular disease, and peripheral vascular disease
IV.	**Familial hypertriglyceridemia (FHTG)**	Increased synthesis and decreased catabolism of endogenous TGs	Autosomal dominant	Hyper pre-beta lipoproteinemia VLDL↑, TG and cholesterol also↑, α- and β-lipoproteins are subnormal (HDL↓ and LDL↓). There is associated impaired glucose tolerance	Presents in early childhood, and is commonly associated with CHD, diabetes mellitus, alcoholism, and obesity
V.	**Combined hyperlipidemia**	Usually secondary to other disorders, such as obesity, excessive alcohol intake, renal failure and pancreatitis. Exact biochemical defect is not known	Autosomal dominant	Complex lipoprotein pattern, increase in both chylomicrons and pre β-lipoproteins (VLDL), TG and cholesterol also↑↑, α and β-lipoproteins are subnormal (HDL↓ and LDL↓).	Xanthomas are frequently present impaired glucose tolerance, frequently found associated with CHD, diabetes mellitus, alcoholism, and obesity

b. **Secondary hyperlipoproteinemia**

Sl. No.	*Hyperlipidemia*	*Conditions*
1.	Secondary hypercholesterolemia	Pregnancy, hypothyroidism, cholestasis, and acute intermittent porphyria
2.	Secondary hypertriglyceridemia	Oral contraceptive use, diabetes mellitus, alcoholism, pancreatitis, gout, sepsis due to gram-negative bacterial organisms, and Type I glycogen storage disease
3.	Combined hypercholesterolemia and hypertriglyceridemia	Nephrotic syndrome, chronic renal failure, and steroid immunosuppressive therapy

(B) Hypolipoproteinemia

Disease	*Biochemical defect*	*Inheritance*	*Laboratory findings*	*Clinical manifestations*
Familial hypobetalipoproteinemia	Inability to synthesize apo B100 and apo B48	Autosomal dominant	LDL between 10% and 50% of normal, cholesterol low but triglycerides and chylomicrons normal	Mostly asymptomatic, but there is decreased risk of CHD
Abetalipoproteinemia	No synthesis or secretion of apo B containing lipoproteins	Rare inherited disease	VLDL↓, LDL↓↓, B-100↓, B-48↓, decrease in TG and a marked ↓in Serum total cholesterol, prolonged prothrombin time	Malabsorption, mental and physical retardation, acanthocytosis, atypical retinitis pigmentosa, fatty infiltration of intestinal mucosal cells and liver
Hypoalphalipoproteinemia	Not known	Autosomal dominant	HDL↓, cholesterol and TGs normal	Increased risk of CHD
Familial alpha lipoprotein deficiency (Tangier's disease)	Deficiency of alpha lipoprotein. Cholesteryl esters are deposited in the reticuloendothelial system, but functions of major organs are not affected	Autosomal recessive	Low or absent HDL, lack of alpha band on electrophoresis	Orange yellow tonsils and adenoids, muscle weakness, atrophy, recurrent peripheral neuropathies and depressed tendon reflexes The pharyngeal and rectal mucosa is also orange colored (the orange color is due to deposition of cholesteryl esters). There is increased predisposition to atherosclerosis

SUMMARY CHART 7

Important Disorders of Fatty Acid Oxidation

Sl. No.	Disease	Biochemical defect	Inheritance	Clinical manifestations	Lab. diagnosis	Treatment
1.	**Refsum disease**	Deficiency of phytanic acid oxidase enzyme Characterized biochemically by the accumulation of phytanic acid in plasma and tissues	**Autosomal recessive**	The disease is characterized by night blindness, loss of smell, deafness, muscle weakness and development of dysmorphic features in children	Serum total cholesterol, HDL and LDL are moderately reduced. Blood phytanic acid levels are elevated Phytanic oxidase activity estimation in skin fibroblast cultures is diagnostic	Eliminate all sources of chlorophyll from diet Plasmapheresis is needed to remove phytanic acid from blood
2.	**Zellweger syndrome**	Zellweger syndrome is characterized by an individual's inability to beta-oxidize very-long chain fatty acids in the Peroxisomes of the cell, due to a genetic disorder in one of the several genes involved with peroxisome biogenesis Zellweger syndrome is the most severe of the PBDs(peroxisome biogenesis Syndrome	**Autosomal recessive**	Symptoms at birth may include a **lack of muscle tone, an inability to move and glaucoma** Other symptoms may include **unusual facial characteristics, mental retardation, seizures, and an inability to suck and/or swallow. Jaundice and gastrointestinal bleeding may** also occur. More than **90% growth failure**	The abnormally **high levels of VLCFA (very long chain fatty acids)** are most diagnostic	There is no cure for Zellweger syndrome, nor is there a standard course of treatment Most treatments are symptomatic and supportive
	Carnitine deficiency	• Inadequate intake • Inability to use carnitine due to enzyme deficiencies (e.g., carnitine palmitoyl transferase deficiency) • Decreased endogenous synthesis of carnitine due to a severe liver disorder • Excess loss of carnitine due to diarrhea, diuresis, or hemodialysis • A hereditary disorder in which carnitine leaks from renal tubules (primary carnitine deficiency) • Increased requirements for carnitine when ketosis is present or demand for fat oxidation is high (e.g., during a critical illness such as sepsis or major burns; after major surgery of the GI tract)	Primary carnitine deficiency—Inheritable	• Muscle aches and fatigue • Muscle necrosis, myoglobinuria • Fasting hypoketotic hypoglycemia • Fatty liver and hyperammonemia, • Cardiomyopathy, heart failure • Coma, and sudden unexpected death	• Extremely reduced carnitine levels in plasma and muscle (1%–2% of normal) • Fasting ketogenesis may be normal if liver carnitine transport is normal, but it may be impaired if dietary carnitine intake is interrupted and there is associated liver disorder	• Pharmacologic doses of oral carnitine are highly effective in correcting the cardiomyopathy and muscle weakness as well as any impairment in fasting ketogenesis • Avoidance of fasting and strenuous exercise • Supplementation with medium-chain triglycerides and essential fatty acids (e.g., linoleic acid and linolenic acid)

SUMMARY CHART 8

Regulatory mechanisms—Lipid metabolism

Enzyme	*Pathway*	*Effect of substrate concentration*	*Allosteric modification/feedback inhibition*	*Induction/ repression*	*Clinical significance*
Acetyl-coA Carboxylase	Fatty acid synthesis	**Activity increases** during well-fed state **Activity** decrease during fasting	**Activator** —citrate, ATP, and acetyl CoA Insulin (by causing dephosphorylation by stimulating protein phosphatase) **Inhibitors**—Long chain fatty acids, epinephrine, glucagon—via changes in phosphorylation state through cAMP-mediated phosphorylation cascade	**Induced by** insulin **Repressed by** glucagon	Activity decreases in diabetes mellitus
Carnitine acyl transferase	**Carnitine shuttle**	**Activity** low in fed state, high during fasting	**Activated by** glucagon through lipolysis and provision of fatty acids for oxidation **Inhibited** by insulin and malonyl CoA		Inherited **CAT-I deficiency** affects only the liver, resulting in reduced fatty acid oxidation and ketogenesis, with hypoglycemia
HMG CoA reductase	**Cholesterol synthesis**	**Activity** low in fasting state,	**Activated by** insulin and thyroid hormone **Inhibited by** glucagon and glucocorticoids (by reversible phosphorylation) Dietary cholesterol (hepatic synthesis) Mevalonate and cholesterol, the products of pathway	Expression of HMG CoA reductase is regulated by sterol regulatory element binding protein Also induced by insulin	Activity high in diabetes mellitus due to availability of excess acetyl CoA Activity inhibited by statins used as cholesterol-lowering drugs

SUMMARY CHART 9

Variations of Serum Sodium and Potassium Levels—A Summary Chart

Electrolyte Imbalance	*Introduction*	*Causes*	*Clinical manifestations*	*Diagnosis*	*Treatment*
Hyponatremia	Decrease in serum sodium concentration <136 mEq/L caused by excess of water relative to solutes	**a). Euvolemic hyponatremia**—Polydipsia, administration of hypotonic fluid, SIADH, Addison's disease, and hypothyroidism **b) Hypovolemic hyponatremia** **i) Renal**—Acute or chronic renal insufficiency, salt wasting nephropathy, and supplementation with diuretics **ii) Extra renal**—Vomiting, diarrhea, excessive sweating, prolonged exercise, sodium and water loss but only water is replaced **c) Hypervolemic hyponatremia** **i) Renal**—Acute or chronic renal failure and nephrotic syndrome **ii) Extra renal**—Cirrhosis of liver and congestive heart failure	Primarily neurological (due to osmotic shift of water in to brain cells) and include headache, confusion, seizures, and coma	**1) Serum and urinary osmolality**—Serum osmolality may be low but urinary osmolality may be high **2) Serum sodium**—Low **3) BUN and creatinine**—Normal but high in renal failure	**a) Euvolemia**—Treat the primary cause **b) Hypovolemia** —0.9% saline **c) Hypervolemia**—Fluid restriction and diuretics
Hypernatremia	Increase in serum sodium concentration > 145 mEq/L caused by a deficit of total body water relative to total body sodium	**a) Euvolemic hypernatremia** **i) Renal** losses—Central diabetes insipidus, nephrogenic diabetes insipidus **ii) Extra renal losses**—Respiratory tract (tachypnea), skin (fever) **iii) Miscellaneous**—Decreased thirst **b) Hypovolemic hypernatremia** **i) GI losses**—Diarrhea, vomiting **ii) Skin**—Burns, excessive sweating **iii) Renal losses**—Interstitial kidney disease, diuretics **c) Hypervolemic hypernatremia**—Administration of hypertonic fluid, saline or sodium bicarbonate, excess mineralocorticoids	Thirst, CNS dysfunction, confusion, seizures or coma, decreased skin turgor in severe cases	1) **Serum sodium**—high **2) BUN, creatinine**— high—if kidneys are involved **3) Urinary sodium**—>20 mEq/L in hypovolemic hypernatremia and <20 mEq/L if there are extra renal losses	**a) Euvolemic hypernatremia**—5% D/W or 0.45% saline **b) Hypovolemic hypernatremia**—0.45% saline or a combination of 0.9% normal saline and 5% D/W **c) Hypervolemic hypernatremia**—5% D/W with loop diuretics **d) Sodium restricted diet**

Electrolyte Imbalance	*Introduction*	*Causes*	*Clinical manifestations*	*Diagnosis*	*Treatment*
Hypokalemia	Serum K concentration <3.5 mEq/L, caused by deficit in total body K or shift of potassium in to the cells	**i) Renal losses**—Renal tubular acidosis **ii) Adrenal steroid excess**—Cushing syndrome, Hyperaldosteronism **iii) GI Losses**—Vomiting, diarrhea, laxative abuse **iv) Drug induced**—Diuretics, beta 2 adrenergic agonists, steroids, theophylline, insulin administration **v) Metabolic** alkalosis **vi) Familial periodic paralysis**	Fatigue, myalgias, weakness, hypoventilation, impaired muscle metabolism, glucose intolerance	**1)Serum potassium** is low **2) ECG findings**—Sagging of ST segment. T wave depression, elevation of U wave AV blocks or Arrhythmias in severe cases **3) BUN and creatinine** may be high, serum calcium high, pH high. Blood glucose may be high	Supplementation by oral route or I/V KCl mixed in normal saline
Hyperkalemia	Serum K concentration >5.5 mEq/L from excess total body potassium stores or abnormal movement of K out of the cells	**a) Pseudohyperkalemia**—Hemolysis, thrombocytosis, leukocytosis **b) Redistribution**—Acidosis, insulin deficiency, beta blocker drugs, digitoxin overdosage, hyperkalemic periodic paralysis **c) Excessive endogenous load**—Hemolysis, rhabdomyolysis, internal hemorrhage **d) Excessive exogenous load**—Parenteral administration, excess in diet, K supplements **e) Diminished excretion**—Renal failure, renal tubular acidosis	Fatigue, paresthesia, paralysis, palpitations, bradycardia, decreased tendon reflexes, decreased motor strength Signs of renal failure or muscle paralysis may be there	**1) Serum K** is low **2) ECG**—Increased PR interval, tall, symmetric, peaked T waves In severe cases—widening of QRS interval, ventricular arrhythmias, ventricular fibrillation **3) BUN, creatinine** may be high **4) Blood glucose** high in diabetes mellitus **5) pH** low in acidosis	1) Supplement with calcium chloride or calcium gluconate To restore resting membrane potential 2) Insulin with glucose supplementation to promote intracellular shift

SUMMARY CHART 10

Vitamins—Functions and Clinical Significance

Vitamin	Function	Deficiency manifestations	Dietary level per day associated with overt deficiency in adults	Contributing factors to deficiency
A Retinol, retinaldehyde, retinoic acid, β-carotene	Retinal (retinaldehyde)—Visual pigments in the retina Retinoic acid—Regulation of gene expression and cell differentiation β-carotene is an antioxidant, also helps in the formation of glycoproteins	**Xerophthalmia**, night blindness, Bitot's spots, follicular hyperkeratosis, impaired embryonic development, immune dysfunction	<300 μg/d	Fat malabsorption, infection, measles, alcoholism, protein-energy malnutrition
D Calciferol, 1,25-dihydroxy vitamin D	Maintenance of calcium balance; enhances intestinal absorption of Ca^{2+} and mobilizes bone mineral; regulation of gene expression cell differentiation and antiproliferative hormone	**Rickets**: Skeletal deformation, frontal bossing, rachitic rosary, Harrison's sulcus, bowed legs, knock knee, widened epiphysis **Osteomalacia in adults** Waddling gate, bone pains, tendency of easy fractures, fragile bones	<2.0 μg/d	Aging, lack of sunlight exposure, fat malabsorption, deeply pigmented skin
E Tocopherols, tocotrienols	Antioxidant, especially in cell membranes; roles in cell signaling	Peripheral neuropathy, spinocerebellar ataxia, skeletal muscle atrophy, retinopathy	Not described unless underlying contributing factor is present	Occurs only with fat malabsorption, or genetic abnormalities of vitamin E metabolism/transport
K Phylloquinone: menaquinones	Coenzyme in formation of γ-carboxyglutamate in enzymes of blood clotting and bone matrix	Elevated prothrombin time, bleeding	<10 μg/d	Fat malabsorption, liver disease, antibiotic use
B_1 Thiamine-pyrophosphate	Coenzyme in pyruvate and α-ketoglutarate dehydrogenases, and transketolase Regulates Cl^- channel in nerve conduction Important in carbohydrate and amino acid metabolism	**Beriberi:** Neuropathy, muscle weakness and wasting, cardiomegaly, edema, ophthalmoplegia, confabulation (**Wernicke's encephalopathy** with **Korsakoff's psychosis)**	<0.3 mg/1000 kcal	Alcoholism, chronic diuretic use, hyper emesis
B_2 Riboflavin Flavin mononucleotide (FMN) and flavin adenine dinucleotide (FAD)	Coenzyme in oxidation and reduction reactions; prosthetic group of flavoproteins	Magenta tongue, angular stomatitis, seborrhea, cheilosis	<0.6 mg	Riboflavin deficiency is widespread but not fatal
B_3 Niacin Nicotinic acid, nicotinamide	Coenzyme in oxidation and reduction reactions, functional part of NAD and NADP; role in intracellular calcium regulation and cell signaling	**Pellagra**: Pigmented rash of sun-exposed areas, bright red tongue, diarrhea, apathy, memory loss, disorientation, death in untreated cases	<9.0 niacin equivalents	Alcoholism, vitamin B_6 deficiency, riboflavin deficiency, tryptophan deficiency, isoniazid therapy, carcinoid syndrome, Hartnup disease.

Vitamin	Function	Deficiency manifestations	Dietary level per day associated with overt deficiency in adults	Contributing factors to deficiency
B_6 Pyridoxine, pyridoxal, pyridoxamine, and the phosphorylated derivatives	Coenzyme in transamination and decarboxylation of amino acids and glycogen phosphorylase; modulation of steroid hormone action	Seborrhea, glossitis convulsions, neuropathy, depression, confusion, microcytic anemia	<0.2 mg	Alcoholism, isoniazid
Folic acid	Coenzyme in transfer of one-carbon fragments in nucleic acid and amino acid metabolism	**Megaloblastic anemia**, atrophic glossitis, depression, homocysteinemia	<100 μg/d	Alcoholism, Sulfasalazine, pyrimethamine, triamterene, methotrexate
B_{12} Cobalamine	Coenzyme in transfer of one-carbon fragments and metabolism	**Megaloblastic anemia,** loss of vibratory and position sense, abnormal gait, dementia, impotence, loss of bladder and bowel control, homocysteinemia methylmalonic aciduria	<1.0 μ g/d	Gastric atrophy (pernicious anemia), terminal ileal disease, strict vegetarianism, acid reducing drugs (e.g., H_2 blockers)
Pantothenic acid	Functional part of CoA and acyl carrier protein: fatty acid synthesis and metabolism	Peripheral nerve damage (nutritional melalgia or "burning foot syndrome")	The vitamin is widely distributed in all food stuffs, and deficiency has not been unequivocally reported in humans	Alcoholism
H Biotin	Coenzyme in carboxylation reactions in gluconeogenesis and fatty acid synthesis; role in regulation of cell cycle	Impaired fat and carbohydrate metabolism, dermatitis		Deficiency is unknown, except total parenteral nutrition, and egg white injury
C Ascorbic acid	Coenzyme in hydroxylation of proline and lysine in collagen synthesis; antioxidant; enhances absorption of iron	**Scurvy:** Petechiae, ecchymoses, coiled hairs, inflamed and bleeding gums, joint effusion, poor wound healing, fatigue	<10 mg/d	Smoking, alcoholism

SUMMARY CHART 11

Clinically Important Hemoglobinopathies

Disease	*Biochemical defect*	*Inheritance*	*Clinical manifestations*	*Diagnosis*	*Treatment*
Sickle cell disease	Point mutation, glutamic acid at the 6th position in β globin chain is replaced by valine	Autosomal recessive Heterozygotes have one normal and one sickle cell gene. The red blood cells of these individuals contain both HbS and HbA. These individuals have **sickle cell trait. They** usually do not show the clinical symptoms and can have a normal life span	1. Painful crisis 2. Chronic hemolytic anemia 3. Organ damage 4. Impaired growth and development 5. Increase susceptibility to infections 6. Chronic skin ulcers 7. Painless hematuria may be there 8. Neurological complications	1. **Peripheral blood film**—Normocytic normochromic, target cells, presence of sickled cells is confirmatory 2. **Positive test for sickling** 3. **Bone marrow** is hyperplasic 4. **Hemoglobin electrophoresis** confirms the diagnosis	A. **Supportive treatment:** 1. Adequate hydration 2. Antibiotics 3. Analgesics 4. Supplementation with iron and folic acid 5. Oxygen administration during attack 6. Blood transfusion B. **Antisickling agents:** 1. Hydroxy urea 2. Recombinant erythropoietin C. **Permanent cure:** 1. Bone marrow transplant 2. Gene therapy
Met hemoglobinemia	1. By exposure to oxidant drugs 2. Exposure to chemicals and poisons, such as—chlorates, acetanilide, nitrites, nitrobenzene, antipyrin, phenacetin, sulfonamide drugs 3. Familial methemoglobinemia deficiency of met hemoglobin reductase enzyme	Autosomal recessive in familial methemoglobinemia	a. **At concentrations of 3%–15%**—A slight discoloration (e.g., pale, gray, blue) of the skin may be present b. **At fractions of 15%–20%**—The patient may be relatively asymptomatic, but cyanosis is likely to be present c. **At fractions of 25%–50%**—Headache, dyspnea, lightheadedness, syncope, weakness, confusion, palpitations and chest pain d. **At fractions of 50%–70%:** i. Cardiovascular—abnormal cardiac rhythms ii. CNS—altered mental status, delirium, seizures, coma iii. Metabolic—profound acidosis	1. Clinical cyanosis in the presence of normal arterial oxygen tensions is highly suggestive of methemoglobinemia ("saturation gap") 2. The diagnosis of methemoglobinemia is confirmed by direct measurement of methemoglobin by a multiple wavelength co-oximeter.	1. Administration of supplemental oxygen 2. Removal of the offending oxidizing agent 3. Methylene blue is the first-line antidotal agent 4. Hyperbaric oxygen therapy or packed RBC exchange transfusions are alternatives

Disease	*Biochemical defect*	*Inheritance*	*Clinical manifestations*	*Diagnosis*	*Treatment*
Alpha thalassemia	Gene deletion	Autosomal recessive	1. **Silent carrier state**—Single gene defect—no hematological abnormality 2. **α-thalassemia**—Two gene deletion—Microcytic hypochromic type of red blood cells, no significant hemolysis 3. **Hb-H disease**—Three gene deletion—The affected individuals have moderate to severe lifelong hemolytic anemia, modest degrees of ineffective erythropoiesis, Splenomegaly, and variable bony changes 4. **Hydrops fetalis—4 gene deletion**—No stable Hb tetramer, most severe form, incompatible with life	1. Hb—low 2. MCV and MCHC—Low depending upon the defect 3. The peripheral blood smear shows severe anisopoikilocytosis, severe hypochromia, and nucleated red blood cells 4. Hb electrophoresis confirms the diagnosis	Symptomatic 1. Iron supplementation is to be avoided 2. Folate supplementation is recommended 3. A blood transfusion is to be administered only if necessary 4. **Rarely, allogeneic stem cell transplantation**
Beta thalassemia	Point or frame shift mutation causing premature termination of the beta globin chain	Autosomal recessive	1. **β-thalassemia minor** —also called beta thalassemia trait—Mild anemia, splenomegaly, mild icterus, no significant manifestations 2. **β-thalassemia major**—also called Cooley's anemia a. Sever anemia b. Marked wasting, malnourished appearance c. Slow growth and development d. Typical skin color—mixture of icterus, pallor and increased melanin deposition e. Skeletal deformities—"Chipmunk Facies" f. Cardiomegaly with signs of CHF g. Marked hepatomegaly and splenomegaly	1. **β-thalassemia minor**—Modest anemia, peripheral blood smear is mildly abnormal, with hypochromia, microcytosis, and target cells Hb electrophoresis confirms the diagnosis 2. **β-thalassemia major** —Severe anemia, and without transfusion the hematocrit may fall to less than 10% The peripheral blood smear shows severe poikilocytosis, hypochromia, microcytosis, target cells, basophilic stippling, and nucleated red blood cells. Little or no hemoglobin A is present. Variable amounts of hemoglobin A_2 are seen, and the major hemoglobin present is hemoglobin F 2. Bone marrow examination to rule out other causes of anemia 3. Skeletal changes can be observed	1. **β-thalassemia minor**—No treatment is recommended 2. **β-thalassemia major** a. Blood transfusions b. **Desferal**—chelation therapy c. Additionally, **splenectomy** (removal of the spleen), bone marrow transplants are being proposed as possible treatments for thalassemia d. Gene reactivation by using **butyrate and hydroxyurea** e. **Gene replacement therapy**

Chapter 29

Normal Laboratory Reference Values

NORMAL LABORATORY REFERENCE VALUES

[Blood (B), Serum (S), Plasma (P), Urine (U)]

Blood gases	
pH	(B-arterial) 7.35–7.45 (H^+ 44.7–45.5 nmol/L)
Partial pressure of CO_2 ($PaCO_2$)	(B-arterial) 35–45 mm Hg (4.7–6 kPa)
Partial pressure of O_2 (PaO_2)	(B-arterial) 80–100 mm Hg (10.67–13.33 kPa)
Bicarbonate (HCO^-)	24–28 mEq/L (24–28 mmol/L)
O_2 saturation % (arterial)	90–95
O_2 saturation % (venous)	40–70
CO_2 content	Total serum 21–30 mmol/L
CO	<5% of hemoglobin
Anion gap	7–16 mmol/L
Hematology	
Hemoglobin Hematocrit (PCV) Red blood count (RBC) Reticulocytes White blood count (WBC) Platelets Mean corpuscular volume (MCV) Mean corpuscular hemoglobin (MCH) Mean corpuscular hemoglobin concentration (MCHC)	(B) Men: 14–18 g/dL (2.09–2.79 mmol/L) Women: 12–16 g/dL (1.86–2.48 mmol/L) (S) 2–3 mg/dL Men: 40–52% (0.4–0.52) Women: 37–47% (0.37–0.47) Men: 4.5–6.2 million/μL ($4.5–6.2 \times 10^{12}$/L) Women: 4–5.5 million/μL ($4–5.5 \times 10^{12}$/L) 0.2–2% of red cells 5000–10,000/μL ($5–10 \times 10^{9}$/L) • Polymorphonuclear (PMN): 35–80% • Immature polys (Bands): 0–10% • Lymphocytes (Lymp): 20–50% • Monocytes (Mono): 2–12% • Eosinophils (Eos): 0–7% • Basophils (Bas): 0–2% 150,000–400,000/μL ($0.15–0.4 \times 10^{12}$/L) Men: 80–94 fL Women: 81–99 fL(By Coulter counter) 27–32 pg 32–36 g/dL, red blood cells (32–36%)
Average diameter of red cell	7.3 μm (5.5–8.8 μm)
Bleeding time	Ivy method, 1–7 minutes (60–420 seconds)
	Template method, 3–9 minutes (180–540 seconds)
Clot retraction	Begins in 1–3 hours: complete in 6–24 hours; no clot lysis in 24 hours
Fragility of red cells	Begins at 0.45–0.38% NaCl, complete at 0.36–0.3% NaCl
Partial thromboplastin time	Activated, 25–37 seconds

Prothrombin time	(P) 11–14.5 seconds, International Normalized Ratio (INR)—
	(P) 2.0–3.0
Erythrocyte sedimentation rate (ESR or Sed-Rate)	Male 1–13 mm/hour Female 1–20 mm/hour
Blood volume	8.5–9.1% of total body weight
Endocrines	
Adrenals hormones and metabolites	
Dopamine	(P) <135 pg/mL
Aldosterone	(U) 2–26 μg/24 hours (5.5–72 nmol/day), values vary with sodium and potassium intake
Catecholamines	(U) Total <100 μg/24 hours
Epinephrine	(U) <10 μg/24 hours (<100 nmol/day)
Norepinephrine	(U) <100 μg/24 hours (<590 nmol/day)
Cortisol	Free (U) 20–100 μg/24 hours (0.55–2.76 μmol/day)
11,17-OH corticoids	(U) Men: 4–12 mg/24 hours
	Women: 4–8 mg/24 hours
17-ketosteroids	(U) <8 years 0–2 mg/24 hours
	Adolescents 2–20 mg/24 hours (1 mg = 3.5 μmol)
Metanephrine	(U) <1.3 mg/24 hours (<6.6 μmol/day) or <2.2 μg/mg creatinine
Vanillylmandelic acid (VMA)	(U) Up–7 mg/24 hours (<35 μmol/day)
Pituitary	
Growth hormone (GH)	(S) Adults 1–10 ng/mL (46–465 pmol/L) by RIA
Thyroid-stimulating hormone (TSH)	(S) <10 μU/mL
Follicle-stimulating hormone (FSH)	(S) Prepubertal 2–12 mIU/mL
	Adult men: 1–15 mIU/mL
	Adult women: 1–30 mIU/mL
Luteinizing hormone (LH)	(S) Prepubertal 2–12 mIU/mL
	Adult men: 1–15 mIU/mL
	Adult women: <30 mIU/mL
Corticotropin (ACTH)	(P) 8.00–10.00 AM, up–100 pg/mL (22 pmol/L)
Prolactin	(S) 1–25 ng/mL (0.4–10 nmol/L)
Somatomedin C Antidiuretic hormone (ADH, vasopressin)	(P) 0.4–2 U/ml (P) Serum osmolality 285 mOsm/kg, 0–2 pg/mL; >290 mOsm/kg, 2–12 + pg/mL
Placenta	
Estriol (E3) Chorionic gonadotropin	(S) Men and nonpregnant women: <0.2 μg/dL (<7 nmol/L) by RIA (S) Beta subunit Men: <9 mIU/mL Pregnant women: >10 mIU/mL
Gonads	
Testosterone, free Testosterone, total	(S) Men: 10–30 ng/dL; Women: 0.3–2 ng/dL (1 ng/dL = 0.035 nmol/L) (S) Prepubertal <100 ng/dL; Adult men: 300–1,000 ng/dL; Adult women: 20–80 ng/dL, luteal phase up to120 ng/dL
Estradiol (E2)	(S) Men: 12–34 pg/mL Women, menstrual cycle 1–10 days, 24–68 pg/mL 11–20 days, 50–300 pg/mL 21–30 days, 73–149 pg/mL by RIA (lpg/mL = 3.6 pmol/L)
Progesterone	(S) Follicular phase 0.2–1.5 ng/mL Luteal phase 6–32 ng/mL Pregnancy >24 ng/mL Men :<1 ng/mL = 3.2 nmol/L

Thyroid	
Thyroxin, free T_4 (FT_4)	(S) 0.8–2.4 ng/dL (10–30 pmol/L)
Thyroxin, total (TT_4)	(S) 5–12 μg/dL (65–156 nmol/L) by RIA
Thyroxin-binding globulin capacity	(S) 12–28 μg T_4/dL (150–360 nmol T_4/dL)
Triiodothyronine (T_3)	(S) 80–220 ng/dL (1.2–3.3 nmol/L)
Reverse triiodothyronine (rT_3)	(S) 30–80 ng/dL (0.45–1.2 nmol/L)
Triiodothyronine uptake (RT_3U)	(S) 25–36% as TBG assessment (RT_3U ratio) 0.85–1.15
Calcitonin	(S) <100 pg/mL (<29.2 pmol/L)
Islets	
Insulin C-peptide Glucagon	(S) 4–25 μU/mL (29–181 pmol/L) (S) 0.9–4.2 ng/mL (S) Fasting 20–100 pg/mL
Parathyroid	
Parathyroid hormone (intact)	(S) 8–51 pg/mL
Stomach	
Gastrin Pepsinogen I	(S) up–100 pg/mL (47 pmol/L) Elevated >200 pg/mL (S) 25–100 ng/mL
Iron studies	
Ferritin	Adult women: 20–120 ng/mL
	Men: 30–300 ng/mL
	Child 15 years, 7–140 ng/mL
Iron	(S) 50–175 μg/dL (9–31.3 μmol/L)
Iron-binding capacity	(S) Total 250–410 μg/dL (44.7–73.4 μmol/L)
	% saturation 20–55%
Transferrin	(S) 200–400 mg/dL (23–45μmol/L)
Haptoglobin	(S) 40–170 mg of Hb-binding capacity
Blood chemistry	
Alanine aminotransferase (ALT); SGPT	0–45 IU/L at 37°C
Aspartate aminotransferase (AST); SGOT	0–41 IU/L at 37°C
Alkaline phosphatase (ALP)	(S) Adults 5–13 units (KA), 0.8–2.3 (Bessey–Lowry): SMA 30–85
	IU/L at 37°C: SMAC 30–115 IU/L at 37°C
Amylase	(S) 80–180 units/dL (Somogyi)
Gamma glutamyl transpeptidase	(S) <30 units/L at 30°C
Lipase	(S) <150 units/L
Acid phosphatase	(S) 1–5 U (KA), 0.1–0.63 U (Bessey–Lowry)
Total creatine kinase (Total CK)	(S) 10–50 IU/L at 30°C
Creatine kinase-MB (CK-MB)	0–3%
Creatine kinase-MM (CK-MM)	97–100%
Creatine kinase-BB (CK-BB)	0%
Lactate dehydrogenase	(S) 55–140 IU/L at 30°C
Aldolase	(S) 1.5–2.0 U/L
Troponin	<0.4 ng/mL

5′-nucleotidase	0–11 U/L
Antistreptolysin O (ASO) titer	Adult: <125
	Child: <250
Glucose	(S or P) 65–110 mg/dL (3.6–6.1 mmol/L)
Impaired glucose tolerance	111–125 mg/dL (6.2–6.9 mmol/L)
Diabetes mellitus	>125 mg/dL (>7.0 mmol/L)
Glucose, 2-hour postprandial	70–120 mg/dL (3.9–6.7 mmol/L)
Fructosamine	<285 μmol/L
Hemoglobin A1c	4.0–6.0%
Urea nitrogen	(S or P) 8–25 mg/dL (2.9–8.9 mmol/L)
Creatinine	(S or P) 0.7–1.5 mg/dL (62–132 μmol/L)
Uric acid	(S or P) Men: 3–9 mg/dL (0.18–0.54 mmol/L) Women: 2.5–7.5 mg/dL (0.15–0.45 mmol/L)
Bicarbonate	(S) 24–28 mEq/L (24–28 mmol/L)
Potassium	(S or P) 3.5–5 mEq/L (3.5–5 mmol/L)
Sodium	(S or P) 136–145 mEq/L (136–145 mmol/L)
Chloride	(S or P) 96–106 mEq/L (96–106 mmol/L)
Magnesium	(S or P) 1.8–3 mg/dL (0.75–1.25 mmol/L)
Copper	(S or P) 100–200 μg/dL (16–31 μmol/L)
Zinc	(S) 50–150 μg/dL (7.65–22.95 μmol/L)
Phosphorus, inorganic	(S–fasting) 3–4.5 mg/dL (1–1.5 mmol/L)
Calcium	(S) 8.5–10.3 mg/dL (2.1–2.6 mmol/L)
Calcium (ionized)	(S) 4.25–5.25 mg/dL; 2.1–2.6 mEq/L (1.05–1.3 mmol/L)
Lead	(U) <80 μg/24 hours (<0.4 μmol/day)
Pyruvate	(B) 0.6–1 mg/dL (70–114 μmol/L)
Lactate	(B) Venous 4–16 mg/dL (0.44–1.8 mmol/L)
Ketone (acetone)	(S) Negative
Acetone and acetoacetate	(S) 0.3–2 mg/dL (3–20 mg/L)
β-hydroxybutyrate	(S) 0–3 mg/dL (0–290 μmol/L)
Serum total protein	(S) 6–8 g/dL (60–80 g/L)
Albumin	(S) 3.5–5.5 g/dL (35–55 g/L)
Prealbumin	170–340 mg/L
Globulins	(S) 2–3.6 g/dL (20–36 g/L)
Fibrinogen	(P) 0.2–0.6 g/dL (2–6 g/L)
Homocysteine	4.4–10.8 μmol/L
α1-antitrypsin	(S) >180 mg/dL
C-reactive protein	0.2–3.0 mg/L
Prostate-specific antigen (PSA)	0–4 ng/mL (likely higher with age)
Ceruloplasmin	(S) 25–43 mg/dL (1.7–2.9 μmol/L)
Bilirubin	(S) Total 0.2–1.2 mg/dL (3.5–20.5 μmol/L)
	Direct (conjugated), 0.1–0.4 mg/dL (<7 μmol/L)
	Indirect 0.2–0.7 mg/dL (<12 μmol/L)
Urobilinogen	(U) 0–2.5 mg/24 hours (70–470 μmol/day)
Urobilinogen (fecal)	40–280 mg/24 hours (70–470 μmol/day)
Porphyrins	1.5–7.5 mg/24 hours (11–57 μmol/day)
Delta aminolevulinic acid (U)	
Porphobilinogen (U)	<2 mg/24 hours (<8.8 μmol/day)
Ammonia	(P) 10–80 μg/dL
Osmolality	(S) 280–296 mOsm/kg water (280–296 mmol/kg water)
Specific gravity	(B) 1.056 (varies with Hb and protein concentration)
	(S) 1.0254–1.0288 (varies with protein concentration)
Fecal fat	<30% dry weight

Lipid profile	
Cholesterol mg/dL (mmol/L) Triglycerides Lipid fractions HDL cholesterol mg/dL (mmol/L) LDL cholesterol mg/dL (mmol/L) VLDL cholesterol Free fatty acid Lipoprotein (a)	(S or P) 150–250 mg/dL (3.9–5.72 mmol/L) <200 (<5.17)—desirable 200–239 (5.17–6.18)—borderline high >240 (>6.21)—high (S) <165 mg/dL (1.9 mmol/L) Desirable levels <40 (<1.03)—low, >60 (>1.55)—high i. <70(<1.81)—Therapeutic option for very high-risk patients ii. <100(<2.59)—Optimal iii. 100–129 (2.59–3.34)—Near optimal/above optimal iv. 130–159 (3.36–4.11)—Borderline high v. 160–189 (4.14–4.89)—High vi. >190(4.91)—Very high <40 mg/dL (P) 200–800 µmol/L 0–30 mg/dL
Vitamins	
Vitamin A	(S) 15–60 µg/dL (0.53–2.1 µmol/L)
β-carotene	(S) Fasting 50–300 µg/dL
Vitamin B_{12}	(S) >200 pg/mL (>148 pmol/L)
Vitamin D	(S) Cholecalciferol (D3); 25-hydroxycholecalciferol, 8–55 ng/mL
	(19.4–137 nmol/L);
	1,25-dihydroxycholecalciferol, 26–65 pg/mL (62–155 pmol/L); 24,25-dihydroxycholecalciferol
	1–5 ng/mL (2.4–12 nmol/L)
Vitamin C (ascorbic acid)	(P) 0.4–1.5 mg/dL (23–85 µmol/L)
Folic acid	(S) 14–34 nmol/L
Vitamin E	(S) 5–18 µg/mL (12–42 µmol/L)
Vitamin K	(S) 0.13–1.19 ng/mL (0.29–2.64 nmol/L)
Vitamin B_6	(P) 5–30 ng/mL (20–121 nmol/L)
Immunoglobulins	
IgA	9.0–33 g/L
IgG	7.2–15.0 g/L
IgM	0.5–2.5 g/L
IgD	0–0.4 g/L
IgE	100–200 µg/L
Renal function tests	
p-aminohippurate (PAH) clearance (RPF) Creatinine clearance, endogenous (GFR) Inulin clearance Filtration fraction (FF) Osmolality Specific gravity of urine	Men: 560–830 mL/min Women: 490–700 mL/min Men: 110–150 mL/min Women: 105–132 mL/min Approximately same as creatinine (corrected to 1.73 m² surface area) Men: 17–21%; women: 17–23% (FF = GFR/RPF) (U) On normal diet and fluid intake: Range 500–850 mOsm/kg water. Achievable range, normal kidney: Dilution 40–80 mOsm; concentration (dehydration) up to 1,400 mOsm/kg water (at least three to four times plasma osmolality) 1.002–1.030
Urinalysis	
Urine volume	0.4–2.0 L/day
Urine pH	5–7
Acidity, titratable	20–40 mEq/day (20–40 mmol/day)
Ammonia	30–50 mEq/day (30–50 mmol/day)
Specific gravity	1.002–1.030

Urine ketone	Negative
Urine blood	Negative
Urine proteins	Negative
Urine nitrites	Negative, traces
Urine bilirubin	Negative
Urobilinogen	0–2.5 mg/24 hours
Urine micro	RBCs: 0–2/HPF WBCs: 0–2/HPF RBC casts: 0/HPF
Urine glucose	<250 mg/dL
Urine creatinine	Men: 1.0–2.0 g/day Women: 0.8–1.8 g/day
Urea nitrogen	6–17 g/day (214–607 mmol/day)
Uric acid (normal diet)	250–800 mg/day (214–607 mmol/day)
Sodium (varies with intake)	100–260 mEq/day (100–260 mmol/day)
Potassium (varies with intake)	25–100 mEq/day (25–100 mmol/day)
Phosphate (phosphorus) (varies with intake)	400–1,300 mg/day (12.9–42.0 mmol/day)
Microalbumin	
Normal	0–30 mg/day (0.0–0.03 g/day)
Microalbuminuria	30–300 mg/day (0.03–0.30 g/day)
Clinical albuminuria	>300 mg/day (>0.3 g/day)
Microalbumin/creatinine ratio	
Normal	0–30 µg/mg creatinine (0–3.4 g/mol creatinine)
Microalbuminuria	30–300 µg/mg creatinine (3.4–34 g/mol creatinine)
Clinical albuminuria	>300 µg/mg creatinine (>34 g/mol creatinine)
Cerebral spinal fluid	
Pressure	60–150 mm Hg
Specific gravity	1.006–1.007
pH	7.3
CSF glucose	45–100 mg/dL
CSF proteins	10–45 mg/dL
CSF chlorides	700–760 mg/dL (120–130 meq/L) as NaCl
CSF urea	20–40 mg/dL
CSF calcium	5.5–6 mg/dL
CSF cells	0–4 mononuclear per cubic mm

TERMINOLOGY

Units

Gram: Common measurements of weight used in this table are: pg (picograms), g (grams), mg (milligrams), etc., per liter.

Micrometer (µm): It is a unit of length. Mean corpuscular volume is expressed in cubic micrometers.

Mole: Also, "gram molecular weight" is a quantity based on the atomic weight of the substance. Many test results in the International System are expressed as the number of moles per liter. In US units, these measurements are usually in grams per liter. Units used in this table are: mmol (millimoles), µmol (micromoles), nmol (nanomoles), pmol (picomoles) per liter.

Some units of measurement include the following fractions and multipliers:

mega (m): 10^6 or ×1,000,000
kilo (k): 10^3 or ×1,000
deca or deka: 10^1 or ×10
deci (d): 10^{-1} or ÷10
milli (m): 10^{-3} or ÷1,000
micro (µ): 10^{-6} or ÷1,000,000
nano (n): 10^{-9} or ÷1,000,000,000
pico (p): 10^{-12} or ÷1,000,000,000,000

Index

Page numbers followed by *f* refer to figure and *t* refer to table.

A

D

H

I

Q

R

T